D0161107

Microbial
Pathogenesis
and the
Intestinal
Epithelial
Cell

Microbial Pathogenesis

and the

Intestinal Epithelial Cell

Gail A. Hecht, *Editor*

Section of Digestive Diseases and Nutrition,
Department of Medicine, University of Illinois at Chicago

ASM Press
Washington, DC

Library of Congress Cataloging-in-Publication Data

Microbial pathogenesis and the intestinal epithelial cell / edited by
Gail A. Hecht.
    p. ; cm.
Includes bibliographical references and index.
    ISBN 1-55581-261-9
1. Intestines—Infections—Pathogenesis.   2. Epithelial cells.   3.
Intestinal mucosa.
[DNLM: 1. Intestinal Diseases—microbiology. 2. Intestinal
Diseases—physiopathology. 3. Intestinal Mucosa—metabolism. 4.
Intestinal Mucosa—microbiology. WI 400 M6266 2003] I. Hecht, Gail A.

RC862.E47M53 2003
616.3′407—dc21
2003009514

10 9 8 7 6 5 4 3 2 1

Address editorial correspondence to: ASM Press, 1752 N St., N.W., Washington, DC 20036-2904, U.S.A.

Send orders to: ASM Press, P.O. Box 605, Herndon, VA 20172, U.S.A.
Phone: 800-546-2416; 703-661-1593
Fax: 703-661-1501
Email: books@asmusa.org
Online: www.asmpress.org

CONTENTS

CONTRIBUTORS

Robert L. Atmar   Departments of Medicine and Molecular Virology and Microbiology, Baylor College of Medicine, Houston, TX 77030-3498

Kim E. Barrett   Department of Medicine, School of Medicine, University of California, San Diego, UCSD Medical Center 8414, 200 West Arbor Drive, San Diego, CA 92103-8414

Lone S. Bertelsen   Department of Medicine, School of Medicine, University of California, San Diego, UCSD Medical Center 8414, 200 West Arbor Drive, San Diego, CA 92103-8414

Robert J. Bloch   Department of Physiology, University of Maryland School of Medicine, Baltimore, MD 21201

Elke Cario   Division of Gastroenterology and Hepatology, University of Essen, Essen, Germany

Crystal Chan   Biotechnology Laboratory, University of British Columbia, Vancouver, B.C., V6T 1Z3, Canada

Bobby J. Cherayil   Combined Program in Pediatric Gastroenterology and Nutrition, Massachusetts General Hospital and Harvard Medical School, Boston, MA 02114

Sean P. Colgan   Center for Experimental Therapeutics, Brigham and Women's Hospital and Harvard Medical School, Boston, MA 02115

Iris Dotan   Mount Sinai School of Medicine, 1425 Madison Avenue, New York, NY 10029

Mary K. Estes   Departments of Molecular Virology and Microbiology and Medicine, Texas Gulf Coast Digestive Diseases Center, Baylor College of Medicine, 1 Baylor Plaza, Mailstop BCM-385, Houston, TX 77030-3498

Alessio Fasano   Center for Vaccine Development, Departments of Pediatrics and Medicine, and Department of Physiology, University of Maryland School of Medicine, Baltimore, MD 21201

M. Isabel Fernandez   Unité de Pathogénie Microbienne Moléculaire, INSERM U389, Institut Pasteur, Rue du Dr. Roux 28, 75724 Paris Cedex 15, France

B. Brett Finlay   Biotechnology Laboratory, University of British Columbia, Vancouver, B.C., V6T 1Z3, Canada

David N. Fredricks   Program in Infectious Diseases, Fred Hutchinson Cancer Research Center, Seattle, WA 98109-1024

Karla Jean Fullner   Department of Microbiology-Immunology, Northwestern University Medical School, 303 E. Chicago Avenue, Morton 6-626, Chicago, IL 60611

Glenn T. Furuta   Combined Program in Pediatric Gastroenterology and Nutrition, Children's Hospital, Harvard Medical School, Boston, MA 02114

Andrew T. Gewirtz   Epithelial Pathobiology Division, Department of Pathology and Laboratory Medicine, Emory University, Atlanta, GA 30322

Gail Hecht   Division of Digestive Diseases and Nutrition, Department of Medicine, University of Illinois at Chicago, Room 714, Clinical Sciences Building (M/C 716), 840 S. Wood Street, Chicago, IL 60612-7323

Dawn A. Israel   Division of Gastroenterology, Department of Medicine, Vanderbilt University Medical Center, Nashville, TN 37232

Martin F. Kagnoff   Department of Medicine, University of California, San Diego, 9500 Gilman Drive (MTF/412), La Jolla, CA 92093-0623

Ciarán P. Kelly   Gastroenterology Division, Dana 601, Beth Israel Deaconess Medical Center, 330 Brookline Avenue, Boston, MA 02215

Jean-Pierre Kraehenbuhl   Swiss Institute for Experimental Cancer Research, Institute of Biochemistry, University of Lausanne, CH-1066 Epalinges, Switzerland

Catherine A. Lee   Department of Microbiology and Molecular Genetics, Harvard Medical School, Boston, MA 02115

Wayne I. Lencer   GI Cell Biology, Children's Hospital/Harvard Medical School, 300 Longwood Avenue, Boston, MA 02115

James L. Madara   Epithelial Pathobiology Division, Department of Pathology and Laboratory Medicine, Emory University, Atlanta, GA 30322

Lloyd Mayer   Mount Sinai School of Medicine, 1425 Madison Avenue, New York, NY 10029

Beth A. McCormick   Department of Pediatric Gastroenterology and Nutrition, Massachusetts General Hospital and Harvard Medical School, Boston, MA 02129

Didier Merlin   Epithelial Pathobiology Division, Department of Pathology and Laboratory Medicine, Emory University, Atlanta, GA 30322

Jiri Mestecky   Department of Microbiology and Department of Medicine, University of Alabama at Birmingham, 845 19th St. South, Birmingham, AL 35294-2170

James P. Nataro   Center for Vaccine Development, Departments of Pediatrics and Medicine, University of Maryland School of Medicine, Baltimore, MD 21201

Andrew S. Neish   Epithelial Pathobiology Unit, Department of Pathology, Emory University School of Medicine, 105F Whitehead Building, 615 Michaels St., Atlanta, GA 30322

Marian R. Neutra   Department of Pediatrics, Harvard Medical School, GI Cell Biology Laboratory, Children's Hospital, Boston, MA 02115

Andre J. Ouellette   Department of Pathology and Department of Microbiology and Molecular Genetics, College of Medicine, University of California, Irvine, CA 92697-4800

Richard M. Peek, Jr.   Division of Gastroenterology, Department of Medicine, Vanderbilt University Medical Center, Nashville, TN 37232

Daniel K. Podolsky   Gastrointestinal Unit, Center for the Study of Inflammatory Bowel Disease, Massachusetts General Hospital, Harvard Medical School, Boston, MA 02114

Charalabos Pothoulakis   Division of Gastroenterology, Beth Israel Deaconess Medical Center, Harvard Medical School, 330 Brookline Ave., Boston, MA 02215

Bärbel Raupach   Department of Cellular Microbiology, Max Planck Institute for Infection Biology, Schumannstrasse 21/22, D-10117 Berlin, Germany

Chiara Rodighiero   GI Cell Biology, Children's Hospital/Harvard Medical School, 300 Longwood Avenue, Boston, MA 02115

Michael W. Russell   Department of Microbiology, University of Buffalo, 138 Farber Hall, 3435 Main St., Buffalo, NY 14214-3000

Philippe J. Sansonetti   Unité de Pathogénie Microbienne Moléculaire, INSERM U389, Institut Pasteur, Rue du Dr. Roux 28, 75724 Paris Cedex 15, France

R. Balfour Sartor   Departments of Medicine, Microbiology and Immunology, University of North Carolina School of Medicine, Chapel Hill, NC 27599-7038

Cynthia Sears   Department of Medicine, The Johns Hopkins School of Medicine, Baltimore, MD 21205

Michael E. Selsted   Department of Pathology and Department of Microbiology and Molecular Genetics, College of Medicine, University of California, Irvine, CA 92697-4800

Shanti V. Sitaraman   Epithelial Pathobiology Division, Department of Pathology and Laboratory Medicine, Emory University, Atlanta, GA 30322

Cormac T. Taylor   Department of Medicine and Therapeutics, The Conway Institute, University College Dublin, Dublin, Ireland

Jerrold R. Turner   Department of Pathology, The University of Chicago, Chicago, IL 60637

Bruce A. Vallance   Biotechnology Laboratory, University of British Columbia, Vancouver, B.C., V6T 1Z3, Canada

V. K. Viswanathan   Division of Digestive Diseases and Nutrition, Department of Medicine, University of Illinois at Chicago, Room 714, Clinical Sciences Building (M/C 716), 840 S. Wood St., Chicago, IL 60612

W. Allan Walker   Combined Program in Pediatric Gastroenterology and Nutrition, Massachusetts General Hospital and Harvard Medical School, Boston, MA 02114

Michel Warny   Acambis, Inc., 38 Sidney Street, Cambridge, MA 02139

Arturo Zychlinsky   Department of Cellular Microbiology, Max Planck Institute for Infection Biology, Schumannstrasse 21/22, D-10117 Berlin, Germany

PREFACE

In August 1991, I was extremely fortunate to attend a unique conference entitled "Molecular Cross Talk between Epithelial Cells and Pathogenic Microorganisms" that was cosponsored by the American Society for Cell Biology (ASCB) and the European Molecular Biology Organization (EMBO). The fact that this meeting was held in a spectacular venue, Arolla, Switzerland, only accentuated the fascinating science that was presented there. The concept that microbes and host cells could be studied in concert was only nascent at that time, yet it attracted premier investigators from a variety of scientific fields including microbiology, cell biology, pharmacology, molecular biology, immunology, infectious disease, and gastroenterology. Now, just over a decade later, meetings concerning host–pathogen interactions are commonplace and even journals dedicated solely to this topic have been created. This stimulating area of investigation is now firmly rooted; as a result, there are a number of scientists committed to this field and the amount of literature published is vast.

While virtually every organ system of the human body is a potential target for infection, one that has received unprecedented attention is the intestinal tract. Gastroenterologically relevant research has often lagged behind that which has focused on more "attractive" organ systems, such as the cardiovascular or central nervous system, so it is very exciting that in the realm of host-microbial interactions, the gastrointestinal tract has taken the lead. The number of recent discoveries regarding enteric pathogens (type III secretion systems, molecular mimicry, exploitation of host molecules for invasion, attachment or initiation of signaling events) and intestinal epithelial cells (the existence of Toll-like receptors, production of antimicrobial peptides, and identification of tight junction proteins as microbial receptors) is remarkable. The additional beauty of these investigations is that, as they reveal mechanisms of microbial pathogenesis, they also unveil mechanisms regulating intestinal epithelial biology and physiology.

It is on this foundation that the concept of a book dedicated to the interactions between microbial pathogens and the intestinal epithelial cell arose. The need for such a volume was underscored by the unanimously high level of enthusiasm from the invited contributors. The thorough and comprehensive nature of this book stems from the diverse backgrounds of the authors, which include microbiology, epithelial cell biology, pathology, immunology, physiology, infectious diseases, and gastroenterology.

The book begins with a comprehensive overview of the morphology of the intestinal tract so that the stage for subsequent chapters is set. The next several chapters focus on unique aspects of the intestine that influence or are influenced by microbial pathogens, such as M cells, intestinal lymphocytes, Toll-like receptors, and the transport of secretory IgA. Advanced methodological approaches for investigating host-pathogen interactions are then covered, followed by a series of contributions that review intestinal epithelial cell responses to microbes, including gene expression, alterations in ion transport and the tight junction barrier, and apoptosis, to name a few. The book then concludes with several chapters dedicated to the effects of specific microbial pathogens on the intestinal epithelium.

I believe that it is unique to have brought together under a single umbrella this level of diversity and expertise. It is a very timely endeavor which I hope will not only be of use as a reference to those already engaged in the field, but also serve as a catalyst to join this area for those who currently work in peripherally related topics. The opportunity to study the interface of two complex biological systems offers tremendous challenge and excitement.

I thank each of the authors who contributed their time and energy to this project. Thanks also go to Greg Payne at ASM Press for advice and for seeing this project through to the end. I also thank my research mentor, Dr. James L. Madara, who has been and continues to be (despite his new position as Dean of Biological Sciences at the Pritzker School of Medicine, University of Chicago) a leader in the field of intestinal epithelial cell biology. I must also thank Dr. James B. Kaper, whom I first met standing at the base of a glacier during a coffee break at that 1991 ASCB/EMBO meeting in Arolla. There, I nervously introduced myself and asked him if he would be willing to send me enteropathogenic *E. coli* (EPEC) strains for some preliminary studies with intestinal epithelial cells. He kindly obliged and has been an unfaltering supporter and collaborator for my studies regarding the impact of EPEC on intestinal epithelial functions ever since.

Finally, I have to say that if this book is viewed by the readers with even a fraction of the enthusiasm that went into its creation, it will be an incredible success.

GAIL HECHT, M.D.

FUNCTIONAL MORPHOLOGY OF THE INTESTINAL MUCOSAE: FROM CRYPTS TO TIPS

Jerrold R. Turner

1

The intestines form a critical interface between the internal milieu and the external environment since, in essence, the luminal space is contiguous with the latter. Thus, like the integument, the intestines must form a barrier to prevent the passage of toxic and otherwise threatening agents that gain access to the lumen. However, unlike the skin, the intestines must also support the digestion and absorption of nutrients, electrolytes, and water from the lumen. Thus, the intestines must form a highly regulated, selectively permeable barrier. Under some conditions, the intestines also manage the secretion of electrolytes and water. Intestinal epithelial cells actively participate in digestion, absorption, and secretion by expressing critical absorptive proteins on their surfaces, including enzymes and transporters, and by directing vectorial transport. Moreover, the intestinal epithelia actively participate in host defense through interaction with critical components of the mucosal immune system. Both a complex structure and a diverse cellular composition are necessary to accomplish this broad range of intestinal func-

tions. The structure and function of the intestinal mucosa and its relevance to absorption, secretion, and microbial pathogenesis are the subject of this chapter. Other chapters in this volume will address the mechanisms by which a wide variety of pathogens exploit the spectrum of unique targets that this cellular specialization affords.

REGIONAL SPECIALIZATION ALONG THE LONGITUDINAL AXIS— PROXIMAL TO DISTAL

The human small intestine is 6 m in length and, along this length, is divided into three regions: the duodenum, the jejunum, and the ileum. These regions are functionally distinctive, although there is some overlap. For example, brush border digestive enzyme function is most important in the duodenum and jejunum, with 90% of absorption occurring within the first 100 cm of the small intestine. The jejunum is the principal site of absorption for Na^+ cotransport of monosaccharides (105) and amino acids and uptake of fatty acids. The duodenum and jejunum are also the primary absorptive sites for water-soluble vitamins, iron, and calcium. In contrast, bile salts and vitamin B_{12} are absorbed in the ileum. The colon, approximately 1 m in length, is pri-

Jerrold R. Turner, Department of Pathology, The University of Chicago, Chicago, IL 60637.

Microbial Pathogenesis and the Intestinal Epithelial Cell, ed. by G. Hecht
© 2003 ASM Press, Washington, D.C.

marily responsible for absorption of Na^+, Cl^-, and water and secretion of K^+ and HCO_3^-.

In addition to regional specialization of function, specific cell types are preferentially localized in different portions of the intestines. For example, Paneth cells are abundant in the small intestine and proximal colon, but their presence in the distal colon is abnormal and represents a metaplastic response, as can be seen in chronic colitides. Regional specialization within the intestines is genetically programmed long before it is phenotypically evident, as isografts of embryonic mouse small intestine implanted into subcutaneous tissues ultimately express features specific to the region from which they originated (88).

As with functional differentiation, there is a gradient of endogenous bacterial flora throughout the intestines (30). The luminal contents of the duodenum and jejunum are often sterile and, on average, contain 100 bacterial organisms per ml. The numbers of bacteria present increase progressively, with averages of 1,000 organisms per ml in the proximal ileum, 10^5 to 10^6 organisms per ml in the distal ileum, and 10^{11} organisms per ml in the colon. In addition to this quantitative gradient, there is significant variation in the relative predominance of individual bacterial species throughout the length of the intestines.

MUCOSAL STRUCTURE

The intestinal mucosa consists of a layer of epithelium; the basement membrane; an underlying supporting layer of stroma, the lamina propria; and a delicate layer of smooth muscle, the muscularis mucosa. In the small intestine, both the mucosa and the underlying submucosa are specialized to increase the absorptive surface area. The submucosa is organized into regular ridges, known as plicae circularis, which have been estimated to increase the available surface area threefold (Fig. 1). Within the mucosa, the lamina propria is arranged into the supporting structure for villi. The villi increase the surface area available for absorption by an additional 10-fold. At the core of each villus is a central arteriole that fans out

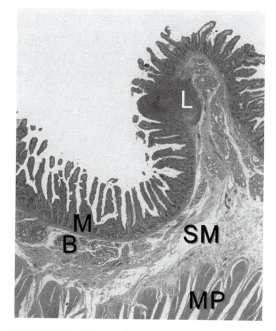

FIGURE 1 Human duodenum. The mucosa (M) and submucosa (SM) are drawn into a prominent ridge, or plica circularis, at the right side of the photomicrograph. The mucosa, composed of epithelium, lamina propria, and muscularis mucosa, is organized into crypts and villi. The submucosa contains numerous Brunner's glands (B), found only in the duodenum. A prominent lymphoid aggregate (L) can also be seen. The epithelium overlying this area lacks villi and assumes a dome-shaped configuration. M cells are found at this site. The inner circular layer of the muscularis propria (MP) can be seen at the bottom of the field. Together with the outer longitudinal layer, these layers of smooth muscle effect peristalsis.

to form an array of capillaries that descend along the lateral surfaces of the villi in close apposition to the basement membrane and epithelia (Fig. 2). The resulting intimate association between the ascending central arteriole and the descending capillaries allows for the countercurrent exchange of solutes, analogous to that occurring in the renal medulla. In the small intestine, this results in the creation of a hypertonic lamina propria in the villus tip during active nutrient absorption (31). When oxygen supply is limited, countercurrent oxygen exchange can also occur, resulting in lower oxygen tension in the villus, as opposed to the

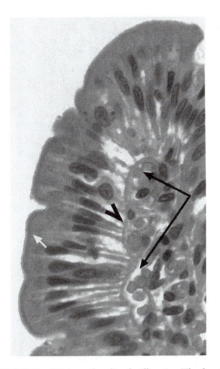

FIGURE 2 Human duodenal villus tip. The lamina propria of the villus core contains a prominent vascular supply (black arrows). Absorptive enterocytes cover the villus tip. At the apical (luminal) edge, the microvillus brush border (see Fig. 4) can be appreciated as a faint fuzzy area. Just beneath the brush border, the terminal bar (white arrow) can be seen as an area of increased density. This structure is composed of the terminal web and apical junctional complex. The epithelial cells rest on a thin layer of collagen, the basement membrane (black arrowhead).

crypt, and greater damage to the villus epithelium, with relative preservation of the crypt epithelium. This has serious consequences for barrier function and nutrient absorption during intestinal ischemia. However, the relative preservation of the crypt zone, where the stem cells are located, affords the possibility of mucosal repair after the acute insult has passed.

The center of each villus core also contains a conduit for lymphatic drainage, known as the lacteal, which is critical for the absorption of chylomicrons and lipoprotein complexes and for the recovery of plasma proteins that have found their way into the lamina propria.

Interestingly, such lymphatics are not present in the colonic lamina propria. This explains the observation that colonic cancers invasive into the lamina propria have a very low metastatic potential, while the same is not true of otherwise similar small intestinal cancers. Obstruction of draining small intestinal lymphatics is associated with profound disease. Examples include infection by *Trophyrema whippelii*, the pathogenic organism of Whipple's disease, and mycobacterial species. Organism-laden macrophages within the lamina propria compress and obstruct draining lymphatics, leading to malabsorption, malnutrition, and vitamin deficiencies.

REGIONAL SPECIALIZATION ALONG THE VERTICAL AXIS—CRYPT TO VILLUS

Similar to the regional compartmentalization that occurs from the proximal small intestine to the distal colon, compartmentalization also exists along the crypt to the villus, or vertical, axis (Fig. 3). In the small intestine, the crypt is populated by stem cells, goblet cells, undifferentiated secretory cells, enteroendocrine cells, Paneth cells, and occasional rarer cell types, such as tuft cells. In contrast, the small intestinal villus is populated by absorptive enterocytes and goblet cells, as well as the rarer tuft and cup cells. This distribution of cell types is responsible for functional compartmentalization in the small intestine. The crypt is responsible for cell renewal, ion and water secretion (see chapters 14 and 15), exocrine secretion of macromolecules such as defensins (see chapter 12) into the crypt lumen, and endocrine/paracrine secretions into capillaries and the lamina propria. In contrast, the villus is primarily responsible for nutrient absorption.

An elegant series of studies using chimeric animals have demonstrated that each crypt is a clonal unit derived from a single progenitor cell (38). In contrast, the villus epithelium is derived from multiple surrounding crypts. Thus, the epithelium covering the surface of each villus is oligoclonal, with cells derived

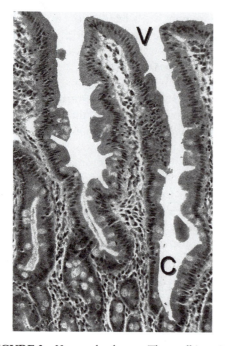

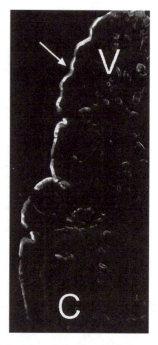

FIGURE 3 Human duodenum. The small intestinal mucosa is organized into villi (V) and crypts (C). Epithelial cell proliferation occurs within the crypt. The crypt is also functionally specialized for water and ion secretion. As enterocytes migrate to the villus, they mature and become specialized for ion and nutrient absorption.

FIGURE 4 Human duodenal villus. Digestive enzyme expression increases during enterocyte migration to the villus. This micrograph shows brush border alkaline phosphatase expression (white band indicated by arrow). Expression increases progressively from crypt (C) to villus (V).

from each crypt arranged in vertical columns along the villus. Differentiation from a secretory to an absorptive phenotype occurs as cells migrate up the villus. Such differentiation is associated with increased expression of nutrient transporters and induction of brush border digestive enzymes (Fig. 4) (41). This process appears to be regulated by position within the villus or the interval since mitosis, as it does not require luminal stimuli. Further evidence that migration and differentiation are linked comes from transgenic overexpression of E-cadherin or expression of a dominant negative N-cadherin within enterocytes under the control of the intestine-specific fatty acid binding protein promoter. Expression of either construct results in altered migration rates and corresponding disruption of enterocyte differentiation (37, 39).

Once the epithelial cells reach the villus tip, apoptosis, or programmed cell death, ensues. This process has been characterized morphologically as the orderly shedding of apoptotic cells with maintenance of cell-cell junctions and barrier function (59). A recent study suggests that early in the process of apoptosis, a rho-mediated activation of actomyosin contraction occurs in cells surrounding the apoptotic cell (86). This allows the remaining cells to form a contractile purse string around the apoptotic cell. It has been proposed that this results in the active extrusion of the apoptotic cell by its neighbors without a significant loss of barrier integrity (86).

SPECIALIZED EPITHELIAL CELL TYPES

Absorptive Enterocytes

Villus absorptive cells are the major constituents of the villus epithelium. They are tall columnar cells that, at the apical (luminal) surface, are lined by a dense brush border of ~1-μm-tall microvilli. These microvilli increase the membrane surface area as much as 20-fold, thereby greatly increasing the efficiency of nutrient absorption by allowing for a greater density of transmembrane transporter proteins. The structural integrity of each microvillus is maintained by a cytoskeletal core composed of actin filaments and associated proteins such as myosin I and villin. As these cytoskeletal cores enter the body of the cell, they encounter a dense mesh of microfilaments, termed the terminal web, that is enriched in myosin II (Fig. 5). Contraction of the terminal web may also be responsible for brush border motility (9, 40). At the periphery of each cell, the terminal web condenses to form a perijunctional actomyosin ring associated with the tight junction and adherens junction and intimately involved in regulation of tight junction permeability and therefore mucosal barrier function (35, 62, 107, 112).

The tight junction also defines the intramembranous fence that prevents diffusional mixing of apical and basolateral membrane domains. Thus, through a combination of targeted postsynthetic delivery, selective membrane retrieval, and prevention of lateral diffusion, the villus absorptive cell maintains the differential composition of apical and basolateral membrane domains (116, 120). This membrane partitioning is critical, since, without it, vectorial transport, both absorptive and secretory, would be impossible.

Villus enterocytes are highly specialized for nutrient absorption. The brush border is enriched in membrane-bound digestive enzymes, such as disaccharidases and peptidases, and nutrient transport proteins. Expression of these proteins increases progressively as enterocytes migrate from crypt to villus (Fig. 4). Diseases that result in villus atrophy or blunting, for example, celiac sprue, are characterized by decreased activity of microvillus membrane enzymes (74, 122). Likely as a result of the dense expression of digestive enzymes, the apical membrane of villus absorptive enterocytes possesses an extraordinarily high protein-lipid ratio and, on freeze fracture electron microscopy, the microvillus P face is heavily covered with the intramembrane particles that represent integral membrane proteins. In addition to this constitutively high expression of digestive enzymes

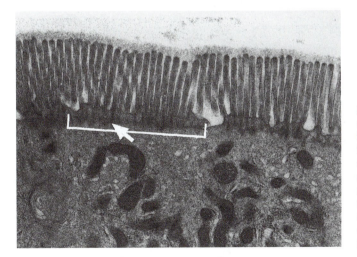

FIGURE 5 Human small intestinal epithelium. This intermediate-magnification electron micrograph of the apical region of absorptive enterocytes emphasizes the dense, well-developed microvillus brush border and overlying mucous gel. Microfilament rootlets can be seen protruding into the apical cytoplasm (arrow), where they become embedded within the terminal web (bracket).

and transport proteins, epidermal growth factor can trigger an acute actin-dependent recruitment of additional membrane with concomitant microvillus lengthening and increases in maximal nutrient transport rates (13, 32). A similar morphological increase in microvillus length has been reported in mice fed a galactose-rich diet (99), suggesting that microvillus length can also be regulated by luminal nutrient composition.

In contrast to the rigid membranes of the apical microvilli, the basolateral membranes have broadly curved contours that interdigitate with those of adjacent cells. As a result, lateral space dimensions are plastic and can be markedly increased in states of active nutrient absorption (61), suggesting critical roles for both the lateral membrane and the paracellular pathway in nutrient transport. The lipid and protein composition of the basolateral membrane domain also differs significantly from that of the apical membrane. Digestive enzymes are conspicuously absent from basolateral membranes. Similarly, the Na^+-coupled nutrient transporters that are so densely expressed in the microvillus membrane are also absent for the most part. However, unlike the microvillus membrane, the Na^+-K^+ ATPase, the facilitated glucose transporter GLUT2, and Na^+-independent amino acid transporters are prevalent in the basolateral membrane. This results in an efficient transcellular transport pathway. For example, glucose and galactose monomers released via brush border disaccharidases are transported by the intestinal Na^+-glucose cotransporter, SGLT1 (43), which depends on the extracellular-to-intracellular Na^+ gradient as its energy source. Intracellular Na^+ is then expelled at the basolateral surface via the Na^+-K^+ ATPase, and glucose exits the cell via basolateral GLUT2. Thus, this transport system, which effects transcellular movement of both Na^+ and glucose, requires the establishment and maintenance of polarized membrane domains. Analogous transport systems also exist for various classes of amino acids.

Undifferentiated Crypt Enterocytes

Undifferentiated cells are derived from the epithelial stem cell and continue to be mitotically active while present within the crypt region. They appear to be the intermediate between the stem cell and all other epithelial cell types. In contrast to villus absorptive cells, undifferentiated crypt cells possess a less well-developed microvillus membrane, with shorter and less dense microvilli and very low expression of digestive enzymes and nutrient transporters. However, despite the "undifferentiated" nomenclature, crypt cells do express a well-developed mechanism for chloride secretion (see chapters 14, 15, and 21). This mechanism requires cell polarity, as four main channels are involved, three on the basolateral surface, Na^+-K^+-$2Cl^-$ cotransporter NKCC1, Na^+-K^+ ATPase, and K^+ channels, as well as the apical Cl^- channels (3). Cl^- enters the epithelial cell from the basolateral surface via NKCC1. This requires the maintenance of a transmembrane Na^+ gradient by the Na^+-K^+ ATPase and an exit pathway for K^+, the basolateral K^+ channels. Cl^- exits the cell apically by one of several apical Cl^- channels. The regulation of Cl^- secretion is discussed in detail in chapter 14.

The physical geometry of the crypt results in crypt cells with narrow apical surfaces and wider bases, more akin to the shape of a pyramid (with the apex removed) than a column. This increased packing of cell profiles at the level of the tight junction results in increased junctional density and increased paracellular permeability. When modeled mathematically, analysis of tight junction density predicts that 73% of ileal paracellular conductance occurs via the crypt, rather than villus, epithelium (63). When analyzed using size-selective probes, an even more striking difference between crypt and villus epithelial tight junctions is apparent. The actively absorbing portion of the villus contains small pores with a radius of less than 6 Å, while pores in the crypts have a radius of 50 to 60 Å (20). An intermediate-size pore with a radius of 10 to

15 Å is present at an intermediate level between the villus and crypt (20). While this distribution of pore sizes may be a direct result of epithelial architecture, the functional consequences are striking. The crypt lumen, which is generally not accessible to luminal contents, is lined by epithelial cells with a porous paracellular pathway. This may enhance the paracellular movement of Na$^+$ and water in response to transcellular Cl$^-$ secretion, thereby facilitating a robust and coordinated secretory response.

Undifferentiated crypt epithelial cells are also specialized for secretion of immunoglobulin A (IgA) into the intestinal lumen. These cells and, to a lesser extent, villus enterocytes (7, 16) express the polymeric immunoglobulin receptor that, at the basolateral surface, binds IgA molecules secreted by lamina propria plasma cells (70). The receptor-IgA complexes are then transported, via vesicular transcytosis, to the apical surface (10), where proteolytic cleavage releases a portion of the receptor, secretory component, with the IgA complex (93) (see chapters 2 and 3).

Goblet Cells

Goblet cells are the mucin-producing cells present in both villus and crypt epithelium. Although their distribution is nonuniform, goblet cells are present throughout the small intestine and colon. In contrast, their presence in the gastric epithelium is indicative of intestinal metaplasia, a consequence of chronic gastritis that is a risk factor for gastric adenocarcinoma (69, 125). Like all other epithelial cell types in the intestines, goblet cells are derived from stem cells via undifferentiated crypt cells (67). Additionally, early goblet cells are also capable of limited mitotic activity (67).

The bulbous apical portion of the goblet cell cytoplasm is filled with ~3-μm-diameter pale granules densely packed with dehydrated mucins (Fig. 6). These are surrounded by a thin layer of organelle-depleted cytoplasm, giving the light-microscopic appearance of the

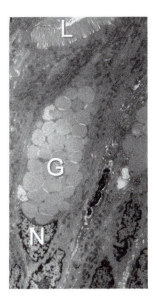

FIGURE 6 Goblet cell. This low-magnification electron micrograph shows abundant mucin granules (G) within the apical cytoplasm of the goblet cell. These granules are ready for discharge into the lumen (L). The nucleus (N) is located basally.

bowl of a wine goblet. The cytoplasmic organelles are located beneath the mucous granules. These include the Golgi complex and endoplasmic reticulum, in which mucins are synthesized as heavily glycosylated glycoproteins in which only 10% of the mass is attributable to the peptide core. The cell appears to narrow in this area, forming a stem, thus enhancing the wine goblet-like configuration. Like villus absorptive and undifferentiated crypt cells, the nucleus is located subjacent to the Golgi complex, adjacent to the basal membrane. Unlike villus absorptive and undifferentiated crypt cells, goblet cells possess irregular microvilli that tend to be found in peripheral perijunctional areas. When analyzed by freeze fracture electron microscopy, goblet cell microvilli do not contain abundant intramembrane particles, reflecting a relative lack of apical membrane specialization for transmembrane transporters. This is consistent with the specialized function of goblet cells, as a well-developed rigid microvillus brush border would likely interfere with and be disrupted by the repeated exocytosis of mucin granules.

Mucin exocytosis appears to occur at a low basal rate. However, it is notable that typical intestinal secretagogues, such as acetylcholine, can dramatically accelerate mucin secretion (101). This may represent a protective response, as *Escherichia coli* and *Vibrio cholerae* toxins can also induce mucin release (53, 68). Consistent with these experimental observations, mucin depletion is frequently noted as a histopathological feature of both infectious (89) and idiopathic (64) inflammatory diseases of the intestines. These and other data have led many to speculate that one function of the apical mucous gel is to form a semipermeable barrier that protects the epithelium from abrasive and toxic luminal contents. In at least one cell culture model of epithelial repair, intestinal mucins also accelerate repair driven by intestinal trefoil factor (50). However, an in vivo transgenic approach that ablated intestinal goblet cells gave the surprising result that transgenic mice were less susceptible to intestinal injury than wild-type littermates, perhaps because the transgenic mice had a compensatory increase in mucosal intestinal trefoil factor (45).

Mucins may also interact with luminal bacteria in several capacities. First, as a diverse array of carbohydrate complexes, mucins provide a plethora of potential binding sites for bacterial glycosidases and adhesins (118). Therefore, mucins may serve as a site of colonization for commensal bacteria (119). Alternatively, the carbohydrate binding sites present on mucins may allow pathogenic bacteria to be trapped within the mucous gel and removed by bulk mucous flow. Production of mucinase and degradation of intestinal mucus may be a mechanism by which *V. cholerae* evades such clearance. Disruption of this mechanism may also explain the protective effect of antibodies against *V. cholerae* mucinase in infant mice (94). Additionally, specific carbohydrate epitopes on intestinal mucins have been described as receptors for several bacterial pathogens, including some verotoxin-producing *E. coli* O157:H7 isolates (92), enterotoxigenic *E. coli* (71), and *Salmonella enterica* serovar Typhimurium (117). Finally, the carbohydrate binding sites present on mucins may also serve as decoys that compete with epithelial binding sites for attachment of pathogenic bacteria (15, 78).

Enteroendocrine Cells

Enteroendocrine cells are found throughout the intestinal mucosa, interspersed among other epithelial cell types, and arise from the same stem cells as enterocytes, goblet cells, and Paneth cells. They are relatively deficient in microvilli and are typically slender at the apex, where they form intercellular junctions with adjacent cells. The distinctive morphological feature of enteroendocrine cells is the presence of numerous cytoplasmic secretory granules that are most concentrated in the basal cytoplasm, subjacent to the nucleus (Fig. 7). The

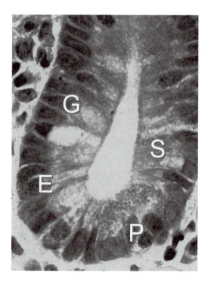

FIGURE 7 Human small intestinal crypt. The most basal portions of the small intestinal crypt are populated by Paneth cells (P). These cells contain an abundance of large apically located granules. In contrast, enteroendocrine cell (E) granules are small and basally oriented. The stem cell zone (S) is located several cell diameters above the crypt base. Goblet cells (G) are also abundant in the crypt.

electron-microscopic morphology of these granules can be used to characterize enteroendocrine cell types, as granule structure tends to correlate with the product secreted. However, this is not always straightforward, as each enteroendocrine cell may secrete more than one peptide or amine (81) and granules with differing morphologies may harbor the same product (8). Some data suggest the existence of two distinct pathways for enteroendocrine cell differentiation. Although cells secreting serotonin, substance P, glucagon-like peptide-1, peptide YY, neurotensin, and cholecystokinin can all arise from a single stem cell, they then diverge into one of two lineages and are able to produce serotonin and substance P or glucagon-like peptide-1, peptide YY, neurotensin, and cholecystokinin (87).

As might be anticipated from their location, the contents of enteroendocrine cell granules are secreted across the basolateral membrane, where they exert their effects by local paracrine action or enter the bloodstream and have endocrine effects. Although enteroendocrine cells are widely distributed, their function is incompletely understood. However, it is notable that enteroendocrine cell number is frequently observed to be increased in longstanding intestinal disease, for example, ulcerative colitis (29). Some have hypothesized that this represents an adaptive response to injury, perhaps by enhancing secretion of the trophic product glucagon-like peptide-2 (5, 127).

Paneth Cells

Paneth cells are a normal constituent of crypt epithelium in the small intestine and proximal colon in most mammals, although they are absent in dogs, cats, and pigs (106). The number of Paneth cells increases from the duodenum to the ileum. Along the vertical axis Paneth cells are restricted to the lower portion of the crypt and are not present in the villus epithelium (Fig. 7). Indeed, the presence of Paneth cells within the villus is a morphological marker of dysplasia (111). Paneth cells are a terminally differentiated cell type derived from the crypt stem cell (12) and are not mitotically

active, although dysplastic Paneth cells may participate in the cell cycle (111). Like goblet cells, the apical cytoplasm of Paneth cells is occupied by secretory granules and microvilli are sparse, although Paneth cell granules are eosinophilic and electron dense. The granules have been described as modified lysosomes that are secreted into the crypt lumen under appropriate conditions. These granules contain lysozyme and antimicrobial peptides and secretagogues, such as cryptdins (see chapter 12). The function, if any, of Paneth cells in digestive function is unknown, and their primary role may be the elaboration of antimicrobial peptides. Consistent with this is the observation that Paneth cell numbers may increase in relation to the luminal bacterial load (17).

M Cells

Follicle-associated epithelial cells, or M (microfold-bearing) cells, are most prominent in the distal ileum, where the follicles aggregate into Peyer's patches, but can be found throughout the intestines. M cells are a unique epithelial cell type specialized for the bulk endocytic sampling of luminal contents. They are present in the flat epithelium overlying lymphoid follicles, although most epithelial cells in these areas are not M cells, and electron microscopy is necessary to distinguish the M cell from the surrounding absorptive cells. Morphological features that can help to identify the M cell are the irregular, short, and relatively sparse microvilli and the poorly developed terminal web. However, the most prominent feature of the M cell is its shape. The basal membrane of the M cell is retracted from the basement membrane to form an intraepithelial cleft surrounded on three sides by the M cell and, at the most basal aspect, by the basement membrane. Lymphocytes and macrophages migrate into this cleft, where the apically derived endocytic vesicles are released by exocytosis. This transcytotic pathway is very rapid, with some particles detectable in the extracellular cleft space of M cells within 10 min of endocytosis. The bulk transport transcytotic pathway mediated by M cells also represents an efficient conduit for infectious organisms and, potentially, mucosal vaccines (73) (see chapter 2).

Stem Cells

Pluripotent small intestinal epithelial cells are located several cells above the base of the crypt in a circumferential ring of approximately 4 to 16 cells (Fig. 7) (83). Colonic pluripotent cells are located at the crypt base. In either case, it is clear that all the pluripotent cells in a given crypt derive from a single original stem cell; that is, each crypt is monoclonal (38). At present there are no known specific morphological markers that characterize the stem cell, although the RNA-binding protein Msi-1 has been proposed as a marker of functional stem cells (6). The progeny of intestinal stem cells ultimately differentiate into enterocytes, goblet cells, Paneth cells, enteroendocrine cells, and M cells. This differentiation is partly regulated by position within the crypt. For example, in the small intestine, enteroendocrine and Paneth cells are primarily found at the crypt base beneath the proliferating stem cell zone. The other cues necessary for lineage-specific differentiation are unknown, but it is possible that determination toward goblet cells, Paneth cells, and enteroendocrine cells occurs early in the process as a single event, since knockout mice deficient in the basic helix-loop-helix transcription factor *Math1* are deficient in all three cell types (128). This implies that *Math1* is necessary for the differentiation of stem cells into goblet cells, Paneth cells, and enteroendocrine cells, but the additional factors necessary for differentiation into these cell types are unknown. Similarly, other data suggest that cells destined to become M cells are committed before they exit the crypt, or at least that surface enterocytes are incapable of transdifferentiation into M cells (54). It is also likely that lymphoid tissue underlying the surface epithelium may, in part, regulate M-cell differentiation (49).

HISTOPATHOLOGY OF SELECTED ENTERIC PATHOGENS IN HUMANS

E. coli

The histopathology of *E. coli*-associated enteritides depends on the organism involved, as pathogenetic mechanisms vary widely (see chapters 13, 14, 15, and 22). Enteropathogenic *E. coli* is noninvasive and does not elaborate enterotoxins. Infection by this pathogen is characterized by the development of attaching and effacing lesions that distort apical actin microfilaments. Subsequently, an inflammatory response and increased tight junction permeability occur via mechanisms that include the actions of several defined bacterial products (see chapters 13, 14, 15, and 22) and, in part, require phosphorylation of myosin II regulatory light chain (discussed below). Given the acute, self-limited nature of the illness, biopsies are not often obtained. Light microscopic examination of small intestinal biopsies generally reveals partial or complete villous atrophy and crypt hyperplasia. Bacteria attached to the apical membrane may be present as microcolonies. However, the overall features are nonspecific, and bacteria are often absent after 10 days of disease.

Enterohemorrhagic *E. coli* is noninvasive and includes the infamous O157:H7 serotype that has been reported widely in the lay press. The primary pathology occurs in the colon, typically involving the ascending and transverse colonic segments. Histopathology seen in biopsy specimens ranges from edema and superficial intraepithelial neutrophil infiltrates to superficial epithelial atrophy, mucosal necrosis, and crypt cell hyperplasia. The last presentation can be difficult to distinguish from ischemic colitis. In the most severe cases, inflammatory pseudomembranes can be present, resulting in a histopathological impression that resembles *Clostridium difficile*-associated pseudomembranous colitis.

Salmonella

Salmonella species (see chapters 11 and 24) include *Salmonella enterica* serovar Typhi, which causes typhoid fever, and a variety of other species that cause self-limited colitides. Serovar Typhi primarily affects mucosal lymphoid tissues, predominantly in the ileum and cecum, with lymphoid hyperplasia, necrosis, and deep mucosal ulcers. Similar lymphoid hyperplasia is present in draining mesenteric lymph nodes. Other *Salmonella* species cause acute, self-limited ileocolitis that is histologically indistinguishable from other acute colitides. Pathologic features are typified by lamina propria edema and intraepithelial neutrophil infiltrates.

Shigella

Very few inoculating organisms are necessary for *Shigella* transmission (see chapter 25), reflecting the relative acid resistance of the organism. *Shigella* sp. is an invasive pathogen that involves the colon to varying degrees. Incomplete involvement is the norm, although in fatal cases disease often involves the entire colon and ileum. The histopathological features may be indistinguishable from those of enteroinvasive *E. coli* and can include lamina propria edema, mucosal capillary congestion and microthrombi, swollen endothelial cells with focal hemorrhage, goblet cell depletion, intraepithelial neutrophils, crypt abscesses, and microscopic ulcers with associated purulent exudates (Fig. 8). Inflammatory pseudomembranes may also be present. Damage to enterocytes and M cells overlying lymphoid follicles may be particularly intense. In severe cases, features of chronic colitis, including branched crypts, may occasionally be present and are evidence of cyclical mucosal injury and regeneration.

V. cholerae

V. cholerae infects via the fecal-oral route. Organisms that survive the harsh gastric environment adhere to the small intestinal mucosa and secrete cholera toxin, which induces a robust Cl^- secretory response (see chapters 14, 21, and 26). Other toxins, for example, zonula occludens toxin, may also participate in disease

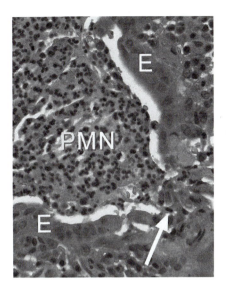

FIGURE 8 Crypt abscess in human colon. The crypt epithelium (E) is damaged and, at the lower right, penetrated (arrow) by a migrating mass of neutrophils (PMN) that fill the crypt lumen.

pathogenesis (see chapters 15 and 25). Upon light-microscopic evaluation, small intestinal biopsies are completely normal. However, electron-microscopic evaluation may demonstrate blebbing of apical microvilli, disrupted apical junctional complexes, and expanded lateral intercellular spaces. Inflammatory infiltrates are not prominent, although degranulation of mucosal mast cells and eosinophils has been reported.

C. difficile

Pseudomembranous, or *C. difficile*-associated, colitis is a major problem in hospitals and long-term-care facilities. Disease-producing infection requires the disruption of normal enteric flora, usually following the administration of broad-spectrum antibiotics. The bacteria elaborate at least two toxins (see chapter 27) that disrupt the actin cytoskeleton and alter tight junction permeability via glucosylation of rho proteins (34, 36, 47). Although biopsy samples may occasionally demonstrate nonspecific intraepithelial neutrophilic infiltrates, the characteristic histopathological lesion of *C. difficile*-associated colitis is the volcano-like eruption of neutrophils, mucus, and adherent inflammatory debris exploding from a severely damaged crypt (Fig. 9). As the infection progresses, these individual punctate lesions may expand and coalesce to form confluent pseudomembranes covering broad areas of colonic mucosa.

STRUCTURE AND REGULATION OF THE PARACELLULAR PATHWAY

The diverse anatomical structures and cell types of the intestines integrate into a precisely regulated organ that is charged with vectorial transport, both secretory and absorptive, and maintenance of the mucosal barrier. Transcellular vectorial transport requires polarization

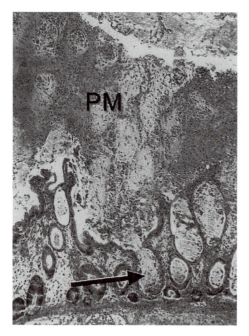

FIGURE 9 *C. difficile*-associated pseudomembranous colitis. The colonic crypt (arrow) is lined by flattened, severely damaged epithelium. The crypt lumen contains purulent debris primarily composed of neutrophils and mucus. This seems to explode from the crypt, forming a volcano-shaped eruption that, at the surface, becomes confluent with exudate from other damaged crypts. Dense sheets of purulent debris, pseudomembranes (PM), cover the mucosal surface.

of membrane domains with specific transporters present on the apical and basolateral membranes, as outlined above and discussed in detail in chapters 2, 4, 6, 12, 14, and 15. In the case of ion and nutrient transport, this cell polarization allows concentration gradients to be established, leading to the transcellular movement of these essential substances. However, larger hydrophilic solutes with hydrodynamic radii of ~4 Å or greater cannot effectively cross cell membranes. In the absence of specific transporters, cell membranes are also impermeable to water, and separate studies suggest roles for transcellular water movement mediated by Na^+-solute cotransporters (66) or aquaporin water channels (27, 33, 51, 95, 121). Alternatively, a large body of data suggests that a significant portion of water movement is paracellular (48, 56, 108). Based on presently available data, it seems most likely that both transcellular and paracellular routes of water movement are operative. Some in vivo data suggest that, in the colon, aquaporins 2 and 4 enhance water permeability and can be upregulated by water deprivation (27, 121). Nonetheless, it is clear that the overall permeability of intestinal mucosae is substantially greater than the permeabilities of apical and basolateral membranes arranged in series. Thus, a major absorptive pathway for large hydrophilic solutes must be paracellular.

The Tight Junction

The rate-limiting barrier that determines the overall permeability of the paracellular pathway is the epithelial tight junction. The tight junction is appreciated morphologically as the uppermost component of the apical junctional complex (Fig. 10). In addition to the tight junction, this complex is composed, in sequence, of the adherens junction and macula adherens (18). This apical junctional complex is intimately associated with the perijunctional actomyosin ring (58, 62). The tight junction itself is a circumferential zone of close membrane apposition that is 100 to 600 nm in depth. Freeze fracture electron microscopy

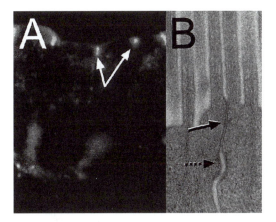

FIGURE 10 (A) Immunofluorescence microscopy of human small intestinal mucosa demonstrates tight junctions to be dot-like areas at the apical portion of each cell-cell junction site (arrows), as shown by immunostaining for occludin. (B) Electron microscopy of the apical junctional complex of a small intestinal enterocyte shows an area of tight membrane apposition, the tight junction (solid arrow) at the most apical region of the lateral membrane. The adherens junction (dashed arrow) is located subapical to the tight junction.

has shown that this zone is composed of a complex anastamosing network of P-face strands and complementary E-face grooves (103). Transmembrane protein components of these strands include claudin isoforms and occludin (26). The precise role of occludin has not been defined, and although occludin knockout mice do have an abnormal phenotype, an initial report suggests that intestinal tight junctions are intact (91). This is not likely to be due to molecular redundancy, as occludin and a splice variant both arise from a single gene and no additional homologous genes have been identified (72). Nonetheless, in vitro studies do point to a critical role for occludin and suggest that occludin may be critical to tight junction assembly and regulation (11, 23, 25, 55, 75, 98, 115, 123, 124).

Claudin Proteins and Paracellular Permeability

It is now clear that the claudin family of proteins forms the core of the tight junction. This point is emphasized by the report that familial hypomagnesemia, a defect in renal tubular paracellular Mg^{2+} reabsorption, is caused by a mutation in a specific isoform, claudin-16 (97). This observation, that a specific claudin appears to be responsible for paracellular permeability of a specific ion, may explain the observation that relative selectivity of the paracellular pathway to different ions is not uniform throughout the gastrointestinal tract. For example, both rabbit jejunum and ileum are slightly more permeable to K^+ than Na^+, with similar P_{K+}/P_{Na+} ratios (84). However, the relative ileal paracellular permeability to Cl^- is greater than in jejunum, with a P_{Cl-}/P_{Na+} ratio that is severalfold higher (84). These observations suggest the hypothesis that a different pattern of claudin family member expression may explain these differences in ion selectivity. Consistent with this hypothesis, the distribution of claudin isoforms throughout the gastrointestinal tract has been mapped, and patterns of expression do vary along both the longitudinal and vertical axes (85). Direct experimental tests of this hypothesis have also been reported, including the observations that expression of claudin-4 induces selective decreases in paracellular Na^+ permeability (114) and expression of claudin-2 results in decreased transepithelial electrical resistance (24), a sensitive measure of tight junction permeability. The essential role of claudins does not appear to have escaped notice as a target for pathogenic organisms. For example, the enterotoxin of *Clostridium perfringens* binds specifically to the second extracellular loop of claudin-3 and claudin-4 (22). This binding results in the selective removal of these claudin isoforms from the cell surface, loss of tight junction strands, and decreased transepithelial electrical resistance (100).

Physiological Regulation of Tight Junction Permeability

When it was first discovered that some epithelia had permeabilities far greater than those explained by the serial conductances of the apical and basolateral membranes, epithelia were classified as leaky (e.g., proximal tubule, gall-bladder, small intestine, and colon) or tight (e.g., skin, urinary bladder). This difference is due to tight junction permeability and likely results from the differential expression of claudin isoforms. However, the permeability of epithelial tight junctions can also be acutely regulated by physiological stimuli. This regulation occurs too quickly to be explained by synthesis of new claudin isoforms. The best example of this regulation occurs in the small intestine as a consequence of Na^+-glucose cotransport (61, 79). A functional role for this acute small intestinal tight junction regulation was proposed and suggested that, at high luminal glucose concentrations, paracellular nutrient absorption could serve to amplify transcellular absorption (80). Although this hypothesis is controversial, subsequent studies using glucose analogs (65) and other nonmetabolizable paracellular tracers (90, 108) in rats and humans support it. Moreover, a detailed analysis of the size, selectivity, number, and location of paracellular pores showed that activation of Na^+-glucose cotransport induced a selective increase in the number of small pores within the villus (20). This is consistent with the location of SGLT1, the intestinal Na^+-glucose cotransporter, in villus, but not crypt, enterocytes. Other studies have failed to document such regulation, but they suffer from a lack of significant water absorption (21, 60, 110, 113) or the use of animals with carbohydrate-poor diets that express little SGLT1 (20, 52).

Regulation of Tight Junctions by Cytoskeletal Contraction

Studies of Na^+-glucose cotransport-dependent tight junction regulation identified two primary morphological changes within the region of the tight junction (61). First, dilatations within the tight junction were identified by transmission electron microscopy (61). These intrajunctional dilatations could be permeated by an oligopeptide added to the apical surface, although the oligopeptide was excluded from tight junctions in the absence

of active Na^+-glucose cotransport, suggesting that the dilatations were the site of enhanced paracellular permeability (2). Additionally, analysis of transmission electron micrographs showed that condensation of the perijunctional actomyosin ring occurred in conjunction with the increases in tight junction permeability (1, 61). This suggested that contraction of perijunctional actin was involved in regulating tight junction permeability.

Subsequent studies of a cultured cell model of Na^+-glucose cotransport-dependent tight junction regulation used a biochemical marker, phosphorylation of myosin II regulatory light chain, to evaluate actomyosin contraction (112). These studies showed that phosphorylation of myosin regulatory light chain occurred as a consequence of Na^+-glucose cotransport (112). Inhibition of myosin light chain kinase prevented myosin regulatory light chain phosphorylation in cultured cells and also blocked tight junction regulation in both the cultured cell model and isolated rodent mucosae (112).

Quantitative immunofluorescent analysis of human jejunal mucosa using antisera specific for myosin regulatory light chain phosphorylated at serine-19, the critical regulatory residue, showed that increased myosin regulatory light chain phosphorylation followed activation of Na^+-glucose cotransport (4). The increase in phosphorylation was localized to the perijunctional ring of villus enterocytes (4). Moreover, dual labeling studies showed that, in contrast to the diffuse distribution of total myosin regulatory light chain within the terminal web, the concentration of phosphorylated myosin regulatory light chain was specifically enhanced in the region of the apical junction complex (4) (Fig. 11).

Myosin Light Chain Kinase and Tight Junction Permeability

Further studies directly evaluated the role of myosin regulatory light chain phosphorylation in tight junction regulation using a truncated myosin light chain kinase construct (35) that lacks the inhibitory domain necessary for

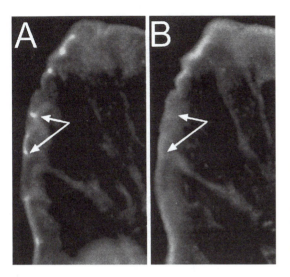

FIGURE 11 Human jejunal mucosae were double-labeled with antiphosphorylated myosin regulatory light chain antisera (A) and antitotal myosin regulatory light chain antisera (B). Focal enrichment of phosphorylated myosin regulatory light chain is obvious at cell-cell junctions (arrows), although total myosin regulatory light chain content is not increased in these areas (B).

kinase regulation (44). This kinase actively phosphorylates myosin regulatory light chain in a calmodulin-independent manner (44). Madin-Darby canine kidney (MDCK) cell monolayers expressing this constitutively active myosin light chain kinase developed transepithelial resistance that was less than 10% of controls (35). Thus, myosin regulatory light chain phosphorylation directly impacted epithelial tight junction permeability. However, since the truncated myosin light chain kinase was expressed continuously, these data do not differentiate between effects of myosin regulatory light chain phosphorylation on tight junction assembly and effects on permeability of assembled tight junctions.

To characterize the effects of myosin regulatory light chain phosphorylation on the function of assembled tight junctions, an inducible expression system was established in the Caco-2 intestinal epithelial cell line (Fig. 12). This model used the same truncated myosin light chain kinase construct, but expression of the kinase was suppressed during monolayer assembly (109). Induction of truncated myosin light chain kinase expression caused a 30% decrease in transepithelial resistance and a comparable increase in transepithelial mannitol flux (109). The decrease in transepithelial resistance was rapidly reversed

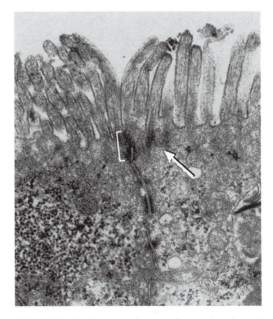

FIGURE 12 In monolayer culture, the Caco-2 human intestinal epithelial cell line has many of the morphological characteristics common to villus enterocytes, including a well-developed microvillus brush border, terminal web (arrow), and mature apical junction complexes (bracket).

by myosin light chain kinase inhibitors (109). Thus, myosin regulatory light chain phosphorylation and the resulting actomyosin contraction acutely regulate the permeability of mature intestinal epithelial tight junctions (109).

Myosin Regulatory Light Chain Phosphorylation by Bacterial Pathogens

A broad range of intestinal pathogens are capable of altering tight junction permeability (14, 19, 28, 34, 36, 76, 77, 82, 102, 104, 126) (see chapters 16, 17, 23, and 27). In many cases, this requires reorganization of perijunctional actin and phosphorylation of myosin regulatory light chain. For example, myosin regulatory light chain phosphorylation is dramatically enhanced after colonization of cultured intestinal epithelial cell monolayers with enteropathogenic *E. coli* (129). This myosin light chain phosphorylation is associated with reorganization of apical F-actin and increased tight junction permeability. Myosin light chain kinase inhibitors blocked both actin reorganization and tight junction regulation (129). Similarly, enterohemorrhagic *E. coli* causes transepithelial electrical resistance to decrease, and this is also partially prevented by myosin light chain kinase inhibitors (82). Thus, myosin regulatory light chain phosphorylation may be a common intermediate in the regulation of tight junctions by both pathogens and nutrients. However, important differences also exist. For example, permeability increases following Na^+-glucose cotransport are tightly regulated and limited to small nutrient-sized molecules (20, 112), while barrier defects induced by bacterial infection are massive and generalized (46, 129).

Myosin Light Chain Kinase as a Therapeutic Target

Based on the evidence that myosin regulatory light chain phosphorylation is associated with physiological and pathophysiological tight junction regulation and that inhibition of myosin light chain kinase can block this reg-

ulation, highly specific inhibitors of myosin light chain kinase were sought as potential therapeutic agents. Unfortunately, the pharmacological inhibitors used in the studies described above compete for the ATP binding site of myosin light chain kinase and, therefore, also inhibit other kinases at only modestly higher doses. Thus, a unique characteristic of myosin light chain kinase was required as a target for therapeutic inhibition. Myosin light chain kinase activity is regulated by interactions between the catalytic domain and the calmodulin-binding inhibitory domain. These interactions are prevented in the presence of Ca^{2+} and calmodulin, resulting in activation of the enzyme. Consistent with this model, a 22-amino-acid peptide from the calmodulin-binding inhibitory domain of smooth muscle myosin light chain kinase effectively inhibits the catalytic domain of smooth muscle myosin light chain kinase (42).

Subsequently, a short linear oligopeptide, derived from that 22-amino-acid sequence, that inhibits myosin light chain kinase but does not significantly inhibit calmodulin-dependent protein kinase II or cyclic AMP (cAMP)-dependent protein kinase was described (57). This peptide also inhibited intestinal epithelial myosin light chain kinase in a dose-dependent, sequence-specific manner (130). Moreover, this oligopeptide contains multiple positively charged residues, analogous to the protein transduction domain of human immunodeficiency virus type 1 (HIV-1) TAT protein (96). Thus, this peptide freely crossed cell membranes and localized to the perijunctional actomyosin ring of cultured intestinal epithelial cells (130).

Consistent with its ability to inhibit myosin light chain kinase in a cell-free biochemical assay, the addition of the oligopeptide to intact cultured cell monolayers caused decreases in intracellular myosin regulatory light chain phosphorylation, reduced paracellular permeability, and increased transepithelial electrical resistance (130). The dose-response and sequence specificity of the effects on transepithelial electrical resistance matched those for myosin light chain kinase inhibition (130).

To evaluate the potential of this oligopeptide as a therapeutic agent, it was applied to cultured cell monolayers after infection with enteropathogenic *E. coli* but before transepithelial electrical resistance fell. The oligopeptide partially prevented the subsequent decline in transepithelial electrical resistance (130). Additionally, the peptide was able to reverse transepithelial electrical resistance defects induced by interferon-γ and tumor necrosis factor-α (130) (see chapter 4), suggesting that the effects of these cytokines on transepithelial electrical resistance are, at least partly, due to activation of myosin light chain kinase (130). Further study of this oligopeptide may lead to the development of a novel class of therapeutic agents that restore intestinal barrier function following noncytolytic epithelial injury.

ACKNOWLEDGMENTS

I greatly appreciate the critical reviews of this chapter provided by John Hart, Randall Mrsny, and Judith Turner. I am also grateful for the expert imaging assistance of Gordon Bowie and Elizabeth Sengupta for use of the clinical electron micrograph collection of The University of Chicago Department of Pathology. Work in my laboratory is supported by NIH grants DK61931 and DK56121.

REFERENCES

1. **Atisook, K., S. Carlson, and J. L. Madara.** 1990. Effects of phlorizin and sodium on glucose-elicited alterations of cell junctions in intestinal epithelia. *Am. J. Physiol.* **258:**C77–C85.
2. **Atisook, K., and J. L. Madara.** 1991. An oligopeptide permeates intestinal tight junctions at glucose-elicited dilatations. Implications for oligopeptide absorption. *Gastroenterology* **100:**719–724.
3. **Barrett, K. E., and S. J. Keely.** 2000. Chloride secretion by the intestinal epithelium: molecular basis and regulatory aspects. *Annu. Rev. Physiol.* **62:**535–572.
4. **Berglund, J. J., M. Riegler, Y. Zolotarevsky, E. Wenzl, and J. R. Turner.** 2001. Regulation of human jejunal transmucosal resistance and MLC phosphorylation by Na$^+$-glucose cotransport. *Am. J. Physiol. Gastrointest. Liver Physiol.* **281:**G1487–G1493.
5. **Bjerknes, M., and H. Cheng.** 2001. Modulation of specific intestinal epithelial progenitors by enteric neurons. *Proc. Natl. Acad. Sci. USA* **98:**12497–12502.
6. **Booth, C., and C. S. Potten.** 2000. Gut instincts: thoughts on intestinal epithelial stem cells. *J. Clin. Invest.* **105:**1493–1499.
7. **Brandtzaeg, P.** 1978. Polymeric IgA is complexed with secretory component (SC) on the surface of human intestinal epithelial cells. *Scand. J. Immunol.* **8:**39–52.
8. **Buchan, A. M., J. M. Polak, E. Solcia, and A. G. Pearse.** 1979. Localisation of intestinal gastrin in a distinct endocrine cell type. *Nature* **277:**138–140.
9. **Burgess, D. R.** 1982. Reactivation of intestinal epithelial cell brush border motility: ATP-dependent contraction via a terminal web contractile ring. *J. Cell Biol.* **95:**853–863.
10. **Casanova, J. E., P. P. Breitfeld, S. A. Ross, and K. E. Mostov.** 1990. Phosphorylation of the polymeric immunoglobulin receptor required for its efficient transcytosis. *Science* **248:**742–745.
11. **Chen, Y., C. Merzdorf, D. L. Paul, and D. A. Goodenough.** 1997. COOH terminus of occludin is required for tight junction barrier function in early *Xenopus* embryos. *J. Cell Biol.* **138:**891–899.
12. **Cheng, H., J. Merzel, and C. P. Leblond.** 1969. Renewal of Paneth cells in the small intestine of the mouse. *Am. J. Anat.* **126:**507–525.
13. **Chung, B. M., J. K. Wong, J. A. Hardin, and D. G. Gall.** 1999. Role of actin in EGF-induced alterations in enterocyte SGLT1 expression. *Am. J. Physiol.* **276:**G463–G469.
14. **Dickman, K. G., S. J. Hempson, J. Anderson, S. Lippe, L. Zhao, R. Burakoff, and R. D. Shaw.** 2000. Rotavirus alters paracellular permeability and energy metabolism in Caco-2 cells. *Am. J. Physiol. Gastrointest. Liver Physiol.* **279:**G757–766.
15. **Drumm, B., A. M. Roberton, and P. M. Sherman.** 1988. Inhibition of attachment of *Escherichia coli* RDEC-1 to intestinal microvillus membranes by rabbit ileal mucus and mucin in vitro. *Infect. Immun.* **56:**2437–2442.
16. **Dura, W. T., and E. Bernatowska.** 1984. Secretory component, alpha 1-antitrypsin and lysozyme in IgA deficient children. An immunohistochemical evaluation of intestinal mucosa. *Histopathology* **8:**747–757.
17. **Elmes, M. E., M. R. Stanton, C. H. Howells, and G. H. Lowe.** 1984. Relation between the mucosal flora and Paneth cell population of human jejunum and ileum. *J. Clin. Pathol.* **37:**1268–1271.

18. **Farquhar, M., and G. Palade.** 1963. Junctional complexes in various epithelia. *J. Cell Biol.* **17:** 375–412.

19. **Fasano, A., C. Fiorentini, G. Donelli, S. Uzzau, J. B. Kaper, K. Margaretten, X. Ding, S. Guandalini, L. Comstock, and S. E. Goldblum.** 1995. Zonula occludens toxin modulates tight junctions through protein kinase C-dependent actin reorganization, in vitro. *J. Clin. Invest.* **96:**710–720.

20. **Fihn, B. M., A. Sjoqvist, and M. Jodal.** 2000. Permeability of the rat small intestinal epithelium along the villus-crypt axis: effects of glucose transport. *Gastroenterology* **119:**1029–1036.

21. **Fine, K. D., C. A. Santa Ana, J. L. Porter, and J. S. Fordtran.** 1994. Mechanism by which glucose stimulates the passive absorption of small solutes by the human jejunum *in vivo. Gastroenterology* **107:**389–395.

22. **Fujita, K., J. Katahira, Y. Horiguchi, N. Sonoda, M. Furuse, and S. Tsukita.** 2000. *Clostridium perfringens* enterotoxin binds to the second extracellular loop of claudin-3, a tight junction integral membrane protein. *FEBS Lett.* **476:**258–261.

23. **Furuse, M., K. Fujimoto, N. Sato, T. Hirase, and S. Tsukita.** 1996. Overexpression of occludin, a tight junction-associated integral membrane protein, induces the formation of intracellular multilamellar bodies bearing tight junction-like structures. *J. Cell Sci.* **109:**429–435.

24. **Furuse, M., K. Furuse, H. Sasaki, and S. Tsukita.** 2001. Conversion of zonulae occludentes from tight to leaky strand type by introducing claudin-2 into Madin-Darby canine kidney I cells. *J. Cell Biol.* **153:**263–272.

25. **Furuse, M., T. Hirase, M. Itoh, A. Nagafuchi, S. Yonemura, S. Tsukita, and S. Tsukita.** 1993. Occludin: a novel integral membrane protein localizing at tight junctions. *J. Cell Biol.* **123:**1777–1788.

26. **Furuse, M., H. Sasaki, K. Fujimoto, and S. Tsukita.** 1998. A single gene product, claudin-1 or -2, reconstitutes tight junction strands and recruits occludin in fibroblasts. *J. Cell Biol.* **143:** 391–401.

27. **Gallardo, P., L. P. Cid, C. P. Vio, and F. V. Sepulveda.** 2001. Aquaporin-2, a regulated water channel, is expressed in apical membranes of rat distal colon epithelium. *Am. J. Physiol. Gastrointest. Liver Physiol.* **281:**G856–G863.

28. **Gerhard, R., G. Schmidt, F. Hofmann, and K. Aktories.** 1998. Activation of Rho GTPases by *Escherichia coli* cytotoxic necrotizing factor 1 increases intestinal permeability in Caco-2 cells. *Infect. Immun.* **66:**5125–5131.

29. **Gledhill, A., P. A. Hall, J. P. Cruse, and D. J. Pollock.** 1986. Enteroendocrine cell hyperplasia, carcinoid tumours and adenocarcinoma in long-standing ulcerative colitis. *Histopathology* **10:**501–508.

30. **Gorbach, S. L., A. G. Plaut, L. Nahas, L. Weinstein, G. Spanknebel, and R. Levitan.** 1967. Studies of intestinal microflora. II. Microorganisms of the small intestine and their relations to oral and fecal flora. *Gastroenterology* **53:**856–867.

31. **Hallback, D. A., M. Jodal, M. Mannischeff, and O. Lundgren.** 1991. Tissue osmolality in intestinal villi of four mammals in vivo and in vitro. *Acta Physiol. Scand.* **143:**271–277.

32. **Hardin, J. A., A. Buret, J. B. Meddings, and D. G. Gall.** 1993. Effect of epidermal growth factor on enterocyte brush-border surface area. *Am. J. Physiol.* **264:**G312–G318.

33. **Hatakeyama, S., Y. Yoshida, T. Tani, Y. Koyama, K. Nihei, K. Ohshiro, J. I. Kamiie, E. Yaoita, T. Suda, K. Hatakeyama, and T. Yamamoto.** 2001. Cloning of a new aquaporin (AQP10) abundantly expressed in duodenum and jejunum. *Biochem. Biophys. Res. Commun.* **287:** 814–819.

34. **Hecht, G., A. Koutsouris, C. Pothoulakis, J. T. LaMont, and J. L. Madara.** 1992. *Clostridium difficile* toxin B disrupts the barrier function of T84 monolayers. *Gastroenterology* **102:** 416–423.

35. **Hecht, G., L. Pestic, G. Nikcevic, A. Koutsouris, J. Tripuraneni, D. D. Lorimer, G. Nowak, V. Guerriero, Jr., E. L. Elson, and P. D. Lanerolle.** 1996. Expression of the catalytic domain of myosin light chain kinase increases paracellular permeability. *Am. J. Physiol.* **271:**C1678–C1684.

36. **Hecht, G., C. Pothoulakis, J. T. LaMont, and J. L. Madara.** 1988. *Clostridium difficile* toxin A perturbs cytoskeletal structure and tight junction permeability of cultured human intestinal epithelial monolayers. *J. Clin. Invest.* **82:**1516–1524.

37. **Hermiston, M. L., and J. I. Gordon.** 1995. Inflammatory bowel disease and adenomas in mice expressing a dominant negative N-cadherin. *Science* **270:**1203–1207.

38. **Hermiston, M. L., R. P. Green, and J. I. Gordon.** 1993. Chimeric-transgenic mice represent a powerful tool for studying how the proliferation and differentiation programs of intestinal epithelial cell lineages are regulated. *Proc. Natl. Acad. Sci. USA* **90:**8866–8870.

39. **Hermiston, M. L., M. H. Wong, and J. I. Gordon.** 1996. Forced expression of E-cadherin in the mouse intestinal epithelium slows cell mi-

gration and provides evidence for nonautonomous regulation of cell fate in a self-renewing system. *Genes Dev.* **10**:985–996.

40. **Hirokawa, N., T. C. Keller 3rd, R. Chasan, and M. S. Mooseker.** 1983. Mechanism of brush border contractility studied by the quick-freeze, deep-etch method. *J. Cell Biol.* **96**:1325–1336.

41. **Hwang, E. S., B. A. Hirayama, and E. M. Wright.** 1991. Distribution of the SGLT1 Na$^+$/glucose cotransporter and mRNA along the crypt-villus axis of rabbit small intestine. *Biochem. Biophys. Res. Commun.* **181**:1208–1217.

42. **Ikebe, M., M. Stepinska, B. E. Kemp, A. R. Means, and D. J. Hartshorne.** 1987. Proteolysis of smooth muscle myosin light chain kinase. Formation of inactive and calmodulin-independent fragments. *J. Biol. Chem.* **262**:13828–13834.

43. **Ikeda, T. S., E.-S. Hwang, M. J. Coady, B. A. Hirayama, M. A. Hediger, and E. M. Wright.** 1989. Characterization of a Na$^+$/glucose cotransporter cloned from rabbit small intestine. *J. Membr. Biol.* **110**:87–95.

44. **Ito, M., V. Guerriero, Jr., X. M. Chen, and D. J. Hartshorne.** 1991. Definition of the inhibitory domain of smooth muscle myosin light chain kinase by site-directed mutagenesis. *Biochemistry* **30**:3498–3503.

45. **Itoh, H., P. L. Beck, N. Inoue, R. Xavier, and D. K. Podolsky.** 1999. A paradoxical reduction in susceptibility to colonic injury upon targeted transgenic ablation of goblet cells. *J. Clin. Invest.* **104**:1539–1547.

46. **Johansen, K., G. Stintzing, K. E. Magnusson, T. Sundqvist, F. Jalil, A. Murtaza, S. R. Khan, B. S. Lindblad, R. Mollby, E. Orusild, et al.** 1989. Intestinal permeability assessed with polyethylene glycols in children with diarrhea due to rotavirus and common bacterial pathogens in a developing community. *J. Pediatr. Gastroenterol. Nutr.* **9**:307–313.

47. **Just, I., J. Selzer, M. Wilm, C. von Eichel-Streiber, M. Mann, and K. Aktories.** 1995. Glucosylation of Rho proteins by *Clostridium difficile* toxin B. *Nature* **375**:500–503.

48. **Karlsson, J., A. Ungell, J. Grasjo, and P. Artursson.** 1999. Paracellular drug transport across intestinal epithelia: influence of charge and induced water flux. *Eur. J. Pharm. Sci.* **9**:47–56.

49. **Kerneis, S., A. Bogdanova, J. P. Kraehenbuhl, and E. Pringault.** 1997. Conversion by Peyer's patch lymphocytes of human enterocytes into M cells that transport bacteria. *Science* **277**:949–952.

50. **Kindon, H., C. Pothoulakis, L. Thim, K. Lynch-Devaney, and D. K. Podolsky.** 1995. Trefoil peptide protection of intestinal epithelial barrier function: cooperative interaction with mucin glycoprotein. *Gastroenterology* **109**:516–523.

51. **Koyama, Y., T. Yamamoto, T. Tani, K. Nihei, D. Kondo, H. Funaki, E. Yaoita, K. Kawasaki, N. Sato, K. Hatakeyama, and I. Kihara.** 1999. Expression and localization of aquaporins in rat gastrointestinal tract. *Am. J. Physiol.* **276**:C621–C627.

52. **Lane, J. S., E. E. Whang, D. A. Rigberg, O. J. Hines, D. Kwan, M. J. Zinner, D. W. McFadden, J. Diamond, and S. W. Ashley.** 1999. Paracellular glucose transport plays a minor role in the unanesthetized dog. *Am. J. Physiol.* **276**:G789–G794.

53. **Leitch, G. J.** 1988. Cholera enterotoxin-induced mucus secretion and increase in the mucus blanket of the rabbit ileum in vivo. *Infect. Immun.* **56**:2871–2875.

54. **Lelouard, H., A. Sahuquet, H. Reggio, and P. Montcourrier.** 2001. Rabbit M cells and dome enterocytes are distinct cell lineages. *J. Cell Sci.* **114**:2077–2083.

55. **Li, D., and R. J. Mrsny.** 2000. Oncogenic Raf-1 disrupts epithelial tight junctions via down-regulation of occludin. *J. Cell Biol.* **148**:791–800.

56. **Lu, H. H., J. D. Thomas, J. J. Tukker, and D. Fleisher.** 1992. Intestinal water and solute absorption studies: comparison of in situ perfusion with chronic isolated loops in rats. *Pharm. Res.* **9**:894–900.

57. **Lukas, T. J., S. Mirzoeva, U. Slomczynska, and D. M. Watterson.** 1999. Identification of novel classes of protein kinase inhibitors using combinatorial peptide chemistry based on functional genomics knowledge. *J. Med. Chem.* **42**:910–919.

58. **Madara, J. L.** 1987. Intestinal absorptive cell tight junctions are linked to cytoskeleton. *Am. J. Physiol.* **253**:C171–C175.

59. **Madara, J. L.** 1990. Maintenance of the macromolecular barrier at cell extrusion sites in intestinal epithelium: physiological rearrangement of tight junctions. *J. Membr. Biol.* **116**:177–184.

60. **Madara, J. L.** 1994. Sodium-glucose cotransport and epithelial permeability. *Gastroenterology* **107**:319–320.

61. **Madara, J. L., and J. R. Pappenheimer.** 1987. Structural basis for physiological regulation of paracellular pathways in intestinal epithelia. *J. Membr. Biol.* **100**:149–164.

62. **Madara, J. L., J. Stafford, D. Barenberg, and S. Carlson.** 1988. Functional coupling of tight junctions and microfilaments in T84 monolayers. *Am. J. Physiol.* **254**:G416-G423.

63. Marcial, M. A., S. L. Carlson, and J. L. Madara. 1984. Partitioning of paracellular conductance along the ileal crypt-villus axis: a hypothesis based on structural analysis with detailed consideration of tight junction structure-function relationships. *J. Membr. Biol.* **80**:59–70.

64. McCormick, D. A., L. W. Horton, and A. S. Mee. 1990. Mucin depletion in inflammatory bowel disease. *J. Clin. Pathol.* **43**:143–146.

65. Meddings, J. B., and H. Westergaard. 1989. Intestinal glucose transport using perfused rat jejunum in vivo: model analysis and derivation of corrected kinetic constants. *Clin. Sci.* (London) **76**:403–413.

66. Meinild, A., D. A. Klaerke, D. D. Loo, E. M. Wright, and T. Zeuthen. 1998. The human Na^+-glucose cotransporter is a molecular water pump. *J. Physiol.* (London) **508**:15–21.

67. Merzel, J., and C. P. Leblond. 1969. Origin and renewal of goblet cells in the epithelium of the mouse small intestine. *Am. J. Anat.* **124**:281–305.

68. Moon, H. W., S. C. Whipp, and A. L. Baetz. 1971. Comparative effects of enterotoxins from *Escherichia coli* and *Vibrio cholerae* on rabbit and swine small intestine. *Lab. Invest.* **25**:133–140.

69. Morson, B. C., L. H. Sobin, E. Grundmann, A. Johansen, T. Nagayo, and A. Serck-Hanssen. 1980. Precancerous conditions and epithelial dysplasia in the stomach. *J. Clin. Pathol.* **33**:711–721.

70. Mostov, K. E. 1994. Transepithelial transport of immunoglobulins. *Annu. Rev. Immunol.* **12**:63–84.

71. Mouricout, M. A., and R. A. Julien. 1987. Pilus-mediated binding of bovine enterotoxigenic *Escherichia coli* to calf small intestinal mucins. *Infect. Immun.* **55**:1216–1223.

72. Muresan, Z., D. L. Paul, and D. A. Goodenough. 2000. Occludin 1B, a variant of the tight junction protein occludin. *Mol. Biol. Cell* **11**:627–634.

73. Neutra, M. R., N. J. Mantis, and J. P. Kraehenbuhl. 2001. Collaboration of epithelial cells with organized mucosal lymphoid tissues. *Nat. Immunol.* **2**:1004–1009.

74. Nieminen, U., A. Kahri, E. Savilahti, and M. A. Farkkila. 2001. Duodenal disaccharidase activities in the follow-up of villous atrophy in coeliac disease. *Scand. J. Gastroenterol.* **36**:507–510.

75. Nusrat, A., J. A. Chen, C. S. Foley, T. W. Liang, J. Tom, M. Cromwell, C. Quan, and R. J. Mrsny. 2000. The coiled-coil domain of occludin can act to organize structural and functional elements of the epithelial tight junction. *J. Biol. Chem.* **275**:29816–29822.

76. Nusrat, A., M. Giry, J. R. Turner, S. P. Colgan, C. A. Parkos, D. Carnes, E. Lemichez, P. Boquet, and J. L. Madara. 1995. Rho protein regulates tight junctions and perijunctional actin organization in polarized epithelia. *Proc. Natl. Acad. Sci. USA* **92**:10629–10633.

77. Obert, G., I. Peiffer, and A. L. Servin. 2000. Rotavirus-induced structural and functional alterations in tight junctions of polarized intestinal Caco-2 cell monolayers. *J. Virol.* **74**:4645–4651.

78. Paerregaard, A., F. Espersen, O. M. Jensen, and M. Skurnik. 1991. Interactions between *Yersinia enterocolitica* and rabbit ileal mucus: growth, adhesion, penetration, and subsequent changes in surface hydrophobicity and ability to adhere to ileal brush border membrane vesicles. *Infect. Immun.* **59**:253–260.

79. Pappenheimer, J. R. 1987. Physiological regulation of transepithelial impedance in the intestinal mucosa of rats and hamsters. *J. Membr. Biol.* **100**:137–148.

80. Pappenheimer, J. R. 1993. On the coupling of membrane digestion with intestinal absorption of sugars and amino acids. *Am. J. Physiol.* **265**:G409–G417.

81. Pearse, A. G., and J. M. Polak. 1975. Immunocytochemical localization of substance P in mammalian intestine. *Histochemistry* **41**:373–375.

82. Philpott, D. J., D. M. McKay, W. Mak, M. H. Perdue, and P. M. Sherman. 1998. Signal transduction pathways involved in enterohemorrhagic *Escherichia coli*-induced alterations in T84 epithelial permeability. *Infect. Immun.* **66**:1680–1687.

83. Potten, C. S., and M. Loeffler. 1990. Stem cells: attributes, cycles, spirals, pitfalls and uncertainties. Lessons for and from the crypt. *Development* **110**:1001–1020.

84. Powell, D. W. 1981. Barrier function of epithelia. *Am. J. Physiol.* **241**:G275–G288.

85. Rahner, C., L. L. Mitic, and J. M. Anderson. 2001. Heterogeneity in expression and subcellular localization of claudins 2, 3, 4, and 5 in the rat liver, pancreas, and gut. *Gastroenterology* **120**:411–422.

86. Rosenblatt, J., M. C. Raff, and L. P. Cramer. 2001. An epithelial cell destined for apoptosis signals its neighbors to extrude it by an actin- and myosin-dependent mechanism. *Curr. Biol.* **11**:1847–1857.

87. Roth, K. A., S. Kim, and J. I. Gordon. 1992. Immunocytochemical studies suggest two pathways for enteroendocrine cell differentiation in the colon. *Am. J. Physiol.* **263**:G174–G180.

88. Rubin, D. C., E. Swietlicki, K. A. Roth, and J. I. Gordon. 1992. Use of fetal intestinal isografts from normal and transgenic mice to study the programming of positional information along the duodenal-to-colonic axis. *J. Biol. Chem.* **267**:15122–15133.

89. Sachdev, H. P., V. Chadha, V. Malhotra, A. Verghese, and R. K. Puri. 1993. Rectal histopathology in endemic *Shigella* and *Salmonella* diarrhea. *J. Pediatr. Gastroenterol. Nutr.* **16**:33–38.

90. Sadowski, D. C., and J. B. Meddings. 1993. Luminal nutrients alter tight-junction permeability in the rat jejunum: an in vivo perfusion model. *Can. J. Physiol. Pharmacol.* **71**:835–839.

91. Saitou, M., M. Furuse, H. Sasaki, J. D. Schulzke, M. Fromm, H. Takano, T. Noda, and S. Tsukita. 2000. Complex phenotype of mice lacking occludin, a component of tight junction strands. *Mol. Biol. Cell* **11**:4131–4142.

92. Sajjan, S. U., and J. F. Forstner. 1990. Characteristics of binding of *Escherichia coli* serotype O157:H7 strain CL-49 to purified intestinal mucin. *Infect. Immun.* **58**:860–867.

93. Schaerer, E., M. R. Neutra, and J. P. Kraehenbuhl. 1991. Molecular and cellular mechanisms involved in transepithelial transport. *J. Membr. Biol.* **123**:93–103.

94. Schneider, D. R., and C. D. Parker. 1982. Purification and characterization of the mucinase of *Vibrio cholerae*. *J. Infect. Dis.* **145**:474–482.

95. Schreiber, R., H. Pavenstadt, R. Greger, and K. Kunzelmann. 2000. Aquaporin 3 cloned from *Xenopus laevis* is regulated by the cystic fibrosis transmembrane conductance regulator. *FEBS Lett.* **475**:291–295.

96. Schwarze, S. R., A. Ho, A. Vocero-Akbani, and S. F. Dowdy. 1999. In vivo protein transduction: delivery of a biologically active protein into the mouse. *Science* **285**:1569–1572.

97. Simon, D. B., Y. Lu, K. A. Choate, H. Velazquez, E. Al-Sabban, M. Praga, G. Casari, A. Bettinelli, G. Colussi, J. Rodriguez-Soriano, D. McCredie, D. Milford, S. Sanjad, and R. P. Lifton. 1999. Paracellin-1, a renal tight junction protein required for paracellular Mg^{2+} resorption. *Science* **285**:103–106.

98. Simonovic, I., J. Rosenberg, A. Koutsouris, and G. Hecht. 2000. Enteropathogenic *Escherichia coli* dephosphorylates and dissociates occludin from intestinal epithelial tight junctions. *Cell Microbiol.* **2**:305–315.

99. Smith, M. W., M. A. Peacock, and P. S. James. 1991. Galactose increases microvillus development in mouse jejunal enterocytes. *Comp. Biochem. Physiol. A* **100**:489–493.

100. Sonoda, N., M. Furuse, H. Sasaki, S. Yonemura, J. Katahira, Y. Horiguchi, and S. Tsukita. 1999. *Clostridium perfringens* enterotoxin fragment removes specific claudins from tight junction strands. Evidence for direct involvement of claudins in tight junction barrier. *J. Cell Biol.* **147**:195–204.

101. Specian, R. D., and M. R. Neutra. 1980. Mechanism of rapid mucus secretion in goblet cells stimulated by acetylcholine. *J. Cell Biol.* **85**:626–640.

102. Spitz, J., R. Yuhan, A. Koutsouris, C. Blatt, J. Alverdy, and G. Hecht. 1995. Enteropathogenic *Escherichia coli* adherence to intestinal epithelial monolayers diminishes barrier function. *Am. J. Physiol.* **268**:G374–G379.

103. Staehelin, L. A., T. M. Mukherjee, and A. W. Williams. 1969. Freeze-etch appearance of the tight junctions in the epithelium of small and large intestine of mice. *Protoplasma* **67**:165–184.

104. Stintzing, G., K. Johansen, K. E. Magnusson, L. Svensson, and T. Sundqvist. 1986. Intestinal permeability in small children during and after rotavirus diarrhoea assessed with different-size polyethyleneglycols (PEG 400 and PEG 1000). *Acta Paediatr. Scand.* **75**:1005–1009.

105. Thomson, A. B. 1984. Effect of region of intestine and unstirred layers on uptake of sugars into rabbit intestine. *Q. J. Exp. Physiol.* **69**:497–505.

106. Trier, J. S. 1966. The Paneth cells: an enigma. *Gastroenterology* **51**:560–562.

107. Turner, J. R. 2000. "Putting the squeeze" on the tight junction: understanding cytoskeletal regulation. *Semin. Cell Dev. Biol.* **11**:301–308.

108. Turner, J. R., D. E. Cohen, R. J. Mrsny, and J. L. Madara. 2000. Noninvasive *in vivo* analysis of human small intestinal paracellular absorption: regulation by Na^+-glucose cotransport. *Dig. Dis. Sci.* **45**:2122–2126.

109. Turner, J. R., V. Guerriero, Jr., E. D. Black, and K. Haelewyn. 2000. Regulated expression of the myosin light chain kinase catalytic domain increases paracellular permeability and alters tight junction structure. *Gastroenterology* **118**:A432.

110. Turner, J. R., and J. L. Madara. 1995. Physiological regulation of intestinal epithelial tight junctions as a consequence of Na^+-coupled nutrient transport. *Gastroenterology* **109**:1391–1396.

111. Turner, J. R., and R. D. Odze. 1996. Proliferative characteristics of differentiated cells in familial adenomatous polyposis-associated duodenal adenomas. *Hum. Pathol.* **27**:63–69.

112. Turner, J. R., B. K. Rill, S. L. Carlson, D. Carnes, R. Kerner, R. J. Mrsny, and J. L. Madara. 1997. Physiological regulation of epithelial tight junctions is associated with myosin light-chain phosphorylation. *Am. J. Physiol.* **273**:C1378–C1385.

113. **Uhing, M. R., and R. E. Kimura.** 1995. The effect of surgical bowel manipulation and anesthesia on intestinal glucose absorption in rats. *J. Clin. Invest.* **95:**2790–2798.

114. **Van Itallie, C., C. Rahner, and J. M. Anderson.** 2001. Regulated expression of claudin-4 decreases paracellular conductance through a selective decrease in sodium permeability. *J. Clin. Invest.* **107:**1319–1327.

115. **Van Itallie, C. M., and J. M. Anderson.** 1997. Occludin confers adhesiveness when expressed in fibroblasts. *J. Cell Sci.* **110:**1113–1121.

116. **Vega-Salas, D. E., P. J. Salas, and E. Rodriguez-Boulan.** 1988. Exocytosis of vacuolar apical compartment (VAC): a cell-cell contact controlled mechanism for the establishment of the apical plasma membrane domain in epithelial cells. *J. Cell Biol.* **107:**1717–1728.

117. **Vimal, D. B., M. Khullar, S. Gupta, and N. K. Ganguly.** 2000. Intestinal mucins: the binding sites for *Salmonella typhimurium*. *Mol. Cell. Biochem.* **204:**107–117.

118. **Wadolkowski, E. A., D. C. Laux, and P. S. Cohen.** 1988. Colonization of the streptomycin-treated mouse large intestine by a human fecal *Escherichia coli* strain: role of adhesion to mucosal receptors. *Infect. Immun.* **56:**1036–1043.

119. **Wadolkowski, E. A., D. C. Laux, and P. S. Cohen.** 1988. Colonization of the streptomycin-treated mouse large intestine by a human fecal *Escherichia coli* strain: role of growth in mucus. *Infect. Immun.* **56:**1030–1035.

120. **Wang, A. Z., J. C. Wang, G. K. Ojakian, and W. J. Nelson.** 1994. Determinants of apical membrane formation and distribution in multicellular epithelial MDCK cysts. *Am. J. Physiol.* **267:**C473–C481.

121. **Wang, K. S., T. Ma, F. Filiz, A. S. Verkman, and J. A. Bastidas.** 2000. Colon water transport in transgenic mice lacking aquaporin-4 water channels. *Am. J. Physiol. Gastrointest. Liver Physiol.* **279:**G463–G470.

122. **Welsh, J. D., O. M. Zschiesche, J. Anderson, and A. Walker.** 1969. Intestinal disaccharidase activity in celiac sprue (gluten-sensitive enteropathy). *Arch. Intern. Med.* **123:**33–38.

123. **Wong, V.** 1997. Phosphorylation of occludin correlates with occludin localization and function at the tight junction. *Am. J. Physiol.* **273:**C1859–C1867.

124. **Wong, V., and B. M. Gumbiner.** 1997. A synthetic peptide corresponding to the extracellular domain of occludin perturbs the tight junction permeability barrier. *J. Cell Biol.* **136:**399–409.

125. **Wu, M. S., C. T. Shun, W. C. Lee, C. J. Chen, H. P. Wang, W. J. Lee, and J. T. Lin.** 1998. Gastric cancer risk in relation to *Helicobacter pylori* infection and subtypes of intestinal metaplasia. *Br. J. Cancer* **78:**125–128.

126. **Wu, S., K. C. Lim, J. Huang, R. F. Saidi, and C. L. Sears.** 1998. *Bacteroides fragilis* enterotoxin cleaves the zonula adherens protein, E-cadherin. *Proc. Natl. Acad. Sci. USA* **95:**14979–14984.

127. **Xiao, Q., R. P. Boushey, M. Cino, D. J. Drucker, and P. L. Brubaker.** 2000. Circulating levels of glucagon-like peptide-2 in human subjects with inflammatory bowel disease. *Am. J. Physiol. Regul. Integr. Comp. Physiol.* **278:**R1057–R1063.

128. **Yang, Q., N. A. Bermingham, M. J. Finegold, and H. Y. Zoghbi.** 2001. Requirement of Math1 for secretory cell lineage commitment in the mouse intestine. *Science* **294:**2155–2158.

129. **Yuhan, R., A. Koutsouris, S. D. Savkovic, and G. Hecht.** 1997. Enteropathogenic *Escherichia coli*-induced myosin light chain phosphorylation alters intestinal epithelial permeability. *Gastroenterology* **113:**1873–1882.

130. **Zolotarevsky, Y., G. Hecht, A. Koutsouris, D. E. Gonzales, C. Quan, J. Tom, R. J. Mrsny, and J. R. Turner.** 2002. A membrane-permeant peptide that inhibits MLC kinase restores barrier function in *in vitro* models of intestinal disease. *Gastroenterology* **123:**163–172.

ROLE OF INTESTINAL M CELLS IN MICROBIAL PATHOGENESIS

Marian R. Neutra, Philippe Sansonetti, and Jean-Pierre Kraehenbuhl

2

THE INTESTINAL EPITHELIUM AND ORGANIZED MUCOSAL LYMPHOID TISSUES

The intestinal epithelium is remarkable in its ability to serve multiple functions simultaneously. While it conducts terminal digestion and absorption of nutrients, it also provides an effective barrier against lumenal microorganisms. This is accomplished by production of secreted defensive factors, including mucins, secretory antibodies, and antibacterial proteins, and by maintenance of a continuous network of tight junctions that exclude macromolecules and microorganisms (94). At the same time the epithelium is responsible for providing the immune system with a continuous stream of information about the contents of the lumen. This immune surveillance function depends on a close collaboration of epithelial cells with antigen-presenting and lymphoid cells, and this collaboration is particularly striking at sites containing organized mucosal

lymphoid follicles (17, 18). A specialized follicle-associated epithelium (FAE) that contains M cells is found only at these sites. Epithelial M cells deliver samples of foreign material through active transepithelial vesicular transport from the intestinal lumen directly to the basolateral side of the epithelium. This tends to restrict the uptake of antigens and microorganisms to organized mucosal lymphoid tissues where mucosal immune responses are initiated (16, 87, 103). M cells can transport noninvasive bacteria, including those of the endogenous flora, and this may result in T-cell-independent immunoglobulin (IgA) antibody responses (92) that are thought to regulate the populations of commensal bacteria in the lumen and to eliminate those that have entered the mucosa. There is recent evidence that lumenal microorganisms can be directly captured by intraepithelial dendritic cells that send processes into the lumen (137). Experiments in mice suggest that antigen presentation and T-cell-independent generation of IgA B cells can occur in the absence of organized mucosal lymphoid tissue (36). However, M cells are known to provide an entry route into the mucosa for a variety of bacterial and viral pathogens and to play an important role in microbial pathogenesis in the intestine (114, 118, 120, 144, 153).

Marian R. Neutra, Department of Pediatrics, Harvard Medical School, GI Cell Biology Laboratory, Children's Hospital, Boston, MA 02115. *Philippe Sansonetti*, Unité de Pathogenie Microbienne Moleculaire, Institut Pasteur, 75724 Paris Cedex 15, France. *Jean-Pierre Kraehenbuhl*, Swiss Institute for Experimental Cancer Research, Institute of Biochemistry, University of Lausanne, CH-1066 Epalinges, Switzerland.

Microbial Pathogenesis and the Intestinal Epithelial Cell, ed. by G. Hecht
© 2003 ASM Press, Washington, D.C.

Mucosal lymphoid follicles with associated FAE are widely distributed in the digestive tract (57, 124). The Peyer's patches have been most extensively studied because they consist of large aggregates of follicles visible on the antimesenteric surface of the intestine. In mice, patches of aggregated follicles are present throughout the small intestine and in the cecum, colon, and rectum (124, 127). In humans, large Peyer's patches are restricted to the ileum, and lymphoid follicles are abundant in the appendix. Single isolated follicles also occur throughout the intestines of all species examined. It is important to note that in humans, isolated lymphoid follicles occur throughout the large intestine, with highest frequency in the rectum (45, 123). In the large intestines of mice and humans, lymphoid follicles are often positioned deep in the mucosa, and their associated FAE is sequestered at the base of a crypt-like epithelial invagination (45, 80, 123, 127).

THE FAE

Taken together, the FAE represents an exceedingly small fraction of the total intestinal surface area. The fact that some pathogens efficiently use the FAE for entry into the mucosa suggests that chemotactic mechanisms may play a role, but these have not been identified. How pathogens recognize the FAE as a potential entry site is poorly understood, but there is evidence that the surface of the entire FAE is biochemically distinct from that of the surrounding epithelium. For example, follicle-associated enterocytes express lower amounts of the membrane-associated digestive hydrolases than do their counterparts on villi (126, 146). There is little mucus production by the FAE (124), and fewer defensin- and lysozyme-producing Paneth cells are present in follicle-associated crypts (54). In addition, the entire FAE is devoid of polymeric immunoglobulin receptors, and this may result in a scarcity of protective IgA on the mucosal surface at these sites (130). All of these features would tend to allow contact of intact antigens and pathogens with the FAE.

Functional assays reveal subtle differences in the FAE and villus epithelial surface chemistry. In mouse and rabbit Peyer's patches, for example, polystyrene microparticles adhere preferentially to the FAE (43, 129), implying a difference in epithelial surface charge. Microorganisms may also recognize the FAE by sensing distinct carbohydrate structures. The glycosylation patterns of epithelial cells in the entire FAE differ from those on villi (49, 53, 54, 149), and in rabbits, lectin-coated microparticles had access to specific carbohydrate binding sites on the FAE but not on villi (96). Although these findings suggest that FAE cells express a distinct array of glycosyltransferases, they may also reflect differences in expression of integral membrane proteins. In current in situ hybridization studies, we have observed that FAE cells in mice and humans contain little or no message for the integral membrane mucins muc 1 and muc 3 (A. Helander, J. Forstner and M. R. Neutra, unpublished data), two highly glycosylated components of the brush border glycocalyx of villus cells (84).

Little is known about expression of specific genes unique to the FAE. An important finding is that the FAE of Peyer's patches expresses a chemokine, CCL20 (MIP-3α), that under normal conditions is not expressed elsewhere in the small intestinal epithelium (29, 71). By release of CCL20, a chemokine that is recognized by cells that express the chemokine receptor CCR6, the FAE may play a role in maintenance of mucosal inductive sites, as discussed below. In mice lacking CCR6, dendritic cells expressing CD11c and CD11b are absent from the subepithelial dome of Peyer's patches, and these mice have an impaired humoral immune response to orally administered antigen and to enteropathogenic rotavirus (29). Studies using transgenic mice have demonstrated that FAE gene expression is indeed distinct from that of the villus epithelium (S. El Bahi, E. Caliot, M. Bens, A. Bogdanova, S. Kerneis, A. Kahn, A. Vandewalle, and E. Pringault, unpublished data). This raises the possibility that there may be an FAE-specific transcription factor that controls the expression of multiple genes in FAE epithelial cells and not elsewhere. The connective tissue scaffold under the FAE also has unusual features: it lacks the subepithelial myofibroblasts that form a sheath under the epithelium of villi, and the basal lamina of the FAE differs from that of villi in that it lacks laminin-2 subunits (155). The FAE basal lamina is unusually porous, containing holes that may reflect frequent migration of cells into and out of the epithelium (102). However, the cardinal feature of the FAE is the presence of M cells.

FACTORS THAT PROMOTE ADHERENCE TO M CELL APICAL SURFACES

The ability of pathogens to exploit the M-cell transport pathway is indeed impressive when one considers the rarity of these cells in the epithelium. M-cell numbers in the FAE vary among species and intestinal regions: while they represent only about 10% of the FAE in mouse Peyer's patches, they constitute 50% of the FAE in rabbit Peyer's patches and appendix. In human ileal patches, 10% or less of FAE cells are M cells and these tend to lie on the lateral margins of the FAE (47). For efficient uptake by M cells, a pathogen must adhere to the cell surface. Apical membranes of M cells seem designed to promote adherence of particles and microorganisms (118). Their microvilli are usually irregular, and the cell surface has many membrane domains involved in endocytosis, described below. Most M cells lack the thick brush border glycocalyx that coats the microvilli of enterocytes (43, 101). Despite the lack of this major diffusion barrier, the M-cell apical membrane is coated with glycoproteins that can prevent access of particles of 100 nm or more to the lipid bilayer (43, 96). M-cell surface glycoconjugates clearly do not prevent microbial binding, however. Both bacteria and viruses have surface proteins that form surface extensions that can presumably penetrate the M-cell surface coat.

It seems likely that M-cell surface glyco- conjugates play a role in the pathogen rec-

ognition of M cells. Studies using lectins or anticarbohydrate antibodies have shown that M-cell membrane glycoconjugates differ from those of enterocytes. In Peyer's patches of BALB/c mice, for example, the lectin UEA-1, which is specific for certain carbohydrate structures containing α(1-2)-fucose, selectively stained all M cells in the FAE (25, 54), and other lectins revealed variations in the glycosylation patterns of individual M cells within a single FAE (54). This heterogeneity might provide an advantage to the host by allowing the FAE to "sample" a variety of microorganisms. M-cell-specific carbohydrate structures differ among species and vary in intestinal regions, as shown in mice (54) and rabbits (49, 74, 90). We observed that in humans, M cells displayed the sialyl Lewis A antigen, defined as Neu5Ac α(2-3) Gal β(1-3) GlcNAc [Fuc α(1-4)], whereas neighboring enterocytes did not (53). Thus, there does not seem to be a single carbohydrate structure common to all M cells. Lectin conjugation of proteins, or lectin coating of particles or liposomes, has been shown to enhance M-cell transport and subsequent mucosal immune responses in experimental animals (23, 52, 73). The practicality of this approach for targeting to M cells is not clear since M-cell carbohydrates are mimicked by the heterogeneous oligosaccharide side chains of secreted mucins. It should also be noted that none of the known M-cell-specific carbohydrates identified to date have been shown to serve as receptors for the pathogens that exploit the M-cell transcytotic pathway.

There is some evidence that the apical surfaces of some M cells display adhesion molecules that are not present on their epithelial neighbors. For example, human colonic (but not Peyer's patch) M cells express intercellular adhesion molecule 1 (ICAM-1) (163). This may reflect the M cell's frequent encounters with microorganisms, since ICAM-1 is also upregulated on apical membranes of intestinal enterocytes under conditions of inflammation and microbial infection (65). In mice, $\alpha4\beta1$ integrin has been detected in the apical membranes of M cells (24, 98), although this adhesion molecule is confined to the basolateral side of other epithelial cells (66). The fact that $\alpha 4\beta 1$ integrin is known to serve as a receptor for the invasin protein of pathogenic *Yersinia* (69, 70) suggests that it is exploited by *Yersinia* spp. to attach to M cells and invade the mucosa (162).

The FAE and M cells do not secrete IgA because they do not express basolateral polymeric immunoglobulin receptors (130). Paradoxically, however, IgA that has been secreted into the lumen adheres selectively to the apical membranes of M cells. This results in accumulation of IgA on apical surfaces of M cells of Peyer's patches in rodents and rabbits (90, 139, 169) as well as in humans (97). Studies in experimental animals have shown that exogenous monoclonal IgA, monoclonal IgA-antigen complexes, and polyclonal secretory IgA can adhere to apical membranes of M cells and be transported into the intraepithelial pocket, and that the interaction is not species specific (167). For example, secretory IgA from human colostrum adheres to mouse M cells (97). How the IgA–M-cell interaction benefits the host is not known. Under experimental conditions, uptake of specific exogenous IgA-antigen complexes by M cells induced secretory immune responses (30, 173), suggesting that specific endogenous IgA could participate in boosting preexisting mucosal immunity. IgA can also interact nonspecifically with certain microorganisms (169); in this case, the IgA–M-cell interaction could possibly promote initial uptake and immune sampling of pathogens. In addition, M-cell uptake of IgA-opsonized commensal microorganisms could play a role in maintenance of the IgA immune responses that control the lumenal microflora. The recently identified, novel Fc alpha/mu receptor on macrophages, B cells, and dendritic cells might play a role in these processes (151). It is also possible that M-cell-associated IgA could sterically hinder binding of certain pathogens to M-cell surfaces in a nonspecific manner.

THE M-CELL TRANSEPITHELIAL TRANSPORT PATHWAY

The M-cell apical membrane, along with its associated cytoplasmic proteins and cytoskeleton, is capable of uptake of macromolecules, particles, bacteria, and viruses using a variety of endocytic strategies (Fig. 1). Ligand-coated particles (43), adherent macromolecules (20, 116), and viruses (119, 152) can be taken up by clathrin-mediated endocytosis. M cells also take up soluble proteins and protein aggregates by pinocytosis (11, 58, 124). M cells can engulf noninvasive microorganisms including *Vibrio cholerae* (128) by actin-dependent phagocytosis (115), while certain pathogens such as *Salmonella* spp. disrupt the M-cell apical cytoskeletal organization and induce macropinocytosis, as described below (76).

M cells have a highly developed vesicular transport system that provides a short and rapid pathway across the epithelial barrier (114, 117). The basolateral cell surface invaginates to form a large intraepithelial "pocket" that brings the apical and basal cell surfaces within a few microns of each other. M cells are unique among epithelial cells in that transepithelial vesicular transport is the major pathway for endocytosed materials. Transport of foreign material involves a system of endosomal tubules and vesicles located in the apical cytoplasm above the intraepithelial pocket (1, 116, 124). Macromolecules and particles taken up at the apical surface of M cells are delivered to endosomes in the apical cytoplasm, some of which acidify their content and contain endosomal proteases (1, 41). The vesicles then fuse with the plasma membrane that lines the pocket to release their content. Whether any antigens or microorganisms are altered in transit is not known, but it is clear that pathogens arrive at the basal side viable and capable of initiating infection. The fact that transported bacteria and viruses are found free in the intraepithelial pocket suggests that uptake involves multiple low-affinity interactions with M-cell membranes that are readily reversible.

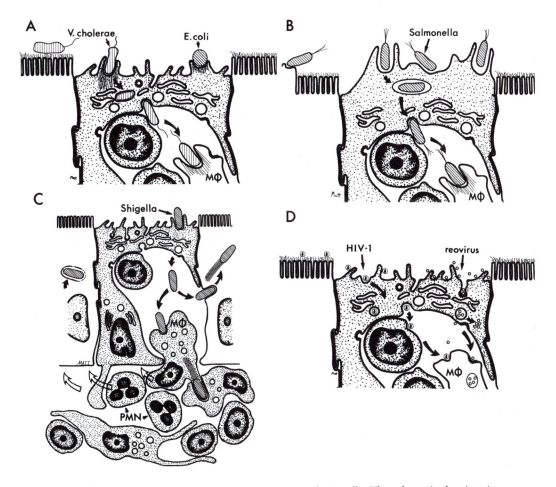

FIGURE 1 Interactions of bacteria and viruses with M cells. The schematic drawings in panels A, B, and D depict the apical pole of an M cell and the brush borders of adjacent enterocytes in the FAE. A portion of the M-cell intraepithelial pocket with lymphocytes and part of a phagocytic cell (Φ) are shown. (C) An entire M cell along with associated cells within the pocket and under the epithelium. (A) *V. cholerae* and enteropathogenic *E. coli* (EPEC) are noninvasive pathogens that colonize enterocyte surfaces but also adhere to M cells. *V. cholerae* is endocytosed and transported to the pocket, but EPEC induces formation of attaching and effacing lesions on the M-cell surface. (B) *S. enterica* serovars Typhi and Typhimurium adhere preferentially (but not exclusively) to M cells. They invade the Peyer's patch by inducing ruffling of the M-cell apical surface and macropinocytosis. (C) *Shigella flexneri* is efficiently transported by M cells. Once on the basolateral side of the epithelium, *S. flexneri* invades both epithelial and subepithelial cells, which in turn release cytokines and chemokines that recruit polymorphonuclear leukocytes (PMNs). (D) Reovirus adheres selectively to M cells in mice. HIV can adhere to the surface of the FAE in experimental animals. M-cell adherence results in transcytosis of virus into the M-cell pocket. (Reproduced with permission from reference 114.)

FATES OF MICROORGANISMS AFTER M-CELL TRANSPORT

Information about the events immediately following M-cell transport is scarce. Early electron microscopy studies showed that pathogens were taken up by subepithelial phagocytic cells, presumed to be macrophages, after transport by M cells (128, 170). It is now clear, however, that the phagocytic cells in the subepithelial dome (SED) region are predominantly dendritic cells (DCs) that form a dense network underlying the FAE (81, 82). DCs in the dome region appear to be immature (71) and thus would be competent for endocytosis of incoming pathogens. M-cell-transported lectins, cholera toxin conjugates, protein tracers, and particles have been detected in cells of the dome, and it is likely that most incoming pathogens are captured by these antigen-presenting cells. For example, attenuated *Salmonella enterica* serovar Typhimurium was detected in SED DCs after oral feeding (63) and orally administered *Listeria monocytogenes* that entered Peyer's patches was taken up by DCs that later appeared in the mesenteric lymph nodes (MLN) (134).

DCs are recognized as key players in capturing antigens peripherally and moving to T-cell areas of organized lymphoid tissues for presentation of antigens to naïve T cells (6). In the Peyer's patches, where the site of antigen uptake in the SED region is in close proximity to the interfollicular T-cell areas, it was predicted that subepithelial DCs would move to adjacent T-cell areas where presentation of antigens would occur (82). There is recent evidence that this occurs. Subepithelial DCs were shown to migrate to adjacent T-cell areas in response to an injected parasite antigen and to express maturation markers in the T-cell zones (71). We recently demonstrated that microorganisms entering via M cells can induce this DC movement; subepithelial DCs that ingested inert fluorescent particles remained in the SED region for long periods, but moved to adjacent T-cell areas in response to live *Salmonella* or cholera toxin (152). DCs may also enter the nearby B-cell follicle and/or leave the mucosa to enter the T-cell areas of draining lymph nodes (82, 93). DC movements and accompanying cellular interactions are likely to be important determinants of mucosal immune responses (6, 95, 138), but they may also facilitate microbial dissemination (99, 134). It is important to note that DCs in the lamina propria, outside of organized lymphoid tissues, carry endocytosed materials, including apoptotic epithelial cells, from the mucosa to mesenteric lymph nodes (64).

M-CELL TRANSPORT OF NONINVASIVE PATHOGENS

Although pathogens can exploit subepithelial antigen-presenting cells and use the migration of these cells to reach local and distant targets, in most cases M-cell-mediated uptake of microorganisms probably results in immune responses that are beneficial to the host. The clearest examples are the responses to bacteria that cause disease by forming colonies on the intestinal mucosal surface such as *V. cholerae* and certain strains of *Escherichia coli*. These organisms do not survive in the mucosa and are efficiently sampled by the mucosal immune system. The resulting secretion of antibacterial secretory IgA (sIgA) antibodies plays a major role in limiting the duration of disease and preventing reinfection.

V. cholerae expresses a group of coregulated proteins including pili and adhesins that mediate initial adherence to the epithelium and formation of colonies on the mucosal surface of the small intestine. Colonization is accompanied by upregulation of toxin genes and by local production of cholera toxin (CT) (89, 105). CT is endocytosed by enterocytes and, via a complex intracellular pathway, induces massive secretion of chloride ions from intestinal epithelial cells, the driving force for severe diarrhea (91). Adherence of *V. cholerae* to enterocytes appears to involve interaction with peripheral sites on the brush border glycocalyx and does not result in close membrane contact or endocytosis. In contrast, *V. cholerae* interacts closely with apical membranes of M cells (4, 115, 168), and this is followed by phagocytosis and transport into the M-cell pocket and Peyer's patch mucosa (128). *V. cholerae* and *Vibrio parahemolyticus* also adhered to the surfaces of M cells in formalin-fixed human mucosal tissue (171, 172). It is likely that uptake by M cells is responsible for the vigorous mucosal immune response, including secretion of IgA antibodies (sIgA) directed primarily against CT and lipopolysaccharide (LPS), that follows experimental feeding of *V. cholerae* or colonization of the intestine in human disease. In support of this, M-cell transport of vibrios in mice resulted in the presence of specific anti-CT and anti-LPS IgA lymphoblasts in Peyer's patches that were recovered and used for generation of IgA hybridomas (4, 168). When these monoclonal IgA antibodies were secreted from "backpack" tumors in suckling mice, the sIgA directed against LPS alone protected against disease, presumably by preventing colonization. This is consistent with studies in humans in which secretion of IgA directed against LPS and CT was associated with protection against subsequent oral challenge (75).

Of the many types of *E. coli* found in the intestine, most do not selectively adhere to epithelial cell surfaces or to M cells. The pathogenic strains that do adhere and colonize and/or invade the mucosa, however, can also interact with M cells. Ultrastructurally, the interaction of such strains with M cells shows dramatic differences. For example, *E. coli* strain O:124, when injected into ligated rabbit appendixes, associated with the surfaces of rabbit M cells, was phagocytosed in large vesicles and then released into the intraepithelial pocket (162). However, the rabbit pathogen *E. coli* RDEC-1, which is analogous to enteropathogenic *E. coli* (EPEC) in humans, induces an elaborate attachment site on M cells that is structurally identical to the attaching and effacing lesions induced on enterocytes (68). These adherence sites are characterized by the presence of submembrane actin assemblies and formation of stable "pedestals" (85). The EPEC-epithelial cell interaction has been elucidated in considerable detail and involves a complex sequence of events orchestrated by the bacterium from a chromosomal pathogenicity island (34). After initial adherence to cell surface carbohydrates, the bacterium uses a type III secretion system to insert a bacterial product (tir) into the host cell membrane. Tir is phosphorylated and then serves as the receptor for the bacterial ligand (intimin). The subsequent cascade of host cell signal transduction events results in formation of an actin-supported pedestal that supports the bacterium (33). The fact that RDEC-1 administered orally to rabbits initially bound preferentially to the surfaces of M cells (68) may reflect the lack of a thick cell glycocalyx on these cells and the accessibility of binding sites for the plasmid-encoded AF/R1 pili that appear to mediate attachment (67, 141). The epitope recognized by AF/R1 pili on M cells is not known, but it may be the sialoglycoprotein complex isolated from rabbit brush border preparations that is thought to act as the receptor on enterocytes (136). Infection of humans with EPEC evokes a vigorous immune response (79), suggesting that in spite of pedestal formation, some M-cell uptake of the bacteria occurs.

EXPLOITATION OF M CELLS BY INVASIVE BACTERIAL PATHOGENS

The range of bacterial pathogens that exploit M-cell transport to invade the mucosa have been reviewed (115). Their interactions with M cells and the FAE and their effects on organized mucosal lymphoid tissues are distinct, however, reflecting their differing pathogenic strategies (145). Translocation across the FAE may be relatively easy, but bacterial survival in the Peyer's patch mucosa is challenging because incoming bacteria find themselves facing a dense network of phagocytic cells in the SED region of the mucosal follicle (81, 82). On the other hand, the activities of phagocytic cells can render the tissue especially vulnerable to infection. In addition, the FAE features that promote microbial adherence make it vulnerable to pathogens that can induce cytokine and chemokine release from epithelial cells, attracting neutrophils and monocytes and setting in motion an inflammatory response that results in the breakdown of the epithelial barrier. The enteroinvasive bacterial pathogens *Salmonella* spp., *Shigella* spp., and *Yersinia* spp. share three major steps in pathogenesis: translocation through the FAE via M cells, survival in the mucosa by evasion of innate defense mechanisms, and establishment of infection. However, their molecular strategies and disease outcomes differ dramatically: infection remains essentially local in the case of *Shigella*, local and regional in the case of *Yersinia*, and systemic in the case of *Salmonella*.

Shigella spp. engage epithelial cells as well as macrophages in a complex molecular cross talk that results in loss of the epithelial barrier, activation and death of phagocytes, influx of neutrophils, and a severe inflammatory cascade in the colonic and rectal mucosa. These events, described in detail elsewhere in this volume, are responsible for the intestinal cramps and bloody diarrhea of shigellosis (56). The mechanism of cell invasion, intracellular motility, and cell-to-cell spread in vitro has been described in detail (15, 141, 142). *Shigella* species use plasmid-encoded virulence factors to invade the large intestinal mucosa in vivo with remarkable efficiency; a bacterial inoculum as low as 10 to 100 CFU can result in mucosal infection (35). This is surprising because *Shigella* spp. invade epithelial cells in vitro through the basolateral but not the apical pole (113, 143). In vivo, however, *Shigella* spp. exploit the FAE for its initial translocation across the epithelium. Involvement of M cells was suspected because in the early stages of *Shigella* infection in patients, small inflammatory lesions were observed in the sigmoid colon and rectum, often at sites of lymphoid follicles (100). Histopathological analysis of mucosal tissues after experimental infection of macaque monkeys and rabbits later confirmed that the FAE is indeed the initial site of *Shigella* entry (141, 142, 166). The limited number of M cells is difficult to reconcile with the efficiency with which low bacterial inocula cause

the disease. So far, no chemotactic or adherence system has been identified in *Shigella* spp. that could account for specific targeting to the M-cell apical surface. Passage through M cells occurs without rupture of the endocytic vacuole membrane; thus, bacteria are rapidly delivered to the intraepithelial pocket and subepithelial space where they may be phagocytosed by macrophages and DCs. To survive macrophage attack, *Shigella* spp. use the invasion protein IpaB that activates caspase-1 and causes the rapid death of macrophages by apoptosis (60, 174). The ability of shigellae to invade the basolateral side of epithelial cells and spread from cell to cell in the epithelium leads to local loss of mucosal barrier function. However, activation of caspase-1 from phagocytes also leads to release of proinflammatory cytokines and the ensuing inflammatory process leads to rapid and widespread disruption of the epithelial barrier, thereby facilitating further *Shigella* invasion (144).

Enteric *Yersinia* species preferentially invade via the FAE overlying lymphoid tissues in the terminal ileum. *Yersinia enterocolitica* and *Yersinia pseudotuberculosis* administered orally to mice and rabbits both cross the intestinal epithelial barrier by adhering to M cells (46, 55, 98). Adherence of *Yersinia* spp. to M cells appears to be mediated in part by invasin, an outer membrane protein that was shown to mediate attachment and invasion of cultured cells, and that uses host cell adhesion molecules $\beta1$ integrins as receptors (69, 70). Invasin-negative *Yersinia* mutants were severely reduced in their capacity to adhere to M cells and colonize Peyer's patches in vivo (24, 98, 133) and to be transported by M-like cells in an epithelial-lymphocyte coculture system (148). On conventional epithelial cells, $\beta1$ integrins are exclusively basolateral (66), but on M cells in vivo, $\beta1$ integrins have been detected on apical surfaces (24), suggesting that these adhesion molecules mediate uptake of *Yersinia* spp. in the intestine. $\beta1$ integrins also appeared on apical surfaces of M-like cells induced in an epithelial-lymphocyte coculture system, and these cells acquired the ability to translocate yersiniae from the apical to the basolateral compartment (124). Like *Shigella* and *Salmonella* spp., *Yersinia* spp. are delivered across the FAE directly to the network of phagocytic cells in the SED region of Peyer's patches. Unlike *Shigella* and *Salmonella* spp., *Yersinia* species, including the plague bacillus *Yersinia pestis*, survive this challenge by inhibiting phagocytosis, using a remarkable strategy. Upon contact with macrophages, the bacterium secretes a set of Yop proteins directly into the host cell cytoplasm via a plasmid-encoded type III secretion system. These proteins block the phagocytic machinery by disrupting the cytoskeleton (37), and eventually cause apoptosis of the macrophage (107, 110, 140). As a result, *Yersinia* spp. remain essentially extracellular in infected mucosa and mesenteric lymph nodes, and eventually cause destruction of the Peyer's patches.

After oral administration in mice, *S. enterica* serovar Typhimurium cells cross the intestinal barrier and cause a lethal septicemia that closely mimicks typhoid fever caused by *Salmonella enterica* serovar Typhi in humans. Following injection into ligated intestinal loops in mice, serovar Typhimurium, like *Shigella* and *Yersinia* spp., shows clear selectivity for M cells of the FAE (26, 76). M cells are a site of rapid entry, but may not represent the exclusive route by which the bacteria enter the mucosa, since there is evidence that *Salmonella* spp. can also enter via the villus epithelium (160, 164). In a recent study of epithelial cell monolayers cocultured with DCs in vitro, luminal salmonellae appeared to be captured by DCs that reached through epithelial tight junctions (137). The most efficient route of entry in vivo is likely to be M-cell transport, however, because initially the infection is localized in Peyer's patches (21, 61). The long Lpf fimbriae seem to mediate somewhat specific adherence to M cells of the murine FAE since *lpf* mutants show reduced colonization of murine Peyer's patches (9). It is likely that M-cell adherence involves multiple systems, however, since *lpf* mutants retain some ability to colonize Peyer's patches, and serovar Typhi

that lacks the *lpf* operon retains the capacity to invade murine M cells (86). The M-cell component that serves as receptor for serovar Typhimurium on M cells is not known, but one candidate is the carbohydrate epitope containing galactose, linked $\beta(1\text{-}3)$ to galactosamine, that serves as a serovar Typhimurium receptor on Caco-2 cells (51). Adherence of Typhimurium to the apical surfaces of M cells is followed by ruffling of the cell membrane that reflects massive reorganization of the cell cytoskeleton and that leads to macropinocytosis, analogous to the entry process observed in cells in vitro (40). Intracellular *Salmonella* spp. are cytotoxic to M cells and this results in destruction of the FAE as well as severe inflammatory lesions in Peyer's patches (76, 86). The invasion machinery, which includes a type III secretion system for cytoplasmic delivery of *Salmonella* invasion proteins, is encoded by the *Salmonella* pathogenicity island 1 (SPI1). This machinery plays a role in M-cell invasion since SPI1 mutants are neither toxic for M cells nor destructive for the FAE (76, 132). The SPI1 appears to be primarily dedicated to the crossing of the intestinal barrier by *Salmonella* spp. since SPI1 mutants are fully virulent when administered intravenously or intraperitoneally instead of orally. After crossing the FAE, salmonellae are captured by subepithelial DCs (63) and can infect mucosal macrophages. Expression of SPI1 is associated with the SipB-dependent apoptotic killing of infected phagocytes (59). Unlike *Shigella* and *Yersinia* spp., however, *Salmonella* spp. can survive inside live phagocytes (106) using SPI2, another pathogenicity island encoding an alternative type III secretion system and its dedicated effector proteins (150), as well as a battery of PhoP/PhoQ-regulated genes (166). Migration of phagocytes out of the mucosa facilitates systemic dissemination (164). Because of the efficiency with which this organism enters the mucosa and interacts with antigen-presenting cells in organized mucosal lymphoid tissues and elsewhere, attenuated *Salmonella* species are prime candidates as vectors for mucosal vaccines (158).

The FAE pathway appears to play a central role in intestinal invasion by other bacterial pathogens as well (153). For example, *Campylobacter jejuni* can selectively associate with and be transported through the FAE of Peyer's patches in rabbits (165). *Mycobacterium paratuberculosis*, inoculated into ligated ileal loops of calves, entered organized mucosal lymphoid tissues (109) and rabbit M cells efficiently transported *Mycobacterium bovis* BCG (bacillus Calmette-Guérin) into mucosal lymphoid tissue (44). M-cell transport of bacteria has important potential applications: genetically attenuated enteroinvasive bacteria may be delivered via M cells directly to the inductive sites of the mucosal immune system and thus are excellent candidate vaccines and vectors for mucosal immunization.

INTERACTION OF INVASIVE VIRUSES WITH M CELLS

Transport of several animal viruses by M cells has been documented. Two closely related viral pathogens—reovirus in mice and poliovirus in humans—have been shown to selectively adhere to M cells and to use this as an invasion route (152, 170). When applied to mucosal explants, human immunodeficiency virus type 1 (HIV-1) adhered to rabbit and mouse M cells (3), but whether M-cell transport plays a role in human transmission is unknown. Although there is evidence for enzymatic activity in viral surface proteins (10, 28) viruses generally depend on one or more key surface proteins to adhere to host cells. In the intestine, adherence of viruses to M cells is sufficient to ensure uptake into the endocytic and transcytotic pathway and delivery into organized mucosal lymphoid tissues.

The mouse pathogen reovirus has served as a valuable model system for study of M-cell-specific viral adherence and uptake. Reovirus selectively binds to mouse M cells not only in the Peyer's patches (2, 8, 170), but also in the colon (125) and airways (111). In the intestine, processing of reovirus by digestive proteases increases viral infectivity (7, 12), and we have shown that such processing is required for M-cell adherence (2). After oral inoculation of

mice, proteases in the intestinal lumen remove the outermost capsid protein (sigma 3), modify a second outer capsid protein (μ1c), and induce a conformational change in the sigma 1 protein that results in its extension up to 45 nm from the viral surface (88, 120, 121). Sigma 1 mediates binding to target neurons and fibroblasts in culture, and is known to contain at least one lectin-like domain that is sialic acid specific in reovirus type 3 (22). Recent studies in this laboratory have shown that reovirus type 1 binding to M cells is mediated by the interaction of sigma 1 with M cells. Viral particles lacking sigma 1 are unable to bind to M cells (A. Helander, K. Silvey, N. J. Mantis, and M. R. Neutra, unpublished data) and antibodies against sigma 1 (but not against other outer capsid proteins) prevented Peyer's patch infection in vivo when fed passively (156) or secreted from IgA hybridoma backpack tumors (A. Hutchings, A. Helander, D. Mielcarz, and M. R. Neutra, unpublished data). The sigma 1 protein of reovirus type 1 recognizes a specific sialic acid-containing determinant on epithelial cell apical surfaces that is present on all epithelial cells in mice and rabbits in vivo (157). The selectivity of reovirus for M cells appears to be due to the fact that the epitope is accessible to virus-sized particles only on these cells (96). Adherent reovirus is endocytosed by M cells in clathrin-coated pits and transcytosed to the intraepithelial pocket and subepithelial tissue where it can infect multiple cell types, primarily phagocytes (88, 120). Although reovirus is unable to adhere to the apical membranes of enterocytes in vivo, after M-cell transport it can infect the entire epithelium from the basolateral side (8). The virus may also infect the M cell during or after transport; cytoplasmic viral factories are seen in M cells after uptake of virus in vivo and M cells are selectively lost during reovirus infection of suckling mice (8).

The pathogenesis of poliovirus in humans parallels that of reovirus in mice in that it enters the body by the oral route and proliferates in Peyer's patches before spreading systemically (135). This helps to explain the efficacy of mucosal immunization with live, attenuated poliovirus that was established decades ago (122), before the ultrastructure and antigen-transporting activity of M cells was first described (11). When wild-type poliovirus type 1 or the attenuated Sabin strain was applied to explants of human Peyer's patches in vitro, the virus was seen by electron microscopy (EM) to adhere to M cells (but not enterocytes) and to be taken up into the mucosa (152). The receptor for poliovirus on neuronal target cell membranes has been identified as a member of the immunoglobulin superfamily, and the cloned gene has been used to create transgenic mice that can be infected by injection of virus (104). It is not known whether the binding site that poliovirus uses to adhere to M cells is the same as or different from that used on target neurons. When the transgenic mice were challenged orally, poliovirus replication was not detected in the intestinal mucosa, perhaps because the transgene was not expressed in this site. The nasal mucosa was infected, however, and the mice developed paralytic disease (135). The ability of poliovirus to use the M-cell pathway for penetration of the epithelial barrier is now being exploited as an oral vaccine strategy. Recombinant poliovirus (31) and empty pseudovirus particles (112) have shown promise as mucosal vaccines.

HIV transmission can clearly occur via the human rectal mucosa (108); this may be due in part to the abundance of mucosal lymphoid follicles and associated M cells at this site (123). Although damage of epithelial barriers presumably facilitates infection, studies of simian immunodeficiency virus (SIV) transmission in monkeys have shown that that free SIV can infect via intact rectal mucosa (27, 131). Indirect evidence that M cells may be involved was obtained by using mouse and rabbit mucosal explants in organ culture, where HIV-1 adhered to M cells and was transported into the M-cell pocket (3). Transport of HIV by M cells would give the virus rapid access to organized mucosal lymphoid tissues rich in target T cells, macrophages, and DCs. Whether free HIV adheres to human rectal epithelial cells in vivo and, if so, what mech-

anism is involved, are unknown. Intestinal epithelial cells of humans and monkeys in vivo do not express CD4, but their membranes do contain galactosylceramide (19, 62), a glycosphingolipid that can mediate HIV infection of neoplastic intestinal epithelial cell lines such as HT29 and Caco-2 cells in culture (38, 48). HIV infection of intestinal or rectal epithelial cells themselves has not been detected in infected humans (42), and to what extent epithelial cells actually transport the virus in vivo is not established. Epithelial monolayers in culture can transport virus derived from attached, infected cells by a transcytotic vesicular pathway (13). Recently one of our laboratories confirmed that free or cell-associated HIV-1 can infect and be transcytosed across poorly differentiated Caco-2 cell monolayers, as well as Caco-2 cells with M-cell-like transcytotic activity induced by co-culture with B cells. However, this occurred only when the Caco-2 cells displayed both CCR5 or CXCR4 chemokine receptors and galactosylceramide (G. Fotopoulos, A. Harari, D. Trono, G. Pantaleo, and J. P. Kraehenbuhl, unpublished data). If transcytosis of HIV-1 across epithelia in vivo is galactosylceramide mediated, the viral envelope must gain access to glycolipids in epithelial cell membranes. Enterocytes in the rectum of humans, like enterocytes throughout the intestine, have brush borders coated with a continuous, 400- to 500-nm-thick glycocalyx that would be expected to block access of particles to enterocyte apical plasma membrane. Indeed, HIV particles failed to penetrate the glycocalyx of enterocytes in mouse and rabbit Peyer's patch mucosa but did adhere to M-cell membranes (3). Further studies are needed to establish whether HIV actually enters the human rectal mucosa via the M-cell route.

ROLE OF MICROORGANISMS IN FORMATION OF FAE AND M CELLS
Organized mucosal lymphoid follicles clearly play an inductive role in the differentiation of the specialized FAE and M cells. Injection of Peyer's patch lymphocytes into the circulation of severe combined immunodeficient (SCID)

mice (146) or into the submucosa of syngeneic normal mice (83) resulted in local assembly of new lymphoid follicles and the appearance of the FAE with M cells. There is evidence in vivo and in vitro that B lymphocytes are important in induction of M cells. In SCID mice, injection of fractions enriched in B cells was most effective in reconstituting mucosal follicles and the FAE (146), and in B-lymphocyte-deficient mice, the size of organized mucosal lymphoid tissues and the FAE, as well as M-cell numbers, is dramatically reduced (32). In addition, migration of B cells into an intestinal epithelial cell monolayer in culture resulted in the appearance of cells with M-cell features (83). The B-cell factors or other signals that induce differentiation of M cells are not known.

Under normal conditions, constitutive differentiation of M cells occurs in the crypts adjacent to mucosal lymphoid follicles. Immature M cells have been identified in the follicle-associated crypts by lectin labeling and EM studies (20, 50, 54). As these cells emerge from the crypts, they acquire typical M-cell features, including endocytic activity, lack of typical brush borders, and clusters of lymphocytes in the characteristic intraepithelial pocket (20, 50). The differentiation of FAE enterocytes in the crypts adjacent to lymphoid follicles is also distinct in that they fail to express polymeric immunoglobulin receptors (130, 167). Thus, inductive factors from the follicle apparently act early in the differentiation pathway, inducing crypt cells to commit to FAE phenotypes. However, FAE enterocyte-like or uncommitted cells may become antigen-transporting M cells after emergence from the crypts, as evidenced by the fact that M-cell numbers can increase within hours after bacterial challenge in vivo (14).

The major organized mucosal lymphoid tissues, such as Peyer's patches, form before birth in animals and humans (reviewed in references 32, 57, and 87). After birth, however, the luminal microflora is required for full development of Peyer's patches and solitary lymphoid follicles. Lymphoid follicles and M cells were shown to rapidly increase in number after the transfer of germ-free mice to a normal animal house environment (159), or even after the introduction of a single bacterial species (14, 147). Intestinal pathogens cause expansion of Peyer's patches and can induce the formation of isolated lymphoid follicles with associated FAE elsewhere in the gut. The sequence of events that leads to formation of new follicles and the FAE in vivo is not clear (39). Microorganisms may initiate the process by inducing epithelial and subepithelial cells to release cytokines and chemokines (71, 77, 78), which in turn may influence traffic of leukocytes (5). For example, expression of the epithelial chemokine CCL20 is transiently induced in epithelial cells in vitro by enteric bacteria, flagellin, and LPS (72, 154, 161). CCL20 can attract DCs and lymphocytes that express CCR6 (29, 71), and influx of such cells may lead to assembly and maintenance of lymphoid follicles.

CONCLUSION

The importance of M cells in invasion of the intestinal mucosa by bacteria and viruses is now widely recognized. However, much remains to be learned about the specific molecular recognition systems and nonspecific adherence mechanisms that allow pathogens to usurp this pathway. A clearer understanding of these mechanisms will facilitate the design of mucosal vaccines that are targeted to organized mucosal lymphoid tissues for efficient induction of protective immune responses.

ACKNOWLEDGMENTS
We are grateful to current and former members of our laboratories who have contributed to the work summarized in this review. The authors are supported by NIH Research Grants HD17557, AI34757, and AI35365 and NIH Center Grant DK34854 to the Harvard Digestive Diseases Center (M.R.N.); the Howard Hughes Medical Institute and European Union Grant CEE QLK2-CT-1999.00973 (P.J.S.); Swiss National Science Foundation Grant 31-56936-99; and Swiss League Against Cancer Grant SKL 635-2—1998 (J.P.K.).

REFERENCES

1. **Allan, C. H., D. L. Mendrick, and J. S. Trier.** 1993. Rat intestinal epithelial M cells contain acidic endosomal lysosomal compartments and express class II major histocompatibility complex determinants. *Gastroenterology* **104:**698–708.
2. **Amerongen, H. M., G. A. R. Wilson, B. N. Fields, and M. R. Neutra.** 1994. Proteolytic processing of reovirus is required for adherence to intestinal M cells. *J. Virol.* **68:**8428–8432.
3. **Amerongen, H. M., R. A. Weltzin, C. M. Farnet, P. Michetti, W. A. Haseltine, and M. R. Neutra.** 1991. Transepithelial transport of HIV-1 by intestinal M cells: a mechanism for transmission of AIDS. *J. Acquir. Immune Defic. Syndr.* **4:**760–765.
4. **Apter, F. M., P. Michetti, L. S. Winner III, J. A. Mack, J. J. Mekalanos, and M. R. Neutra.** 1993. Analysis of the roles of anti-lipopolysaccharide and anti-cholera toxin IgA antibodies in protection against *Vibrio cholerae* and cholera toxin using monoclonal IgA antibodies in vivo. *Infect. Immun.* **61:**5279–5285.
5. **Baggiolini, M.** 1998. Chemokines and leukocyte traffic. *Nature* **392:**565–568.
6. **Banchereau, J., and R. M. Steinman.** 1998. Dendritic cells and the control of immunity. *Nature* **392:**245–252.
7. **Bass, D. M., D. Bodkin, R. Dambrauskas, J. S. Trier, B. N. Fields, and J. L. Wolf.** 1990. Intraluminal proteolytic activation plays an important role in replication of type 1 reovirus in the intestines of neonatal mice. *J. Virol.* **64:**1830–1833.
8. **Bass, D. M., J. S. Trier, R. Dambrauskas, and J. L. Wolf.** 1988. Reovirus type 1 infection of small intestinal epithelium in suckling mice and its effect on M cells. *Lab. Invest.* **55:**226–235.
9. **Baumler, A. J., R. M. Tsolis, and F. Heffron.** 1996. The *lpf* fimbrial operon mediates adhesion of *Salmonella typhimurium* to murine Peyer's patch. *Proc. Natl. Acad. Sci. USA* **93:**279–283.
10. **Bisaillon, M., L. Bernier, S. Sénéchal, and G. Lemay.** 1999. A glycosyl hydrolase activity of mammalian reovirus sigma1 protein can contribute to viral infection through a mucus layer. *J. Mol. Biol.* **286:**759–773.
11. **Bockman, D. E., and M. D. Cooper.** 1973. Pinocytosis by epithelium associated with lymphoid follicles in the bursa of Fabricius, appendix, and Peyer's patches. An electron microscopic study. *Am. J. Anat.* **136:**455–478.
12. **Bodkin, D. K., M. L. Nibert, and B. N. Fields.** 1989. Proteolytic digestion of reovirus in the intestinal lumen of neonatal mice. *J. Virol.* **63:**4676–4681.
13. **Bomsel, M.** 1997. Transcytosis of infectious human immunodeficiency virus across a tight human epithelial cell line barrier. *Nature Med.* **3:**42–47.
14. **Borghesi, C., M. J. Taussig, and C. Nicoletti.** 1999. Rapid appearance of M cells after microbial challenge is restricted at the periphery of the follicle-associated epithelium of Peyer's patch. *Lab. Invest.* **79:**1393–1401.
15. **Bourdet-Sicard, R., C. Egile, P. J. Sansonetti, and G. Tran Van Nhieu.** 2000. Diversion of cytoskeletal processes by *Shigella* during invasion of epithelial cells. *Microbes Infect.* **2:**813–819.
16. **Brandtzaeg, P., and I. N. Farstad.** 1999. The human mucosal B cell system, p. 439–468. *In* R. Ogra, J. Mestecky, J. McGhee, J. Bienenstock, M. Lamm, and W. Strober (ed.), *Mucosal Immunology.* Academic Press, Inc., New York, N.Y.
17. **Brandtzaeg, P., E. S. Baekkevold, I. N. Farstad, F. L. Jahnsen, F. E. Johansen, E. M. Nilsen, and T. Yamanaka.** 1999. Regional specialization in the mucosal immune system: what happens in the microcompartments? *Immunol. Today* **20:**141–151.
18. **Brandtzaeg, P., I. N. Farstad, and G. Haraldsen.** 1999. Regional specialization in the mucosal immune system: primed cells do not always home along the same track. *Immunol. Today* **20:**267–277.
19. **Butor, C., A. Couedel-Courteille, J. G. Guilet, and A. Venet.** 1996. Differential distribution of galactosylceramide, H antigen, and carcinoembryonic antigen in rhesus macaque digestive mucosa. *J. Histochem. Cytochem.* **44:**1021–1031.
20. **Bye, W. A., C. H. Allan, and J. S. Trier.** 1984. Structure, distribution and origin of M cells in Peyer's patches of mouse ileum. *Gastroenterology* **86:**789–801.
21. **Carter, P. B., and F. M. Collins.** 1974. The route of enteric infection in normal mice. *J. Exp. Med.* **139:**1189–1203.
22. **Chappell, J. D., J. L. Duong, B. A. Wright, and T. S. Dermody.** 2000. Identification of carbohydrate-binding domains in the attachment proteins of type 1 and type 3 reoviruses. *J. Virol.* **74:**8472–8479.
23. **Chen, H., V. Torchilin, and R. Langer.** 1996. Lectin-bearing polymerized liposomes as potential oral vaccine carriers. *Pharm. Res.* **13:**1378–1383.
24. **Clark, M. A., B. H. Hirst, and M. A. Jepson.** 1998. M-cell surface β1 integrin expression and invasin-mediated targeting of *Yersinia pseudotuberculosis* to mouse Peyer's patch M cells. *Infect. Immun.* **66:**1237–1244.

25. **Clark, M. A., M. A. Jepson, N. L. Simmons, T. A. Booth, and B. H. Hirst.** 1993. Differential expression of lectin-binding sites defines mouse intestinal M-cells. *J. Histochem. Cytochem.* **41:**1679–1687.

26. **Clark, M. A., M. A. Jepson, N. L. Simmons, and B. H. Hirst.** 1994. Preferential interaction of *Salmonella typhimurium* with mouse Peyer's patch M cells. *Res. Microbiol.* **145:**543–552.

27. **Clerici, M., E. A. Clark, P. Polacino, I. Axberg, L. Kuller, N. I. Casey, W. R. Morton, G. M. Shearer, and R. E. Benveniste.** 1994. T-cell proliferation to subinfectious SIV correlates with lack of infection after challenge of macaques. *AIDS* **8:**1391–1395.

28. **Colman, P. M., J. N. Varghese, and W. G. Laver.** 1983. Structure of the catalytic and antigenic sites in influenza virus neuraminidase. *Nature* (London) **303:**41–47.

29. **Cook, D. N., D. M. Prosser, R. Forster, J. Zhang, N. A. Kuklin, S. J. Abbondanzo, X. D. Niu, S. C. Chen, D. J. Manfra, M. T. Wiekowski, L. M. Sullivan, S. R. Smith, H. B. Greenberg, S. K. Narula, M. Lipp, and S. A. Lira.** 2000. CCR6 mediates dendritic cell localization, lymphocyte homeostasis, and immune responses in mucosal tissue. *Immunity* **12:**495–503.

30. **Corthésy, B., M. Kaufmann, A. Phalipon, M. C. Peitsch, M. R. Neutra, and J.-P. Kraehenbuhl.** 1996. A pathogen-specific epitope inserted into recombinant secretory immunoglobulin A is immunogenic by the oral route. *J. Biol. Chem.* **271:**33670–33677.

31. **Crotty, S., C. J. Miller, B. L. Lohman, M. R. Neagu, L. Compton, D. Lu, F. X. Lu, L. Fritts, J. D. Lifson, and R. Andino.** 2001. Protection against simian immunodeficiency virus vaginal challenge by using Sabin poliovirus vectors. *J. Virol.* **75:**7435–7452.

32. **Debard, N., F. Sierro, J. Browning, and J.-P. Kraehenbuhl.** 2001. Effect of mature lymphocytes and lymphotoxin on the development of the follicle-associated epithelium and M cells in mouse Peyer's patches. *Gastroenterology* **120:** 1173–1182.

33. **DeVinney, R., D. G. Knoechel, and B. B. Finlay.** 1999. Enteropathogenic *Escherichia coli:* cellular harrassment. *Curr. Opin. Microbiol.* **2:**83–88.

34. **Donnenberg, M. S., J. B. Kaper, and B. B. Finlay.** 1997. Interactions between enteropathogenic *Escherichia coli* and host epithelial cells. *Trends Microbiol.* **5:**109–114.

35. **Dupont, H. L., M. M. Levine, R. B. Hornick, and S. B. Formal.** 1989. Inoculum size in shigellosis and implications for expected mode of transmission. *J. Infect. Dis.* **159:**1126–1128.

36. **Fagarasan, S., K. Kinoshita, M. Muramatsu, K. Ikuta, and T. Honjo.** 2001. In situ class switching and differentiation to IgA-producing cells in the gut lamina propria. *Nature* **413:**639–643.

37. **Fällmann, M., C. Persson, and H. Wolf-Watz.** 1997. *Yersinia* proteins that target host-cell signaling pathways. *J. Clin. Invest.* **99:**1153–1157.

38. **Fantini, J., D. G. Cook, N. Nathanson, S. L. Spitalnik, and F. Gonzalez-Scarano.** 1993. Infection of colonic epithelial cell lines by type 1 human immunodeficiency virus (HIV-1) is associated with cell surface expression of galactosyl ceramide, a potential alternative gp120 receptor. *Proc. Natl. Acad. Sci. USA* **90:**2700–2704.

39. **Finke, D., and J.-P. Kraehenbuhl.** 2001. Formation of Peyer's patches. *Curr. Opin. Gen. Dev.* **11:**562–569.

40. **Finlay, B. B., and S. Falkow.** 1990. *Salmonella* interactions with polarized human intestinal Caco-2 epithelial cells. *J. Infect. Dis.* **162:**1096–1106.

41. **Finzi, G., M. Cornaggia, C. Capella, R. Fiocca, F. Bosi, E. Solcia, and I. M. Samloff.** 1993. Cathepsin E in follicle associated epithelium of intestine and tonsils: localization to M cells and possible role in antigen processing. *Histochemistry* **99:**201–211.

42. **Fox, C. H., D. Kotler, A. Tierney, C. S. Wilson, and A. S. Fauci.** 1989. Detection of HIV-1 RNA in the lamina propria of patients with AIDS and gastrointestinal disease. *J. Infect. Dis.* **159:**467–471.

43. **Frey, A., K. T. Giannasca, R. Weltzin, P. J. Giannasca, H. Reggio, W. I. Lencer, and M. R. Neutra.** 1996. Role of the glycocalyx in regulating access of microparticles to apical plasma membranes of intestinal epithelial cells—implications for microbial attachment and oral vaccine targeting. *J. Exp. Med.* **184:**1045–1059.

44. **Fujimura, Y.** 1986. Functional morphology of microfold cells (M cells) in Peyer's patches. Phagocytosis and transport of BCG by M cells into rabbit Peyer's patches. *Gastroenterol. Jpn.* **21:**325–335.

45. **Fujimura, Y., M. Hosobe, and T. Kihara.** 1992. Ultrastructural study of M cells from colonic lymphoid nodules obtained by colonoscopic biopsy. *Digest. Dis. Sci.* **37:**1089–1098.

46. **Fujimura, Y., T. Kihara, and H. Mine.** 1992. Membranous cells as a portal of *Yersinia pseudotuberculosis* entry into rabbit ileum. *J. Clin. Electron Microsc.* **25:**35–45.

47. **Fujimura, Y., T. Kihara, K. Ohtani, R. Kamoi, T. Kato, K. Kojuka, N. Miyashima,**

and J. Uchida. 1990. Distribution of microfold cells (M cells) in human follicle-associated epithelium. *Gastroenterol. Jpn.* **25**:130.

48. **Furuta, Y., K. Erikkson, B. Svennerholm, P. Fredman, P. Horal, S. Jeansson, A. Vahlne, J. Holmgren, and C. Czerkinsky.** 1994. Infection of vaginal and colonic epithelial cells by the human immunodeficiency virus type 1 is neutralized by antibodies raised against conserved epitopes in the envelope glycoprotein gp120. *Proc. Natl. Acad. Sci. USA* **91**:12559–12563.

49. **Gebert, A., and G. Hach.** 1993. Differential binding of lectins to M cells and enterocytes in the rabbit cecum. *Gastroenterology* **105**:1350–1361.

50. **Gebert, A., S. Fassbender, K. Werner, and A. Weissferdt.** 1999. The development of M cells in Peyer's patches is restricted to specialized dome-associated crypts. *Am. J. Pathol.* **154**:1573–1582.

51. **Giannasca, K. T., P. J. Giannasca, and M. R. Neutra.** 1996. Adherence of *Salmonella typhimurium* to Caco-2 cells: identification of a glycoconjugate receptor. *Infect. Immun.* **64**:135–145.

52. **Giannasca, P. J., J. A. Boden, and T. P. Monath.** 1997. Targeted delivery of antigen to hamster nasal lymphoid tissue with M-cell-directed lectins. *Infect. Immun.* **65**:4288–4298.

53. **Giannasca, P. J., K. T. Giannasca, A. M. Leichtner, and M. R. Neutra.** 1999. Human intestinal M cells display the sialyl Lewis A antigen. *Infect. Immun.* **67**:946–953.

54. **Giannasca, P. J., K. T. Giannasca, P. Falk, J. I. Gordon, and M. R. Neutra.** 1994. Regional differences in glycoconjugates of intestinal M cells in mice: potential targets for mucosal vaccines. *Am. J. Physiol.* **267**:G1108–G1121.

55. **Grutzkau, A., C. Hanski, H. Hahn, and E. O. Riecken.** 1990. Involvement of M cells in the bacterial invasion of Peyer's patches: a common mechanism shared by *Yersinia enterocolitica* and other enteroinvasive bacteria. *Gut* **31**:1011–1015.

56. **Hale, T. L.** 1998. Bacillary dysentery. *In* W. J. Hausler and M. Sussman (ed.), *Topley and Wilson's Microbiology and Microbial Infections. Bacterial Infections*, vol. 3. Arnold, London, United Kingdom.

57. **Hein, W. R.** 1999. Organization of mucosal lymphoid tissue. *Curr. Top. Microbiol. Immunol.* **236**:1–15.

58. **Heppner, F. L., A. D. Christ, M. A. Klein, M. Prinz, M. Fried, J.-P. Kraehenbuhl, and A. Aguzzi.** 2001. Transepithelial prion transport by M cells. *Nature Med.* **7**:1–2.

59. **Hersh, D., D. M. Monack, M. R. Smith, N. Ghori, S. Falkow, and A. Zychlinsky.** 1999. The *Salmonella* invasin SipB induces macrophage apoptosis by binding to caspase-1. *Proc. Natl. Acad. Sci. USA* **96**:2396–2401.

60. **Hilbi, H., J. E. Moss, D. Hersh, Y. Chen, J. Arondel, S. Banerjee, P. J. Sansonetti, and A. Zychlinsky.** 1998. *Shigella*-induced apoptosis is dependent on caspase-1 which binds to IpaB. *J. Biol. Chem.* **273**:32895–32900.

61. **Hohmann, A. W., G. Schmidt, and D. Rowley.** 1978. Intestinal colonization and virulence of *Salmonella* in mice. *Infect. Immun.* **22**:763–770.

62. **Holgersson, J., N. Stromberg, and M. E. Breimer.** 1988. Glycolipids of human large intestine: differences in glycolipid expression related to anatomical localization, epithelial/nonepithelial tissue and the ABO, Le and Se phenotypes of the donors. *Biochemie* **70**:1565–1574.

63. **Hopkins, S., F. Niedergang, I. E. Corthésy-Theulaz, and J.-P. Kraehenbuhl.** 2000. A recombinant *Salmonella typhimurium* vaccine strain is taken up and survives within murine Peyer's patch dendritic cells. *Cell. Microbiol.* **2**:56–68.

64. **Huang, F. P., N. Platt, M. Wykes, J. R. Major, T. J. Powell, C. D. Jenkins, and G. G. MacPherson.** 2000. A discrete subpopulation of dendritic cells transports apoptotic intestinal epithelial cells to T cell areas of mesenteric lymph nodes. *J. Exp. Med.* **191**:435–443.

65. **Huang, G. T. J., L. Eckmann, T. C. Savidge, and M. F. Kagnoff.** 1996. Infection of human intestinal epithelial cells with invasive bacteria upregulates apical intercellular adhesion molecule-1 (ICAM-1) expression and neutrophil adhesion. *J. Clin. Invest.* **98**:572–583.

66. **Hynes, R. O.** 1992. Integrins: versatility, modulation and signalling in cell adhesion. *Cell* **69**:11–25.

67. **Inman, L. R., and J. R. Cantey.** 1984. Peyer's patch lymphoid follicle epithelial adherence of a rabbit enteropathogenic *Escherichia coli* (strain RDEC-1). Role of plasmid-mediated pili in initial adherence. *J. Clin. Invest.* **74**:90–95.

68. **Inman, L. R., and J. R. Cantey.** 1983. Specific adherence of *Escherichia coli* (strain RDEC-1) to membranous (M) cells of the Peyer's patch in *Escherichia coli* diarrhea in the rabbit. *J. Clin. Invest.* **71**:1–8.

69. **Isberg, R. R., and D. L. Voorhis.** 1987. Identification of invasin, a protein that allows enteric bacteria to penetrate mammalian cells. *Cell* **50**:769–778.

70. **Isberg, R. R., and J. M. Leong.** 1990. Multiple β1 chain integrins are receptors for invasin,

a protein that promotes bacterial penetration into mammalian cells. *Cell* **60**:861–871.

71. **Iwasaki, A., and B. L. Kelsall.** 2000. Localization of distinct Peyer's patch dendritic cell subsets and their recruitment by chemokines macrophage inflammatory protein (MIP)-3α, MIP-3β, and secondary lymphoid organ chemokine. *J. Exp. Med.* **191**:1381–1393.

72. **Izadpanah, A., M. B. Dwinell, L. Eckmann, N. M. Varki, and M. F. Kagnoff.** 2001. Regulated MIP-3alpha/CCL20 production by human intestinal epithelium: mechanism for modulating mucosal immunity. *Am. J. Physiol.* **280**:G710–G719.

73. **Jepson, M. A., M. A. Clark, N. Foster, C. M. Mason, M. K. Bennett, N. L. Simmons, and B. H. Hirst.** 1996. Targeting to intestinal M cells. *J. Anat.* **189**:507–516.

74. **Jepson, M. A., M. A. Clark, N. L. Simmons, and B. H. Hirst.** 1993. Epithelial M cells in the rabbit caecal lymphoid patch display distinctive surface characteristics. *Histochemistry* **100**:441–447.

75. **Jertborn, M., A.-M. Svennerholm, and J. Holmgren.** 1986. Saliva, breast milk, and serum antibody responses as indirect measures of intestinal immunity after oral cholera vaccination. *J. Clin. Microbiol.* **24**:203–209.

76. **Jones, B. D., N. Ghori, and S. Falkow.** 1994. *Salmonella typhimurium* initiates murine infection by penetrating and destroying the specialized epithelial M cells of the Peyer's patches. *J. Exp. Med.* **180**:15–23.

77. **Jung, H. C., L. Eckmann, S. K. Yang, A. Panja, J. Fierer, E. Morzycka-Wroblewska, and M. F. Kagnoff.** 1995. A distinct array of proinflammatory cytokines is expressed in human colon epithelial cells in response to bacterial invasion. *J. Clin. Invest.* **95**:55–65.

78. **Kagnoff, M. F., and L. Eckmann.** 1997. Epithelial cells as sensors for microbial infection. *J. Clin. Invest.* **100**:S51–S55.

79. **Karch, H., J. Heesemann, R. Laufs, H. P. Kroll, J. B. Kaper, and M. M. Levine.** 1987. Serological response to type 1-like somatic fimbriae in diarrheal infection due to classical enteropathogenic *Escherichia coli. Microb. Pathogen* **2**:425–434.

80. **Kealy, W. F.** 1976. Colonic lymphoid-glandular complex (microbursa): nature and morphology. *J. Clin. Pathol.* **29**:241–244.

81. **Kelsall, B. L., and W. Strober.** 1996. Distinct populations of dendritic cells are present in the subepithelial dome and T cell regions of murine Peyer's patches. *J. Exp. Med.* **183**:237–247.

82. **Kelsall, B., and W. Strober.** 1999. Gut-associated lymphoid tissue: antigen handling and T cell responses, p. 293–318. *In* R. Ogra, J. Mestecky, J. McGhee, J. Bienenstock, M. Lamm, and W. Strober (ed.), *Mucosal Immunology.* Academic Press Inc., New York, N.Y.

83. **Kernéis, S., A. Bogdanova, J.-P. Kraehenbuhl, and E. Pringault.** 1997. Conversion by Peyer's patch lymphocytes of human enterocytes into M cells that transport bacteria. *Science* **277**:948–952.

84. **Khatri, I. A., C. Ho, R. D. Specian, and J. F. Forstner.** 2001. Characteristics of rodent intestinal mucin Muc3 and alterations in a mouse model of human cystic fibrosis. *Am. J. Physiol. Gastrointest. Liver Physiol.* **280**:G1321–G1330.

85. **Knutton, S., D. R. Lloyd, and A. S. McNeish.** 1987. Adhesion of enteropathogenic *Escherichia coli* to human intestinal enterocytes and cultured human intestinal mucosa. *Infect. Immun.* **55**:69–77.

86. **Kohbata, S., H. Yokobata, and E. Yabuuchi.** 1986. Cytopathogenic effect of *Salmonella typhi* GIFU 10007 on M cells of murine ileal Peyer's patches in ligated ileal loops: an ultrastructural study. *Microbiol. Immunol.* **30**:1225–1237.

87. **Kraehenbuhl, J.-P., and M. R. Neutra.** 2000. Epithelial M cells: differentiation and function. *Annu. Rev. Cell Dev. Biol.* **16**:301–332.

88. **Lee, P. W. K., and R. Gilmore.** 1998. Reovirus cell attachment protein s1: structure-function relationships and biogenesis, p. 137–153. *In* K. L. Tyler and M. B. A. Oldstone (ed.), *Reoviruses. I: Structure, Proteins, and Genetics.* Springer-Verlag, Berlin, Germany.

89. **Lee, S. H., D. L. Hava, M. K. Waldor, and A. Camilli.** 1999. Regulation and temporal expression patterns of *Vibrio cholerae* virulence genes during infection. *Cell* **99**:625–634.

90. **Lelouard, H., H. Reggio, P. Mangeat, M. R. Neutra, and P. Montcourrier.** 1999. Mucin related epitopes distinguish M cells and enterocytes in rabbit appendix and Peyer's patches. *Infect. Immun.* **67**:357–367.

91. **Lencer, W. I., T. R. Hirst, and R. K. Holmes.** 1999. Membrane traffic and the cellular uptake of cholera toxin. *Biochim. Biophys. Acta* **1450**:177–190.

92. **MacPherson, A. J., D. Gatto, E. Sainsbury, G. R. Harriman, H. Hengartner, and R. M. Zinkernagel.** 2000. A primitive T cell-independent mechanism of intestinal mucosal IgA responses to commensal bacteria. *Science* **288**:2222–2226.

93. **MacPherson, G. G., and L. M. Liu.** 1999. Dendritic cells and Langerhans cells in the uptake of mucosal antigens. *Curr. Top. Microbiol. Immunol.* **256**:33–54.

94. **Madara, J. L., S. Nash, R. Moore, and K. Atisook.** 1990. Structure and function of the intestinal epithelial barrier in health and disease. *Monogr. Pathol.* 306–324.

95. **Maldonado-Lopez, R., T. De Smedt, P. Michel, J. Godfroid, B. Pajak, C. Hierman, K. Thielemans, O. Leo, J. Urbain, and M. Moser.** 1999. CD8 alpha$^+$ and CD8 alpha- subclasses of dendritic cells direct the development of distinct T helper cells in vivo. *J. Exp. Med.* **189:**587–592.

96. **Mantis, N. J., A. Frey, and M. R. Neutra.** 2000. Accessibility of glycolipid and oligosaccharide epitopes on apical surfaces of rabbit villus and follicle-associated epithelium. *Am. J. Physiol. Gastrointest. Liver Physiol.* **278:**G915–G929.

97. **Mantis, N. J., M. C. Cheung, K. R. Chintalacharuvu, J. Rey, B. Corthesy, and M. R. Neutra.** 2002. Selective adherence of IgA to murine Peyer's patch M cells: evidence for a novel IgA receptor. *J. Immunol.* **169:**1844–1851.

98. **Marra, A., and R. R. Isberg.** 1997. Invasin-dependent and invasin-independent pathways for translocation of *Yersinia pseudotuberculosis* across the Peyer's patch intestinal epithelium. *Infect. Immun.* **65:**3412–3421.

99. **Masurier, C., B. Salomon, N. Guettari, N. Pioche, F. Lachapelle, M. Guigon, and D. Klatzmann.** 1998. Dendritic cells route human immunodeficiency virus to lymph nodes after vaginal or intravenous administration to mice. *J. Virol.* **72:**7822–7829.

100. **Mathan, M. M., and V. I. Mathan.** 1991. Morphology of rectal mucosa of patients with shigellosis. *Rev. Infect. Dis.* **13**(Suppl. 4):S314–S318.

101. **Maury, J., C. Nicoletti, L. Guzzo-Chambraud, and S. Maroux.** 1995. The filamentous brush border glycocalyx, a mucin-like marker of enterocyte hyper-polarization. *Eur. J. Biochem.* **228:**323–331.

102. **McClugage, S. G., F. N. Low, and M. L. Zimmy.** 1986. Porosity of the basement membrane overlying Peyer's patches in rats and monkeys. *Gastroenterology* **91:**1128–1133.

103. **McGhee, J. R., M. E. Lamm, and W. Strober.** 1999. Mucosal immune responses, p. 485–506. *In* R. Ogra, J. Mestecky, J. McGhee, J. Bienenstock, M. Lamm, and W. Strober (ed.), *Mucosal Immunology*, 2nd ed. Academic Press Inc., New York, N.Y.

104. **Mendelsohn, C. L., E. Wimmer, and V. R. Racaniello.** 1989. Cellular receptor for poliovirus: molecular cloning, nucleotide sequence, and expression of a new member of the immunoglobulin superfamily. *Cell* **56:**855–865.

105. **Miller, J. F., J. J. Mekalanos, and S. Falkow.** 1989. Coordinate regulation and sensory transduction in the control of bacterial virulence. *Science* **243:**916–921.

106. **Miller, S. I.** 1991. PhoP/PhoQ: macrophage-specific modulator of *Salmonella* virulence? *Molec. Microbiol.* **5:**2073–2078.

107. **Mills, S., A. Boland, M. P. Sory, P. Van der Smissen, C. Kerbourch, B. B. Finlay, and G. Cornelis.** 1997. *Yersinia enterocolitica* induces apoptosis in macrophages by a process requiring functional type III secretion and translocation mechanism and involving YopP presumably acting as an effector protein. *Proc. Natl. Acad. Sci. USA* **94:**12638–12643.

108. **Milman, G., and O. Sharma.** 1994. Mechanisms of HIV/SIV mucosal transmission. *AIDS Res. Human Retrovir.* **10:**1305–1312.

109. **Momotani, E., D. L. Whipple, A. B. Thiermann, and N. F. Cheville.** 1988. Role of M cells and macrophages in the entrance of *Mycobacterium paratuberculosis* into domes of ileal Peyer's patches in calves. *Vet. Pathol.* **25:**131–137.

110. **Monack, D. M., J. Mecsas, N. Ghori, and S. Falkow.** 1997. *Yersinia* signals macrophages to undergo apoptosis and Yop J is necessary for the cell death. *Proc. Natl. Acad. Sci. USA* **94:**10385–10390.

111. **Morin, M. J., A. Warner, and B. N. Fields.** 1994. A pathway for entry of reoviruses into the host through M cells of the respiratory tract. *J. Exp. Med.* **180:**1523–1527.

112. **Morrow, C. D., M. J. Novak, D. C. Ansardi, D. C. Porter, and Z. Moldoveanu.** 1998. Recombinant viruses as vectors for mucosal immunity. *Curr. Top. Microbiol. Immunol.* **236:**255–274.

113. **Mounier, J., T. Vasselon, R. Hellio, M. Lesourd, and P. J. Sansonetti.** 1992. *Shigella flexneri* enters human colonic Caco-2 cells through the basolateral pole. *Infect. Immun.* **60:**237–248.

114. **Neutra, M. R., A. Frey, and J.-P. Kraehenbuhl.** 1996. Epithelial M cells: gateways for mucosal infection and immunization. *Cell* **86:**345–348.

115. **Neutra, M. R., P. J. Giannasca, K. T. Giannasca, and J.-P. Kraehenbuhl.** 1995. M cells and microbial pathogens, p. 163–178. *In* M. Blaser, P. D. Smith, J. I. Ravdin, H. B. Greenberg, and R. L. Guerrant (ed.), *Infections of the Gastrointestinal Tract.* Raven Press, New York, N.Y.

116. **Neutra, M. R., T. L. Phillips, E. L. Mayer, and D. J. Fishkind.** 1987. Transport of membrane-bound macromolecules by M cells in

follicle-associated epithelium of rabbit Peyer's patch. *Cell Tiss. Res.* **247:**537–546.

117. **Neutra, M. R., E. Pringault, and J. P. Kraehenbuhl.** 1996. Antigen sampling across epithelial barriers and induction of mucosal immune responses. *Annu. Rev. Immunol.* **14:**275–300.

118. **Neutra, M. R., N. J. Mantis, A. Frey, and P. J. Giannasca.** 1999. The composition and function of M cell apical membranes: implications for microbial pathogenesis. *Sem. Immunol.* **11:**171–181.

119. **Neutra, M. R., P. Sansonetti, and J. P. Kraehenbuhl.** 2002. M cells and microbial pathogens, p. 141–156. *In* M. J. Blaser, P. D. Smith, J. I. Ravdin, H. B. Greenberg, and L. Guerrant (ed.), *Infections of the Gastrointestinal Tract.* Raven Press, New York, N.Y.

120. **Nibert, M. L.** 1998. Structure of mammalian orthoreovirus particles, p. 1–30. *In* K. L. Tyler and M. B. A. Oldstone (ed.), *Reoviruses I: Structure, Proteins, and Genetics.* Springer-Verlag, Berlin, Germany.

121. **Nibert, M. L., D. B. Furlong, and B. N. Fields.** 1991. Mechanisms of viral pathogenesis. Distinct forms of reoviruses and their roles during replication in cells and host. *J. Clin. Invest.* **88:**727–734.

122. **Ogra, P. L., and D. T. Karzon.** 1969. Distribution of poliovirus antibody in serum, nasopharynx and alimentary tract following segmental immunization of lower alimentary tract with polio-vaccine. *J. Immunol.* **102:**1423–1430.

123. **O'Leary, A. D., and E. C. Sweeney.** 1986. Lymphoglandular complexes of the colon: structure and distribution. *Histopathology* **10:**267–283.

124. **Owen, R.** 1999. Uptake and transport of intestinal macromolecules and microorganisms by M cells in Peyer's patches—a personal and historic perspective. *Semin. Immunol.* **11:**1–7.

125. **Owen, R. L., D. M. Bass, and A. J. Piazza.** 1990. Colonic lymphoid patches. A portal of entry in mice for type I reovirus administered anally. *Gastroenterology* **98:**A468.

126. **Owen, R. L., and D. K. Bhalla.** 1983. Cytochemical analysis of alkaline phosphatase and esterase activities and of lectin-binding and anionic sites in rat and mouse Peyer's patch M cells. *Am. J. Anat.* **168:**199–212.

127. **Owen, R. L., A. J. Piazza, and T. H. Ermak.** 1991. Ultrastructural and cytoarchitectural features of lymphoreticular organs in the colon and rectum of adult BALB/c mice. *Am. J. Anat.* **190:**10–18.

128. **Owen, R. L., N. F. Pierce, R. T. Apple, and W. C. J. Cray.** 1986. M cell transport of *Vibrio cholerae* from the intestinal lumen into Peyer's patches: a mechanism for antigen sampling and for microbial transepithelial migration. *J. Infect. Dis.* **153:**1108–1118.

129. **Pappo, J., and T. H. Ermak.** 1989. Uptake and translocation of fluorescent latex particles by rabbit Peyer's patch follicle epithelium: a quantitative model for M cell uptake. *Clin. Exp. Immunol.* **76:**144–148.

130. **Pappo, J., and R. L. Owen.** 1988. Absence of secretory component expression by epithelial cells overlying rabbit gut-associated lymphoid tissue. *Gastroenterology* **95:**1173–1177.

131. **Pauza, C. D., P. Emau, M. S. Salvato, P. Trivedi, D. MacKensie, M. Malkovsky, H. Uno, and K. T. Schultz.** 1993. Pathogenesis of SIV mac51 after atraumatic inoculation of the rectal mucosa in rhesus monkeys. *J. Med. Primatol.* **22:**154–161.

132. **Penheiter, K. L., N. Mathur, D. Giles, T. Fahlen, and B. D. Jones.** 1997. Non-invasive *Salmonella typhimurium* mutants are avirulent because of an inability to enter and destroy M cells of ileal Peyer's patches. *Mol. Microbiol.* **24:**697–709.

133. **Pepe, J. C., and V. L. Miller.** 1993. *Yersinia enterocolitica* invasin: a primary role in the initiation of infection. *Proc. Natl. Acad. Sci. USA* **90:**6473–6477.

134. **Pron, B., C. Boumalia, F. Jaubert, P. Berche, G. Milon, F. Geissman, and J. L. Gaillard.** 2001. Dendritic cells are early cellular targets of *Listeria monocytogenes* after intestinal delivery and are involved in bacterial spread in the host. *Cell. Microbiol.* **3:**331–340.

135. **Racaniello, V. R., and R. Ren.** 1996. Poliovirus biology and pathogenesis. *Curr. Top. Microbiol. Immunol.* **206:**305–325.

136. **Rafiee, P., H. Leffler, J. C. Byrd, F. J. Cassels, E. C. Boedeker, and Y. S. Kim.** 1991. A sialoglycoprotein complex linked to the microvillus cytoskeleton acts as a receptor for pilus (AF/R1) mediated adhesion of enteropathogenic *Escherichia coli* (RDEC-1) in rabbit small intestine. *J. Cell Biol.* **115:**1021–1029.

137. **Rescigno, M., M. Urbano, B. Valzasina, M. Francolini, G. Rotta, R. Bonasio, F. Granucci, J.-P. Kraehenbuhl, and P. Ricciardi-Castagnoli.** 2001. Dendritic cells express tight junction proteins and penetrate gut epithelial monolayers to sample bacteria. *Nature Immunol.* **2:**361–367.

138. **Rissoan, M. C., V. Soumelis, N. Kadowaki, G. Grouard, F. Briere, R. W. Malefyt, and Y. J. Liu.** 1999. Reciprocal control of

T helper cell and dendritic cell differentiation. *Science* **283**:1183–1186.

139. **Roy, M. J., and M. Varvayanis.** 1987. Development of dome epithelium in gut-associated lymphoid tissues: association of IgA with M cells. *Cell Tissue Res.* **248**:645–651.

140. **Ruckdeschel, K., A. Roggenkamp, V. Lafont, P. Mangeat, J. Heesemann, and B. Rouot.** 1997. Interaction of *Yersinia enterocolitica* with macrophages leads to macrophage cell death through apoptosis. *Infect. Immun.* **65**:4813–4821.

141. **Sansonetti, P. J.** 1991. Genetic and molecular basis of epithelial cell invasion by *Shigella* species. *Rev. Infect. Dis.* **13**:S285–S292.

142. **Sansonetti, P. J., J. Arondel, J. R. Cantey, M. C. Prevost, and M. Huerre.** 1996. Infection of rabbit Peyer's patches by *Shigella flexneri*: effect of adhesive or invasive bacterial phenotypes on follicle-associated epithelium. *Infect. Immun.* **64**:2752–2764.

143. **Sansonetti, P. J., J. Mounier, M. C. Prevost, and R. M. Mege.** 1994. Cadherin expression is required for the spread of *Shigella flexneri* between epithelial cells. *Cell* **76**:829–839.

144. **Sansonetti, P. J., A. Phalipon, J. Arondel, K. Thirumalai, S. Banerjee, S. Akira, K. Takeda, and A. Zychlinsky.** 2000. Caspase-1 activation of IL-1b and IL-18 are essential for *Shigella flexneri*-induced inflammation. *Immunity* **12**:581–590.

145. **Sansonetti, P. J., and A. Phalipon.** 1999. M cells as ports of entry for enteroinvasive pathogens: mechanisms of interaction, consequences for the disease process. *Semin. Immunol.* **11**:193–203.

146. **Savidge, T. C., and M. W. Smith.** 1995. Evidence that membranous (M) cell genesis is immunoregulated. *Adv. Exp. Med. Biol.* **371**:239–241.

147. **Savidge, T. C., M. W. Smith, P. S. James, and P. Aldred.** 1991. *Salmonella*-induced M-cell formation in germ-free mouse Peyer's patch tissue. *Am. J. Pathol.* **139**:177–184.

148. **Schulte, R., S. Kernéis, S. Klinke, H. Bartels, S. Preger, J.-P. Kraehenbuhl, E. Pringault, and I. B. Autenrieth.** 2000. Translocation of *Yersinia enterocolitica* across reconstituted intestinal epithelial monolayers is triggered by *Yersinia* invasin binding to beta 1 integrins apically expressed on M-like cells. *Cell Microbiol.* **2**:173–185.

149. **Sharma, R., E. J. M. Van Damme, W. J. Peumans, P. Sarsfield, and U. Schumacher.** 1996. Lectin binding reveals divergent carbohydrate expression in human and mouse Peyer's patches. *Histochem. Cell Biol.* **105**:459–465.

150. **Shea, J., M. Hensel, C. Gleeson, and D. Holden.** 1996. Identification of a virulence locus encoding a second type III secretion system in *Salmonella typhimurium*. *Proc. Natl. Acad. Sci. USA* **93**:2593–2597.

151. **Shibuya, A., N. Sakamoto, Y. Shimizu, K. Shibuya, M. Osawa, T. Hiroyama, H. J. Eyre, G. R. Sutherland, Y. Endo, T. Fujita, T. Miyabayashi, S. Sakano, T. Tsuji, E. Nakayama, J. H. Phillips, L. L. Lanier, and H. Nakauchi.** 2000. Fc alpha/mu receptor mediates endocytosis of IgM-coated microbes. *Nat. Immunol.* **1**:441–446.

152. **Shreedhar, V. K., B. L. Kelsall, and M. R. Neutra.** 2003. Cholera toxin induces migration of dendritic cells from the subepithelial dome region to T- and B-cell areas of Peyer's patches. *Infect. Immun.* **71**:504–509.

153. **Sicinski, P., J. Rowinski, J. B. Warchol, Z. Jarzcabek, W. Gut, B. Szczygiel, K. Bielecki, and G. Koch.** 1990. Poliovirus type 1 enters the human host through intestinal M cells. *Gastroenterology* **98**:56–58.

154. **Sierro, F., B. Dubois, A. Coste, D. Kaiserlian, J.-P. Kraehenbuhl, and J. C. Sirard.** 2001. Flagellin stimulation of intestinal epithelial cells triggers CCL20-mediated migration of dendritic cells. *Proc. Natl. Acad. Sci. USA* **98**:13722–13727.

155. **Sierro, F., E. Pringault, P. Simon Assman, J.-P. Kraehenbuhl, and N. Debard.** 2000. Transient expression of M cell phenotype by enterocyte-like cells of the follicle-associated epithelium of mouse Peyer's patches. *Gastroenterology* **119**:734–743.

156. **Silvey, K. J., A. B. Hutchings, M. Vajdy, M. M. Petzke, and M. R. Neutra.** 2001. Role of IgA in protection against reovirus entry into murine Peyer's patches. *J. Virol.* **75**:10870–10879.

157. **Silvey, K. J., M. Vajdy, N. J. Mantis, and M. R. Neutra.** 1999. Reovirus: a model to study M cell specific interactions and secretory antibody function in the intestine. *Immunol. Lett.* **69**:65.

158. **Sirard, J. C., F. Niedergang, and J.-P. Kraehenbuhl.** 1999. Live attenuated *Salmonella*: a paradigm of mucosal vaccines. *Immunol. Rev.* **171**:5–26.

159. **Smith, M. W., P. S. James, and D. R. Tivey.** 1987. M cell numbers increase after transfer of SPF mice to a normal animal house environment. *Am. J. Pathol.* **128**:385–389.

160. **Takeuchi, A.** 1967. Electron microscope studies of experimental *Salmonella* infection. I. Pen-

etration into the intestinal epithelium by *Salmonella typhimurium*. *Am. J. Pathol.* **50:**109–136.

161. **Tanaka, Y., T. Imai, M. Baba, I. Ishikawa, M. Uehira, H. Nomiyama, and O. Yoshie.** 1999. Selective expression of liver and activation-regulated chemokine (LARC) in intestinal epithelium in mice and humans. *Eur. J. Immunol.* **29:**633–642.

162. **Uchida, J.** 1987. An ultrastructural study on active uptake and transport of bacteria by microfold cells (M cells) to the lymphoid follicles in the rabbit appendix. *J. Clin. Electron Microsc.* **20:**379–394.

163. **Ueki, T., M. Mizuno, T. Ueso, T. Kiso, and T. Tsuji.** 1995. Expression of ICAM-1 on M cells covering isolated lymphoid follicles of the human colon. *Acta Med. Okayama* **49**(3):145–151.

164. **Vasquez-Torres, A., J. Jones-Carson, A. J. Baumler, S. Falkow, R. Valdivia, W. Brown, M. Le, R. Berggren, W. T. Parks, and F. Fang.** 1999. Extraintestinal dissemination of *Salmonella* by CD18-expressing phagocytes. *Nature* **401:**804–808.

165. **Walker, R. I., E. A. Schauder-Chock, and J. L. Parker.** 1988. Selective association and transport of *Campylobacter jejuni* through M cells of rabbit Peyer's patches. *Can. J. Microbiol.* **34:**1142–1147.

166. **Wassef, J. S., D. F. Keren, and J. L Mailloux.** 1989. Role of M cells in initial antigen uptake and in ulcer formation in the rabbit intestinal loop model of shigellosis. *Infect. Immun.* **57:**858–863.

167. **Weltzin, R. A., P. Lucia, P. Jandris, P. Michetti, B. N. Fields, J.-P. Kraehenbuhl, and M. R. Neutra.** 1989. Binding and transepithelial transport of immunoglobulins by intestinal M cells: demonstration using monoclonal IgA antibodies against enteric viral proteins. *J. Cell Biol.* **108:**1673–1685.

168. **Winner, L. S. III, J. Mack, R. A. Weltzin, J. J. Mekalanos, J.-P. Kraehenbuhl, and M. R. Neutra.** 1991. New model for analysis of mucosal immunity: intestinal secretion of specific monoclonal immunoglobulin A from hybridoma tumors protects against *Vibrio cholerae* infection. *Infect. Immun.* **59:**977–982.

169. **Wold, A. E., J. Mestecky, M. Tomana, A. Kobata, H. Ohbayashi, T. Endo, and C. Svanborg-Eden.** 1990. Secretory immunoglobulin A carries oligosaccharide receptors for *Escherichia coli* type 1 fimbrial lectin. *Infect. Immun.* **58:**3073–3077.

170. **Wolf, J. L., D. H. Rubin, R. Finberg, R. S. Kauffman, A. H. Sharpe, J. S. Trier, and B. N. Fields.** 1981. Intestinal M cells: a pathway for entry of reovirus into the host. *Science* **212:**471–472.

171. **Yamamoto, T., and T. Yokota.** 1989. Adherence targets of *Vibrio parahaemolyticus* in human small intestines. *Infect. Immun.* **57:**2410–2419.

172. **Yamamoto, T., and T. Yokota.** 1989. *Vibrio cholerae* O1 adherence to human small intestinal M cells *in vitro. J. Infect. Dis.* **160:**168–169.

173. **Zhou, F., J.-P. Kraehenbuhl, and M. R. Neutra.** 1995. Mucosal IgA response to rectally administered antigen formulated in IgA-coated liposomes. *Vaccine* **13:**637–644.

174. **Zychlinsky, A., M. C. Prévost, and P. J. Sansonetti.** 1992. *Shigella flexneri* induces apoptosis in infected macrophages. *Nature* **358:**167–169.

INTESTINAL IMMUNITY

Iris Dotan and Lloyd Mayer

3

Intestinal immunity is a relatively new term in relation to events and processes that precede human biology. Microorganisms inhabited the Earth before humans. The evolution of intestinal immunity was therefore influenced by its interaction with these microorganisms. The intestinal tract successfully faces challenges that no other defense system handles. It encounters an enormous load of antigens while maintaining a normal homeostatic environment. Most of these antigens are beneficial to the host, such as dietary antigens and symbiotic bacteria, and some are harmless, such as commensals. On the other hand, pathogenic microorganisms need to be recognized and eliminated before damage occurs. Upon exposure, the systemic immune system elicits an aggressive immune response to any nonself antigen. The intestinal immune system, however, needs to be more flexible. Antigens need to be sampled, processed, and presented in such a way that enables the destruction of pathogens and tolerance of nonpathogens. Therefore, the rules governing intestinal immunity differ from those observed in systemic immunity. The challenges of facing billions of bacteria, limitless dietary antigens, and the largest pool of lymphocytes in the body (i.e., "controlled inflammation") necessitated the development of unique cells, mediators, and regulatory processes.

Cells of the gut-associated lymphoid tissue (GALT) include conventional cells of the innate and adaptive immune system such as B and T lymphocytes, macrophages, and dendritic cells (DC), as well as more unusual antigen-presenting cells (APC) and lymphocytes unique to the GALT, such as intestinal epithelial cells (IEC), lamina propria lymphocytes (LPL), and intraepithelial lymphocytes (IEL). These cells have unique activation requirements, and they secrete, and are influenced by, a special array of cytokines and mediators. These unique cells and phenomena are the focus of this chapter. The phenomena characterizing mucosal immunity reflect the unusual challenges facing this immune system and the nature of the unique interacting cell types. Each component will be discussed and placed into the context of these phenomena. As this book focuses on interactions of the IEC with microbial pathogens, a special emphasis is on the IEC in intestinal immunity. In each section, an attempt has been made to associate histology and phenotypic observations with function in the GALT.

Iris Dotan and Lloyd Mayer, Mount Sinai School of Medicine, 1425 Madison Avenue, New York, NY 10029.

Microbial Pathogenesis and the Intestinal Epithelial Cell, ed. by G. Hecht
© 2003 ASM Press, Washington, D.C.

CONTROLLED/PHYSIOLOGIC INFLAMMATION—MECHANISMS

As alluded to above, one of the remarkable features of the immune system within the gastrointestinal (GI) tract is its capacity to remain controlled in the setting of an enormous antigenic load. The term physiologic inflammation has been used to define the state of activation and number of cells in the lamina propria (LP) under normal, nonstressed conditions. Within a short time after birth, the LP of the gut is replete with memory/activated T cells, B cells, and macrophages. These cells express activation markers (e.g., interleukin-2R [IL-2R]) and spontaneously secrete cytokines. If one were to superimpose this histologic picture on any other epithelial organ (e.g., liver, pancreas, thyroid), it would be considered a chronic inflammatory disease. In the gut, however, this picture is the norm. The GALT becomes activated to a point and remains at a steady state. Even with acute infections there is a transient increase in the inflammatory cell infiltrate, with a rapid restoration of the baseline-activated state. This is clearly a tightly regulated process. Every aspect of the cellular and soluble microenvironment is geared toward either facilitating a nonresponse or inhibiting a response.

The research focus in this area has emphasized regulatory networks within the GALT itself. However, these studies ignore the much larger component, nonimmune and innate immune factors, that may play a much greater role than previously appreciated. One hypothesis is that nonimmune, innate, and adaptive immune responses all contribute to immunologic nonresponsiveness and it is the coordination of these specific components that optimizes controlled or physiologic inflammation.

To understand this regulated state, it is important to address the contribution of both nonimmune and immune factors. Nonimmune factors consist of a variety of barriers and factors produced or constituted by nonimmune cells (Table 1). By sheer size and by the physical and chemical barriers to antigen, entry cannot be trivialized. Mucins and related compounds exist throughout mucous membranes in the gut, lung, genitourinary (GU) tract, and so forth. The functions of these large-molecular-weight glycoproteins are multifold: trapping bacteria and viruses, preventing them from gaining initial access to the host, serving as a microenvironment for the accumulation of bacteriocidal and bacteriostatic chemicals and enzymes, and acting as a scaffold for secreted immunoglobulin A (IgA) molecules, which trap potentially harmful antigens in this mucus layer and facilitate their exit from the gut lumen. In the absence of a mucus barrier, inflammatory responses to noxious stimuli are enhanced. If potential antigens are either physically prevented from gaining access to the underlying lymphoid tissue or physically or chemically altered to the point

TABLE 1 Innate and adaptive immunity in the gut

Innate immunity		Adaptive immunity
Physicochemical	Cellular	
Mucus	NK cells (?some IEL)	IEL
Tight junctions	Macrophages	LPL
Epithelial membranes	Polymorphonuclear leukocytes	Regulatory cytokines
Luminal/brush border enzymes	PRRs (Toll-like receptors)	sIgA
Bile salts	Epithelial cells	PP
pH ranges		Epithelial cells; antigen presentation
Somatostatin		
Trefoil factors		

of nonantigenicity, the result is the same—the lack of a response to that antigen. The source of the mucin is specialized epithelial cells that differentiate in a microenvironment which promotes their development. The mechanisms regulating this differentiation process are not well characterized, but a number of laboratories have provided growing evidence that cytokines and lymphoepithelial cell (cognate?) interactions are involved. Other barrier functions are clearly affected by changes in the microenvironment. Tight junctions between epithelial cells function as potent exclusion barriers for large macromolecules or pathogens. Specialized proteins and cytoskeletal organization come together to form these junctions in a highly regulated manner. Gamma interferon (IFN-γ) treatment of epithelial cell monolayers disrupts tight junctions and alters cytoskeletal structure. Animal models of barrier dysfunction have been reported to exhibit a defect in maintenance of controlled/physiologic inflammation. Further, N-cadherin-dominant negative mutations in transgenic mice result in a mild but evident colitis (28).

It is plausible that the normally established microenvironment composed of components of innate and adaptive immunity as well as nonimmune factors is actually responsible for establishing the physical barriers in the first place (19). In this scenario, factors (such as IL-10, transforming growth factor β [TGF-β], somatostatin) produced locally by these various constituents would promote not only epithelial cell differentiation and mucin production but also tight junction formation, actin/cytoskeletal rearrangements, and the establishment of transporters and channels. While this might be overstating the point, there is ample published evidence to support this concept.

ORAL TOLERANCE

Oral tolerance (OT) is defined as the specific suppression of cellular and/or humoral immune responses to an antigen administered via the oral route (78). Four responses are classically associated with OT. These are soluble IgA (sIgA) production, suppression of delayed-type hypersensitivity (DTH) and T-cell proliferation, and characteristic cytokine production. OT is a phenomenon unique to mucosal-associated lymphoid tissue (MALT). It is a complex process, made up of at least two fundamentally different mechanisms—clonal deletion/anergy and active suppression (9, 77). These mechanisms exist in parallel, and determination of the mechanism employed is related first and foremost to the amount of antigen presented. Other factors, however, may also be of major significance. These include the nature of the antigen—particulate versus soluble (soluble antigens are more tolerogenic)—the age and genetic background of the host, and the presence of mucosal adjuvants.

High-dose oral tolerance (HD OT) is characterized by clonal anergy/deletion of potentially immunoreactive T cells, both Th1 and Th2 lymphocytes, induced by feeding high doses of antigen. In contrast, low-dose oral tolerance (LD OT) is an active, antigen-driven activation of regulatory T cells predominantly tolerizing Th1 cells while activating IL-4 and IL-10 secreting Th2, as well as TGF-β-secreting Th3 cells (11). Of note, while the inductive phase is antigen specific, the effector arm is antigen nonspecific, mediated by cytokines. This accounts for what has been termed bystander suppression of naïve T cells. The major regulatory cells identified in LD OT are CD4$^+$ T cells. Currently, at least three regulatory T-cell subpopulations have been defined: Th3, Tr1, and CD4$^+$ CD25$^+$ CD45RB^{low} (22, 23, 67, 72, 73). Th3 and Tr1 cells are defined by the cytokine profile secreted, with TGF-β being the dominant cytokine secreted by Th3 CD4$^+$ T cells and IL-10 being the dominant cytokine secreted by Tr1 cells, while CD4$^+$ CD25$^+$ CD45Rb^{low} are defined by their regulatory function. T cells that are specifically CD4$^+$ CD25$^+$ have been shown to prevent autoimmune diseases in rodents and to suppress proliferation and cytokine secretion of CD4$^+$ CD25$^-$ cells in vitro (56, 62) via a contact-mediated mechanism. The cytokine milieu required for each differentiation pathway is also different. IL-10 is a differentiation factor and IL-15 is a growth factor for Tr1 cells (reviewed in reference 61) while IL-4 and TGF-β promote Th3 differentiation (78). The growth and differentiation factors for CD4$^+$ CD25$^+$ T cells are less well characterized.

Early studies suggested a role for CD8$^+$ T cells in OT as well. Increasing evidence suggests that CD8$^+$ regulatory T cells are stimulated in the GALT after interaction with IEC or DC.

The cells responsible for the presentation of antigen in both LD and HD OT are, according to the majority of studies, DC. Even these most potent APC share many peculiarities of intestinal immunity, reflecting the multifaceted nature of the cells of the GALT; on the one hand, they must be prepared to fight potentially harmful antigens, while on the other hand, they must deal with an enormous load of harmless antigens, which should elicit tolerance to the benefit of the host. The importance of DC in OT induction is especially compelling in studies in mice treated with the hemopoietic growth factor flt3L (76). This factor induces expansion of DC with a resting phenotype (i.e., without increasing costimulatory molecule expression) in vivo. Mice treated with flt3L were significantly more susceptible to OT induction. Others (1a) have shown that DC were required for OT induction, whereas M cells and B cells were not.

The major site of OT induction, both low and high dose, is believed to be the Peyer's patches (PP). Several groups (9, 47) have shown this in murine models. These groups used adoptive transfer of T-cell receptor (TCR) transgenic T cells that could be tracked after antigen recognition in vivo. The fact that immunoregulatory cytokines were detected in the PP of mice early (1 to 6 h) after oral antigen feeding (20) further supported the concept that the PP is the site of OT induction. It should be noted, however, that recent studies have indicated that PP may not be necessary for the induction of OT. Lymphotoxin-β (LTβ) knockout (KO) mice, or mice without PP because of prenatal treatment with soluble LTβ receptor, had normal OT responses (70). Further, μMT mice that do not contain B cells because of a targeted mutation in the transmembrane region of the IgM heavy chain and fail to develop M cells and PP because of B-cell deficiency, were able to mount a normal tolerant response to oral antigen. This was shown to be a DC-dependent process and implicated the DC as the most important cell in OT (1a). Alternative sites for OT induction are the mesenteric lymph nodes (MLN)s and LP. Systemic induction of OT may occur as well, but data on the mechanism of OT induction in these alternative sites are modest. An intriguing possibility is that IEC, which are nonprofessional APC, when exposed to high doses of luminal antigens activate CD4$^+$ T cells without sufficient costimulation, thereby causing anergy/deletion of the affected CD4$^+$ T-cell clone.

The cytokine milieu in the PP (or in the MLN) has been shown to be crucial for determining the type of regulatory cell generated in response to fed antigens. Interestingly, PP DC have been shown to produce IL-10 and TGF-β, thus priming naïve T cells to produce IL-10 (36), in contrast to splenic DC, which promote IFN-γ production. Further, MLN DC activate T cells producing IL-4 and TGF-β, but not IFN-γ. Therefore the immunologic tone required for OT induction as well as effector function is that of a Th2/Th3 pathway, in contrast to the immunologic tone in the systemic immune system.

After activation by APC, regulatory cells may exert their effect by one of two basic mechanisms: cytokine-mediated inhibition or suppression mediated by cognate interaction. The major regulatory cytokine implicated in OT is TGF-β. In addition to its role in the IgA switch in the PP, it also known for its potent suppressive effects on immune responses. Moreover, the importance of this cytokine has been documented in several OT models where either increased TGF-β production was reported or the effects of regulatory $CD4^+$ T cells in vivo and in vitro were blocked by anti-TGF-β antibodies (11) (even though this was not a universal finding) (16).

The other major cytokine implicated in OT is IL-10. This cytokine, secreted by Tr1 cells, Th3 cells, and Th2 cells, suppresses Th1-mediated immune responses by decreasing costimulatory molecule expression and IL-12 production by APC, as well as by promoting the generation of Tr1 cells. The immuno-regulatory effect of IL-10 in the GALT is supported by several observations. First, clones of IL-10-secreting cells were isolated from animals tolerized by oral antigens (11). Second, IL-10 KO mice develop severe colitis. Third, transferred $CD4^+RB^{low}$ cells in the $CD45Rb^{high} \rightarrow$ severe combined immuno-deficient (SCID) transfer model fail to prevent colitis when they are generated from IL-10 KO mice (2) (wild-type $CD45Rb^{low}$ cells prevent colitis development).

IL-4 has also been implicated in oral tolerance, although these data are less compelling, as Th2 $CD4^+$ T cells that were isolated from orally tolerized mice secrete this cytokine (11). IL-4 was initially thought to be a growth factor for Th3 cells, but $IL4^{-/-}$ mice can develop LD OT normally (82).

Controversy exists concerning a possible role for IFN-γ in OT. The controversy is due to both confounding data and the complex kinetics of IFN-γ secretion in OT. Specifically, IFN-γ is increased in intestinal tissues early after OT induction (10), but it is down-regulated in later stages. This observation and studies demonstrating a relationship between increased IFN-γ in PP and MLN and de-creased T-cell migration to the skin suggested a mechanistic role for IFN-γ in at least one of the processes in OT, i.e., DTH (44). This was supported by studies showing a lack of, or partial, OT induction in IFN-$\gamma^{-/-}$ mice fed ovalbumin (OVA) (B-cell responses were af-fected more than T-cell responses). Others, however, have disputed these results by show-ing normal OT induction in IFN-$\gamma R^{-/-}$ mice, IFN-γ-depleted mice, and IL-12 P40

KO mice (40, 50). Therefore, much remains to be studied with regard to IFN-γ in OT. Most probably, kinetics and cytokine ratios will be shown to have an additive role, that is, early higher and late lower amounts, where "some IFN-γ is good and too much is bad." With regard to kinetics and the amount of IFN-γ secretion in OT, Strober et al. (71) suggested an intriguing hypothesis. In studies conducted in OVA-specific TCR transgenic mice, increased IFN-γ and no TGF-β pro-duction in PP were demonstrated. However, when IL-12 was administered in parallel with OVA feeding, Th1 responses were blocked and PP TGF-β production increased. The conclusion that Th1 responses block TGF-β production led to the hypothesis that in LD OT the level of IFN-γ produced is not enough to inhibit TGF-β production or, alternatively, that other cytokines, such as IL-10, are produced and inhibit IFN-γ pro-duction, thereby leading to increased TGF-β production.

In addition to cytokine-mediated tolerance, OT may also be induced by cognate interac-tions of APC and T-regulatory cells. This may be a bidirectional event—APC interact with T cells and promote their regulatory functions, while conversely, T cells may interact with APC and stimulate them to become "regula-tory lymphocyte promoting" APC in their subsequent interactions. This was specifically shown for interactions of DC and lympho-cytes mediated by CD40-CD40L (25, 43).

The importance of CD40-CD40L interac-tion in OT was further shown in $CD40L^{-/-}$ mice. These mice were resistant to HD OT, and their splenic $CD4^+$ T cells proliferated in response to the tolerizing antigen, in contrast to splenic $CD4^+$ T cells from $CD40L^{+/+}$ mice (42). Their Th1/Th2 cytokine responses were not downregulated. This suggested that T-cell unresponsiveness, which is normally induced by HD administration of oral antigen, did not occur in mice deficient in the CD40L-CD40 pathway. Further, the ability of $CD4^+$ T cells to support antigen-specific B-cell responses was shown to be CD40-CD40L mediated. Interestingly, it is believed that when T cells are activated without costimulation, anergy results. These studies show, however, that OT could not be induced in the absence of a form of costimulation.

The CD40-CD40L costimulatory pathway in OT may be related to CD80-CD86 interactions with CTLA-4. It has already been shown that ligation of CD40-CD40L mediates CD80-CD86 expression and that binding of CTLA-4-immunoglobulin (Ig) fusion protein to CD80-CD86 decreases T-cell proliferation in mixed lymphocyte reaction (55). Direct evidence for the significance of CTLA-4 in HD OT has also been reported. Mice that were tolerized with HD oral antigen after CD28 and CTLA-4 signals were blocked were partially tolerized to the antigen, while selective blocking of CTLA-4 completely abrogated HD OT (63). Thus, costimulation by the CTLA-4-B7 pathway may be directly involved in HD OT.

Others, however, have found that CD40-CD40L signaling is not required for induction of OT and that OT could be induced in the absence of CD40. This was shown in genetically unmanipulated mice in whom CTLA-4 was transiently blocked, or in CD40$^{-/-}$ chimeric mice. The problem in using this approach is that CD40$^{-/-}$ mice have several other immune defects that may interfere with OT induction, such as failure to form GC, activate memory B cells, and induce Ig class switching (38).

UNIQUE APC: IEC

The IEC is part of the columnar epithelium lining the intestinal tract from the duodenum to the rectum. This epithelium is single layered and has important functions in absorption and secretion of nutrients and ions that are beyond the scope of this chapter. Its function in the mucosal immune system is incompletely defined, but accumulated data suggest that this cell may function as an important APC in the mucosal immune system, both in health and in disease. The "immunophysiologic rationale" of such a function is clear, as this cell is at the interface of the largest antigenic load in the body and the largest population of lymphocytes. In addition, it outnumbers the antigen-sampling M cell and is better equipped than M cells for antigen processing and presentation—expressing more lysosomal structures and relevant cell surface molecules. The epithelial cell is a highly polarized cell, with distinct apical (luminal) and basolateral surfaces joined together by tight junctions.

Under normal circumstances, these structures are very efficient in preventing the passage of molecules. In certain inflammatory states, however, the function of tight junctions is disturbed, thus enabling the transit of charged molecules, bacteria, and nutrients across the epithelium (18, 45, 64). The apical surface is composed of the glycocalyx and microvillus brush border and covered with specialized mucus. The basolateral surface is capable of forming pseudopods, which pass through the 0.3- to 3-μm pores of the basement membrane, enabling direct contact of IEC with cells of the LP (26). In addition, human IEC, similar to professional APC, have been shown to secrete exosome-like vesicles (75). These are 30- to 90-nm-diameter vesicles, containing major histocompatibility complex (MHC) class I and class II molecules, an observation that suggests that IEC may influence antigen presentation to LPL even without direct contact.

IEC as APC in the GALT

Since the 1980s, the expression by IEC of several surface molecules that are involved in antigen presentation was noted (Table 2). This has led several groups to investigate the potential role of IEC as APC. In contrast to bone marrow-derived, professional APC, IEC are not equipped with the full armamentarium of antigen-presenting and costimulatory molecules. Therefore, it was assumed that they are capable of providing lymphocytes with "signal 1"—activation via TCR—only. In such a case, anergy, not stimulation, would be the expected result. However, the rules of the mucosal immune system are different from

TABLE 2 IEC express surface molecules that are relevant to antigen processing and presentation to T cells

Molecules	Polarized expression	Constitutive (C)/ induced (I)	References
Antigen-presenting molecules			
HLA class I		C	
HLA A, B, C	Basolateral>>apical		30
HLA E	ND[a]		5
CD1d		C+I[b]	68
β2-m associated	Basolateral>apical		
Non β2-m associated	Apical>basolateral		
MICA/MICB	ND	I	21
HLA class II	Basolateral>>apical	C+I	29, 31
Costimulatory molecules			
CD58	Basolateral	C	14
CD86	ND	I (UC only)	52
gp180		C	80
PI-linked form	Apical>basolateral		
Transmembrane form	Basolateral>apical		
ICAM-I	Apical	I	32
Receptors for antigen internalization			
FcRn		C	34
Villous	Apical>basolateral		
Crypt	Apical=basolateral		
DEC-205	ND	C	79
Polymeric Ig receptor	Basolateral>apical	C	6

[a] ND, not done.
[b] L. Shao and L. Mayer, unpublished data.

those of the systemic immune system. First, it has long been known that most of the LPL, as well as the IEL, are memory cells requiring less (or no) costimulation than naïve T cells for activation. More important, it was discovered that in addition to the constitutive expression of classical MHC class I and II molecules, IEC express several unique costimulatory molecules, whether constitutively or during inflammatory conditions, thereby allowing for the capacity of providing both "signal 1" and "signal 2." Normal IEC do not express B7-1 (CD80), B7-2 (CD86), or CD40, but do express LFA-3 (CD58) (14) and gp180 (80), a CD8 ligand. In contrast, inflammatory bowel disease (IBD) (ulcerative colitis [UC]) IEC express B7-2 (CD86) (52) and infected IEC express intercellular adhesion mol-

ecule-1 (ICAM-1) (32). Taken together, the location of IEC, separating antigens from lymphocytes, the expression of surface molecules required for lymphocyte activation and costimulation, and the ability to interact with LPL as well as IEL make the IEC a prime candidate for antigen presentation in the mucosal immune system.

IEC Interactions with CD8[+] T Cells

The observation that normal IEC stimulate CD8[+] regulatory T-cell proliferation in vitro (3, 49) was unexplained until 1997, when gp180, a 180-kDa molecule present on the apical as well as the basolateral membrane of IEC, was identified (80). When the association between gp180 and the nonclassical class I molecule CD1d on IEC was subsequently described (8), a model for the interaction between IEC and the CD8+ regulatory T cell was proposed. In this model, gp180 binds to CD8 and CD1d binds to the TCR. This interaction forms an MHC class I-like complex on the IEC surface, thereby promoting suppressor CD8+ T-cell activation. While the inductive phase may be antigen specific, the effector phase is antigen nonspecific, in contrast to class I-restricted CD8+ T cells activated by conventional APC, which are antigen specific. The nature of the antigen presented to CD8+ T cells by the MHC class I-like complex composed of gp180 and CD1d is as yet unknown. Both human and murine CD1d molecules have been shown to present the synthetic acylphytosphingolipid originally isolated from a marine sponge, α-galactosylceramide (α-GalCer) (39, 69), and murine natural killer (NK) T cells (NKT cells) recognize cellular phospholipids presented by CD1d (24). It was also suggested, based on crystallographic studies, that the deep hydrophobic pocket of the CD1d molecule allowed it to present microbial lipid components. In any case, it remains to be determined whether the antigen presented by CD1d to cells (either CD8+ CD4− or double negative) in the GALT will drive the stimulation of cells with regulatory functions.

A population of T cells that are stimulated by normal IEC are CD8+ CD28− T cells with regulatory activity (M. Allez and L. Mayer, manuscript submitted). The vast majority of IEL are CD8+ T cells, some with an NKT phenotype. Thus, an interaction between IEC and the interspersed IEL is plausible. However, as will be discussed in the IEL section of this chapter, the function of these intriguing cells in mucosal immune responses, as well as their stimulation requirements is as yet undefined.

Taken together, the observations on the interaction of IEC and CD8+ T cells suggest that in the normal intestine, antigen (probably bacterial) presented to CD8+ T cells by an MHC class I-like complex on the IEC surface stimulates an immune response that is of the antigen-nonspecific, suppressor type, thus contributing to the general tone in the GALT, which is normally that of tolerance.

IEC Interactions with CD4+ T Cells

The prerequisite for CD4+ T-cell stimulation by APC is the presence of MHC class II molecules. Normal IEC constitutively express human leukocyte antigen (HLA)-DR, and this expression increases in inflammatory conditions (48). The potential for interaction of IEC and CD4+ T cells therefore exists. It was subsequently shown that human IEC—both freshly isolated and cell lines—are capable of stimulating CD4+ T-cell proliferation and cytokine production (30). A central issue is what subtype of CD4+ T cells is stimulated by IEC. In IBD, where MHC class II expression is increased, and costimulatory molecules such as CD86 (in UC patients) are coexpressed, the stimulation of Th1/Th2-biased CD4+ T cells may occur. In the normal state, however, where no CD80, CD86, CD40, or other costimulatory molecules such as LFA3 (CD58) are expressed, different subsets of CD4+ T cells may proliferate. The stimulation of naïve CD4+ T cells through the TCR without provision of "signal 2" is expected to result in anergic CD4+ T cells. As mentioned above, this situation is the exception rather than the rule in the LP, where most CD4+ T cells are memory cells. Whether normal IEC are responsible for the stimulation of regulatory CD4+ T cells remains to be determined; however, the potential of IEC to activate different CD4+ T-cell subpopulations in health and disease exists. A suggested model for the interactions of IEC with CD4 and CD8+ T cells in the normal and inflamed mucosa is depicted in Fig. 1.

Mediators Secreted by IEC

The epithelium may also contribute positively or negatively to mucosal immune homeostasis in other ways. Its functions as a barrier between the luminal antigenic load and the mucosal immune system and as a nonprofessional APC have been discussed earlier. In addition,

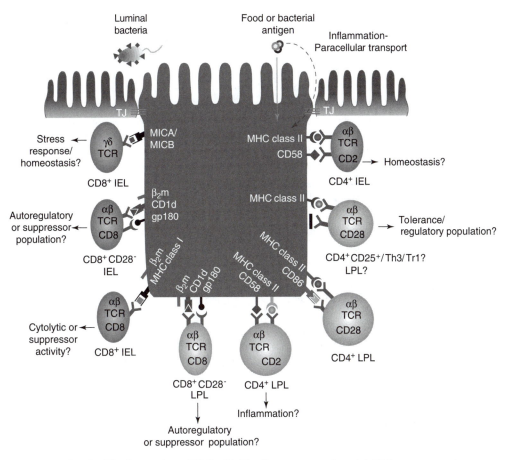

FIGURE 1 The interaction of IEC with T cells—a suggested model. IEC express a variety of surface molecules relevant for antigen presentation and stimulation of T cells (see Table 2). Luminal antigens derived from food or bacteria may be internalized via the apical surface. In the presence of inflammation, paracellular transport of antigens and presentation by basolateral surface molecules may occur. The amount and type of antigen, as well as the combination of antigen-presenting molecules with costimulatory molecules, determine the population of T cells that will expand. CD8$^+$ IEL and LPL may be stimulated by classical MHC class I molecules. Stimulation by class I-like molecules, such as the complex gp180:CD1d and MICA/MICB, may also occur. The antigen presented in the IEC:CD8$^+$ T-cell interaction is of nonpeptide origin. When presented by CD1d, data suggest it is a bacterial-derived phospholipid. The nature of antigen presented to CD8$^+$ T cells by MICA/MICB expressing IEC remains hypothetical at this point. CD8$^+$ T cells activated by IEC have a suppressor activity and may function in regulating mucosal homeostasis. Peptide antigens can be presented to CD4$^+$ T cells by MHC class II molecules, which are constitutively expressed on IEC. Different CD4$^+$ T-cell populations may expand when the antigen is taken up via the apical or the basolateral surface. In normal mucosal homeostasis, regulatory CD4$^+$ T cells, activated via MHC class II without costimulation, may contribute to controlled inflammation. In inflammatory states, upregulation of MHC class II as well as costimulatory molecules such as CD86 may promote the expansion of TH1/TH2 cells and contribute to uncontrolled inflammation.

IEC secrete mediators that influence cells in their vicinity. Several chemokines and cytokines have recently been shown to be expressed by IEC. IEC-derived chemokines can induce the migration of inflammatory cells toward the epithelium. Therefore, their production by IEC demonstrates the potential for active participation in intestinal innate and adaptive immune responses.

In regard to adaptive immunity, IEC secrete the CXC chemokines, monokine induced by IFN-γ (MIG), IFN-γ-inducible protein 10 (IP-10), and I-TAC (13, 66). Importantly, fresh human IEL, as well as CD4$^+$ Th1 lymphocytes, express CXCR3, the common receptor for these chemokines. By attracting CD4$^+$ Th1 cells that produce IFN-γ, upregulation of expression and secretion of CXC chemokines occurs and contributes to a positive feedback loop that may be relevant in inflammatory states, specifically IBD. In contrast to the "inflammation-related" CXCR3, a "tissue-specific" chemokine receptor—CCR9—is expressed on IEL and LPL, and its ligand TECK (thymus-expressed chemokine) is differentially expressed in the small bowel mucosa (41). Finally, a CC chemokine that attracts immature dendritic cells, macrophage inflammatory protein-3α (MIP-3α), is also expressed and produced by human IEC (mainly in the follicle-associated epithelium [FAE]) (53). Mucosal T cells as well as IEC express CCR6, the cognate receptor for MIP-3α. It is intriguing to speculate that FAE IEC attract DC and lymphocytes to the place where positive immune responses occur and where the highest possibility for interaction with antigen takes place. Another interesting finding is that CCR6 and CCR9 are coexpressed in T cells with the $\alpha4\beta7$ integrin that is characteristic of mucosa-homing lymphocytes. Therefore, in inflammatory states and to some degree in the normal state, MIP-3α and TECK expression attract CCR9$^+$ or CCR6$^+$ lymphocytes that are activated in MLN, enter the peripheral blood, and then are recruited to the intestinal mucosa where they undergo activation-induced apoptosis or differentiation.

Other cytokines produced by IEC may play a role in the expansion or differentiation of mucosal lymphocytes. The accessory cytokine IL-6 was shown to be produced constitutively by fresh human IEC (54) as well as by malignant epithelial cell lines. This cytokine promotes T-cell growth and B-cell differentiation.

The common γc receptor cytokines IL-7 and IL-15 were also reported to be expressed in human IEC. IL-7 is a growth and differentiation factor for early B and T cells, specifically for $\gamma\delta$-TCR and CD8$^+$ T cells, which interestingly are enriched among the IEL. The expression and secretion of IL-7 were detected in fresh human small intestinal IEC as well as colonic tumor cell lines (46). Earlier studies demonstrated the expression of functional IL-7R on colonic tumor epithelial cell lines and on fresh human IEC (58).

IL-15 expression was demonstrated in fresh human IEC as well as in epithelial cell lines (57). Moreover, IEC also express functional receptors for IL-15 (common γc IL-2 receptor) (58). IL-15 affects both T- and B-cell differentiation and IEC proliferation and migration (through TGF-β expression) and thus, restitution. IL-15 is used by CD8$^+$ T-cell populations for growth. The ability of IEC to express and interact with IL-7 and IL-15 adds support to their potential function in intestinal immunity.

Reports on other cytokines secreted by IEC, such as TGF-β and tumor necrosis factor alpha (TNF-α), have been inconsistent. However, they emphasize the ability of the IEC to influence its vicinity and to participate in immune regulation in the mucosa.

APC IN THE SUBEPITHELIAL DOME AND PP

DC

DC are the most potent professional APC known. They are found in the gut in both organized and diffuse lymphoid compartments. Their ability to sense a luminal antigen was recently demonstrated (60). This makes their role in the GALT even more central, as from within the LP they are capable of sampling, processing, and presenting antigens. Their existence in the subepithelial dome (SED) where the vast majority of DC are immature (i.e., not expressing the markers DEC-205 and the intracellular antigen recognized by antibody 342) is especially prominent. In addition, SED DC are "double negative" cells, expressing CD11c without CD11b or CD8α. This fact may be functionally significant as double negative as well as CD11c$^+$ CD8α^+ DC produce high concentrations of IL-12p70 in vitro, in contrast to CD11c$^+$ 11b$^+$ DC, which produce higher concentrations of IL-10 and are more prominent in the PP. DC in the SED can move bidirectionally, i.e., toward the FAE as well as toward the PP. The movement of DC toward the FAE and the maintenance of immature DC in the SED are dependent on MIP-3α expression by enterocytes in the FAE, as well as the expression of CCR6 on DC. Interestingly, enteric bacteria, LPS, and flagellin upregulate MIP-3α expression by IEC (37). This may suggest that increased expression of this chemokine after exposure to bacterial components attracts DC from the SED to the epithelium where they come into close contact with the antigen and with lymphocytes within the epithelial pocket, thus generating a rapid immune response. However, the main site of antigen capture by immature DC is probably the SED. DC then carry the engulfed antigens to adjacent T-cell zones (interfollicular regions), where DC maturation and antigen presentation to T cells occur. An important issue that remains unresolved is how DC sense whether the antigen is pathogenic, thereby requiring presentation that will lead to an active immune response, or harmless, requiring tolerance. Few data exist regarding this crucial question. However, it is assumed that factors such as the amount of antigen (low dose versus high dose) delivered by the FAE to the DC, as well as the cytokine milieu in the PP (IL-10 and TGF-β versus IL-12), play an impor-

tant role in determining the result of the immune response.

Unique Lymphocytes in the GALT

Two distinct lymphocyte populations are separated by the thin basement membrane separating the epithelium and the LP. These are the IEL and the LPL. Both are different from systemic lymphocytes with regard to phenotype and activation requirements, and they differ from one another by phenotype and function.

IEL. IEL are among the most intriguing lymphocytes that exist. It is surprising that despite their numbers (epithelial lymphocytes are one of the major lymphocyte populations in the body) and the fact that they are the focus of intense research, their function is as yet undefined. This is attributed in part to difficulty in their isolation and to the intrinsic heterogeneity of IEL subsets. Virtually all IEL are T cells, most of which are CD8$^+$ T cells ($\sim$70%), at least in the small bowel. In contrast to their systemic counterparts, the majority of CD8$^+$ IEL in young mice express the CD8$\alpha\alpha$ homodimer. Two phenotypes that are rare in the circulation are expressed in IEL: CD4$^-$CD8$^-$ double negative ($\sim$10%) and CD4$^+$ 8$\alpha\alpha^+$ (5 to 15%). Another unique characteristic of IEL is their TCR usage, whether $\alpha\beta$ or $\gamma\delta$. In young mice there is a skewing toward the usage of a $\gamma\delta$ TCR, but this is not seen in humans. However, in both species there is a bias in TCR usage, with clonal populations present in the small bowel and colon. Since different TCR phenotypes are associated with different functional characteristics, to simplify characterization, Hayday et al. (27) suggested a classification of type a and type b IEL. According to this classification, type a IEL are TCR$\alpha\beta^+$ CD8$\alpha\beta^+$. Their proportion in the human small and large intestine is $\sim$50% and $\sim$100%, respectively. Type a IEL are cytolytic cells, with an oligoclonal repertoire that partially overlaps that of the LP and thoracic duct CD8$^+$ T cells. These observations support the hypothesis that type a IEL are primed in the MALT, migrate via the MLN and the thoracic duct to the systemic circulation, and home back to the LP, from where they pass into the epithelium. In that regard, IEL express the integrin $\alpha4\beta7$, which binds to the mucosal addressin MAdCAM-1. Homing of IEL is also directed by chemokines expressed by IEC such as IP-10, MIG, and I-TAC. IEL express CXCR3, the cognate receptor for these chemokines, as well as CCR9, the receptor for TECK that is expressed in small bowel IECs (81). Furthermore, mostly all IEL express $\alpha E\beta7$. This integrin binds to E-cadherin on IEC and may trigger the accumulation of IEL within the epithelium. Type b IEL are TCR$\alpha\beta^+$ CD8$\alpha\alpha^+$, TCR$\gamma\delta^+$ CD8$\alpha\alpha^+$, and TCR$\gamma\delta$ "double negative" T cells. Several criteria distinguish type b IEL from type a IEL. They have different gene expression, failing to express several T-cell maturation markers such as CD2, CD28, and CD5 (reviewed in reference 27). They differ by MHC restriction, with type a being conventionally restricted while type b is not, and they have different immunological memory. In humans, type b IEL make up ~50% of small intestinal IEL and are rare in the large intestine, possibly due to the overrepresentation of the antigenic-primed type a IEL in this bacterial-antigenic-loaded part of the gastrointestinal tract. Type b IEL are less MHC dependent than are type a and may develop in athymic mice, leading to the hypothesis that these cells may be autoreactive, peripherally positively selected regulatory cells. IEL may recognize nonpolymorphic restriction elements, such as human CD1 or murine TL, or surface proteins, such as MICA or MICB on IEC. The role of the TCR in these interactions, and of these molecules in activating specific IEL subsets, remains to be determined. Current data suggest that type b IEL have a role in promoting epithelial repair and healing and in eliminating infected or transformed epithelial cells. Carrying out this role of "epithelial sanitation" is dependent on the cytolytic properties of type b IEL and on cytokine secretion, specifically IFN-γ.

LPL. Another peculiar lymphocyte population of the intestinal immune system is that residing within the LP. LPL are a very heterogeneous group composed of T and B cells, as well as plasma and mast cells and macrophages. In contrast to IEL, LP CD4:CD8 T-cell ratios are similar to those in the blood, and they express the $\alpha\beta$ TCR. Similar to IEL, most of LPL are memory cells. Interestingly, when stimulated via the TCR their responses are poor, and they seem to depend on CD2/CD28-mediated stimulation to proliferate and secrete cytokines (4, 74). The propensity for stimulation via the CD2 pathway may be one explanation for the increased tendency toward apoptotic cell death in comparison to peripheral blood lymphocytes. Increased susceptibility to apoptosis may be related to the fact that the vast majority of LPL express Fas antigen and a subset also expresses Fas ligand. Again, this is a peculiarity of mucosal intestinal lymphocytes, as only 50% of peripheral blood lymphocytes are Fas positive (12). Not only are LPL more Fas positive than their peripheral counterparts, but also upon Fas ligation, cell death is induced more effectively in LPL, suggesting that they are "death prone" (12).

The significance of LPL preprogrammed cell death for intestinal mucosal homeostasis is seen in conditions in which this homeostasis is disturbed. In IBD, mucosal inflammation is associated with decreased sensitivity of LPL to cell death induced by Fas ligation (or by other cell-death inducers such as deprivation of IL-2 and exposure to nitric oxide). Differences between normal LPL and those generated from inflamed mucosa tell us that apoptosis-associated genes such as *bax* and *bcl-2* are differentially expressed in the normal versus inflamed mucosa. Specifically, increased expression of the anti-apoptotic Bcl-2 protein, increased Bcl/Bax ratio in the mucosa, and decreased Bax expression in LPL were reported in Crohn's disease (33, 35). This suggests, again, that normal LPL are an activated, apoptosis-prone population and that dysregulation of this death propensity may lead to intestinal inflammation. Inconsistent reports exist regarding the issue of the nature of cytokines secreted by LPL. This inconsistency is related to methodological differences in both cytokine detection and manipulation of LPL. However, it has been shown that IFN-γ is produced by LPL both in the normal state and in inflammatory conditions. Other cytokines produced under various conditions and stimuli are IL-5 (UC), TNF-α (Crohn's disease), and IL-10 (7, 15, 51, 59, 65). The targets of these cytokines are other immune cells (CD4$^+$ T cells, macrophages), the IEC themselves, and even endothelial cells. A cytokine network is thus created in which activated LPL activate additional cells in the LP-regulating (or dysregulating) mucosal homeostasis.

It is interesting to note that the LP is relatively sparse, in terms of LPL, in mice reared in a germ-free environment. These mice are fed comparable diets to those reared in conventional facilities, so dietary antigens are not likely to be the stimulus for LPL activation and recruitment. When germfree mice are "conventionalized," given normal flora, there is a rapid influx of activated LPL that quickly establish a controlled/physiologic inflammatory state. Thus, bacteria are the driving force for this phenomenon. How they do this is unknown.

SUMMARY

Unique challenges call for unique responses, and that may be the mantra of the mucosal immune system. The GALT has evolved to use a wide variety of exclusionary processes, novel mechanisms of antigen sampling, and new pathways of cellular activation to form an interactive, tightly regulated system. The most abundant antigen exists in the form of bacteria, and the role that these bacteria play in establishing the GALT is not understood. We do know that the epithelium plays a key role in this process, in all aspects. It is the challenge of the immediate future to define the interactions between luminal contents and epithelial surfaces in an attempt to understand the mechanisms involved in intestinal homeostasis and how these are disrupted in disease.

REFERENCES

1. **Allez, M., J. Brimnes, I. Dotan, and L. Mayer.** 2002. Expansion of CD8+ T cells with regulatory function after interaction with intestinal epithelial cells. *Gastroenterology* **123**:1516–1526.

1a. **Alpan, O., G. Rudomen, and P. Matzinger.** 2001. The role of dendritic cells, B cells, and M cells in gut-oriented immune responses. *J. Immunol.* **166**:4843–4852.

2. **Asseman, C., S. Mauze, M. W. Leach, R. L. Coffman, and F. Powrie.** 1999. An essential role for interleukin 10 in the function of regulatory T cells that inhibit intestinal inflammation. *J. Exp. Med.* **190**:995–1004.

3. **Bland, P. W., and L. G. Warren.** 1986. Antigen presentation by epithelial cells of the rat small intestine. II. Selective induction of suppressor T cells. *Immunology* **58**:9–14.

4. **Boirivant, M., M. Marini, G. Di Felice, A. M. Pronio, C. Montesani, R. Tersigni, and W. Strober.** 1999. Lamina propria T cells in Crohn's disease and other gastrointestinal inflammation show defective CD2 pathway-induced apoptosis. *Gastroenterology* **116**:557–565.

5. **Braud, V. M., D. S. Allan, and A. J. McMichael.** 1999. Functions of nonclassical MHC and non-MHC-encoded class I molecules. *Curr. Opin. Immunol.* **11**:100–108.

6. **Breitfeld, P. P., J. M. Harris, and K. E. Mostov.** 1989. Postendocytotic sorting of the ligand for the polymeric immunoglobulin receptor in Madin-Darby canine kidney cells. *J. Cell Biol.* **109**:475–486.

7. **Camoglio, L., A. A. te Velde, A. J. Tigges, P. K. Das, and S. J. van Deventer.** 1998. Altered expression of interferon-gamma and interleukin-4 in inflammatory bowel disease. *Inflamm. Bowel Dis.* **4**:285–290.

8. **Campbell, N. A., H. S. Kim, R. S. Blumberg, and L. Mayer.** 1999. The nonclassical class I molecule CD1d associates with the novel CD8 ligand gp180 on intestinal epithelial cells. *J. Biol. Chem.* **274**:26259–26265.

9. **Chen, Y., J. Inobe, R. Marks, P. Gonnella, V. K. Kuchroo, and H. L. Weiner.** 1995. Peripheral deletion of antigen-reactive T cells in oral tolerance. *Nature* **376**:177–180.

10. **Chen, Y., J. Inobe, and H. L. Weiner.** 1997. Inductive events in oral tolerance in the TCR transgenic adoptive transfer model. *Cell Immunol.* **178:**62–68.

11. **Chen, Y., V. K. Kuchroo, J. Inobe, D. A. Hafler, and H. L. Weiner.** 1994. Regulatory T cell clones induced by oral tolerance: suppression of autoimmune encephalomyelitis. *Science* **265:**1237–1240.

12. **De Maria, R., M. Boirivant, M. G. Cifone, P. Roncaioli, M. Hahne, J. Tschopp, F. Pallone, A. Santoni, and R. Testi.** 1996. Functional expression of Fas and Fas ligand on human gut lamina propria T lymphocytes. A potential role for the acidic sphingomyelinase pathway in normal immunoregulation. *J. Clin. Invest.* **97:** 316–322.

13. **Dwinell, M. B., N. Lugering, L. Eckmann, and M. F. Kagnoff.** 2001. Regulated production of interferon-inducible T-cell chemoattractants by human intestinal epithelial cells. *Gastroenterology* **120:**49–59.

14. **Framson, P. E., D. H. Cho, L. Y. Lee, and R. M. Hershberg.** 1999. Polarized expression and function of the costimulatory molecule CD58 on human intestinal epithelial cells. *Gastroenterology* **116:**1054–1062.

15. **Fuss, I. J., M. Neurath, M. Boirivant, J. S. Klein, M. C. de La, S. A. Strong, C. Fiocchi, and W. Strober.** 1996. Disparate CD4$^+$ lamina propria (LP) lymphokine secretion profiles in inflammatory bowel disease. Crohn's disease LP cells manifest increased secretion of IFN-gamma, whereas ulcerative colitis LP cells manifest increased secretion of IL-5. *J. Immunol.* **157:**1261–1270.

16. **Garside, P., and A. M. Mowat.** 2001. Oral tolerance. *Semin. Immunol.* **13:**177–185.

17. **Gasche, C., S. Bakos, C. Dejaco, W. Tillinger, S. Zakeri, and W. Reinisch.** 2000. IL-10 secretion and sensitivity in normal human intestine and inflammatory bowel disease. *J. Clin. Immunol.* **20:**362–370.

18. **Gassler, N., C. Rohr, A. Schneider, J. Kartenbeck, A. Bach, N. Obermuller, H. F. Otto, and F. Autschbach.** 2001. Inflammatory bowel disease is associated with changes of enterocytic junctions. *Am. J. Physiol. Gastrointest. Liver Physiol.* **281:**G216–G228.

19. **Goke, M., and D. K. Podolsky.** 1996. Regulation of the mucosal epithelial barrier. *Baillieres Clin. Gastroenterol.* **10:**393–405.

20. **Gonnella, P. A., Y. Chen, J. Inobe, Y. Komagata, M. Quartulli, and H. L. Weiner.** 1998. In situ immune response in gut-associated lymphoid tissue (GALT) following oral antigen in TCR-transgenic mice. *J. Immunol.* **160:**4708–4718.

21. **Groh, V., S. Bahram, S. Bauer, A. Herman, M. Beauchamp, and T. Spies.** 1996. Cell stress-regulated human major histocompatibility complex class I gene expressed in gastrointestinal epithelium. *Proc. Natl. Acad. Sci. USA* **93:**12445–12450.

22. **Groux, H., A. O'Garra, M. Bigler, M. Rouleau, S. Antonenko, J. E. de Vries, and M. G. Roncarolo.** 1997. A CD4$^+$ T-cell subset inhibits antigen-specific T-cell responses and prevents colitis. *Nature* **389:**737–742.

23. **Groux, H., and F. Powrie.** 1999. Regulatory T cells and inflammatory bowel disease. *Immunol. Today* **20:**442–445.

24. **Gumperz, J. E., C. Roy, A. Makowska, D. Lum, M. Sugita, T. Podrebarac, Y. Koezuka, S. A. Porcelli, S. Cardell, M. B. Brenner, and S. M. Behar.** 2000. Murine CD1d-restricted T cell recognition of cellular lipids. *Immunity* **12:**211–221.

25. **Hanninen, A., N. R. Martinez, G. M. Davey, W. R. Heath, and L. C. Harrison.** 2002. Transient blockade of CD40 ligand dissociates pathogenic from protective mucosal immunity. *J. Clin. Invest.* **109:**261–267.

26. **Hashimoto, Y., and T. Komuro.** 1988. Close relationships between the cells of the immune system and the epithelial cells in the rat small intestine. *Cell Tissue Res.* **254:**41–47.

27. **Hayday, A., E. Theodoridis, E. Ramsburg, and J. Shires.** 2001. Intraepithelial lymphocytes: exploring the Third Way in immunology. *Nat. Immunol.* **2:**997–1003.

28. **Hermiston, M. L., and J. I. Gordon.** 1995. In vivo analysis of cadherin function in the mouse intestinal epithelium: essential roles in adhesion, maintenance of differentiation, and regulation of programmed cell death. *J. Cell Biol.* **129:**489–506.

29. **Hershberg, R. M., D. H. Cho, A. Youakim, M. B. Bradley, J. S. Lee, P. E. Framson, and G. T. Nepom.** 1998. Highly polarized HLA class II antigen processing and presentation by human intestinal epithelial cells. *J. Clin. Invest.* **102:**792–803.

30. **Hershberg, R. M., P. E. Framson, D. H. Cho, L. Y. Lee, S. Kovats, J. Beitz, J. S. Blum, and G. T. Nepom.** 1997. Intestinal epithelial cells use two distinct pathways for HLA class II antigen processing. *J. Clin. Invest.* **100:** 204–215.

31. **Hirata, I., L. L. Austin, W. H. Blackwell, J. R. Weber, and W. O. Dobbins III.** 1986. Immunoelectron microscopic localization of HLA-DR antigen in control small intestine and

colon and in inflammatory bowel disease. *Dig. Dis. Sci.* **31:**1317–1330.

32. **Huang, G. T., L. Eckmann, T. C. Savidge, and M. F. Kagnoff.** 1996. Infection of human intestinal epithelial cells with invasive bacteria upregulates apical intercellular adhesion molecule-1 (ICAM-1) expression and neutrophil adhesion. *J. Clin. Invest.* **98:**572–583.

33. **Ina, K., J. Itoh, K. Fukushima, K. Kusugami, T. Yamaguchi, K. Kyokane, A. Imada, D. G. Binion, A. Musso, G. A. West, G. M. Dobrea, T. S. McCormick, E. G. Lapetina, A. D. Levine, C. A. Ottaway, and C. Fiocchi.** 1999. Resistance of Crohn's disease T cells to multiple apoptotic signals is associated with a Bcl-2/Bax mucosal imbalance. *J. Immunol.* **163:**1081–1090.

34. **Israel, E. J., S. Taylor, Z. Wu, E. Mizoguchi, R. S. Blumberg, A. Bahn, and N. E. Sinister.** 1997. Expression of the neonatal Fc receptor, FcRn, on human intestinal epithelial cells. *Immunology* **92:**69–74.

35. **Itoh, J., M. C. de La, S. A. Strong, A. D. Levine, and C. Fiocchi.** 2001. Decreased Bax expression by mucosal T cells favours resistance to apoptosis in Crohn's disease. *Gut* **49:**35–41.

36. **Iwasaki, A., and B. L. Kelsall.** 1999. Freshly isolated Peyer's patch, but not spleen, dendritic cells produce interleukin 10 and induce the differentiation of T helper type 2 cells. *J. Exp. Med.* **190:**229–239.

37. **Izadpanah, A., M. B. Dwinell, L. Eckmann, N. M. Varki, and M. F. Kagnoff.** 2001. Regulated MIP-3alpha/CCL20 production by human intestinal epithelium: mechanism for modulating mucosal immunity. *Am. J. Physiol. Gastrointest. Liver Physiol.* **280:**G710–G719.

38. **Kawabe, T., T. Naka, K. Yoshida, T. Tanaka, H. Fujiwara, S. Suematsu, N. Yoshida, T. Kishimoto, and H. Kikutani.** 1994. The immune responses in CD40-deficient mice: impaired immunoglobulin class switching and germinal center formation. *Immunity* **1:**167–178.

39. **Kawano, T., J. Cui, Y. Koezuka, I. Toura, Y. Kaneko, K. Motoki, H. Ueno, R. Nakagawa, H. Sato, E. Kondo, H. Koseki, and M. Taniguchi.** 1997. CD1d-restricted and TCR-mediated activation of valpha14 NKT cells by glycosylceramides. *Science* **278:**1626–1629.

40. **Kjerrulf, M., D. Grdic, L. Ekman, K. Schon, M. Vajdy, and N. Y. Lycke.** 1997. Interferon-gamma receptor-deficient mice exhibit impaired gut mucosal immune responses but intact oral tolerance. *Immunology* **92:**60–68.

41. **Kunkel, E. J., J. J. Campbell, G. Haraldsen, J. Pan, J. Boisvert, A. I. Roberts, E. C. Ebert, M. A. Vierra, S. B. Goodman, M. C.** Genovese, A. J. Wardlaw, H. B. Greenberg, C. M. Parker, E. C. Butcher, D. P. Andrew, and W. W. Agace. 2000. Lymphocyte CC chemokine receptor 9 and epithelial thymus-expressed chemokine (TECK) expression distinguish the small intestinal immune compartment: epithelial expression of tissue-specific chemokines as an organizing principle in regional immunity. *J. Exp. Med.* **192:**761–768.

42. **Kweon, M. N., K. Fujihashi, Y. Wakatsuki, T. Koga, M. Yamamoto, J. R. McGhee, and H. Kiyono.** 1999. Mucosally induced systemic T cell unresponsiveness to ovalbumin requires CD40 ligand-CD40 interactions. *J. Immunol.* **162:**1904–1909.

43. **Kweon, M. N., and H. Kiyono.** 2002. CD40L in autoimmunity and mucosally induced tolerance. *J. Clin. Invest.* **109:**171–173.

44. **Lee, H. O., S. D. Miller, S. D. Hurst, L. J. Tan, C. J. Cooper, and T. A. Barrett.** 2000. Interferon gamma induction during oral tolerance reduces T-cell migration to sites of inflammation. *Gastroenterology* **119:**129–138.

45. **Madara, J. L.** 1998. Regulation of the movement of solutes across tight junctions. *Annu. Rev. Physiol.* **60:**143–159.

46. **Madrigal-Estebas, L., R. McManus, B. Byrne, S. Lynch, D. G. Doherty, D. Kelleher, D. P. O'Donoghue, C. Feighery, and C. O'Farrelly.** 1997. Human small intestinal epithelial cells secrete interleukin-7 and differentially express two different interleukin-7 mRNA transcripts: implications for extrathymic T-cell differentiation. *Hum. Immunol.* **58:**83–90.

47. **Marth, T., W. Strober, and B. L. Kelsall.** 1996. High dose oral tolerance in ovalbumin TCR-transgenic mice: systemic neutralization of IL-12 augments TGF-beta secretion and T cell apoptosis. *J. Immunol.* **157:**2348–2357.

48. **Mayer, L., D. Eisenhardt, P. Salomon, W. Bauer, R. Plous, and L. Piccinini.** 1991. Expression of class II molecules on intestinal epithelial cells in humans. Differences between normal and inflammatory bowel disease. *Gastroenterology* **100:**3–12.

49. **Mayer, L., and R. Shlien.** 1987. Evidence for function of Ia molecules on gut epithelial cells in man. *J. Exp. Med.* **166:**1471–1483.

50. **Mowat, A. M., M. Steel, A. J. Leishman, and P. Garside.** 1999. Normal induction of oral tolerance in the absence of a functional IL-12-dependent IFN-gamma signaling pathway. *J. Immunol.* **163:**4728–4736.

51. **Murch, S. H., C. P. Braegger, J. A. Walker-Smith, and T. T. MacDonald.** 1993. Location of tumour necrosis factor alpha by immunohis-

tochemistry in chronic inflammatory bowel disease. *Gut* **34:**1705–1709.

52. **Nakazawa, A., M. Watanabe, T. Kanai, T. Yajima, M. Yamazaki, H. Ogata, H. Ishii, M. Azuma, and T. Hibi.** 1999. Functional expression of costimulatory molecule CD86 on epithelial cells in the inflamed colonic mucosa. *Gastroenterology* **117:**536–545.

53. **Neutra, M. R., N. J. Mantis, and J. P. Kraehenbuhl.** 2001. Collaboration of epithelial cells with organized mucosal lymphoid tissues. *Nat. Immunol.* **2:**1004–1009.

54. **Panja, A., E. Siden, and L. Mayer.** 1995. Synthesis and regulation of accessory/proinflammatory cytokines by intestinal epithelial cells. *Clin. Exp. Immunol.* **100:**298–305.

55. **Ranheim, E. A., and T. J. Kipps.** 1993. Activated T cells induce expression of B7/BB1 on normal or leukemic B cells through a CD40-dependent signal. *J. Exp. Med.* **177:**925–935.

56. **Read, S., V. Malmstrom, and F. Powrie.** 2000. Cytotoxic T lymphocyte-associated antigen 4 plays an essential role in the function of CD25(+)CD4(+) regulatory cells that control intestinal inflammation. *J. Exp. Med.* **192:**295–302.

57. **Reinecker, H. C., R. P. MacDermott, S. Mirau, A. Dignass, and D. K. Podolsky.** 1996. Intestinal epithelial cells both express and respond to interleukin 15. *Gastroenterology* **111:**1706–1713.

58. **Reinecker, H. C., and D. K. Podolsky.** 1995. Human intestinal epithelial cells express functional cytokine receptors sharing the common gamma c chain of the interleukin 2 receptor. *Proc. Natl. Acad. Sci. USA* **92:**8353–8357.

59. **Reinecker, H. C., M. Steffen, T. Witthoeft, I. Pflueger, S. Schreiber, R. P. MacDermott, and A. Raedler.** 1993. Enhanced secretion of tumour necrosis factor-alpha, IL-6, and IL-1 beta by isolated lamina propria mononuclear cells from patients with ulcerative colitis and Crohn's disease. *Clin. Exp. Immunol.* **94:**174–181.

60. **Rescigno, M., M. Urbano, B. Valzasina, M. Francolini, G. Rotta, R. Bonasio, F. Granucci, J. P. Kraehenbuhl, and P. Ricciardi-Castagnoli.** 2001. Dendritic cells express tight junction proteins and penetrate gut epithelial monolayers to sample bacteria. *Nat. Immunol.* **2:**361–367.

61. **Roncarolo, M. G., R. Bacchetta, C. Bordignon, S. Narula, and M. K. Levings.** 2001. Type 1 T regulatory cells. *Immunol. Rev.* **182:**68–79.

62. **Sakaguchi, S., N. Sakaguchi, M. Asano, M. Itoh, and M. Toda.** 1995. Immunologic self-tolerance maintained by activated T cells expressing IL-2 receptor alpha-chains (CD25). Breakdown of a single mechanism of self-tolerance causes various autoimmune diseases. *J. Immunol.* **155:**1151–1164.

63. **Samoilova, E. B., J. L. Horton, H. Zhang, S. J. Khoury, H. L. Weiner, and Y. Chen.** 1998. CTLA-4 is required for the induction of high dose oral tolerance. *Int. Immunol.* **10:**491–498.

64. **Schneeberger, E. E., and R. D. Lynch.** 1992. Structure, function, and regulation of cellular tight junctions. *Am. J. Physiol.* **262:**L647–L661.

65. **Schreiber, S., S. Nikolaus, J. Hampe, J. Hamling, I. Koop, B. Groessner, H. Lochs, and A. Raedler.** 1999. Tumour necrosis factor alpha and interleukin 1beta in relapse of Crohn's disease. *Lancet* **353:**459–461.

66. **Shibahara, T., J. N. Wilcox, T. Couse, and J. L. Madara.** 2001. Characterization of epithelial chemoattractants for human intestinal intraepithelial lymphocytes. *Gastroenterology* **120:**60–70.

67. **Singh, B., S. Read, C. Asseman, V. Malmstrom, C. Mottet, L. A. Stephens, R. Stepankova, H. Tlaskalova, and F. Powrie.** 2001. Control of intestinal inflammation by regulatory T cells. *Immunol. Rev.* **182:**190–200.

68. **Somnay-Wadgaonkar, K., A. Nusrat, H. S. Kim, W. P. Canchis, S. P. Balk, S. P. Colgan, and R. S. Blumberg.** 1999. Immunolocalization of CD1d in human intestinal epithelial cells and identification of a beta2-microglobulin-associated form. *Int. Immunol.* **11:**383–392.

69. **Spada, F. M., Y. Koezuka, and S. A. Porcelli.** 1998. CD1d-restricted recognition of synthetic glycolipid antigens by human natural killer T cells. *J. Exp. Med.* **188:**1529–1534.

70. **Spahn, T. W., A. Fontana, A. M. Faria, A. J. Slavin, H. P. Eugster, X. Zhang, P. A. Koni, N. H. Ruddle, R. A. Flavell, P. D. Rennert, and H. L. Weiner.** 2001. Induction of oral tolerance to cellular immune responses in the absence of Peyer's patches. *Eur. J. Immunol.* **31:**1278–1287.

71. **Strober, W., B. Kelsall, I. Fuss, T. Marth, B. Ludviksson, R. Ehrhardt, and M. Neurath.** 1997. Reciprocal IFN-gamma and TGF-beta responses regulate the occurrence of mucosal inflammation. *Immunol. Today* **18:**61–64.

72. **Suri-Payer, E., A. Z. Amar, A. M. Thornton, and E. M. Shevach.** 1998. CD4+CD25+ T cells inhibit both the induction and effector function of autoreactive T cells and represent a unique lineage of immunoregulatory cells. *J. Immunol.* **160:**1212–1218.

73. **Takahashi, T., Y. Kuniyasu, M. Toda, N. Sakaguchi, M. Itoh, M. Iwata, J. Shimizu,**

and S. Sakaguchi. 1998. Immunologic self-tolerance maintained by CD25$^+$CD4$^+$ naturally anergic and suppressive T cells: induction of autoimmune disease by breaking their anergic/suppressive state. *Int. Immunol.* **10**:1969–1980.

74. Targan, S. R., R. L. Deem, M. Liu, S. Wang, and A. Nel. 1995. Definition of a lamina propria T cell responsive state. Enhanced cytokine responsiveness of T cells stimulated through the CD2 pathway. *J. Immunol.* **154**:664–675.

75. van Niel, G., G. Raposo, C. Candalh, M. Boussac, R. Hershberg, N. Cerf-Bensussan, and M. Heyman. 2001. Intestinal epithelial cells secrete exosome-like vesicles. *Gastroenterology* **121**:337–349.

76. Viney, J. L., A. M. Mowat, J. M. O'Malley, E. Williamson, and N. A. Fanger. 1998. Expanding dendritic cells in vivo enhances the induction of oral tolerance. *J. Immunol.* **160**:5815–5825.

77. Weiner, H. L. 1997. Oral tolerance: immune mechanisms and treatment of autoimmune diseases. *Immunol. Today* **18**:335–343.

78. Weiner, H. L. 2001. Oral tolerance: immune mechanisms and the generation of Th3-type TGF-beta-secreting regulatory cells. *Microbes Infect.* **3**:947–954.

79. Witmer-Pack, M. D., W. J. Swiggard, A. Mirza, K. Inaba, and R. M. Steinman. 1995. Tissue distribution of the DEC-205 protein that is detected by the monoclonal antibody NLDC-145. II. Expression in situ in lymphoid and nonlymphoid tissues. *Cell Immunol.* **163**:157–162.

80. Yio, X. Y., and L. Mayer. 1997. Characterization of a 180-kDa intestinal epithelial cell membrane glycoprotein, gp180. A candidate molecule mediating t cell-epithelial cell interactions. *J. Biol. Chem.* **272**:12786–12792.

81. Zabel, B. A., W. W. Agace, J. J. Campbell, H. M. Heath, D. Parent, A. I. Roberts, E. C. Ebert, N. Kassam, S. Qin, M. Zovko, G. J. LaRosa, L. L. Yang, D. Soler, E. C. Butcher, P. D. Ponath, C. M. Parker, and D. P. Andrew. 1999. Human G protein-coupled receptor GPR-9-6/CC chemokine receptor 9 is selectively expressed on intestinal homing T lymphocytes, mucosal lymphocytes, and thymocytes and is required for thymus-expressed chemokine-mediated chemotaxis. *J. Exp. Med.* **190**:1241–1256.

82. Zhang, W., and Y. C. Kong. 1998. Noninvolvement of IL-4 and IL-10 in tolerance induction to experimental autoimmune thyroiditis. *Cell Immunol.* **187**:95–102.

CYTOKINES AND EPITHELIAL FUNCTION

Sean P. Colgan, Glenn T. Furuta, and Cormac T. Taylor

4

BACKGROUND

Epithelial cells that line many organs are uniquely positioned to serve as a direct line of communication between the immune system and the external environment. In their normal state, mucosal surfaces of the alimentary tract are exposed on the lumenal surface to high concentrations of foreign antigens, while at the same time, they are intimately associated with the immune system via subepithelial lymphoid tissue (5). Consequently, the epithelium forms an important barrier, preventing the free mixing of lumenal antigenic material with the lamina propria, which houses the mucosal immune system (40, 64). This latter capability is attributable to intercellular tight junctions, present as gaskets which circumferentially join epithelial cells at their apices. Tight junctions regulate the passive permeation of hydrophilic solutes through the "paracellular" space. Tight junctions are dynamic structures, the permeability of which is a highly regulated process (65). A second important function of the epithelium is the maintenance of mucosal hydration (89). A coordinated series of signaling events to epithelial stimuli (secretagogues) result in the activation of membrane ion channels and transporters (90). Depending on the net effect of such events (absorption or secretion of ions), an epithelial osmotic gradient is established and provides the driving force for paracellular water transport (4). Like many aspects of cell biology and immunology, this view has changed dramatically in the past decade. The epithelium is now viewed as an active player in normal homeostatic mechanisms of mucosal immunity, and in some instances, the epithelium may orchestrate mucosal responses in a variety of diseases.

The observation that epithelial cells express and respond to cytokines has contributed significantly to the burgeoning area of mucosal immunology (74). In the past, it was broadly accepted that mucosal immunity differed from other classical immune responses, and that the difference likely rested on the ability of mucosal tissues to separate and distinguish themselves from the outside world. The observations that epithelial cells respond to and provide an available reservoir of cyto-

Sean P. Colgan, Center for Experimental Therapeutics, Brigham and Women's Hospital and Harvard Medical School, Boston, MA 02115. *Glenn T. Furuta*, Combined Program in Pediatric Gastroenterology and Nutrition, Children's Hospital, Harvard Medical School, Boston, MA 02114. *Cormac T. Taylor*, Department of Medicine and Therapeutics, The Conway Institute, University College, Dublin, Ireland.

Microbial Pathogenesis and the Intestinal Epithelial Cell, ed. by G. Hecht
© 2003 ASM Press, Washington, D.C.

kines, chemokines, and growth factors have ushered in a new view of the epithelium as a functionally dynamic cell population. Here, we will review the recent literature with regard to epithelial cytokine responses, with particular emphasis on functional consequences. With some unavoidable exceptions, we will keep the discussion primarily to cytokines, since other chapters in this book will review the role of epithelial cells in chemokine and growth factor liberation and function.

INTESTINAL EPITHELIAL CYTOKINE RECEPTORS

The microenvironment surrounding intestinal epithelial cells is particularly enriched with cytokine-liberating cell types. In close proximity, and even juxtaposed against the basolateral epithelial membrane, are intraepithelial lymphocytes, dendritic cells, and resident eosinophils. During disease states, the number and composition of these cells can dramatically change, providing a new array of signals to which epithelial cells must adapt. As such, in both health and disease, cytokines can be delivered directly to the epithelial plasma membrane. Important in this regard, the cytokine receptors studied to date are expressed in a polarized fashion. Almost without exception, cytokine receptors are expressed on the basolateral surface, in close physiologic proximity to cytokine sources.

One of the first cytokines studied with regard to paracrine activation of intestinal epithelia was gamma interferon (IFN-γ) (67). This was particularly interesting given that IFN-γ production is readily detectable in the mucosa, and the mucosa is one of the more enriched sources of IFN-γ (91). During numerous disease states, the number of lymphocytes increases (55), and upon antigenic challenge of mucosal T-lymphocytes, the IFN-γ signal is markedly enhanced in the mucosa (91). The biological effects of IFN-γ are pleiotropic and have been most extensively studied in its role as a modulator of the immune system (117). IFN-γ-elicited immunomodulation may extend to cell types not

classically associated with the immune system. For example, this lymphokine elicits major histocompatibility complex (MHC) class II molecule expression on both endothelial (27, 117) and epithelial cells (17, 72, 104), and, as a result, these cells may become endowed with the ability to present antigen (17, 73). Moreover, recent studies have suggested that IFN-γ may influence basic physiological functions of such nonimmune cells as epithelial cells (49, 67), fibroblasts (117), and keratinocytes (117).

Since these initial studies with IFN-γ, functional receptors for a wide variety of cytokines (as well as those for growth factors and chemokines, discussed in more detail within this book) have been described. Included among the epithelial cytokine receptors are interleukin-1 (IL-1), IL-2, IL-4, IL-6, IL-7, IL-9, IL-10, IL-11, IL-13, and tumor necrosis factor alpha (TNF-α) (74, 108). The expression of these receptors can also be regulated. For example, endotoxin and IFN-γ have been shown to regulate the IL-1 and IL-6R (81), IFN-γ induces TNF-αR II (114), and bacterial invasion appears to modulate the IL-7R (121). Some redundancy also exists among the expression and function of these cytokine receptors. For instance, functional IL-2 receptors are expressed on epithelia (18, 92). Signaling by IL-2 requires the dimerization of the IL-2 receptor beta chain and a common gamma chain, the latter of which is also a component of the receptor for IL-4, IL-7, and IL-9 (29). Similarly, the IL-4 and IL-13 receptors share common structures, in that the IL-4 alpha chain is critical for IL-13 signaling (127) (also see below). Although such studies largely analyze single cytokine-elicited modulations on cell surfaces/secreted proteins, in aggregate, these results suggest a more global phenotypic switch from cells expressing classic epithelial function (e.g., barrier, ion transport) to those with significant immune function (regulated MHC function, chemokine and cytokine balance, coordination of leukocyte trafficking) (24).

PARACRINE ACTIVATION PATHWAYS

In any discussion of paracrine activation pathways, it is important to define the architectural playing field. The intestinal mucosa is a particularly complicated tissue in this regard. The complex nature of the intact intestinal mucosa (many cell types including epithelia, endothelia, smooth muscle, nerves, etc.), as well as those cells which traffic through the intestinal mucosa (monocytes, dendritic cells, lymphocytes, eosinophils, and neutrophils), is organized in a three-dimensional fashion and contributes to the dynamic nature of these tissues. Each individual cell type can be a source of cytokine, and each expresses its own array of cytokine responses. An additional aspect of this problem has been the need for primary cultures of native epithelial cells. Indeed, until recently, problems of the complex architecture and issues of cell separation have prohibited addressing specific and focused questions regarding single cells/single cell populations. To circumvent this complexity of the intact mucosa, the majority of studies have relied on cultured epithelial cell lines, a number of which form polarized cell monolayers with high barrier and ion transport properties that recapitulate native epithelia in both structure and function. Here, we will discuss the direct consequences of cytokines on aspects of epithelial function.

Epithelial Barrier Function

The loss of epithelial barrier function, with concomitant increases in paracellular permeability, has been reported in a number of enteropathies, including the inflammatory bowel diseases (IBD), Crohn's disease, and ulcerative colitis (75). Debates still occur as to whether decreased barrier function is associated with the etiology of IBD or, rather, as a potentiating factor of ongoing disease (48, 75). Nonetheless, of particular interest is the observation that epithelial barrier function is markedly attenuated upon exposure to IFN-γ in vitro (67). A number of elegant studies have addressed the molecular details of this response.

For instance, Mankertz et. al. (70) demonstrated that TNF-α and IFN-γ independently and synergistically downregulate transcription of occludin, one of the transmembrane "sealing" proteins localized to the tight junction (36). This transcriptional response mapped within the occludin promoter to a ~200-bp fragment upstream from the transcription start site, an area rich in binding sites for the transcription factors AP2 and NFIL6. In addition to these studies, it has been reported that IFN-γ downregulates other tight junction proteins such as ZO-1 (123), and recent studies indicate that TNF-α and IFN-γ synergistically alter the overall expression of tight junctions (98). Other cytokines also influence intestinal epithelial barrier function. For example, both IL-4 and IL-13 attenuate barrier function in vitro (126), and compelling evidence exists that IL-4 significantly enhances transepithelial transport of lumenal antigens in vivo (8, 124).

Epithelial Ion Transport

A number of cytokines have also been shown to influence epithelial electrogenic chloride secretion, the transport event responsible for mucosal hydration (89). This aspect of epithelial function has been studied in detail using IFN-γ (7, 24, 94, 111). Epithelial exposure to IFN-γ elicits a marked attenuation in stimulated Cl$^-$ secretion, as measured by generation of short circuit current (Isc). Importantly, the observed downregulation of Cl$^-$ secretion is not simply a reflection of altered barrier function of IFN-γ-treated monolayers. The IFN-γ-mediated attenuation of Cl$^-$ secretion was demonstrated at times that predated any alteration in barrier function, and even after 48-h exposure times, transepithelial resistance was substantial (>500 ohm·cm^2), though less than that of controls. The global nature of IFN-γ-mediated downregulation of Cl$^-$ secretion is further highlighted by the fact that agonists acting through differing signaling pathways and exerting primary effects at differing membrane channels (Ca^{2+}, receptor-mediated and non-receptor-mediated cyclic AMP [cAMP] pathways) were all markedly downregulated. The influence of IFN-γ on chloride secretion was documented using rate constant measurements of uptake/efflux experiments that delineate the specific transport proteins involved independent of monolayer confluency. Interestingly, these later studies demonstrated that functionally defined surface expression of all transporters, pumps, and channels contributing to Cl⁻ secretion were downregulated by IFN-γ. These include an apical Cl⁻ channel, basolateral K⁺ channels, Na-K-2Cl cotransporters, and Na-K-ATPase. These studies also demonstrate that surface expression of the Na-K-2Cl⁻ cotransporter is downregulated as shown by ^{3}H-bumetanide binding. Downregulation of the ubiquitous Na-K-ATPase activity is consistent with the notion of less ATPase activity being required in cells that do not vectorially transport ions in an Na⁺-dependent fashion, but rather chiefly require this pump for maintenance of homeostasis. Extensions of these studies revealed that IL-4 and IFN-γ posttranscriptionally downregulate expression of the cystic fibrosis transmembrane regulator (CFTR) in intestinal cell lines (7, 126) and a recent hypothesis suggests that a primary mechanism of IFN-γ-mediated activity in vitro and in vivo may be mediated by decreased Na⁺ absorption via diminished expression of Na⁺/H⁺ exchangers NHE2 and NHE3 (94, 111). Interestingly, it was recently found that postcolitis epithelial responses may be selectively impaired. Indeed, using a rat model of colitis, Asfaha et al. demonstrated that at 6 weeks after colitis induction, barrier function defects had resolved but colonic secretory dysfunction persisted (1). These findings paralleled increased bacterial translocation and increased colonic aerobes, suggesting that prolonged secretory impairment may underlie the chronic nature of enteropathies such as IBD.

An interesting exception with regard to cytokine influences on ion transport is that of IL-4 and IL-13. While these cytokines share common receptor subunits and in most cases display overlapping functions (e.g., attenuation of barrier function) (126), only IL-4

appears to influence electrogenic chloride secretion (126). This finding was one of the first divergent functions ascribed to these apparently redundant cytokines, although recent studies suggest no differences between IL-4 and IL-13 with regard to proximal receptor activation (16). Nonetheless, a number of discernible differences between IL-4 and IL-13 have now been documented (12). These differences lie in activity associated with two novel proteins, termed IL-13R alpha 1 and 2 (37, 76), recently cloned and demonstrated as important in IL-13R signaling, suggesting that IL-13 signaling may be more complicated than first appreciated. More work is required to definitively define the relative role of IL-13 and IL-4 in epithelial responses.

Antigen Processing and Presentation

The overwhelming majority of antigen encounters occur at mucosal surfaces, particularly those associated with the intestine. Moreover, this surface is constitutively bathed in a heterogeneous population of microorganisms made up of the so-called autochthonous flora. Receptor- and non-receptor-mediated processes of antigen uptake have the capability of delivering macromolecules into endosomal compartments in association with MHC class II antigen presentation. MHC class II is constitutively expressed by villous epithelial cells of the small intestine of rodents and humans and upregulated by inflammation, presumably in response to cytokines such as IFN-γ. Upon exposure to IFN-γ in vitro, MHC class II is distributed predominantly on the basolateral surface consistent with a presentation function to CD4⁺ intraepithelial and lamina propria lymphocytes (43). Although little is known of the MHC class II-associated antigen processing machinery in intestinal epithelial cells (IEC), it is clear that IEC may express invariant chain, cathepsins, and process soluble antigens for presentation to T cells (45). In modeling MHC class II function, Hershberg et al. provided strong evidence for epithelial uptake of soluble antigen, either apically or basolaterally, and presentation from the basolateral surface (44). Interestingly, in this system, antigen presentation was more efficient as a consequence of receptor-mediated uptake when antigen was coupled to the cholera toxin B subunit, which targets uptake by granulocyte macrophage-1 (GM-1) gangliosides. Since IEC take up antigen poorly, receptor-mediated uptake may be of major importance to such a process. In addition, basal processing, which models antigen delivered paracellularly, revealed T-cell responses to neoepitopes not observed when processing proceeded from the apical surface. Taken together, these studies suggest that antigen uptake under noninflammatory (antigen uptake apical) and inflammatory (antigen uptake basal) conditions may have different outcomes. The consequences of MHC class II presentation are, however, unclear. Some evidence exists in support of MHC class II function in vivo (45), and recent work suggests that the costimulatory molecule CD58, but not CD80 or CD86, was observed to be expressed constitutively on both native epithelia and in T84 and HT-29 cell lines (35). Surface expression of CD58 was polarized to the basolateral surface of the cell, and antibodies directed against CD58, but not CD80 or CD86, inhibited the stimulation of $CD4^+$ T-cell proliferation mediated by epithelia.

In addition to MHC class I and II antigens, intestinal epithelia constitutively express the nonclassical MHC molecule CD1d, a transmembrane molecule with a short cytoplasmic tail expressed as a β_2-microglobulin-associated 48-kD glycoprotein and novel β_2-microglobulin-independent 37-kDa nonglycosylated protein on intestinal epithelia (2). Like MHC class I and II, epithelial CD1d is induced by IFN-γ (22). Moreover, this response appears to be specific for IFN-γ, since exogenous administration of IL-2, IL-4, IL-5, IL-6, TNF-α, or granulocyte and monocyte colony-stimulating factor (GM-CSF) resulted in no observable change in CD1-d expression (22). Recently, mouse CD1 and human CD1d have been shown to present a model glycolipid antigen α-galactosyl-ceramide (α-GalCer) to a specialized subset of T cells (NK-T cells) that expresses both the T-cell receptor (TCR)/CD3 complex and CD161 (32). NK-T cells use an invariant TCR-α chain paired with a limited set of TCR-β chains. In mice, this semi-invariant TCR is composed of Vα14-Jα281 paired predominantly with Vβ8.2, while in humans, a homologous TCR is found that is composed of Vα24-JαQ paired with Vβ11 (32). NK-T cells appear to play an important role in regulating immune responses through their rapid production of large amounts of IL-4 and IFN-γ upon stimulation. As such, CD1d–NK-T-cell cross talk in the intestinal mucosa may significantly impact epithelial function, such as barrier.

Cytokines and PMN Trafficking

Neutrophils. Neutrophil (polymorphonuclear leukocyte, PMN) accumulation on the lumenal side of intestinal epithelia, termed the crypt abscess, is one of the pathological hallmarks of inflammatory intestinal disease (122). PMN migration into and across intestinal epithelia is a result of an orchestrated series of steps (52). In the late 1960s, it was observed that mice colonized with pathogenic bacterial strains resulted in the large-scale accumulation of PMN at the epithelial surface (112). Such morphologic observations lead to a burgeoning area of research into defining mechanism(s) of bacterial-epithelial-PMN interactions (87). While related studies are too numerous to review here, a few of those highlighted provide important insight into basic mechanisms of inflammation. First, it is clear that pathogenic bacteria have evolved complex mechanisms to use host machinery to successfully invade and colonize the epithelium. The interaction of *Shigella* spp. with epithelial cells, for example, includes interactions of bacteria with the epithelial cell surface and release of Ipa proteins through a specialized type III secretion system. A complex signaling process involving activation of small GTPases of the Rho family and c-src results in dramatic rearrangements of the subcortical cytoskeleton. Actin-mediated motility promotes efficient colonization of the host cell cytoplasm and rapid cell-to-cell dissemination through protrusions that are engulfed by adjacent cells in a cadherin-dependent process (96). Recent work suggests that blockade of *Shigella* interaction with the cytoskelton using the polyamine cadaverine severely abrogates epithelial signaling to PMN (33). Second, successful bacterial invasion transforms infected cells into strongly proinflammatory cells, not the least of which includes the liberation of numerous factors for recruitment of large numbers of PMN to the epithelial surface. These factors include chemokines, cytokines, cell adhesion molecules, and lipid mediators (56), and some evidence indicates that PMN themselves may directly promote cytokine and chemokine induction in intestinal epithelia in vivo (106). Third, some pathogenic bacterial strains have developed mechanisms to defend against host inflammatory elements. For example, studies addressing oral epithelial-PMN interactions have indicated that active bacterial infection (e.g., *Porphyromonas gingivalis*) may "paralyze" chemokine generation (28), and it has been proposed that this aspect may serve as a pathogenic mechanism for such oral pathogens (28).

The molecular details of PMN-epithelial interactions have evolved over the past decade. It is now appreciated that adhesion-based interactions, involving specific cell adhesion epitopes, are the primary means by which PMN interact with epithelial cells (82). For example, initial adhesion events between PMN and epithelia are dependent on PMN β_2 integrins (23, 83, 86). These integrins, like others, are heterodimeric glycoproteins that exist in four forms on the PMN. Each displays a unique α-subunit (CD11a, b, c, or d) and an identical β-subunit (CD18) (105, 118). The epithelial counter-receptor for PMN β_2 integrins remains elusive, and functional mapping studies of this β_2 integrin-dependent pathway have suggested that the profile of inhibition is distinct from that of other known ligands of CD11b/CD18 (3). Such data suggest novel pathways for PMN trafficking

across the epithelium, and discovery of such pathways provides a potential therapeutic target.

A number of studies have demonstrated that intercellular adhesion molecule-1 (ICAM-1), unlike endothelial cells, is not an epithelial ligand during transmigration (20, 23, 68, 84, 86), although under some conditions, ICAM-1 may function as an apical anchor for PMN (84). Indeed, studies using either enteric bacterial strains or IFN-γ as activating stimuli resulted in induction of ICAM-1 exclusively to the apical membrane domain (50, 84). These studies were verified in tissue sections from IBD patients (84). Studies directed at defining the influence of cytokines on PMN transepithelial migration revealed that IFN-γ significantly modulates PMN transmigration, and does so in a polarized manner (23). Both IFN-γ and IL-4 markedly downregulate transepithelial migration of PMN in the physiologic (basolateral-to-apical) direction (23, 25). This IFN-γ influence on transmigration was specifically due to cytokine-mediated events on epithelial cells and was not secondary to IFN-γ influences on epithelial tight junction permeability. Moreover, this downregulation of PMN migration in the physiologic direction was not due to the failure of PMN to move into epithelial monolayers. Indeed, IFN-γ exposure to epithelia increased the number of PMN that had moved into the paracellular space of the epithelium. Specifically, it appeared that in naturally directed migration, IFN-γ enhanced the retention time of the recruited PMN in the paracellular space below tight junctions, and did so, at least in part, by inducing a basolateral ligand on the membrane of intestinal epithelia. Later studies identified a functionally inhibitory monoclonal antibody (MAb) that blocks PMN transmigration, but not PMN adhesion, to epithelia (85). Subsequent experiments revealed that the antigen recognized by this MAb is CD47 (also termed integrin-associated protein), a previously cloned protein with homology to the immunoglobulin supergene family (13) and with multiple ligands and a number of demonstrated leukocyte functions (11). As predicted by the above-described experiments, epithelial CD47 surface expression was induced by IFN-γ (85). Thus, it would appear that CD47 is critically important to mucosal inflammation and that cytokine regulation of this process provides a potential therapeutic target.

Eosinophils. Much recent attention has been paid to understanding the role of eosinophils in gastrointestinal disease (95). Eosinophils reside in the normal intestine and accumulate during inflammatory disease (95). Some studies have been done with regard to cytokines and trafficking of eosinophils to and across the intestinal mucosa. For example, initial in vitro studies suggested that unactivated eosinophils failed to migrate across cultured epithelial monolayers (93). In contrast, activation of eosinophils GM-CSF enabled subsequent transepithelial migration in response to platelet-activating factor (PAF), but not to C5a or formyl-methionyl-leucyl-phenylalanine (FMLP) gradients. Addition of functionally inhibitory MAbs to CD11b, but not CD11a, VLA-4, or ICAM-1 inhibited PAF-driven transepithelial migration of eosinophils. Since epithelial cells release GM-CSF under modeled inflammatory conditions (54), it is possible that epithelial-derived cytokines may coordinate eosinophil function at the mucosal surface. Eotaxin, an eosinophil-selective chemokine, is constitutively expressed by intestinal epithelial cells (95). Moreover, studies with eotaxin null mice have suggested that eotaxin is critical to the maintenance of eosinophil levels in nonhematopoietic tissues, including the intestine (71). Indeed, while eosinophils were readily detectable in the mouse jejunum, eotaxin null mice showed a selective reduction in resident eosinophil numbers, indicating that mucosal-derived eotaxin maintains a homeostatic function in the intestine. In conditions of ongoing inflammation, recruitment signals for eosinophils may be enhanced. For example, both IL-4 and IFN-γ have been shown to transcriptionally induce eotaxin in intestinal epithelia (120), and recent studies with IL-5 null mice suggest that IL-5 may function primarily in recruitment, as opposed to activation, of intestinal eosinophils (109). These latter studies with IL-5 were independently confirmed in human IBD patients (58).

In murine models of gastrointestinal eosinophilia, both eotaxin and IL-5 significantly influence eosinophil trafficking. For instance, mice receiving an oral challenge of ovalbumin develop significant gastric and small intestinal eosinophilia (46, 47). This eosinophilia was dependent on eotaxin, as demonstrated with the use of eotaxin null mice. In addition, investigators recently generated enterocyte-specific transgenic mice using fatty acid binding promoter to overexpress eotaxin and IL-5 (77). While both mice demonstrated significant small intestinal eosinophilia when compared to nontransgenic controls, eotaxin transgenic mice developed significantly more intestinal eosinophilia. As such, these findings demonstrate the significant contribution of epithelial-derived eotaxin in intestinal eosinophilic inflammation.

AUTOCRINE ACTIVATION PATHWAYS
With regard to the influence of autocrine cytokine networks, it is important to consider that the surface area of the intestine covered by epithelial cells is orders of magnitude larger than that covered by T cells; thus, even with smaller amounts produced per epithelial cell, the total quantity of epithelial-derived cytokine can be quite large and physiologically important in this regard. Additionally, given the architecture of the paracellular space of the intact epithelium (long cylindrical space sealed by the tight junction), it is probable that epithelial cell-derived mediators (growth factors, cytokines, lipids) concentrate within this space, and with cytokine delivered directly to the receptor in this fashion (autocrine), the relative bioactivity for these mediators may be enhanced manyfold.

Transforming Growth Factors (TGF)
Epithelial cells have long been known to produce TGF (TGF-α and -β), and their expression is controlled in an autocrine manner

(74). Both TGF-β (antiproliferative) and TGF-α (mitogenic) regulate epithelial differentiation along the crypt-villous axis (88), but TGF may also function during wound repair and in the inflammatory response. For example, TGF-β enhances cell migration, cells migrating into "wounds" in vitro express increased amounts of TGF-β, and IL-2 has been reported to increase expression of TGF-β (6). Moreover, recent studies also indicate an interesting role for epidermal growth factor (EGF), a homolog of TGF-α, in inhibition of Ca^{2+}-mediated epithelial chloride secretion. For instance, Keely et al. reported that transactivation of the epithelial EGF receptor by the muscarinic agonist carbachol may mediate inhibitory influences on electrogenic chloride secretion (57), and as such, may provide an "off switch" for chloride secretion under some circumstances.

IL-6

One of the first recognized autocrine pathways in intestinal epithelia was that of IL-6 (108). Functionally, both IL-6 and IFN-γ downregulate sucrase isomaltase expression in small intestinal epithelia (78, 125) and induce sodium glucose transport, with resultant increased glucose uptake (42). In addition, a recent study indicated that adenosine A_{2b} receptor activation, such as occurs through PMN interactions with intestinal epithelial cells (66), results in the transcriptional induction of epithelial IL-6, which through paracrine mechanisms can modulate PMN functional responses (103). These studies included the novel observation that IL-6 release occurs predominantly through the apical (lumenal) aspect of epithelial cells.

TNF-α

Intestinal epithelial cells can produce and respond to TNF-α. Epithelial TNF-α production is transcriptionally regulated and can be induced by a diverse array of activators, including bacterial infection, tumor promoters, and hypoxia (54, 114) (see Fig. 1). Receptors for TNF-α are expressed on the basolateral surface (114), and ligation of these receptors results in increased epithelial permeability, induction of chemokine generation, and, under some circumstances, induction of apoptosis (108) (discussed elsewhere in this book).

We have studied autocrine signaling in epithelial cells with regard to hypoxia. Epithelial surfaces, including the intestine, support a rich and extensive underlying vasculature. Episodes of diminished blood flow, such as occur with ischemia, vasculitis, or chronic inflammation, can result in significant tissue hypoxia (119). It is now appreciated that epithelial cells subjected to hypoxia are rich sources of proinflammatory cytokines and chemokines that can serve as directives for phenotypic changes to the epithelium (113). In particular, we hypothesized that inflammatory cytokine signaling may be differentially regulated by hypoxia. Using a T84 cell model, our initial experiments revealed a hypoxia-elicited increase in epithelial responsiveness to IFN-γ. Such enhanced responses to IFN-γ during hypoxia were found to be conferrable in a conditioned media supernatant from hypoxic epithelia, and subsequent experiments identified this transferable factor as TNF-α (114). In separate studies addressing mechanisms of hypoxia-induced TNF-α, a novel transcriptional pathway entailing proteolytic degradation of cyclic AMP response element binding protein (CREB) was identified (115, 116). These studies identified a previously unappreciated proteasomal-targeting motif in CREB (DSVTDS), which functions as a substrate for protein phosphatase-1 gamma (PP-1γ). Ambient hypoxia resulted in temporally sequential CREB serine phosphorylation, ubiquitination, and degradation in vitro and in vivo. HIV-*tat* peptide-facilitated loading of intact epithelia with phosphopeptides corresponding to this proteasome-targeting motif resulted in inhibition of CREB ubiquitination. Further studies revealed that PP-1 inhibitors mimicked hypoxia-induced gene expression, while proteasome inhibitors reversed the hypoxic phenotype. Thus, hypoxia establishes conditions

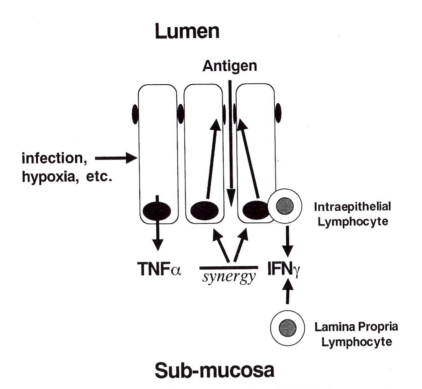

FIGURE 1 Epithelial-derived TNF-α synergizes with IFN-γ in an autocrine manner. In response to a number of stimuli, including bacterial invasion and hypoxia, epithelial cells become a source of TNF-α. The polarized release (basolateral) of TNF-α synergizes with immune-derived cytokines, especially IFN-γ, resulting in influences on a number of epithelial functions, including decreased barrier function, diminished electrogenic chloride secretion, induction of MHC molecules, and liberation of proinflammatory chemokines.

that target CREB to proteasomal degradation and result in transcriptional TNF-α induction.

IL-10

Epithelial cells are demonstrated sources of IL-10 (47, 48), and significant evidence exists that IL-10 contributes to the development of mucosal tolerance. For instance, IL-10-deficient mice develop an IBD-like condition, administration of IL-10 restores tolerance to indigenous flora in mice with IBD, and IL-10 accompanies the induction of IL-4 in animals tolerized to low-dose antigen (49). Given the further role of IL-10 in regulating important subsets of T cells dedicated to IL-10 production and downregulation of colitis, IEC responses to lumenal and/or T-cell stimuli may

directly regulate this important population of cells (45). In support of this concept, it was recently shown that glycosphingolipids induce T-cell IL-10 production and that such induction parallels findings with tyrosine-kinase dependency (50). Moreover, in vitro studies addressing CD1d function on epithelia indicated that antibody cross-linking transcriptionally induces IL-10 and, through autocrine means, may dampen proinflammatory cytokine-mediated barrier disruption (21). These studies, taken together with the proposed role of CD1d in lipid binding and processing, unveil the unique possibility that CD1d contributes significantly to the regulation of IFN-γ-mediated epithelial responses (barrier function, ion transport, MHC molecule expression, etc.) and potentially to oral tolerance directed toward lipid antigens in the intestine.

COUNTERREGULATORY PATHWAYS

Cytokine Networks

Some work has also been done with regard to counterregulatory influences of cytokine signaling in epithelia. IL-10 is particularly interesting in this regard. For instance, epithelial IFN-γ responses (specifically increased permeability) are dampened by recombinant IL-10 in cultured intestinal epithelia (69), and superantigen-elicited influences may be similarly attenuated by IL-10 (63). At present, it is not clear how IL-10 modulates IFN-γ bioactivity, but it was recently demonstrated that IL-10 specifically suppresses tyrosine phosphorylation of signal transducer and activator of transcription-1 (STAT-1), a component of the IFN-γ-induced DNA complex (51).

A number of studies have suggested that intestinal epithelial cells can modulate pre- and postreceptor events as an adaptive pathway to dampen inflammation. While epithelial cells are both a source of and responder to IL-1 (108), they express relatively high levels of IL-1 receptor antagonist (IL-1ra) (15, 107), and such expression is regulated by proinflammatory stimuli (10). The balance of mucosal IL-1 and IL-1ra has been studied in detail using animal models of colitis and in human IBD patient samples (15, 34), and the data are clear that a decrease in IL-1ra/IL-1 ratio correlates with disease severity and chronicity. Similarly, a number of interesting studies by Jobin et al. have reported that IL-1-activated IkBα degradation in freshly isolated epithelia is delayed, resulting in an overall decrease in NF-κB activation (53). A related study recently showed that some enteric organisms (e.g., nonvirulent strains of *Salmonella* spp.) may attenuate epithelial responses to prokaryotic organisms through inhibition of IkBα degradation (80), providing new insight into the unique tolerance of mucosal epithelial cells to proinflammatory signals.

Lipid Mediator Networks

Prostaglandins are derived from arachidonic acid metabolism through the action of cyclooxygenase-1 and -2 (COX-1 and -2). COX-1 is expressed in constitutive fashion in most cell types along the gastrointestinal tract (30). The expression of COX-2 is induced by proinflammatory cytokines such as IL-1 and TNF-α (39) and by invasive bacterial species (e.g., *Shigella, Salmonella*, enteroinvasive *Escherichia coli*) (31). The major product appears to be prostaglandin E$_2$ (PGE$_2$), a potent epithelial secretagogue (4). Such conditions of COX-2 activation can also result in endothelial liberation of PGI$_2$, which through nonmetabolic hydrolysis can form the stable intermediate 6-keto-PGF$_{1\alpha}$, also an epithelial secretagogue (9). COX-2 induction by invasive bacteria may not require direct bacterial-epithelial interaction, since some evidence indicates liberation of an as yet unknown paracrine factor in parallel with activation of NF-κB (31). Taken together, these studies indicate the likelihood that COX-2-derived epithelial products may mediate symptomatic diarrhea associated with both infection and inflammation.

Much recent attention has been paid to understanding the innate "dampening" mechanisms involved in inhibition of inflammation at mucosal sites. Of particular interest are a group of lipid mediators termed the lipoxins (100). Lipoxins are bioactive eicosanoids derived from membrane arachidonic acid by the combined action of 5-lipoxygenase (LO) and 12-LO or 15-LO (99). A number of recent in vitro and in vivo studies have revealed that lipoxins, and specifically lipoxin A$_4$ (LXA$_4$), function as an innate "stop signal," functioning to control local inflammatory processes (19, 26, 38, 101). The action of LXA$_4$ is mediated by a G-protein-coupled surface receptor (102). Studies using intestinal epithelial cell lines revealed that a diverse panel of proinflammatory cytokines, as well as endotoxin, transcriptionally induces the LXA$_4$ receptor (39), suggesting that lipoxins may mediate an adaptive pathway for resolution of ongoing inflammation. This conceptual paradigm was recently confirmed (60).

Very recent work indicates that LXA$_4$ may promote bacterial clearance and inhibition of endotoxin signaling by intestinal epithelial cells (14). Initial studies profiling human epithelial gene expression in response to LXA$_4$ stimulation revealed the induction of bactericidal/permeability-increasing protein (BPI), a 55- to 60-kDa protein previously associated only with neutrophils and, to a lesser extent, eosinophils (61). BPI selectively exerts multiple anti-infective actions against gram-negative bacteria, including cytotoxicity through damage to bacterial inner/outer membranes and neutralization of bacterial lipopolysaccharide (LPS) (endotoxin), as well as serves as an opsonin for phagocytosis of gram-negative bacteria by neutrophils (61). Epithelial BPI functioned to promote the killing of *Salmonella enterica* serovar Typhimurium, and to inhibit LPS signaling. In addition, analysis of normal human esophagus and colon sections revealed dominant localization of BPI to the epithelium. In the case of esophageal tissue, BPI was most strongly expressed at the transition zone between epithelia and the lamina propria, with graded decreasing expression toward surface epithelia. In the colon, BPI was expressed dominantly in crypt and villous epithelia, with less expression along the crypt-villous transition. These results contribute to the present knowledge of mucosal defense mechanisms and define a previously unappreciated expression of BPI on the surface of alimentary tract epithelia. Since infectious agents have been implicated as etiologic agents in IBD (97), and attempts to attribute individual diseases to single specific bacterial strains have failed, BPI may be an important expression marker. For example, high levels of neutrophil-associated BPI are found in the colonic mucosa of patients with ulcerative colitis (41, 79), and autoantibodies directed against BPI are proposed seromarkers for IBD (110). Moreover, BPI congeners are currently being

evaluated as novel therapies for diseases in which endotoxin is thought to play a role (59), including Crohn's disease (62). As such, these observations provide further support for the notion that BPI and other antimicrobial agents play important anti-infective roles in the gastrointestinal tract, particularly as a molecular shield to dampen the inflammatory influence of endotoxin. Regulated expression of BPI by lipid mediators such as LXA$_4$ provides additional clues to the potent nature of these anti-inflammatory agents and provides for the possible therapeutic induction of BPI in the treatment of mucosal infections.

CONCLUSIONS

In recent years, much attention has been paid to epithelial responses to cytokines and the impact of such activation pathways on the development and resolution of mucosal inflammation. In the intestine, cytokine influences on epithelial function may best be exemplified through the study of enteric infections, specifically related to acute responses following initial microorganism-epithelial interaction. In this review, we have attempted to highlight some of the consistent observations in this ever-growing area. As such, a putative model is shown in Fig. 2 to summarize the salient features of this review and to highlight the central role of cytokines in the development and resolution of inflammation. In this model, five response phases are identified, but it should be noted that these are dynamic and overlapping phases within the responses. Nonetheless, following initial microorganism interaction with the epithelium (phase 1), rapid induction and epithelial release of PMN chemokines (phase 2) elicit the recruitment of PMN to the epithelial surface and across the lumenal aspect of the epithelium. PMN at the lumenal surface initiates a Cl$^-$ secretory response and fluid transport that functionally flushes the surface of the epithelium. As part of phase 3 of this response, epithelial-derived cytokines (e.g., TNF-α) synergize with cytokines liberated in the intraepithelial and lamina

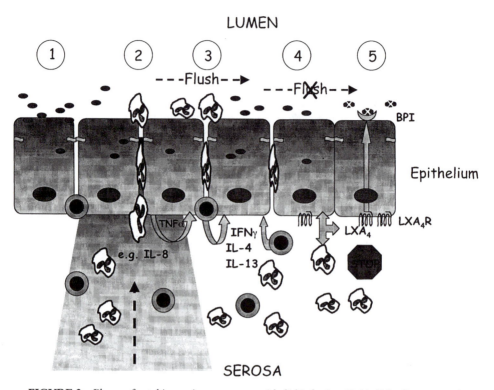

FIGURE 2 Phases of cytokine actions on acute epithelial infection. Epithelial cells are central to the coordinated response to microorganism infection (phase 1). Rapid induction and release of PMN chemokines (phase 2) elicit the accumulation of PMN within and across the epithelial surface. PMN at the lumenal surface initiates a Cl⁻ secretory response and fluid transport which functionally flushes the surface of the epithelium. In phase 3 of the response, epithelial-derived cytokines (e.g., TNF-α) synergize with cytokines liberated in the intraepithelial and lamina propria compartments (e.g., IFN-γ) to attenuate fluid transport. In phase 4, intraepithelial and lamina propria lymphocyte-derived cytokines (e.g., IFN-γ, IL-4, and IL-13) induce epithelial lipoxin receptors, the ligation of which results in attenuation of PMN accumulation. In phase 5, lipoxin-induced epithelial BPI provides a protective antimicrobial action for the resolution of acute inflammation.

propria compartments (e.g., IFN-γ) to attenuate fluid transport and prevent excessive fluid loss associated with enteric infections. Phases 4 and 5 represent the resolution phase of acute inflammation. Intraepithelial and lamina propria lymphocyte–derived cytokines (e.g., IFN-γ, IL-4, and IL-13) induce epithelial lipoxin receptors (phase 4), the ligation of which results in attenuation of PMN accumulation through downregulation of chemokine generation. In phase 5, lipoxin-induced epithelial antimicrobials (e.g., BPI) provide a protective action for the resolution of inflammation, in-

cluding both bactericidal activities and endotoxin neutralization functions.

ACKNOWLEDGMENTS

This work was supported by grants RO-1 DK50189 and PO-1 DE13499 from the National Institutes of Health.

REFERENCES

1. **Asfaha, S., W. K. MacNaughton, C. B. Appleyard, K. Chadee, and J. L. Wallace.** 2001. Persistent epithelial dysfunction and bacterial translocation after resolution of intestinal inflam-

mation. *Am. J. Physiol. Gastrointest. Liver Physiol.* **281**:G635–G644.

2. **Balk, S. P., S. Burke, J. E. Polischuk, M. E. Frantz, L. Yang, S. Porcelli, S. P. Colgan, and R. S. Blumberg.** 1994. β_2-microglobulin-independent MHC class Ib molecule expressed by human intestinal epithelium. *Science* **265**:259–262.

3. **Balsam, L. B., T. W. Liang, and C. A. Parkos.** 1998. Functional mapping of CD11b/CD18 epitopes important in neutrophil-epithelial interactions: a central role of the I domain. *J. Immunol.* **160**:5058–5065.

4. **Barrett, K. E.** 1993. Positive and negative regulation of chloride secretion in T84 cells. *Am. J. Physiol.* **265**:C859–C868.

5. **Beagley, K. W., and A. J. Husband.** 1998. Intraepithelial lymphocytes: origins, distribution, and function. *Crit. Rev. Immunol.* **18**:237–254.

6. **Beck, P. L., and D. K. Podolsky.** 1999. Growth factors in inflammatory bowel disease. *Inflamm. Bowel Dis.* **5**:44–60.

7. **Bensancon, F., G. Przewlocki, I. Baro, A.-S. Hongre, D. Escande, and A. Edelman.** 1994. Interferon-γ downregulates CFTR gene expression in epithelial cells. *Am. J. Physiol.* **267**:C1398–C1404.

8. **Berin, M. C., P.-C. Yang, L. Ciok, S. Waserman, and M. H. Perdue.** 1999. Role of IL-4 in macromolecular transport across human intestinal epithelium. *Am. J. Physiol. (Cell Physiol.)* **276**:C1046–C1052.

9. **Blume, E. D., C. T. Taylor, P. F. Lennon, G. L. Stahl, and S. P. Colgan.** 1998. Activated endothelial cells elicit paracrine induction of epithelial chloride secretion: 6-keto-PGF$_{1\alpha}$ is an epithelial secretagogue. *J. Clin. Invest.* **102**:1161–1172.

10. **Bocker, U., A. Damiao, L. Holt, D. S. Han, C. Jobin, A. Panja, L. Mayer, and R. B. Sartor.** 1998. Differential expression of interleukin 1 receptor antagonist isoforms in human intestinal epithelial cells. *Gastroenterology* **115**:1426–1438.

11. **Brown, E. J., and W. A. Frazier.** 2001. Integrin-associated protein (CD47) and its ligands. *Trends Cell Biol.* **11**:130–135.

12. **Brubaker, J. O., and L. J. Montaner.** 2001. Role of interleukin-13 in innate and adaptive immunity. *Cell Mol. Biol.* **47**:637–651.

13. **Cambell, I. G., P. S. Freemont, W. Foulkes, and J. Trowsdale.** 1992. An ovarian tumor marker with homology to vaccinia virus contains an IgV-like region and multiple transmembrane domains. *Cancer Res.* **52**:5416–5420.

14. **Canny, G., O. Levy, G. T. Furuta, S. Narravula-Alipati, R. B. Sisson, C. N. Serhan, and S. P. Colgan.** 2002. Lipid mediator-induced expression of bactericidal/permeability-increasing protein (BPI) in human mucosal epithelia. *Proc. Nat. Acad. Sci. USA* **99**:3902–3907.

15. **Casini-Raggi, V., L. Kam, Y. J. Chong, C. Fiocchi, T. T. Pizarro, and F. Cominelli.** 1995. Mucosal imbalance of IL-1 and IL-1 receptor antagonist in inflammatory bowel disease. A novel mechanism of chronic intestinal inflammation. *J. Immunol.* **154**:2434–2440.

16. **Ceponis, P. J., F. Botelho, C. D. Richards, and D. M. McKay.** 2000. Interleukins 4 and 13 increase intestinal epithelial permeability by a phosphatidylinositol 3-kinase pathway. Lack of evidence for STAT 6 involvement. *J. Biol. Chem.* **275**:29132–29137.

17. **Cerf-Bensussan, N., A. Quaroni, J. T. Kurnick, and A. K. Bahn.** 1984. Intraepithelial lymphocytes modulate Ia expression by intestinal epithelial cells. *J. Immunol.* **132**:2244–2252.

18. **Ciacci, C., Y. R. Mahida, A. Dignass, M. Koizumi, and D. K. Podolsky.** 1993. Functional IL-2 receptors on intestinal epithelial cells. *J. Clin. Invest.* **92**:527–532.

19. **Claria, J., M. H. Lee, and C. N. Serhan.** 1996. Aspirin-triggered lipoxins (15-epi-LX) are generated by the human lung adenocarcinoma cell line (A549)-neutrophil interactions and are potent inhibitors of cell proliferation. *Mol. Med.* **2**:583–596.

20. **Colgan, S. P., A. L. Dzus, and C. A. Parkos.** 1996. Epithelial exposure to hypoxia modulates neutrophil transepithelial migration. *J. Exp. Med.* **184**:1003–1015.

21. **Colgan, S. P., R. M. Hershberg, G. T. Furuta, and R. S. Blumberg.** 1999. Ligation of intestinal epithelial CD1d induces bioactive IL-10: critical role of the cytoplasmic tail in autocrine signaling. *Proc. Natl. Acad. Sci. USA* **96**:13938–13943.

22. **Colgan, S. P., V. M. Morales, J. L. Madara, S. P. Balk, and R. S. Blumberg.** 1996. IFN-γ modulates CD1d expression on intestinal epithelia. *Am. J. Physiol.* **271**:C276–C283.

23. **Colgan, S. P., C. A. Parkos, C. Delp, M. A. Arnaout, and J. L. Madara.** 1993. Neutrophil migration across cultured intestinal epithelial monolayers is modulated by epithelial exposure to interferon-gamma in a highly polarized fashion. *J. Cell Biol.* **120**:785–795.

24. **Colgan, S. P., C. A. Parkos, J. B. Matthews, L. D'Andrea, C. S. Awtrey, A. Lichtman, C. Delp, and J. L. Madara.** 1994. Interferon-γ induces a surface phenotype switch in intestinal epithelia: downregulation of ion transport and upregulation of immune accessory ligands. *Am. J. Physiol.* **267**:C402–C410.

25. Colgan, S. P., M. B. Resnick, C. A. Parkos, C. Delp-Archer, A. E. Bacarra, P. F. Weller, and J. L. Madara. 1994. Interleukin-4 directly modulates function of a model human intestinal epithelium. *J. Immunol.* **153:**2122–2129.

26. Colgan, S. P., C. N. Serhan, C. A. Parkos, C. Delp-Archer, and J. L. Madara. 1993. Lipoxin A₄ modulates transmigration of human neutrophils across intestinal epithelial monolayers. *J. Clin. Invest.* **92:**75–82.

27. Collins, T., A. J. Korman, C. T. Wake, J. M. Boss, D. J. Kappes, W. Fiers, K. A. Ault, M. A. Gimbrone, J. L. Strominger, and J. S. Pober. 1988. Immune interferon activates multiple class II major histocompatibility complex genes and the associated invariant chain gene in human endothelial cells and dermal fibroblasts. *Proc. Nat. Acad. Sci. USA* **81:**4917–4921.

28. Darveau, R. P., C. M. Belton, R. A. Reife, and R. J. Lamont. 1998. Local chemokine paralysis, a novel pathogenic mechanism for *Porphyromonas gingivalis*. *Infect. Immun.* **66:**1660–1665.

29. Demoulin, J. B., and J. C. Renauld. 1998. Signalling by cytokines interacting with the interleukin-2 receptor gamma chain. *Cytokines Cell Mol. Ther.* **4:**243–256.

30. Dubois, R. N., S. B. Abramson, L. Crofford, R. A. Gupta, L. S. Simon, L. B. Van De Putte, and P. E. Lipsky. 1998. Cyclooxygenase in biology and disease [see comments]. *FASEB J.* **12:**1063–1073.

31. Eckmann, L., W. F. Stenson, T. C. Savidge, D. C. Lowe, K. E. Barrett, J. Fierer, J. R. Smith, and M. F. Kagnoff. 1997. Role of intestinal epithelial cells in host secretory response to infection by invasive bacteria: bacterial entry induces epithelial prostaglandin H synthase-2 expression and prostaglandin E₂ and F₂α production. *J. Clin. Invest.* **100:**296–309.

32. Elewaut, D., and M. Kronenberg. 2000. Molecular biology of NK T cell specificity and development. *Semin. Immunol.* **12:**561–568.

33. Fernandez, I. M., M. Silva, R. Schuch, W. A. Walker, A. M. Siber, A. T. Maurelli, and B. A. McCormick. 2001. Cadaverine prevents the escape of *Shigella flexneri* from the phagolysosome: a connection between bacterial dissemination and neutrophil transepithelial signaling. *J. Infect. Dis.* **184:**743–753.

34. Ferretti, M., V. Casini-Raggi, T. T. Pizarro, S. P. Eisenberg, C. C. Nast, and F. Cominelli. 1994. Neutralization of endogenous IL-1 receptor antagonist exacerbates and prolongs inflammation in rabbit immune colitis. *J. Clin. Invest.* **94:**449–453.

35. Framson, P. E., D. H. Cho, L. Y. Lee, and R. M. Hershberg. 1999. Polarized expression and function of the costimulatory molecule CD58 on human intestinal epithelial cells. *Gastroenterology* **116:**1054–1062.

36. Furuse, M., T. Hirase, M. Itoh, A. Nagafuchi, S. Yonemura, S. Tsukita, and S. Tsukita. 1993. Occludin: a novel integral membrane protein localizing at tight junctions. *J. Cell Biol.* **123:**1777–1788.

37. Gauchat, J. F., E. Schlagenhauf, N. P. Feng, R. Moser, M. Yamage, P. Jeannin, S. Alouani, G. Elson, L. D. Notarangelo, T. Wells, H. P. Eugster, and J. Y. Bonnefoy. 1997. A novel 4-kb interleukin-13 receptor alpha mRNA expressed in human B, T, and endothelial cells encoding an alternate type-II interleukin-4/interleukin-13 receptor. *Eur. J. Immunol.* **27:**971–978.

38. Gewirtz, A. T., B. A. McCormick, A. S. Neisch, N. A. Petasis, K. Gronert, C. N. Serhan, and J. L. Madara. 1998. Pathogen-induced chemokine secretion from model intestinal epithelium is inhibited by lipoxin A₄ analogs. *J. Clin. Invest.* **101:**1860–1869.

39. Gronert, K., A. Gewirtz, J. L. Madara, and C. N. Serhan. 1998. Identification of a human enterocyte lipoxin A4 receptor that is regulated by interleukin (IL)-13 and interferon gamma and inhibits tumor necrosis factor alpha-induced IL-8 release. *J. Exp. Med.* **187:**1285–1294.

40. Gumbiner, B. M. 1993. Breaking through the tight junction barrier. *J. Cell Biol.* **123:**1631–1633.

41. Haapamaki, M. M., J. O. Haggblom, J. M. Gronroos, E. Pekkala, K. Alanen, and T. J. Nevalainen. 1999. Bactericidal/permeability-increasing protein in colonic mucosa in ulcerative colitis. *Hepatogastroenterology* **46:**2273–2277.

42. Hardin, J., K. Kroeker, B. Chung, and D. G. Gall. 2000. Effect of proinflammatory interleukins on jejunal nutrient transport. *Gut* **47:**184–191.

43. Hershberg, R. M., D. H. Cho, A. Youakim, M. B. Bradley, J. S. Lee, P. E. Framson, and G. T. Nepom. 1998. Highly polarized HLA class II antigen processing and presentation by human intestinal epithelial cells. *J. Clin. Invest.* **102:**792–803.

44. Hershberg, R. M., P. E. Framson, D. H. Cho, L. Y. Lee, S. Kovats, J. Beitz, J. S. Blum, and G. T. Nepom. 1997. Intestinal epithelial cells use two distinct pathways for HLA class II antigen processing. *J. Clin. Invest.* **100:**204–215.

45. Hershberg, R. M., and L. F. Mayer. 2000. Antigen processing and presentation by intestinal

epithelial cells—polarity and complexity. *Immunol. Today* **21:**123–128.

46. **Hogan, S. P., A. Mishra, E. B. Brandt, P. S. Foster, and M. E. Rothenberg.** 2000. A critical role for eotaxin in experimental oral antigen-induced eosinophilic gastrointestinal allergy. *Proc. Natl. Acad. Sci. USA* **97:**6681–6686.

47. **Hogan, S. P., A. Mishra, E. B. Brandt, M. P. Royalty, S. M. Pope, N. Zimmermann, P. S. Foster, and M. E. Rothenberg.** 2001. A pathological function for eotaxin and eosinophils in eosinophilic gastrointestinal inflammation. *Nat. Immunol.* **2:**353–360.

48. **Hollander, D.** 1999. Intestinal permeability, leaky gut, and intestinal disorders. *Curr. Gastroenterol. Rep.* **1:**410–416.

49. **Holmgren, J., J. Fryklund, and H. Larsson.** 1989. Gamma-interferon-mediated down regulation of electrolyte secretion by intestinal epithelial cells: a local immune mechanism? *Scand. J. Immunol.* **30:**499–503.

50. **Huang, G. T., L. Eckmann, T. C. Savidge, and M. F. Kagnoff.** 1996. Infection of human intestinal epithelial cells with invasive bacteria up-regulates apical intercellular adhesion molecule-1 (ICAM-1) expression and neutrophil adhesion. *J. Clin. Invest.* **98:**572–583.

51. **Ito, S., P. Ansari, M. Sakatsume, H. Dickensheets, N. Vazquez, R. P. Donnelly, A. C. Larner, and D. S. Finbloom.** 1999. Interleukin-10 inhibits expression of both interferon alpha- and interferon gamma-induced genes by suppressing tyrosine phosphorylation of STAT1. *Blood* **93:**1456–1463.

52. **Jaye, D. L., and C. A. Parkos.** 2000. Neutrophil migration across intestinal epithelium. *Ann. N.Y. Acad. Sci.* **915:**151–161.

53. **Jobin, C., and R. B. Sartor.** 2000. The I kappa B/NF-kappa B system: a key determinant of mucosal inflammation and protection. *Am. J. Physiol. Cell Physiol.* **278:**C451–C462.

54. **Jung, H. C., L. Eckmann, S.-K. Yang, A. Panja, J. Fierer, E. Morzycka-Wroblewska, and M. F. Kagnoff.** 1995. A distinct array of proinflammatory cytokines is expressed in human colon epithelial cells in response to bacterial invasion. *J. Clin. Invest.* **95:**55–65.

55. **Kagnoff, M.** 1978. Immunology and disease of the gastrointestinal tract, p. 114–144. *In* S. A. Fordtran (ed.), *Gastrointestinal Disease.* W.B. Saunders Co., Philadelphia, Pa.

56. **Kagnoff, M. F., and L. Eckmann.** 1997. Epithelial cells as sensors for microbial infection. *J. Clin. Invest.* **100:**6–10.

57. **Keely, S. J., J. M. Uribe, and K. E. Barrett.** 1998. Carbachol stimulates transactivation of epidermal growth factor receptor and mitogen-activated protein kinase in T84 cells. Implications for carbachol-stimulated chloride secretion. *J. Biol. Chem.* **273:**27111–27117.

58. **Lampinen, M., M. Carlson, P. Sangfelt, Y. Taha, M. Thorn, L. Loof, Y. Raab, and P. Venge.** 2001. IL-5 and TNF-alpha participate in recruitment of eosinophils to intestinal mucosa in ulcerative colitis. *Dig. Dis. Sci.* **46:**2004–2009.

59. **Levin, M., P. A. Quint, B. Goldstein, P. Barton, J. S. Bradley, S. D. Shemie, T. Yeh, S. S. Kim, D. P. Cafaro, P. J. Scannon, B. P. Giroir, and the rBPI21 Meningococcal Sepsis Study Group.** 2000. Recombinant bactericidal/permeability-increasing protein (rBPI21) as adjunctive treatment for children with severe meningococcal sepsis: a randomised trial. *Lancet* **356:**961–967.

60. **Levy, B. D., C. B. Clish, B. Schmidt, K. Gronert, and C. N. Serhan.** 2001. Lipid mediator class switching during acute inflammation: signals in resolution. *Nat. Immunol.* **2:**612–619.

61. **Levy, O.** 2000. Antimicrobial proteins and peptides of blood: templates for novel antimicrobial agents. *Blood* **96:**2664–2672.

62. **Levy, O., and P. Elsbach.** 2001. Bactericidal/permeability-increasing protein in host defense and its efficacy in the treatment of sepsis. *Curr. Infect. Dis. Rep.* **3:**407–412.

63. **Lu, J., D. J. Philpott, P. R. Saunders, M. H. Perdue, P. C. Yang, and D. M. McKay.** 1998. Epithelial ion transport and barrier abnormalities evoked by superantigen-activated immune cells are inhibited by interleukin-10 but not interleukin-4. *J. Pharmacol. Exp. Ther.* **287:**128–136.

64. **Madara, J. L.** 1990. Pathobiology of the intestinal epithelial barrier. *Am. J. Path.* **137:**1273–1278.

65. **Madara, J. L.** 2000. Modulation of tight junctional permeability. *Adv. Drug Deliv. Rev.* **41:**251–253.

66. **Madara, J. L., T. W. Patapoff, B. Gillece-Castro, S. P. Colgan, C. A. Parkos, C. Delp, and R. J. Mrsny.** 1993. 5′-adenosine monophosphate is the neutrophil-derived paracrine factor that elicits chloride secretion from T84 intestinal epithelial cell monolayers. *J. Clin. Invest.* **91:**2320–2325.

67. **Madara, J. L., and J. Stafford.** 1989. Interferon-gamma directly affects barrier function of cultured intestinal epithelial monolayers. *J. Clin. Invest.* **83:**724–727.

68. **Madianos, P. N., P. N. Papapanou, and J. Sandros.** 1997. *Porphyrimonas gingivalis* infection of oral epithelium inhibits neutrophil transepithelial migration. *Infect. Immun.* **65:**3983–3990.

69. **Madsen, K. L., S. A. Lewis, M. N. Taverini, J. Hibbard, and R. N. Fedorak.** 1997. Interleukin 10 prevents cytokine induced disruption of T84 monolayer barrier integrity and limits chloride secretion. *Gastroenterology* **113**:151–159.

70. **Mankertz, J., S. Tavalali, H. Schmitz, A. Mankertz, E. O. Riecken, M. Fromm, and J. D. Schulzke.** 2000. Expression from the human occludin promoter is affected by tumor necrosis factor alpha and interferon gamma. *J. Cell Sci.* **113**:2085–2090.

71. **Matthews, A. N., D. S. Friend, N. Zimmermann, M. N. Sarafi, A. D. Luster, E. Pearlman, S. E. Wert, and M. E. Rothenberg.** 1998. Eotaxin is required for the baseline level of tissue eosinophils. *Proc. Natl. Acad. Sci. USA* **95**:6273–6278.

72. **Mayer, L., D. Eisenhardt, P. Salomon, W. Bauer, R. Plous, and L. Piccinini.** 1991. Expression of class II molecules on intestinal epithelial cells in humans: differences between normal and inflammatory bowel disease. *Gastroenterology* **100**:3–12.

73. **Mayer, L., and R. Shlien.** 1987. Evidence for function of Ia molecules on gut epithelial cells in man. *J. Exp. Med.* **166**:1471–1483.

74. **McGee, D. W.** 1999. Inflammation and mucosal cytokine production, p. 559–573. *In* J. Mestecky, P. L. Ogra, M. E. Lamm, W. Strober, J. Bienenstock, and J. R. McGhee (ed.), *Mucosal Immunology.* Academic Press, Inc., San Diego, Calif.

75. **Meddings, J. B.** 1997. Review article: Intestinal permeability in Crohn's disease. *Aliment. Pharmacol. Ther.* **3**:47–53; discussion, 53–56.

76. **Miloux, B., P. Laurent, O. Bonnin, J. Lupker, D. Caput, N. Vita, and P. Ferrara.** 1997. Cloning of the human IL-13R alpha1 chain and reconstitution with the IL4R alpha of a functional IL-4/IL-13 receptor complex. *FEBS Lett.* **401**:163–166.

77. **Mishra, A., S. P. Hogan, E. B. Brandt, N. Wagner, M. W. Crossman, P. S. Foster, and M. E. Rothenberg.** 2002. Enterocyte expression of the eotaxin and IL-5 transgenes induces compartmentalized dysregulation of eosinophil trafficking. *J. Biol. Chem.* **277**:4406–4412.

78. **Molmenti, E. P., T. Ziambaras, and D. H. Perlmutter.** 1993. Evidence for an acute phase response in human intestinal epithelial cells. *J. Biol. Chem.* **268**:14116–14124.

79. **Monajemi, H., J. Meenan, R. Lamping, D. O. Obradov, S. A. Radema, P. W. Trown, G. N. Tytgat, and S. J. Van Deventer.** 1996. Inflammatory bowel disease is associated with increased mucosal levels of bactericidal/permeability-increasing protein. *Gastroenterology* **110**:733–739.

80. **Neish, A. S., A. T. Gewirtz, H. Zeng, A. N. Young, M. E. Hobert, V. Karmali, A. S. Rao, and J. L. Madara.** 2000. Prokaryotic regulation of epithelial responses by inhibition of IkappaB-alpha ubiquitination. *Science* **289**:1560–1563.

81. **Panja, A., S. Goldberg, L. Eckmann, P. Krishen, and L. Mayer.** 1998. The regulation and functional consequence of proinflammatory cytokine binding on human intestinal epithelial cells. *J. Immunol.* **161**:3675–3684.

82. **Parkos, C. A.** 1997. Molecular events in neutrophil transepithelial migration. *BioEssays* **19**:865–873.

83. **Parkos, C. A., S. P. Colgan, D. Delp, M. A. Arnaout, and J. L. Madara.** 1992. Neutrophil migration across a cultured epithelial monolayer elicits a biphasic resistance response representing sequential effects on transcellular and paracellular pathways. *J. Cell Biol.* **117**:757–764.

84. **Parkos, C. A., S. P. Colgan, M. S. Diamond, A. Nusrat, T. Liang, T. A. Springer, and J. L. Madara.** 1996. Expression and polarization of intercellular adhesion molecule-1 on human intestinal epithelia: consequences for CD11b/18-mediated interactions with neutrophils. *Molec. Med.* **2**:489–505.

85. **Parkos, C. A., S. P. Colgan, A. Liang, A. Nusrat, A. E. Bacarra, D. K. Carnes, and J. L. Madara.** 1996. CD 47 mediates postadhesive events required for neutrophil migration across polarized intestinal epithelia. *J. Cell Biol.* **132**:437–450.

86. **Parkos, C. A., C. Delp, M. A. Arnaout, and J. L. Madara.** 1991. Neutrophil migration across a cultured intestinal epithelium: dependence on a CD11b/CD18-mediated event and enhanced efficiency in the physiologic direction. *J. Clin. Invest.* **88**:1605–1612.

87. **Phalipon, A., and P. J. Sansonetti.** 1999. Microbial-host interactions at mucosal sites. Host response to pathogenic bacteria at mucosal sites. *Curr. Top. Microbiol. Immunol.* **236**:163–189.

88. **Podolsky, D. K.** 1997. Healing the epithelium: solving the problems from two sides. *J. Gastroenterol.* **32**:122–126.

89. **Powell, D. W.** 1987. Intestinal water and electrolyte transport, p. 1267–1291. *In* L. R. Johnson (ed.), *Physiology of the Gastrointestinal Tract.* Raven Press, New York, N.Y.

90. **Powell, D. W.** 1991. Immunophysiology of intestinal electrolyte transport. p. 591–641. *In Handbook of Physiology.* American Physiological Society, New York, N.Y.

91. **Quiding, M., I. Nordstrom, A. Kilander, G. Andersson, L. A. Hanson, J. Holmgren, and C. Czerkinsky.** 1991. Intestinal immune re-

sponses in humans: oral cholera vaccination induces strong intestinal antibody responses and interferon-gamma production and evokes local immunological memory. *J. Clin. Invest.* **88:**143–148.

92. **Reinecker, H. C., and D. K. Podolsky.** 1995. Human intestinal epithelial cells express functional cytokine receptors sharing the common γc chain of the interleukin 2 receptor. *Proc. Natl. Acad. Sci. USA* **92:**8353–8357.

93. **Resnick, M. B., S. P. Colgan, C. A. Parkos, C. Delp-Archer, D. McGuirk, P. F. Weller, and J. L. Madara.** 1995. GM-CSF primed eosinophils migrate across a model intestinal epithelium in response to a platelet-activating factor gradient. *Gastroenterology* **108:**409–416.

94. **Rocha, F., M. W. Musch, L. Lishanskiy, C. Bookstein, K. Sugi, Y. Xie, and E. B. Chang.** 2001. IFN-gamma downregulates expression of Na(+)/H(+) exchangers NHE2 and NHE3 in rat intestine and human Caco-2/bbe cells. *Am. J. Physiol. Cell Physiol.* **280:**C1224–C1232.

95. **Rothenberg, M. E., A. Mishra, E. B. Brandt, and S. P. Hogan.** 2001. Gastrointestinal eosinophils. *Immunol. Rev.* **179:**139–155.

96. **Sansonetti, P. J.** 2000. Microbes and microbial toxins: paradigms for microbial-mucosal interactions III. Shigellosis: from symptoms to molecular pathogenesis. *Am. J. Physiol. Gastrointest. Liver Physiol.* **280:**G319–G323.

97. **Sartor, R. B.** 1995. Microbial factors in the pathogenesis of Crohn's disease, ulcerative colitis, and experimental intestinal inflammation, p. 96–124. *In* J. B. Kirsner and R. J. Shorter (ed.), *Inflammatory Bowel Disease.* Williams and Wilkins, Baltimore, Md.

98. **Schmitz, H., M. Fromm, C. J. Bentzel, P. Scholz, K. Detjen, J. Mankertz, H. Bode, H. J. Epple, E. O. Riecken, and J. D. Schulzke.** 1999. Tumor necrosis factor-alpha (TNF-alpha) regulates the epithelial barrier in the human intestinal cell line HT-29/B6. *J. Cell Sci.* **112:**137–146.

99. **Serhan, C. N.** 1994. Lipoxin biosynthesis and its impact in inflammatory and vascular events. *Biochim. Biophys. Acta* **1212:**1–25.

100. **Serhan, C. N., J. Z. Haeggstrom, and C. C. Leslie.** 1996. Lipid mediator networks in cell signaling: update and impact of cytokines. *FASEB J.* **10:**1147–1158.

101. **Serhan, C. N., J. F. Maddox, N. Petasis, I. Akritopoulou-Zanze, A. Papayianni, H. R. Brady, S. P. Colgan, and J. L. Madara.** 1995. Design of lipoxin A$_4$ stable analogs that block human neutrophil transmigration and adhesion. *Biochemistry* (USA) **34:**14609–14615.

102. **Serhan, C. N., T. Takano, and J. F. Maddox.** 1999. Aspirin-triggered 15-epi-lipoxin A4 and stable analogs on lipoxin A4 are potent inhibitors of acute inflammation. Receptors and pathways. *Adv. Exp. Med. Biol.* **447:**133–149.

103. **Sitaraman, S. V., D. Merlin, L. Wang, M. Wong, A. T. Gewirtz, M. Si-Tahar, and J. L. Madara.** 2001. Neutrophil-epithelial crosstalk at the intestinal lumenal surface mediated by reciprocal secretion of adenosine and IL-6. *J. Clin. Invest.* **107:**861–869.

104. **Sollid, L. M., G. Gaudernack, G. Markussen, D. Kvale, P. Brandtzaeg, and E. Thorsby.** 1987. Induction of various HLA class II molecules in a human colonic adenocarcinoma cell line. *Scand. J. Immunol.* **25:**175–180.

105. **Springer, T. A.** 1990. Adhesion receptors of the immune system. *Nature* **346:**425–430.

106. **Stadnyk, A. W., C. D. Dollard, and A. C. Issekutz.** 2000. Neutrophil migration stimulates rat intestinal epithelial cell cytokine expression during helminth infection. *J. Leukoc. Biol.* **68:**821–827.

107. **Stadnyk, A. W., G. R. Sisson, and C. C. Waterhouse.** 1995. IL-1 alpha is constitutively expressed in the rat intestinal epithelial cell line IEC-6. *Exp. Cell Res.* **220:**298–303.

108. **Stadnyk, A. W., and C. M. Waterhouse.** 1997. Epithelial cytokines in intestinal inflammation and mucosal immunity. *Curr. Opin. Gastroenterol.* **13:**510–517.

109. **Stevceva, L., P. Pavli, A. Husband, K. I. Matthaei, I. G. Young, and W. F. Doe.** 2000. Eosinophilia is attenuated in experimental colitis induced in IL-5 deficient mice. *Genes Immun.* **1:**213–218.

110. **Stoffel, M. P., E. Csernok, C. Herzberg, T. Johnson, S. F. Carroll, and W. L. Gross.** 1996. Anti-neutrophil cytoplasmic antibodies (ANCA) directed against bactericidal/permeability increasing protein (BPI): a new seromarker for inflammatory bowel disease and associated disorders. *Clin. Exp. Immunol.* **104:**54–59.

111. **Sugi, K., M. W. Musch, M. Field, and E. B. Chang.** 2001. Inhibition of Na$^+$,K$^+$-ATPase by interferon gamma down-regulates intestinal epithelial transport and barrier function. *Gastroenterology* **120:**1393–1403.

112. **Takeuchi, A.** 1967. Electron microscope studies of experimental *Salmonella* infection. *Am. J. Pathol.* **50:**109–119.

113. **Taylor, C. T., and S. P. Colgan.** 1999. Therapeutic targets for hypoxia-elicited pathways. *Pharm. Res.* **16:**1498–1505.

114. Taylor, C. T., A. L. Dzus, and S. P. Colgan. 1998. Autocrine regulation of intestinal epithelial permeability induced by hypoxia: role for basolateral release of tumor necrosis factor-α (TNF-α). *Gastroenterology* **114:**657–668.

115. Taylor, C. T., N. Fueki, A. Agah, R. M. Hershberg, and S. P. Colgan. 1999. Critical role of cAMP response element binding protein expression in hypoxia-elicited induction of epithelial TNF-α. *J. Biol. Chem.* **274:**19447–19450.

116. Taylor, C. T., G. T. Furuta, K. Synnestvedt, and S. P. Colgan. 2000. Phosphorylation-dependent targeting of cAMP response element binding protein to the ubiquitin/proteasome pathway in hypoxia. *Proc. Natl. Acad. Sci. USA* **97:**12091–12096.

117. Trinchier, G., and B. Perussia. 1985. Immune interferon: a pleiotropic lymphokine with multiple effects. *Immunol. Today* **6:**131–137.

118. Van der Vieren, M., H. Le Trong, C. L. Wood, P. F. Moore, T. St. John, D. E. Staunton, and W. M. Gallatin. 1995. A novel leukointegrin, alpha d beta 2, binds preferentially to ICAM-3. *Immunity* **3:**683–690.

119. Waxman, K. 1996. Shock: ischemia, reperfusion and inflammation. *New Horizons* **4:**153–160.

120. Winsor, G. L., C. C. Waterhouse, R. L. MacLellan, and A. W. Stadnyk. 2000. Interleukin-4 and IFN-gamma differentially stimulate macrophage chemoattractant protein-1 (MCP-1) and eotaxin production by intestinal epithelial cells. *J. Interferon Cytokine Res.* **20:**299–308.

121. Yamada, K., M. Shimaoka, K. Nagayama, T. Hiroi, H. Kiyono, and T. Honda. 1997. Bacterial invasion induces interleukin-7 receptor expression in colonic epithelial cell line, T84. *Eur. J. Immunol.* **27:**3456–3460.

122. Yardley, J. H., and M. Donowitz. 1977. Colo-rectal biopsies in inflammatory bowel disease, p. 57–94. *In* J. H. Yardley and B. C. Morson (ed.), *The Gastrointestinal Tract.* The Williams and Wilkins Co., Baltimore, Md.

123. Youakim, A., and M. Ahdieh. 1999. Interferon-γ decreases barrier function in T84 cells by reducing ZO-1 levels and disrupting apical actin. *Am. J. Physiol. Gastrointest. Liver Physiol.* **276:**G1279–G1288.

124. Yu, L. C., P. C. Yang, M. C. Berin, V. Di Leo, D. H. Conrad, D. M. McKay, A. R. Satoskar, and M. H. Perdue. 2001. Enhanced transepithelial antigen transport in intestine of allergic mice is mediated by IgE/CD23 and regulated by interleukin-4. *Gastroenterology* **121:**370–381.

125. Ziambaras, T., D. C. Rubin, and D. H. Perlmutter. 1996. Regulation of sucrase-isomaltase gene expression in human intestinal epithelial cells by inflammatory cytokines. *J. Biol. Chem.* **271:**1237–1242.

126. Zünd, G., J. L. Madara, A. L. Dzus, C. S. Awtrey, and S. P. Colgan. 1996. Interleukin 4 and interleukin 13 differentially regulate epithelial chloride secretion. *J. Biol. Chem.* **271:** 7460–7464.

127. Zurawski, S. M., F. J. Vega, B. Huyghe, and G. Zurawski. 1993. Receptors for interleukin-13 and interleukin-4 are complex and share a novel component that functions in signal transduction. *EMBO J.* **12:**2663–2670.

ROLE OF TOLL-LIKE RECEPTORS IN INNATE IMMUNITY OF THE INTESTINE

Elke Cario and Daniel K. Podolsky

5

The intestinal epithelium serves as an essential defensive barrier that forms a bipolar interface between the diverse populations of lumenal microbes and the subjacent cellular elements present in the lamina propria. Recent studies have demonstrated the important role of the intestinal epithelium as a key component of the mucosal immune system—exhibiting both adaptive and innate immune characteristics (16, 41, 54, 68, 91). However, relatively little is known about the mechanisms mediating the constant host-microbial interactions in differential recognition and sorting of the lumenal microbial products by these frontline "nonclassical" immune cells.

Most of the bacteria that constitute the resident microflora of the gut are commensals that, by definition, coexist with intestinal epithelial cells (IEC) without harming them. The normal intestinal epithelium must maintain hyporesponsiveness toward the commensal bacteria that are constantly present in the lumen (126). It has recently been demonstrated that commensal bacteria and their nonpathogenic constituents (commensal-associated molecular patterns [CAMP]) may directly "switch off" downstream signal transduction pathways in IEC via NF-κB to maintain mucosal homeostasis and prevent excessive inflammatory responses (83). Other bacteria are obligate pathogens that either directly invade the intestinal epithelial mucosa or produce toxins that damage it. Pathogenic bacteria are also able to directly deposit their toxic and proinflammatory constituents including their cell-wall-specific signatures (pathogen-associated molecular patterns [PAMP]) such as lipopolysaccharide (LPS), a glycolipid derived from the outermost membrane of pathogenic gram-negative bacteria, at the intestinal epithelial apical surface. LPS may then be internalized, recycled, or transcytosed from the apical to the basolateral pole of the intestinal epithelium (7, 8).

To coexist with the milieu of the gut, the host has evolved survival and active defense features that are incompletely defined so far (126). The pre-epithelial mucous layer at the apical epithelial surface—consisting of mucin glycoproteins, trefoil peptides, and, in the small intestine, defensins—significantly contributes to efficient protection of the underlying host (91, 92). However, the intestine's

Elke Cario, Division of Gastroenterology and Hepatology, University of Essen, Essen, Germany. *Daniel K. Podolsky*, Gastrointestinal Unit, Center for the Study of Inflammatory Bowel Disease, Massachusetts General Hospital, Harvard Medical School, Boston, MA 02114.

Microbial Pathogenesis and the Intestinal Epithelial Cell, ed. by G. Hecht
© 2003 ASM Press, Washington, D.C.

primary protection from this broad microbial ecosystem is likely the highly selective *anatomic barrier* formed by the intestinal epithelium with its intracellular tight junctions that effectively restricts penetration of deleterious lumenal constituents. In addition to this anatomic barrier, the intestinal epithelium functions as a highly efficient *immunologic barrier* exhibiting a combination of adaptive immune features and maintaining lumenal homeostasis through controlled inflammatory responses in vivo. Thus, IEC as nonprofessional antigen-presenting cells express various major histocompatibility complex class I and II molecules, enabling them to mediate adaptive immune responses to pathogenic bacterial products (17, 71, 72). In response to apical pathogenic bacteria, the intestinal epithelial cell can produce a variety of pro- and anti-inflammatory cytokines and chemokines that may be secreted at its basolateral pole to "instruct" the underlying lamina propria (52, 104, 117, 125, 128).

In contrast to the adaptive immune system that responds to antigens with exquisite specificity, the innate immune system senses more generic molecular signatures that are broadly conserved. Innate immune recognition is mediated by a structurally diverse set of receptors, so-called pattern-recognition receptors (PRR) that belong to several distinct protein families (75). Among these, the family of so-called Toll-like receptors (TLR) seems to be especially important. Recognition of their importance emerged from efforts to define the molecular basis of response to the prototypic PAMP, LPS. Earlier studies demonstrated that LPS-induced activation of monocytes, macrophages, or polymorphonuclear neutrophils is mediated in part through CD14, a glycosylphosphatidylinositol (GPI)-anchored membrane receptor structurally unrelated to the TLR (22, 101). Soluble CD14 is present in serum and may facilitate binding of LPS to cells that do not express membrane CD14, including epithelial and endothelial cells (20, 95). However, recognition that membrane-bound CD14 lacks an intracellular signaling domain implied the requirement for at least

one additional receptor molecule to trigger cellular responses. Subsequent studies demonstrated that actual signal transduction is effected by the mammalian homologue of the *Drosophila* Toll protein (48, 76, 99). Of interest, the *Drosophila* Toll pathway has been found to mediate the immune response of insects to microbial infection.

Ten human TLR have now been cloned (24, 25, 113). Mammalian TLR appear to play a central role in host defense against microbial infection, mirroring the role of Toll in *Drosophila*. All mammalian TLR contain several common structural features that include multiple leucine-rich repeats (LRR) and a cysteine-rich domain in the very large and divergent ligand-binding ectodomain (>500 amino acids), a short transmembrane region, and a highly conserved cytoplasmic domain. The last is highly homologous among the individual TLR (approximately 80%) and similar to the cytoplasmic domain of the interleukin-1 (IL-1) receptor (Toll/IL-1-receptor homologous region, or TIR). Human TLR interact via TIR with downstream signaling partners (87, 127).

TLR IN IEC

Initial studies of TLR focused almost exclusively on cells of myeloid lineage, and their expression was presumed to be relatively restricted to these cell populations. In mononuclear cells present in intestinal mucosa and blood, TLR can be classified based on expression pattern as ubiquitous (TLR1), restricted (TLR2, TLR4, and TLR5 in myelomonocytic cells), and specific (TLR3 in dendritic cell [DC]) molecules (80). Moreover, monocytes preferentially express TLR1, TLR2, TLR4, TLR5, and TLR8, whereas plasmacytoid precursor DC strongly express TLR7 and TLR9 (53). As expected, monocytes respond to the known microbial ligands for TLR2 and TLR4 by producing tumor necrosis factor-alpha (TNF-α) and IL-6. In contrast, plasmacytoid precursor DC respond only to the TLR9-microbial ligand, CpG DNA, producing alpha interferon (IFN-α). CD11c$^+$

iDC (immature dendritic cells) preferentially express TLR1, TLR2, and TLR3 and respond to TLR2-ligand peptidoglycan (PGN) by producing large amounts of TNF-α and to TLR3-ligand viral double-stranded RNA by producing IFN-α and IL-12 (53).

We and others have recently demonstrated that intestinal epithelial cells also express most TLR, enabling them to detect specific bacterial signatures and to initiate and regulate diverse innate immune responses (1, 11, 18–20, 29, 34, 35, 117). Indeed, TLR are found expressed by many cell types throughout the whole gastrointestinal tract in vitro and in vivo, e.g., several IEC lines of the small intestine and colon (19, 20, 35, 117), gastric pit cells (58, 59), fetal intestinal cells (34), intestinal macrophages of the lamina propria (108), and intestinal myofibroblasts (38).

Mammalian TLR may enable IEC to participate in innate immunity to microbial pathogens in at least four ways: (i) recognition of molecular patterns present on commensals and pathogens; (ii) expression at the interface with the "environment" of the gastrointestinal lumen; (iii) induction of secretion of pro- or anti-inflammatory cytokines and chemokines that link to the adaptive immune system; and (iv) induction of antimicrobial effector pathways.

TLR LIGANDS
Different PAMP selectively activate different TLR (Fig. 1). The specificity of TLR2 and TLR4 as mediators of cellular immune responses to distinct PAMP has been intensively studied (64, 73). Genetic and biochemical approaches have provided compelling evidence that TLR4 serves as the major receptor for LPS activation in vitro and in vivo using MD-2, which may be secreted in a soluble form, as an accessory protein (23, 27, 42, 62, 112, 115, 119). Among the observations that support this conclusion was the finding that C3H/HeJ mice have naturally occurring mutations in the TLR4 gene that render them hyporesponsive to LPS (96, 121). On the basis of studies using genetic complementation of

C3H/HeJ mice with either human or mouse TLR4, it has been suggested that direct binding interaction between TLR4 and LPS occurs (93). However, gene products other than TLR4 may also participate in the receptor complex that mediates immune responses to LPS (67). Thus, the protein moesin functions as a secondary low-affinity LPS receptor on human monocytes (4). There is a potentially relevant precedent in *Drosophila*, where Toll does not bind bacterial products directly. Instead, infection results in the activation of a protease cascade leading to the extracellular cleavage of the Toll ligand, *Spätzle*, which is regulated by endogenous proteases (66). To date, an equivalent endogenous human TLR ligand/protease has not been identified.

PAMP from, e.g., *Neisseria meningitidis* (94), *Staphylococcus aureus* (111), *Leptospira interrogans* (123), or *zymosan* (118) have been found to serve as ligands for TLR2. In contrast, double-stranded RNA, an intermediate of viral replication, has recently been implicated as a ligand for TLR3, which seems to play a crucial role in dendritic maturation (2, 56, 79, 120). Flagellin has just recently been identified as a ligand for TLR5 (39) and bacterial CpG DNA as a ligand for TLR9 (43, 110).

Of note, TLR can also bind nonbacterial and even nonmicrobial ligands, e.g., respiratory syncytial virus (40, 65), taxol (62, 90), heat shock protein 60 (85), fibronectin (86), or cytokines, including IL-4 (109), IL-1 (70), IL-2 or IL-15 (69), or IFN (78). The ligands of TLR6, -7, -8, and -10 remain to be identified.

MORPHOLOGICAL FEATURES OF TLRS IN IEC
We recently demonstrated that TLR2 and TLR4 are present at the apical pole of differentiated IEC in vitro and in vivo and thus are well positioned to monitor the lumenal milieu of CAMP (18). In contrast, TLR5 appears to be preferentially expressed at the basolateral pole in vitro (35) and in vivo (19). Of note, immature IEC do not exhibit stringent apical polarization of TLR2 or TLR4, suggesting

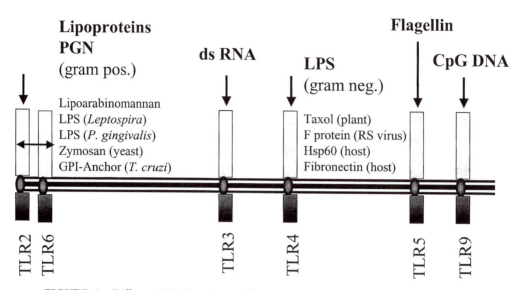

FIGURE 1 Different PAMPs activate different TLRs. TLRs recognize specifically a restricted number of PAMP or CAMP. TLR2 interacts with TLR1 and TLR6 in recognition of a variety of ligands, mainly gram-positive bacterial cell wall components. Aided by at least three other molecules, including CD14, LPS-binding-protein (LBP), and MD-2, TLR4 mainly detects LPS. Double-stranded RNA is recognized by TLR3, and TLR5 binds flagellin. TLR9 is a receptor for abundant bacterial CpG DNA. The ligands for TLR7, TLR8, and TLR10 remain to be determined.

that regionalization of these receptors is dependent on differentiation. Interestingly, immature IEC do not respond adequately to LPS in vitro, in contrast to differentiated IEC, which exhibit serum-dependent activation of p42/p44 mitogen–activated protein kinase (MAPK) and NF-κB in response to LPS (20). The lack of responsiveness of immature IEC to bacterial products could reflect the lack of LPS access to TLR4 in nondifferentiated IEC because of its intracytoplasmic distribution and overall low level of expression (18). Minimal expression and altered localization of TLR could explain hyporesponsiveness in nondifferentiated IEC to LPS as well (1, 81).

The state of cell differentiation also appears to influence TLR expression in primary immune cells. Expression of mRNA for some TLR decreases as monocytes differentiate into iDC, while mRNA encoding TLR3 and MD2 markedly increases during iDC formation. In contrast, in iDC induced to mature

with LPS or TNF-α, expression of most TLR transiently increases and then nearly disappears, although actual leukocyte cellular responsiveness does not seem to change (120).

Deployment of intestinal epithelial TLR may be dynamically influenced by their specific ligands. We recently found that LPS induces redistribution of TLR4 in vitro. In response to simultaneous LPS stimulation, TLR4 is redistributed from its apical location to intracytoplasmic compartments near the basolateral membrane (18). After basolateral stimulation of IEC with LPS, TLR4 undergoes transcytotic redistribution from the apical to the basolateral cytoplasmic domain of differentiated T84 cells, seemingly trafficking directly toward the basolateral stimulus. In contrast, TLR2 does not traffic in response to LPS, and TLR4 distribution is not altered in the presense of PGN, respectively, suggesting that the observed effects of induced redistribution must be ligand specific. Taken together, these findings imply that TLR trafficking may reflect polarized cell-specific responses to their respective ligands, indicating that despite rigid cell polarity, the intestinal epithelial cell is uniquely adapted to dynamically monitor its perimeter.

In the context of the dynamic changes in distribution of TLR4, we have found that TLR4 appears in "vesicular" structures in the apical cytoplasm of IEC after exposure to LPS (18). We speculate that these TLR4-positive vesicles carry endocytosed LPS as "cargo." It is well known that macrophages eliminate pathogens by phagocytosis and that TLR2 is specifically recruited to macrophage phagosomes in response to yeast (89, 118). Ongoing studies should determine the functional role of these TLR4-coated vesicles in IEC. It is possible they function to sample and detoxify LPS in IEC, perhaps acting as IEC-specific "phagosomes." It remains unclear whether cytoplasmic TLR are capable of specifically recognizing endocytosed LPS to activate downstream signaling effects. The eukaryotic endoplasmic reticulum chaperone gp96 appears to be essential for folding and dynamic assembly of newly synthesized TLR on the cell surface. In the absence of gp96, TLR are retained intracellularly and recognition of PAMP is dysfunctional (97). Preliminary data demonstrate that long-term stimulation of IEC with LPS leads to immune hyporesponsiveness to CAMP when reexposed, suggesting that cytoplasmic redistribution of TLR may indeed functionally downregulate cells (unpublished observation). It remains unclear whether gp96 or other chaperones play a regulatory role in dynamic TLR redistribution in IEC—"switching on and off" immune responses to CAMP in these cell populations.

TLR-ACTIVATED SIGNAL TRANSDUCTION PATHWAYS AND CELLULAR RESPONSES

The mammalian TLR signaling pathway has been found to be similar to that activated by Toll in *Drosophila*. Thus, PAMP activation of most TLR induces a "classical" intracellular signaling cascade (122) involving the adapter protein MyD88 (114, 124), IL-1R accessory protein kinase (IRAK) (36), transforming growth factor beta-activated kinase 1 (TAK-1) (59), TNFR-associated factor 6 (TRAF-6) (129), and NF-κB-inducing kinase (NIK), leading to activation of NF-κB (31) and subsequent gene transcription, resulting in cytokine and chemokine production (Fig. 2). Rac1/Akt controls a second, IκB-independent pathway to NF-κB activation and is essential in innate immune cell signaling via TLR2 (6). In addition, TLR2 may also promote apoptosis through MyD88 via a pathway involving Fas-associated death domain protein (FADD) and caspase 8 (3).

Of note, activation of neither NF-κB nor the MAPK family is abolished in MyD88 knockout mice in response to LPS, suggesting the presence of a second and MyD88-*independent* signaling cascade (60). Kawai et al. demonstrated a MyD88/TRAF6-*independent* pathway that regulates induction of IP-10 via IRF3 (61). In addition, Kupffer cells lacking MyD88 secrete IL-18 after stimulation with LPS via activation of endogenous caspase-1 in a MyD88-*independent* fashion (102). LPS also induces functional maturation of MyD88-deficient DC, including upregulation of costimulatory molecules and enhancement of antigen-presenting cell activity, whereas CpG DNA binds TLR9 and induces DC maturation in a MyD88-*dependent* manner (55). It remains unclear whether lipopeptide-induced DC maturation via TLR2 involves MyD88 (44). "TIR domain-containing adapter protein" (TIRAP, identical to the recently identified Mal [32]) has been shown to control activation of MyD88-*independent* signaling pathways downstream of TLR4 (46). In contrast, LPS-induced cytokine production from DC is dependent on functional MyD88 (56). Thus, involvement of the "checkpoint" MyD88 is only partially necessary for TLR-mediated distinct downstream signaling effects.

Numerous pro- and anti-inflammatory cytokines are produced in response to bacterial

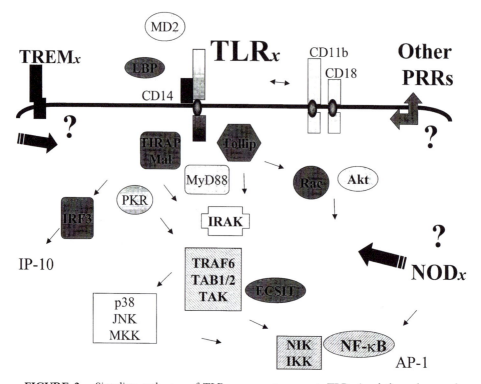

FIGURE 2. Signaling pathways of TLRx—current concept. TLR signal through several signaling components, including the adapter protein MyD88, Toll-interacting protein (Tollip), IL-1R-associated kinase (IRAK), and TNF receptor-associated factor 6 (TRAF-6), leading to liberation of the transcription factor NF-κB and activation of MKK and the JNK-p38 pathways. All these events lead downstream to the transcription of various cytokine/chemokine genes. TLR4 also signals through an MyD88-independent pathway via another adapter, recently identified as TIRAP (or Mal). The interactions among TLR versus MyD88, TIRAP, and Tollip are complex and remain unresolved. The protein kinase PKR is possibly positioned between TIRAP and TRAF-6. Rho GTPase Rac-1 and Akt have also been shown to mediate TLR2-dependent activation. The roles of other PRR, such as TREM or Nods, possibly interacting with TLR signaling proteins and thus regulating innate immune responses to bacterial ligands, remain to be defined.

ligands via activation of TLRs, for example, IL-1, IL-6, IL-8, IL-10, IL-12, and TNF-α (26, 74, 100, 116, 122). Nitric oxide secretion and cyclooxygenase-2 (Cox-2) gene expression can also be induced (85, 90). Binding of CpGDNA to TLR9 selectively induces expression of "suppressor of cytokine signaling" (SOCS), which acts as a cytokine-inducible negative feedback regulator of c-Jun-N-terminal kinase (JNK)/STAT signaling in hematopoietic cells (28).

CD14, TLR4, and CD11b/CD18 appear to be coordinately engaged to yield optimal

signaling in blood macrophages (90). In contrast, intestinal macrophages as well as epithelial cells appear to lack constitutive expression of mCD14 (107, 108). Expression of CD14 among intestine cell lines varies; while some tumor-cell-derived IEC lines do express CD14 constitutively at the mRNA and protein level in vitro, others lack CD14 expression (20, 33). Of note, CD14 expression may be induced by proinflammatory challenges in vivo (77). Consistent with their CD14 null phenotype, lamina propria macrophages and epithelial cells display reduced LPS-induced stress responses and cytokine production compared to blood mononuclear cells (20, 108).

p42/p44 MAPK and NF-κB are central to pathways mediating LPS activation of IEC (20). Interestingly, CAMP-induced stimulation of different IEC lines involves selective activation of MAPK/JNK/p38 pathways and downstream cytokine gene expression. These findings may reflect cell-specific features, including the state of differentiation or idiosyncratic alterations of signal transduction pathways among colon cancer cell lines, but also overall differences in signaling events via different PRR and adapters among cell types.

As noted, activation of p42/p44 MAPK and NF-κB to LPS in IEC model cell lines in response is less strong than that observed after other stress stimuli, e.g., phorbol myristate acetate (PMA) or IL-1β in IEC, and in comparison to primary immune cells such as monocytes or macrophages. Preliminary data suggest that constant exposure to low-concentration LPS may block any activation of MAPK or NF-κB in IEC when restimulated with LPS at any concentration (unpublished observation). This suggests that IEC may be partially desensitized or "tolerant" of LPS, limiting activation of the underlying immune cells in the face of constant exposure to LPS at the apical surface of the epithelium. Responsiveness and ability to induce such "tolerance to LPS" appear to be acquired in association with IEC differentiation.

It remains unclear which component(s) of the TLR-signaling pathway is responsible for the development of LPS tolerance in IEC. General hyporesponsiveness may reflect the absence of MD-2 (1). In classical models of cell tolerance, a cell surface receptor is downregulated or uncoupled from downstream signaling. We recently demonstrated that TLR2 and TLR4 are normally present in small amounts on IEC in vivo, thus minimizing lumenal CAMP recognition in the healthy intestine (19). Decreased expression of TLR4 surface protein may correlate with inhibition of downstream cytokine production in intestinal epithelial LPS tolerance, as recently demonstrated by Abreu et al. (1). In this study,

various IEC lines failed to respond to purified, protein-free LPS. However, overexpression of both TLR4 and MD-2 conferred LPS responsiveness to IEC.

Mutations that result in functional alterations of TLR4 lead to LPS hyporesponsiveness and tolerance, as illustrated by C3H/HeJ mice, which have a single point mutation of the LPS gene product TLR4 (121). However, it appears that this mutation is not necessary to induce LPS tolerance in the related C3H/HeN strain. Ex vivo macrophages from C3H/HeN mice also render LPS tolerant by low-dose LPS pretreatment; in contrast to C3H/HeJ mice, they have alterations in activation of NF-κB, suggesting that disruptions elsewhere within the TLR-signaling pathway may all lead to the same LPS-tolerant phenotype.

Based on initial studies in Drosophila (105), cotransfection studies have recently demonstrated that TLR may functionally interact and communicate in heteromeric multireceptor complexes (37, 88, 89). Tyrosine phosphorylation of TLR2 is required for assembly of a multiprotein complex that is necessary for subsequent induction of NF-κB transcriptional activity (6). We have also recently obtained preliminary evidence from the cross-linking of surface proteins of IEC that endogenously expressed intestinal epithelial TLR functionally interact in a ligand-sensitive, tyrosine-phosphorylated multireceptor complex that may be dynamically modulated by CAMP in vitro and in vivo, expanding the plasticity of this family of receptors to maximize innate pattern recognition (unpublished observation). Plevy et al. have also recently shown that cotransfection of TLR1 and TLR2 may lead to functional and synergistic interaction in order to activate NF-κB and expression of inflammatory genes in IEC (29). These complexes presumably contain secondary interacting partners of monomeric TLR, including downstream signaling proteins. Identification of the components of the TLR multireceptor complex and its cross talk with other pathways (e.g., via TRAF-6), as well as the details of the subsequent functional cellular activation pathways in IEC and other cell types, is needed.

Several additional components of the TLR/IL-1R signaling cascade have recently been identified in other cell types, including Tollip (14, 15) and ECSIT (63). The double-stranded RNA (dsRNA)-binding protein kinase PKR is a component of both the TIRAP- and MyD88-dependent signaling pathways (46) and could potentially mediate cross talk between signaling pathways. Further studies should reveal whether these adapters or adapter-like proteins play a role in intestinal epithelial immune recognition of CAMP/PAMP.

ALTERATION OF TLR EXPRESSION IN HUMAN IBD

Recent studies have demonstrated that TLR are expressed in normal human intestinal mucosa: mRNA for TLR1-TLR4, but not TLR5, was detected in isolated primary IEC (11). It appears that epithelial cells rather than macrophages and other lamina propria populations are the predominant cells expressing TLR, with differential expression of various members of this receptor family (19). Thus, primary IEC of normal, nondiseased mucosa may constitutively express TLR3 and TLR5 protein, whereas TLR2 and TLR4 appear to be present in much lower amounts as assessed by immunohistochemistry.

Expression of TLR may be selectively altered in association with inflammatory bowel disease (IBD), and further, some of these alterations may be specific to the form of IBD. Thus, TLR3 and TLR4 appear to be differentially modulated in the intestinal epithelium of patients with IBD. While TLR3 expression by IEC of ulcerative colitis (UC) patients is comparable to that of normal controls, TLR3 expression is significantly downregulated in Crohn's disease (CD). Of interest, reduced expression of TLR3 on IEC seems to be consistent in CD, irrespective of location or inflammatory activity. This implies that reduced TLR3 may not simply reflect the local effect of inflammatory mediators. Inflamma-

tory cells of the lamina propria remain positive for cell surface expression of TLR3, suggesting that decreased TLR3 may be a distinctive feature of CD but not UC and could reflect a divergent dimension of pathophysiological mechanisms involved in these two disorders.

In contrast to human IBD, when murine colitis is induced by either dextran sodium sulfate (DSS) or trinitrobenzene sulfonic acid (TNBS) in various wild-type strains (C57BL/6, C3H/HeJ, C3H/SnJ), TLR expression seems to remain unchanged in intact IEC during the early stages of disease. However, both TLR3 and TLR4 are diminished in IEC in spontaneous chronic colitis of mice with targeted gene deletion of T-cell receptor alpha (TCR-α) (E. Cario, E. Mizoguchi, A. Mizoguchi, A. K. Bhan, and D. K. Podolsky, unpublished observation). TLR2 is not significantly modulated in either colitis model. Reduced TLR3 and TLR4 could reflect the local effect of some inflammatory mediator in TCR-$\alpha^{-/-}$ colitis, such as IL-4. These data suggest that chronic colitis in TCR-$\alpha^{-/-}$ mice may be mechanistically distinct from other forms of murine colitis or human IBD and may be sustained by a dysregulated host defense response to lumenal bacteria resulting from endo- and exogenously induced selective alteration of TLR3 and TLR4 expression.

These findings in the murine model contrast with the results of the studies of human tissue mentioned above; in patients with UC, TLR3 remains unchanged and TLR4 is significantly increased in IEC throughout the lower gastrointestinal tract, regardless of whether assessed during active or inactive disease. This disparity may reflect mechanistic differences between this form of murine colitis model and human UC despite similarities in histopathological and clinical features. Contrasting TLR expression patterns may result from species-specific differences reflecting diverse genetic, evolutionary, or environmental factors that need to be elucidated in further studies.

It is important to note that the functional role of either human or murine TLR3 in mediating innate immune responses to specific microbes and their toxic constituents in vivo has not yet been established. Mammalian TLR3 is thought to recognize dsRNA—a molecular pattern associated with viral infection because most viruses produce dsRNA at some point during their replication. Activation of TLR3 induces production of type 1 IFNs (2). To date, it is not known whether TLR3-deficient (TLR3$^{-/-}$) mice are more susceptible or resistant to developing spontaneous or chemically induced (DSS/TNBS) colitis. So far, viral dsRNA has not been found to play a pathophysiological role as a ligand in IBD. Interestingly, TLR3 is localized on chromosome 4 (q35) at the border of a large region suspected to contain an IBD susceptibility gene on the basis of linkage analysis, suggesting a potential pathogenic association of IBD with the TLR3 gene. Identification and characterization of polymorphisms in the TLR3 gene may provide insight into IEC-specific dysregulation of the receptor in CD. In addition, further studies are needed to clarify the functional role of TLR3 in IEC as a specific PRR, its interaction with other receptor molecules, its regulation by cytokines in the intestinal epithelium as well as inflammatory cells, and, finally, its relevance in the differential pathogenesis of IBD.

In contrast to TLR3, TLR4 appears to be significantly increased in IEC throughout the lower gastrointestinal tract in both CD and UC patients (19). This observation could result from a "gain-of-function" mutation in this receptor, which could functionally exhibit proinflammatory effects in response to physiological concentrations of LPS. However, Plevy and coworkers, using other anti-TLR4 antisera, found that TLR4 expression is markedly increased in CD, but not in UC (11).

In general, these changes could play an important linking role in enhancing hyperresponsiveness of the intestinal mucosa to LPS in IBD. It is possible that spontaneous mutations of TLR4 prime individuals experiencing acute infections to develop especially severe disease. In active IBD, variant alleles in the TLR4 gene could induce functional dysregulation of the receptor to LPS. The two tissue-restricted transcription factors PU.1 and IFN consensus sequence-binding protein have been found to participate in the basal regulation of human TLR4 in myeloid cells (98), although it remains to be determined whether they may also play a similar modulatory role in IEC.

TLR2 and TLR5 expression in IEC remain unchanged in active IBD (19). Neither control nor IBD tissues exhibit significant TLR2 expression in IEC. Upregulation of TLR2 is restricted to scattered inflammatory cells of the lamina propria in active IBD, findings compatible with the observations of Hausmann et al. (38). Similar to TLR2, TLR5 did not appear to be significantly regulated in acute intestinal inflammation in IBD (19). Thus, TLR2, which serves as a receptor for ligands derived from gram-positive bacteria, and TLR5, which binds flagellin protein, do not play an obvious role in the pathobiology of IBD.

It remains unclear whether immune imbalance in IBD may either lead to or result from TLR dysregulation in IEC. Further studies are needed to focus on the direct pathogenetic relevance and immune consequences of TLR dysregulation in active IBD and other gastrointestinal disorders.

TLR DYSREGULATION IN INFECTIOUS DISEASES

The detection of TLR has provided new insights into the mechanism underlying serious infectious diseases (10). Thus, products of *Hemophilus influenzae* may directly upregulate TLR2 in epithelial cells, leading to exaggerated immune responses via NF-κB (106). In human immunodeficiency virus (HIV)-infected patients, opportunistic infections with coliform bacteria that cause enteritis may lead to increases in local and circulating levels of biologically active lumenal LPS activating IEC cells via TLR4.

TLR mutations may modify the detection of pathogens, leading to increased susceptibility to pneumococcal severe infections, gram-negative and gram-positive bacterial septic shock, lepromatous leprosy, and meningococcal disease (21, 57). However, such defects are difficult to identify and mutations may have short evolutionary durability. In a recent analysis of TLR mutations in meningococcal septicemia, it was observed that patients with meningococcal sepsis have an excess of rare coding mutations at the TLR4 locus. It was concluded that approximately 6% of meningococcal disease in the European population can be explained by mutations altering TLR4 structure (9).

Detailed identification of such mutations in populations and causal, direct linkage to certain pathogens could provide insight into individual susceptibility and prognosis in both infectious and noninfectious diseases (such as autoimmune disorders).

TARGETING TLR FOR THERAPEUTIC EFFECT— FUTURE PERSPECTIVES

Different strategies could be used to modulate sensing and signal transduction effects via TLR and MyD88: (i) soluble TLR that bind the respective class of ligands, thus preventing recognition through the host; (ii) anti-TLR that neutralize specific TLR, thus preventing ligand-induced activation; and (iii) cell-permeable agents that block binding of specific TLR or downstream signaling partners, thus preventing exaggerated inflammatory responses. Finally, a restricted, desired immune response could be induced via a TLR by applying purified low-dose, attenuated PAMP locally or systemically. This approach has already been successfully applied in the therapy of superficial bladder cancer using attenuated BCG (103). However, not enough is known about the functional roles of TLR and their downstream consequences via MyD88 or other cascades under physiological and, more importantly, pathophysiological conditions, to define an optimal therapeutic strategy for targeting components of the TLR signaling pathway.

CONCLUSIONS

Recent studies have begun to elucidate the mechanisms by which TLR initiate innate immune responses in IEC. Future research will identify further TLR ligands, specify interconnective signaling cascades activated by TLR, and clarify the potential role of intestinal epithelial TLR in the pathogenesis of IBD and other aberrant inflammatory processes in the gastrointestinal tract. In addition, other receptor families have recently been added to the list of key regulators in innate immunity to microbial invasion, such as TREM-1 (12, 13, 82) and Nod1/2 (49, 50). Genetic studies have recently implicated Nods in innate immune responses to bacterial components, and variants of Nod2 are associated with the risk of CD (47, 84). It will be essential to determine how these families of proteins and other—as yet unknown—kinases cross talk with TLR in regulatory feedback loops in monitoring the vast array of lumenal CAMP/PAMP in IEC and how an imbalance of signaling events may lead to disease. Identifying the physiological mechanisms through which intestinal TLR and other PRR modulate host defense in the gastrointestinal tract could lead to new therapeutic approaches to combat microbial-associated gastrointestinal disorders, such as infectious diseases and perhaps IBD.

REFERENCES

1. **Abreu, M. T., P. Vora, E. Faure, L. S. Thomas, E. T. Arnold, and M. Arditi.** 2001. Decreased expression of Toll-like receptor-4 and MD-2 correlates with intestinal epithelial cell protection against dysregulated proinflammatory gene expression in response to bacterial lipopolysaccharide. *J. Immunol.* **167:**1609–1616.
2. **Alexopoulou, L., A. C. Holt, R. Medzhitov, and R. A. Flavell.** 2001. Recognition of double-stranded RNA and activation of NF-kappaB by Toll-like receptor 3. *Nature* **413:**732–738.
3. **Aliprantis, A. O., R. B. Yang, D. S. Weiss, P. Godowski, and A. Zychlinsky.** 2000. The apoptotic signaling pathway activated by Toll-like receptor-2. *EMBO J.* **19:**3325–3336.
4. **Amar, S., K. Oyaisu, L. Li, and T. Van Dyke.** 2001. Moesin: a potential LPS receptor

on human monocytes. *J. Endotoxin Res.* **7:**281–286.

5. **Anderson, K. V.** 2000. Toll signaling pathways in the innate immune response. *Curr. Opin. Immunol.* **12:**13–19.

6. **Arbibe, L., J. P. Mira, N. Teusch, L. Kline, M. Guha, N. Mackman, P. J. Godowski, R. J. Ulevitch, and U. G. Knaus.** 2000. Toll-like receptor 2-mediated NF-kappa B activation requires a Rac1-dependent pathway. *Nat. Immunol.* **1:**533–540.

7. **Beatty, W. L., S. Meresse, P. Gounon, J. Davoust, J. Mounier, P. J. Sansonetti, and J. P. Gorvel.** 1999. Trafficking of *Shigella lipopolysaccharide* in polarized intestinal epithelial cells. *J. Cell Biol.* **145:**689–698.

8. **Beatty, W. L., and P. J. Sansonetti.** 1997. Role of lipopolysaccharide in signaling to subepithelial polymorphonuclear leukocytes. *Infect. Immun.* **65:**4395–4404.

9. **Beutler, B.** 2001. Sepsis begins at the interface of pathogen and host. *Biochem. Soc. Trans.* **29:**853–859.

10. **Beutler, B., and R. J. Ulevitch.** 2001. Genetic analysis of host responses in sepsis. *Curr. Infect. Dis. Rep.* **3:**419.

11. **Bogunovic, M., S. Reka, K. N. Evans, L. F. Mayer, K. Sperber, and S. E. Plevy.** 2000. Functional Toll-like receptors (TLR) are expressed on intestinal epithelial cells (IEC) *Gastroenterology* **118:**A804.

12. **Bouchon, A., J. Dietrich, and M. Colonna.** 2000. Cutting edge: inflammatory responses can be triggered by TREM-1, a novel receptor expressed on neutrophils and monocytes. *J. Immunol.* **164:**4991–4995.

13. **Bouchon, A., F. Facchetti, M. A. Weigand, and M. Colonna.** 2001. TREM-1 amplifies inflammation and is a crucial mediator of septic shock. *Nature* **410:**1103–1107.

14. **Bulut, Y., E. Faure, L. Thomas, O. Equils, and M. Arditi.** 2001. Cooperation of Toll-like receptor 2 and 6 for cellular activation by soluble tuberculosis factor and *Borrelia burgdorferi* outer surface protein A lipoprotein: role of Toll-interacting protein and IL-1 receptor signaling molecules in Toll-like receptor 2 signaling. *J. Immunol.* **167:**987–994.

15. **Burns, K., J. Clatworthy, L. Martin, F. Martinon, C. Plumpton, B. Maschera, A. Lewis, K. Ray, J. Tschopp, and F. Volpe.** 2000. Tollip, a new component of the IL-1RI pathway, links IRAK to the IL-1 receptor. *Nat. Cell Biol.* **2:**346–351.

16. **Campbell, N., X. Y. Yio, L. P. So, Y. Li, and L. Mayer.** 1999. The intestinal epithelial cell: processing and presentation of antigen to the mucosal immune system. *Immunol. Rev.* **172:**315–324.

17. **Campbell, N. A., H. S. Kim, R. S. Blumberg, and L. Mayer.** 1999. The nonclassical class I molecule CD1d associates with the novel CD8 ligand gp180 on intestinal epithelial cells. *J. Biol. Chem.* **274:**26259–26265.

18. **Cario, E., D. Brown, M. McKee, K. Lynch-Devaney, G. Gerken, and D. K. Podolsky.** 2002. Commensal-associated molecular pattern molecules induce selective toll-like receptor-trafficking from apical membrane to cytoplasmic compartments in polarized intestinal epithelium. *Am. J. Pathol.* **160:**165–173.

19. **Cario, E., and D. K. Podolsky.** 2000. Differential alteration in intestinal epithelial cell expression of Toll-like receptor 3 (TLR3) and TLR4 in inflammatory bowel disease. *Infect. Immun.* **68:**7010–7017.

20. **Cario, E., I. M. Rosenberg, S. L. Brandwein, P. L. Beck, H. C. Reinecker, and D. K. Podolsky.** 2000. Lipopolysaccharide activates distinct signaling pathways in intestinal epithelial cell lines expressing Toll-like receptors. *J. Immunol.* **164:**966–972.

21. **Charpentier, J., and J. P. Mira.** 2001. Role of host response during severe bacterial infection. *Arch. Pediatr.* **8**(Suppl. 4):689S–696S.

22. **Chen, T. Y., M. G. Lei, T. Suzuki, and D. C. Morrison.** 1992. Lipopolysaccharide receptors and signal transduction pathways in mononuclear phagocytes. *Curr. Top. Microbiol. Immunol.* **181:**169–188.

23. **Chow, J. C., D. W. Young, D. T. Golenbock, W. J. Christ, and F. Gusovsky.** 1999. Toll-like receptor-4 mediates lipopolysaccharide-induced signal transduction. *J. Biol. Chem.* **274:**10689–10692.

24. **Chuang, T. H., and R. J. Ulevitch.** 2000. Cloning and characterization of a sub-family of human Toll-like receptors: hTLR7, hTLR8 and hTLR9. *Eur. Cytokine Netw.* **11:**372–378.

25. **Chuang, T. H., and R. J. Ulevitch.** 2001. Identification of hTLR10: a novel human Toll-like receptor preferentially expressed in immune cells. *Biochim. Biophys. Acta* **1518:**157–161.

26. **Chung, C. S., G. Y. Song, L. L. Moldawer, I. H. Chaudry, and A. Ayala.** 2000. Neither Fas ligand nor endotoxin is responsible for inducible peritoneal phagocyte apoptosis during sepsis/peritonitis. *J. Surg. Res.* **91:**147–153.

27. **da Silva Correia, J., K. Soldau, U. Christen, P. S. Tobias, and R. J. Ulevitch.** 2001. Lipopolysaccharide is in close proximity to each of the proteins in its membrane receptor complex. Transfer from CD14 to TLR4 and MD-2. *J. Biol. Chem.* **276:**21129–21135.

28. **Dalpke, A. H., S. Opper, S. Zimmermann, and K. Heeg.** 2001. Suppressors of cytokine signaling (SOCS)-1 and SOCS-3 are induced by CpG-DNA and modulate cytokine responses in APCs. *J. Immunol.* **166:**7082–7089.

29. **Edwards, E. W., M. Bogunovic, J. Yager, and S. E. Plevy.** 2001. Toll-like receptor expression and function in intestinal epithelial cells: an epithelial cell type co-expressing TLR1 and TLR2. *FASEB J.* **2001:**abstract.

30. **Equils, O., E. Faure, L. Thomas, Y. Bulut, S. Trushin, and M. Arditi.** 2001. Bacterial lipopolysaccharide activates HIV long terminal repeat through Toll-like receptor 4. *J. Immunol.* **166:**2342–2347.

31. **Faure, E., O. Equils, P. A. Sieling, L. Thomas, F. X. Zhang, C. J. Kirschning, N. Polentarutti, M. Muzio, and M. Arditi.** 2000. Bacterial lipopolysaccharide activates NF-kappaB through Toll-like receptor 4 (TLR-4) in cultured human dermal endothelial cells. Differential expression of TLR-4 and TLR-2 in endothelial cells. *J. Biol. Chem.* **275:**11058–11063.

32. **Fitzgerald, K. A., E. M. Palsson-McDermott, A. G. Bowie, C. A. Jefferies, A. S. Mansell, G. Brady, E. Brint, A. Dunne, P. Gray, M. T. Harte, D. McMurray, D. E. Smith, J. E. Sims, T. A. Bird, and L. A. O'Neill.** 2001. Mal (MyD88-adapter-like) is required for Toll-like receptor-4 signal transduction. *Nature* **413:**78–83.

33. **Funda, D. P., L. Tuckova, M. A. Farre, T. Iwase, I. Moro, and H. Tlaskalova-Hogenova.** 2001. CD14 is expressed and released as soluble CD14 by human intestinal epithelial cells in vitro: lipopolysaccharide activation of epithelial cells revisited. *Infect. Immun.* **69:**3772–3781.

34. **Fusunyan, R. D., N. N. Nanthakumar, M. E. Baldeon, and W. A. Walker.** 2001. Evidence for an innate immune response in the immature human intestine: Toll-like receptors on fetal enterocytes. *Pediatr. Res.* **49:**589–593.

35. **Gewirtz, A. T., T. A. Navas, S. Lyons, P. J. Godowski, and J. L. Madara.** 2001. Cutting edge: bacterial flagellin activates basolaterally expressed tlr5 to induce epithelial proinflammatory gene expression. *J. Immunol.* **167:**1882–1885.

36. **Hacker, H., R. M. Vabulas, O. Takeuchi, K. Hoshino, S. Akira, and H. Wagner.** 2000. Immune cell activation by bacterial CpG-DNA through myeloid differentiation marker 88 and tumor necrosis factor receptor-associated factor (TRAF)6. *J. Exp. Med.* **192:**595–600.

37. **Hajjar, A. M., D. S. O'Mahony, A. Ozinsky, D. M. Underhill, A. Aderem, S. J. Klebanoff, and C. B. Wilson.** 2001. Cutting edge: functional interactions between Toll-like receptor (TLR) 2 and TLR1 or TLR6 in response to phenol-soluble modulin. *J. Immunol.* **166:**15–19.

38. **Hausmann, M., T. Spoettl, J. Schoelmerich, W. Falk, T. Andus, and G. Rogler.** 2000. Induction of Toll-like Receptor 2 in human intestinal myofibroblasts by interferon gamma. *Gastroenterology* **118:**A791.

39. **Hayashi, F., K. D. Smith, A. Ozinsky, T. R. Hawn, E. C. Yi, D. R. Goodlett, J. K. Eng, S. Akira, D. M. Underhill, and A. Aderem.** 2001. The innate immune response to bacterial flagellin is mediated by Toll-like receptor 5. *Nature* **410:**1099–1103.

40. **Haynes, L. M., D. D. Moore, E. A. Kurt-Jones, R. W. Finberg, L. J. Anderson, and R. A. Tripp.** 2001. Involvement of Toll-like receptor 4 in innate immunity to respiratory syncytial virus. *J. Virol.* **75:**10730–10737.

41. **Hecht, G.** 1999. Innate mechanisms of epithelial host defense: spotlight on intestine. *Am. J. Physiol.* **277:**C351–C358.

42. **Heine, H., C. J. Kirschning, E. Lien, B. G. Monks, M. Rothe, and D. T. Golenbock.** 1999. Cutting edge: cells that carry A null allele for Toll-like receptor 2 are capable of responding to endotoxin. *J. Immunol.* **162:**6971–6975.

43. **Hemmi, H., O. Takeuchi, T. Kawai, T. Kaisho, S. Sato, H. Sanjo, M. Matsumoto, K. Hoshino, H. Wagner, K. Takeda, and S. Akira.** 2000. A Toll-like receptor recognizes bacterial DNA. *Nature* **408:**740–745.

44. **Hertz, C. J., S. M. Kiertscher, P. J. Godowski, D. A. Bouis, M. V. Norgard, M. D. Roth, and R. L. Modlin.** 2001. Microbial lipopeptides stimulate dendritic cell maturation via Toll-like receptor 2. *J. Immunol.* **166:**2444–2450.

45. **Hirschfeld, M., Y. Ma, J. H. Weis, S. N. Vogel, and J. J. Weis.** 2000. Cutting edge: repurification of lipopolysaccharide eliminates signaling through both human and murine Toll-like receptor 2. *J. Immunol.* **165:**618–622.

46. **Horng, T., G. M. Barton, and R. Medzhitov.** 2001. TIRAP: an adapter molecule in the Toll signaling pathway. *Nat. Immunol.* **2:**835–841.

47. **Hugot, J. P., M. Chamalliard, H. Zouali, S. Lesage, J. P. Cézard, J. Belaiche, S. Almer, C. Tysk, C. A. O'Morain, M. Gassull, V. Binder, Y. Finkel, A. Cortot, R. Modigliani, P. Laurent-Preig, C. Gower-Rousseau, J. Macry, J. F. Colomvel, M. Sahbatou, and G. Thomas.** 2001. Association of NOD2 leucine-rich repeat variants with susceptibility to Crohn's disease. *Nature* **411:**599–603.

48. **Imler, J. L., and J. A. Hoffmann.** 2000. Signalling mechanisms in the antimicrobial host de-

fense of *Drosophila*. *Curr. Opin. Microbiol.* **3**:16–22.

49. **Inohara, N., T. Koseki, J. Lin, L. del Peso, P. C. Lucas, F. F. Chen, Y. Ogura, and G. Nunez.** 2000. An induced proximity model for NF-kappa B activation in the Nod1/RICK and RIP signaling pathways. *J. Biol. Chem.* **275:** 27823–27831.

50. **Inohara, N., Y. Ogura, F. F. Chen, A. Muto, and G. Nunez.** 2001. Human nod1 confers responsiveness to bacterial lipopolysaccharides. *J. Biol. Chem.* **276**:2551–2554.

51. **Janeway, C. A.** 1992. The immune system evolved to discriminate infectious nonself from noninfectious self. *Immunol. Today* **13**:11.

52. **Jung, H. C., L. Eckmann, S. K. Yang, A. Panja, J. Fierer, E. Morzycka-Wroblewska, and M. F. Kagnoff.** 1995. A distinct array of proinflammatory cytokines is expressed in human colon epithelial cells in response to bacterial invasion. *J. Clin. Invest.* **95**:55–65.

53. **Kadowaki, N., S. Ho, S. Antonenko, R. W. Malefyt, R. A. Kastelein, F. Bazan, and Y. J. Liu.** 2001. Subsets of human dendritic cell precursors express different Toll-like receptors and respond to different microbial antigens. *J. Exp. Med.* **194**:863–869.

54. **Kagnoff, M. F., and L. Eckmann.** 1997. Epithelial cells as sensors for microbial infection. *J. Clin. Invest.* **100**:6–10.

55. **Kaisho, T., and S. Akira.** 2001. Dendritic-cell function in Toll-like receptor- and MyD88-knockout mice. *Trends Immunol.* **22**:78–83.

56. **Kaisho, T., O. Takeuchi, T. Kawai, K. Hoshino, and S. Akira.** 2001. Endotoxin-induced maturation of myd88-deficient dendritic cells. *J. Immunol.* **166**:5688–5694.

57. **Kang, T. J., and G. T. Chae.** 2001. Detection of Toll-like receptor 2 (TLR2) mutation in the lepromatous leprosy patients. *FEMS Immunol. Med. Microbiol.* **31**:53–58.

58. **Kawahara, T., Y. Kuwano, S. Teshima-Kondo, T. Kawai, T. Nikawa, K. Kishi, and K. Rokutan.** 2001. Toll-like receptor 4 regulates gastric pit cell responses to *Helicobacter pylori* infection. *J. Med. Invest.* **48**:190–197.

59. **Kawahara, T., Y. Kuwano, S. Teshima-Kondo, T. Sugiyama, T. Kawai, T. Nikawa, K. Kishi, and K. Rokutan.** 2001. *Helicobacter pylori* lipopolysaccharide from type I, but not type II strains, stimulates apoptosis of cultured gastric mucosal cells. *J. Med. Invest.* **48**:167–174.

60. **Kawai, T., O. Adachi, T. Ogawa, K. Takeda, and S. Akira.** 1999. Unresponsiveness of MyD88-deficient mice to endotoxin. *Immunity* **11**:115–122.

61. **Kawai, T., O. Takeuchi, T. Fujita, J. Inoue Ji, P. F. Muhlradt, S. Sato, K. Hoshino, and S. Akira.** 2001. Lipopolysaccharide stimulates the MyD88-independent pathway and results in activation of IFN-regulatory factor 3 and the expression of a subset of lipopolysaccharide-inducible genes. *J. Immunol.* **167**:5887–5894.

62. **Kawasaki, K., K. Gomi, and M. Nishijima.** 2001. Cutting edge: gln(22) of mouse MD-2 is essential for species-specific lipopolysaccharide mimetic action of taxol. *J. Immunol.* **166**:11–14.

63. **Kopp, E., R. Medzhitov, J. Carothers, C. Xiao, I. Douglas, C. A. Janeway, and S. Ghosh.** 1999. ECSIT is an evolutionarily conserved intermediate in the Toll/IL-1 signal transduction pathway. *Genes Dev.* **13**:2059–2071.

64. **Krutzik, S. R., P. A. Sieling, and R. L. Modlin.** 2001. The role of Toll-like receptors in host defense against microbial infection. *Curr. Opin. Immunol.* **13**:104–108.

65. **Kurt-Jones, E. A., L. Popova, L. Kwinn, L. M. Haynes, L. P. Jones, R. A. Tripp, E. E. Walsh, M. W. Freeman, D. T. Golenbock, L. J. Anderson, and R. W. Finberg.** 2000. Pattern recognition receptors TLR4 and CD14 mediate response to respiratory syncytial virus. *Nat. Immunol.* **1**:398–401.

66. **Levashina, E. A., E. Langley, C. Green, D. Gubb, M. Ashburner, J. A. Hoffmann, and J. M. Reichhart.** 1999. Constitutive activation of Toll-mediated antifungal defense in serpin-deficient *Drosophila*. *Science* **285**:1917–1919.

67. **Lorenz, E., M. Jones, C. Wohlford-Lenane, N. Meyer, K. L. Frees, N. C. Arbour, and D. A. Schwartz.** 2001. Genes other than TLR4 are involved in the response to inhaled LPS. *Am. J. Physiol. Lung Cell Mol. Physiol.* **281**:L1106–L1114.

68. **MacDonald, T. T., and S. Pettersson.** 2000. Bacterial regulation of intestinal immune responses. *Inflamm. Bowel Dis.* **6**:116–122.

69. **Matsuguchi, T., K. Takagi, T. Musikacharoen, and Y. Yoshikai.** 2000. Gene expressions of lipopolysaccharide receptors, Toll-like receptors 2 and 4, are differently regulated in mouse T lymphocytes. *Blood* **95**:1378–1385.

70. **Matsumura, T., A. Ito, T. Takii, H. Hayashi, and K. Onozaki.** 2000. Endotoxin and cytokine regulation of Toll-like receptor (TLR) 2 and TLR4 gene expression in murine liver and hepatocytes. *J. Interferon Cytokine Res.* **20**:915–921.

71. **Mayer, L.** 2000. Mucosal immunity and gastrointestinal antigen processing. *J. Pediatr. Gastroenterol. Nutr.* **30**:S4–S12.

72. **Mayer, L., D. Eisenhardt, P. Salomon, W. Bauer, R. Plous, and L. Piccinini.** 1991. Ex-

pression of class II molecules on intestinal epithelial cells in humans: differences between normal and inflammatory bowel disease. *Gastroenterology* **100:**3.

73. **Means, T. K., D. T. Golenbock, and M. J. Fenton.** 2000. Structure and function of Toll-like receptor proteins. *Life Sci.* **68:**241–258.

74. **Medvedev, A. E., K. M. Kopydlowski, and S. N. Vogel.** 2000. Inhibition of lipopolysaccharide-induced signal transduction in endotoxin-tolerized mouse macrophages: dysregulation of cytokine, chemokine, and Toll-like receptor 2 and 4 gene expression. *J. Immunol.* **164:**5564–5574.

75. **Medzhitov, R., and C. A. Janeway.** 2000. Innate immunity. *N. Engl. J. Med.* **343:**338–344.

76. **Medzhitov, R., P. Preston-Hurlburt, and C. A. Janeway.** 1997. A human homologue of the *Drosophila* Toll protein signals activation of adaptive immunity. *Nature* **388:**394–397.

77. **Meijssen, M. A., S. L. Brandwein, H. C. Reinecker, A. K. Bhan, and D. K. Podolsky.** 1998. Alteration of gene expression by intestinal epithelial cells precedes colitis in interleukin-2-deficient mice. *Am. J. Physiol.* **274:**G472–G479.

78. **Miettinen, M., T. Sareneva, I. Julkunen, and S. Matikainen.** 2001. IFNs activate Toll-like receptor gene expression in viral infections. *Genes Immun.* **2:**349–355.

79. **Muzio, M., D. Bosisio, N. Polentarutti, G. D'Amico, A. Stoppacciaro, R. Mancinelli, C. van't Veer, G. Penton-Rol, L. P. Ruco, P. Allavena, and A. Mantovani.** 2000. Differential expression and regulation of Toll-like receptors (TLR) in human leukocytes: selective expression of TLR3 in dendritic cells. *J. Immunol.* **164:**5998–6004.

80. **Muzio, M., N. Polentarutti, D. Bosisio, M. K. Prahladan, and A. Mantovani.** 2000. Toll-like receptors: a growing family of immune receptors that are differentially expressed and regulated by different leukocytes. *J. Leukoc. Biol.* **67:**450–456.

81. **Naik, S., E. J. Kelly, L. Meijer, S. Pettersson, and I. R. Sanderson.** 2001. Absence of Toll-like receptor 4 explains endotoxin hyporesponsiveness in human intestinal epithelium. *J. Pediatr. Gastroenterol. Nutr.* **32:**449–453.

82. **Nathan, C., and A. Ding.** 2001. TREM-1: A new regulator of innate immunity in sepsis syndrome. *Nat. Med.* **7:**530–532.

83. **Neish, A. S., A. T. Gewirtz, H. Zeng, A. N. Young, M. E. Hobert, V. Karmali, A. S. Rao, and J. L. Madara.** 2000. Prokaryotic regulation of epithelial responses by inhibition of IkappaB-alpha ubiquination. *Science* **289:**1560–1563.

84. **Ogura, Y., D. K. Bonen, N. Inohara, D. L. Nicolae, F. F. Chen, R. Ramos, H. Britton, T. Moran, R. Karaliuskas, R. H. Duerr, J. P. Aklar, S. R. Brant, T. M. Bayless, B. S. Kirschner, S. B. Hanauer, G. Nunez, and J. H. Cho.** 2001. A frameshift mutation in NOD2 associated with susceptibility to Crohn's disease. *Nature* **411:**603–608.

85. **Ohashi, K., V. Burkart, S. Flohe, and H. Kolb.** 2000. Cutting edge: heat shock protein 60 is a putative endogenous ligand of the Toll-like receptor-4 complex. *J. Immunol.* **164:**558–561.

86. **Okamura, Y., M. Watari, E. S. Jerud, D. W. Young, S. T. Ishizaka, J. Rose, J. C. Chow, and J. F. Strauss 3rd.** 2001. The extra domain A of fibronectin activates Toll-like receptor 4. *J. Biol. Chem.* **276:**10229–10233.

87. **O'Neill, L.** 2000. The Toll/interleukin-1 receptor domain: a molecular switch for inflammation and host defence. *Biochem. Soc. Trans.* **28:**557–563.

88. **O'Neill, L.** 2001. Specificity in the innate response: pathogen recognition by Toll-like receptor combinations. *Trends Immunol.* **22:**70.

89. **Ozinsky, A., D. M. Underhill, J. D. Fontenot, A. M. Hajjar, K. D. Smith, C. B. Wilson, L. Schroeder, and A. Aderem.** 2000. The repertoire for pattern recognition of pathogens by the innate immune system is defined by cooperation between Toll-like receptors. *Proc. Natl. Acad. Sci. USA* **97:**13766–13771.

90. **Perera, P. Y., T. N. Mayadas, O. Takeuchi, S. Akira, M. Zaks-Zilberman, S. M. Goyert, and S. N. Vogel.** 2001. CD11b/CD18 acts in concert with CD14 and Toll-like receptor (TLR) 4 to elicit full lipopolysaccharide and taxol-inducible gene expression. *J. Immunol.* **166:**574–581.

91. **Podolsky, D. K.** 1999. Mucosal immunity and inflammation. V. Innate mechanisms of mucosal defense and repair: the best offense is a good defense. *Am. J. Physiol.* **277:**G495–G499.

92. **Podolsky, D. K.** 2000. Review article: healing after inflammatory injury—coordination of a regulatory peptide network. *Aliment. Pharmacol. Ther.* **14**(Supp. 1):87–93.

93. **Poltorak, A., P. Ricciardi-Castagnoli, S. Citterio, and B. Beutler.** 2000. Physical contact between lipopolysaccharide and Toll-like receptor 4 revealed by genetic complementation. *Proc. Natl. Acad. Sci. USA* **97:**2163–2167.

94. **Pridmore, A. C., D. H. Wyllie, F. Abdillahi, L. Steeghs, P. van der Ley, S. K. Dower, and R. C. Read.** 2001. A lipopolysaccharide-deficient mutant of *Neisseria meningitidis* elicits attenuated cytokine release by human macrophages

and signals via Toll-like receptor (TLR) 2 but not via TLR4/MD2. *J. Infect. Dis.* **183:**89–96.

95. **Pugin, J., C. C. Schurer-Maly, D. Leturcq, A. Moriarty, R. J. Ulevitch, and P. S. Tobias.** 1993. Lipopolysaccharide activation of human endothelial and epithelial cells is mediated by lipopolysaccharide-binding protein and soluble CD14. *Proc. Natl. Acad. Sci. USA* **90:** 2744–2748.

96. **Qureshi, S. T., P. Gros, and D. Malo.** 1999. The Lps locus: genetic regulation of host responses to bacterial lipopolysaccharide. *Inflamm. Res.* **48:**613–620.

97. **Randow, F., and B. Seed.** 2001. Endoplasmic reticulum chaperone gp96 is required for innate immunity but not cell viability. *Nat. Cell Biol.* **3:**891–896.

98. **Rehli, M., A. Poltorak, L. Schwarzfischer, S. W. Krause, R. Andreesen, and B. Beutler.** 2000. PU.1 and interferon consensus sequence-binding protein regulate the myeloid expression of the human Toll-like receptor 4 gene. *J. Biol. Chem.* **275:**9773–9781.

99. **Rock, F. L., G. Hardiman, J. C. Timans, R. A. Kastelein, and J. F. Bazan.** 1998. A family of human receptors structurally related to *Drosophila* Toll. *Proc. Natl. Acad. Sci. USA* **95:** 588–593.

100. **Sato, S., F. Nomura, T. Kawai, O. Takeuchi, P. F. Muhlradt, K. Takeda, and S. Akira.** 2000. Synergy and cross-tolerance between Toll-like receptor (TLR) 2- and TLR4-mediated signaling pathways. *J. Immunol.* **165:** 7096–7101.

101. **Schumann, R. R.** 1992. Function of lipopolysaccharide (LPS)-binding protein (LBP) and CD14, the receptor for LPS/LBP complexes: a short review. *Res. Immunol.* **143:**11–15.

102. **Seki, E., H. Tsutsui, H. Nakano, N. M. Tsuji, K. Hoshino, O. Adachi, K. Adachi, S. Futatsugi, K. Kuida, O. Takeuchi, H. Okamura, J. Fujimoto, S. Akira, and K. Nakanishi.** 2001. Lipopolysaccharide-induced IL-18 secretion from murine Kupffer cells independently of MyD88 that is critically involved in induction of production of IL-12 and IL-1β. *J. Immunol.* **166:**2651–2657.

103. **Seya, T., M. Matsumoto, S. Tsuji, N. A. Begum, M. Nomura, I. Azuma, A. Hayashi, and K. Toyoshima.** 2001. Two receptor theory in innate immune activation: studies on the receptors for bacillus Callmette-Guérin-cell wall skeleton. *Arch. Immunol. Ther. Exp.* (Warszawa) **49:**S13–S21.

104. **Seydel, K. B., E. Li, P. E. Swanson, and S. L. Stanley, Jr.** 1997. Human intestinal epithelial cells produce proinflammatory cytokines in response to infection in a SCID mouse-human intestinal xenograft model of amebiasis. *Infect. Immun.* **65:**1631–1639.

105. **Shen, B., and J. L. Manley.** 1998. Phosphorylation modulates direct interactions between the Toll receptor, Pelle kinase and Tube. *Development* **125:**4719–4728.

106. **Shuto, T., H. Xu, B. Wang, J. Han, H. Kai, X. X. Gu, T. F. Murphy, D. J. Lim, and J. D. Li.** 2001. Activation of NF-kappa B by nontypeable *Hemophilus influenzae* is mediated by Toll-like receptor 2-TAK1-dependent NIK-IKK alpha/beta-I kappa B alpha and MKK3/6-p38 MAP kinase signaling pathways in epithelial cells. *Proc. Natl. Acad. Sci. USA* **98:** 8774–8779.

107. **Smith, P. D., E. N. Janoff, M. Mosteller-Barnum, M. Merger, J. M. Orenstein, J. F. Kearney, and M. F. Graham.** 1997. Isolation and purification of CD14-negative mucosal macrophages from normal human small intestine. *J. Immunol. Methods* **202:**1–11.

108. **Smith, P. D., L. E. Smythies, M. Mosteller-Barnum, D. A. Sibley, M. W. Russell, M. Merger, M. T. Sellers, J. M. Orenstein, T. Shimada, M. F. Graham, and H. Kubagawa.** 2001. Intestinal macrophages lack CD14 and CD89 and consequently are down-regulated for LPS- and IgA-mediated activities. *J. Immunol.* **167:**2651–2656.

109. **Staege, H., A. Schaffner, and M. Schneemann.** 2000. Human Toll-like receptors 2 and 4 are targets for deactivation of mononuclear phagocytes by interleukin-4. *Immunol. Lett.* **71:** 1–3.

110. **Takeshita, F., C. A. Leifer, I. Gursel, K. J. Ishii, S. Takeshita, M. Gursel, and D. M. Klinman.** 2001. Cutting edge: role of Toll-like receptor 9 in CpG DNA-induced activation of human cells. *J. Immunol.* **167:**3555–3558.

111. **Takeuchi, O., K. Hoshino, and S. Akira.** 2000. Cutting edge: TLR2-deficient and MyD88-deficient mice are highly susceptible to *Staphylococcus Aureus* infection. *J. Immunol.* **165:** 5392–5396.

112. **Takeuchi, O., K. Hoshino, T. Kawai, H. Sanjo, H. Takada, T. Ogawa, K. Takeda, and S. Akira.** 1999. Differential roles of TLR2 and TLR4 in recognition of gram-negative and gram-positive bacterial cell wall components. *Immunity* **11:**443–451.

113. **Takeuchi, O., T. Kawai, H. Sanjo, N. G. Copeland, D. J. Gilbert, N. A. Jenkins, K. Takeda, and S. Akira.** 1999. TLR6: a novel member of an expanding Toll-like receptor family. *Gene* **231:**59–65.

114. **Takeuchi, O., K. Takeda, K. Hoshino, O. Adachi, T. Ogawa, and S. Akira.** 2000. Cellular responses to bacterial cell wall components are mediated through MyD88-dependent signaling cascades. *Int. Immunol.* **12:**113–117.

115. **Tapping, R. I., S. Akashi, K. Miyake, P. J. Godowski, and P. S. Tobias.** 2000. Toll-like receptor 4, but not Toll-like receptor 2, is a signaling receptor for *Escherichia* and *Salmonella* lipopolysaccharides. *J. Immunol.* **165:**5780–5787.

116. **Thoma-Uszynski, S., S. M. Kiertscher, M. T. Ochoa, D. A. Bouis, M. V. Norgard, K. Miyake, P. J. Godowski, M. D. Roth, and R. L. Modlin.** 2000. Activation of Toll-like receptor 2 on human dendritic cells triggers induction of IL-12, but not IL-10. *J. Immunol.* **165:**3804–3810.

117. **Uehara, A., S. Sugawara, R. Tamai, and H. Takada.** 2001. Contrasting responses of human gingival and colonic epithelial cells to lipopolysaccharides, lipoteichoic acids and peptidoglycans in the presence of soluble CD14. *Med. Microbiol. Immunol.* (Berlin) **189:**185–192.

118. **Underhill, D. M., A. Ozinsky, A. M. Hajjar, A. Stevens, C. B. Wilson, M. Bassetti, and A. Aderem.** 1999. The Toll-like receptor 2 is recruited to macrophage phagosomes and discriminates between pathogens. *Nature* **401:**811–815.

119. **Visintin, A., A. Mazzoni, J. A. Spitzer, and D. M. Segal.** 2001. Secreted MD-2 is a large polymeric protein that efficiently confers lipopolysaccharide sensitivity to Toll-like receptor 4. *Proc. Natl. Acad. Sci. USA* **98:**12156–12161.

120. **Visintin, A., A. Mazzoni, J. H. Spitzer, D. H. Wyllie, S. K. Dower, and D. M. Segal.** 2001. Regulation of Toll-like receptors in human monocytes and dendritic cells. *J. Immunol.* **166:**249–255.

121. **Vogel, S. N., D. Johnson, P. Y. Perera, A. Medvedev, L. Lariviere, S. T. Qureshi, and D. Malo.** 1999. Cutting edge: functional characterization of the effect of the C3H/HeJ defect in mice that lack an Lpsn gene: in vivo evidence for a dominant negative mutation. *J. Immunol.* **162:**5666–5670.

122. **Wang, Q., R. Dziarski, C. J. Kirschning, M. Muzio, and D. Gupta.** 2001. Micrococci and peptidoglycan activate TLR2→MyD88→IRAK→TRAF→NIK→IKK→NF-kappaB signal transduction pathway that induces transcription of interleukin-8. *Infect. Immun.* **69:**2270–2276.

123. **Werts, C., R. I. Tapping, J. C. Mathison, T. H. Chuang, V. Kravchenko, I. Saint Girons, D. A. Haake, P. Godowski, F. Hayashi, A. Ozinsky, D. M. Underhill, C. J. Kirschning, H. Wagner, A. Aderem, P. S. Tobias, and R. J. Ulevitch.** 2001. Leptospiral lipopolysaccharide activates cells through a TLR2-dependent mechanism. *Nat. Immunol.* **2:**346–352.

124. **Wesche, H., W. J. Henzel, W. Shillinglaw, S. Li, and Z. Cao.** 1997. MyD88: an adapter that recruits IRAK to the IL-1 receptor complex. *Immunity* **7:**837–847.

125. **Witthoft, T., L. Eckmann, J. M. Kim, and M. F. Kagnoff.** 1998. Enteroinvasive bacteria directly activate expression of iNOS and NO production in human colon epithelial cells. *Am. J. Physiol.* **275:**G564–G571.

126. **Xavier, R. J., and D. K. Podolsky.** 2000. Microbiology. How to get along—friendly microbes in a hostile world [comment]. *Science* **289:**1483–1484.

127. **Xu, Y., X. Tao, B. Shen, T. Horng, R. Medzhitov, J. L. Manley, and L. Tong.** 2000. Structural basis for signal transduction by the Toll/interleukin-1 receptor domains. *Nature* **408:**111–115.

128. **Yang, S. K., L. Eckmann, A. Panja, and M. F. Kagnoff.** 1997. Differential and regulated expression of C-X-C, C-C, and C-chemokines by human colon epithelial cells *Gastroenterology* **113:**1214–1223.

129. **Zhang, F. X., C. J. Kirschning, R. Mancinelli, X. P. Xu, Y. Jin, E. Faure, A. Mantovani, M. Rothe, M. Muzio, and M. Arditi.** 1999. Bacterial lipopolysaccharide activates nuclear factor-kappaB through interleukin-1 signaling mediators in cultured human dermal endothelial cells and mononuclear phagocytes. *J. Biol. Chem.* **274:**7611–7614.

INTESTINAL IMMUNOGLOBULIN A: ROLE IN HOST DEFENSE

Jiri Mestecky and Michael W. Russell

6

IMPORTANCE OF IgA IN INTESTINAL PROTECTION

The major source of stimulation of the entire immune system is the external environment, comprising potentially pathogenic microorganisms, many species of the commensal mucosal microbiota, food antigens, and allergens, all of which are encountered primarily at mucosal surfaces that cover an enormous surface area. This evolutionary selective pressure has resulted in a strategically and functionally advantageous distribution of cells involved in the handling of antigens and the initiation of immune responses in mucosal tissues. The mucosal immune system contains the onslaught of such antigens by mechanisms that do not compromise the integrity of the mucosal barrier by providing antigen-specific protection through antibodies and mucosal T cells. Characteristic features of all antibodies include their ability to react specifically with a very wide variety of antigens. However, the subsequent fate of antigen-antibody complexes depends largely on the Fc regions of immunoglobulins (Ig), which determine the biological properties of the different isotypes. The outcomes of antigen-antibody union may be dramatically different and range from life-saving protection (e.g., neutralization of tetanus toxin) to death of the individual (e.g., anaphylactic reaction to insect bites). The characteristic distribution of antibodies in body fluids of higher vertebrates is reflected in the functional advantages of the various Ig isotypes.

Readers of this brief review may be surprised to learn that the majority of antibodies are produced in mucosal lymphoid tissues, particularly in the intestine, rather than in the spleen, lymph nodes, or bone marrow, and that more than half of total antibodies produced appear in the secretions of mucosal tissues and their associated glands (71). When the daily synthesis of all isotypes of Ig is taken into account, the production of IgA far exceeds the combined synthesis of IgG, IgM, IgD, and IgE; however, more than two-thirds of total IgA finishes its short life span in the external secretions (71). Quantitative studies of the origin of IgA in the human intestinal lumen have convincingly demonstrated that ~99% is of local origin and only trace amounts are derived from the circulation (37).

This volume of IgA production and the selectivity of its distribution raise the question

Jiri Mestecky, Department of Microbiology and Department of Medicine, University of Alabama at Birmingham, 845 19th St. South, Birmingham, AL 35294-2170. *Michael W. Russell*, Department of Microbiology, University of Buffalo, 138 Farber Hall, 3435 Main St., Buffalo, NY 14214-3000.

Microbial Pathogenesis and the Intestinal Epithelial Cell, ed. by G. Hecht
© 2003 ASM Press, Washington, D.C.

of Ig function, particularly IgA, in external secretions. It should be emphasized that the mucosal microbiota, epithelial cells, and the immune system, especially its humoral component predominantly represented by IgA, constitute an interdependent "tripod" which, under normal conditions, stabilizes the mucosal microenvironment by complex mechanisms. This basic concept and the essential protective role of intestinal antibodies in survival were most convincingly demonstrated almost 40 years ago in a unique model of germfree, colostrum- and milk-deprived newborn piglets (86). The essential features of this model include the placental barrier and absence of Ig Fc receptors on placental cells so that piglets, unlike humans, are born without any transplacentally acquired antibodies. For about the first 36 h, the intestinal epithelium of a newborn piglet is permeable and allows absorption of colostral/milk antibodies, predominantly IgG rather than IgA, into the circulation. Colostrum- and milk-deprived piglets invariably die within ~72 h of septicemia usually caused by *Escherichia coli*, whereas milk-fed animals survive. The argument that protection is mediated by circulating antibodies absorbed from milk that, in concert with complement, kill invading *E. coli* was contravened by infecting animals *after* closure of the epithelial barrier so that milk antibodies were no longer absorbed but remained in the gut lumen. Although all control animals given *E. coli* orally succumbed to infection, experimental animals that also orally received immune milk or serum (or isolated antibodies) survived irrespective of the source or isotype of Ig provided. These elegant experiments clearly demonstrate that antibodies act locally within the intestinal lumen and prevent otherwise fatal infection with normally commensal bacteria.

Further support for the operation of IgA-mediated protection within the intestinal lumen has more recently been provided in the mouse IgA antibody-secreting tumor "backpack" model (49, 74). In this model, a polymeric (p) IgA hybridoma specific for a selected pathogen is implanted subcutaneously on the back of mice, and the pIgA antibody secreted into the circulation is transported into the intestine by hepatobiliary transport, since mice express the polymeric Ig receptor (pIgR) on their hepatocytes. Pathogen-specific IgA hybridoma antibodies thus transported into the intestine have been demonstrated to protect mice against oral challenge with *Salmonella enterica* serovar Typhimurium, *Vibrio cholerae*, or rotavirus, whereas IgG antibodies that are not transported are not protective (92). J-chain-knockout mice, which cannot assemble secretory IgA (S-IgA), are not protected against enteric challenge with cholera toxin despite the presence of circulating IgG and IgA antibodies (58).

An important observation is that indigenous mucosal bacteria are coated in vivo with corresponding antibodies without any apparent functional impairment (5, 101, 112). It is probably significant that mucosal immunity does not result in intestinal sterility, since the complete destruction of the commensal microbiota would be detrimental, as these organisms are essential for the physiological function of epithelial cells and the intestinal immune system, as well as a source of certain beneficial products (e.g., butyric acid, vitamin K) (98). However, IgG or IgM antibodies may functionally substitute for IgA in some experimental systems. This may be one major reason for the relatively unimpaired health of humans with the most common immunodeficiency disorder, selective IgA deficiency (13).

STRUCTURAL FEATURES IMPORTANT IN IgA FUNCTION

IgA and IgG, which are confined to birds and mammals, presumably evolved from earlier Ig isotypes with the phylogenetic divergence of these vertebrate classes from the reptiles (82). Some of the structural and functional features of IgM are also seen in IgA molecules. Sequence homologies between the Fc regions of μ and α chains include the C-terminal 18-amino-acid extension relative to other isotypes; this short "tail" is structurally required for IgM and IgA to form polymers and to bind the glycoprotein J chain, a characteristic component of polymeric Ig (71). IgM in the sera and secretions of lower vertebrates occurs in tetrameric (four subunits comprising two heavy and two light chains) or pentameric configurations, and IgA occurs in dimeric or tetrameric forms as well as monomers. In addition to the presence of multiple antigen-binding sites (see below), the polymeric configuration and presence of J chain are essential for the ability of IgM or IgA to interact with the pIgR that is expressed on epithelial cells (and hepatocytes in some species) and that transports IgM and pIgA through epithelial cells (77). Interestingly, the transport of IgM represents an important compensatory mechanism that protects the mucosae of IgA-deficient individuals (13). The ability to generate IgM and mucosal IgA responses develops shortly after birth concomitantly with extensive stimulation of the mucosal immune system with exogenous antigens (18, 56, 66).

The interplay between the epithelium and immune cells is a distinct and important feature of the mucosal immune system. Thus, epithelial cells transport pIgA and IgM into the lumen and in so doing contribute the secretory component (SC), the extracellular part of pIgR, to the secretory Ig as a one-trip receptor that also enhances their functional properties (see below). Expression of pIgR on the basolateral surface of epithelial cells is regulated by cytokines, particularly gamma interferon (IFN-γ), tumor necrosis factor alpha (TNF-α), and interleukin 4 (IL-4), secreted by lymphocytes or macrophages (77, 81). Epithelial cells express major histocompatibility complex (MHC) class II molecules under regulation by these cytokines, as well as non-classical MHC class I molecules, and have been demonstrated to present antigens to T cells in vitro (62), although debate continues over whether this results in IgA- or T-cell-mediated immunity, or tolerance in vivo. Moreover, epithelial cells secrete inflammatory cytokines and chemokines (including IL-1, IL-6, IL-7, IL-8, IL-10, and transforming growth factor beta (TGF-β), especially in response to microbial challenge, which are involved in the influx, activation, and differentiation of lymphoid and myeloid cells (27). Indeed, some of these cytokines may be responsible for the selective differentiation of pIgA-secreting plasma cell precursors after they home to the lamina propria.

In humans and hominoid primates, further diversification of IgA forms and functions has occurred. In contrast to the dominance of pIgA in secretions including tears; saliva; nasal, intestinal, and vaginal washes; bile; semen; and milk, the major proportion of circulating IgA is monomeric (mIgA). Molecular size analysis of pIgA in selected external secretions (e.g., saliva and milk) has shown the presence of both dimers and tetramers in a ratio of ~3:2 (9, 68, 122). Furthermore, two subclasses, IgA1 and IgA2, have evolved and are distributed differently in various body fluids (72). Approximately equal amounts of IgA1 and IgA2 are found in the large intestine and female genital tract (sometimes IgA2 levels are slightly higher), whereas higher proportions of IgA1 occur in other external secretions (71). The distribution of pIgA/mIgA and IgA1/IgA2 in these fluids parallels the distribution of cells involved in their production (8, 71). Analyses of IgA molecular forms in perfusates of human intestinal explants and in supernatants of intestinal plasma cells, and immuno-histochemical evaluation using markers of pIgA production (the presence of J chain and ability to bind SC), show that the clear majority of IgA cells in the gut are engaged in the production of pIgA (8, 71). By the same criteria, IgA-producing cells in the bone marrow, the major source of plasma IgA, secrete almost exclusively mIgA (3). Staining of mucosal tissues and immunochemical studies of intestinal fluids with IgA subclass-specific antibodies show that, in the small intestine, ~60 to 80% of cells produce IgA1 and 20 to 40% produce IgA2, while in the large intestine ~60% produce IgA2 and ~40% produce IgA1; ~90% of IgA cells in the bone marrow produce IgA1 (17, 41).

IgM and pIgA have certain functional advantages in comparison to mIgA and IgG. Although the intrinsic affinity of the antigen-binding sites on IgM or pIgA is usually lower than that of IgG, the presence of multiple antigen-binding sites in pentameric IgM and in IgA dimers or tetramers confers enhanced antigen-binding ability and greater neutralizing activity due to the bonus effect of multivalency, which increases functional avidity. Furthermore, the binding of pIgA to SC renders the resultant S-IgA more resistant to proteolytic enzymes (19, 55), which is of obvious advantage for its functionality in secretions rich in proteolytic enzymes such as intestinal fluids. Although Fab and Fc fragments can be generated in vitro, for example, using trypsin, nonphysiological conditions (increased temperature and salt concentration) are required for optimal cleavage (67, 122). However, IgA1 is uniquely sensitive to proteolysis by bacterial IgA1 proteases because of the presence of an unusual hinge region containing susceptible Pro-Ser or Pro-Thr sequences (45) (for details, see below).

Recently, the glycans associated with cell surfaces and soluble glycoproteins, including Ig, have received considerable attention with respect to function (2, 88a, 90). For example, cell-surface glycoproteins are involved in intercellular communication, such as the homing of lymphocytes to various tissues, and in cell activation. Glycan moieties on IgA, as well as on the Fcα receptor, play an important role in IgA binding and its subsequent internalization and catabolism (70, 75). Ig-associated glycans greatly influence the ability of different isotypes to activate complement by the alternative and lectin pathways (80) and thus initiate inflammatory responses.

In human IgA, glycans contribute approximately 6 to 11% of total molecular mass, with marked structural variation between IgA1, IgA2, and S-IgA (71). N-Linked glycans are present on all IgA molecules, and a larger number occur on IgA2 and S-IgA (owing to the heavily glycosylated SC) than on IgA1. The constant regions of IgA2 heavy chains each contain four or five N-linked glycan chains compared to two in IgA1, and the hinge region of each IgA1 heavy chain also contains three to five short O-linked glycan chains (61). Detailed studies of several human IgA1 and IgA2 myeloma proteins have revealed marked variability in the total content, composition, and number of glycans (24). High-mannose-type N-linked glycans in both IgA1 and IgA2 and sialyloligosaccharides on S-IgA may be involved in the inhibition of adherence of certain species of bacteria to receptors expressed on intestinal epithelial cells (2, 99, 118). This concept has been recently expanded to O-linked glycans in the hinge region of IgA1 and N-glycans on SC, which are likely to display additional epitopes potentially involved as bacteria-binding sites (88a). Thus, in addition to the protective functions of S-IgA mediated by the specific antigen binding through the variable regions of heavy and light chains, O- and N-linked glycans endow IgA and particularly S-IgA molecules with further nonspecific or innate bacteria-binding sites. Furthermore, N-linked glycans within the variable region may also play a role in polyreactivity of IgA, as discussed below.

FUNCTIONS OF IgA ANTIBODIES AT INTESTINAL EPITHELIAL SURFACES

Direct Functions

The most widely recognized protective mechanism of S-IgA antibodies against pathogens at mucosal surfaces is inhibition of adherence (Fig. 1), which has been demonstrated with S-IgA antibodies to microbial surface antigens in the context of pharyngeal, intestinal, and genitourinary tract epithelia as well as tooth surfaces (31, 92). The Fc.SC part of S-IgA in particular confers a negatively charged, hydrophilic shell on microbes that repels attachment to a mucosal surface. In addition, agglutination of microorganisms by polymeric S-IgA antibodies facilitates their removal in flowing secretions. Human IgA may also be able to bind bacteria by means of its glycan chains and

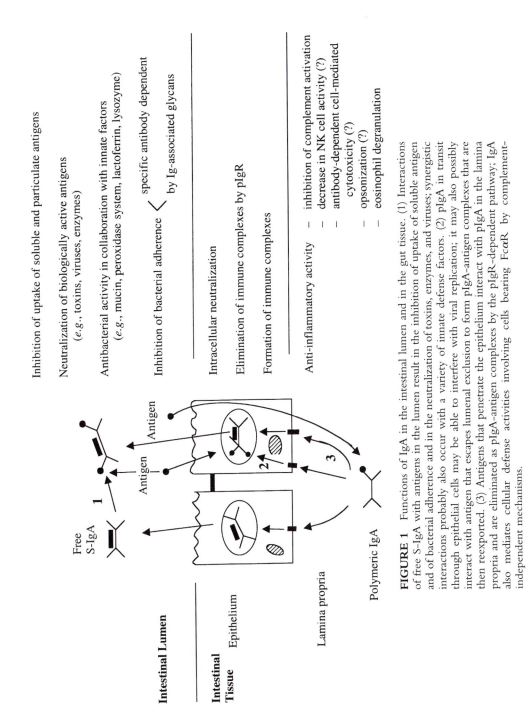

Inhibition of uptake of soluble and particulate antigens

Neutralization of biologically active antigens
(e.g., toxins, viruses, enzymes)

Antibacterial activity in collaboration with innate factors
(e.g., mucin, peroxidase system, lactoferrin, lysozyme)

Inhibition of bacterial adherence < specific antibody dependent
by Ig-associated glycans

Intracellular neutralization

Elimination of immune complexes by pIgR

Formation of immune complexes

Anti-inflammatory activity – inhibition of complement activation
                             – decrease in NK cell activity (?)
                             – antibody–dependent cell-mediated
                                cytotoxicity (?)
                             – opsonization (?)
                             – eosinophil degranulation

FIGURE 1 Functions of IgA in the intestinal lumen and in the gut tissue. (1) Interactions of free S–IgA with antigens in the lumen result in the inhibition of uptake of soluble antigen and of bacterial adherence and in the neutralization of toxins, enzymes, and viruses; synergistic interactions probably also occur with a variety of innate defense factors. (2) pIgA in transit through epithelial cells may be able to interfere with viral replication; it may also possibly interact with antigen that escapes lumenal exclusion to form pIgA–antigen complexes that are then reexported. (3) Antigens that penetrate the epithelium interact with pIgA in the lamina propria and are eliminated as pIgA–antigen complexes by the pIgR–dependent pathway; IgA also mediates cellular defense activities involving cells bearing FcαR by complement–independent mechanisms.

thereby agglutinate them or inhibit their adherence (88a, 91, 99, 118). This has been demonstrated in vitro with *E. coli* type 1 (mannose-dependent) pilus-mediated adherence to epithelial cells and the mannose-rich glycans found especially on IgA2 (118). In analogous experiments, human colostral S-IgA inhibited the adherence of S-fimbriated *E. coli* to human epithelial cells by sialyloligosaccharides (sialyl [α2,3]galactose) present in *N*- and *O*-linked glycans (99). Similar binding of IgA1 has been reported by oral actinomycetes and streptococci and may, therefore, also be effective inhibitors of bacterial attachment (91). As *Lactobacillus plantarum* has been shown to adhere to HT-29 intestinal epithelial cells in vitro through mannose-specific mechanisms, it is possible that its adherence would also be inhibitable by high-mannose glycans on IgA (2).

The binding of S–IgA antibodies to biologically active molecules may neutralize such activity (Fig. 1), whether by directly occluding the active site, by steric hindrance of access to the site, or by inducing allosteric conformational change in the molecule. Several instances of neutralization of enzymes and toxins have been reported (reviewed in reference 92). In some cases, such neutralization is independent of antibody isotype or even the presence of the Fc region, so that, for example, the cleaved Fabα fragments of IgA1 antibodies against IgA1 proteases retain enzyme-inhibiting activity. In contrast, *Clostridium difficile* toxin A is more effectively neutralized by pIgA than by mIgA or IgG antibodies bearing the same antigen-binding site (109).

Viruses can also be neutralized by S–IgA antibodies through several mechanisms, such as inhibition of binding to cellular receptors or of internalization and intracellular replication. Antibody isotype and molecular form may play a role, as S–IgA antibodies are more effective than IgG in mediating cross-protective immunity against different antigenic variants of influenza virus, and dimeric IgA antibody neutralizes transmissible gastroenteritis virus more effectively than monomeric IgG (14, 53, 87). In contrast, polymeric IgA antibodies

have been shown to promote the uptake of Epstein-Barr virus (EBV) by pIgR-expressing epithelial cells, although any isotype of antibody can neutralize its infectivity for B cells (105). Similarly, infection of FcαR-expressing monocytes by human immunodeficiency virus (HIV) can be enhanced by IgA antibodies, whereas they interfere with infection of T cells (35, 48). However, the state of the cells is an important factor, as *polarized* epithelial cells or hepatocytes transport pIgA-coated EBV (28).

During pIgR-mediated transport across epithelial cells, pIgA antibodies may be able to neutralize viruses invading from the apical surface (Fig. 1). This has been demonstrated in vitro with Sendai and influenza viruses and pIgR-expressing polarized MDCK cells (63, 64), and some evidence suggests that IgA antibodies can similarly neutralize invading rotavirus or hepatitis viruses in vivo (32). However, given the speed with which pIgA traverses the epithelium (~30 min), S-IgA antibodies will inevitably be present in the lumen, where they may interact with the virus and then subsequently inhibit its replication within the epithelial cells. Moreover, the cells through which IgA is transported (mainly in the crypts) do not always coincide with the cells through which the viruses invade, which in the case of rotavirus is through the villus tips. Furthermore, for a virus to encounter specific IgA antibody in a particular epithelial cell, there would need to be a plasma cell secreting IgA of that specificity located in the immediately adjacent part of the lamina propria. As even in the most favorable circumstances (e.g., recent mucosal immunization with potent immunogens such as cholera toxin) specific IgA antibody-secreting cells account for 0.1 to 10% of all IgA-secreting cells in the lamina propria or salivary glands (120), this necessary condition will not often be met.

Absorption of food antigens is diminished by intestinal S-IgA antibodies induced by previous exposure (116) (Fig. 1). IgA-deficient subjects show increased absorption of food antigens and formation of circulating immune complexes (20), and it is thought that diminished immune exclusion could contribute to increased susceptibility to atopic allergies or autoimmune disease displayed by such individuals. It has further been proposed that S-IgA-mediated intestinal immunity could be exploited to inhibit the absorption of environmental carcinogens (103). The hepatobiliary transport and elimination of pIgA-complexed antigens, for example, undegradable bacterial polysaccharides, has been demonstrated in mice and rats. In this way, IgA antibodies, in contrast to IgM or IgG, can form immune complexes and dispose of antigens without inducing complement-mediated inflammation and consequent collateral damage to nearby tissues (12). This may be especially important in the preservation of mucosal integrity, since IgG antibodies against one antigen can promote the uptake of an unrelated bystander antigen through mucosal epithelia (10). An analogous pIgR-mediated transport of pIgA through epithelial cells has been demonstrated in vitro and proposed to remove absorbed antigens that become complexed with pIgA antibody in the lamina propria (39). However, as discussed in connection with intracellular viral neutralization, pIgA is transported mainly through crypt cells, whereas food materials are absorbed through the villi usually directly into the lacteals (89) and so are unlikely to come into contact with IgA secreted by plasma cells in the lamina propria.

Counterintuitively in light of the generally accepted view that S-IgA antibodies inhibit antigen absorption, S-IgA has been proposed to promote the uptake of antigens into Peyer's patch M cells (117) and thereby enhance mucosal immune responses to antigens complexed with it (16). These reports, however, conflict with the finding that S-IgA antibodies inhibit the entry of reovirus into M cells (104). However, it does appear that pneumococci are able to bind to pIgR and reverse the normal direction of its transcytosis, thereby exploiting it to gain entry across the respiratory epithelium (38, 121).

It is estimated that a large proportion of naturally occurring antibodies display a high degree of polyreactivity against many, often unrelated, antigens (85). Although the generation of such polyreactivity depends on somatic mutations, particularly in the third complementarity-determining region of the Ig heavy chains and multiple reassortment of heavy and light chain variable segments, more recent studies suggest that additional potential N-glycosylation sites are generated by somatic hypermutation in the heavy chain variable regions (21, 25, 26). As a consequence of increased (or decreased) variable region glycosylation, specificity or affinity for antigens may be substantially altered (21). While human intestinal plasma cells may lose potential glycosylation sites because of the high frequency of somatic mutation, IgA (and IgG) cells also have the greatest tendency to create such sites, and it is speculated that this broadens the antibody repertoire of intestinal IgA, perhaps particularly toward carbohydrate-containing antigens. Large amounts of polyreactive S-IgA antibodies that recognize a variety of self and microbial antigens have been described in human colostrum and saliva (85). Although such "natural" antibodies, possibly produced by B-1 cells, fail to detect major virulence factor antigens or toxins, they may afford a first line of defense against pathogens, perhaps in concert with protein Fv, prior to the development of more specific antibodies from conventional B-2 cells (7).

Indirect Functions

The original concept that S-IgA specifically associates with mucus to form an immunological "fly-paper" has been difficult to substantiate fully, and recent findings suggest that uncomplexed S-IgA can diffuse freely through mucus (96). Several observations, however, indicate that microorganisms coated with S-IgA antibodies become less hydrophobic and more easily entrapped in the mucus layer, thereby enhancing the activities of both S-IgA and mucin as inhibitors of bacterial adherence to epithelia (60). An interaction between salivary mucins and S-IgA is suggested by the finding that IgA colocalizes with high-molecular-weight mucin fractions, and S-IgA has been found to bind to mucin MG2 (4). The findings that spermatozoa coated with S-

IgA antibodies have impaired ability to penetrate cervical mucus and that treatment of the coated spermatozoa with IgA1 protease restores mobility (11), however, imply an interaction between the Fc.SC region of S-IgA and mucus.

Most mucosal secretions contain numerous humoral innate defense factors that kill or inhibit microorganisms. Given the variety of molecules involved and their diverse modes of action, there is wide scope for synergism between them and with S-IgA antibodies (Fig. 1), but these have received scant attention and few interactions have been described in molecular detail (reviewed in reference 92). S-IgA can form complexes and synergize with lactoferrin, possibly by antibody-mediated inhibition of alternative iron acquisition mechanisms in bacteria. The inhibition of bacterial metabolism by the lactoperoxidase-H_2O_2-thiocyanate system is enhanced by IgA, but this may be due to stabilization of enzyme activity. Lysis of *E. coli* by colostral S-IgA antibody, complement, and lysozyme has been difficult to confirm and may have been due to other contaminating isotypes of antibody. IgA is prone to form complexes with several other plasma and mucosal proteins, e.g., albumin, α1-antitrypsin, chymotrypsin, and also fibronectin, a glycoprotein having pronounced ability to inhibit the adherence of bacteria to cells (73).

The question of whether, and how, IgA interacts with the complement system has been a matter of some controversy (reviewed in reference 92). It is clear that IgA does not bind C1q or activate the classical complement pathway (CCP), as the C1q-binding motif is not present in IgA. However, the notion that IgA activates the alternative complement pathway (ACP) derives from experiments performed under nonphysiological conditions. Denatured, artificially aggregated, chemically crosslinked, or deglycosylated human IgA can activate the ACP in vitro. Constructs of human IgA2 and rat antibody complexed with a haptenated protein antigen, and IgA antibodies against certain encapsulated bacteria are

also reported to activate the ACP. However, carefully prepared human IgA antibodies complexed with corresponding antigen fail to activate the ACP. These conflicting findings may be due to several factors, such as whether the native conformation of IgA is fully preserved after purification, whether the IgA (especially if produced in nonhuman cells) is completely and correctly glycosylated, and whether the antigens themselves directly activate the ACP. In contrast, native IgA antibodies and Fabα fragments inhibit complement-dependent cytolysis induced by IgG or IgM antibody (Fig. 1). Recent reports suggest that IgA may initiate complement activation through the lectin pathway (88), but as with ACP activation, this presumably depends upon the glycan chains in IgA and whether these are intact, abnormal, or degraded by glycosidases. In general, human IgA antibodies physiologically complexed with antigen have poor to no complement-activating ability, whereas ACP activation is associated with denaturation or conformational change unrelated to antigen binding. Abnormal structural changes resulting from pathological conditions, such as aberrant synthesis or microbial degradation, however, may lead to complement activation, for example, in IgA nephropathy. Under normal physiological conditions, however, the abundance of IgA antibodies in mucosal tissues may aid in controlling complement-dependent inflammation where the maintenance of the epithelial barrier is important. It should also be noted that while some complement components can often be detected in secretions, they may not all be present in sufficiently high concentrations to constitute an active system.

Early reports described inhibition of neutrophil chemotaxis by myeloma IgA (114), and various concentration-dependent effects of IgA have been observed on the chemotaxis or chemokinesis of neutrophils in vitro (102). Numerous instances of complement-independent opsonization or antibody-dependent cellular cytotoxicity mediated by IgA antibodies have been reported (reviewed in references 40 and 92). The Fc receptor for IgA, FcαR (CD89), has been demonstrated in human neutrophils, eosinophils, and monocytes or macrophages (76), but curiously a murine homolog has not been identified. Although expressed constitutively, FcαR is upregulated on exudative neutrophils (e.g., from the gingival crevice), or on activation by cytokines (TNF-α, IL-8, and granulocyte and monocyte colony-stimulating factor [GM-CSF]), lipopolysaccharide (LPS), or IgA (reviewed in reference 92). In contrast, macrophages isolated from human intestine appear to lack FcαR (106). FcαR mediates phagocytosis and killing of bacteria opsonized by serum IgA of either subclass, but apparently not by S-IgA (113, 115), and also the postphagocytic respiratory burst in neutrophils in vitro (108). Conversely, IgA has been found to suppress the release of inflammatory cytokines (IL-1, IL-6, and TNF-α) and enhance the production of IL-1 receptor antagonist in human monocytes exposed to bacterial LPS (119). This finding is held to account for the beneficial (though controversial) effect of orally treating infants suffering necrotizing enterocolitis with an IgA-enriched Ig preparation (23).

Because IgA inhibits IgG-mediated complement activation, the complement-dependent opsonizing effects of IgA and IgG antibodies will be different (79). However, when FcαR is upregulated on neutrophils by treatment with TNF-α, IL-8, or GM-CSF, phagocytosis of IgA-opsonized particles is enhanced (reviewed in reference 92). This may be relevant at mucosal surfaces such as the intestine, when in the event of bacterial invasion cytokines produced by epithelial cells attract and activate neutrophils, which must then operate in an IgA-rich environment. Consistent with this, Janoff et al. (34) have shown that pIgA antibodies against capsular polysaccharide promote the phagocytosis of pneumococci in an FcαR-dependent manner, especially when the phagocytes are preactivated by C5a and TNF-α.

Although several reports have described the binding of IgA by T cells, the presence of an IgA receptor on lymphocytes remained controversial, as the receptor was not characterized or cloned. Recently, however, a receptor capable of binding the Fc of both IgM and IgA (Fcα/μR) and apparently related to pIgR (83) has been identified on human and murine B cells (95), although its biological significance remains to be established. IgA-mediated killing of bacteria by intestinal T cells has been reported (110), possibly involving IgA receptor-bearing γ/δ CD8$^+$ intraepithelial cells (97). Furthermore, S-IgA may in certain experimental systems synergize with IgG in promoting antibody-dependent cell-mediated cytotoxicity by human polymorphonuclear leukocytes, monocytes, and lymphocytes (100). In contrast, the finding that NK cell activity was inhibited by IgA2 is probably due to interaction with carbohydrate-specific receptors (47).

A novel receptor for IgA, distinct from pIgR, FcαR, asialoglycoprotein receptor, or galactosyltransferase, has been described on human intestinal epithelial cell lines (46). It binds mIgA but not other isotypes, and its function is unknown; whether it might account for the presence of mIgA that is found in some secretions (mIgA cannot be transported by pIgR) remains speculative.

IgA is a potent stimulus for eosinophil degranulation (1) and mediates the killing of schistosomes by eosinophils (22, 29). Human eosinophils are also reported to bind S-IgA and SC and consequently degranulate through a 15-kDa receptor that is unrelated to FcαR but otherwise uncharacterized (52). In contrast, IgA antibodies can inhibit IgE-mediated hypersensitivity (33, 94). The interaction of IgA with these systems and its potential in defense against parasites and in the amelioration of atopic allergy deserve more attention.

On most mucosal surfaces where S-IgA is the predominant Ig, functionally active complement and intact phagocytes are not normally present; therefore, S-IgA cannot activate either system. However, when mucosal barriers are breached or inflammation develops, S-IgA in the secretions or pIgA present in the tissue could be important for anti-inflammatory control in a complex interplay of factors that may provide damage-limiting capability as well as immune defense.

FUNCTIONAL SIGNIFICANCE OF HUMAN IgA1 AND IgA2 SUBCLASSES; "NATURAL" IgA ANTIBODIES

The most obvious structural difference between IgA1 and IgA2 is the presence in the IgA1 hinge of a tandem 8-residue repeat containing peptide bonds susceptible to cleavage by bacterial IgA1 proteases, described below, and an insertion of 13 residues in IgA1. Otherwise, the entire constant region sequences of the α1 and α2 heavy chains comprising 340 to 353 amino acids differ at only 21 residues (84). Differences also occur in the number and arrangement of N-linked glycans and of O-linked glycans (only in the IgA1 hinge region). Yet antibodies of IgA1 and IgA2 isotypes display subtle functional differences.

Functionally important differences pertain to the distribution of specific antibody activity to various types of exogenous antigens (69). Examination of naturally occurring or immunization-induced serum and S-IgA antibodies to a broad spectrum of antigens reveals several important principles. Thus, serum and S-IgA antibodies to food-protein antigens and viral glycoproteins (e.g., influenza virus and HIV) are found predominantly in the IgA1 isotype in most individuals. In contrast, S-IgA antibodies to bacterial LPS, lipoteichoic acid, and pneumococcal polysaccharide are predominantly of the IgA2 isotype, especially after systemic immunization of adults (57). In serum, however, anti-LPS antibodies are predominantly IgA1 associated. This finding may be due to the fact that, in contrast to secretions, serum IgA1 represents 85% of total IgA, or that serum IgA and S-IgA anti-LPS antibodies originate from different sources and may have been induced by different stimulatory pathways.

These differences in IgA subclass distribution of specific antibodies become accentuated upon local or systemic immunization. For example, IgA responses to live attenuated influenza virus and its hemagglutinin administered mucosally or systemically, respectively, are almost entirely accounted for by increases in IgA1 antibodies. However, systemic immunization with polysaccharides from *Streptococcus pneumoniae*, *Haemophilus influenzae*, or *Neisseria meningitidis* induces vigorous IgA2 responses manifested by the appearance of antibody-secreting cells in peripheral blood and S-IgA2 antibodies in external secretions (111). Thus, the character of antigen and the site of its encounter with the immune system greatly influence the IgA subclass of the immune response, but the mechanisms responsible remain speculative.

Although IgA1 and IgA2 subclasses exist in hominoid primates (e.g., chimpanzee and gorilla), functional differences, apart from the susceptibility of chimpanzee IgA1 to bacterial proteases (15), have not been examined. There are 13 IgA subclasses present in lagomorphs (e.g., rabbits and hares) with distinct structural features (107), but their functional properties have not been explored.

Although other common species of laboratory animals (e.g., mice and rats) express a single IgA isotype that is structurally more similar to human IgA2 than to IgA1, there are apparently some functional differences in IgA molecules produced by B-1 (CD5$^+$) and B-2 cell subpopulations (51). B-1 cells display distinctive phenotypic markers (Ly-1 in mice and CD5 in humans), unique anatomical location within the peritoneal cavity, early appearance in ontogeny, and extensive ability for self-renewal (78). Cells of the B-1 lineage preferentially produce antibodies of the IgM, IgA, and IgG3 isotypes with low affinity and broad specificity for common bacterial antigens such as phosphocholine, LPS, and dextrans. Studies performed in mice demonstrate that a large proportion of IgA-secreting cells in the intestinal lamina propria originate in the peritoneal cavity from surface-IgM$^+$ cells that switch to

IgA-secreting cells in the peritoneal cavity and gut, probably under the influence of T-cell-derived cytokines. It has been proposed that a large proportion of intestinal specific IgA antibodies to commensal organisms and the mucosal B-1 cells that produce them in mice may be generated in the absence of T cells (59). However, this may overlook the role of polyclonal stimulation of intestinal IgA production by bacterial products such as LPS, and the contribution of B-cell-regulatory cytokines by cells other than T lymphocytes (6). In either case, it is clear that "natural" mucosal IgA antibodies do not exist prior to microbial colonization, in contrast to the occurrence of natural systemic IgM antibodies before exogenous antigenic challenge.

Nevertheless, conventional B-2 cells are generated in organized gut-associated lymphoid tissues, especially Peyer's patches, and their switching and differentiation is T-cell dependent (65). Examination of the intestinal microbiota in mice that are selectively deficient in B-1 or B-2 cells suggests that the effector functions of IgA produced by B-1 and B-2 IgA plasma cells are different. It appears that commensal bacteria, particularly intestinal anaerobes, are coated in vivo with IgA produced most likely by B-1 cells without being eliminated (101, 112). In contrast, IgA derived from conventional B-2 cells has the capacity to eliminate pathogenic bacteria such as *S. enterica* serovar Typhimurium or *V. cholerae* as amply documented in the "back-pack" murine model (see above). These marked differences in effector functions of IgA derived from B-1 and B-2 cells may be due to differences in their V-region-dependent affinities, specificities, or perhaps glycosylation patterns, even if their C_H regions may be identical (50). Although B-1 and B-2 cells exist in humans, no evidence is currently available for functional differences in mucosal IgA derived from these two B-cell populations. However, based on the findings indicating that antibodies to basic bacterial antigens such as LPS, lipoteichoic acid, and polysaccharides are associated in humans with the phylogenetically older IgA2,

while antiprotein, antiglycoprotein, and antiviral antibodies occur predominantly in IgA1, and that IgA2-producing cells are dominant in the heavily colonized large intestine, it is tempting to speculate that mucosal IgA2 plasma cells are primarily derived from the B-1 precursors.

BACTERIAL IgA PROTEASES

Several medically important bacteria produce highly specialized proteases that cleave human IgA1 at one of the Pro-Ser or Pro-Thr bonds in the hinge region, yielding Fabα and Fcα fragments (44). Although Fabα fragments possess full antigen-binding activity, Fcα-dependent defensive properties are lost. Bacteria that produce IgA1 proteases include pathogens of the respiratory tract (*H. influenzae, N. meningitidis,* and *S. pneumoniae*), which also cause bacterial meningitis, and of the genital and urinary tracts (*Neisseria gonorrhoeae* and *Ureaplasma urealyticum*); oral commensals (*Streptococcus sanguis, Streptacoccus oralis,* and some strains of *Streptococcus mitis*), which are considered to be pioneering colonizers; and some gram-negative anaerobes implicated in periodontal disease (*Prevotella* and *Capnocytophaga* species). At least three biochemically and genetically distinct types of IgA1 protease have evolved in widely different groups of bacteria: the *Haemophilus-Neisseria* enzymes are homologous serine proteases, the streptococcal enzymes are metalloproteases, the *Prevotella-Capnocytophaga* enzymes are thought to be thiol proteases, and the *Ureaplasma* enzyme is probably a different serine protease. The separate evolution of these enzymes is strong evidence of their importance as virulence factors, but given their remarkable specificity for human IgA1 (only the anthropoid apes have IgA1 that is cleavable by IgA1 proteases), this has been very difficult to establish experimentally. Certain strains of *Clostridium ramosum,* which colonizes the large intestine but is of unknown pathological significance, produce another enzyme that cleaves both IgA1 and IgA2 of allotype A2(m)1 at a proline-valine bond near the junction of the Cα1 domain and the hinge. Although S–IgA is quite resistant to most common proteases, largely on account of the protection afforded by SC, other bacteria, notably the urinary tract pathogen *Proteus mirabilis* and the highly proteolytic periodontal pathogen *Porphyromonas gingivalis*, can also degrade IgA and other Ig isotypes. However, this results in the complete destruction of the antibodies. The unique effect of IgA1 proteases is thought to consist of coating the organisms with Fabα fragments that have little or no protective value but yet block the binding of other functional antibodies, thereby facilitating colonization and invasion (43). This hypothesis is supported by the finding that Fabα antibody fragments interfere with IgG antibody-mediated complement activation and bacteriolysis (36, 93). Moreover, IgA1 proteases from some species are antigenically variable: more than 30 antigenic types of enzyme from *H. influenzae* and four to five types from the pathogenic *Neisseria* species have been described (44). As antibodies against these proteases inhibit their activity, antigenic variation affords an escape mechanism from host responses. Mucosal immunity to these pathogens may therefore partly depend on the balance between S-IgA1 antibodies to bacterial surface antigens and inhibitory antibodies against IgA1 proteases. However, the streptococcal IgA1 proteases display little or no antigenic variation and do not induce significant inhibitory antibodies.

As IgA1 proteases are secreted into the environment of the bacteria, they can presumably cleave IgA1 molecules regardless of specificity, giving rise to a local antibody deficiency, which might permit other organisms or antigens to penetrate the mucosal epithelium. In support of this concept, it has been found that the pharyngeal microbiota of infants who develop atopic allergies contains a higher proportion of IgA1 protease-producing bacteria than that of nonatopic infants (42). Diminished mucosal protection in the upper airway resulting from the activity of IgA1 proteases would then allow the uptake of potential allergens and consequent atopic sensitization.

Further mechanisms of action of IgA1 proteases have been suggested by the recent finding that the neisserial enzymes can cleave LAMP-1, a protein found in lysosomes and early endosomes (30, 54). It is thought that such cleavage results in greater survival of the bacteria within phagocytic cells. Other unusual substrates of IgA1 proteases have been proposed but not confirmed, and the significance of such activity is not known (45).

CONCLUDING REMARKS

The gut has been thought of as existing in a perpetual state of controlled inflammation because of the huge load of foreign antigenic material in the form of food, as well as the potentially harmful onslaught of enteric microorganisms, both commensal and pathogenic. The predominant isotype of Ig found in this location, both at the surface and within the mucosal tissues, is IgA, and its essentially noninflammatory nature is of great importance for the maintenance of the integrity of the mucosae. While inflammation is a physiological response, involving numerous cells and effector molecules, to damage inflicted by infectious or noninfectious agents, and may be important in the initiation of the immune response in generating "second signals" to lymphocytes, it is also a consequence of systemic immune effector mechanisms in combating infection, and the collateral damage to tissues may be even greater than that caused by the pathogens themselves. Thus, the principal role of IgA in the intestine and other mucosae is to maintain protection of these surfaces against microbial attack and to control inflammation.

REFERENCES

1. **Abu-Ghazaleh, R. I., T. Fujisawa, J. Mestecky, R. A. Kyle, and G. J. Gleich.** 1989. IgA-induced eosinophil degranulation. *J. Immunol.* 142:2393–2400.
2. **Adlerberth, I., S. Ahrne, M. L. Johansson, G. Molin, L. Å. Hanson, and A. E. Wold.** 1996. A mannose-specific adherence mechanism in *Lactobacillus plantarum* conferring binding to the

human colonic cell line HT-29. *Appl. Environ. Microbiol.* **62**:2244–2251.

3. **Alley, C. D., G. S. Nash, and R. P. Mac-Dermott.** 1982. Marked *in vitro* spontaneous secretion of IgA by human rib bone marrow mononuclear cells. *J. Immunol.* **128**:2604–2608.

4. **Biesbrock, A. R., M. S. Reddy, and M. J. Levine.** 1991. Interaction of a salivary mucin-secretory immunoglobulin A complex with mucosal pathogens. *Infect. Immun.* **59**:3492–3497.

5. **Bos, N. A., J. J. Cebra, and F. G. Kroese.** 2000. B-1 cells and the intestinal microflora. *Curr. Top. Microbiol. Immunol.* **252**:211–220.

6. **Bos, N. A., H. Q. Jiang, and J. J. Cebra.** 2001. T cell control of the gut IgA response against commensal bacteria. *Gut* **48**:762–764.

7. **Bouvet, J.-P., and V. A. Fischetti.** 1999. Diversity of antibody-mediated immunity at the mucosal barrier. *Infect. Immun.* **67**:2687–2691.

8. **Brandtzaeg, P., I. N. Farstad, F. E. Johansen, H. C. Morton, I. N. Norderhaug, and T. Yamanaka.** 1999. The B-cell system of human mucosae and exocrine glands. *Immunol. Rev.* **171**:45–87.

9. **Brandtzaeg, P., I. Fjellanger, and S. T. Gjeruldsen.** 1970. Human secretory immunoglobulins. I. Salivary secretions from individuals with normal or low levels of serum immunoglobulins. *Scand. J. Haematol.* **S12**:3–83.

10. **Brandtzaeg, P., and K. Tolo.** 1977. Mucosal penetrability enhanced by serum-derived antibodies. *Nature* **266**:262–263.

11. **Bronson, R. A., G. W. Cooper, D. L. Rosenfeld, J. V. Gilbert, and A. G. Plaut.** 1987. The effect of an IgA1 protease on immunoglobulins bound to the sperm surface and sperm cervical mucus penetrating ability. *Fertil. Steril.* **47**:985–991.

12. **Brown, T. A., M. W. Russell, and J. Mestecky.** 1982. Hepatobiliary transport of IgA immune complexes: molecular and cellular aspects. *J. Immunol.* **128**:2183–2186.

13. **Burrows, P. D., and M. D. Cooper.** 1997. IgA deficiency. *Adv. Immunol.* **65**:245–276.

14. **Castilla, J., I. Sola, and L. Enjuanes.** 1997. Interference of coronavirus infection by expression of immunoglobulin G (IgG) or IgA virus-neutralizing antibodies. *J. Virol.* **71**:5251–5258.

15. **Cole, M. F., and C. A. Hale.** 1991. Cleavage of chimpanzee secretory immunoglobulin A by *Haemophilus influenzae* IgA1 protease. *Microb. Pathog.* **11**:39–46.

16. **Corthésy, B., M. Kaufmann, A. Phalipon, M. Peitsch, M. R. Neutra, and J. P. Kraehenbuhl.** 1996. A pathogen-specific epitope inserted into recombinant secretory immunoglobulin A is immunogenic by the oral route. *J. Biol. Chem.* **271**:33670–33677.

17. **Crago, S. S., W. H. Kutteh, I. Moro, M. R. Allansmith, J. Radl, J. J. Haaijman, and J. Mestecky.** 1984. Distribution of IgA1-, IgA2- and J chain-containing cells in human tissues. *J. Immunol.* **132**:16–18.

18. **Cripps, A. W., and M. Gleeson.** 1999. Ontogeny of mucosal immunity and aging, p. 253–266. *In* P. L. Ogra, J. Mestecky, M. E. Lamm, W. Strober, J. Bienenstock, and J. R. McGhee (ed.), *Mucosal Immunology*, 2nd ed. Academic Press, Inc., San Diego, Calif.

19. **Crottet, P., and B. Corthésy.** 1998. Secretory component delays the conversion of secretory IgA into antigen-binding competent F(ab')$_2$: a possible implication for mucosal defense. *J. Immunol.* **161**:5445–5453.

20. **Cunningham-Rundles, C., W. E. Brandeis, R. A. Good, and N. K. Day.** 1978. Milk precipitins, circulating immune complexes, and IgA deficiency. *Proc. Natl. Acad. Sci. USA* **75**:3387–3389.

21. **Dunn-Walters, D., L. Boursier, and J. Spencer.** 2000. Effect of somatic hypermutation on potential N-glycosylation sites in human immunoglobulin heavy chain variable regions. *Mol. Immunol.* **37**:107–113.

22. **Dunne, D. W., B. A. Richardson, F. M. Jones, M. Clark, K. J. I. Thorne, and A. E. Butterworth.** 1993. The use of mouse/human chimaeric antibodies to investigate the roles of different antibody isotypes, including IgA2, in the killing of *Schistosoma mansoni* schistosomula by eosinophils. *Parasite Immunol.* **15**:181–185.

23. **Eibl, M., H. M. Wolf, H. Fürnkranz, and A. Rosenkranz.** 1988. Prevention of necrotizing enterocolitis in low-birth-weight infants by IgA-IgG feeding. *N. Engl. J. Med.* **319**:1–7.

24. **Endo, T., J. Mestecky, R. Kulhavy, and A. Kobata.** 1994. Carbohydrate heterogeneity of human myeloma proteins of the IgA1 and IgA2 subclasses. *Mol. Immunol.* **31**:1415–1422.

25. **Fernandez, C., M. E. Alarcon-Riquelme, M. Abedi-Valugerdi, E. Sverremark, and V. Cortez.** 1997. Polyreactive binding to antibodies generated by polyclonal B cell activation. I. Polyreactivity could be caused by differential glycosylation of immunoglobulins. *Scand. J. Immunol.* **43**:231–239.

26. **Fernandez, C., M. E. Alarcon-Riquelme, and E. Sverremark.** 1997. Polyreactive binding to antibodies generated by polyclonal B cell activation. II. Crossreactive and monospecific antibodies can be generated from an identical Ig rearrangement by differential glycosylation. *Scand. J. Immunol.* **45**:240–247.

27. Fujihashi, K., and P. B. Ernst. 1999. A mucosal internet. Epithelial cell-immune cell interactions, p. 619–630. In P. L. Ogra, J. Mestecky, M. E. Lamm, W. Strober, J. Bienenstock, and J. R. McGhee (ed.), Mucosal Immunology, 2nd ed. Academic Press, Inc., San Diego, Calif.

28. Gan, Y. J., J. Chodosh, A. Morgan, and J. W. Sixbey. 1997. Epithelial cell polarization is a determinant in the infectious outcome of immunoglobulin A-mediated entry by Epstein-Barr virus. J. Virol. 71:519–526.

29. Grezel, D., M. Capron, J.-M. Grzych, J. Fontaine, J.-P. Lecocq, and A. Capron. 1993. Protective immunity induced in rat schistosomiasis by a single dose of the Sm28GST recombinant antigen: effector mechanisms involving IgE and IgA antibodies. Eur. J. Immunol. 23:454–460.

30. Hauck, C. R., and T. F. Meyer. 1997. The lysosomal/phagosomal membrane protein h-lamp-1 is a target of the IgA1 protease of Neisseria gonorrhoeae. FEBS Lett. 405:86–90.

31. Heremans, J. F. 1974. Immunoglobulin A, p. 365–522. In M. Sela (ed.), The Antigens, vol. 2. Academic Press Inc., New York, N.Y.

32. Huang, D. S., S. N. Emancipator, M. E. Lamm, T. L. Karban, F. H. Blatnik, H. M. Tsao, and M. B. Mazanec. 1997. Virus-specific IgA reduces hepatic viral titers in vivo on mouse hepatitis virus (MHV) infection. Immunol. Cell Biol. 75(Suppl. 1):A12.

33. Ishizaka, K., T. Ishizaka, and M. M. Hornbrook. 1963. Blocking of Prausnitz-Küstner sensitization with reagin by normal human β_{2A} globulin. J. Allergy 34:395–403.

34. Janoff, E. N., C. Fasching, J. M. Orenstein, J. B. Rubins, N. L. Opstad, and A. P. Dalmasso. 1999. Killing of Streptococcus pneumoniae by capsular polysaccharide-specific polymeric IgA, complement, and phagocytes. J. Clin. Invest. 104:1139–1147.

35. Janoff, E. N., S. M. Wahl, K. Thomas, and P. D. Smith. 1995. Modulation of human immunodeficiency virus type 1 infection of human monocytes by IgA. J. Infect. Dis. 172:855–858.

36. Jarvis, G. A., and J. M. Griffiss. 1991. Human IgA1 blockade of IgG-initiated lysis of Neisseria meningitidis is a function of antigen-binding fragment binding to the polysaccharide capsule. J. Immunol. 147:1962–1967.

37. Jonard, P. P., J. C. Rambaud, C. Dive, J. P. Vaerman, A. Galian, and D. L. Delacroix. 1984. Secretion of immunoglobulins and plasma proteins from the jejunal mucosa. Transport data and origin of polymeric immunoglobulin A. J. Clin. Invest. 74:525–535.

38. Kaetzel, C. S. 2001. Polymeric Ig receptor: defender of the fort or Trojan horse? Curr. Biol. 11: R35–R38.

39. Kaetzel, C. S., J. K. Robinson, K. R. Chintalacharuvu, J.-P. Vaerman, and M. E. Lamm. 1991. The polymeric immunoglobulin receptor (secretory component) mediates transport of immune complexes across epithelial cells: A local defense function for IgA. Proc. Natl. Acad. Sci. USA 88:8796–8800.

40. Kerr, M. A. 1990. The structure and function of human IgA. Biochem. J. 271:285–296.

41. Kett, K., P. Brandtzaeg, J. Radl, and J. J. Haaijman. 1986. Different subclass distribution of IgA-producing cells in human lymphoid organs and various secretory tissues. J. Immunol. 136:3631–3635.

42. Kilian, M., S. Husby, A. Host, and S. Halken. 1995. Increased proportions of bacteria capable of cleaving IgA1 in the pharynx of infants with atopic disease. Pediatr. Res. 38:182–186.

43. Kilian, M., and J. Reinholdt. 1987. A hypothetical model for the development of invasive infection due to IgA1 protease-producing bacteria. Adv. Exp. Med. Biol. 216B:1261–1269.

44. Kilian, M., J. Reinholdt, H. Lomholt, K. Poulsen, and E. V. G. Frandsen. 1996. Biological significance of IgA1 proteases in bacterial colonization and pathogenesis: critical evaluation of experimental evidence. APMIS 104:321–338.

45. Kilian, M., and M. W. Russell. 1999. Bacterial evasion of mucosal immune defenses, p. 241–251. In P. L. Ogra, J. Mestecky, M. E. Lamm, W. Strober, J. Bienenstock, and J. R. McGhee (ed.), Mucosal Immunology, 2nd ed. Academic Press, Inc., San Diego, Calif.

46. Kitamura, T., R. P. Garofalo, A. Kamijo, D. K. Hammond, J. A. Oka, C. R. Caflisch, M. Shenoy, A. Casola, P. H. Weigel, and R. M. Goldblum. 2000. Human intestinal epithelial cells express a novel receptor for IgA. J. Immunol. 164:5029–5034.

47. Komiyama, K., S. S. Crago, K. Itoh, I. Moro, and J. Mestecky. 1986. Inhibition of natural killer cell activity by IgA. Cell. Immunol. 101:143–155.

48. Kozlowski, P. A., D. Chen, J. H. Eldridge, and S. Jackson. 1994. Contrasting IgA and IgG neutralization capacities and responses to HIV type 1 gp120 V3 loop in HIV-infected individuals. AIDS Res. Hum. Retrovir. 10:813–822.

49. Kraehenbuhl, J. P., and M. R. Neutra. 1994. Monoclonal secretory IgA for protection of the intestinal mucosa against viral and bacterial pathogens, p. 403–410. In P. L. Ogra, J. Mestecky, M. E. Lamm, W. Strober, J. R. McGhee, and J.

Bienenstock (ed.), *Handbook of Mucosal Immunology*. Academic Press, Inc., San Diego, Calif.

50. **Kroese, F. G. M., R. de Ward, and N. A. Bos.** 1996. B-1 cells and their reactivity with the murine intestinal microflora. *Semin. Immunol.* **8:**11–18.

51. **Kroese, F. G. M., A. B. Kantor, and L. A. Herzenberg.** 1994. The role of B-1 cells in mucosal immune responses, p. 217–224. *In* P. L. Ogra, J. Mestecky, M. E. Lamm, W. Strober, J. R. McGhee, and J. Bienenstock (ed.), *Handbook of Mucosal Immunology*. Academic Press, Inc., San Diego, Calif.

52. **Lamkhioued, B., A. S. Gounni, V. Gruart, A. Pierce, A. Capron, and M. Capron.** 1995. Human eosinophils express a receptor for secretory component. Role in secretory IgA-dependent activation. *Eur. J. Immunol.* **25:**117–125.

53. **Liew, F. Y., S. M. Russell, G. Appleyard, C. M. Brand, and J. Beale.** 1984. Cross protection in mice infected with influenza A virus by the respiratory route is correlated with local IgA antibody rather than serum antibody or cytotoxic T cell reactivity. *Eur. J. Immunol.* **14:**350–356.

54. **Lin, L., P. Ayala, J. Larson, M. Mulks, M. Fukuda, S. R. Carlsson, C. Enns, and M. So.** 1997. The *Neisseria* type 2 IgA1 protease cleaves LAMP1 and promotes survival of bacteria within epithelial cells. *Mol. Microbiol.* **24:**1083–1094.

55. **Lindh, E.** 1975. Increased resistance of immunoglobulin A dimers to proteolytic degradation after binding of secretory component. *J. Immunol.* **114:**284–286.

56. **Lodinová-Zádníková, R., H. Tlaskalová, B. Korych, and Z. Bartáková.** 1995. The antibody response in infants after oral administration of inactivated and living *E. coli* vaccines and their protective effect against nosocomial infections. *Adv. Exp. Med. Biol.* **371B:**1431–1438.

57. **Lue, C., A. Tarkowski, and J. Mestecky.** 1988. Systemic immunization with pneumococcal polysaccharide vaccine induces a predominant IgA2 response of peripheral blood lymphocytes and increases of both serum and secretory anti-pneumococcal antibodies. *J. Immunol.* **140:**3793–3800.

58. **Lycke, N., L. Erlandsson, L. Ekman, K. Schön, and T. Leanderson.** 1999. Lack of J chain inhibits the transport of gut IgA and abrogates the development of intestinal antitoxic protection. *J. Immunol.* **163:**913–919.

59. **Macpherson, A. J., D. Gatto, E. Sainsbury, G. R. Harriman, H. Hengartner, and R. M. Zinkernagel.** 2000. A primitive T cell-independent mechanism of intestinal mucosal IgA responses to commensal bacteria. *Science* **288:**2222–2226.

60. **Magnusson, K.-E., and I. Stjernström.** 1982. Mucosal barrier systems. Interplay between secretory IgA (SIgA), IgG and mucins on the surface properties and association of salmonellae with intestine and granulocytes. *Immunology* **45:**239–248.

61. **Mattu, T. S., R. J. Pleass, A. C. Willis, M. Kilian, M. R. Wormald, A. C. Lellouch, P. M. Rudd, J. M. Woof, and R. A. Dwek.** 1998. The glycosylation and structure of human serum IgA1, Fab, and Fc regions and the role of N-glycosylation on Fcα receptor interactions. *J. Biol. Chem.* **273:**2260–2272.

62. **Mayer, L., and R. S. Blumberg.** 1999. Antigen-presenting cells. Epithelial cells, p. 365–379. *In* P. L. Ogra, J. Mestecky, M. E. Lamm, W. Strober, J. Bienenstock, and J. R. McGhee (ed.), *Mucosal Immunology*, 2nd ed. Academic Press, Inc., San Diego, Calif.

63. **Mazanec, M. B., C. L. Coudret, and D. R. Fletcher.** 1995. Intracellular neutralization of influenza virus by immunoglobulin A anti-hemagglutinin monoclonal antibodies. *J. Virol.* **69:**1339–1343.

64. **Mazanec, M. B., C. S. Kaetzel, M. E. Lamm, D. Fletcher, and J. G. Nedrud.** 1992. Intracellular neutralization of virus by immunoglobulin A antibodies. *Proc. Natl. Acad. Sci. USA* **89:**6901–6905.

65. **McIntyre, T. M., and W. Strober.** 1999. Gut-associated lymphoid tissue: regulation of IgA B-cell development, p. 319–356. *In* P. L. Ogra, J. Mestecky, M. E. Lamm, W. Strober, J. Bienenstock, and J. R. McGhee (ed.), *Mucosal Immunology*, 2nd ed. Academic Press, Inc., San Diego, Calif.

66. **Mellander, L., B. Carlsson, F. Jalil, T. Söderström, and L. Å. Hanson.** 1985. Secretory IgA antibody response against *Escherichia coli* antigens in infants in relation to exposure. *J. Pediatr.* **107:**430–433.

67. **Mestecky, J., and M. Kilian.** 1985. Immunoglobulin A (IgA). *Methods Enzymol.* **116:**37–75.

68. **Mestecky, J., R. Kulhavy, and F. W. Kraus.** 1972. Studies on human secretory immunoglobulin A. II. Subunit structure. *J. Immunol.* **108:**738–747.

69. **Mestecky, J., C. Lue, A. Tarkowski, I. Ladjeva, J. Peterman, Z. Moldoveanu, M. W. Russell, T. A. Brown, J. Radl, J. J. Haaijman, H. Kiyono, and J. R. McGhee.** 1989. Comparative studies of the biological properties of human IgA subclasses. *Protides Biol. Fluids* **36:**173–182.

70. Mestecky, J., Z. Moldoveanu, M. Tomana, J. M. Epps, S. R. Thorpe, J. O. Phillips, and R. Kulhavy. 1989. The role of the liver in catabolism of mouse and human IgA. *Immunol. Invest.* **18**:313–324.

71. Mestecky, J., I. Moro, and B. J. Underdown. 1999. Mucosal immunoglobulins, p. 133–152. *In* P. L. Ogra, J. Mestecky, M. E. Lamm, W. Strober, J. Bienenstock, and J. R. McGhee (ed.), *Mucosal Immunology*, 2nd ed. Academic Press, Inc., San Diego, Calif.

72. Mestecky, J., and M. W. Russell. 1986. IgA Subclasses. *Monogr. Allergy* **19**:277–301.

73. Mestecky, J., M. Tomana, C. Czerkinsky, A. Tarkowski, S. Matsuda, F. B. Waldo, Z. Moldoveanu, B. A. Julian, J. H. Galla, M. W. Russell, and S. Jackson. 1987. IgA-associated renal diseases: immunochemical studies of IgA1 proteins, circulating immune complexes, and cellular interactions. *Semin. Nephrol.* **7**:332–335.

74. Michetti, P., M. J. Mahan, J. M. Slauch, J. J. Mekalanos, and M. R. Neutra. 1992. Monoclonal secretory immunoglobulin A protects mice against oral challenge with the invasive pathogen *Salmonella typhimurium*. *Infect. Immun.* **60**:1786–1792.

75. Monteiro, R. C., H. Kubagawa, and M. D. Cooper. 1990. Cellular distribution, regulation, and biochemical nature of an Fcα receptor in humans. *J. Exp. Med.* **171**:597–613.

76. Morton, H. C., M. Van Egmond, and J. G. J. Van de Winkel. 1996. Structure and function of human IgA Fc receptors (FcαR). *Crit. Rev. Immunol.* **16**:423–440.

77. Mostov, K., and C. S. Kaetzel. 1999. Immunoglobulin transport and the polymeric immunoglobulin receptor, p. 181–211. *In* P. L. Ogra, J. Mestecky, M. E. Lamm, W. Strober, J. Bienenstock, and J. R. McGhee (ed.), *Mucosal Immunology*, 2nd ed. Academic Press, Inc., San Diego, Calif.

78. Murakami, M., and T. Honjo. 1995. Involvement of B-1 cells in mucosal immunity and autoimmunity. *Immunol. Today* **16**:534–539.

79. Nikolova, E. B., and M. W. Russell. 1995. Dual function of human IgA antibodies: inhibition of phagocytosis in circulating neutrophils and enhancement of responses in IL-8-stimulated cells. *J. Leuk. Biol.* **57**:875–882.

80. Nikolova, E. B., M. Tomana, and M. W. Russell. 1994. The role of the carbohydrate chains in complement (C3) fixation by solid-phase-bound human IgA. *Immunology* **82**:321–327.

81. Norderhaug, I. N., F. E. Johansen, H. Schjerven, and P. Brandtzaeg. 1999. Regulation of the formation and external transport of secretory immunoglobulins. *Crit. Rev. Immunol.* **19**:481–508.

82. Peppard, J. V., and M. W. Russell. 1999. Phylogenetic development and comparative physiology of IgA, p. 163–179. *In* P. L. Ogra, J. Mestecky, M. E. Lamm, W. Strober, J. Bienenstock, and J. R. McGhee (ed.), *Mucosal Immunology*, 2nd ed. Academic Press, Inc., San Diego, Calif.

83. Phillips-Quagliata, J. M., S. Patel, J. K. Han, S. Arakelov, T. D. Rao, M. J. Shulman, S. Fatal, R. B. Corley, M. Everett, M. H. Klein, B. J. Underdown, and B. Corthésy. 2000. The IgA/IgM receptor expressed on a murine B cell lymphoma is poly-Ig receptor. *J. Immunol.* **165**:2544–2555.

84. Putnam, F. W. 1989. Structure of the human IgA subclasses and allotypes. *Protides Biol. Fluids* **36**:27–37.

85. Quan, C. P., A. Berneman, R. Pires, S. Avrameas, and J.-P. Bouvet. 1997. Natural polyreactive secretory immunoglobulin A autoantibodies as a possible barrier to infection in humans. *Infect. Immun.* **65**:3997–4004.

86. Rejnek, J., J. Trávnícek, J. Kostka, J. Sterzl, and A. Lanc. 1968. Study of the effect of antibodies in the intestinal tract of germ-free baby pigs. *Folia Microbiol.* **13**:36–42.

87. Renegar, K. B., G. D. F. Jackson, and J. Mestecky. 1998. *In vitro* comparison of the biologic activities of monoclonal monomeric IgA, polymeric IgA, and secretory IgA. *J. Immunol.* **160**:1219–1223.

88. Ross, A., L. H. Bouwman, D. J. van Gijlswijk-Janssen, M. C. Faber-Krol, G. L. Stahl, and M. R. Daha. 2001. Human IgA activates the complement system via the mannan-binding lectin pathway. *J. Immunol.* **167**:2861–2868.

88a. Royle, L., A. Roos, D. J. Harvey, M. R. Wormald, D. van Gijlswijk-Janssen, E.-R. M. Redwan, I. A. Wilson, M. R. Daha, R. A. Dwek, and P. M. Rudd. Secretory IgA N- and O-glycans provide a link between the innate and adaptive immune systems. *J. Biol. Chem.*, in press.

89. Rubas, W., and G. M. Grass. 1991. Gastrointestinal lymphatic absorption of peptides and proteins. *Adv. Drug Deliv. Rev.* **7**:15–69.

90. Rudd, P. M., and R. A. Dwek. 1998. The importance of sugars for the function of antibodies. *Immunol. News* **5**:84–89.

91. Ruhl, S., A. L. Sandberg, M. F. Cole, and J. O. Cisar. 1996. Recognition of immunoglobulin A1 by oral actinomyces and streptococcal lectins. *Infect. Immun.* **64**:5421–5424.

92. **Russell, M. W., M. Kilian, and M. E. Lamm.** 1999. Biological activities of IgA, p. 225–240. *In* P. L. Ogra, J. Mestecky, M. E. Lamm, W. Strober, J. Bienenstock, and J. R. McGhee (ed.), *Mucosal Immunology*, 2nd ed. Academic Press, Inc., San Diego, Calif.

93. **Russell, M. W., J. Reinholdt, and M. Kilian.** 1989. Anti-inflammatory activity of human IgA antibodies and their Fabα fragments: inhibition of IgG-mediated complement activation. *Eur. J. Immunol.* **19:**2243–2249.

94. **Russell-Jones, G. J., P. L. Ey, and B. L. Reynolds.** 1981. Inhibition of cutaneous anaphylaxis and Arthus reactions in the mouse by antigen-specific IgA. *Int. Arch. Allergy Appl. Immunol.* **66:**316–325.

95. **Sakamoto, N., K. Shibuya, Y. Shimizu, K. Yotsumoto, T. Miyabayashi, S. Sakano, T. Tsuji, E. Nakayama, H. Nakauchi, and A. Shibuya.** 2001. A novel Fc receptor for IgA and IgM is expressed on both hematopoietic and non-hematopoietic tissues. *Eur. J. Immunol.* **31:**1310–1316.

96. **Saltzman, W. M., M. L. Radomsky, K. J. Whaley, and R. A. Cone.** 1994. Antibody diffusion in human cervical mucus. *Biophys. J.* **66:**508–515.

97. **Sandor, M., B. Houlden, J. Bluestone, S. M. Hedrick, J. Weinstock, and R. G. Lynch.** 1992. *In vitro* and *in vivo* activation of murine γ/δ T cells induces the expression of IgA, IgM, and IgG Fc receptors. *J. Immunol.* **148:**2363–2369.

98. **Savage, D. C.** 1999. Mucosal microbiota, p. 19–30. *In* P. L. Ogra, J. Mestecky, M. E. Lamm, W. Strober, J. Bienenstock, and J. R. McGhee (ed.), *Mucosal Immunology*, 2nd ed. Academic Press, Inc., San Diego, Calif.

99. **Schroten, H., C. Stapper, R. Plogmann, H. Köhler, J. Hacker, and F.-G. Hanisch.** 1998. Fab-independent antiadhesion effects of secretory immunoglobulin A on S-fimbriated *Escherichia coli* are mediated by sialyloligosaccharides. *Infect. Immun.* **66:**3971–3973.

100. **Shen, L., and M. W. Fanger.** 1981. Secretory IgA antibodies synergize with IgG in promoting ADCC by human polymorphonuclear cells, monocytes, and lymphocytes. *Cell. Immunol.* **59:**75–81.

101. **Shroff, K. E., K. Meslin, and J. J. Cebra.** 1995. Commensal enteric bacteria engender a self-limiting humoral mucosal immune response while permanently colonizing the gut. *Infect. Immun.* **63:**3904–3913.

102. **Sibille, Y., D. L. Delacroix, W. W. Merill, B. Chatelain, and J. P. Vaerman.** 1987. IgA-induced chemokinesis of human polymorpho-nuclear neutrophils: requirement of their Fc-α receptor. *Mol. Immunol.* **24:**551–559.

103. **Silbart, L. K., and D. F. Keren.** 1989. Reduction of intestinal carcinogen absorption by carcinogen-specific secretory immunity. *Science* **243:**1462–1464.

104. **Silvey, K. J., A. B. Hutchings, M. Vajdy, M. M. Petzke, and M. R. Neutra.** 2001. Role of immunoglobulin A in protection against reovirus entry into murine Peyer's patches. *J. Virol.* **75:**10870–10879.

105. **Sixbey, J. W., and Q. Yao.** 1992. Immunoglobulin A-induced shift of Epstein-Barr virus tissue tropism. *Science* **255:**1578–1580.

106. **Smith, P. D., L. E. Smythies, M. Mosteller-Barnum, D. A. Sibley, M. W. Russell, M. Merger, M. T. Sellers, J. M. Orenstein, T. Shimada, M. F. Graham, and H. Kubagawa.** 2001. Intestinal macrophages lack CD14 and CD89 and consequently are down-regulated for LPS- and IgA-mediated activities. *J. Immunol.* **167:**2651–2656.

107. **Spieker-Polet, H., P.-C. Yam, and K. L. Knight.** 1993. Differential expression of 13 IgA-heavy chain genes in rabbit lymphoid tissues. *J. Immunol.* **150:**5457–5465.

108. **Stewart, W. W., and M. A. Kerr.** 1991. The measurement of respiratory burst induced in polymorphonuclear neutrophils by IgA and IgG anti-gliadin antibodies isolated from coeliac serum. *Immunology* **73:**491–497.

109. **Stubbe, H., J. Berdoz, J. P. Kraehenbuhl, and B. Corthésy.** 2000. Polymeric IgA is superior to monomeric IgA and IgG carrying the same variable domain in preventing *Clostridium difficile* toxin A damaging of T84 monolayers. *J. Immunol.* **164:**1952–1960.

110. **Tagliabue, A., L. Villa, M. T. De Magistris, M. Romano, S. Silvestri, D. Boraschi, and L. Nencioni.** 1986. IgA-driven T cell-mediated anti-bacterial immunity in man after live oral Ty21a vaccine. *J. Immunol.* **137:**1504–1510.

111. **Tarkowski, A., C. Lue, Z. Moldoveanu, H. Kiyono, J. R. McGhee, and J. Mestecky.** 1990. Immunization of humans with polysaccharide vaccines induces systemic, predominantly polymeric-IgA2 subclass antibody responses. *J. Immunol.* **144:**3770–3778.

112. **Van der Waaij, L. A., P. C. Limburg, G. Mesander, and D. Van der Waaij.** 1996. *In vivo* IgA coating of anaerobic bacteria in human faeces. *Gut* **38:**348–354.

113. **Van Egmond, M., E. Van Garderen, A. B. Van Spriel, C. A. Damen, E. S. Van Amersfoort, G. Van Zandbergen, J. Van Hattum, J. Kuiper, and J. G. J. Van de**

Winkel. 2000. FcαRI-positive liver Kupffer cells: reappraisal of the function of immuno-globulin A in immunity. *Nat. Med.* **6:**680–685.

114. **Van Epps, D. E., and S. L. Brown.** 1981. Inhibition of formylmethionyl-leucyl-phenylalanine-stimulated neutrophil chemilu-minescence by human immunoglobulin A paraproteins. *Infect. Immun.* **34:**864–870.

115. **Vidarsson, G., W.-L. van der Pol, J. M. H. van den Elsen, H. Vilé, M. Jansen, J. Duijs, H. C. Morton, E. Boel, M. R. Daha, B. Corthésy, and J. G. J. Van de Winkel.** 2001. Activity of human IgG and IgA subclasses in immune defense against *Neisseria meningitidis* serogroup B. *J. Immunol.* **166:**6250–6256.

116. **Walker, W. A., K. J. Isselbacher, and K. J. Bloch.** 1972. Intestinal uptake of macromole-cules: effect of oral immunization. *Science* **177:**608–610.

117. **Weltzin, R., P. Lecia-Jandris, P. Michetti, B. N. Fields, J. P. Kraehenbuhl, and M. R. Neutra.** 1989. Binding and transepithelial trans-port of immunoglobulins by intestinal M cells: demonstration using monoclonal IgA antibodies against enteric viral proteins. *J. Cell. Biol.* **108:**1673–1685.

118. **Wold, A., J. Mestecky, M. Tomana, A. Ko-bata, H. Ohbayashi, T. Endo, and C. Svan-**

borg Edén. 1990. Secretory immunoglobulin A carries oligosaccharide receptors for *Escherichia coli* type 1 fimbrial lectin. *Infect. Immun.* **58:**3073–3077.

119. **Wolf, H. M., I. Hauber, H. Gulle, A. Sam-stag, M. B. Fischer, R. U. Ahmad, and M. M. Eibl.** 1996. Anti-inflammatory proper-ties of human serum IgA: induction of IL-1 re-ceptor antagonist and FcαR (CD89)-mediated down regulation of tumor necrosis factor-alpha (TNF-α) and IL-6 in human monocytes. *Clin. Exp. Immunol.* **105:**537–543.

120. **Wu, H.-Y., and M. W. Russell.** 1993. In-duction of mucosal immunity by intranasal ap-plication of a streptococcal surface protein antigen with the cholera toxin B subunit. *Infect. Immun.* **61:**314–322.

121. **Zhang, J. R., K. E. Mostov, M. E. Lamm, M. Nanno, S. Shimida, M. Ohwaki, and E. Tuomanen.** 2000. The polymeric immuno-globulin receptor translocates pneumococci across human nasopharyngeal epithelial cells. *Cell* **102:**827–837.

122. **Zikan, J., J. Mestecky, R. E. Schrohen-loher, M. Tomana, and R. Kulhavy.** 1972. Studies on human immunoglobulin A V. Tryp-sin hydrolysis at elevated temperatures. *Immu-nochemistry* **9:**1185–1193.

SEQUENCE-BASED METHODS FOR INVESTIGATING INTESTINAL MICROBES

David N. Fredricks

7

Our rapidly expanding knowledge of microbial genes and genomes has created new molecular tools for studying how microbes interact with each other and with host cells. This chapter focuses on the use of microbial nucleic acid sequences for the detection, localization, and characterization of microbes in the human intestine, with emphasis on cultivation-resistant pathogens and commensals.

The traditional approach for studying microbes in the gastrointestinal tract relies on cultivation. Organisms are recovered from diseased tissues by inoculating axenic media and classified based on their ability to grow, using defined substrates at particular temperatures and atmospheres. Isolated microbes are then inoculated into susceptible hosts or cell culture systems to study interactions with host cells. Although this approach works well for cultivable microbes, it obviously fails for microbes that resist attempts at laboratory propagation. The traditional approach for localizing microbes relies on light or electron microscopy, frequently in conjunction with labeled antibodies for the specific detection of particular

organisms. Having a cultivated microbe is again critical for making antibodies for serological or immunohistochemical detection of infection. For an organism such as *Salmonella enterica*, the traditional approach for studying infection works very well. Indeed, having a cultivated microbe creates many more opportunities for scientific investigation. For an organism such as *Tropheryma whippelii*, which is difficult to propagate in the laboratory, this approach is not as facile.

A nucleic acid sequence-based approach to microbial detection, classification, characterization, and localization does not require that the organism be cultivated in the laboratory. Thus, both cultivated and cultivation-resistant microbes are suitable substrates for investigation. Rather than growing microbes in the laboratory, microbial nucleic acid sequences can be "grown" using PCR. For instance, consensus sequence PCR of the bacterial 16S rRNA gene can be used to directly detect and classify bacteria present in the intestine. Quantitative reverse transcriptase PCR (RT-PCR) of bacterial mRNA can be used to measure gene expression of microbes during infection. Fluorescence in situ hybridization can be used to localize microbes to cells in the intestine by targeting microbial nucleic acid sequences with fluorescently labeled probes and visualizing them with fluorescence microscopy.

David N. Fredricks, Program in Infectious Diseases, Fred Hutchinson Cancer Research Center, Seattle, WA 98109-1024.

Microbial Pathogenesis and the Intestinal Epithelial Cell, ed. by G. Hecht
© 2003 ASM Press, Washington, D.C.

BACTERIAL DIVERSITY IN THE INTESTINE: A MOLECULAR CENSUS

The intestine is home to many different species of bacteria that exist in commensal or symbiotic relationships with their host. Some of these microbes are capable of becoming pathogens if provided with an opportunity, such as through perforation of the intestinal wall or migration to another niche (e.g., urinary tract). The microflora in the intestinal niche has been well characterized using cultivation methods, identifying *Escherichia, Bacteroides, Eubacteria, Clostridia, Bifidobacteria*, and other genera (8). What role do sequence-based methods have for defining the bacterial diversity within the human intestine? Studies of natural microbial ecosystems show that cultivation detects only a small fraction of the microbes detected by direct microscopy or sequence-based approaches (1, 13, 18). Is the same true for the microbial ecosystem of the human intestine?

Wilson and Blitchington analyzed a single fecal sample from a 40-year-old man (31). The sample was divided; 1 ml was cultured anaerobically after dilution in tryptic soy broth and plated on modified medium 10, and 1 ml was digested to lyse bacteria and liberate DNA for PCR. Consensus sequence PCR was used to amplify 300-bp segments of bacterial 16S rRNA genes present in the fecal sample, and these PCR products were cloned into *Escherichia coli* to identify individual 16S rDNA sequences from the mixture of bacteria. In this method, PCR primers are used that anneal to highly conserved regions of the bacterial 16S rDNA gene during PCR, amplifying the intervening variable sequence. This variable sequence can be used to identify bacteria, since unique bacterial phylotypes have unique 16S rDNA. The investigators compared the results from direct PCR of the fecal sample with results from PCR analysis of isolates obtained by cultivation on axenic media. Forty-eight culture isolates were compared to 50 PCR clones generated with nine cycles of PCR. In the culture isolates, 21 distinct rDNA sequences were found. In the PCR clones, 27 distinct rDNA sequences were found. Some sequences were found only by culture, and some sequences were found only by PCR. Nevertheless, greater bacterial diversity was detected by PCR than by cultivation. Several bacteria were detected by PCR that had never been isolated from human feces, including a planctomycete and *Lachnospira pectinoschiza*. Almost 75% of the 16S rDNA sequences generated by PCR were more than 2 bp different from sequences in public databases. Interestingly, 69% of the cultivated bacteria also had 16S rDNA sequences that were more than two bases different from 16S rDNA sequences in public databases. It is not clear if these differences were due to identification of novel microbes, sequencing/Taq misincorporation errors, or poor representation of fecal flora in public 16S rDNA databases.

Suau and colleagues also used sequence-based methods to study the fecal flora of a 40-year-old man (28). Although they used PCR to amplify most of the 16S rRNA gene from bacteria in the sample (~1,500 bp), they sequenced only about 500 bp from each clone. They were able to cultivate 2.2×10^{11} bacteria per g (dry weight) of feces. Using 4′,6-diamidino-2-phenylindole (DAPI) staining of bacteria and fluorescence microscopy, they counted 10.6×10^{11} bacteria per g in the same sample. Using fluorescence in situ hybridization with a 16S rRNA probe, they counted 7.1×10^{11} bacteria per g of feces. Thus, fecal colony counts represented only 21 to 32% of the bacteria detected with direct microscopy. These results are analogous to what is routinely found when attempts are made to culture bacteria from environmental niches such as ocean water or soil. The cultivated bacteria represent only a small proportion of the bacteria detected by cultivation-independent methods.

Suau and colleagues analyzed 284 clones from their 16S rDNA PCR (28). There were 82 distinct phylotypes represented in the clone library. Ninety-five percent of these phylotypes belonged to one of three major phylogenetic groups: the *Bacteroides* group, the

Clostridium coccoides group, and the *Clostridium leptum* group. Again, about 75% of all clone sequences did not match sequences in public databases, suggesting the presence of novel species. Several bacteria appeared to be only distantly related to known bacteria. For instance, phylogenetic analysis showed that some clones branched deeply with the *Mycoplasma*. Other clones were related to *Phasocolarctobacterium faecium, Atopobium, Verrucomicrobium*, and *Eubacterium* groups. These data confirm that sequence-based methods reveal a surprising degree of bacterial diversity in human feces that is not appreciated using cultivation-based methods.

The previous studies examined a single fecal sample from one individual. Zoetendal and colleagues also used 16S rDNA and rRNA profiles to catalog bacteria present in human feces, but analyzed multiple samples (32). They employed temperature gradient gel electrophoresis to compare 16S rDNA profiles among fecal samples from several individuals, and also performed cloning with sequence analysis of bacterial 16S rDNA, as in previous studies. These investigators found that each individual had a unique complement of bacteria in his or her feces, and these assemblages of bacteria were stable over time. Again, the investigators found that most of the bacterial 16S rDNA sequences analyzed by cloning and sequencing represented novel bacteria.

Leser and colleagues performed an exhaustive study of the bacterial flora of pig intestines using PCR of bacterial 16S rDNA with cloning and sequence analysis (14). Fifty-two samples of ileum, cecum, and colon were sampled from 24 pigs, generating 4,270 clones. Leser et al. identified 375 different phylotypes of bacteria, defining a phylotype as a group of bacteria that is less than 97% similar in 16S rDNA to other bacteria. Only 17% of the clones represented well-defined, cultivated bacteria, thus showing that the microbial inhabitants of animal intestines are also poorly characterized.

These sequence-based studies provide a consistent picture of the bacteria that colonize the intestine. It is a picture in which many of the subjects are hard to identify and poorly understood. Defining the whole assemblage of microbes in the human intestine, not just the cultivated members, is necessary for understanding this important niche.

A MICROBE'S VIEW OF THE INTESTINAL EPITHELIAL CELL

Why is it important to define all the microbes that colonize the human intestine? Microbes may play a major role in determining how the intestine develops and functions. Recent studies suggest that an intestine without microbes is like bread without yeast—underdeveloped and flat. The intestine has evolved in step with microbes as a fermentation chamber, allowing the host to digest foods and absorb critical nutrients.

Hooper and colleagues recently highlighted the nature of this finely tuned relationship using *Bacteroides thetaiotaomicron* and germfree mice (12). When developing mice are raised in germfree conditions, they stop expressing fucosylated glycans on intestinal epithelial cells, but resume expression when colonized with *B. thetaiotaomicron*. *B. thetaiotaomicron* scavenges fucose for metabolism and appears to signal the intestinal cells to produce hydrolyzable fucosylated glycans. The bacteria use a repressor, FucR, as a sensor of fucose availability. FucR controls expression of enzymes used in bacterial fucose metabolism, and controls another locus that appears to play a role in signaling host epithelial cells to manufacture fucose. The bacterial signal that promotes production of fucosylated glycans on intestinal cells has not been elucidated.

Hooper et al. extended this work by using DNA microarrays and quantitative RT-PCR to monitor gene expression in the intestine of germfree mice inoculated with *B. thetaiotaomicron* (11). *B. thetaiotaomicron* causes a shift in the intestinal transcriptional response beyond that used for glycan production, modulating genes involved in nutrient absorption, mucosal barrier formation, metabolism, and development. For instance, *B. thetaiotaomicron* induces upregulation of intestinal sodium-glucose transporter, pancreatic lipase-related protein, colipase, fatty acid-binding protein, apolipoprotein A-IV, and high-affinity epithelial copper transporter. Stimulation of intestinal nutrient transport mechanisms by bacteria may explain a curious observation. Germfree mice require about 30% more calories to maintain weight than mice with normal intestinal microflora do. These studies show that there is an intricate interaction between the intestinal epithelial cell and *B. thetaiotaomicron* and that both microbe and host depend on each other for normal function and development in the intestine.

These data provide evidence that the intestine is no passive receptacle for microbes, but actively promotes colonization with selected microbes or microbial communities for mutual benefit (9, 10). By "feeding" *B. thetaiotaomicron*, for instance, the intestine may help exclude pathogenic microbes from the intestinal niche. Given the hundreds of bacteria present in the human intestine, the number of potential interactions between host and bacterium is large indeed. Understanding the exquisite orchestration between commensal microbes and host cells may provide additional insights on how pathogens interfere to cause disease. For instance, do any pathogens disrupt the normal signaling between *B. thetaiotaomicron* and intestinal epithelial cells, thereby terminating the supply of fucose used for maintenance of normal flora?

WHIPPLE'S DISEASE: USING NUCLEIC ACIDS TO DETECT AND CHARACTERIZE PATHOGENS

In 1907 Whipple described a fatal wasting disease in a 36-year-old physician (29). Notable features of this illness include migratory polyarthritis, fever, weight loss, diarrhea, abdominal pain, lymphadenopathy, and hyperpigmentation of the skin. Although the clinical characteristics of Whipple's disease overlap with other conditions such as tuberculosis and cancer, the histological findings in the small intestine are distinct. Patients with

intestinal involvement usually have short, blunted intestinal villi, which are infiltrated with abundant foamy histiocytes. Staining with periodic acid-Schiff (PAS) reagent reveals magenta inclusions within the histiocytes infiltrating the intestine. Although Whipple noted bacterial structures in a silver-stained section of abdominal lymph node from his initial case, he attributed the pathological abnormalities to a derangement in fat metabolism, since neither culture nor animal inoculation revealed a pathogen.

The microbial cause of Whipple's disease was first revealed by studies showing that this fatal disease could be cured with antibiotics (19). Confirmation that a bacterium was responsible came from studies using electron microscopy to visualize affected tissues (16). A small, monomorphic bacterium with a characteristic cell wall was seen in both intracellular and extracellular sites of diseased tissue. Clumps of partially degraded bacteria were noted to form the PAS-positive macrophage inclusions noted on histologic sections of intestine. Antibiotic treatment resulted in clearance of bacteria, while relapse was associated with the reappearance of bacteria. Although this bacterium was visualized in diseased tissues, multiple attempts to cultivate the organism failed.

The identity of the Whipple bacillus was first revealed not through cultivation, but through identification of a bacterial nucleic acid sequence in affected tissues, specifically the 16S rRNA gene. In 1991–1992 two groups used consensus sequence PCR to amplify segments of the bacterial 16S rRNA gene directly from the tissues of patients with Whipple's disease (25, 30). Phylogenetic analysis of these amplified gene fragments revealed that the Whipple bacillus belongs to the actinobacteria clade of the actinomycetes. This bacterium is sufficiently different from other known bacteria to suggest that it deserves its own genus designation, and the name *Tropheryma whippelii* was proposed. PCR shows that the unique 16S rDNA sequence from this bacterium is consistently found in tissues from patients with Whipple's disease and disappears with effective antibiotic treatment (20, 22).

In 1997, Schoedon and colleagues reported the successful propagation of *T. whippelii* in human macrophages by using cytokines to deactivate intracellular killing of bacteria (26). A continuous culture of bacteria was not achieved, however. In 2000, Raoult and colleagues successfully passaged *T. whippelii* by cocultivation with a human fibroblast cell line (23). Although the prolonged doubling time and fastidious nature of this organism make routine cultivation impractical in the clinical microbiology laboratory, propagation of bacteria in the research laboratory may create a system for determining in vitro antibiotic susceptibility and allow development of a serologic assay for infection.

The relationship between *T. whippelii* and intestinal epithelial cells is poorly understood. Although *T. whippelii* has been detected by electron microscopy within some intestinal epithelial cells, most bacteria are found in other compartments (2, 3, 27). Ultrastructural studies show intact bacteria are most prevalent in the lamina propria just basal to epithelial cells. Both intact and degraded bacteria are found within macrophages of the lamina propria. Where do bacteria multiply, and how can one measure this? One approach is to label bacterial rRNA with a fluorescent probe and visualize the distribution of bacteria directly in affected tissues. Intact bacteria require intact rRNA for synthesis of proteins. Bacteria also regulate rRNA levels depending on growth conditions, with levels of rRNA mirroring the metabolic state of the organism (21). Thus, binding of fluorescent probes to bacterial rRNA has been used as an indirect measure of metabolic activity in bacteria.

A *T. whippelii*-specific DNA probe targeting 16S rRNA was synthesized for use in a fluorescence in situ hybridization assay (FISH). Hybridization of this probe to sections of fixed, paraffin-embedded intestinal biopsies obtained from Whipple's disease patients showed an interesting pattern of uptake (6). Most of the probe hybridized to bacteria located in the lamina propria at the tips of blunted intestinal villi, just underneath the intestinal epithelial cells (Color Plate 1). Staining of the intracellular human cytoskeletal protein vimentin confirmed that most of the bacterial rRNA signal occurred in the extracellular compartment (Color Plate 2). In contrast, most of the PAS staining in these tissues occurred within macrophages in the lamina propria, and there was very little uptake of rDNA probe within these cells. Taken together, these data suggest that *T. whippelii* is metabolically active in the extracellular compartment of the lamina propria, and bacteria that are engulfed by macrophages are mostly destroyed.

Many questions are left unanswered. How does *T. whippelii* get into the lamina propria to initiate infection? The most appealing explanation is that this bacterium is ingested and passes through intestinal epithelial cells or M cells and is deposited in the lamina propria. Without an animal model of Whipple's disease, it is difficult to test these hypotheses. If bacteria replicate in the extracellular spaces of the lamina propria and are killed by macrophages, then why does disease ensue? Do patients with Whipple's disease have an immune defect that prevents destruction of this microbe? Patients with Whipple's disease develop a malabsorptive diarrhea with steatorrhea. Intestinal epithelial cells appear intact. How does *T. whippelii* orchestrate this change in intestinal function? Whipple's disease is a systemic illness which commonly involves the joints, lung, brain, heart, and other organs. Intact bacteria have been detected in these tissues. How does *T. whippelii* disseminate in the body? Is this bacterium an intracellular passenger within macrophages, or does it travel in the extracellular environment?

C. CAYETANENSIS: TAXONOMY OF AN INTESTINAL PARASITE

Cyclospora cayetanensis is an obligate intracellular parasite of the intestinal epithelial cell that has thus far defied attempts at laboratory propagation (7). *C. cayetanensis* infection causes prolonged diarrhea and is treated with trimethoprim-sulfamethoxazole. Cyclosporiasis is found throughout the world, with recent outbreaks in North America linked to imported raspberries. Diagnosis is usually made by detecting the large, spherical, 8- to 10-μm, acid-fast oocysts in stool. The taxonomic history of this organism reflects the difficulties posed by using morphological characteristics alone to classify organisms. Although first labeled a coccidian protozoan parasite when detected in 1977 in Papua New Guinea, the organism has also been called a fungus, a cyanobacterium-like body, and blue-green algae.

PCR, sequencing, and phylogenetic analysis of the small subunit rRNA gene from purified oocysts showed that *C. cayetanensis* clusters with the *Eimeria* family (24), a group of intestinal pathogens of animals that were first described in moles but have also been found in other mammals, birds, snakes, and insects. Each *Eimeria* species tends to infect a single host species. Other species of *Cyclospora* have been detected in stool samples from non-human primates (4, 15). *Cyclospora papionis* infects baboons, *Cyclospora colobi* infects colobus monkeys, and *Cyclospora cercopitheci* infects green monkeys. These *Cyclospora* species have unique rRNA sequences and form a distinct clade with *C. cayetanensis*. The presence of a single 18S rDNA profile in human fecal samples and the failure to find another animal host suggest that *C. cayetanensis* has evolved as a human pathogen (5). Analysis of the *C. cayetanensis* internal transcribed spacer region 1 (ITS-1) of the rRNA operon shows that there is great diversity among human strains in this sequence, but there is no geographical clustering of particular ITS-1 types (17).

Nucleic acid sequence-based methods have been used to develop PCR assays for *Cyclospora* species. These assays have been used to test fecal samples for diagnosis of infection and to screen food to identify sources of contamination. PCR has also been used to study the epidemiology of cyclosporiasis and the evolutionary relationships between *C. cayetanensis* and other pathogens with similar appearance—all without having a cultivated supply of organisms. These advances highlight the potential for using nucleic acid sequences to study intestinal pathogens.

REFERENCES

1. **Amann, R. I., W. Ludwig, and K. H. Schleifer.** 1995. Phylogenetic identification and in situ detection of individual microbial cells without cultivation. *Microbiol. Rev.* **59:**143–169.
2. **Denholm, R. B., P. R. Mills, and I. A. More.** 1981. Electron microscopy in the long-term follow-up of Whipple's disease. Effect of antibiotics. *Am. J. Surg. Pathol.* **5:**507–516.
3. **Dobbins, W. O. 3rd, and J. M. Ruffin.** 1967. A light- and electron-microscopic study of bacterial invasion in Whipple's disease. *Am. J. Pathol.* **51:**225–242.
4. **Eberhard, M. L., A. J. da Silva, B. G. Lilley, and N. J. Pieniazek.** 1999. Morphologic and molecular characterization of new *Cyclospora* species from Ethiopian monkeys: *C. cercopitheci* sp.n., *C. colobi* sp.n., and *C. papionis* sp.n. *Emerg. Infect. Dis.* **5:**651–658.
5. **Eberhard, M. L., Y. R. Ortega, D. E. Hanes, E. K. Nace, R. Q. Do, M. G. Robl, K. Y. Won, C. Gavidia, N. L. Sass, K. Mansfield, A. Gozalo, J. Griffiths, R. Gilman, C. R. Sterling, and M. J. Arrowood.** 2000. Attempts to establish experimental *Cyclospora cayetanensis* infection in laboratory animals. *J. Parasitol.* **86:** 577–582.
6. **Fredricks, D. N., and D. A. Relman.** 2001. Localization of *Tropheryma whippelii* rRNA in tissues from patients with Whipple's disease. *J. Infect. Dis.* **183:**1229–1233.
7. **Herwaldt, B. L.** 2000. *Cyclospora cayetanensis*: a review, focusing on the outbreaks of cyclosporiasis in the 1990s. *Clin. Infect. Dis.* **31:**1040–1057.
8. **Holdeman, L. V., I. J. Good, and W. E. Moore.** 1976. Human fecal flora: variation in bacterial composition within individuals and a possible effect of emotional stress. *Appl. Environ. Microbiol.* **31:**359–375.
9. **Hooper, L. V., and J. I. Gordon.** 2001. Commensal host-bacterial relationships in the gut. *Science* **292:**1115–1118.
10. **Hooper, L. V., and J. I. Gordon.** 2001. Glycans as legislators of host-microbial interactions: spanning the spectrum from symbiosis to pathogenicity. *Glycobiology* **11:**1R–10R.
11. **Hooper, L. V., M. H. Wong, A. Thelin, L. Hansson, P. G. Falk, and J. I. Gordon.** 2001. Molecular analysis of commensal host-microbial

relationships in the intestine. *Science* 291:881–884.

12. **Hooper, L. V., J. Xu, P. G. Falk, T. Midtvedt, and J. I. Gordon.** 1999. A molecular sensor that allows a gut commensal to control its nutrient foundation in a competitive ecosystem. *Proc. Natl. Acad. Sci. USA* **96**:9833–9838.

13. **Hugenholtz, P., B. M. Goebel, and N. R. Pace.** 1998. Impact of culture-independent studies on the emerging phylogenetic view of bacterial diversity. *J. Bacteriol.* **180**:4765–4774.

14. **Leser, T. D., J. Z. Amenuvor, T. K. Jensen, R. H. Lindecrona, M. Boye, and K. Moller.** 2002. Culture-independent analysis of gut bacteria: the pig gastrointestinal tract microbiota revisited. *Appl. Environ. Microbiol.* **68**:673–690.

15. **Lopez, F. A., J. Manglicmot, T. M. Schmidt, C. Yeh, H. V. Smith, and D. A. Relman.** 1999. Molecular characterization of *Cyclospora*-like organisms from baboons. *J. Infect. Dis.* **179**:670–676.

16. **Maiwald, M., and D. Relman.** 2001. Whipple's disease and *Tropheryma whippelii*: secrets slowly revealed. *Clin. Infect. Dis.* **32**:457–463.

17. **Olivier, C., S. van de Pas, P. W. Lepp, K. Yoder, and D. A. Relman.** 2001. Sequence variability in the first internal transcribed spacer region within and among *Cyclospora* species is consistent with polyparasitism. *Int. J. Parasitol.* **31**:1475–1487.

18. **Pace, N. R.** 1997. A molecular view of microbial diversity and the biosphere. *Science* **276**:734–740.

19. **Paulley, J. W.** 1952. A case of Whipple's disease. *Gastroenterology* 22:128–133.

20. **Petrides, P. E., J. Muller-Hocker, D. N. Fredricks, and D. A. Relman.** 1998. PCR analysis of *T. whippelii* DNA in a case of Whipple's disease: effect of antibiotics and correlation with histology. *Am. J. Gastroenterol.* **93**:1579–1582.

21. **Poulsen, L. K., G. Ballard, and D. A. Stahl.** 1993. Use of rRNA fluorescence in situ hybridization for measuring the activity of single cells in young and established biofilms. *Appl. Environ. Microbiol.* **59**:1354–1360.

22. **Ramzan, N. N., E. Loftus, Jr., L. J. Burgart, M. Rooney, K. P. Batts, R. H. Wiesner, D. N. Fredricks, D. A. Relman, and D. H. Persing.** 1997. Diagnosis and monitoring of Whipple disease by polymerase chain reaction. *Ann. Intern. Med.* **126**:520–527.

23. **Raoult, D., M. L. Birg, B. La Scola, P. E. Fournier, M. Enea, H. Lepidi, V. Roux, J. C. Piette, F. Vandenesch, D. Vital-Durand, and T. J. Marrie.** 2000. Cultivation of the bacillus of Whipple's disease. *N. Engl. J. Med.* **342**:620–625.

24. **Relman, D. A., T. M. Schmidt, A. Gajadhar, M. Sogin, J. Cross, K. Yoder, O. Sethabutr, and P. Echeverria.** 1996. Molecular phylogenetic analysis of *Cyclospora*, the human intestinal pathogen, suggests that it is closely related to *Eimeria* species. *J. Infect. Dis.* **173**:440–445.

25. **Relman, D. A., T. M. Schmidt, R. P. MacDermott, and S. Falkow.** 1992. Identification of the uncultured bacillus of Whipple's disease. *N. Engl. J. Med.* **327**:293–301.

26. **Schoedon, G., D. Goldenberger, R. Forrer, A. Gunz, F. Dutly, M. Hochli, M. Altwegg, and A. Schaffner.** 1997. Deactivation of macrophages with interleukin-4 is the key to the isolation of *Tropheryma whippelii*. *J. Infect. Dis.* **176:**672–677.

27. **Silva, M. T., P. M. Macedo, and J. F. Moura Nunes.** 1985. Ultrastructure of bacilli and the bacillary origin of the macrophagic inclusions in Whipple's disease. *J. Gen. Microbiol.* **131**(Pt. 5):1001–1013.

28. **Suau, A., R. Bonnet, M. Sutren, J. J. Godon, G. R. Gibson, M. D. Collins, and J. Dore.** 1999. Direct analysis of genes encoding 16S rRNA from complex communities reveals many novel molecular species within the human gut. *Appl. Environ. Microbiol.* **65**:4799–4807.

29. **Whipple, G. H.** 1907. A hitherto undescribed disease characterized anatomically by deposits of fat and fatty acids in the intestinal mesenteric lymphatic tissues. *Johns Hopkins Hosp. Bull.* **18**:382–391.

30. **Wilson, K. H., R. Blitchington, R. Frothingham, and J. A. Wilson.** 1991. Phylogeny of the Whipple's-disease-associated bacterium. *Lancet* **338**:474–475.

31. **Wilson, K. H., and R. B. Blitchington.** 1996. Human colonic biota studied by ribosomal DNA sequence analysis. *Appl. Environ. Microbiol.* **62**:2273–2278.

32. **Zoetendal, E. G., A. D. Akkermans, and W. M. De Vos.** 1998. Temperature gradient gel electrophoresis analysis of 16S rRNA from human fecal samples reveals stable and host-specific communities of active bacteria. *Appl. Environ. Microbiol.* **64**:3854–3859.

APPLICATION OF MICROARRAY ANALYSIS TO THE INVESTIGATION OF HOST-PATHOGEN INTERACTIONS

Dawn A. Israel and Richard M. Peek, Jr.

8

The gastrointestinal tract is a dynamic, interactive barrier that normally segregates microbial populations from their cognate human hosts. A potential aberrant consequence of contact between microbes and gut epithelial cells is the development of mucosal inflammation, which may lead to clinically apparent sequelae in a subset of affected individuals. Disease risk likely involves specific and choreographed interactions (signature responses) between pathogen and host, which, in turn, are dependent upon strain-specific bacterial factors and/or host characteristics governed by genetic polymorphisms. Since epithelial cells represent the first sites of contact for most bacteria within the gut lumen, detailed characterization of both bacterial and host determinants that regulate microbial:epithelial cell interactions will likely generate a molecular portrait of events important in pathogenesis.

Researchers have traditionally identified pathogenesis-related bacterial genes using molecular fingerprinting techniques such as restriction fragment length polymorphisms (RFLP) and random arbitrarily primed PCR

(RAP PCR) to compare virulent and avirulent isolates. Similarly, investigations that focused on changes in bacterial or host gene expression under environmental conditions designed to approximate events occurring in vivo (i.e., bacterial adherence to epithelial cells) have relied on differential screening or differential display techniques. A significant limitation of these approaches, however, is that only a small fraction of the genome or transcriptome can be evaluated. A more comprehensive approach to understanding the different pathogenic effects of diverse bacteria on their hosts requires that each gene within the bacterial genome be interrogated simultaneously. The availability of 95 complete genome sequences from 83 different microbial species and the development of microarrays containing representations of genes for many of these pathogens provide both of the prerequisites required for this approach (Table 1). Eukaryotic arrays that are now readily available also offer the potential to define specific host responses to a particular pathogen (Table 1).

HIGH-DENSITY DNA MICROARRAYS
Microarrays contain thousands of ordered DNAs of known sequence attached to a physical support. The two most common forms are high-density DNA arrays and oligonucleotide

Dawn A. Israel and Richard M. Peek, Jr., Division of Gastroenterology, Department of Medicine, Vanderbilt University Medical Center, Nashville, TN 37232.

Microbial Pathogenesis and the Intestinal Epithelial Cell, ed. by G. Hecht
© 2003 ASM Press, Washington, D.C.

TABLE 1 Summary of published studies using microarray analysis to investigate host-pathogen interactions

Field of study	Authors	Array type	Bacterial species	Eukaryotic cell type	Type of analysis	Comment	Reference
Bacterial genome assessment	Salama et al.	Prokaryotic	*H. pylori*	N/A	DNA	Genome comparison	59
	Israel et al.	Prokaryotic	*H. pylori*	N/A	DNA	Genome comparison	33
	Dorrell et al.	Prokaryotic	*C. jejuni*	N/A	DNA	Genome comparison	21
	Bjorkholm et al.	Prokaryotic	*H. pylori*	N/A	DNA	Genome comparison	9
	Israel et al.	Prokaryotic	*H. pylori*	N/A	DNA	Genome comparison	34
In vitro bacterial gene expression in response to signals that reflect the host environment	Tao et al.	Prokaryotic	*E. coli*	N/A	RNA	Rich *vs.* minimal medium	66
	Selinger et al.	Prokaryotic	*E. coli*	N/A	RNA	Log vs. stationary phase	62
	DeLisa et al.	Prokaryotic	*E. coli*	N/A	RNA	Quorum sensing	18
	Zheng et al.	Prokaryotic	*E. coli*	N/A	RNA	Oxidative stress	74
	Ang et al.	Prokaryotic	*H. pylori*	N/A	RNA	Acid growth	6
	Allan et al.	Prokaryotic	*H. pylori*	N/A	RNA	Acid exposure	4
	Donahue et al.	Prokaryotic	*H. pylori*	AGS gastric epithelial cells	RNA	Adherence	20

Eukaryotic gene expression in vitro following contact with microbial pathogens

Author		Organism	Cell line	Sample	Comparison	Ref.
Rosenberger et al.	Eukaryotic	S. enterica serovar Typhimurium	Macrophages	RNA	Compared wild-type bacteria and purified LPS	57
Detweiler et al.	Eukaryotic	S. enterica serovar Typhimurium	Macrophages	RNA	Compared wild-type and isogenic phoP mutant	19
Eckmann et al.	Eukaryotic	S. dublin	HT29 and T84 intestinal epithelial cells	RNA	Infection	22
Chiou et al.	Eukaryotic	H. pylori	AGS gastric epithelial cells	RNA	Coculture	12
Cox et al.	Eukaryotic	H. pylori	KATO 3 gastric epithelial cells	RNA	Compared wild-type cag^+ and wild-type cag^- strains	14
Maeda et al.	Eukaryotic	H. pylori	MKN45, AGS gastric epithelial cells	RNA	Compared wild-type and isogenic cagE mutant	40
Maeda et al.	Eukaryotic	H. pylori	MKN45 gastric epithelial cells, THP-1 monocytes	RNA	Compared wild-type and cagE mutant in two different cell types	39
Bach et al.	Eukaryotic	H. pylori	AGS gastric epithelial cells	RNA	Compared wild-type and isogenic cagA mutants	8

Characterization of host gene expression in response to bacterial colonization in vivo

Author		Organism	Cell line	Sample	Comparison	Ref.
Hooper et al.	Eukaryotic	B. thetaiotaomicron	Small intestinal cells	RNA	In vivo	32

arrays (24, 29). For DNA arrays, DNA from cloned, synthesized, or PCR-amplified substrate is robotically printed onto glass slides or nylon membranes. For completely sequenced microbial pathogens with small genomes, all the open reading frames (ORFs) are typically included as separate spots on an individual array (often in duplicate or triplicate). In contrast, most eukaryotic arrays contain only a subset of the total ORFs (200 to 15,000) present in that organism. Custom glass arrays can be designed and constructed in conjunction with a biotechnology company or within an individual academic facility, contributing to their flexibility. However, quality control is critical and discrepancies in the amounts of DNA mechanically placed on the slides, length and composition of sequences, and hybridization issues each can reduce the accuracy of replicate experiments. In contrast, primer-based arrays contain short overlapping oligonucleotides representing different genes and are currently available only through commercial manufacturers (38). High-density oligonucleotide arrays yield more reproducible results than arrays containing PCR products because multiple oligonucleotides interrogate each gene, but these systems are less malleable owing to their more stringent design. Although each type of array has particular advantages and disadvantages, both forms can rapidly compare differences in genomic content between bacterial strains by measuring the relative abundance of DNA (Fig. 1). Microarrays can also identify global patterns of transcriptional events that underpin host-microbial interactions relevant to pathogenesis by comparing levels of prokaryotic and eukaryotic RNA that are present under different conditions (Fig. 1).

H. PYLORI AS A PARADIGM FOR USING MICROARRAY TO STUDY GENETIC DIVERSITY AND HOST-MICROBIAL INTERACTIONS

The human stomach was long regarded as a biological sanctuary site that was inhospitable for bacterial growth. Although curved gram-negative bacilli had occasionally been visualized adjacent to the gastric epithelium, their relationship to clinical disease remained inapparent until Marshall and Warren's seminal report relating the presence of these organisms to peptic ulceration (41). *Helicobacter pylori* persists within the stomachs of humans and primates for the life span of its host, and, once established, it has no major bacterial competitors. *H. pylori* induces gastric inflammation in all hosts, and such gastritis increases the risk for peptic ulceration, distal gastric adenocarcinoma, and gastric mucosal lymphoproliferative disease (Fig. 2) (46, 51, 52, 56). In contrast to infection with other mucosal pathogens such as *Shigella* sp. and *Salmonella* sp., however, only a small percentage (<15%) of persons carrying *H. pylori* ever develop clinical sequelae. These observations suggest that disease outcome is likely dependent upon differentially represented bacterial determinants, host characteristics, and/or the specific interactions between a particular strain and its host that occur during decades of coexistence.

H. pylori is tremendously diverse, with virtually each isolate from a different patient being unique (2, 3, 26, 36, 69). Two strains of

FIGURE 1 Identification of differences in bacterial genomic content (A) or gene expression following host-microbial interactions (B). (A) Genomic DNA isolated from a reference and a clinical strain is labeled by incorporating one of two fluorescent nucleotide analogs (Cy3 or Cy5) into the DNA. Differentially labeled DNA samples are then mixed and cohybridized to a whole-genome microbial microarray. Resulting signal intensities from each fluorophore are then compared for each ORF represented on the array, thus allowing one to identify differences in gene content between strains. (B) RNA is isolated from broth-exposed and cocultured bacteria and host cells, reverse transcribed into cDNA, and fluorescently labeled with Cy3 or Cy5. Differentially labeled cDNA samples are then mixed and cohybridized to either a microbial or eukaryotic microarray. Resulting signal intensities from each fluorophore are then compared to identify differences in pathogen and host gene expression that occur following contact.

A

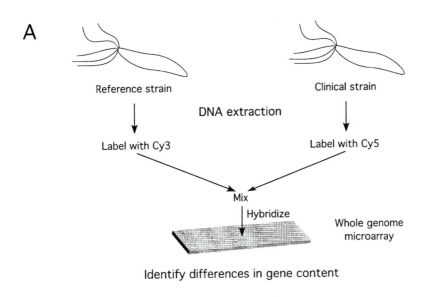

Reference strain

Clinical strain

DNA extraction

Label with Cy3

Label with Cy5

Mix

Hybridize

Whole genome microarray

Identify differences in gene content

B

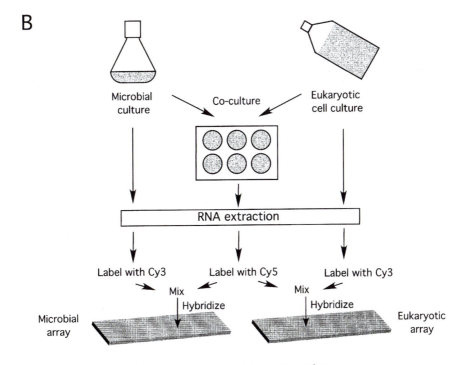

Microbial culture

Co-culture

Eukaryotic cell culture

RNA extraction

Label with Cy3

Label with Cy5

Label with Cy3

Mix

Hybridize

Mix

Hybridize

Microbial array

Eukaryotic array

Identify changes in gene expression

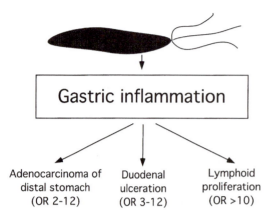

Gastric inflammation

Adenocarcinoma of distal stomach (OR 2-12)

Duodenal ulceration (OR 3-12)

Lymphoid proliferation (OR >10)

FIGURE 2 Relationship of *H. pylori*-induced gastric inflammation with variable disease outcomes. OR, odds ratios.

H. pylori (26695 and J99) have now been completely sequenced, and genomic comparison has revealed that between 6 and 7% of the genes are strain specific, reflecting a high level of genetic diversity. In addition, isolates within an individual may gradually change over time because of recombination between strains, gene rearrangements, or deletions. The most important distinguishing factor among *H. pylori* strains is the presence of the *cag* pathogenicity island, a locus of approximately 40 kb that contains 31 genes (5, 67). Compared with *cag⁻* strains, *H. pylori cag⁺* strains significantly increase the risk for severe gastritis, peptic ulcer disease, and distal gastric cancer (10, 13, 16, 17, 37, 50, 53). The terminal gene in the island, *cagA*, is commonly used as a marker for the entire *cag* locus, and several *cag* island genes have homology to genes encoding type IV secretion system proteins, which export proteins from bacterial cells, raising the hypothesis that interaction between *cag⁺* strains and epithelial cells may instigate aberrant host responses. In point of fact, following *H. pylori* adherence to gastric epithelial cells, the type IV secretion homologs translocate the CagA protein from *H. pylori* into the host cell, where it undergoes c-Src-dependent tyrosine phosphorylation and activates a eukaryotic phosphatase (SHP-2), leading to dephos-

phorylation of host cell proteins (7, 31, 47, 61, 65) and host cell morphological changes (Fig. 3) (60).

Genes within the *cag* island (but not *cagA*) are also required for contact-mediated *H. pylori*-induced release of proinflammatory cytokines, such as interleukin-8 (IL-8), from gastric epithelial cells (25, 64, 68) through activation of the NF-κB and mitogen-activated protein kinase (MAPK) signal transduction cascades (Fig. 3) (25, 35, 42, 44, 63). These in vitro observations mirror in vivo events, as *cag⁺* strains are associated with increased mucosal expression of IL-8 and inflammation in human gastric tissue (53, 72), and loss of genes within the *cag* locus attenuates the severity of gastritis in *H. pylori*-infected Mongolian gerbils (33, 48). The majority of individuals colonized by *cag⁺* strains, however, remain asymptomatic, suggesting that additional *H. pylori* genes may also be important in disease pathogenesis. Collectively, the genetic diversity and availability of complete sequence data from two different strains, the ability to induce disease in a fraction of infected individuals, and the presence of strain-specific virulence determinants in this organism combined with its ability to singularly colonize the gastric niche in the majority of individuals make *H. pylori* an attractive model for studying signature microbial and host interactions relevant to pathogenesis through the use of microarray-based systems.

BACTERIAL GENOME ASSESSMENT

A comprehensive comparison of genetic content among isolates from the same species can distinguish different strains, provide insights into mechanisms of transmission, and delineate relationships between genetic composition and phenotype. The most complete method for determining the genetic composition of an organism is to completely sequence its genome. Although there are now numerous bacterial species for which multiple genome sequences are available, this approach is time-consuming and expensive if applied to more than a few isolates of a single species. Microar-

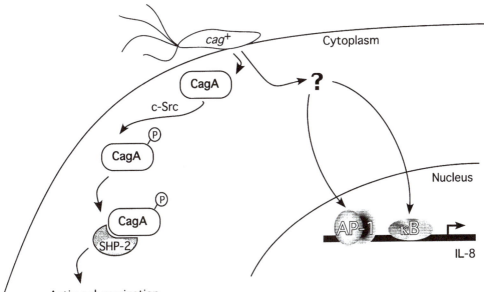

FIGURE 3 Hypothetical model by which *H. pylori cag⁺* strains activate multiple pathways following contact with gastric epithelial cells. Following adherence, CagA is internalized and phosphorylated within the host cell by c-Src. Phospho-CagA then binds to and activates the host phosphatase SHP-2 and induces actin polymerization. A CagA-independent consequence of *cag*-mediated cellular interactions is translocation of an unknown factor ("?"), which then regulates pathways involved in the activation of transcription factors, such as AP-1 and NF-κB, which subsequently stimulate production of IL-8, a proinflammatory cytokine.

ray is a viable and attractive alternative method by which the genetic content of multiple strains can be compared to sequenced genomes from standard strains to assess for the presence or absence of known ORFs. Further, since evolutionary pressures tend to select for the coinheritance of genes involved in common pathways, microarray-based identification of genes that segregate with known virulence-related loci can reveal functional relationships that are not evident from sequence data alone. For this approach, arrays are constructed that contain virtually all the known ORFs of the organism of interest. Genomic DNA isolated from different strains of that particular species is then labeled by incorporating one of two fluorescent nucleotide analogues (generally Cy3- or Cy5-dUTP) into the DNA (Fig. 1). The two differentially labeled DNA samples are then mixed and cohybridized to the whole-genome microarray, and resulting signal intensities from each fluorophore are compared for each ORF represented on the array, allowing one to identify differences in gene content between strains (Fig. 1).

Such a whole-genome approach was recently used to successfully identify *H. pylori* strain-specific genes in multiple isolates (59). Using a microarray containing representations of each gene present in the two completely sequenced *H. pylori* strains (5, 67), Salama et al. compared the genetic content of 15 clinical *H. pylori* isolates and identified 1,281 "core" *H. pylori* genes that were present in all the strains. These investigators also determined that 22% of *H. pylori* genes are nonessential (i.e., strain specific) (59) and that a subset of these covaried with the presence of the *cag* island, including two that encode predicted outer membrane proteins: omp-27 and babA (59). In addition to providing important information regarding the extent of genetic diversity that exists among different isolates, these results have direct clinical ramifications. For example, if certain differentially represented genes are found in future studies to be related to distinct disease outcomes, they may represent novel molecular epidemiologic markers that could identify colonized persons at increased risk for clinical sequelae, who then might be considered for eradication therapy.

Integrating bacterial genomic data with clinical information is another promising application of microarray. Our laboratory recently described two H. pylori strains that induced distinct patterns of host inflammatory responses in vivo and in vitro (33). One strain (B128) rapidly induced pangastritis (i.e., inflammation that involved the entire stomach), ulcerations, and premalignant lesions within the gastric mucosa of Mongolian gerbils, while the other strain (G1.1) merely induced a mild inflammatory response that was localized to the distal stomach. Consistent with its ability to augment gastric mucosal inflammation and injury, B128 also significantly enhanced the production of proinflammatory cytokines from gastric epithelial cells in vitro compared to G1.1. DNA isolated from these two prototype strains was analyzed by hybridization with an H. pylori whole-genome microarray (33), and several strain-specific differences were identified, including a large deletion of the cag pathogenicity island in the less virulent G1.1 strain. Subsequent studies confirmed that absence of these cag island sequences was responsible for differences in the intensity of the host response elicited by these strains, indicating that microarray is an effective method to identify biologically relevant differences in gene content between H. pylori strains that induce distinct pathological outcomes.

The studies described above used an array containing PCR-generated representations of each ORF of the complete H. pylori genome. A modification of this approach is to construct microarrays using amplicons from a genomic library as probes. The disadvantage of this approach is that multiple ORFs may be present in a single clone, thereby complicating interpretation of hybridization data. However, this method takes advantage of preexisting libraries that contain all genomic sequences, which increases the speed in which an array can be developed and reduces the initial expense. Dorrell et al. used such an approach to compare sequence diversity among isolates of Campylobacter jejuni, an organism that is closely related evolutionarily to H. pylori and which is the principal cause of human bacterial gastroenteritis worldwide (21). The C. jejuni array was developed from the clone library of sequenced strain NCTC11168 (49) and was used to compare the genetic composition of 11 C. jejuni strains obtained from a variety of sources. The results of this study were remarkably similar to those initially reported by Salama et al. for H. pylori (59), even though different types of arrays were used. Approximately 21% of the ORFs of the sequenced C. jejuni strain were absent in at least one of the clinical strains tested, indicating that these genes are nonessential and strain specific. Thus, extensive genetic diversity is also present among C. jejuni strains, and these results have provided a framework to correlate differences in gene content with pathogenic outcomes.

In addition to comparing the genomic content of unrelated strains, microarray has also been used to ascertain the extent of bacterial genetic diversity within the biological niche of a single human host to address questions regarding microbial evolution and population dynamics in vivo. In one report, two H. pylori isolates harvested from a single patient were initially compared by macroscale analyses (RFLP and RAP PCR), and were found to be closely related (9, 23). However, comprehensive analysis using microarray revealed that approximately 2% of the ORFs were variably present in these two isolates and that they differed with regard to the presence of the cag island, indicating that they were not identical. To determine whether in vivo adaptation resulted in the gain or loss of virulence genes, the *cag*⁺ isolate was then used to infect conventionally raised and germ-free mice and, after as many as 10 months of colonization, DNA from recovered *H. pylori* isolates was analyzed by microarray to assess the integrity of the *cag* island. There were no differences in *cag* island gene content when the input strain was compared to the recovered isolates, suggesting either that longer periods of colonization are required for such changes to occur, or that this particular mouse model does not exert the same selective pressures found within the human stomach.

Our laboratory also used *H. pylori* whole-genome microarray to examine the genetic diversity of numerous isolates ($n = 14$) harvested from a single patient and to investigate changes in genetic composition that occur over time by comparing DNA content of recent isolates to that from an archival isolate obtained 6 years earlier (34). These isolates were unique in that they were derived from the source patient from whom the fully sequenced *H. pylori* J99 originated. Microarray analysis demonstrated that all 14 isolates examined (archival and 13 recent) were distinct (Fig. 4), varying in the presence or absence of 3% of the genome and that the 13 recent isolates possessed ORFs not present in the archival J99 strain. These results suggest that the *H. pylori* population within the gastric niche of this individual appears to be in a state of genetic flux, which may allow the bacteria to rapidly adapt to changing conditions within its current host, as well as to be poised to colonize a new host. Collectively, these studies demonstrate the utility of microarray technology for analyzing the genetic composition of unrelated members of a bacterial species, identifying potential virulence factors, and defining the population structure of a particularly diverse species.

BACTERIAL GENE EXPRESSION IN RESPONSE TO IN VITRO CONDITIONS THAT REFLECT ELEMENTS OF THE IN VIVO HOST ENVIRONMENT

A central challenge for microbial pathogens is to adapt to changing conditions within the

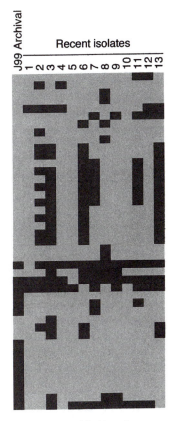

FIGURE 4 Absence (black) and presence (gray) of ORF in archival and recent *H. pylori* strain J99 isolates as determined by microarray analysis. DNA from 13 recent isolates was compared with that from archival strain J99 by hybridization to a whole-genome microarray. Variably present ORFs are shown vertically for each of the isolates.

host, a process that involves regulating gene expression in response to distinct environmental cues. Since microarrays provide the capacity to examine not only global patterns of gene content but also gene expression (Fig. 1), this technique has recently been used to investigate microbial transcriptional responses under well-defined conditions. An additional advantage is that by elucidating the repertoire of genes coexpressed at specific times or under particular physiologic conditions, insights into function can be postulated, with the underpinning assumption being that genes with similar expression profiles likely have similar functions.

Tao et al. used a whole-genome *Escherichia coli* array to analyze differences in gene expression during growth on either rich or minimal medium (66). As expected, genes involved in biosynthesis were not highly expressed when cells were grown in rich medium, whereas those involved in protein synthesis were highly expressed. In contrast, genes involved in biosynthetic pathways, stress responses, and regulatory pathways were highly expressed in minimal medium. From these data, several genes were newly assigned to functional groups based on their coregulation with related genes, and a putative regulatory sequence was identified by comparing the promoter regions of such coregulated genes. In another study, a 25-mer oligonucleotide array that spanned the entire *E. coli* genome, including intergenic regions, was used to assess differences in transcript levels between log and stationary phase cells (62). This global analysis demonstrated that >1,500 genes were differentially expressed under these conditions, including some that were not previously recognized to be growth phase regulated. An additional advantage of this study was that the array design allowed for detection of small and antisense RNAs that would have been undetectable using conventional ORF-limited arrays, which may be important for small regulatory transcripts that have not been previously identified.

Many bacteria such as *E. coli* regulate gene expression in response to cell density or growth rate by the secretion and detection of low-molecular-weight pheromones called autoinducers, a phenomenon known as quorum sensing. Based on these observations, DeLisa and colleagues used microarray hybridization experiments to identify *E. coli* genes that were regulated in response to the signaling molecule autoinducer-2 (AI-2) (18). More than 200 genes were found to have altered expression patterns in response to the presence of AI-2, and many of these genes had quorum-regulated orthologs in other bacteria, including genes involved in cell division, DNA processing, and virulence. Numerous genes of unknown function were also determined to be regulated in response to AI-2 and may be of interest for further study based on their inclusion in this regulon. Another study assessed changes in *E. coli* gene expression in response to oxidative stress by exposing cells to hydrogen peroxide (74). Hybridization of RNA isolated from controls and hydrogen peroxide-exposed bacteria to an *E. coli* microarray identified 140 genes that were strongly induced by oxidative stress, including genes that had previously been shown to be regulated under these conditions using more rudimentary techniques. OxyR is a global regulator of genes induced during oxidative stress, and the use of an *oxyR* isogenic mutant in these experiments identified new members of the OxyR regulon as well as genes induced independently of OxyR, suggesting the existence of a previously unrecognized regulatory pathway.

Microarrays have also been used to identify virulence genes that are required for establishment of colonization and/or tissue damage. As described above, a presupposition is that virulence-associated genes are more likely to be coregulated. This approach is also dependent upon establishing environmental conditions that mirror events occurring within the host ecological niche. *H. pylori* is unique among bacterial pathogens in that it persists for decades in the acidic environment of the human stomach. Exposure to acid in vitro may therefore mimic conditions that these organisms experience in vivo, and two laboratories have now examined *H. pylori* gene expression at neutral and acidic pH. In the first study, RNA from a duodenal ulcer strain grown at pH 7.2 and pH 5.5 for 48 h was reverse transcribed and hybridized with membrane arrays (6). Eighty transcripts were increased and four transcripts were decreased by growth at low pH. Upregulated genes included those encoding an outer membrane protein (*omp-11*), arginase (*rocF*), and an iron ATP-binding cassette (ABC) transporter. The second study analyzed RNA isolated from a different *H. pylori* strain (26695) exposed to neutral (pH 7.0) and acidic (pH 4.0) conditions for only a brief period of time (30 min) (4). Hybridization of cDNA to a membrane array constructed from an *H. pylori* clone library demonstrated that only 11 genes were induced by acid exposure, and this induction was confirmed for 7 of the genes by RNA slot blot hybridizations. Additionally, four genes were repressed under acidic conditions. Highly expressed transcripts originated from genes involved in protein export (*secF*), lipid A biosynthesis (*lpxC*), and *cagA*, while repressed genes included *hopA*, which encodes an outer membrane protein, and *fliS*, encoding a flagellar protein. Interestingly, none of the *H. pylori* genes identified in these two studies as being acid regulated were concordant. The most likely explanation for this discrepancy is a difference in experimental design, including *H. pylori* strain differences, acid growth (48 h) versus acid exposure (30 min), varying acidic pH values (5.5 versus 4.0), and different types of arrays used for analysis. These differences exemplify some of the limitations in attempting to compare results between microarray-based studies, and they emphasize that caution should be taken when drawing broad conclusions from these types of data.

Attachment to underlying gastrointestinal epithelium is critical for colonization, survival, and induction of disease for a number of mucosal pathogens, and, not surprisingly, contact with eukaryotic cells is another stimulus that has been used to investigate regulation of bacterial virulence gene expression. Prior to the advent of bacterial microarrays, studies used random primer-based approaches to successfully identify virulence genes induced by interactions with eukaryotic cells in *Salmonella enterica* serovar Typhimurium (71), *Legionella pneumophila* (1), uropathogenic *E. coli* (73), *Yersinia pseudotuberculosis* (58), and *H. pylori* (54). However, these techniques sample only a small fraction of the total transcriptional pool and are dependent upon the G+C content of the interrogating primers and the particular microbial genome. Recently, Donahue et al. used microarrays to address the same question

more comprehensively (20). In this study, *H. pylori* strain J166 was allowed to adhere to AGS gastric epithelial cells for 1 h. RNA was then extracted from adherent and broth-exposed control *H. pylori*, reverse transcribed, and hybridized with a membrane array. The expression of several *H. pylori* genes was found to be increased following adherence (20), indicating that contact with epithelial cells is an important stimulus for *H. pylori* genes that may be related to pathogenesis. For example, transcript levels of *prfA*, encoding peptide chain release factor, were found to be low in broth-exposed bacteria, but increased following adherence. Experiments involving exposure of bacteria to conditions that are similar to those encountered in vivo followed by assessment of the transcriptional responses using microarrays will undoubtedly become more common as investigators continue to elucidate bacterial signaling pathways that are involved in pathogenic host-microbial interactions.

EUKARYOTIC GENE EXPRESSION IN RESPONSE TO BACTERIAL CONTACT

Contact between a host and a specific microbial pathogen not only alters bacterial gene expression but also results in dramatic changes in eukaryotic gene expression. The commercial availability of a variety of human, murine, and rat DNA and oligonucleotide arrays has now provided the ability to monitor host gene expression in response to different pathogens. This approach can also be used to compare cellular responses to wild-type and isogenic mutant strains in which well-defined virulence genes have been inactivated, which can provide more detailed insights into mechanisms of pathogenesis. These types of studies should, however, be supplemented with confirmatory experiments to verify the role of particular virulence determinants in inducing a specific host expression profile. One approach to confirm microarray-derived results is to use genetic complementation studies that restore the wild-type phenotype. For example, bacterial genes identified by isogenic mutagenesis as being associated with a particular host transcriptional response can be replaced on the bacterial chromosome of a knockout mutant strain adjacent to a strong promoter for single copy expression. Alternatively, genes can be placed downstream of a promoter on a plasmid for multicopy expression (30). These complemented strains can then be tested for their ability to restore host gene expression profiles induced by wild-type bacteria using microarray, Northern analysis, RNA slot-blot hybridizations, or quantitative reverse transcriptase (qRT)-PCR. These same constructs can also be transfected into avirulent strains to determine whether the addition of single genes can alter the phenotype such that recombinant strains might gain the ability to induce specific host genes that are upregulated by virulent strains. Purified virulence components (i.e., lipopolysaccharide [LPS], toxins) can also be tested to further establish that particular host expression patterns are induced by specific bacterial constituents per se.

Most studies that have examined eukaryotic gene expression in response to pathogens used isolated in vitro systems in which host cell gene expression is measured before and following infection with a microorganism (Fig. 1). Patterns of gene expression can be followed temporally, allowing one to elucidate which host genes are up- or downregulated over the course of infection. Two studies have used microarrays to examine alterations in macrophage gene expression in response to infection with S. enterica serovar Typhimurium, an invasive pathogen that induces a robust mucosal inflammatory response and is a major cause of diarrhea (19, 57). In the first study, serovar Typhimurium infection of murine macrophages in vitro for 4 h resulted in the induction of 40 and suppression of 3 genes on a 588-gene membrane array compared with control cells (57). Transcripts that were present at higher levels included those encoding IL-1β, the tumor necrosis factor-alpha (TNF-α) receptor, CD40, and IκBβ. This study also demonstrated that alterations in macrophage gene expression observed following coculture

with viable serovar Typhimurium were remarkably similar to changes seen when cells were stimulated by bacterial LPS alone, implicating this bacterial determinant as a virulence component.

Detweiler and colleagues examined a similar question more comprehensively by using a 22,571 human cDNA microarray to assess the effect of infection of human macrophages with wild-type and isogenic mutant S. enterica serovar Typhimurium strains (19). Sixty-eight transcripts were increased to levels twofold or greater as a result of infection with the wild-type Salmonella strain, and 55 (81%) of these have known functions. Since the S. enterica gene phoP encodes the transcriptional activator component of a two-component response-regulator system involved in control of gene expression in response to particular environmental conditions and is required for virulence in mice (27, 43), the investigators next sought to determine whether different macrophage gene expression profiles were induced by wild-type serovar Typhimurium versus an isogenic phoP mutant. Thirty-four mRNAs were present at lower levels in cells infected with the phoP mutant, including six that encoded proteins involved in cell cycle regulation or cell death. These observational data were elegantly confirmed by functional studies, demonstrating that twice as many macrophages were killed after 4 h of coculture with the wild-type strain compared with the phoP mutant, and this increased to a three-fold difference after 24 h. Thus, in these experiments, the use of microarrays led to the identification of a direct role for PhoP in macrophage cell death.

Although studies of the effects of Salmonella spp. on macrophage gene expression have provided important insights into potential mechanisms of pathogenesis in vivo, the interaction between enteric pathogens and intestinal epithelial cells is often the first step in establishment of mucosal and ultimately systemic infection of the host. Emphasizing the utility of in vitro model systems to study the interaction between Salmonella spp. and intestinal epithelial cells, Eckmann et al. compared the transcription profiles of uninfected and *Salmonella dublin*-infected HT-29 and T84 cells using two different membrane arrays that contained >4,000 cDNAs (22). In general, there was high concordance in the results from the two arrays, and genes that were upregulated by infection included cytokines (granulocyte-stimulating factor, IL-8, macrophage inflammatory protein-2α), kinases, transcription factors, and human leukocyte antigen (HLA) class I genes. The authors next repeated these studies following inhibition of NF-κB activation and demonstrated that many of the bacterial-induced genes were repressed, underscoring the pivotal role of NF-κB signaling in the inflammatory response to *Salmonella* spp. That only a fraction of epithelial cell transcripts were increased after infection also suggested that the epithelial cell response to *Salmonella* spp. was specific.

Adherence of *H. pylori* to gastric epithelial cells is critical for colonization and survival, and epithelial cells undergo transcriptional and morphological alterations following binding of these organisms. To date, five studies have examined the transcriptional responses of gastric epithelial cells to *H. pylori* (8, 12, 14, 39, 40). These studies were similar in design to the *Salmonella* experiments described above, as they involved coculture of *H. pylori* with gastric epithelial cells that was followed by assessment of differences in epithelial cell gene expression using arrays. However, these studies used various strains of *H. pylori*, different gastric epithelial cell lines, varying times of coculture, and different arrays. Chiou et al. used a 588-gene array to examine gene expression in AGS cells following 24 h of coculture with a single strain of *H. pylori*. Twenty-one genes were overexpressed and 17 genes were downregulated by *H. pylori*. Upregulated genes included transcription factors (*c*-jun), signal transduction components (ERK1, MKK3, MKK4), and epidermal growth factors (EGF). Importantly, the authors then attempted to confirm that a subset of these genes ($n = 5$) had similar expression patterns within *H.*

pylori-infected compared to uninfected gastric mucosa. Three of the five genes analyzed (*ERCC3*, *Id-2*, *NM23-H2*) were downregulated in both *H. pylori*-infected AGS cells and colonized gastric tissue; however, 2/5 (*c*-jun, *CDC25B*) were differentially altered in AGS cells as determined by microarray, but levels were no different than controls in vivo. These results underscore an inherent limitation of in vitro systems and emphasize that restraint must be exercised when one attempts to extrapolate results obtained in isolated bacterial:epithelial cell models to events that occur within an infected host.

Another study using multiple arrays that contained 57,800 represented eukaryotic genes examined a much more extensive spectrum of differences in gene expression induced by a wild-type *H. pylori* cag$^+$ strain and a wild-type cag$^-$ strain. Using multiple time points (45 min, 3 h, 24 h), the authors identified 208 genes with known predicted functions and 48 novel genes that were differentially expressed following *H. pylori* infection. Further, 92 known genes and 15 novel cDNAs were differentially expressed by the cag$^+$ versus the cag$^-$ strain. Expression levels of three genes (encoding ADAM 10, amphiregulin, HPYR1), which were found to be upregulated by array analysis, were also quantitated within colonized and normal gastric tissue by RT-PCR. All three transcripts were increased in infected versus uninfected mucosa, and investigations are continuing to more completely verify differential expression levels of microarray-identified *H. pylori* genes.

A more limited study reported by Maeda et al. used an array containing only 2,304 represented genes (40). An *H. pylori* cag$^+$ isolate was incubated with either AGS or MKN45 gastric epithelial cells for 3 h and expression profiles were determined. Only eight transcripts were found to be increased by *H. pylori*, and these included genes encoding IL-8, IκBα, and glutathione peroxidase. In six of the eight genes, enhanced expression was confirmed by RT-PCR. The authors then repeated the experiments using an isogenic *H.*

pylori cagE mutant derivative and found that, in contrast to the wild-type strain, no genes were significantly upregulated, suggesting that genes within the *cag* island are required for induction of these transcripts. These same investigators have recently extended these findings by using membrane-based arrays specific for cytokines and their receptors to examine differences in immune response genes in gastric epithelial cells and monocytes following incubation with *H. pylori* (39). They identified 15 genes whose expression increased in both cell types following *H. pylori* coculture, including precursors of IL-8, IL-6, and IL-1β. Interestingly, there were also genes for which increased expression was lineage specific, including genes that encode neuromodulin and bone morphogenetic protein 4 (epithelial cells), as well as macrophage inflammatory protein 2-α (MIP2-α), precursors for the IL-4 and IL-7 receptors, and vascular endothelial growth factor (VEGF) (monocytes). When these experiments were repeated using an *H. pylori cagE* isogenic mutant strain, induction of epithelial cell, but not monocyte, gene expression was abrogated, suggesting that *H. pylori* regulates gene expression in these cell types by independent mechanisms.

The last study used a 588-human-cDNA array to examine AGS gastric epithelial cell gene expression in response to a 4.5-h incubation with wild-type and isogenic *cagA* mutant *H. pylori* strains (8). Transcription levels of LIM kinase (LIMK), bone morphogenetic protein 1, and MIP2-α were increased, while focal adhesion kinase (FAK), Y-box protein 1, and c-*myc* were decreased by wild-type *H. pylori* compared to the *cagA⁻* mutants, and altered levels of expression for LIMK and FAK were confirmed by Northern blots. Although limited by differences in methodologic design, these studies have set the stage for further delineation of cellular processes altered by *H. pylori* infection.

COMPREHENSIVE CHARACTERIZATION AND VERIFICATION OF MICROBIALLY INITIATED HOST GENE EXPRESSION IN VIVO

The studies described above demonstrate the utility of microarray-based approaches for investigating pathogen-induced changes in host gene expression; however, they also exemplify limitations of this approach. These include the use of different strains, varying cell lines, multiple time points, distinct arrays, and limited analyses for verification of array data. Even if a single strain is used to infect one cell type for a specific time period, the growth characteristics of that organism on particular days may not be exactly comparable, leading to differences in nutrient utilization or pH of the growth medium. Another limitation is that ex vivo systems are isolated compared to the host environment where epithelial cells exist in a complex milieu with luminal bacteria, lamina propria cells, and cytokines each exerting an influence on transcriptional events. Therefore, although in vitro experiments can yield a wealth of information and provide promising leads regarding host-pathogen interactions, complete effects of microbes on their hosts can be studied only in vivo. To this end, Hooper et al. used microarrays complemented by real-time RT-PCR and laser capture microdissection to examine the global transcriptome response of mouse ileal cells to colonization by a commensal organism, *Bacteroides thetaiotaomicron* (32). Germfree mice were colonized with *B. thetaiotaomicron* and, following 10 days of infection, mRNA from ileal tissue was harvested from treated and untreated animals and hybridized to an oligonucleotide array designed to approximately 25,000 murine sequences. mRNAs representing 95 probe sets increased and those representing 23 probe sets decreased as a result of colonization. Because of redundancies in the probe set, 71 known genes and 34 uncharacterized genes were actually differentially expressed. Changes in the abundance of selected transcripts ($n = 12$) were subsequently verified by real-time qRT-PCR, and very consistent results were obtained using the two modalities. Genes with increased expression levels included those encoding acute phase proteins, serum amyloid A, a C-reactive protein homolog, and proteins associated with nutrient utilization. The investigators also assessed cellular responses by supplementing qRT-PCR with laser-capture microdissection (LCM) to compare expression in crypt epithelial cells, epithelial cells overlying villi, and mesenchymal cells beneath the crypt-villus axis. By combining these techniques, the authors were able to distinguish differences in gene expression, not only in colonized versus germfree mice, but also among host cell types.

Of interest, colonization by *B. thetaiotaomicron* did not activate genes associated with inflammation or immune stimulation, which is congruent with this organism's postulated role as a component of the commensal flora. The ability of nonpathogenic bacteria to contribute to the normal development of digestive and immunological functions within the gut is becoming increasingly recognized, and specific mechanisms that may underpin these events have recently been delineated. For example, nonpathogenic *Salmonella* spp. attenuate IL-8 secretion induced by pathogenic strains by inhibiting the ubiquitination of IκBα, a novel mechanism for dampening the inflammatory response (45). These concepts can also be extended to extraintestinal microbial-host interactions. An intriguing characteristic of *H. pylori*-induced gastritis is its capacity to persist for decades without causing serious damage in most cases. This is in marked contrast to inflammatory reactions induced by other gram-negative pathogens, which either resolve over a limited time span or progress to eliminate the host. Clinical complications of *H. pylori* colonization, such as peptic ulcer disease and gastric cancer, therefore likely represent imbalances in gastric homeostasis that are disadvantageous for both microbe and host, particularly if death of the host ensues. A hypothesis based on these microecological perspectives is that *H. pylori* possesses mechanisms to subdue the host inflammatory response, a requirement seemingly inherent for an infectious microbe that persists for the lifetime of its host. In support of this, Crabtree and colleagues have found that inactivation of a *cag* island gene (*cag-10*) results in a paradoxical increase in IL-8 secretion compared to levels induced by wild-type *H. pylori* (15). *H. pylori* infection is associated with increased mucosal levels of IL-10 (11, 28, 53, 72), an anti-inflammatory cytokine that inhibits secretion of proinflammatory chemokines from macrophages and neutrophils. When compared with LPS from the *Enterobacteriaceae*, *H. pylori* LPS is 1,000-fold less active and only weakly activates macrophages (55). The failure of *H. pylori* to invade the mucosa may contribute to its long-term persistence. It is tempting to speculate that *H. pylori* can also orchestrate the host response by negatively regulating intracellular eukaryotic signaling pathways, as has recently been described in *S. enterica* serovar Typhimurium (45). This can be determined more definitively in the future through the use of global assay systems such as microarray, with an additional benefit being the identification of prokaryotic factors required for these phenomena.

CONCLUSIONS

Microarray analysis of bacterial and host gene expression provides a powerful and comprehensive method of examining microbial pathogenesis from a novel perspective. The explosive increase in the amount of genomic sequence available in the past few years has now been coupled with bioinformatic approaches that contain great promise for predicting the role of specific genes differentially altered by the interaction between a pathogen and its host. The ability to survey responses of complete (bacterial) or a large subset (host) of genomes and to identify signature transcriptional profiles from bacteria and hosts will allow fundamental questions to be addressed regarding the basis of pathogen recognition and mechanisms of host defense and microbial virulence. Another fertile area is identification of novel targets for antimicrobial agents and determination of their mechanism of action. For this approach, expression profiles of microorganisms are compared in the presence or absence of a specific drug. This has now been used successfully in *Mycobacterium tuberculosis*, as exposure to isoniazid upregulated expression of both known and novel bacterial genes, including a gene encoding an efflux protein that was present only in virulence-related strains, making this a particularly attractive pharmacologic target (70).

There are caveats, however, to complete reliance on microarray-based studies. Much of the existing microarray data has been obtained using in vitro systems, and both pathogen and host gene expression patterns can be influenced by the particular model used. Microarray experiments should always be complemented by an independent assay, such as Northern hybridization or qRT-PCR. Even if microarray-based gene alterations are confirmed, there is an inconsistent correlation between levels of mRNA and protein expression, and in the future, microarray analyses will be supplemented with proteomic approaches, which will likely provide a plethora of additional insights. Viewed in this context, microarrays will simply augment and not replace more traditional techniques for investigating host-pathogen interactions. However, the ability to simultaneously analyze hundreds of thousands of genes, a high-throughput capacity, and a relative ease of use will undoubtedly place microarray analysis at the forefront for dissecting mechanisms of disease that develop within the context of microbially initiated inflammatory states.

NOTE ADDED IN PROOF

Since the initial authoring of this chapter and its publication, there have been dramatic changes in the literature that could not be included. Remarkably, the number of published studies focused on microarray analysis of host-pathogen interactions has escalated from those shown in Table 1 to over 160. These numbers will undoubtedly continue to increase as the availability of genome sequences and accessibility to microarray technology become more universal.

REFERENCES

1. Abu Kwaik, Y., and L. L. Pederson. 1996. The use of differential display-PCR to isolate and characterize a *Legionella pneumophila* locus induced during the intracellular infection of macrophages. *Mol. Microbiol.* 21:543–556.
2. Achtman, M., T. Azuma, D. E. Berg, Y. Ito, G. Morelli, Z. J. Pan, S. Suerbaum, S. A. Thompson, A. van der Ende, and L. J. van Doorn. 1999. Recombination and clonal groupings within *Helicobacter pylori* from different geographical regions. *Mol. Microbiol.* 32:459–470.
3. Akopyanz, N., N. O. Bukanov, T. U. Westblom, S. Kresovich, and D. E. Berg. 1992. DNA diversity among clinical isolates of *Helicobacter pylori* detected by PCR-based RAPD fingerprinting. *Nucleic Acids Res.* 20:5137–5142.
4. Allan, E., C. L. Clayton, A. McLaren, D. M. Wallace, and B. W. Wren. 2001. Characterization of the low-pH responses of *Helicobacter pylori* using genomic DNA arrays. *Microbiology* 147(Pt. 8):2285–2292.
5. Alm, R. A., L. S. Ling, D. T. Moir, B. L. King, E. D. Brown, P. C. Doig, D. R. Smith, B. Noonan, B. C. Guild, B. L. deJonge, G. Carmel, P. J. Tummino, A. Caruso, M. Uria-Nickelsen, D. M. Mills, C. Ives, R. Gibson, D. Merberg, S. D. Mills, Q. Jiang, D. E. Taylor, G. F. Vovis, and T. J. Trust. 1999. Genomic-sequence comparison of two unrelated isolates of the human gastric pathogen *Helicobacter pylori*. *Nature* 397(6715):176–180.
6. Ang, S., C. Z. Lee, K. Peck, M. Sindici, U. Matrubutham, M. A. Gleeson, and J. T. Wang. 2001. Acid-induced gene expression in *Helicobacter pylori*: study in genomic scale by microarray. *Infect. Immun.* 69:1679–1686.
7. Asahi, M., T. Azuma, S. Ito, Y. Ito, H. Suto, Y. Nagai, M. Tsubokawa, Y. Tohyama, S. Maeda, M. Omata, T. Suzuki, and C. Sasakawa. 2000. *Helicobacter pylori* CagA protein can be tyrosine phosphorylated in gastric epithelial cells. *J. Exp. Med.* 191:593–602.
8. Bach, S., A. Makristathis, M. Rotter, and A. M. Hirschl. 2002. Gene expression profiling in AGS cells stimulated with *Helicobacter pylori* isogenic strains (*cagA* positive or *cagA* negative). *Infect. Immun.* 70:988–992.
9. Bjorkholm, B., A. Lundin, A. Sillen, K. Guillemin, N. Salama, C. Rubio, J. I. Gordon, P. Falk, and L. Engstrand. 2001. Comparison of genetic divergence and fitness between two subclones of *Helicobacter pylori*. *Infect. Immun.* 69:7832–7838.
10. Blaser, M. J., G. I. Perez-Perez, H. Kleanthous, T. L. Cover, R. M. Peek, P. H. Chyou, G. N. Stemmermann, and A. Nomura. 1995. Infection with *Helicobacter pylori* strains possessing *cagA* is associated with an increased risk of developing adenocarcinoma of the stomach. *Cancer Res.* 55:2111–2115.
11. Bodger, K., J. I. Wyatt, and R. V. Heatley. 1997. Gastric mucosal secretion of interleukin-10: relations to histopathology, *Helicobacter pylori* status, and tumour necrosis factor-alpha secretion. *Gut* 40:739–744.

12. **Chiou, C. C., C. C. Chan, D. L. Sheu, K. T. Chen, Y. S. Li, and E. C. Chan.** 2001. *Helicobacter pylori* infection induced alteration of gene expression in human gastric cells. *Gut* **48:** 598–604.

13. **Cover, T. L., C. P. Dooley, and M. J. Blaser.** 1990. Characterization of and human serologic response to proteins in *Helicobacter pylori* broth culture supernatants with vacuolizing cytotoxin activity. *Infect. Immun.* **58:**603–610.

14. **Cox, J. M., C. L. Clayton, T. Tomita, D. M. Wallace, P. A. Robinson, and J. E. Crabtree.** 2001. cDNA array analysis of *cag* pathogenicity island-associated *Helicobacter pylori* epithelial cell response genes. *Infect. Immun.* **69:**6970–6980.

15. **Crabtree, J. E., D. Kersulyte, S. D. Li, I. J. Lindley, and D. E. Berg.** 1999. Modulation of *Helicobacter pylori* induced interleukin-8 synthesis in gastric epithelial cells mediated by *cag* PAI encoded VirD4 homologue. *J. Clin. Pathol.* **52:** 653–657.

16. **Crabtree, J. E., J. D. Taylor, J. I. Wyatt, R. V. Heatley, T. M. Shallcross, D. S. Tompkins, and B. J. Rathbone.** 1991. Mucosal IgA recognition of *Helicobacter pylori* 120 kDa protein, peptic ulceration, and gastric pathology. *Lancet* **338:**332–335.

17. **Crabtree, J. E., J. I. Wyatt, G. M. Sobala, G. Miller, D. S. Tompkins, J. N. Primrose, and A. G. Morgan.** 1993. Systemic and mucosal humoral responses to *Helicobacter pylori* in gastric cancer. *Gut* **34:**1339–1343.

18. **DeLisa, M. P., C. F. Wu, L. Wang, J. J. Valdes, and W. E. Bentley.** 2001. DNA microarray-based identification of genes controlled by autoinducer 2-stimulated quorum sensing in *Escherichia coli*. *J. Bacteriol.* **183:**5239–5247.

19. **Detweiler, C. S., D. B. Cunanan, and S. Falkow.** 2001. Host microarray analysis reveals a role for the *Salmonella* response regulator *phoP* in human macrophage cell death. *Proc. Natl. Acad. Sci. USA* **98:**5850–5855.

20. **Donahue, J. P., D. A. Israel, V. J. Torres, A. S. Necheva, and G. G. Miller.** 2002. Inactivation of a *Helicobacter pylori* DNA methyltransferase alters *dnaK* operon expresion following host cell adherence. *FEMS Microbiol. Lett.* **208:**295–301.

21. **Dorrell, N., J. A. Mangan, K. G. Laing, J. Hinds, D. Linton, H. Al-Ghusein, B. G. Barrell, J. Parkhill, N. G. Stoker, A. V. Karlyshev, P. D. Butcher, and B. W. Wren.** 2001. Whole genome comparison of *Campylobacter jejuni* human isolates using a low-cost microarray reveals extensive genetic diversity. *Genome Res.* **11:**1706–1715.

22. **Eckmann, L., J. R. Smith, M. P. Housley, M. B. Dwinell, and M. F. Kagnoff.** 2000. Analysis by high density cDNA arrays of altered gene expression in human intestinal epithelial cells in response to infection with the invasive enteric bacteria *Salmonella*. *J. Biol. Chem.* **275:** 14084–14094.

23. **Enroth, H., O. Nyren, and L. Engstrand.** 1999. One stomach—one strain: does *Helicobacter pylori* strain variation influence disease outcome? *Dig. Dis. Sci.* **44:**102–107.

24. **Gerhold, D., T. Rushmore, and C. T. Caskey.** 1999. DNA chips: promising toys have become powerful tools. *Trends Biochem. Sci.* **24:** 168–173.

25. **Glocker, E., C. Lange, A. Covacci, S. Bereswill, M. Kist, and H. L. Pahl.** 1998. Proteins encoded by the *cag* pathogenicity island of *Helicobacter pylori* are required for NF-kappaB activation. *Infect. Immun.* **66:**2346–2348.

26. **Go, M. F., V. Kapur, D. Y. Graham, and J. M. Musser.** 1996. Population genetic analysis of *Helicobacter pylori* by multilocus enzyme electrophoresis: extensive allelic diversity and recombinational population structure. *J. Bacteriol.* **178:** 3934–3938.

27. **Groisman, E. A.** 2001. The pleiotropic two-component regulatory system PhoP-PhoQ. *J. Bacteriol.* **183:**1835–1842.

28. **Haeberle, H. A., M. Kubin, K. B. Bamford, R. Garofalo, D. Y. Graham, F. El-Zaatari, R. Karttunen, S. E. Crowe, V. E. Reyes, and P. B. Ernst.** 1997. Differential stimulation of interleukin-12 (IL-12) and IL-10 by live and killed *Helicobacter pylori in vitro* and association of IL-12 production with gamma interferon-producing T cells in the human gastric mucosa. *Infect. Immun.* **65:**4229–4235.

29. **Harrington, C. A., C. Rosenow, and J. Retief.** 2000. Monitoring gene expression using DNA microarrays. *Curr. Opin. Microbiol.* **3(3):** 285–291.

30. **Heuermann, D., and R. Haas.** 1998. A stable shuttle vector system for efficient genetic complementation of *Helicobacter pylori* strains by transformation and conjugation. *Mol. Gen. Genet.* **257:**519–528.

31. **Higashi, H., R. Tsutsumi, S. Muto, T. Sugiyama, T. Azuma, M. Asaka, and M. Hatakeyama.** 2002. SHP-2 tyrosine phosphatase as an intracellular target of *Helicobacter pylori* CagA protein. *Science* **295:**683–686.

32. **Hooper, L. V., M. H. Wong, A. Thelin, L. Hansson, P. G. Falk, and J. I. Gordon.** 2001. Molecular analysis of commensal host-microbial relationships in the intestine. *Science* **291:**881–884.

33. **Israel, D. A., N. Salama, C. N. Arnold, S. F. Moss, T. Ando, H. P. Wirth, K. T. Tham, M. Camorlinga, M. J. Blaser, S. Falkow, and R. M. Peek, Jr.** 2001. *Helicobacter pylori* strain-specific differences in genetic content, identified by microarray, influence host inflammatory responses. *J. Clin. Invest.* **107**:611–620.

34. **Israel, D. A., N. Salama, U. Krishna, U. M. Rieger, J. C. Atherton, S. Falkow, and R. M. Peek, Jr.** 2001. *Helicobacter pylori* genetic diversity within the gastric niche of a single human host. *Proc. Natl. Acad. Sci. USA* **98**:14625–14630.

35. **Keates, S., A. C. Keates, M. Warny, R. M. Peek, Jr., P. G. Murray, and C. P. Kelly.** 1999. Differential activation of mitogen-activated protein kinases in AGS gastric epithelial cells by cag^+ and cag^- *Helicobacter pylori*. *J. Immunol.* **163**:5552–5559.

36. **Kuipers, E. J., D. A. Israel, J. G. Kusters, M. M. Gerrits, J. Weel, J. van Der Ende, R. W. van Der Hulst, H. P. Wirth, J. Hook-Nikanne, S. A. Thompson, and M. J. Blaser.** 2000. Quasispecies development of *Helicobacter pylori* observed in paired isolates obtained years apart from the same host. *J. Infect. Dis.* **181**(1):273–282.

37. **Kuipers, E. J., G. I. Perez-Perez, S. G. Meuwissen, and M. J. Blaser.** 1995. *Helicobacter pylori* and atrophic gastritis: importance of the *cagA* status. *J. Natl. Cancer Inst.* **87**:1777–1780.

38. **Lipshutz, R. J., S. P. Fodor, T. R. Gingeras, and D. J. Lockhart.** 1999. High density synthetic oligonucleotide arrays. *Nat. Genet.* **21**(Suppl. 1):20–24.

39. **Maeda, S., M. Akanuma, Y. Mitsuno, Y. Hirata, K. Ogura, H. Yoshida, Y. Shiratori, and M. Omata.** 2001. Distinct mechanism of *Helicobacter pylori*-mediated NF-kappa B activation between gastric cancer cells and monocytic cells. *J. Biol. Chem.* **276**:44856–44864.

40. **Maeda, S., M. Otsuka, Y. Hirata, Y. Mitsuno, H. Yoshida, Y. Shiratori, Y. Masuho, M. Muramatsu, N. Seki, and M. Omata.** 2001. cDNA microarray analysis of *Helicobacter pylori*-mediated alteration of gene expression in gastric cancer cells. *Biochem. Biophys. Res. Commun.* **284**(2):443–449.

41. **Marshall, B. J., and J. R. Warren.** 1984. Unidentified curved bacilli in the stomach of patients with gastritis and peptic ulceration. *Lancet* **i**:1311–1315.

42. **Meyer-ter-Vehn, T., A. Covacci, M. Kist, and H. L. Pahl.** 2000. *Helicobacter pylori* activates mitogen-activated protein kinase cascades and induces expression of the proto-oncogenes c-*fos* and c-*jun*. *J. Biol. Chem.* **275**:16064–16072.

43. **Miller, S. I., A. M. Kukral, and J. J. Mekalanos.** 1989. A two-component regulatory system (*phoP phoQ*) controls *Salmonella typhimurium* virulence. *Proc. Natl. Acad. Sci. USA* **86**:5054–5058.

44. **Naumann, M., S. Wessler, C. Bartsch, B. Wieland, A. Covacci, R. Haas, and T. F. Meyer.** 1999. Activation of activator protein 1 and stress response kinases in epithelial cells colonized by *Helicobacter pylori* encoding the *cag* pathogenicity island. *J. Biol. Chem.* **274**:31655–31662.

45. **Neish, A. S., A. T. Gewirtz, H. Zeng, A. N. Young, M. E. Hobert, V. Karmali, A. S. Rao, and J. L. Madara.** 2000. Prokaryotic regulation of epithelial responses by inhibition of IkappaB-alpha ubiquitination. *Science* **289**:1560–1563.

46. **Nomura, A., G. N. Stemmermann, P. H. Chyou, I. Kato, G. I. Pérez-Pérez, and M. J. Blaser.** 1991. *Helicobacter pylori* infection and gastric carcinoma among Japanese Americans in Hawaii. *N. Engl. J. Med.* **325**:1132–1136.

47. **Odenbreit, S., J. Puls, B. Sedlmaier, E. Gerland, W. Fischer, and R. Haas.** 2000. Translocation of *Helicobacter pylori* CagA into gastric epithelial cells by type IV secretion. *Science* **287**:1497–1500.

48. **Ogura, K., S. Maeda, M. Nakao, T. Watanabe, M. Tada, T. Kyutoku, H. Yoshida, Y. Shiratori, and M. Omata.** 2000. Virulence factors of *Helicobacter pylori* responsible for gastric diseases in Mongolian gerbil. *J. Exp. Med.* **192**:1601–1610.

49. **Parkhill, J., B. W. Wren, K. Mungall, J. M. Ketley, C. Churcher, D. Basham, T. Chillingworth, R. M. Davies, T. Feltwell, S. Holroyd, K. Jagels, A. V. Karlyshev, S. Moule, M. J. Pallen, C. W. Penn, M. A. Quail, M. A. Rajandream, K. M. Rutherford, A. H. van Vliet, S. Whitehead, and B. G. Barrell.** 2000. The genome sequence of the food-borne pathogen *Campylobacter jejuni* reveals hypervariable sequences. *Nature* **403**:665–668.

50. **Parsonnet, J., G. D. Friedman, N. Orentreich, and H. Vogelman.** 1997. Risk for gastric cancer in people with CagA positive or CagA negative *Helicobacter pylori* infection. *Gut* **40**(3):297–301.

51. **Parsonnet, J., G. D. Friedman, D. P. Vandersteen, Y. Chang, J. H. Vogelman, N. Orentreich, and R. K. Sibley.** 1991. *Helicobacter pylori* infection and the risk of gastric carcinoma. *N. Engl. J. Med.* **325**:1127–1131.

52. **Parsonnet, J., S. Hansen, L. Rodriguez, A. B. Gelb, R. A. Warnke, E. Jellum, N.**

Orentreich, J. H. Vogelman, and G. D. Friedman. 1994. *Helicobacter pylori* infection and gastric lymphoma. *N. Engl. J. Med.* **330:**1267–1271.

53. Peek, R. M., Jr., G. G. Miller, K. T. Tham, G. I. Perez-Perez, X. Zhao, J. C. Atherton, and M. J. Blaser. 1995. Heightened inflammatory response and cytokine expression in vivo to *cagA+ Helicobacter pylori* strains. *Lab. Invest.* **73:** 760–770.

54. Peek, R. M., Jr., S. A. Thompson, J. P. Donahue, K. T. Tham, J. C. Atherton, M. J. Blaser, and G. G. Miller. 1998. Adherence to gastric epithelial cells induces expression of a *Helicobacter pylori* gene, *iceA*, that is associated with clinical outcome. *Proc. Assoc. Am. Physic.* **110**(6):531–544.

55. Perez-Perez, G. I., V. L. Shepherd, J. D. Morrow, and M. J. Blaser. 1995. Activation of human THP-1 cells and rat bone marrow-derived macrophages by *Helicobacter pylori* lipopolysaccharide. *Infect. Immun.* **63:**1183–1187.

56. Peterson, W. L. 1991. *Helicobacter pylori* and peptic ulcer disease. *N. Engl. J. Med.* **324:**1043–1048.

57. Rosenberger, C. M., M. G. Scott, M. R. Gold, R. E. Hancock, and B. B. Finlay. 2000. *Salmonella typhimurium* infection and lipopolysaccharide stimulation induce similar changes in macrophage gene expression. *J. Immunol.* **164:** 5894–5904.

58. Rosqvist, R., K. E. Magnusson, and H. Wolf-Watz. 1994. Target cell contact triggers expression and polarized transfer of *Yersinia* YopE cytotoxin into mammalian cells. *EMBO J.* **13:** 964–972.

59. Salama, N., K. Guillemin, T. K. McDaniel, G. Sherlock, L. Tompkins, and S. Falkow. 2000. A whole-genome microarray reveals genetic diversity among *Helicobacter pylori* strains. *Proc. Natl. Acad. Sci. USA* **97:**14668–14673.

60. Segal, E. D., J. Cha, J. Lo, S. Falkow, and L. S. Tompkins. 1999. Altered states: involvement of phosphorylated CagA in the induction of host cellular growth changes by *Helicobacter pylori. Proc. Natl. Acad. Sci. USA* **96:**14559–14564.

61. Selbach, M., S. Moese, C. R. Hauck, T. F. Meyer, and S. Backert. 2002. Src is the kinase of the *Helicobacter pylori* CagA protein in vitro and in vivo. *J. Biol. Chem.* **277:**6775–6778.

62. Selinger, D. W., K. J. Cheung, R. Mei, E. M. Johansson, C. S. Richmond, F. R. Blattner, D. J. Lockhart, and G. M. Church. 2000. RNA expression analysis using a 30 base

pair resolution *Escherichia coli* genome array. *Nat. Biotechnol.* **18:**1262–1268.

63. Sharma, S. A., M. K. Tummuru, M. J. Blaser, and L. D. Kerr. 1998. Activation of IL-8 gene expression by *Helicobacter pylori* is regulated by transcription factor nuclear factor-kappa B in gastric epithelial cells. *J. Immunol.* **160:**2401–2407.

64. Sharma, S. A., M. K. Tummuru, G. G. Miller, and M. J. Blaser. 1995. Interleukin-8 response of gastric epithelial cell lines to *Helicobacter pylori* stimulation in vitro. *Infect. Immun.* **63:** 1681–1687.

65. Stein, M., R. Rappuoli, and A. Covacci. 2000. Tyrosine phosphorylation of the *Helicobacter pylori* CagA antigen after *cag*-driven host cell translocation. *Proc. Natl. Acad. Sci. USA* **97:** 1263–1268.

66. Tao, H., C. Bausch, C. Richmond, F. R. Blattner, and T. Conway. 1999. Functional genomics: expression analysis of *Escherichia coli* growing on minimal and rich media. *J. Bacteriol.* **181:**6425–6440.

67. Tomb, J. F., O. White, A. R. Kerlavage, R. A. Clayton, G. G. Sutton, R. D. Fleischmann, K. A. Ketchum, H. P. Klenk, S. Gill, B. A. Dougherty, K. Nelson, J. Quackenbush, L. Zhou, E. F. Kirkness, S. Peterson, B. Loftus, D. Richardson, R. Dodson, H. G. Khalak, A. Glodek, K. McKenney, L. M. Fitzegerald, N. Lee, M. D. Adams, J. C. Venter, et al. 1997. The complete genome sequence of the gastric pathogen *Helicobacter pylori. Nature* **388:**539–547.

68. Tummuru, M. K., S. A. Sharma, and M. J. Blaser. 1995. *Helicobacter pylori picB*, a homologue of the *Bordetella pertussis* toxin secretion protein, is required for induction of IL-8 in gastric epithelial cells. *Mol. Microbiol.* **18:**867–876.

69. van Doorn, N. E., F. Namavar, J. G. Kusters, E. P. van Rees, E. J. Kuipers, and J. de Graaff. 1998. Genomic DNA fingerprinting of clinical isolates of *Helicobacter pylori* by REP-PCR and restriction fragment end-labelling. *FEMS Microbiol. Lett.* **160**(1):145–150.

70. Wilson, M., J. DeRisi, H. H. Kristensen, P. Imboden, S. Rane, P. O. Brown, and G. K. Schoolnik. 1999. Exploring drug-induced alterations in gene expression in *Mycobacterium tuberculosis* by microarray hybridization. *Proc. Natl. Acad. Sci. USA* **96:**12833–12838.

71. Wong, K. K., and M. McClelland. 1994. Stress-inducible gene of *Salmonella typhimurium* identified by arbitrarily primed PCR of RNA. *Proc. Natl. Acad. Sci. USA* **91:**639–643.

72. **Yamaoka, Y., M. Kita, T. Kodama, N. Sawai, and J. Imanishi.** 1996. *Helicobacter pylori cagA* gene and expression of cytokine messenger RNA in gastric mucosa. *Gastroenterology* **110:** 1744–1752.

73. **Zhang, J. P., and S. Normark.** 1996. Induction of gene expression in *Escherichia coli* after pilus-mediated adherence. *Science* **273:**1234–1236.

74. **Zheng, M., X. Wang, L. J. Templeton, D. R. Smulski, R. A. LaRossa, and G. Storz.** 2001. DNA microarray-mediated transcriptional profiling of the *Escherichia coli* response to hydrogen peroxide. *J. Bacteriol.* **183:**4562–4570.

PATHOGEN-INITIATED INFLAMMATORY RESPONSE IN INTESTINAL EPITHELIAL CELLS: CROSS TALK WITH NEUTROPHILS

Andrew T. Gewirtz, Shanti V. Sitaraman, Didier Merlin, and James L. Madara

9

The human intestine is colonized by a diverse microbial ecosystem, whose constituents have only recently begun to be described. Specifically, the colon contains more than 10^{11} microbes per ml of lumenal contents, comprising more than 400 known species as well as many others that cannot yet be cultured via existing techniques (27). While perhaps this host-microbial relationship does not meet the definition of symbiosis to the same extent as that of ruminant mammals with their microflora, the microbes of the healthy human intestine certainly provide some benefit, particularly by generating important metabolites (especially folates) and by reducing the colonization efficiency of dietary pathogens via occupying their potential niches. However, these "commensal" microbes have the potential to cause disease, especially upon gaining systemic access to the host. Moreover, the human intestine can also be colonized by pathogens that have evolved a variety of mechanisms to disturb the host-prokaryotic equilibrium, presumably acquiring a selective advantage. This chapter considers the interactions of bacteria and their metabolites with the intestinal epithelium, how neutrophil-mediated inflammation results, and how perturbing microbes are cleared and homeostasis is restored. While our own work provides the foundation for this chapter, we relate our findings to the many other mechanisms that others have shown to regulate intestinal homeostasis and inflammation.

THE INTESTINAL EPITHELIUM—AN INTERACTIVE BARRIER

The epithelial cells that line the gastrointestinal tract are the front line of defense against the diverse population of commensal and potentially pathogenic microbes that thrive within the lumen of the intestine (27). The intestine's primary protection from the lumenal flora is the highly selective barrier formed by the epithelial cells lining this organ. Specifically, intestinal epithelial cells (IEC) form intercellular tight junctions that effectively restrict transepithelial movement of particulates and even hydrophilic molecules of molecular mass higher than ~2,000 Da, thus barring not only bacteria but also many of their metabolites from access to the host (38). However, the defensive function of the intestinal epithelium is not merely limited to providing a barrier. Rather, the intestinal ep-

Andrew T. Gewirtz, Shanti V. Sitaraman, Didier Merlin, and James L. Madara, Epithelial Pathobiology Division, Department of Pathology and Laboratory Medicine, Emory University, Atlanta, GA 30322.

Microbial Pathogenesis and the Intestinal Epithelial Cell, ed. by G. Hecht
© 2003 ASM Press, Washington, D.C.

ithelium is interactive in that it secretes molecules that affect both microbes and immune cells. Specifically, the intestinal epithelium secretes peptides such as defensins with direct antimicrobial activity. Furthermore, the epithelium secretes cytokines and chemokines that recruit and regulate immune cells. The importance of such epithelial cell secretory pathways is demonstrated via the recently created intestinal epithelial-specific IκB kinase β (IKKβ)-knockout mouse which is unable to activate gut epithelial proinflammatory gene expression and thus is extremely susceptible to infection (12). How such gut epithelial secretion is regulated is discussed below.

In addition to the secretion of cytokines and chemokines, the intestinal epithelium transports both products of bacteria and immune cells. For example, it has long been known that immunoglobulin A (IgA) produced by B cells is transcytosed by IEC into the intestinal lumen and that such IgA is protective of the host, presumably via neutralizing important molecules on the microbial surface. More recently, it has been realized that IEC possess an Fc receptor isoform (FcRn) formerly thought to be restricted to neonates and that this receptor is capable of bidirectionally transporting IgG (10). Lumenal to serosal (i.e., apical to basolateral) transport of IgG (and potentially attached epitopes) could perhaps be a method of immunosurveillance, while basolateral to apical IgG transport could serve to mark microbes for engulfment by innate immune cells (e.g., neutrophil FcgR-mediated phagocytosis).

The intestinal epithelium, long assumed to play only a passive role in immunity, has recently been shown to be actively involved. Specifically, bacteria release N-formylated peptides that are potent chemoattractants for neutrophils and monocytes. Such N-formylated peptides likely play a role in directing neutrophil movement across the gut epithelium, which defines the formation of a crypt abscess. It has generally been assumed that such peptides simply diffuse across epithelial tight junctions and through the epithelial paracellular space, thus forming a chemotactic gradient. However, it has now been demonstrated that the apical membrane transporter hPepT1 transports N-formylated tripeptides (along with the other di- and tripeptides carried by this transporter) and that this transport may help establish or at least optimize a chemoattractant gradient (45). Furthermore, gut epithelial cells respond to such intracellular dipeptides by altering gene expression, specifically upregulation of major histocompatibility complex (MHC) class II molecules (46). Interestingly, hPepT1 expression is normally restricted to the small intestine where the bacterial load is, compared to the colon, relatively small but is upregulated in the latter under certain conditions, including inflammatory bowel disease (IBD). The role of hPepT1 and MHC expression as an epithelial immune accessory function and in inflammatory bowel disease is currently under investigation.

NF-κB: THE CENTRAL REGULATOR OF EPITHELIAL ANTIMICROBIAL GENE EXPRESSION

While epithelial transport of products from microbes and immune cells likely plays a key role in maintaining intestinal homeostasis, it is not a sufficient defense against intestinal pathogens. Rather, colonization of the gut by pathogens alters epithelial gene expression, resulting in the coordination of an immune inflammatory response. One of the primary means by which gut epithelial cells activate expression of the genes involved in such a host defense is via activation of the proinflammatory transcription factor NF-κB. Thus, understanding microbial-epithelial-immune cell cross talk demands extensive consideration of this signaling pathway. While this transcription factor plays a central role in many host defense-signaling pathways, certain aspects of regulation of NF-κB and the consequences of its activation are unique to the gut epithelium, and these unique aspects of the NF-κB pathway will be emphasized here.

NF-κB is composed of two subunits, both heterodimers and homodimers, of various members of the Rel family of DNA-binding transcription factors (7, 33). However, as there appears to be nothing unique about the specific NF-κB isoforms used by the intestinal epithelium, this chapter will refer to classic NF-κB isoforms (p50/p65 heterodimers and p65 homodimers). Such NF-κB dimers are held in an inactivated state by the so-called inhibitor of κB, IκB, which binds NF-κB and sequesters it in the cytosol. Upon generation of appropriate signals, IκB is phosphorylated and degraded, thus resulting in NF-κB translocation to the nucleus and activation of NF-κB-responsive genes. Such signal-activated IκB phosphorylation is largely mediated by IKKβ (11), thus explaining the inability of gut epithelial-IKKβ knockout mice to express its NF-κB-mediated genes discussed above.

Activation of NF-κB

A variety of stimuli, including cytokines, bacteria, viruses, bacterial products, ionizing radiation, and oxidant stress, can activate NF-κB. This chapter limits its focus to bacterially mediated pathways of activation. In contrast to most other cell types, intestinal epithelial cells are relatively unresponsive, in terms of proinflammatory gene expression, to large quantities of commensal bacteria and their products. However, a number of enteropathogenic bacteria and, under some specialized circumstances, opportunistic commensal bacteria, will provoke NF-κB activation and subsequently intestinal inflammation. The broad categories of mechanisms by which microbes activate epithelial cell NF-κB are via (i) receptor-mediated detection of soluble extracellular ligands, (ii) direct activation of host-signaling protein by bacterial products translocated into the host cell cytoplasm, or (iii) detection of intact intracellular organisms by intracellular receptors. While these mechanisms are clearly interrelated, this categorization is nonetheless a useful starting point to understanding the proinflammatory aspects of microbial-epithelial interactions.

The surfaces of microbes are composed of complex macromolecules, often with a number of repeated structural motifs. Although microbes have tremendous mutability, certain structural features permit relatively little variation in their structure to maintain their function. Such critical microbial structural motifs have been termed pathogen-associated molecular patterns or PAMP (43). PAMP appear to be a primary means by which gut epithelial cells, and the innate immune system in general, recognize pathogens and activate NF-κB. PAMP characterized to date include N-formylated peptides, lipopolysaccharides (LPS), and lipopeptides, as well as the more recently described PAMP flagellin (20) and unmethylated segments of CpG DNA (41). Although the latter is not a surface structure, it is nonetheless a feature that distinguishes microbes from the host. While the former are generally part of the bacterial surface, it is clear that bacteria also release these PAMP, although whether release is purposeful or unavoidable is not yet clear.

Some PAMP, particularly N-formylated peptides, are potent chemoattractants and thus play a direct role in recruiting and activating inflammatory cells. The receptors for this class of PAMP are of the heterotrimeric G-protein-coupled receptor class. In contrast, PAMP that activate the NF-κB pathway do so via Toll-like receptors (TLR) (44). TLR are so named because of their homology to the Toll receptor in *Drosophila melanogaster*, a protein involved in early embryonic patterning that also plays a critical role in the insect innate immune system. The human genome contains at least 10 known TLR (2). Biochemically, TLR are transmembrane receptors defined by the presence of leucine rich repeats (LRR) in the extracellular portion of the molecule and a TIR (Toll/interleukin-1R [IL-1R]/resistance) cytoplasmic domain. The extracellular LRR domain is thought to function in ligand recognition, while the TIR domain functions in signaling (26). LRR domains are common to proteins involved in the recognition of foreign proteins and are even instrumental in plant antibacterial responses (8). It has been hypothesized that TLR (and the innate immune system in general) originally evolved as a mechanism to recognize a limited number of surface determinants that are likely to remain invariant across large classes of potentially pathogenic organisms (28). Because of the efficiency of eukaryotic recognition of PAMP such as LPS, bacteria have evolved effective means to modify these structures (62).

Recent progress has been made in identifying ligands for mammalian TLR. A significant amount of in vitro and in vivo evidence indicates that TLR4 functions as a receptor for LPS. For example, cells transfected with TLR4 acquire the ability to activate NF-κB in response to LPS (6). Moreover, mice lacking a functional TLR are highly resistant to LPS-induced sepsis (52). In vitro evidence has identified potential ligands of other TLR. For example, cells expressing TLR2 respond to lipoprotein and the lipoteichoic acid (peptidoglycan) component of gram-positive cell walls (57). Expression of TLR5 confers cells with the ability to respond to flagellin (18, 24), while expression of TLR9 does so for CpG DNA (3). TLR exist as dimers, and recent discoveries indicate that responses to some ligands (e.g., soluble tuberculosis factor and *Borrelia burgdorferi* outer surface protein A lipoprotein) require a specific TLR combination, thus greatly increasing both the specificity and potential ligands of TLR activation (4).

TLR appear to be widely expressed on host tissues (or at least detectable at the mRNA level in many tissues). While they presumably generate similar signals in different cell types, the biology of their activation has a unique aspect in the gut epithelium. Clearly, TLR must not be routinely activated by commensal microflora, as to do so would result in a constant state of gut inflammation. The mechanism by which one TLR, TLR5, accomplishes this feat has recently been elucidated (18, 20). Specifically, gut epithelial cells express TLR5 only on their basolateral surfaces. Thus, only bacteria that have breached the epithelia, or have translocated flagellin across the epithelia, will activate this receptor. Whether this mechanism of restricting activation through polarity will be true of other TLR awaits further investigation. Most investigators find gut epithelial cells do not respond to LPS,

whether applied to the apical or basolateral surface (20) and references therein. However, whether these cells express significant amounts of TLR4 is controversial at this time, with some investigators detecting it (5) and other studies finding little (1) or none (48) of this molecule. In any case, additional mechanisms of desensitizing TLR may exist.

Many gram-negative pathogens such as *Salmonella* spp., *Yersinia* spp., and enteropathogenic *Escherichia coli* (EPEC) are able to translocate (i.e., inject) proteins into gut epithelia that directly activate host-signaling pathways; for example, *Salmonella* inserts SopB protein in epithelial cells which activates small GTP-binding proteins (67), perhaps eventuating in activation of the mitogen-activated protein (MAP) kinase cascade (25). While a direct signaling link between these prokaryotic proteins and the NF-κB pathway has not been demonstrated under physiological conditions, it is likely that mechanisms of activating host signals exist and play a role in activation of this proinflammatory transcription factor. The translocation of gram-negative effector proteins is accomplished by the type III secretion apparatus reviewed in chapter 22 (14). EPEC, for example, uses this apparatus to activate tyrosine kinase pathways and deliver its own receptor into host cells. It may also play a role in the subsequent NF-κB activation (32).

Most recently, it has become apparent that epithelial cells have a means of detecting intracellular bacteria and activating NF-κB in response (21). Studies regarding *Shigella flexneri* led to this finding. This pathogen cannot adhere efficiently to or invade the apical surface (47) and, being nonmotile, expresses no flagellins. However, *Shigella* spp. can invade through the basolateral surface, thrive within the cytoplasm (nonvacuolar), and, in the process, activate the NF-κB pathway in an LPS-dependent manner. Interestingly, an intracellular LRR-containing protein, NOD1, may mediate this intracellular recognition. NOD1 and perhaps other LRR repeat-containing proteins presumably act to monitor the cell cytoplasm for PAMP present on intracellular pathogens, thus providing a means of detecting invasive bacteria not perceived by cell surface receptors.

Not surprisingly, there is redundancy in the mechanisms of activation of the NF-κB pathway, and gut epithelia can likely use more than one pathway to detect specific pathogens. For example, while intestinal epithelia have developed basolateral detection of extracellular flagellin as a means of activating an inflammatory response to *Salmonella* spp., there is also likely direct activation, perhaps type III secretion system mediated, of cells in physical contact with this microbe. Further, the mechanisms discussed above can be interrelated. For example, detection of basolateral flagellin requires bacteria or at least its flagellin to cross the epithelial barrier (Fig. 1). *Salmonella enterica* serovar Typhimurium can translocate flagellin across epithelia in an invasion-independent manner. While such translocation does not appear to require the type III secretory apparatus (20), it nonetheless does require direct interaction of the apical epithelial surface with live intact *Salmonella* spp. Analogously, while *Shigella* spp. can be detected intracellularly, its invasion requires bacterial activation of host-signaling pathways that can potentially themselves mediate activation of the NF-κB pathway. Such redundancy would seem to provide a more thorough host defense system.

Intracellular Signals Regulating NF-κB Activation

As discussed above, NF-κB is activated by a rapid posttranslational pathway (31). Specifically, this requires loss of IκB, allowing free NF-κB dimers to translocate to the nucleus and activate transcription. IκB degradation is preceded by phosphorylation mediated by IKK, a large, multisubunit complex that is generally viewed as the key rate-limiting step in the activation pathway. Multiple proinflammatory signals activate various signal transduction pathways that are integrated by this complex(es).

The signaling pathways by which bacteria activate IKK are beginning to be unraveled,

particularly via TLR (Fig. 2) (29, 59). Specifically, binding of an appropriate ligand to a TLR results in the sequential recruitment of the adaptor proteins MyD88 and IRAK to the TIR cytoplasmic domain on the TLR. IRAK, a serine kinase, then activates the cytoplasmic intermediate TRAF6, probably by phosphorylation. TRAF6 then undergoes an unusual modification, lysine-63 ubiquitination catalyzed by the action of two other proteins Ubc13 and Uev1a (9, 65). Upon activation by lysine-63 ubiquitination, TRAF6 in turn activates TAK1 (a kinase of the MEKKK group), in complex with TAB1 and TAB2. The TAK1/TAB1/TAB2 complex functions as an IKK (65).

There appear to be a variety of signaling pathways that result in IKK activation and thus IKK has been suggested to function as an integrator of many signaling pathways (40). Aside from TLR-mediated signals, many stimuli activate the IKK complex, such as the proinflammatory cytokines tumor necrosis factor-α (TNF-α) and IL-1, both of which have dedicated receptors and IKK proximal signaling intermediates (30). Additionally, activation of Ca^{2+} mobilization can serve as a sufficient signal to activate these pathways (19). Bacterial effector proteins may directly activate the kinase or upstream signaling intermediates (25). In each case, signaling converges on IKK. The IKK complex is composed of many subunits, and its exact composition has yet to be defined. The main catalytic subunits of the complex have been identified as IKK-α and IKK-β, which recognize a conserved 6-amino-acid motif present on all IκB isoforms and phosphorylate two serine residues within the motif (30). IKK knockout mice exhibit a complete deficiency in NF-κB activation in response to proinflammatory stimuli, while IKK-α null mice show early lethality and developmental defects (31). Degradation of IκB results in exposure of the NF-κB nuclear localization signal leading to translocation across the nuclear membrane, subsequent DNA binding to NF-κB elements, and ultimate transcription of these genes.

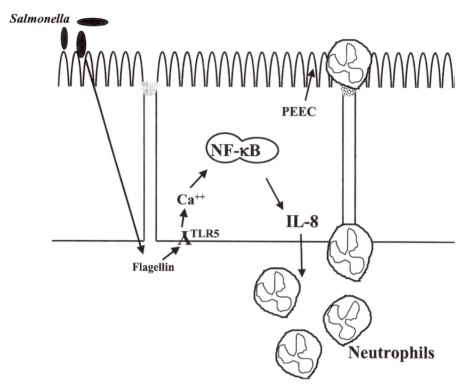

FIGURE 1 Mechanism of *Salmonella*-induced active intestinal inflammation. Serovar Ty-phimurium colonization of model epithelia results in translocation of the microbes' flagellin across the epithelium. Such flagellin can activate, via a Ca^{2+}-dependent pathway, the tran-scription factor NF-κB. This will result in an influx of polymorphonuclear leukocytes and their subsequent pathogen-elicited epithelial chemoattractant (PEEC)-driven migration across the epithelium, resulting in a crypt abscess. While such neutrophils clear the infection, they are also responsible for the clinical manifestations of pathogen-induced gastroenteritis.

CONSEQUENCES OF PATHOGEN-INDUCED CHANGES IN GENE EXPRESSION

Pathogen-Induced Epithelial Orchestration of the Inflammatory Response

Pathogen-induced changes in epithelial gene expression encompass a remarkable panel of effects designed to lead to the clearance of the perturbing organism. Some NF-κB-activated genes are directly antibacterial (e.g, defensins) and thus the consequences of their upregul-ation are straightforward. NF-κB-activated genes also include proinflammatory mediators that cause further activation of NF-κB in other cells, thus amplifying the response. Per-haps most important is the induction of NF-κB genes that directly result in the recruitment of inflammatory cells (13), the soldiers of the innate immune system. Such immune cell re-cruitment is mediated by epithelial expression of adhesion molecules and chemokines, both of which are NF-κB regulated. Examples of the former are intercellular adhesin molecule 1 (ICAM-1) and vascular cell adhesion mol-ecule (VCAM), while chemokines include IL-8, epithelial neutrophil-activating peptide 78 (ENA-78), and monocyte chemotactic protein (MCP). Chemokine secretion is absolutely critical to the recruitment of neutrophils. A consequence of exposure to prolonged pro-inflammatory stimuli is the NF-κB-induced

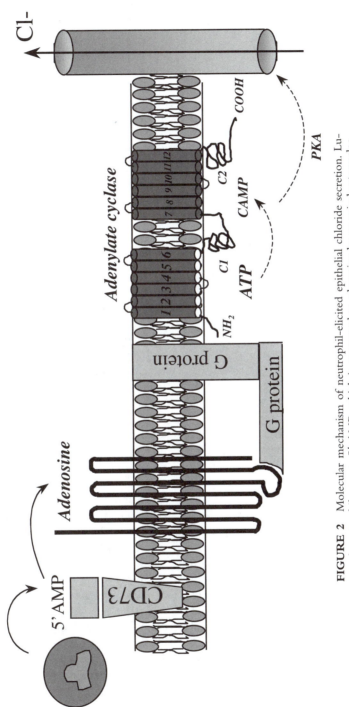

FIGURE 2   Molecular mechanism of neutrophil-elicited epithelial chloride secretion. Luminal neutrophils secrete 5'-AMP, which is converted to adenosine by an apical ectonucleotidase. Such adenosine activates the A2B receptor, leading to apical chloride secretion that provides the driving force for secretory diarrhea.

activation of mediators of lymphocytic infiltration (MCP, ICAM).

Epithelial expression of NF-κB-mediated chemokines and adhesion markers leads to the recruitment of immune cells (especially neutrophils). Recruited neutrophils then transmigrate across the epithelium to the intestinal lumen, resulting in the formation of an intestinal crypt abscess, a histopathologic finding characteristic of acute inflammation of the intestine (37). Neutrophils "on site" contain and clear most infections; mucosal neutrophil recruitment has been clearly demonstrated in vivo to reduce the number of bacteria that reach the systemic circulation (55). In addition to being able to directly destroy bacteria, polymorphonuclear leukocytes (PMN) induce lumenally directed epithelial chloride secretion that acts as the driving force for secretory diarrhea (50). Secretory diarrhea is believed to act as a flushing mechanism in the intestinal tract, thus clearing a wide variety of infections.

Lumenal Neutrophils Aid in Pathogen Clearance

Neutrophil-epithelial interactions have important functional sequelae. Upon entry into the lumenal compartment, neutrophils are stimulated by activating factors that are naturally present in the intestinal lumen (such as LPS and fMLP [n-formyl-leucyl-methionine]) to release numerous compounds via exocytosis of intracellular granules or directly across the cellular membrane. An important consequence of neutrophil activation is the induction of epithelial ion transport, resulting in the movement of isotonic fluid into the intestinal lumen. In fact, conditioned supernatants from activated neutrophils have been shown to induce a significant short circuit current representing the activation of transepithelial chloride secretion (50). With the use of high-performance liquid chromatography and Raman spectroscopy techniques, the neutrophil-derived secretogogue has been identified as 5′-AMP (39). Subsequent studies have shown that this classic intracellular metabolite interfaces, in a paracrine fashion, with

the apical membrane of intestinal epithelial cells and is converted to authentic adenosine by epithelial 5′ ectonucleotidase CD73, a glycosylphosphotidylinositol (GPI)-anchored protein (63). Inhibition of CD73 activity attenuates both the conversion of neutrophil-derived 5′-AMP to adenosine and a 5′-AMP-elicited endogenous transepithelial chloride secretion. 5′-AMP is not only secreted in physiologically significant concentration (micromolar range) but also accounts for the bulk of secretory bioactivity derived from apically positioned neutrophils. Like model intestinal epithelia, native intestinal epithelial cells have been shown to express CD73 on their surface in a preferentially apically polarized fashion (Fig. 2).

Studies performed using intestinal mucosal sheets or cultured human IEC indicate that adenosine, by interacting with a specific adenosine receptor, mediates chloride secretion induced by 5′-AMP (64). Adenosine receptor subtypes may be classified as A1, A2a, A2b, and A3 depending on their coupling to specific G proteins. Using molecular, pharmacologic, and biochemical approaches, we have characterized the intestinal adenosine receptor to be of the A2b subtype in both model intestinal epithelial cells and native intestinal epithelium (64). The A2b receptor, a seven-transmembrane G-protein-coupled cell-surface receptor, is functionally coupled to Gαs, and stimulation of the apical or basolateral surface with adenosine results in increased cyclic AMP (cAMP) in a polarized manner that in turn, via the cAMP-protein kinase A pathway, elicits chloride secretion by regulated gating of apical membrane chloride conductive pathways. The A2b receptor seems to be the only adenosine receptor in the colonic cells and is present in both apical and basolateral membranes (61). Like CD73, the A2b receptor is localized predominantly in the apical membrane as visualized by confocal microscopy (S. V. Sitaraman and J. L. Madara, unpublished observation). In addition, adenosine in the concentration generated from 5′-AMP is only a secretogogue when applied apically. Recently, a similar paradigm of apical localization of CD73, generation of adenosine from neutrophil-derived 5′-AMP, and chloride efflux via the interaction of adenosine with the A2b receptor has also been shown to occur in endothelial cells (35). In this model, adenosine also upregulates CD73, forming a "feed-forward" loop (49).

In addition to regulating ion transport in a variety of epithelia, adenosine is also a well-known mediator of inflammation in many tissues through its potent and selective regulation of proinflammatory or anti-inflammatory cytokines. For example, adenosine induces IL-10 and suppresses IL-12 secretion in monocytes, induces IL-8 release by mast cells, and stimulates IL-6 secretion by astrocytes (36). We have recently shown that adenosine, acting via the activation of the A2b receptor, causes substantial and polarized IL-6 secretion into the luminal compartment of intestinal epithelial cells (60). IL-6 is an important proinflammatory cytokine that is consistently seen in high levels in the serum and tissues of patients with IBD. Interestingly, adenosine, whether placed apically or basolaterally, induces IL-6 secretion into the apical/luminal compartment. Such apical polarization of IL-6 secretion is also induced by other stimuli, such as *Salmonella* infection and TNF-α. The IL-6 secretion induced by adenosine is transcriptionally mediated by activation of the IL-6 promoter through phosphorylated cAMP response element binding (CREB) protein.

IL-6 is the only known proinflammatory cytokine that is secreted apically. When potential targets are considered intestinal lumen, neutrophils seem to be logical candidates because epithelial cell IL-6 receptors are localized to the basolateral membrane (Sitaraman and Madara, unpublished observation). Indeed, IL-6 interacts with neutrophil IL-6 receptors to activate calcium flux in neutrophils, a classic early signal in neutrophil activation. This specific signaling event is consistent with studies of downstream events in which IL-6 exposure has been shown to induce elastase release, platelet-activating factor (PAF) pro-

duction, and oxygen free radicals in neutrophils that may potentially be involved in killing pathogens (Fig. 3). In addition to its effect on intestinal epithelial cells, adenosine has also been shown to interact with neutrophil adenosine receptors to downregulate neutrophil activation, adherence, and neutrophil-mediated inflammation in endothelial cells (7, 53).

Negative Consequences of Epithelial Promotion of Neutrophil Movement

Inflammation is a double-edged sword; neutrophil transepithelial migration also results in a reduction of epithelial barrier function (51). This can lead to opportunistic infections of microorganisms that would normally not be able to breach the epithelial barrier. For example, neutrophil-mediated disruption of epithelial barrier function has been specifically demonstrated to allow *Shigella* spp. (54) and *Yersinia* spp. (42) to breach mucosal defenses. Furthermore, such epithelial disruption allows the noxious, PAMP-laden contents of the intestinal lumen to reach the basolateral epithelial surface, leading to further NF-κB activation/inflammation. In addition to the risk of opportunistic infection and dehydration, the oxidants and proteases released by neutrophils can cause lasting tissue damage and likely play a role in the early development of neoplasia. Therefore, it is extremely important for the host to activate the inflammatory process sparingly. Interestingly though, some degree of low level "surveillance" NF-κB activation may be physiological. The one IBD susceptibility gene (NOD-2) cloned to date is an isoform of an intracellular LPS detector that is unable to activate NF-κB in response to LPS. Thus, it is possible that the failure to activate low levels of NF-κB in response to normally harmless intracellular pathogens leads to chronic infection with subsequent severe and global proinflammatory activation. Several studies have shown marked upregulated expression of NF-κB-mediated genes in IBD (56). In the dextran sodium sulfate (DSS) models of IBD, blockade of NF-κB via in

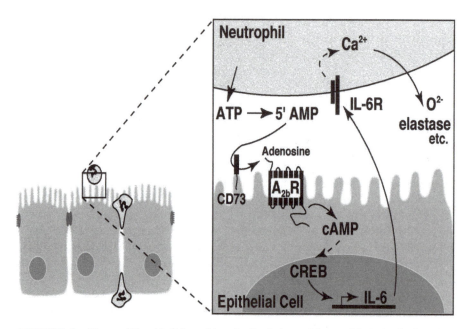

FIGURE 3 Neutrophil-epithelial positive feedback loop. Neutrophil-derived adenosine elicits epithelial secretion of IL-6, which will activate lumenal neutrophils to secrete oxidants and other antibacterial products.

vivo expression of a dominant-negative iso-form of IκBα led to worse disease than in control mice (54a). Thus, NF-κB activation plays an essential role in both maintaining the well-being of the intestine through a low level of inflammation and inducing excessive activation of inflammation, which can lead to pathology.

RESOLUTION OF INFLAMMATION

Clearly, given the deleterious effects of uncontrolled inflammation, tight control over the NF-κB activation pathway is critical. It is perhaps not surprising that there are also specific mechanisms of downregulating the activity of this proinflammatory transcription factor. Just as there are many ways of activating this pathway, there are multiple ways of repressing it. Chapter 11 by Neish discusses how bacteria can repress activation of the NF-κB pathway for their benefit. There are also endogenous means of downregulating epithelial proinflammatory signaling. For example,

the anti-inflammatory cytokine IL-10 down-regulates NF-κB activation and subsequently chemokine secretion (66). The potential importance of the counterregulatory role of this cytokine is illustrated by the fact that IL-10 mice develop spontaneous colitis (34). Select members of the lipoxin class of lipid mediators also downregulate NF-κB-mediated responses. Specifically, lipoxin A4 and its stable analogs downregulate IL-8 expression by epithelial cells (17, 23). Recent studies have shown that this eicosanoid ligates its receptor and results in inhibition of IκBα degradation but not phosphorylation (15). LXA$_4$ also acts on neutrophils, resulting in reduced secretion of preformed granule mediators such as the protease elastase (16). Interestingly, lipoxins are primarily made through cell-cell interactions that occur only during inflammation (e.g., neutrophil-epithelial interactions); thus, their synthesis likely provides a natural negative feedback loop to help resolve inflammation (58). Thus, the end result of the definitive hallmark of active inflammation is the biosynthesis of eicosanoids that will reduce the inflammatory signaling. Furthermore, recent studies have demonstrated that lipoxins not only block activation of proinflammatory pathways but also actively aid in the resolution of inflammation by stimulating nonphlogistic phagocytosis of apoptotic neutrophils by macrophages (22). Such apoptosis occurs without further release of proinflammatory mediators and thus sequesters the neutrophil contents, thus reducing tissue damage to the host and allowing healing to occur. Several laboratories are investigating whether synthetic lipoxin analogs that mimic the bioactivity of the native eicosanoid can be used to treat inappropriate intestinal inflammation.

CONCLUSIONS

Over the last 10 years, it has become clear that the intestinal epithelium is not a passive barrier, but rather the central mediator in the complex interactions between the residents of its external and internal environments; i.e., the commensal microbiota and the immune cells that underlie the intestinal epithelium. In vitro and in vivo evidence indicates that the gut epithelium's ability to sense dangerous pathogens among this complex milieu and to act appropriately is an essential aspect of innate immunity, even if it results in unpleasant consequences (i.e., diarrhea) for the host. Conversely, inappropriate or unwarranted activation of such stress response pathways can also have serious detrimental consequences, such as perhaps IBD.

The NF-κB pathway is clearly a critical mediator of immune and inflammatory responses in the intestinal tract, and, as such, its regulation is both germane to innate immunity and also very likely central to the pathogenesis of idiopathic IBD (as evidenced by the fact that all genetic models of IBD are absolutely dependent on the presence of "commensal" microbes). Studies of the mechanisms that regulate activation of the NF-κB reveal some of the mechanisms by which epithelia can distinguish between commensal and pathogenic microbes and also suggest means by which defects in basic epithelial physiology (i.e., a leaky epithelium) can result in an inflammatory response. Further knowledge of the basic mechanisms that regulate the activation of this and other proinflammatory transcription factors will be essential for improved understanding and subsequent pharmacological manipulation of intestinal inflammation.

REFERENCES

1. **Abreu, M. T., P. Vora, E. Faure, L. S. Thomas, E. T. Arnold, and M. Arditi.** 2001. Decreased expression of Toll-like receptor-4 and MD-2 correlates with intestinal epithelial cell protection against dysregulated proinflammatory gene expression in response to bacterial lipopolysaccharide. *J. Immunol.* **167:**1609–1616.

2. **Aderem, A., and R. Ulevitch.** 2000. Toll-like receptors in the induction of the innate immune response. *Nature* **406:**782–787.

3. **Bauer, S., C. J. Kirschning, H. Hacker, V. Redecke, S. Hausmann, S. Akira, H. Wagner, and G. B. Lipford.** 2001. Human TLR9 confers responsiveness to bacterial DNA via species-specific CpG motif recognition. *Proc. Natl. Acad. Sci. USA* **98:**9237–9242.

4. **Bulut, Y., E. Faure, L. Thomas, O. Equils, and M. Arditi.** 2001. Cooperation of Toll-like receptor 2 and 6 for cellular activation by soluble tuberculosis factor and *Borrelia burgdorferi* outer surface protein A lipoprotein: role of Toll-interacting protein and IL-1 receptor signaling molecules in Toll-like receptor 2 signaling. *J. Immunol.* **167:**987–994.

5. **Cario, E., I. M. Rosenberg, S. L. Brandwein, P. L. Beck, H. C. Reinecker, and D. K. Podolsky.** 2000. Lipopolysaccharide activates distinct signaling pathways in intestinal epithelial cell lines expressing Toll-like receptors. *J. Immunol.* **164:**966–972.

6. **Chow, J. C., D. W. Young, D. T. Golenbock, W. J. Christ, and F. Gusovsky.** 1999. Toll-like receptor-4 mediates lipopolysaccharide-induced signal transduction. *J. Biol. Chem.* **274:**10689–10692.

7. **Cronstein, B. N.** 1995. A novel approach to the development of anti-inflammatory agents: adenosine release at inflamed sites. *J. Investig. Med.* **43:**50–57.

8. **Dangl, J., and J. Jones.** 2001. Plant pathogens and integrated defence responses to infection. *Nature* **411:**826–833.

9. **Deng, L., C. Wang, E. Spencer, L. Yang, A. Braun, X. You, C. Slaughter, C. Pickart,**

and Z. Chen. 2000. Activation of the IkB kinase complex by TRAF6 requires a dimeric ubiquitin-conjugating enzyme complex and a unique polyubiquitin chain. *Cell* **103**:351–361.

10. Dickinson, B. L., K. Badizadegan, Z. Wu, J. C. Ahouse, X. Zhu, N. E. Simister, R. S. Blumberg, and W. I. Lencer. 1999. Bidirectional FcRn-dependent IgG transport in a polarized human intestinal epithelial cell line. *J. Clin. Invest.* **104**:903–911.

11. DiDonato, J. A., M. Hayakawa, D. M. Rothwarf, E. Zandi, and M. Karin. 1997. A cytokine-responsive IkappaB kinase that activates the transcription factor NF-kappaB. *Nature* **388**: 548–554.

12. Egan, L., L. Eckmann, Z.-W. Li, F. Greten, M. Karin, S. Robine, and M. Kagnoff. 2002. Systemic inflammation and decreased survival in conditional intestinal epithelial cell IKKβ knockout mice generated using a villin-cre transgenic mouse line. *Gastroenterology* **122**:172.

13. Elewaut, D., J. DiDonato, J. Kim, F. Truong, L. Eckmann, and M. Kagnoff. 1999. NF-κB is a central regulator of the intestinal epithelial cell innate immune response induced by infection with enteroinvasive bacteria. *J. Immunol.* **163**:1457–1466.

14. Galan, J. E. 1998. Interactions of *Salmonella* with host cells: encounters of the closest kind. *Proc. Natl. Acad. Sci. USA* **95**:14006–14008.

15. Gewirtz, A. T., L. S. Collier-Hyams, A. N. Young, T. Kucharzik, W. J. Guilford, J. F. Parkinson, I. R. Williams, A. S. Neish, and J. L. Madara. 2002. Lipoxin A4 analogs attenuate induction of intestinal epithelial proinflammatory gene expression and reduce the severity of dextran sodium sulfate-induced colitis. *J. Immunol.* **168**:5260–5267.

16. Gewirtz, A. T., V. V. Fokin, N. A. Petasis, C. N. Serhan, and J. L. Madara. 1999. LXA$_4$, aspirin-triggered 15-epi LXA$_4$, and their stable analogs selectively down-regulate PMN azurophilic degranulation. *Am. J. Phys.* (*Cell*) **276**: C988–C994.

17. Gewirtz, A. T., B. McCormick, A. S. Neish, N. A. Petasis, K. Gronert, C. N. Serhan, and J. L. Madara. 1998. Pathogen-induced chemokine secretion from model intestinal epithelium is inhibited by lipoxin A4 analogs. *J. Clin. Invest.* **101**:1860–1869.

18. Gewirtz, A. T., T. A. Navas, S. Lyons, P. J. Godowski, and J. L. Madara. 2001. Cutting edge: bacterial flagellin activates basolaterally expressed tlr5 to induce epithelial proinflammatory gene expression. *J. Immunol.* **167**:1882–1885.

19. Gewirtz, A. T., A. S. Rao, P. O. Simon, Jr., D. Merlin, D. Carnes, J. L. Madara, and

A. S. Neish. 2000. *Salmonella typhimurium* induces epithelial IL-8 expression via Ca(2$^+$)-mediated activation of the NF-kappaB pathway. *J. Clin. Invest.* **105**:79–92.

20. Gewirtz, A. T., P. O. Simon, Jr., C. K. Schmitt, L. J. Taylor, C. H. Hagedorn, A. D. O'Brien, A. S. Neish, and J. L. Madara. 2001. *Salmonella typhimurium* translocates flagellin across intestinal epithelia, inducing a proinflammatory response. *J. Clin. Invest.* **107**: 99–109.

21. Girardin, S. E., R. Tournebize, M. Mavris, A. L. Page, X. Li, G. R. Stark, J. Bertin, P. S. DiStefano, M. Yaniv, P. J. Sansonetti, and D. J. Philpott. 2001. CARD4/Nod1 mediates NF-kappaB and JNK activation by invasive *Shigella flexneri*. *EMBO Rep.* **2**:736–742.

22. Godson, C., S. Mitchell, K. Harvey, N. A. Petasis, N. Hogg, and H. R. Brady. 2000. Cutting edge: lipoxins rapidly stimulate nonphlogistic phagocytosis of apoptotic neutrophils by monocyte-derived macrophages. *J. Immunol.* **164**: 1663–1667.

23. Gronert, K. G., A. T. Gewirtz, J. L. Madara, and C. N. Serhan. 1998. Identification of a human enterocyte lipoxin A4 receptor that is regulated by IL-13 and INF-γ that inhibits TNF-α-induced IL-8 release. *J. Exp. Med.* **187**:1285–1294.

24. Hayashi, F., K. D. Smith, A. Ozinsky, T. R. Hawn, E. C. Yi, D. R. Goodlett, J. K. Eng, S. Akira, D. M. Underhill, and A. Aderem. 2001. The innate immune response to bacterial flagellin is mediated by Toll-like receptor 5. *Nature* **410**:1099–1103.

25. Hobbie, S., L. Chen, R. Davis, and J. Galan. 1997. Involvement of mitogen-activated protein kinase pathways in the nuclear responses and cytokine production induced by *Salmonella typhimurium* in cultured intestinal epithelial cells. *J. Immunol.* **159**:5550–5559.

26. Hoffman, J., F. Kafatos, C. Janeway, and R. Ezekowitz. 1999. Phylogenetic perspectives in innate immunity. *Science* **284**:1313–1318.

27. Hooper, L. V., L. Bry, P. G. Falk, and J. I. Gordon. 1998. Host-microbial symbiosis in the mammalian intestine: exploring an internal ecosystem. *Bioessays* **20**:336–343.

28. Janeway, C. A., Jr. 2001. How the immune system works to protect the host from infection: a personal view. *Proc. Natl. Acad. Sci. USA.* **98**: 7461–7468.

29. Jobin, C., and R. Sartor. 2000. The IkB/NF-kB system; a key determinant of mucosal inflammation and protection. *Am. J. Physiol. Cell Physiol.* **278**:451–462.

30. **Karin, M.** 1999. The beginning of the end: Ikb kinase (IKK) and NF-kB activation. *J. Biol. Chem.* **274**:27339–27342.

31. **Karin, M., and Y. Ben-Neriah.** 2000. Phosphorylation meets ubiquitination: the control of NF-kB activity. *Annu. Rev. Immunol.* **18**:621–663.

32. **Kenny, B., R. DeVinney, M. Stein, D. J. Reinscheid, E. A. Frey, and B. B. Finlay.** 1997. Enteropathogenic *E. coli* (EPEC) transfers its receptor for intimate adherence into mammalian cells. *Cell* **91**:511–520.

33. **Kopp, E., and S. Ghosh.** 1995. NF-kB and Rel proteins in innate immunity. *Adv. Immunol.* **58**:1–12.

34. **Kuhn, R., J. Lohler, D. Rennick, K. Rajewsky, and W. Muller.** 1993. Interleukin-10-deficient mice develop chronic enterocolitis [see comments]. *Cell* **75**:263–274.

35. **Lennon, P. F., C. T. Taylor, G. L. Stahl, and S. P. Colgan.** 1998. Neutrophil-derived 5′-adenosine monophosphate promotes endothelial barrier function via CD73-mediated conversion to adenosine and endothelial A2B receptor activation. *J. Exp. Med.* **188**:1433–1443.

36. **Link, A. A., T. Kino, J. A. Worth, J. L. McGuire, M. L. Crane, G. P. Chrousos, R. L. Wilder, and I. J. Elenkov.** 2000. Ligand-activation of the adenosine A2a receptors inhibits IL-12 production by human monocytes. *J. Immunol.* **164**:436–442.

37. **Madara, J. L.** 1990. Pathobiology of the intestinal epithelial barrier. *Am. J. Pathol.* **137**:1273–1281.

38. **Madara, J. L., C. A. Parkos, A. Nusrat, K. Atisook, and P. Kaoutzani.** 1992. The movement of solutes and cells across tight junctions. *N.Y. Acad. of Sci.* **664**:47–60.

39. **Madara, J. L., T. W. Patapoff, B. Gillece-Castro, S. P. Colgan, C. A. Parkos, C. Delp, and R. J. Mrsny.** 1993. 5′-Adenosine monophosphate is the neutrophil-derived paracrine factor that elicits chloride secretion from T84 intestinal epithelial cells. *J. Clin. Invest.* **91**:2320–2325.

40. **May, M., and S. Ghosh.** 1999. IkB kinases: kinsmen with different crafts. *Science* **284**:271–273.

41. **Mayer, L.** 1993. *Immunophysiology of the Gut.* Academic Press, Inc., New York, N.Y.

42. **McCormick, B. A., A. Nusrat, C. A. Parkos, L. D'Andrea, P. M. Hofman, D. Carnes, T. W. Liang, and J. L. Madara.** 1997. Unmasking of intestinal epithelial lateral membrane beta1 integrin consequent to transepithelial neutrophil migration in vitro facilitates inv-mediated invasion by *Yersinia pseudotuberculosis. Infect. Immun.* **65**:1414–1421.

43. **Medzhitov, R., and C. Janeway, Jr.** 2000. Innate immunity. *N. Engl. J. Med.* **343**:338–344.

44. **Medzhitov, R., and C. Janeway, Jr.** 2000. The Toll receptor family and microbial recognition. *Trends Microbiol.* **8**:452–456.

45. **Merlin, D., A. Steel, A.T. Gewirtz, M. Sitahar, M. A. Hediger, and J. L. Madara.** 1998. hPepT1-mediated epithelial transport of bacteria derived chemotactic peptides enhances neutrophil epithelial interactions. *J. Clin. Invest.* **102**:2011–2018.

46. **Merlin, D., M. Si-Tahar, S. V. Sitaraman, K. Eastburn, I. Williams, X. Liu, M. A. Hediger, and J. L. Madara.** 2001. Colonic epithelial hPepT1 expression occurs in inflammatory bowel disease: transport of bacterial peptides influences expression of MHC class 1 molecules. *Gastroenterology* **120**:1666–1679.

47. **Mounier, J., T. Vasselon, R. Hellio, M. Lesourd, and P. J. Sansonetti.** 1992. *Shigella flexneri* enters human colonic Caco-2 epithelial cells through the basolateral pole. *Infect. Immun.* **60**:237–248.

48. **Naik, S., E. J. Kelly, L. Meijer, S. Pettersson, and I. R. Sanderson.** 2001. Absence of Toll-like receptor 4 explains endotoxin hyporesponsiveness in human intestinal epithelium. *J. Pediatr. Gastroenterol. Nutr.* **32**:449–453.

49. **Narravula, S., P. F. Lennon, B. U. Mueller, and S. P. Colgan.** 2000. Regulation of endothelial CD73 by adenosine: paracrine pathway for enhanced endothelial barrier function. *J. Immunol.* **165**:5262–5268.

50. **Nash, S., C. A. Parkos, A. Nusrat, C. Delp, and J. L. Madara.** 1991. In vitro model of intestinal crypt abcess: a novel neutrophil-derived secretagogue activity. *J. Clin. Invest.* **87**:1474–1477.

51. **Nash, S., J. Stafford, and J. L. Madara.** 1987. Effects of polymorphonuclear leukocyte transmigration on barrier function of cultured intestinal epithelial monolayers *J. Clin. Invest.* **80**:1104–1113.

52. **Poltorak, A., X. He, I. Smirnova, M. Y. Liu, C. V. Huffel, X. Du, D. Birdwell, E. Alejos, M. Silva, C. Galanos, M. Freudenberg, P. Ricciardi-Castagnoli, B. Layton, and B. Beutler.** 1998. Defective LPS signaling in C3H/HeJ and C57BL/10ScCr mice: mutations in Tlr4 gene. *Science* **282**:2085–2088.

53. **Revan, S., M. C. Montesinos, D. Naime, S. Landau, and B. N. Cronstein.** 1996. Adenosine A2 receptor occupancy regulates stimulated neutrophil function via activation of a serine/

threonine protein phosphatase. *J. Biol. Chem.* **271**:17114–17118.

53a. Russo, M. P., F. Boubreau, F. L. Li, A. Panja, P. G. Traber, R. G. Sartor, and C. Jobin. 2001. NF-kappa B blockade exacerbates experimental colitis in transgenic mice expressing an intestinal epithelial cell specific I kappa B super-repressor. *Gastroenterology* **120**(Suppl. 1): 369.

54. Sansonetti, P. J. 2001. Rupture, invasion and inflammatory destruction of the intestinal barrier by *Shigella*, making sense of prokaryote-eukaryote cross-talks. *FEMS Microbiol Rev.* **25**:3–14.

55. Sansonetti, P. J., J. Arondel, M. Huerre, A. Harada, and K. Matsushima. 1999. Interleukin-8 controls bacterial transepithelial translocation at the cost of epithelial destruction in experimental shigellosis. *Infect. Immun.* **67**:1471–1480.

56. Schreiber, S., S. Nikolaus, and J. Hampe. 1998. Activation of nuclear factor kappa B inflammatory bowel disease. *Gut* **42**:477–484.

57. Schwandner, R., R. Dziarski, H. Wesche, M. Rothe, and C. J. Kirschning. 1999. Peptidoglycan- and lipoteichoic acid-induced cell activation is mediated by Toll-like receptor 2. *J. Biol. Chem.* **274**:17406–17409.

58. Serhan, C. N. 1997. Lipoxins and novel aspirin-triggered 15-epi-lipoxins (ATL): a jungle of cell-cell interactions or a therapeutic opportunity? *Prostaglandins* **53**:107–137.

59. Silverman, N., and T. Maniatis. 2001. NF-kB signaling pathways in mammalian and insect immunity. *Gene Dev.* **15**:2321–2342.

60. Sitaraman, S. V., D. Merlin, L. Wang, M. Wong, A. T. Gewirtz, M. Si-Tahar, and J. L. Madara. 2001. Neutrophil-epithelial cross-talk at the intestinal lumenal surface mediated by reciprocal secretion of adenosine and IL-6. *J. Clin. Invest.* **107**:861–869.

61. Sitaraman, S. V., M. Si-Tahar, D. Merlin, G. R. Strohmeier, and J. L. Madara. 2000. Polarity of A2b adenosine receptor expression determines characteristics of receptor desensitization. *Am. J. Physiol. Cell. Physiol.* **278**:C1230–C1236.

62. Smirnova, I., A. Poltorak, E. K. Chan, C. McBride, and B. Beutler. 2000. Phylogenetic variation and polymorphism at the Toll-like receptor 4 locus (TLR4). *Genome Biol.* **1**:1–11.

63. Strohmeier, G. R., W. I. Lencer, T. W. Patapoff, L. F. Thompson, S. L. Carlson, S. J. Moe, D. K. Carnes, R. J. Mrsny, and J. L. Madara. 1997. Surface expression, polarization, and functional significance of CD73 in human intestinal epithelia. *J. Clin. Invest.* **99**:2588–2601.

64. Strohmeier, G. R., S. M. Reppert, W. I. Lencer, and J. L. Madara. 1995. The A2b adenosine receptor mediates cAMP responses to adenosine receptor agonists in human intestinal epithelia. *J. Biol. Chem.* **270**:2387–2394.

65. Wang, C., L. Deng, M. Hong, G. Akkaraju, J.-I. Inoue, and Z. Chen. 2001. Tak1 is a ubiquitin-dependent kinase of MKK and IKK. *Nature* **412**:346–351.

66. Wang, P., P. Wu, M. I. Siegel, R. W. Egan, and M. M. Billah. 1995. Interleukin (IL)-10 inhibits nuclear factor kappa B (NF kappa B) activation in human monocytes. IL-10 and IL-4 suppress cytokine synthesis by different mechanisms. *J. Biol. Chem.* **270**:9558–9563.

67. Zhou, D., L. M. Chen, L. Hernandez, S. B. Shears, and J. E. Galan. 2001. A *Salmonella* inositol polyphosphatase acts in conjunction with other bacterial effectors to promote host cell actin cytoskeleton rearrangements and bacterial internalization. *Mol. Microbiol.* **39**:248–259.

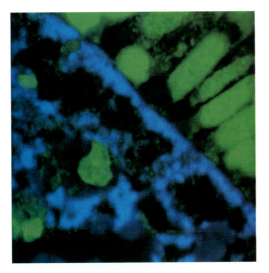

Color Plate 1 (chapter 7)   A section of small intestine from a patient with Whipple's disease examined with confocal fluorescence microscopy at 3,000× magnification. Intestinal epithelial cells are located in the upper right corner of these images, with the mucosa in the lower left. Yo-Pro nucleic acid stain (green) highlights host cell nuclei and bacterial nucleic acids, revealing multiple small bacillary bodies free in the lamina propria. A *T. whippelii*-specific rDNA probe labeled with Cy-5 and targeting bacterial rRNA (blue) reveals clumps of bacteria in the lamina propria. Most bacteria appear just basal to the intestinal epithelial cells, forming a continuous band.

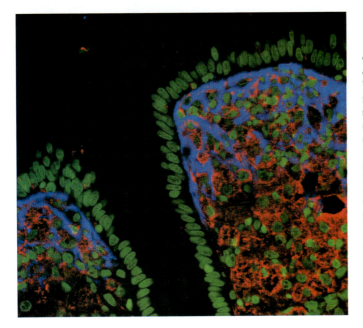

Color Plate 2 (chapter 7)   A section of small intestine from a patient with Whipple's disease subjected to fluorescence in situ hybridization and visualized at 400× magnification using a confocal microscope. Nucleic acids are stained green with Yo-Pro dye, *T. whippelii* rRNA appears blue using a Cy-5-labeled rDNA probe, and the human intracellular cytoskeletal protein vimentin appears red using a Texas red-labeled antivimentin antibody. Only cells of mesenchymal origin have vimentin; hence, epithelial cells do not stain with the antivimentin antibody, but macrophages in the lamina propria do contain vimentin. Most of the rRNA signal from bacteria appears in the extracellular compartment.

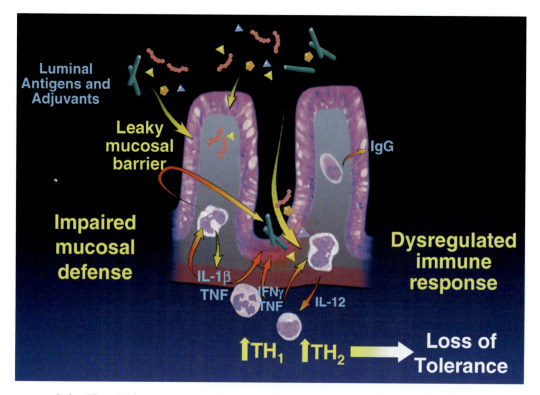

Color Plate 3 (chapter 13) Activation of pathogenic mucosal immune responses leading to chronic intestinal inflammation in genetically susceptible hosts. Acquired or intrinsic enhanced mucosal permeability enhances uptake of luminal bacterial adjuvants and antigens, which activate lamina propria innate and cognate immune cells. Resultant proinflammatory cytokines cause tissue injury, which initiates a self-perpetuating inflammatory response driven by an ever-increasing uptake of microbial antigens. Genetic susceptibility is mediated by defective immunoregulation or barrier function. Used with permission from the AGA.

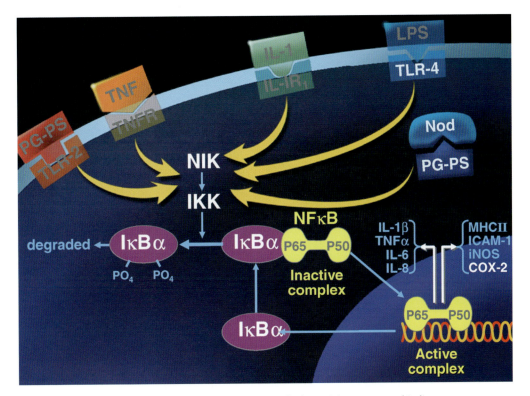

Color Plate 4 (chapter 13)   Activation of NF-κB by bacterial components binding to pattern recognition receptors. Bacterial cell wall polymers selectively bind to membrane TLR or intracytoplasmic NOD-1 and NOD-2 to initiate signaling of a cascade of kinases resulting in activation of NF-κB. PG-PS bind to TLR-2 while LPS binds to TLR-4; both LPS and PG-PS bind to NOD-1 and NOD-2. Signal transduction activates NF-κB to induce transcription of a number of proinflammatory gene products. Used with permission from the AGA.

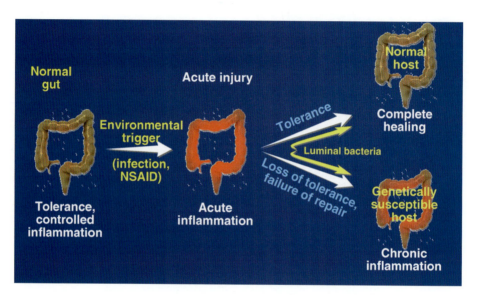

Color Plate 5 (chapter 13)   Induction of self-limited versus chronic intestinal inflammation in normal versus genetically susceptible hosts, respectively, following a transient injury. Non-specific injury due to an acute infection or exposure to nonsteroidal anti-inflammatory drugs (NSAID) leads to acute inflammation in all hosts. Genetically resistant (normal) hosts rapidly heal mucosal injury with no residual damage. In contrast, genetically susceptible hosts with dysregulated immune responses or defective mucosal barrier function/healing develop chronic inflammation due to constant antigenic stimulation of aggressive immune responses. Used with permission from the AGA.

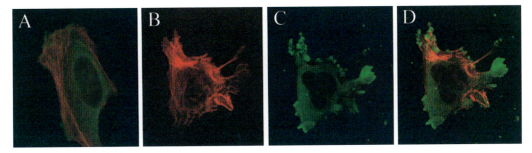

Color Plate 6 (chapter 17)   Effect of the SPATE toxin Pet on the epithelial cytoskeleton. Hep-2 cells were incubated with 30 nM purified Pet toxin on ice, then shifted to 37°C for 2 h. Cells were then fixed and stained with rhodamine-phalloidin and with mouse anti-spectrin monoclonals, followed by fluorescein isothiocyanate (FITC)-conjugated anti-mouse immunoglobulin. Cells were visualized under confocal microscopy. Actin stress fibers appear red and spectrin green. (A) Merge of images for unintoxicated Hep-2 cells. Spectrin localizes to the membrane cytoskeleton and therefore stains diffusely. (B through D) Pet-intoxicated cell. (B) When visualized for actin, stress fibers are still apparent, although the cell has begun to manifest actin-containing lamellipodium-like structures. (C) Spectrin appears condensed and peripherally localized, with formation of spectrin-containing blebs. (D) Merge of images B and C. Actin filaments are seen condensed in areas of bleb formation. (R. Cappello and J. Nataro, unpublished observations.)

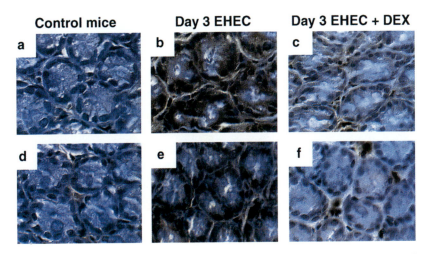

Color Plate 7 (chapter 19)   Immunohistochemical localization of Gal1 receptors and the p65 subunit of NF-κB on mouse colonic epithelium in EHEC-infected mice. Colonic epithelium of noninfected mice (a and d) shows no evidence of either Gal1 receptor or NF-κB p65 subunit immunoreactivity. However, 3 days after infection with EHEC, increased expression of both Gal1 receptors and NF-κB is evident (b and e). Administration of the NF-κB inhibitor dexamethasone during EHEC infection diminishes expression of Gal1 receptor and NF-κB activation in colonic epithelial cells, indicating that Gal1 receptor upregulation in response to EHEC is mediating via NF-κB. Magnification, ×400. (From reference 39, with permission.)

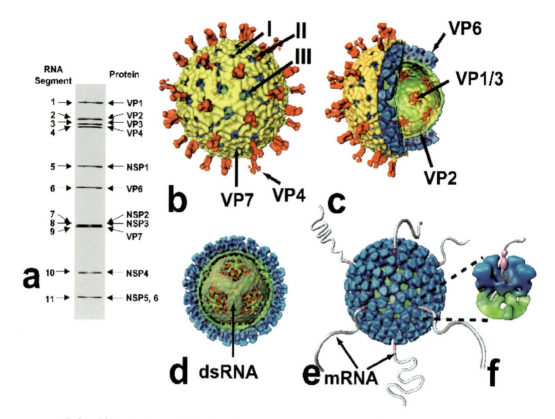

Color Plate 8 (chapter 28) Rotavirus genes, proteins, and viral structure. (a) Pattern of separation of the 11 segments of rotavirus RNA after electrophoresis on a polyacrylamide gel, giving the names of the proteins encoded in each segment. Proteins found in virus particles (VP1 through 7) and nonstructural proteins (NSP1 through NSP6) found only in infected cells are shown. (b) Surface representation of the rotavirus structure. Three types of channels (I, II, III), the VP4 spikes, and the VP7 capsid layer are highlighted by arrows. (c) Cutaway structure illustrating the internal VP6 and VP2 layers. The flower-shaped VP1/VP3 complex, attached to the inside of the VP2 layer, is also shown. (d) Structural organization of the genomic double-stranded RNA. The outer layer of RNA has a dodecahedral appearance. (e) Structure of double-layered particles transcribing mRNAs that exit the virus through the type I channels at the fivefold vertices. (f) Cutaway view depicting the exit pathway of mRNA in one of the channels. Viral structures provided by B. V. V. Prasad.

Color Plate 9 (chapter 28) Norwalk virus structure. VLPs (top left) visualized by negative-stain electron microscopy have a surface structure that consists of 90 dimeric arches that emanate from the surface of the particles (top right). A ribbon diagram of a monomer of the capsid protein (lower right) shows it is composed of a shell domain connected to a protruding domain that has two subdomains. The N terminus is inside particles, while the C terminus is exposed in the hollows made by dimers of the capsid protein (lower left). Viral structures kindly provided by B. V. V. Prasad.

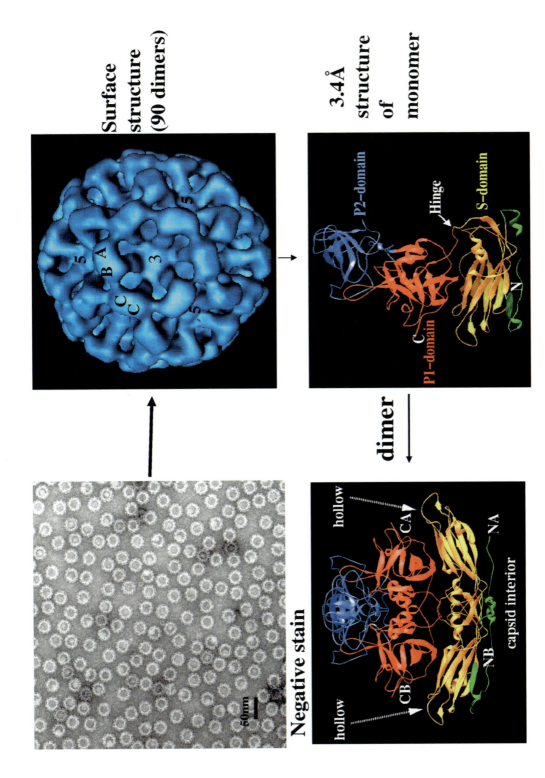

Surface structure (90 dimers)

3.4Å structure of monomer

dimer

Negative stain

UPREGULATION OF INNATE DEFENSE MECHANISMS BY ENTERIC INFECTIONS

Martin F. Kagnoff

10

The mucosa that lines the human colon and small intestine is a site of chronic, regulated, "physiologic" inflammation. This contrasts with other mucosal sites and the skin. If the numbers of T and B lymphocytes, eosinophils, mast cells, macrophages, and dendritic cells that are present in the human intestinal tract were to be present in other sites, those sites would be considered to be chronically inflamed. In addition to intermittent encounters with enteric microbial pathogens, the intestinal mucosa is continuously exposed to an abundant, and normally nonpathogenic, commensal bacterial flora. Consistent with this, the epithelium requires mechanisms to distinguish the presence of pathogens from nonpathogenic commensals that are constitutively present and do not represent a threat to the host. Normal epithelial cell barrier function and constitutively produced epithelial products, such as antimicrobial peptides, likely play an important role in producing effective host defense to nonpathogenic commensal microbes. Moreover, the intestinal epithelium functions to maintain its barrier function while concur-

rently mediating absorptive and secretory functions that are essential to host survival.

The intestinal mucosa is lined by a single layer of epithelial cells that separates the host's internal milieu from the intestinal lumen and the external environment. From time to time these epithelial cells are exposed to pathogenic bacterial, viral, and protozoan microbial pathogens. Innate epithelial defense mechanisms provide a rapid response whereby microbial pathogens in the host are quickly detected and signals are generated that activate mucosal antimicrobial defense mechanisms. The intestinal epithelium functions as a microbial detector, signal integrator, and central relay system in a communications network that transmits signals from pathogenic microbes and their products to cells in the underlying lamina propria. In addition to their key role in signaling innate mucosal defense, intestinal epithelial cells produce mediators with antimicrobial activity (e.g., defensins, nitric oxide).

In contrast to innate immune defense mechanisms, the generation of adaptive T- and B-cell-mediated immune defense is delayed and results in a protective primary host response only several days after an encounter with the pathogen. In the absence of effective innate immune defense mechanisms, many enteric pathogens can cause severe disease and

Martin F. Kagnoff, Department of Medicine, University of California, San Diego, 9500 Gilman Dr. (MTF/412), La Jolla, CA 92093-0623.

Microbial Pathogenesis and the Intestinal Epithelial Cell, ed. by G. Hecht
© 2003 ASM Press, Washington, D.C.

even death during this lag period. Moreover, the initiation of adaptive immune defense requires the activation of T cells by antigen-presenting cells of the innate immune system. When viewed in this context, it is evident that innate defense mechanisms are essential for host survival during encounters with many enteric pathogens.

Over the past decade, intestinal epithelial cells have been reported to express, either constitutively or in a regulated manner, receptors that are important for both innate and adaptive immunity (e.g., interleukin-1 [IL-1], IL-4, IL-6, IL-7, IL-9, IL-10, IL-15, and IL-17, gamma interferon [IFN-γ], granulocyte-macrophage colony-stimulating factor [GM-CSF], and tumor necrosis factor-α [TNF-α]) (21, 24, 35, 94, 95, 114, 118), receptors for a selected group of chemokines (e.g., CXCR4, CCR5, CCR6, CX3CR1) (11, 23, 26, 60), Toll-like receptors (15, 16, 43), major histocompatibility complex (MHC) class II molecules, and non-classical MHC class I molecules (20, 47, 108). This chapter examines the role of the intestinal epithelium in innate immune defense against enteric microbial pathogens. It focuses on in vitro and in vivo model systems that can be used to define epithelial cell innate immune defense mechanisms that are activated in response to microbial infection and a spectrum of intestinal epithelial innate defense mechanisms that can be activated by microbial pathogens that use different strategies to interact with the host.

MODEL SYSTEMS TO STUDY HOST EPITHELIAL CELL INNATE DEFENSE TO MICROBIAL PATHOGENS

Interactions between enteric microbial pathogens and intestinal epithelial cells involve, by definition, two major players: the pathogen and the host epithelial cell. Several approaches can be used to study the constitutive and regulated epithelial innate host defense mechanisms. One of the simplest reductionist approaches is to ask the question, What host genes are upregulated and what epithelial cell

mediators are produced by intestinal epithelial cells when they encounter a microbial pathogen in a tissue culture plate in vitro? As many of the human intestinal epithelial cells available for such studies are long-term cell lines generated from colon carcinomas, the cellular responses of a single cell line to a given microbial pathogen should be verified using several different cell lines and, even then, the results should be interpreted with caution as they may not always accurately reflect the response of normal intestinal epithelial cells. Nonetheless, this approach has provided a great deal of data, much of which has subsequently been confirmed with normal epithelial cells using in vivo models.

In addition to studies focused on individual epithelial cell mediators, cultured human colon epithelial cell lines have been used in studies employing high-density cDNA arrays to probe the upregulated expression of thousands of genes in intestinal epithelial cells in response to infection with enteroinvasive bacteria (5, 32, 62, 98). Notably, those studies revealed that infection of intestinal epithelial cell lines with enteric pathogens (e.g., *Salmonella* spp.) upregulates mRNA expression of a relatively small fraction of all genes tested, and, as will be discussed later, one group of genes that is upregulated is the NF-κB responsive genes. mRNA expression profiles obtained using microarray analysis provide a powerful approach to characterizing and understanding epithelial cell-pathogen interactions, and lead to the discovery of epithelial cell products upregulated by microbial pathogens, which would not have been otherwise predicted. In contrast to colon carcinoma cell lines, few, if any, representative human small intestinal epithelial cell lines are available for study using in vitro model systems.

The ability to grow several human colon cancer-derived epithelial cell lines as a polarized epithelium on microporous supports in in vitro culture adds another useful tool for exploring epithelial cell-microbial interactions. At least three human colon cancer epithelial cell lines, T84, Caco-2, and HCA-7, can be grown in this reductionist system as a "model epithelium" (27, 28, 58, 71, 80, 117). This model system more closely approximates the epithelium in vivo, which is polarized into apical and basolateral domains. Thus, in vivo the intestinal epithelium variably interacts with microbial pathogens at the apical and basolateral surface and vectorally secretes innate defense molecules from the basolateral or apical membrane. Delineating the apical versus basolateral secretion of innate defense molecules is clearly important when considering intestinal epithelial cell mediators that must signal effective host defense responses and defend against luminal dwelling noninvasive pathogens, compared to enteroinvasive pathogens. Such model epithelia grown on permeable supports can also be used to generate more complex cellular systems where one examines interactions between microbes, epithelial cells, and an additional cell type, for example, by the addition of dendritic cells or lymphocytes (97, 105). Nonetheless, these model epithelia are generated using colon cancer cell lines and the same cautions regarding generalizing results to normal epithelium, as outlined above, also apply here.

Studies of epithelial cell innate defense mechanisms against enteric pathogens in humans in vivo are markedly limited for ethical reasons. Further, it is often not possible to examine the very early epithelial cell events following natural infection with enteric pathogens, as patients present to the clinic only several hours to days after the onset of infection. Moreover, in areas where enteric microbial infections are common, patients are often infected with multiple pathogens.

This led researchers to establish a model system in which one could examine very early intestinal epithelial cell innate defense mechanisms that are activated by microbial infection in vivo. The human fetal intestinal xenograft model provides such a model and an opportunity to study the responses of an intact human intestinal epithelium in vivo to a range of human microbial pathogens (27, 33, 56, 71, 101). In this model, human fetal small intestine or colon is transplanted subcutaneously in immunodeficient mice (i.e., either severe combined immunodeficient [SCID] or Rag$^{-/-}$ mice) that cannot reject the xenograft (Fig. 1). In the initial period after transplantation, the graft undergoes degeneration, but over a 10-week period the xenograft subsequently regrows a small segment of intestine. The mature xenograft contains a fully regenerated intestinal mucosa characteristic of either the colon or the small intestine, and is lined by an epithelium that is strictly of human origin. The xenografts can be infected intraluminally with microbes or stimulated by systemic injection of mice carrying xenografts with cytokines or mediators of human origin that, in some cases (e.g., human IFN-γ), act only on their cognate receptors on human cells in the xenograft, and not on murine cells. Infected or cytokine-stimulated xenografts can be removed from mice and analyzed using molecular or histopathological tools. Alternatively, unstimulated xenografts can be harvested and used as a source of intact, nontransformed human intestinal epithelium for ex vivo studies (e.g., the mucosa can be mounted in Ussing chambers for studies of mucosal secretion or barrier function). No model is a panacea for all studies, and this is also the case for the human intestinal xenograft model. For example, the usefulness of xenografts is limited in human-to-mouse myeloid cell transfers since the vasculature of the xenografts is of mouse origin, limiting the normal entry of human cells into the xenografts. Nonetheless, some cytokines, such as human CXCL8 (also termed IL-8) produced by human epithelial cells in the xenograft, are functional on murine myeloid cell populations. For example, following infection of the xenografts, CXCL8 produced by human epithelium in the xenografts was shown to chemoattract murine neutrophils into the lamina propria and subepithelial region of the infected xenografts (71).

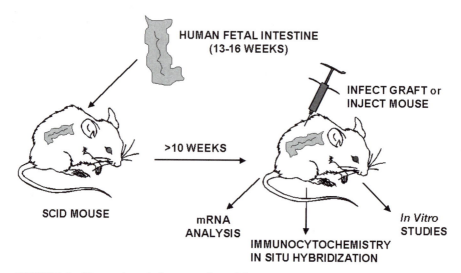

FIGURE 1 Human intestinal xenograft model. Human fetal intestine (small intestine or colon) is transplanted subcutaneously onto the backs of SCID adult mice and allowed to mature for 10 or more weeks. The mature xenograft contains a fully regenerated intestinal mucosa lined by an epithelium that is of human origin, and the lumen is sterile as assessed by the absence of 16S rRNA. Early epithelial cell signaling events in the xenografts in response to microbial infection can be studied in mice infected intraluminally with human enteric pathogens (33, 71, 89). In another approach, mice can be injected with human recombinant cytokines known to act on human intestinal epithelial cells to study intestinal epithelial cell signaling events and responses to human mediators in an in vivo model that has an intact human intestinal epithelium (27, 58). Tissue responses can be studied using histological and molecular approaches. Tissues can also be removed and studied ex vivo (e.g., in modified Ussing chambers).

Murine models have been a mainstay for studies of innate defense mechanisms and adaptive immunity. This, in part, reflects the ability to readily generate genetic models in mice in which the products of selected genes are overexpressed or specific genes are knocked out. In general, murine models have not been broadly applied to studies of intestinal mucosal infection by human enteric pathogens, as the infection in mice has not paralleled that in humans. Thus, some pathogens such as *Salmonella* spp. that cause gastroenteritis in humans cause systemic disease with little if any gastroenteritis in mice, whereas other pathogens, like *Cryptosporidium parvum* and rotavirus, that readily infect neonatal mice do not efficiently infect the intestinal mucosa of adult mice. Nonetheless, recent genetic approaches have proven, in principle, that murine models can be rendered more suitable for studies of the role of the epithelium in innate host defense to microbial pathogens that cause human disease. For example, the enteric pathogen *Listeria monocytogenes* does not infect murine intestinal epithelial cells. E-cadherin is the intestinal epithelial cell receptor for *Listeria* internalin A, and internalin A is essential for epithelial cell invasion by *L. monocytogenes* (38, 83). It is now known that murine E-cadherin has an amino acid mutation at position 16 that interferes with binding to internalin A (72). However, transgenic mice can be engineered whose epithelium expresses the human E-cadherin molecule. This renders *L. monocytogenes* invasive for mouse intestinal epithelium, with resulting mucosal inflammation in response to infection (73). Thus, novel strategies can be applied to render murine models more useful for studies of epithelial cell-mediated innate host defense to human microbial pathogens.

MICROBIAL PRODUCTS CAN ACTIVATE EPITHELIAL CELL SIGNALING PATHWAYS THAT ARE IMPORTANT IN INNATE MUCOSAL DEFENSE

Invasive and noninvasive pathogens can activate epithelial cell signaling cascades that are essential for the development of innate defense. This involves a number of sophisticated evolutionary coevolved strategies on the part of the microbes and the host epithelial cells that are the targets of infection. Pathogen-associated molecular patterns (PAMP) that are expressed by microbial products can activate signaling pathways that are important for epithelial cell innate defense mechanisms. PAMP are highly conserved and characteristic of various microbes (59) and include the bacterial cell wall component lipopolysaccharide (LPS), peptidoglycans and lipoteichoic acid (LTA), bacterial flagellin, nonmethylated bacterial DNA (also termed immunostimulatory DNA or ISS-DNA), and double-stranded RNA (dsRNA). PAMP are recognized by receptors called pattern-recognition receptors (PRR). PRR in turn activate host cellular signal transduction pathways that trigger innate defense mechanisms (59, 82).

Relevant to the activation of innate mucosal defense by intestinal epithelial cells, some of the members of one family of PRR, the Toll-like receptors (TLR) (82), are expressed by intestinal epithelial cells (15, 16, 43). These include TLR2, which is involved in recognizing a broad range of PAMP, including peptidoglycans and bacterial lipoproteins from gram-positive bacteria, mycobacterial cell wall components, atypical LPS from certain gram-negative bacteria, and yeast cell wall components (2, 13, 112). In contrast, TLR4 is mostly involved in recognition of LPS (92, 109). TLR3, which is also expressed by intestinal epithelial cell lines, mediates responses to dsRNA (1). The TLR family also includes

TLR5, which is involved in recognition of bacterial flagellin (50) and which is emerging as important for microbial-epithelial cell interactions, as well as TLR9, which mediates responses to nonmethylated, CpG-containing-bacterial DNA (51).

Signaling through TLR activates genes whose products play a key role in further activating or mediating innate defense mechanisms. TLR signaling leads to activation of NF-κB and mitogen-activated protein kinase (MAPK) (82). Whereas all TLRs appear to use a "shared" signaling mechanism, based on recruitment of the MyD88 adaptor protein, the protein kinase IL-1 receptor-associated kinase (IRAK) (85, 116), and TNF receptor-associated factor 6 (TRAF6) (14) with downstream activation of NF-κB and the MAPK cascades, there may also be TLR receptor-specific signaling mechanisms that account for receptor-specific biological responses (3, 12, 36, 55, 82, 85, 110). Thus far, the consequences of cellular activation through TLR have been studied most extensively in non-epithelial cell types key for innate immunity (i.e., macrophages and dendritic cells), but emerging evidence suggests that engagement of TLR on intestinal epithelial cells (e.g., TLR5 by bacterial flagellin) may also play a key functional role in epithelial cell signaling of innate immune defense (44, 106, 107).

PAMP such as bacterial LPS and unmethylated bacterial DNA are not unique to enteric pathogens and are also present in commensal microorganisms that populate the gastrointestinal tract. A key question is why does the host tolerate the presence of commensal microbes, yet activate an innate immune and inflammatory response to enteric pathogens? Several possibilities may explain this apparent paradox. For example, intestinal epithelial cells may not express certain TLR or may not effectively signal through some of those receptors (e.g., intestinal epithelial cell lines do not appear to express CD14 and MD2 important for signaling through TLR4). However, bacterial peptidoglycan components that enter the host epithelial cell consequent to epithelial cell invasion by a pathogen have the potential to activate epithelial cell signaling pathways, including the NF-κB pathway, through interacting, for example, with cytoplasmic binding molecules (e.g., NOD1) (45, 57). In addition, the site of cellular expression of certain TLR may favor interactions with membrane adherent or invasive pathogens, as has been suggested for TLR5 (43). Further, mechanisms that maintain the integrity and barrier functions of epithelial surfaces likely play a key role in the host's ability to discriminate between commensal and pathogenic microorganisms, with pathogenic microbes having strategies to breach this barrier and better activate PRR on underlying cells important for innate host defense. Moreover, it is also possible that exposure to microbial products such as LPS or unmethylated DNA associated with commensal bacteria may activate different signaling pathways from the ones activated by enteric pathogens, and lead to the induction of different gene programs.

ENTEROINVASIVE, NONINVASIVE, AND MINIMALLY INVASIVE PATHOGENS AS PROBES OF EPITHELIAL CELL INNATE DEFENSE MECHANISMS

One can operationally define three general classes of microbial pathogens from the perspective of the epithelial cell that lines the mucosa, and use members of those classes to probe the epithelial cell response to infection. One class of enteric pathogens includes those that invade intestinal epithelial cells, pass through the epithelial cell, infect deeper layers of the intestinal mucosa, and spread systemically. Examples include *Salmonella* spp., *Shigella* spp., *Listeria* spp., enteroinvasive *Escherichia coli*, and *Yersinia* spp. As a general consideration, signaling responses to those pathogens must be rapid if the intestinal epithelial cell is to play a meaningful role in innate mucosal defense and provide an effective warning to other targets in the host following infection. However, to the extent that infection of the epithelium is not long lasting, the

duration of those signaling responses can be relatively short-lived. These pathogens may activate epithelial cell signaling pathways important for host innate defense through interactions with the cell membrane (e.g., PAMP signaling through TLR), through the injection of microbial proteins into the host cell through type III secretory mechanisms (40, 113), or through microbial virulence factors interacting with components of the host cytosol (e.g., NOD proteins) (45, 57).

A second class of enteric pathogen is the "minimally invasive" enteric pathogen. These pathogens invade the intestinal epithelium, where they reside and replicate. Although they frequently activate a relatively low level of intestinal inflammation, they do not invade deeper layers of the intestinal mucosa. Some minimally invasive microbial pathogens have two or more stages in their life cycle (e.g., *C. parvum* in the intestinal or biliary epithelium, *Chlamydia trachomatis* in the genital tract or rectal epithelium). In this case, one of the life stages infects the intestinal epithelium, after which it proliferates and/or differentiates within the intestinal epithelial cells (i.e., the epithelial cell acts as an incubator and nutrition source for the pathogen's development). The newly emerged stage in the life cycle may lyse the epithelial cell, gain its release, and move on to infect neighboring epithelial cells. An important strategy for epithelial pathogens that must replicate and differentiate in epithelial cells, as part of their life cycle, is to keep the epithelial cell alive long enough to complete the essential part of the pathogen's reproductive cycle. In the case of minimally invasive pathogens like *C. parvum*, signaling pathways activated by the pathogen that delay epithelial cell death may be the same as those that can also activate innate immune responses.

A third class of enteric pathogens is generally noninvasive for the gastrointestinal tract epithelium (although some may invade at a low level). These pathogens reside in the intestinal tract, often in association with the epithelial cell apical membrane, and engage in cross talk with the epithelium. Depending on the nature of the virulence factors they produce, these microbial pathogens have a wide spectrum of activities with respect to signaling host innate defense mechanisms. For example, enterohemorrhagic *E. coli* (EHEC), through its virulence factors, can signal a marked acute mucosal inflammatory response, even though it is largely an intraluminal pathogen. In contrast, the protozoan parasite *Geordia lamblia* interacts closely with the epithelial cell apical membrane for prolonged periods, mostly in the upper small intestine, but does not activate epithelial signals that initiate a mucosal inflammatory response. On the other hand, the microbial pathogen *Helicobacter pylori* associates with the gastric epithelium and initiates a low-grade, prolonged inflammatory response that likely is sufficient for the transudation of host nutrients essential for its survival.

ROLE OF HUMAN EPITHELIAL CELL DEFENSINS AND THE CATHELICIDIN LL-37/hCAP18 IN INNATE MUCOSAL DEFENSE

Antimicrobial peptides and proteins are highly conserved in evolution and appear to play an important role in intestinal epithelial cell innate defense. Two classes of human antimicrobial peptides produced by the gastrointestinal tract epithelium are discussed here briefly, as antimicrobial peptides are the subject of a subsequent chapter. The defensins are one major class of antimicrobial peptides produced by the human gastrointestinal epithelium (75). Human defensins can be divided into two major families, the α-defensins and the β-defensins, both of which have three disulfide bonds and a β-sheet structure. α-Defensins are produced by specialized cells, the Paneth cells, in the small intestinal crypts and consist of two members, human defensin (HD)5 and HD6 (91). In contrast, the β-defensins are ubiquitously expressed throughout the epithelium in the stomach, small intestine, and colon. Although there are several reported subfamilies of β-defensins (41, 104), most currently available information regarding the intestinal epithelium relates to human β-defensin 1 (hBD-1) and hBD-2 (25, 37, 48, 88, 89). hBD-1 is constitutively expressed in the stomach, small intestine, and colon. It is not upregulated by proinflammatory stimuli or microbial infection, as shown in studies using intestinal epithelial cell lines, human intestinal xenografts, and human gastrointestinal tissue (89). In marked contrast, there is little constitutive expression of hBD-2 in the epithelium of normal gastrointestinal mucosa (89). Instead, hBD-2 is specifically upregulated in response to epithelial cell infection with enteric pathogens or stimulation of intestinal epithelial cells with proinflammatory mediators such as IL-1. hBD-2 functions as an NF-κB target gene (88, 89).

The cathelicidins are another class of antimicrobial peptide, in which a cathelin domain is linked to a peptide that has antimicrobial activity (74). The only known cathelicidin in humans is LL-37/hCAP18. LL-37, the carboxy-terminal part of the molecule that is cleaved and has antimicrobial activity, has a linear amphipathic α-helical structure. In addition to its antimicrobial activity, LL-37 has binding activity for bacterial LPS and monocyte chemotactic activity (22, 70). LL-37/hCAP18 has a restricted distribution in the human gastrointestinal tract, being expressed by the more differentiated surface and upper crypt epithelial cells in the human colon, with little or no expression within the deeper colon crypts, or within epithelial cells of the small intestine (49) (Fig. 2). Studies using cell lines, human intestinal xenografts, and human colon tissue have shown that LL-37 is constitutively produced by the colon epithelium and that its expression does not require commensal microflora (49). Moreover, its expression by human intestinal epithelial cells is not upregulated by several proinflammatory mediators and other cytokines including TNF-α, IL-1, IFN-γ, IL-6, and bacterial LPS. Consistent with the latter findings, LL-37 expression was similar in healthy and inflamed human colon (49). Nonetheless, studies using cell lines suggest LL-37/hCAP18 may be modestly

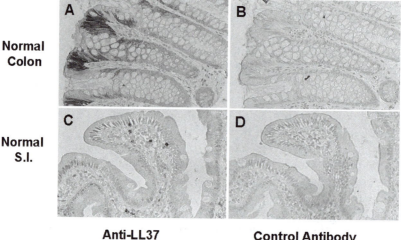

Anti-LL37   **Control Antibody**

FIGURE 2 Immunohistochemical detection of LL-37/hCAP18 in the epithelium of normal human colon and small intestine. Biopsy specimens from normal human colon (A and B) and proximal human small intestine (C and D) were examined for LL-37/hCAP18 using indirect immunoperoxidase staining. In normal colon, LL37/hCAP18 is expressed mainly by the surface epithelium and adjacent epithelium in the upper crypts (A). There is little or no expression of LL37/hCAP18 in the villus or crypt epithelium in proximal small intestine (C), although in some specimens staining is seen in duodenal Brunner's glands (not shown).

upregulated in intestinal epithelial cells infected with *Salmonella* spp. or enteroinvasive *E. coli* (49). Based on the above studies, a paradigm is emerging wherein the distribution and regulation of a variety of antimicrobial peptides differ in the epithelium in various regions of the human gastrointestinal tract, suggesting that the various antimicrobial peptides have distinct functional niches in mucosal innate defense.

EPITHELIAL CELL SIGNALS CHEMOATTRACT NEUTROPHILS AND MACROPHAGES THAT ARE ESSENTIAL FOR INNATE MUCOSAL DEFENSE

Chemokines are small-molecular-weight cytokines (8 to 10 kDa) that have a broad range of activities on the recruitment and function of populations of leukocytes at sites of microbial infection or inflammation. The chemokines can be categorized into four families based on the structural arrangement of their amino-terminal cysteines and intervening amino acids (i.e., CXC, CC, CX3C, and C chemokines) (69, 87). Several of the CXC chemokines have an ELR (glutamic acid, leucine, arginine) motif near their amino terminus, and these CXC chemokines function as neutrophil chemoattractants, the prototype being CXCL8/IL8. Human intestinal epithelial cells can produce several CXC ELR-motif neutrophil chemoattractants in response to bacterial infection. These include CXCL8 as well as members of the GRO family of CXC chemokines (29, 61, 119). CXCL8 and GRO family members (CXCL1, CXCL2, CXCL3) are rapidly, but transiently, upregulated following bacterial infection of intestinal epithelial cells (29, 61, 119). Human intestinal epithelial cells also produce another CXC ELR-motif chemokine, CXCL5 (also termed ENA78) (119). However, the regulation of CXCL5 differs from that of CXCL8 and the GRO family members (65). Thus, the upregulated expression of CXCL5 is slower than that of CXCL8, but its production is more long-lived (67, 119). Such findings suggest a model in which the epithelium produces an array of chemokines that can establish spatial and temporal chemokine gradients in the underlying mucosa (119). For example, CXCL8, which is produced rapidly and in relatively large amounts by intestinal epithelial cells, but whose duration of production is short-lived, might function to rapidly chemoattract neutrophils into the proximity of epithelial cells from more distant sites. In contrast, CXCL5, with its delayed onset of expression, lower potency, and more long-lived production, may imprint chemotactic gradients that bring neutrophils into closer contact with the epithelium and maintain neutrophils in that location for longer periods of time (119). In addition to neutrophil chemoattractants, microbial infection of intestinal epithelial cells can upregulate the production of CC chemokines that act as macrophage/monocyte chemoattractants (e.g., CCL2, which is also termed MCP-1) (119).

Substantial information is available regarding the repertoire of innate defense molecules produced by the intestinal epithelium, yet less is known regarding their in vivo functional importance. Consistent with the importance of these molecules, studies of the role of CXCL8 in a rabbit model of intestinal invasion by *Shigella flexneri* showed that CXCL8, which is largely produced by intestinal epithelial cells, acts as a major mediator in the recruitment of polymorphonuclear leukocytes (PMN) to the subepithelial area and in the transmigration of those cells through the epithelial lining (100). Neutralization of CXCL8 in this model resulted in a decrease in the numbers of PMN entering the lamina propria and the epithelium, and decreased the severity of epithelial lesions in areas of bacterial invasion. However, concurrently there was increased transepithelial translocation of bacteria, as well as bacterial overgrowth in the lamina propria and increased passage of bacteria into the mesenteric blood. By mediating eradication of bacteria at their epithelial entry site,

although at the cost of severe epithelial destruction, intestinal epithelial cell-produced neutrophil chemoattractants appear to be important as an innate defense mechanism for the control of bacterial translocation (100).

ROLE OF EPITHELIAL CELL-PRODUCED NITRIC OXIDE IN INNATE MUCOSAL DEFENSE

Bacterial infection of human colon epithelial cells rapidly upregulates expression of inducible nitric oxide synthase (iNOS) and nitric oxide (NO) production (117). This suggests that NO and/or its redox products are an important component of the intestinal epithelial cell response to microbial infection (117). In addition to epithelial invasive pathogens, NO may also play a role in epithelial innate defense to minimally invasive and noninvasive pathogens. Thus, recent studies demonstrated interactions between NO produced by human intestinal epithelial cells and the noninvasive lumen-dwelling protozoan pathogen *G. lamblia* (30). NO was shown to be cytostatic for *G. lamblia* and to inhibit giardial differentiation. However, *G. lamblia* was not a passive target for host-produced NO. Rather, *G. lamblia* has strategies to evade this potential innate host defense (30). Thus, in model human intestinal epithelia in vitro, *G. lamblia* inhibited epithelial NO production by consuming arginine, the crucial substrate used by epithelial cell NO synthase to produce NO (30). It will be important to determine whether such mechanisms alone, or in concert with other innate host defense mechanisms, also play a role in host defense to these enteric pathogens in vivo.

ROLE OF CCL20, AN EPITHELIAL CELL CHEMOKINE, IN LINKING INNATE AND ADAPTIVE HOST DEFENSE

Dendritic cells (DC) play a key role in linking innate and adaptive immunity through their role in antigen uptake and presentation to T lymphocytes (79). Recent studies using cultured human intestinal epithelial cell lines, including those grown as model polarized epithelia on permeable supports, suggest that DC-intestinal epithelial cell interactions may have a central role in the activation of host innate immune defense and the later signaling of adaptive immune responses to enteric microbial pathogens. The CC chemokine CCL20 (also termed MIP3α or LARC) is chemotactic for immature DC (46) that express the receptor CCR6 (4), which is the cognate chemokine receptor for CCL20 (58). Recent studies showed that CCL20 production is markedly upregulated in human intestinal cell lines in response to infection with enteric microbial pathogens or stimulation with the proinflammatory mediators (e.g., IL-1 or TNF-α) (58). Moreover, CCL20 is basolaterally secreted from polarized model intestinal epithelium infected with bacterial enteric pathogens or stimulated with proinflammatory cytokines (58). In vivo human intestinal xenografts stimulated with proinflammatory mediators and inflamed human intestinal mucosa showed a marked upregu-

lation of epithelial cell CCL20, suggesting that under conditions of microbial infection or intestinal inflammation CCL20 produced by intestinal epithelial cells may chemoattract immature DC into the proximity of the intestinal epithelium (58).

DC recruited by CCL20 produced by intestinal epithelial cells in response to microbial infection may be involved in bacterial uptake across the intestinal epithelium. Recent studies suggest that DC can open tight junctions between intestinal epithelial cells and send their dendrites into the intestinal lumen and sample luminal bacteria (Fig. 3). During this process, the integrity of the epithelial barrier is thought to be preserved because DC express tight junction proteins, such as occludin, claudin 1, and junctional adhesion molecule (JAM), and can establish tight junction-like structures with neighboring epithelial cells. Following bacterial uptake, the dendrites recede and the tight junction is once again re-formed by interactions between adjacent epithelial cells (96, 97). These studies offer a mechanism by which

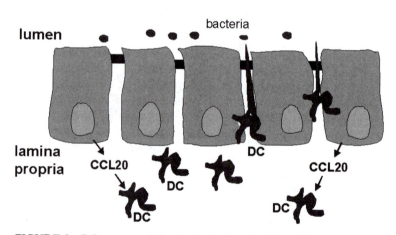

FIGURE 3 DC may sample luminal microbes. In this model, epithelial cells are proposed to produce CCL20 (MIP3α) that can chemoattract DC, a key cell type required for antigen presentation to T cells. DC subsequently send out dendrites that cross the epithelial layer and extend into the intestinal lumen where they can sample luminal bacteria. The passage of dendrites across the epithelium is thought to involve an unsealing and resealing of epithelial cell tight junctions and involves interactions between proteins expressed by DC and intestinal epithelial cells (e.g., occludin, claudin-1, JAM) (97).

DC-epithelial cell interactions can play a key role in the linking of mucosal innate and adaptive immune responses.

EPITHELIAL CELL SECRETORY RESPONSES IN INNATE HOST DEFENSE

Interactions between microbial pathogens and intestinal epithelial cells may play a role in the early onset of diarrhea after infection with microbial pathogens like *Salmonella* spp. Increased intestinal fluid secretion is an important host innate defense mechanism, as, coupled with intestinal motility, it plays a key role in "flushing" the enteric pathogen from the intestinal tract. Concurrently, this allows the enteric pathogen to escape the host and infect additional hosts.

Infection of intestinal epithelial cells with *Salmonella* spp. results in increased epithelial cell chloride secretion, a parameter that reflects increased fluid secretion. One pathway leading to increased chloride secretion was revealed by demonstrating the upregulated expression of cyclooxygenase 2 (COX2) in vitro and in vivo in response to infection of intestinal epithelial cells with *Salmonella* spp., with subsequent upregulated production of prostaglandin E_2 (PGE$_2$) (33). PGE$_2$ released by intestinal epithelial cells in response to infection was shown to act in an autocrine/paracrine manner and activate epithelial chloride secretion, a process that occurs via a cyclic AMP (cAMP)-mediated pathway (33). A second pathway leading to increased chloride secretion was revealed through studies showing that *Salmonella* infection of intestinal epithelial cells can also alter Ca^{2+}-mediated chloride secretion (31, 86). Those investigations focused on inositol-containing compounds that are known to play a key role in receptor-mediated signaling events. Infection of intestinal epithelial cells with *Salmonella* spp., but not other invasive enteric bacteria, induced a rapid multifold increase in D-*myo*-inositol 1,4,5,6-tetrakisphosphate [Ins(1,4,5,6)P$_4$] levels in cultured human intestinal epithelial cells (33).

Moreover, Ins(1,4,5,6)P$_4$ was shown to antagonize epidermal growth factor-induced inhibition of calcium-mediated chloride secretion (33). The underlying mechanism involves Sop B, a protein secreted by the *Salmonella* type III secretory system (86). Sop B acts as an inositol polyphosphate phosphatase, resulting in increased cellular levels of Ins(1,4,5,6)P$_4$ that, in turn, abrogate inhibition by epidermal growth factor of a basolateral potassium channel that is essential for Ca^{2+}-activated chloride secretion (86). Thus, a bacterial protein can directly counteract a host cell inhibitory pathway, with the net result being increased epithelial cell chloride secretion. Additional pathways by which intestinal fluid secretion is increased in response to microbial infection are discussed in later chapters.

EPITHELIAL CELL SIGNALS THAT ACTIVATE MUCOSAL INNATE DEFENSE: CENTRAL ROLE OF NF-κB

NF-κB is a term used to collectively refer to dimeric transcription factors that belong to the Rel family. NF-κB dimers are held in the cytoplasm through interactions with specific inhibitors, the IκBs, which mask the nuclear localization domains of the NF-κB proteins. In response to microbes and their products, or in response to cell stimulation with proinflammatory stimuli like TNF-α and IL-1, IκBs are phosphorylated, which triggers their polyubiquitination and proteasomal degradation (63). The inducible phosphorylation of IκBs is mediated by the IκB kinase (IKK) complex (99), which contains two catalytic subunits, IKKα and IKKβ. Most signal-induced phosphorylation of the IκBs that is relevant to the activation of innate defense mechanisms is mediated by IKKβ. Thus, IKKβ is required for activation of the prevalent p50:RelA(p65) heterodimers in response to enteric microbes, PAMP, and proinflammatory cytokines (such as IL-1 and TNF-α) (18, 19, 34, 76, 77).

Activation of the NF-κB signaling via IKKβ has two major physiological functions: the activation of genes whose products are important for signaling and mediating innate immune defense and inflammation (6, 7) and the activation of genes whose products are important for the suppression of apoptosis (64). Thus, many of the genes that encode cytokines, chemokines, and adhesion molecules that are produced and regulated in intestinal epithelial cells and involved in innate defense and inflammatory reactions, as discussed above, contain NF-κB binding sites in their promoters (e.g., CXCL8, CXCL1, CCL2, CCL20, CCL22, COX2, NOS2, ICAM-1, TNF-α, hBD2) (6, 8, 34, 58, 88, 89). These genes, and genes that encode enzymes that produce secondary inflammatory mediators, such as NOS2 and COX2, which also contain NF-κB binding sites in their promoters, are induced in the intestinal epithelium during the course of microbial infection and mucosal inflammatory responses (33, 71, 117).

NF-κB is a central regulator of intestinal epithelial cell innate defense (34). Enteric pathogens use different strategies and mechanisms to interact with or invade intestinal epithelial cells and have various PAMP and virulence factors. Nonetheless, downstream, each of these microbes, PAMP, and many of the virulence factors activate NF-κB and NF-κB target genes that play a key role in epithelial cell responses that are essential for innate defense (34, 66, 102). In this way, the diverse signals that are activated by enteric bacterial pathogens can be integrated by a common signaling pathway that culminates in the activation of a conserved set of proinflammatory genes in infected host cells. Although NF-κB is required for activation of host innate defense, other signal transduction pathways are also important, most notably MAPK pathways (54, 68, 102, 103). Whereas some target genes important for innate defense appear to be regulated mainly by NF-κB, the expression of other target genes that are dependent on NF-κB are also modulated by additional signal transduction pathways such as those mediated by the MAPK.

A newly described pathway for the activation of NF-κB was elucidated by investigators who noted the presence in mammalian cells of intracellular proteins with structural homology to apoptosis regulators and a class of plant disease-resistant gene products. These proteins in mammalian cells are termed NOD or CARD proteins (10, 57). At least one of the NOD proteins (NOD1) can bind bacterial peptidoglycan components in the cell and activate IKK and NF-κB by a pathway independent from TLR4. This provides a possible pathway by which bacterial products that enter the intestinal epithelial cell in association with invasive enteric microbes can activate NF-κB, its target genes, and innate epithelial cell defense mechanisms (45, 57).

EVASION OF INNATE HOST DEFENSE BY BACTERIAL PATHOGENS

Enteric pathogens can avoid host innate mucosal defense mechanisms by inducing apoptosis of key immune cells. This can prevent detection of the microbe and its subsequent destruction by innate host defenses (115). The induction of macrophage apoptosis is an important strategy used by a number of mucosal pathogens to evade and paralyze innate mucosal defense. By eliminating macrophages through the action of specialized virulence determinants, pathogenic bacteria can destroy one of the major cell types responsible for detecting the presence of infectious organisms and for alerting other components of both innate and adaptive immunity to their presence.

Bacteria like *L. monocytogenes* use poreforming toxins to kill host myeloid, epithelial, and lymphoid cells. *Shigella dysenteriae* and Shiga toxin-producing *E. coli* use shiga toxins to inhibit protein synthesis and kill host cells (111). Another mechanism used by *Shigella* spp. (e.g., *S. dysenteriae* and *S. flexneri*) to induce macrophage death involves their secretion of the IpaB protein, which causes activation of caspase-1, the IL-1-converting enzyme (53). Caspase-1-deficient macrophages are resistant to *Shigella*-induced death, while caspase-3- or caspase-11-deficient macrophages are fully sensitive (53). *Yersinia* sp.

uses a more sophisticated mechanism to cause macrophage death by interfering with host cell pro-survival-signaling mechanisms (84). Thus, *Yersinia* sp. produces the YopJ gene product, which is a ubiquitin-like protease that interacts with MAPK kinase kinases (MKKK) to inhibit MAPK and IKK activation (90). This results in inhibition of NF-κB-dependent pro-survival pathways in macrophages. *Salmonella* spp. secrete invasion proteins, encoded by the *Salmonella* pathogenicity island-1 (SPI-1) locus, into the host cell to promote bacterial uptake (39). The SipB invasion protein, a homolog of IpaB from *Shigella* spp., acts in a similar manner as IpaB to activate caspase-1 and induces rapid macrophage death by a process that has generally been termed apoptosis, although it has atypical features such as early loss of cell membrane integrity (52). SipB-dependent cell death may have a role in the intestine, where caspase-1 activation would also lead to proinflammatory effects by activating IL-1 and IL-18, although SipB is not required for the systemic phase of *Salmonella* infection (39).

Enteric pathogens like *Salmonella* spp. and enteroinvasive *E. coli* also induce apoptosis of human intestinal epithelial cells. Apoptosis of human intestinal epithelial cell lines in *Salmonella*-infected cells is delayed for 18 to 24 h after infection and is accompanied by a loss of F-actin and activation of caspase 3. Moreover, bacterial products produced during the initial phase of intracellular infection, and that are related to the activity of *Salmonella spv* and SPI-2 genes, have a key role in the delayed execution phase of apoptosis in intestinal epithelial cell lines. Apoptosis of intestinal epithelial cells in response to bacterial infection may function in innate host defense by deleting infected and damaged epithelial cells and restoring epithelial cell growth regulation and epithelial integrity that are altered during the course of enteric infection. The delay in onset of epithelial cell apoptosis after bacterial invasion may be important to both the host and the invading pathogen. Thus, it would provide sufficient time for host epithelial cells to

generate signals important for the activation of mucosal innate and downstream acquired immune defense systems. However, the delay concurrently would allow invading bacteria time to adapt to the intracellular host environment before invading deeper mucosal layers. A similar theme has emerged from studies of *C. parvum* infection of intestinal epithelial cells (71). Thus, *C. parvum* activates NF-κB in intestinal and biliary epithelial cells (17, 71). This activates innate defense mechanisms such as upregulated expression of the neutrophil chemoattractant CXCL8, which results in the mucosal influx of neutrophils. The latter can prevent dissemination of the pathogen at the cost of a degree of mucosal damage and altered barrier function (71). On the other hand, NF-κB has antiapoptotic functions and a delay in epithelial cell apoptosis can allow sufficient time for this pathogen to undergo the development and life cycle changes essential for its replication and survival (81).

EPITHELIAL CELL SIGNALS THAT CHEMOATTRACT T CELLS

T cells are a central component of host mucosal adaptive immunity. In addition to signaling neutrophils, macrophages, and DC, as examples of host cell types that are essential for mediating mucosal innate defense, epithelial cells produce mediators important for chemoattracting subpopulations of T cells into the intestinal mucosa (Fig. 4). CXCL9 (Mig), CXCL10 (IP-10), and CXCL11 (I-TAC) are CXC chemokines that do not have the ELR motif mentioned earlier, and the expression of these chemokines is upregulated by IFN-γ (42). They function as chemoattractants for CXCR3 expressing CD4$^+$ T cells that produce the cytokine IFN-γ (i.e., Th-1-type cytokine) that is essential for host resistance to a broad array of microbial pathogens (78, 93). CXCL9, 10, and 11 are constitutively expressed by normal human colon epithelium, and their cognate receptor, CXCR3, is expressed on mucosal mononuclear cells (27), including intraepithelial lymphocytes (105). As in other cell types, intestinal epithe-

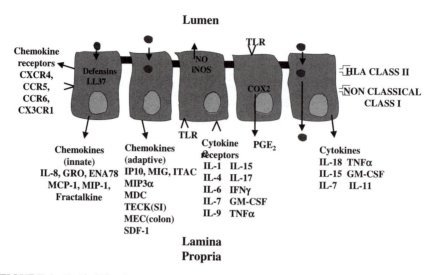

FIGURE 4 Epithelial cells produce mediators and express receptors important in innate and adaptive mucosal immunity.

lial cell–produced CXCL9, 10, and 11 mRNA and protein production are upregulated in response to stimulation with IFN-γ (27). Whereas infection of intestinal epithelial cells with enteroinvasive bacteria or proinflammatory cytokines minimally, if at all, affects epithelial cell CXCL9, 10, or 11 production, microbial infection or proinflammatory cytokines strongly potentiate IFN-γ-induced epithelial cell production of CXCL10 and, to a lesser extent, CXCL11, as shown in studies using intestinal epithelial cell lines or human intestinal xenografts in vivo (27). Taken together, studies suggest that IFN-γ-inducible CXC chemokines produced by intestinal epithelial cells may function as chemoattractants for intraepithelial and lamina propria CXCR3-expressing T cells. This may be particularly important under conditions that activate mucosal inflammation, most notably during enteric microbial infection.

The normal intestinal mucosa predominantly contains CD4 T-cell populations that produce a Th1 pattern of cytokines. Nonetheless, it also contains a smaller subset of T lymphocytes that produce Th2 cytokines. Recent studies revealed that intestinal epithelial cells produce CCL22/MDC, a chemo-kine known to chemoattract Th2 cytokine-producing CD4 T cells that express the chemokine receptor CCR4 (8). Human colon epithelium in healthy individuals and the epithelium of human intestinal xenografts constitutively produce CCL22 (8). Moreover, CCL22 mRNA levels and CCL22 protein secretion are upregulated in colon epithelial cell lines infected with enteroinvasive bacteria or stimulated with proinflammatory cytokines (8). Whereas IFN-γ synergizes with TNF-α to upregulate CCL22 production, the Th2 cytokines IL-4 and IL-13 downregulate TNF-α-induced CCL22 production. CCL22 produced by intestinal epithelial cells is basolaterally secreted and manifests functional activity with respect to chemoattracting CCR4-expressing T cells, as shown in studies using polarized model intestinal epithelium (8). Of note, intestinal epithelial cells do not produce another chemokine, CCL17/TARC, that acts on the same receptor. However, studies using cultured human airway epithelial cells and human fetal lung xenografts demonstrated that CCL17/TARC, but not CCL22/MDC, is abundantly expressed and regulated by human bronchial epithelial cells (9). Although both CCL22/MDC and

CCL17/TARC function as NF-κB responsive genes (8, 9) and act on the same receptor, these chemokines are differentially expressed by the intestinal epithelium compared to the bronchial epithelium, suggesting that they may have different functional roles in defense of the intestine and airways.

SUMMARY

Intestinal epithelial cells are an integral component of innate mucosal defense. In this role, they can produce antimicrobial peptides, chemokines, cytokines, NO, and eicosanoids and express receptors for cytokines and PAMP, each of which can play a role in epithelial cell innate defense mechanisms. In addition, epithelial cells express, or can be induced to express, human leukocyte antigen (HLA) class II molecules and nonclassical HLA class I molecules that can play a role in innate and adaptive immune responses. The function of several chemokine receptors (e.g., CXCR4, CCR5, CCR6, CX3CR1) on intestinal epithelial cells (11, 26) is not fully known. Figure 4 shows examples of mediators and receptors that are important for innate and acquired mucosal defense and that are either expressed constitutively or upregulated by intestinal epithelial cells in response to enteric microbial infection.

REFERENCES

1. **Alexopoulou, L., A. C. Holt, R. Medzhitov, and R. A. Flavell.** 2001. Recognition of double-stranded RNA and activation of NF-κB by Toll-like receptor 3. *Nature* **413**:732–738.
2. **Aliprantis, A., R.-B. Yang, M. Mark, S. Suggett, B. Devaux, J. Radolf, G. Klimpel, P. Godowski, and A. Zychlinsky.** 1999. Cell activation and apoptosis by bacterial lipoproteins through Toll-like receptor-2. *Science* **285**:736–739.
3. **Arbibe, L., J. P. Mira, N. Teusch, L. Kline, M. Guha, N. Mackman, P. J. Godowski, R. J. Ulevitch, and U. G. Knaus.** 2000. Toll-like receptor 2-mediated NF-κB activation requires a Rac1-dependent pathway. *Nat. Immunol.* **1**:533–540.
4. **Baba, M., T. Imai, M. Nishimura, M. Kakizaki, S. Takagi, K. Hieshima, H. Nomiyama, and O. Yoshie.** 1997. Identification of CCR6, the specific receptor for a novel lymphocyte-directed CC chemokine LARC. *J. Biol. Chem.* **272**:14893–14898.
5. **Bach, S., A. Makristathis, M. Rotter, and A. M. Hirschl.** 2002. Gene expression profiling in AGS cells stimulated with *Helicobacter pylori* isogenic strains (cagA positive or cagA negative). *Infect. Immun.* **70**:988–992.
6. **Baeuerle, P. A., and T. Henkel.** 1994. Function and activation of NF-kB in the immune system. *Annu. Rev. Immunol.* **12**:141–179.
7. **Barnes, P. J., and M. Karin.** 1997. NF-κB—a pivotal transcription factor in chronic inflammatory diseases. *New Engl. J. Med.* **336**:1066–1071.
8. **Berin, M. C., M. B. Dwinell, L. Eckmann, and M. F. Kagnoff.** 2001. Production of MDC/CCL22 by human intestinal epithelial cells. *Am. J. Physiol. Gastrointest. Liver Physiol.* **280**:G1217–G1226.
9. **Berin, M. C., L. Eckmann, D. H. Broide, and M. F. Kagnoff.** 2001. Regulated production of the T helper 2-type T-cell chemoattractant TARC by human bronchial epithelial cells in vitro and in human lung xenografts. *Am. J. Respir. Cell Mol. Biol.* **24**:382–389.
10. **Bertin, J., W. J. Nir, C. M. Fischer, O. V. Tayber, P. R. Errada, J. R. Grant, J. J. Keilty, M. L. Gosselin, K. E. Robison, G. H. Wong, M. A. Glucksmann, and P. S. DiStefano.** 1999. Human CARD4 protein is a novel CED-4/Apaf-1 cell death family member that activates NF-κB. *J. Biol. Chem.* **274**:12955–12958.
11. **Brand, S., T. Sakaguchi, X. Gu, S. P. Colgan, and H. C. Reinecker.** 2002. Fractalkine-mediated signals regulate cell-survival and immune-modulatory responses in intestinal epithelial cells. *Gastroenterology* **122**:166–177.
12. **Burns, K., J. Clatworthy, L. Martin, F. Martinon, C. Plumpton, B. Maschera, A. Lewis, K. Ray, J. Tschapp, and F. Volpe.** 2000. Tollip, a new component of the IL-1RI pathway, links IRAK to the IL-1 receptor. *Nat. Cell Biol.* **2**:346–351.
13. **Campos, M. A., I. C. Almeida, O. Takeuchi, S. Akira, E. P. Valente, D. O. Procopio, L. R. Travassos, J. A. Smith, D. T. Golenbock, and R. T. Gazzinelli.** 2001. Activation of Toll-like receptor-2 by glycosylphosphatidylinositol anchors from a protozoan parasite. *J. Immunol.* **167**:416–423.
14. **Cao, Z., J. Xiong, M. Takeuchi, T. Kurama, and D. V. Goeddel.** 1996. TRAF6 is a signal transducer for interleukin-1. *Nature* **383**:443–446.

15. **Cario, E., and D. K. Podolsky.** 2000. Differential alteration in intestinal epithelial cell expression of Toll-like receptor 3 (TLR3) and TLR4 in inflammatory bowel disease. *Infect. Immun.* **68:**7010–7017.

16. **Cario, E., I. M. Rosenberg, S. L. Brandwein, P. L. Beck, H. C. Reinecker, and D. K. Podolsky.** 2000. Lipopolysaccharide activates distinct signaling pathways in intestinal epithelial cell lines expressing Toll-like receptors. *J. Immunol.* **164:**966–972.

17. **Chen, X. M., S. A. Levine, P. L. Splinter, P. S. Tietz, A. L. Ganong, C. Jobin, G. J. Gores, C. V. Paya, and N. F. LaRusso.** 2001. *Cryptosporidium parvum* activates nuclear factor κB in biliary epithelia preventing epithelial cell apoptosis. *Gastroenterology* **120:**1774–1783.

18. **Chu, W. M., X. Gong, Z. W. Li, K. Takabayashi, H. H. Ouyang, Y. Chen, A. Lois, D. J. Chen, G. C. Li, M. Karin, and E. Raz.** 2000. DNA-PKcs is required for activation of innate immunity by immunostimulatory DNA. *Cell* **103:**909–918.

19. **Chu, W.-M., D. Ostertag, Z.-W. Li, L. Chang, Y. Chen, Y. Hu, J. Perrault, and M. Karin.** 1999. JNK2 and IKKβ are required for activating the innate response to viral infection. *Immunity* **11:**721–731.

20. **Colgan, S. P., R. M. Hershberg, G. T. Furuta, and R. S. Blumberg.** 1999. Ligation of intestinal epithelial CD1d induces bioactive IL-10: critical role of the cytoplasmic tail in autocrine signaling. *Proc. Natl. Acad. Sci USA* **96:**13938–13943.

21. **Colgan, S. P., M. B. Resnick, C. A. Parkos, C. Delp-Archer, D. McGuirk, A. E. Bacarra, P. F. Weller, and J. L. Madara.** 1994. IL-4 directly modulates function of a model human intestinal epithelium. *J. Immunol.* **153:**2122–2129.

22. **De, Y., Q. Chen, A. P. Schmidt, G. M. Anderson, J. M. Wang, J. Wooters, J. J. Oppenheim, and O. Chertov.** 2000. LL-37, the neutrophil granule- and epithelial cell-derived cathelicidin, utilizes formyl peptide receptor-like 1 (FPRL1) as a receptor to chemoattract human peripheral blood neutrophils, monocytes, and T cells. *J. Exp. Med.* **192:**1069–1074.

23. **Delezay, O., N. Koch, N. Yahi, D. Hammache, C. Tourres, C. Tamalet, and J. Fantini.** 1997. Co-expression of CXCR4/fusin and galactosylceramide in the human intestinal epithelial cell line HT-29. *AIDS* **11:**1311–1318.

24. **Denning, T. L., N. A. Campbell, F. Song, R. P. Garofalo, G. R. Klimpel, V. E. Reyes, and P. B. Ernst.** 2000. Expression of IL-10 receptors on epithelial cells from the murine small and large intestine. *Int. Immunol.* **12:**133–139.

25. **Dunsche, A., Y. Acil, H. Dommisch, R. Siebert, J. M. Schroder, and S. Jepsen.** 2002. The novel human beta-defensin-3 is widely expressed in oral tissues. *Eur. J. Oral Sci.* **110:**121–124.

26. **Dwinell, M. B., L. Eckmann, J. D. Leopard, N. M. Varki, and M. F. Kagnoff.** 1999. Chemokine receptor expression by human intestinal epithelial cells. *Gastroenterology* **117:**359–367.

27. **Dwinell, M. B., N. Lugering, L. Eckmann, and M. F. Kagnoff.** 2001. Regulated production of interferon-inducible T-cell chemoattractants by human intestinal epithelial cells. *Gastroenterology* **120:**49–59.

28. **Eckmann, L., H. C. Jung, C. Schurer-Maly, A. Panja, E. Morzycka-Wroblewska, and M. F. Kagnoff.** 1993. Differential cytokine expression by human intestinal epithelial cell lines: regulated expression of interleukin 8. *Gastroenterology* **105:**1689–1697.

29. **Eckmann, L., M. F. Kagnoff, and J. Fierer.** 1993. Epithelial cells secrete the chemokine interleukin-8 in response to bacterial entry. *Infect. Immun.* **61:**4569–4574.

30. **Eckmann, L., F. Laurent, T. D. Langford, M. L. Hetsko, J. R. Smith, M. F. Kagnoff, and F. D. Gillin.** 2000. Nitric oxide production by human intestinal epithelial cells and competition for arginine as potential determinants of host defense against the lumen-dwelling pathogen *Giardia lamblia. J. Immunol.* **164:**1478–1487.

31. **Eckmann, L., M. T. Rudolf, A. Ptasznik, C. Schultz, T. Jiang, N. Wolfson, R. Tsien, J. Fierer, S. B. Shears, M. F. Kagnoff, and A. E. Traynor-Kaplan.** 1997. D-myo-Inositol 1,4,5,6-tetrakisphosphate produced in human intestinal epithelial cells in response to *Salmonella* invasion inhibits phosphoinositide 3-kinase signaling pathways. *Proc. Natl. Acad. Sci. USA* **94:**14456–14460.

32. **Eckmann, L., J. R. Smith, M. P. Housley, M. B. Dwinell, and M. F. Kagnoff.** 2000. Analysis by high density cDNA arrays of altered gene expression in human intestinal epithelial cells in response to infection with the invasive enteric bacteria *Salmonella. J. Biol. Chem.* **275:**14084–14094.

33. **Eckmann, L., W. F. Stenson, T. C. Savidge, D. C. Lowe, K. E. Barrett, J. Fierer, J. R. Smith, and M. F. Kagnoff.** 1997. Role of intestinal epithelial cells in the host secretory response to infection by invasive bacteria. Bacterial entry induces epithelial prostaglandin h synthase-2 expression and prostaglandin E2 and F2α production. *J. Clin. Invest.* **100:**296–309.

34. Elewaut, D., J. A. DiDonato, J. M. Kim, F. Truong, L. Eckmann, and M. F. Kagnoff. 1999. NF-κB is a central regulator of the intestinal epithelial cell innate immune response induced by infection with enteroinvasive bacteria. *J. Immunol.* **163:**1457–1466.

35. Fish, S. M., R. Proujansky, and W. W. Reenstra. 1999. Synergistic effects of interferon γ and tumour necrosis factor α on T84 cell function. *Gut* **45:**191–198.

36. Fitzgerald, K. A., E. M. Palsson-McDermott, A. G. Bowie, C. A. Jefferies, A. S. Mansell, G. Brady, E. Brint, A. Dunne, P. Gray, M. T. Harte, D. McMurray, D. E. Smith, J. E. Sims, T. A. Bird, and L. A. O'Neill. 2001. Mal (MyD88-adapter-like) is required for Toll-like receptor-4 signal transduction. *Nature* **413:**78–83.

37. Frye, M., J. Bargon, B. Lembcke, T. O. Wagner, and R. Gropp. 2000. Differential expression of human α- and β-defensins mRNA in gastrointestinal epithelia. *Eur. J. Clin. Invest.* **30:** 695–701.

38. Gaillard, J. L., P. Berche, C. Frehel, E. Gouin, and P. Cossart. 1991. Entry of *L. monocytogenes* into cells is mediated by internalin, a repeat protein reminiscent of surface antigens from gram-positive cocci. *Cell* **65:**1127–1141.

39. Galan, J. E. 2001. *Salmonella* interactions with host cells: type III secretion at work. *Annu. Rev. Cell Dev. Biol.* **17:**53–86.

40. Galan, J. E., and A. Collmer. 1999. Type III secretion machines: bacterial devices for protein delivery into host cells. *Science* **284:**1322–1328.

41. Garcia, J. R., F. Jaumann, S. Schulz, A. Krause, J. Rodriguez-Jimenez, U. Forssmann, K. Adermann, E. Kluver, C. Vogelmeier, D. Becker, R. Hedrich, W. G. Forssmann, and R. Bals. 2001. Identification of a novel, multifunctional β-defensin (human β-defensin 3) with specific antimicrobial activity. Its interaction with plasma membranes of *Xenopus oocytes* and the induction of macrophage chemoattraction. *Cell Tissue Res.* **306:**257–264.

42. Gasperini, S., M. Marchi, F. Calzetti, C. Laudanna, L. Vicentini, H. Olsen, M. Murphy, F. Liao, J. Farber, and M. A. Cassatella. 1999. Gene expression and production of the monokine induced by IFN-γ (MIG), IFN-inducible T cell α chemoattractant (I-TAC), and IFN-γ-inducible protein-10 (IP-10) chemokines by human neutrophils. *J. Immunol.* **162:**4928–4937.

43. Gewirtz, A. T., T. A. Navas, S. Lyons, P. J. Godowski, and J. L. Madara. 2001. Cutting edge: bacterial flagellin activates basolaterally expressed TLR5 to induce epithelial proinflammatory gene expression. *J. Immunol.* **167:**1882–1885.

44. Gewirtz, A. T., P. O. Simon, Jr., C. K. Schmitt, L. J. Taylor, C. H. Hagedorn, A. D. O'Brien, A. S. Neish, and J. L. Madara. 2001. *Salmonella typhimurium* translocates flagellin across intestinal epithelia, inducing a proinflammatory response. *J. Clin. Invest.* **107:** 99–109.

45. Girardin, S. E., R. Tournebize, M. Mavris, A. L. Page, X. Li, G. R. Stark, J. Bertin, P. S. DiStefano, M. Yaniv, P. J. Sansonetti, and D. J. Philpott. 2001. CARD4/Nod1 mediates NF-kappaB and JNK activation by invasive *Shigella flexneri*. *EMBO Rep.* **2:**736–742.

46. Greaves, D. R., W. Wang, D. J. Dairaghi, M. C. Dieu, B. Saint-Vis, K. Franz-Bacon, D. Rossi, C. Caux, T. McClanahan, S. Gordon, A. Zlotnik, and T. J. Schall. 1997. CCR6, a CC chemokine receptor that interacts with macrophage inflammatory protein 3α and is highly expressed in human dendritic cells. *J. Exp. Med.* **186:**837–844.

47. Groh, V., A. Steinle, S. Bauer, and T. Spies. 1998. Recognition of stress-induced MHC molecules by intestinal epithelial γδ T cells. *Science* **279:**1737–1740.

48. Hamanaka, Y., M. Nakashima, A. Wada, M. Ito, H. Kurazono, H. Hojo, Y. Nakahara, S. Kohno, T. Hirayama, and I. Sekine. 2001. Expression of human β-defensin 2 (hBD-2) in *Helicobacter pylori* induced gastritis: antibacterial effect of hBD-2 against *Helicobacter pylori*. *Gut* **49:**481–487.

49. Hase, K., L. Eckmann, J. D. Leopard, N. Varki, and M. F. Kagnoff. 2002. Cell differentiation is a key determinant of cathelicidin LL-37/human cationic antimicrobial protein 18 expression by human colon epithelium. *Infect. Immun.* **70:**953–963.

50. Hayashi, F., K. D. Smith, A. Ozinsky, T. R. Hawn, E. C. Yi, D. R. Goodlett, J. K. Eng, S. Akira, D. M. Underhill, and A. Aderem. 2001. The innate immune response to bacterial flagellin is mediated by Toll-like receptor 5. *Nature* **410:**1099–1103.

51. Hemmi, H., O. Takeuchi, T. Kawai, T. Kaisho, S. Sato, H. Sanjo, M. Matsumoto, K. Hoshino, H. Wagner, K. Takeda, and S. Akira. 2000. A Toll-like receptor recognizes bacterial DNA. *Nature* **408:**740–745.

52. Hersh, D., D. M. Monack, M. R. Smith, N. Ghori, S. Falkow, and A. Zychlinsky. 1999. The *Salmonella* invasin SipB induces macrophage apoptosis by binding to caspase-1. *Proc. Natl. Acad. Sci. USA* **96:**2396–2401.

53. Hilbi, H., J. E. Moss, D. Hersh, Y. Chen, J. Arondel, S. Banerjee, R. A. Flavell, J. Yuan, P. J. Sansonetti, and A. Zychlinsky. 1998. *Shigella*-induced apoptosis is dependent on caspase-1 which binds to IpaB. *J. Biol. Chem.* **273:**32895–32900.

54. Hobbie, S., L. M. Chen, R. J. Davis, and J. E. Galan. 1997. Involvement of mitogen-activated protein kinase pathways in the nuclear responses and cytokine production induced by *Salmonella typhimurium* in cultured intestinal epithelial cells. *J. Immunol.* **159:**5550–5559.

55. Horng, T., G. M. Barton, and R. Medzhitov. 2001. TIRAP: an adapter molecule in the Toll signaling pathway. *Nat. Immunol.* **2:**835–841.

56. Huang, G. T., L. Eckmann, T. C. Savidge, and M. F. Kagnoff. 1996. Infection of human intestinal epithelial cells with invasive bacteria upregulates apical intercellular adhesion molecule-1 (ICAM-1) expression and neutrophil adhesion. *J. Clin. Invest.* **98:**572–583.

57. Inohara, N., Y. Ogura, F. F. Chen, A. Muto, and G. Nunez. 2001. Human Nod1 confers responsiveness to bacterial lipopolysaccharides. *J. Biol. Chem.* **276:**2551–2554.

58. Izadpanah, A., M. B. Dwinell, L. Eckmann, N. M. Varki, and M. F. Kagnoff. 2001. Regulated MIP-3α/CCL20 production by human intestinal epithelium: mechanism for modulating mucosal immunity. *Am. J. Physiol. Gastrointest. Liver Physiol.* **280:**G710–G719.

59. Janeway, C. A., Jr. 1992. The immune system evolved to discriminate infectious nonself from noninfectious self. *Immunol. Today* **13:**11–16.

60. Jordan, N. J., G. Kolios, S. E. Abbot, M. A. Sinai, D. A. Thompson, K. Petraki, and J. Westwick. 1999. Expression of functional CXCR4 chemokine receptors on human colonic epithelial cells. *J. Clin. Invest.* **104:**1061–1069.

61. Jung, H. C., L. Eckmann, S. K. Yang, A. Panja, J. Fierer, E. Morzycka-Wroblewska, and M. F. Kagnoff. 1995. A distinct array of proinflammatory cytokines is expressed in human colon epithelial cells in response to bacterial invasion. *J. Clin. Invest.* **95:**55–65.

62. Kagnoff, M. F., and L. Eckmann. 2001. Analysis of host responses to microbial infection using gene expression profiling. *Curr. Opin. Microbiol.* **4:**246–250.

63. Karin, M., and Y. Ben-Neriah. 2000. Phosphorylation meets ubiquitination: the control of NF-κB activity. *Annu. Rev. Immunol.* **18:**621–663.

64. Karin, M., and A. Lin. 2002. NF-κB at the crossroads of life and death. *Nat. Immunol.* **3:**221–227.

65. Keates, A. C., S. Keates, J. H. Kwon, K. O. Arseneau, D. J. Law, L. Bai, J. L. Merchant, T. C. Wang, and C. P. Kelly. 2001. ZBP-89, Sp1, and nuclear factor-κ B regulate epithelial neutrophil-activating peptide-78 gene expression in Caco-2 human colonic epithelial cells. *J. Biol. Chem.* **276:**43713–43722.

66. Keates, S., Y. S. Hitti, M. Upton, and C. P. Kelly. 1997. *Helicobacter pylori* infection activates NF-κB in gastric epithelial cells. *Gastroenterology* **113:**1099–1109.

67. Keates, S., A. C. Keates, E. Mizoguchi, A. Bhan, and C. P. Kelly. 1997. Enterocytes are the primary source of the chemokine ENA-78 in normal colon and ulcerative colitis. *Am. J. Physiol. Gastrointest. Liver Physiol.* **273:**G75–G82.

68. Keates, S., A. C. Keates, M. Warny, R. M. Peek, Jr., P. G. Murray, and C. P. Kelly. 1999. Differential activation of mitogen-activated protein kinases in AGS gastric epithelial cells by cag$^+$ and cag$^-$ *Helicobacter pylori*. *J. Immunol.* **163:**5552–5559.

69. Kunkel, E. J., and E. C. Butcher. 2002. Chemokines and the tissue-specific migration of lymphocytes. *Immunity* **16:**1–4.

70. Larrick, J. W., M. Hirata, R. F. Balint, J. Lee, J. Zhong, and S. C. Wright. 1995. Human CAP18: a novel antimicrobial lipopolysaccharide-binding protein. *Infect. Immun.* **63:**1291–1297.

71. Laurent, F., L. Eckmann, T. C. Savidge, G. Morgan, C. Theodos, M. Naciri, and M. F. Kagnoff. 1997. *Cryptosporidium parvum* infection of human intestinal epithelial cells induces the polarized secretion of C-X-C chemokines. *Infect. Immun.* **65:**5067–5073.

72. Lecuit, M., S. Dramsi, C. Gottardi, M. Fedor-Chaiken, B. Gumbiner, and P. Cossart. 1999. A single amino acid in E-cadherin responsible for host specificity towards the human pathogen *Listeria monocytogenes*. *EMBO J.* **18:**3956–3963.

73. Lecuit, M., S. Vandormael-Pournin, J. Lefort, M. Huerre, P. Gounon, C. Dupuy, C. Babinet, and P. Cossart. 2001. A transgenic model for listeriosis: role of internalin in crossing the intestinal barrier. *Science* **292:**1722–1725.

74. Lehrer, R. I., and T. Ganz. 2002. Cathelicidins: a family of endogenous antimicrobial peptides. *Curr. Opin. Hematol.* **9:**18–22.

75. Lehrer, R. I., and T. Ganz. 2002. Defensins of vertebrate animals. *Curr. Opin. Immunol.* **14:**96–102.

76. Li, Q., D. Van Antwerp, F. Mercurio, K.-F. Lee, and I. M. Verma. 1999. Severe liver degeneration in mice lacking the IκB kinase 2 gene. *Science* **284:**321–325.

77. **Li, Z.-W., W. Chu, Y. Hu, M. Delhase, T. Deerinck, M. Ellisman, R. Johnson, and M. Karin.** 1999. The IKK subunit of IκB kinase (IKK) is essential for NF-κB activation and prevention of apoptosis. *J. Exp. Med.* **189:**1839–1845.

78. **Loetscher, M., B. Gerber, P. Loetscher, S. A. Jones, L. Piali, I. Clark-Lewis, M. Baggiolini, and B. Moser.** 1996. Chemokine receptor specific for IP10 and mig: structure, function, and expression in activated T-lymphocytes. *J. Exp. Med.* **184:**963–969.

79. **Luster, A. D.** 2002. The role of chemokines in linking innate and adaptive immunity. *Curr. Opin. Immunol.* **14:**129–135.

80. **Maaser, C., L. Eckmann, G. Paesold, H. S. Kim, and M. F. Kagnoff.** 2002. Ubiquitous production of macrophage migration inhibitory factor by human gastric and intestinal epithelium. *Gastroenterology* **122:**667–680.

81. **McCole, D. F., L. Eckmann, F. Laurent, and M. F. Kagnoff.** 2000. Intestinal epithelial cell apoptosis following *Cryptosporidium parvum* infection. *Infect. Immun.* **68:**1710–1713.

82. **Medzhitov, R.** 2001. Toll-like receptors and innate immunity. *Nat. Rev. Immunol.* **1:**135–145.

83. **Mengaud, J., H. Ohayon, P. Gounon, R. M. Mege, and P. Cossart.** 1996. E-cadherin is the receptor for internalin, a surface protein required for entry of *L. monocytogenes* into epithelial cells. *Cell* **84:**923–932.

84. **Monack, D. M., J. Mecsas, D. Bouley, and S. Falkow.** 1998. *Yersinia*-induced apoptosis *in vivo* aids in the establishment of a systemic infection of mice. *J. Exp. Med.* **188:**2127–2137.

85. **Muzio, M., J. Ni, P. Feng, and V. M. Dixit.** 1997. IRAK (Pelle) family member IRAK-2 and MyD88 as proximal mediators of IL-1 signaling. *Science* **278:**1612–1615.

86. **Norris, F. A., M. P. Wilson, T. S. Wallis, E. E. Galyov, and P. W. Majerus.** 1998. SopB, a protein required for virulence of *Salmonella dublin*, is an inositol phosphate phosphatase. *Proc. Natl. Acad. Sci. USA* **95:**14057–14059.

87. **Olson, T. S., and K. Ley.** 2002. Chemokines and chemokine receptors in leukocyte trafficking. *Am. J. Physiol. Regul. Integr. Comp. Physiol.* **283:**R7–R28.

88. **O'Neil, D. A., S. P. Cole, E. Martin-Porter, M. P. Housley, L. Liu, T. Ganz, and M. F. Kagnoff.** 2000. Regulation of human β-defensins by gastric epithelial cells in response to infection with *Helicobacter pylori* or stimulation with interleukin-1. *Infect. Immun.* **68:**5412–5415.

89. **O'Neil, D. A., E. M. Porter, D. Elewaut, G. M. Anderson, L. Eckmann, T. Ganz, and M. F. Kagnoff.** 1999. Expression and regulation of the human β-defensins hBD-1 and hBD-2 in intestinal epithelium. *J. Immunol.* **163:**6718–6724.

90. **Orth, K., Z. Xu, M. B. Mudgett, Z. Q. Bao, L. E. Palmer, J. B. Bliska, W. F. Mangel, B. Staskawicz, and J. E. Dixon.** 2000. Disruption of signaling by *Yersinia* effector YopJ, a ubiquitin-like protein protease. *Science* **290:**1594–1597.

91. **Ouellette, A. J., and C. L. Bevins.** 2001. Paneth cell defensins and innate immunity of the small bowel. *Inflamm. Bowel Dis.* **7:**43–50.

92. **Poltorak, A., X. He, I. Smirnova, M.-Y. Liu, C. Van Huffel, X. Du, D. Birdwell, E. Alejos, M. Silva, C. Galanos, M. Freudenberg, P. Ricciardi-Castagnoli, B. Layton, and B. Beutler.** 1998. Defective LPS signaling in C3H/HeJ and C57BL/10ScCr mice: mutations in *Tlr4* gene. *Science* **282:**2082–2088.

93. **Qin, S., J. B. Rottman, P. Myers, N. Kassam, M. Weinblatt, M. Loetscher, A. E. Koch, B. Moser, and C. R. Mackay.** 1998. The chemokine receptors CXCR3 and CCR5 mark subsets of T cells associated with certain inflammatory reactions. *J. Clin. Invest.* **101:**746–754.

94. **Reinecker, H. C., R. P. MacDermott, S. Mirau, A. Dignass, and D. K. Podolsky.** 1996. Intestinal epithelial cells both express and respond to interleukin 15. *Gastroenterology* **111:**1706–1713.

95. **Reinecker, H. C., and D. K. Podolsky.** 1995. Human intestinal epithelial cells express functional cytokine receptors sharing the common γ c chain of the interleukin 2 receptor. *Proc. Natl. Acad. Sci. USA* **92:**8353–8357.

96. **Rescigno, M., G. Rotta, B. Valzasina, and P. Ricciardi-Castagnoli.** 2001. Dendritic cells shuttle microbes across gut epithelial monolayers. *Immunobiology* **204:**572–581.

97. **Rescigno, M., M. Urbano, B. Valzasina, M. Francolini, G. Rotta, R. Bonasio, F. Granucci, J. P. Kraehenbuhl, and P. Ricciardi-Castagnoli.** 2001. Dendritic cells express tight junction proteins and penetrate gut epithelial monolayers to sample bacteria. *Nat. Immunol.* **2:**361–367.

98. **Rosenberger, C. M., A. J. Pollard, and B. B. Finlay.** 2001. Gene array technology to determine host responses to *Salmonella*. *Microbes Infect.* **3:**1353–1360.

99. **Rothwarf, D. M., and M. Karin.** 1999. The NF-kB activation pathway: a paradigm in information transfer from membrane to nucleus. *Science's STKE.* www.stke.org/cgi/content/fullOC_sigtrans;1999/5/re1.

100. **Sansonetti, P. J., J. Arondel, M. Huerre, A. Harada, and K. Matsushima.** 1999. Interleukin-8 controls bacterial transepithelial translocation at the cost of epithelial destruction in experimental shigellosis. *Infect. Immun.* **67:**1471–1480.

101. **Savidge, T. C., D. C. Lowe, and W. A. Walker.** 2001. Developmental regulation of intestinal epithelial hydrolase activity in human fetal jejunal xenografts maintained in severe-combined immunodeficient mice. *Pediatr. Res.* **50:**196–202.

102. **Savkovic, S. D., A. Koutsouris, and G. Hecht.** 1997. Activation of NF-κB in intestinal epithelial cells by enteropathogenic *Escherichia coli. Am. J. Physiol.* **273:**C1160–C1167.

103. **Savkovic, S. D., A. Ramaswamy, A. Koutsouris, and G. Hecht.** 2001. EPEC-activated ERK1/2 participate in inflammatory response but not tight junction barrier disruption. *Am. J. Physiol. Gastrointest. Liver Physiol.* **281:**G890–G898.

104. **Schutte, B. C., J. P. Mitros, J. A. Bartlett, J. D. Walters, H. P. Jia, M. J. Welsh, T. L. Casavant, and P. B. McCray, Jr.** 2002. Discovery of five conserved β-defensin gene clusters using a computational search strategy. *Proc. Natl. Acad. Sci. USA* **99:**2129–2133.

105. **Shibahara, T., J. N. Wilcox, T. Couse, and J. L. Madara.** 2001. Characterization of epithelial chemoattractants for human intestinal intraepithelial lymphocytes. *Gastroenterology* **120:**60–70.

106. **Sierro, F., B. Dubois, A. Coste, D. Kaiserlian, J. P. Kraehenbuhl, and J. C. Sirard.** 2001. Flagellin stimulation of intestinal epithelial cells triggers CCL20-mediated migration of dendritic cells. *Proc. Natl. Acad. Sci. USA* **98:**13722–13727.

107. **Steiner, T. S., J. P. Nataro, C. E. Poteet-Smith, J. A. Smith, and R. L. Guerrant.** 2000. Enteroaggregative *Escherichia coli* expresses a novel flagellin that causes IL-8 release from intestinal epithelial cells. *J. Clin. Invest.* **105:**1769–1777.

108. **Steinle, A., V. Groh, and T. Spies.** 1998. Diversification, expression, and $\gamma\delta$ T cell recognition of evolutionarily distant members of the MIC family of major histocompatibility complex class I-related molecules. *Proc. Natl. Acad. Sci. USA* **95:**12510–12515.

109. **Takeuchi, O., K. Hoshino, T. Kawai, H. Sanjo, H. Takada, T. Ogawa, K. Takeda, and S. Akira.** 1999. Differential roles of TLR2 and TLR4 in recognition of gram-negative and gram-positive bacterial cell wall components. *Immunity* **11:**443–451.

110. **Takeuchi, O., A. Kaufmann, K. Grote, T. Kawai, K. Hoshino, M. Morr, P. F. Muhlradt, and S. Akira.** 2000. Cutting edge: preferentially the R-stereoisomer of the mycoplasmal lipopeptide macrophage-activating lipopeptide-2 activates immune cells through a Toll-like receptor 2- and MyD88-dependent signaling pathway. *J. Immunol.* **164:**554–557.

111. **Tesh, V. L., and A. D. O'Brien.** 1991. The pathogenic mechanisms of Shiga toxin and the Shiga-like toxins. *Mol. Microbiol.* **5:**1817–1822.

112. **Underhill, D. M., A. Ozinsky, K. D. Smith, and A. Aderem.** 1999. Toll-like receptor-2 mediates mycobacteria-induced proinflammatory signaling in macrophages. *Proc. Natl. Acad. Sci. USA* **96:**14459–14463.

113. **Vallance, B. A., and B. B. Finlay.** 2000. Exploitation of host cells by enteropathogenic *Escherichia coli. Proc. Natl. Acad. Sci. USA* **97:**8799–8806.

114. **Varilek, G. W., G. A. Neil, and W. P. Bishop.** 1994. Caco-2 cells express type I interleukin-1 receptors: ligand binding enhances proliferation. *Am. J. Physiol.* **267:**G1101–G1107.

115. **Weinrauch, Y., and A. Zychlinsky.** 1999. The induction of apoptosis by bacterial pathogens. *Annu. Rev. Microbiol.* **53:**155–187.

116. **Wesche, H., W. J. Henzel, W. Shillinglaw, S. Li, and Z. Cao.** 1997. MyD88: an adapter that recruits IRAK to the IL-1 receptor complex. *Immunity* **7:**837–847.

117. **Witthoft, T., L. Eckmann, J. M. Kim, and M. F. Kagnoff.** 1998. Enteroinvasive bacteria directly activate expression of iNOS and NO production in human colon epithelial cells. *Am. J. Physiol.* **275:**G564–G571.

118. **Yamada, K., M. Shimaoka, K. Nagayama, T. Hiroi, H. Kiyono, and T. Honda.** 1997. Bacterial invasion induces interleukin-7 receptor expression in colonic epithelial cell line, T84. *Eur. J. Immunol.* **27:**3456–3460.

119. **Yang, S. K., L. Eckmann, A. Panja, and M. F. Kagnoff.** 1997. Differential and regulated expression of C-X-C, C-C, and C-chemokines by human colon epithelial cells. *Gastroenterology* **113:**1214–1223.

MICROBIAL INTERFERENCE WITH HOST INFLAMMATORY RESPONSES

Andrew S. Neish

11

Virtually all life forms are potential targets of pathogens. Pathogens, whether viral, prokaryotic, or eukaryotic, are parasites; their own life cycle requires exploitation of other organisms in a manner that is deleterious to that host. Potential hosts have necessarily evolved physical and biochemical defenses to prevent or limit damage from would-be parasites. Whether it is as simple as the prokaryotic restriction endonuclease systems or as sophisticated as the mammalian innate and adaptive immune systems, all life forms possess some type of defensive response. Thus, a successful parasite must deploy mechanisms to overcome host defenses. In addition, more benign interactions between eukaryotes and prokaryotes have been present since the beginning of unicellular life. These relationships, especially if longstanding, can be mutually indispensable at various cellular, organismal, and ecological levels, as illustrated by the endosymbiotic nature of mitochondria, the gut-dwelling,

cellulose-digesting bacteria of ruminants, and the nitrogen-fixing bacteria in leguminous plants, respectively. Commensals and symbionts face the same host defenses as frank parasites; thus, they too must be able to modulate host defenses as part of a "give and take" between both parties to establish a mutually beneficial (nonparasitic) arrangement.

The human gastrointestinal tract, home to vast numbers and a vast diversity of microbial life, maintains complex physical and chemical barriers that allow normal physiological functioning amidst a large and complex bacterial community. However, as is well known, certain bacteria have evolved mechanisms to breach these barriers and gain systemic access. This highly deleterious situation (from our point of view) is usually avoided by the innate and adaptive immune systems, which use specialized cells to fight off invading microorganisms. The initial and usually adequate phase of the immune response is inflammation. This basic pathological process is characteristically elicited by most enteric infections, including *Salmonella, Shigella,* certain pathogenic *Escherichia coli, Yersinia, Entamoeba,* and others. Even usually benign gut flora can elicit inflamma-

Andrew S. Neish, Epithelial Pathobiology Unit, Department of Pathology, Emory University School of Medicine, 105F Whitehead Building, 615 Michaels St., Atlanta GA 30322.

Microbial Pathogenesis and the Intestinal Epithelial Cell, ed. by G. Hecht
© 2003 ASM Press, Washington, D.C.

tion if the physical and/or functional integrity of the epithelial barriers are compromised. Interestingly, recent research has shown that many organisms have evolved mechanisms to suppress inflammation as a critical phase of their parasitic life cycles. This chapter discusses recent findings that may shed light on how pathogens circumvent the usually effective intestinal inflammatory defenses. Additionally, it discusses how nonpathogens and commensals may also have developed signals that inhibit or dampen host inflammatory pathways. While immune suppression by pathogens is intuitively understandable, similar effects by nonpathogens are more difficult to conceptualize. Yet such relationships may play a role in immune tolerance in the gastrointestinal (GI) tract, affect normal physiology, and even have significant clinical implications.

ENTERIC INFLAMMATION AND PATHOGENS

Bacteria and bacterial products (e.g., lipopolysaccharide [LPS], flagellin) are well-studied and potent exogenous inducers of inflammation. As mentioned in chapter 1 of this volume, the enterocytes (lumen-lining intestinal epithelial cells) have evolved highly selective barriers to protect against cellular injury from the resident luminal flora and their products. Only when these barriers are breached or when proinflammatory signals emanate from the abluminal (systemic) side do mucosal tissues respond with a typical inflammatory response. Enterocytes play an active role in orchestrating an inflammatory response because they possess batteries of "pattern recognition receptors" such as the extracellular Toll-like receptors (TLR) and the intracellular Nod proteins. These pattern recognition receptors collectively act as a microbial monitoring and surveillance system (described in chapter 5). These cells can respond to the detection of microbes by activating proinflammatory signaling pathways that result in synthetic upregulation and secretion of neutrophil- and lymphocyte-specific chemokines, adhesion molecules, and other inflam-

matory effector molecules. These effector molecules cooperatively direct the spatial and temporal leukocyte movement that defines the inflammatory process (described in chapter 9). While necessary for the initial control of infection and for repair of tissue injury, acute inflammation and increased epithelial permeability can result in potentially life-threatening secretory diarrhea, whereas sustained, repeated, or inappropriate inflammation can result in tissue scarring, loss of function, or even neoplasia (15). Thus, while the intestine is uniquely tolerant of agents highly proinflammatory to other cells, enterocytes can and do manifest the full spectrum of the inflammatory process.

It is now well known that most enteropathogens possess a so-called type III secretion system (TTSS) (see chapter 22). This multicomponent "machine" (structurally related to the flagellar apparatus) spans the bacterial cell wall and is thought to mediate the translocation of bacterial effector proteins from the interior of the bacterium into an external environment, possibly into the cytoplasm of the host animal (or, in some cases, plant) cells (14). The component structural, effector, and regulatory genes of the TTSS tend to be clustered contiguously on "pathogenicity islands." Organisms bearing mutations in components of this apparatus are often deficient to varying degrees in in vivo and in vitro assays of pathogenicity.

Presumably, an ancestral E. coli-like gram-negative bacterium actively colonized the intestines of early land vertebrates. The acquisition of genes encoding structures and machinery necessary for firm adhesion and invasion, probably acquired via horizontal transmission from prokaryotes already adapted to other eukaryotic hosts, enabled a subset of enteric bacteria to gain a competitive advantage over organisms literally "just passing through" the enteric tract (5, 30).

Certain proteins translocated via the TTSS, such as SipA (44) and SopB (28) from Salmonella enterica serovar Typhimurium, may have proinflammatory effects, such that their absence renders the organisms nonpathogenic, and the isolated protein may activate cellular proinflammatory pathways in vitro. However, the teleology of these events is unclear. Do proinflammatory prokaryotic effector proteins elicit inflammation as a finely tuned virulence mechanism, possibly to produce diarrhea and increase the environmental dissemination of the responsible organism? Alternatively, these proteins may have other, not yet defined functions, and proinflammatory signaling results from the cellular detection of these translocated proteins by cytoplasmic pattern recognition receptors. The efficiency of neutrophil killing of most enteric bacteria during a bout of inflammatory (as opposed to secretory) diarrhea may lend support to the latter hypothesis.

The deleterious effects of uncontrolled or sustained inflammation necessitate tight control over the process. Thus, mediators of inflammation are not constitutively expressed. A large body of research indicates that most proinflammatory cytokines, chemotactic chemokines, and leukocyte adhesion molecules are regulated by the de novo synthesis of new mRNA (transcription). The process of transcriptional activation is mediated by the action of soluble nuclear transcription factors that bind DNA in a site-specific fashion and assemble on the promoters of target genes. Transcription factors themselves are under strict regulatory control, often synthetic or posttranslational, to prevent inappropriate gene expression. The DNA binding proteins that interact with the promoters of inflammatory regulatory genes represent a relatively small subset of transcription factors. Recent research indicates that NF-κB is a central factor in all inflammatory modulatory genes.

THE NF-κB
PROINFLAMMATORY PATHWAY

NF-κB is the generic term for members of the Rel family of DNA binding transcription factors (23, 38, 42). This family of proteins is typically regulated by rapid protein synthesis-independent activation, and is characteristi-

cally involved in the transcriptional activation of many genes of the innate immune and inflammatory responses. As such, the NF-κB system is critical to host cell pathogen responses (23). Indeed, orthologs of the NF-κB proteins are structurally and functionally conserved in insects and are critical mediators of antimicrobial responses (34, 45). Murine loss-of-function studies have confirmed key in vivo roles for NF-κB in mammalian immune and inflammatory processes. Mice null for one NF-κB subunit (p50) display a range of abnormal immune functions and hypersensitivity to infectious organisms (67). Mice null for the p65 subunit in a genetic background that permits normal development are similarly deficient in their ability to mount an inflammatory reaction in response to bacterial infection (2). Promoter mutagenesis studies clearly demonstrate the critical role that NF-κB binding motifs play in the promoters of a wide array of genes involved in stress, immune, inflammatory, and antiapoptotic functions (13). Expression profiling by microarray has been performed on cultured human epithelial cells infected with a variety of pathogenic bacteria, including *S. enterica* serovar Typhimurium, *Pseudomonas aeruginosa,* and *Helicobacter pylori* (16, 61). One realization from these studies is that NF-κB responsive genes as a class are consistently activated (often de novo) by these infections.

Structure of NF-κB

The designation NF-κB was originally applied to a site-specific DNA binding activity present in B lymphocytes (4, 70). Determination of the genomic structure of two dimeric proteins that makeup NF-κB defined the Rel domain, a 300-amino-acid DNA binding motif. It is now known that the Rel domain defines a family of proteins including RelA, RelB, and cRel (Fig. 1). These proteins contain potent activation domains (the protein motif involved in recruiting and stabilizing the basal transcriptional apparatus), as well as p50 (NF-κB1) and p49 (NF-κB2), which lack an activation domain but have a stronger affinity for the DNA

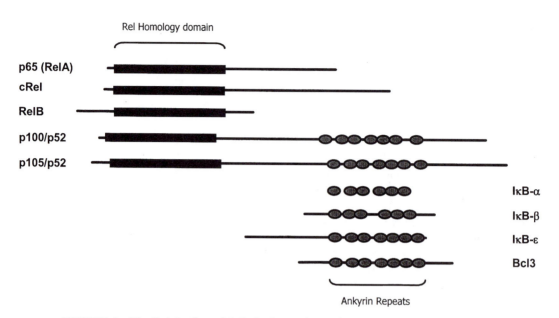

FIGURE 1 The Rel family and IκB family. Each member is a separate gene. The 300-amino-acid Rel homology domain is shown as a black rectangle; the 33-amino-acid ankyrin repeats are shown as gray ovals.

binding motif. Both p50 and p49 are proteolytically processed forms of larger precursors, p105 and p100, respectively. These genes both have C-terminal domains composed of multimerized ankyrin repeats.

Another family of genes typified by repeats of ankyrin domains is the IκB family (inhibitor of κB), which consists of four identified members (39) (Fig. 1). Each IκB family protein is the product of a distinct gene. IκB proteins form a complex with NF-κB in the cytoplasm, retaining it in an inactive state. Additionally, IκB imposes a conformational change on the dimeric partners, rendering them unable to bind DNA. IκB-like function can also be provided by the C-terminal ankyrin repeat-containing region of the p105 and p100 genes. NF-κB is activated by a rapid posttranslational mechanism, accomplished by loss of either the IκB free protein or the C terminus, which will be discussed in detail below. The existence of two inhibitory proteins, free IκB and IκB-like C termini, may suggest separate activation pathways.

Classical NF-κB is generally understood to be composed of heterodimeric p65 and p50,

though other homo- and heterodimeric combinations of cRel, RelB, and p49 have been described, at least in vitro (70). Binding of various dimeric combinations may be influenced by variation in the DNA binding motif, a potential mechanism for varying promoter-specific interactions. The generic κB binding motif, GGGAANNTTCC (N = any nucleotide), shows the partial dyad symmetry that is typical of dimeric transcription factors. Optimal interaction with this motif occurs with p50/p65 heterodimers. However, homodimeric p65 preferentially interacts with a GGAAANNTCC motif, which is found in the promoters of the interleukin 8 (IL-8) and IL-6 promoters (43). The functional consequences of different dimeric combinations are not fully established. Most studies using epithelial cells have detected homo- and heterodimeric combinations of p50 and p65 (23, 29).

Activation of NF-κB

Activation of the NF-κB pathway can be initiated by a myriad of stimuli, including endogenous cytokines, bacteria, viruses, bacterial products, ionizing radiation, and oxidant stress. It is apparent that NF-κB activation follows acute stress or "danger signals." Extensive research has characterized the initial signaling by which endogenous proinflammatory mediators such as tumor necrosis factor (TNF) stimulate NF-κB. Additionally, the mechanisms by which bacteria and other exogenous threats activate NF-κB are beginning to be unraveled (Fig. 2) (38, 68). As currently understood, binding of an appropriate ligand (e.g., prokaryotic surface structure) to a transmembrane TLR results in the sequential recruitment of the adaptor proteins MyD88 and IRAK to the Toll/interleukin-1 receptor (TIR) cytoplasmic domain on the TLR.

IRAK, a serine kinase, then activates the cytoplasmic intermediate TRAF6 by inducing an unusual modification; the lysine-63 ubiquitination catalyzed by the action of two other proteins, Ubc13 and Uev1a (20, 73). Ubiquitin, a highly conserved 76-amino-acid peptide, is commonly used to modify cellular proteins by covalent linkage through lysine-48 residues (65). Originally, ubiquitination of proteins was assumed to target the modified protein for regulated destruction by the cellular proteasome organelle. Recent discoveries of alternative ubiquitin linkages, such as lysine-63 and families of ubiquitin-like proteins (e.g. SUMO [sentrin] and Nedd8) have

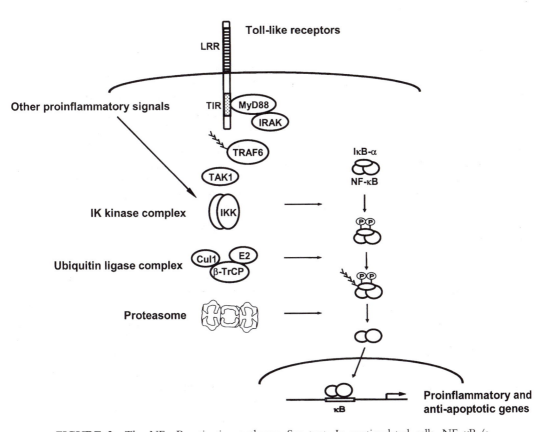

FIGURE 2 The NF-κB activation pathway. See text. In unstimulated cells, NF-κB (a heterodimer of p50/p65) is sequestered in the cytoplasm by IκB. Activation of proinflammatory signaling receptors, such as the TLR, sets in motion a series of enzymatic modifications of IκB: phosphorylation, ubiquitination, and degradation. Loss of IκB allows NF-κB to translocate to the nucleus, bind to the promoters of numerous proinflammatory effector genes, and activate the epithelial proinflammatory program. Perturbation of any of these enzymatic steps could inhibit the entire pathway.

revealed that modifications by these molecules play a role in diverse processes such as intracellular trafficking and potential enzymatic activation, as in the case of TRAF6 (79). Once activated by lysine-63 ubiquitination, TRAF6 in turn activates TAK1 (a kinase of the MEKKK group) in complex with TAB1 and TAB2. The TAK1/TAB1/TAB2 complex functions to induce phosphorylation and activation of the terminal IκB kinase complex, IKK (73).

IKK is a signaling nexus, receiving and integrating signals from multiple proinflammatory signal transduction pathways, of which the Toll pathway is only one example (49). In addition to TLR-mediated signals, many stimuli activate the IKK complex, such as the proinflammatory cytokines TNF and IL-1. Both TNF and IL-1 have dedicated receptors and IKK proximal signaling intermediates (39). Additionally, activation of Ca^{2+} mobilization can serve as a sufficient signal to activate these pathways (29). Bacterial effector proteins may directly activate either the kinase or upstream signaling intermediates (33). In each case, signaling converges on IKK, which acts as an "integrator." The IKK complex is composed of a bewildering combination of subunits, and the exact composition is the subject of considerable debate. The main catalytic subunits of the complex have been identified as IKK-α and IKK-β, which recognize a conserved 6-amino-acid motif present on all IκB isoforms and phosphorylate two serine residues within the motif (11, 21, 39). Murine knockout studies revealed that IKK-β null mice are defective in NF-κB activation in response to proinflammatory stimuli, while IKK-α null mice show early lethality and developmental defects (40). Interestingly, marrow transplantation studies that transferred IKK-α null bone marrow precursor cells to a normal background to circumvent these developmental effects found that IKK-α plays a role in processing p105 (NF-κB2), while having no effect on the degradation of IκB heterotrimerized with p50/p65 (66). These results define differential utilization of IKK

isoforms and may imply distinct functions of the different types of NF-κB dimers.

The serine-phosphorylated IκB isoforms are subjected to a second rapid covalent modification by another multicomponent enzymatic complex—polyubiquitination. IκB-α polyubiquitination is mediated by the action of a recently described ubiquitin ligase complex designated β-TrCP-SCF (69, 78). β-TrCP is the protein that physically interacts with the phospho-domain of IκB-α and on a highly similar domain on the transcriptional activator and structural protein β-catenin (47). Several other components make up the complex, including the actual ubiquitin-conjugating enzyme and a subunit, Cul1, which is itself regulated by covalent modification of the ubiquitin-like molecule Nedd8 (58).

Unlike the lysine-63–linked ubiquitination implicated in the activation of TRAF6, IκB polyubiquitination occurs at lysine-48. The results of polyubiquitination is the recognition of the modified IκB by the 18S regulatory subunit of the proteasome, followed by the proteolytic digestion of the IκB molecule (10, 11, 56). Interestingly, although ubiquitinated IκB is totally degraded by the proteasome, it is able to specifically degrade only the C termini of ubiquitinated p100/105 (32). How this limited proteolysis occurs is not known. Degradation of all forms of IκB is necessary for NF-κB activation. Small molecule inhibitors of the catalytic activity of the proteasome block IκB degradation and subsequent proinflammatory signaling (59). Following IκB degradation, the NF-κB nuclear localization signal is exposed, allowing regulated translocation across the nuclear membrane, with subsequent DNA binding to relevant promoters and transcriptional activation of proinflammatory effector genes.

One distinctly recognizable subset of NF-κB inducible genes are antiapoptotic effector proteins such as A20 and the IAP (inhibitor of apoptosis) family of inhibitors, suggesting that NF-κB activation is globally antiapoptotic (26, 74). Indeed, the initial analysis of p65 null mice showed that embryonic lethality was secondary to massive apoptosis in the liver, suggesting that transcriptional activation of NF-κB-dependent genes is necessary (at least in embryonic stages) to allow cell survival (6). Overlap is clearly evident in the protein machinery necessary for intracellular transmission of proapoptotic and proinflammatory signaling. Both events can be mediated by TNF-receptor proteins and use adaptor proteins of the TRAF/TRADD family (74). As mentioned, NF-κB is activated by "danger signals." The proximal aspects of the NF-κB pathway may have coevolved with the apoptotic machinery to ensure that activation of NF-κB proceeds in parallel with initiation of the apoptotic death program. The NF-κB-mediated induction of antiapoptotic genes thus aborts the sequence of events leading to self-destruction. This intertwined arrangement may have evolved to protect the whole organism from microbe-mediated inhibition of immune and inflammatory pathways by committing individual infected cells to apoptotic destruction. Not surprisingly, some pathogens have acquired the ability to exploit this system to eliminate immune cells (54).

ACTIVE SUPPRESSION OF INFLAMMATORY PATHWAYS

Pathogens

Immune and inflammatory evasion by pathogens is an expected facet of parasitic life cycles, especially those that involve invasion into the corpus of the host. The common enteropathogen S. enterica serovar Typhimurium is fully capable of epithelial invasion and characteristically provokes an intense neutrophilic infiltrate that accounts for its clinical manifestations (19). In contrast, Salmonella enterica serovar Typhi, an enteric pathogen that also invades through the epithelia, gains systemic access and proliferates within the cells of the reticuloendothelial system, but does not elicit inflammation. The Vi surface antigen of serovar Typhi may endow the organism with the stealth necessary to escape certain aspects of

innate immune detection (46). Some bacteria establish intracellular niches transparent to host defenses, even cytoplasmic pattern recognition receptors (22, 25). Pathogenic strategies based on evading host detection can be termed passive.

Recently it has become apparent that certain microbes may take a more proactive approach by suppressing host responses. As reviewed by Wilson et al. (77), pathogens as diverse as *Bacillus anthracis*, *Brucella suis*, *Actinomyces actinomycetemcomitans*, and several members of the *Enterobacteriaceae* secrete soluble toxins that inhibit the production of cytokines from cocultured lymphocytes and macrophages. Several pathogens, often those whose infection elicits little inflammation in vivo, have been shown to reduce synthesis of inflammatory mediators in vitro from epithelial and endothelial cells. For example, *Mycobacterium avium* preinfection of cultured human intestinal epithelial cells has been shown to block subsequent induction of IL-8 secretion in response to S. enterica serovar Typhimurium, although no mechanisms have been described (63). Similarly, the fungal pathogen *Cryptococcus neoformans* fails to elicit proinflammatory cytokine secretion from cultured human endothelial cells (50).

Direct microbial inhibition of NF-κB activation is being reported with increasing frequency. Yuk et al. showed that colonization of cultured respiratory epithelial cells with *Bordetella bronchiseptica* inhibited cytoplasmic to nuclear translocation of the NF-κB subunit p65 in response to TNF-α (80). Intracytoplasmic "aggregates" of p65 immunoreactivity were detected in cells thus colonized. The mechanism of formation and composition of these aggregates is unknown. It is of interest that the effects observed could not be mediated by a strain bearing mutations in the type III secretion apparatus, implying the existence of a translocated effector protein. Notably, *B. bronchiseptica* is generally regarded as a long-term, chronic pathogen, if not a commensal organism, in contrast to *Bordetella pertussis*, a strain that mediates acute inflammatory disease. A possibly similar phenomenon was observed in an in vitro culture system using murine peritoneal macrophages infected with *Toxoplasma* trophozooites. This host-pathogen interaction was marked by inhibition of the typical upregulation of inflammatory effector molecules following LPS administration. The infected cells exhibited typical IκB phosphorylation, ubiquitination, and degradation; however, cytoplasmic-to-nuclear translocation of NF-κB did not occur (9). The data in both of these reports imply interference with the regulation of nuclear import. One could also speculate that inhibition of the proteasomal enzymatic activity would lead to cytoplasmic aggregation of NF-κB complexed to phosphorylated and ubiquitinated IκB.

A potentially different mechanism of NF-κB inhibition was reported in uropathogenic strains of *E. coli* (41). This pathogen has been shown to inhibit NF-κB and mitogen-activated protein kinase (MAPK) activation in cultured urothelial cells. These bacteria blocked LPS-stimulated IκB degradation and were shown to be proapoptotic to these cells, consistent with the antiapoptotic role of NF-κB. Similar observations have been made with *Yersinia enterocolitica* and *Yersinia pseudotuberculosis*, enteropathogens that are known to inhibit TNF production in infected macrophages and induce apoptosis (55, 64). This ability is mediated by the type III-secreted effector molecule YopP/J (62). Mutation of this gene renders *Yersinia* less virulent in vivo in murine models and blocks the ability to induce apoptosis in macrophages in vitro. Orth and others showed that YopJ blocks the NF-κB (and MAPK) pathway by physically associating with the IKK-β subunit and inhibiting the subsequent phosphorylation of IκB-α (53). Abrogation of IκB phosphorylation would prevent subsequent ubiquitination, degradation, and NF-κB translocation. Because inhibition of NF-κB is potently proapoptotic, *Yersinia* has apparently evolved a mechanism to eliminate the threat of phagocytic cells by blocking their proinflammatory responses and ultimately inducing apoptotic destruction.

Some insight into the biochemical mechanisms of NF-κB inhibition can be gleaned from the study of viral pathogens. African swine fever virus is a large DNA virus that causes a lethal hemorrhagic infection of domestic pigs. The viral genome encodes an ankyrin repeat containing molecule A238L, with significant homology to mammalian IκB. Live virus or overexpressed A238L was shown to inhibit NF-κB activation and proinflammatory gene expression in a variety of in vitro assays (57, 60). Mechanistically, the viral IκB acts as an IκB substitute, maintaining the NF-κB in a cytoplasmic location, even if the endogenous IκB is degraded.

Certain poxviruses are able to inhibit proinflammatory gene expression in vitro. While the responsible gene or protein has not been identified, work has shown that viral infection prevents IκB degradation in response to proinflammatory activators. Interestingly, IκB phosphorylation is not inhibited, suggesting inhibition at the level of ubiquitination (52). Inhibition of IκB ubiquitination has been implicated in human immunodeficiency virus (HIV) pathogenesis. The HIV-encoded Vpu protein in HIV-infected HeLa cells interfered with degradation of IκB by binding to and inactivating the β-TrCP component of the IκB SCF complex. In this model, phosphorylated Vpu binds to the SCF complex but is not degraded, thus acting as a competitive inhibitor of the IκB ubiquitin ligase complex (7). A phosphorylation-defective mutant could not mediate the repressive effect.

Epithelial Interactions with Nonpathogens

Prokaryotic life has an understandable affinity for intimate relationships with eukaryotic organisms. Beginning with the earliest endosymbiotic interaction of bacteria and blue-green algae within eukaryotes, leading to modern mitochondria and chloroplasts, prokaryotic organisms have exploited and thrived in these environments, which provide a generally nutrient-rich and thermostable environment, courtesy of the host. Classic examples of a prokaryote maintaining a symbiotic relationship with a metazoan host are the soil bacteria that colonize the roots of leguminous plants. Infection or colonization by *Rhizobium* sp. induces a defensive "nodulation" reaction by the plant, providing a focus for colonization (27). The end result is that the bacteria establish a stable niche and carbohydrate supply, while the plants (and animals throughout the food web) benefit from the nitrogen-fixing abilities of this prokaryote. Similarly, in animals, cellulolytic bacteria found in the guts of termites and ruminant mammals (*Ruminococcus* spp., *Fibrobacter* spp.) enjoy a benign local environment and are necessary for the animal's nutritional use of an otherwise undigestible substance (71). These relationships coevolved over hundreds of millions of years, spanning the development of the innate and adaptive immune systems.

With the evolution of vertebrates, the intestinal tract, with its steady supply of partially digested macromolecules, clearly represented an attractive niche for long-term colonization, particularly in terrestrial animals. It has been commented that >90% of the total cells of a healthy human are actually bacterial cells, present as intestinal flora (76). This rich ecosystem is composed of approximately 10^{14} bacterial cells, representing 30 known genera and 500 species, with many more suspected that may have fastidious culture requirements and are currently undescribed. The enteric flora colonizes infants immediately after birth and is necessary for normal development of immune surveillance and perhaps other vital functions. Limited symbiosis does exist in the human GI tract, as intestinal bacteria have clearly established a comfortable niche for themselves while providing the human host with the metabolism of bile acids, bilirubin, cholesterol, and short-chain fatty acids and assisting in the synthesis of nutrients such as menaquinones (vitamin K) (24, 35, 36).

Recent experiments with rodents raised under lifelong sterile conditions ("gnotobiotic") demonstrate a significant role that the microflora play in the normal physiologic processes in the gut. Gnotobiotic mice exhibit hypoplasia of the intestinal villi and cuboidal morphology of the enterocytes, as well as a lack of development of lymphoid follicles and the physiological presence of lymphocytes and plasma cells in the lamina propria. Germfree mice develop luminal mucus inspissation, presumably a result of the lack of flora that normally serve to digest secreted mucus glycoproteins. Recolonization of the mice with members of the normal murine flora reverses this condition (24). Furthermore, Bry et al. have found that the intestinal commensal *Bacteroides thetaiotaomicron* is able to deliver a signal to the host epithelium, inducing the epithelial upregulation of carbohydrate components (fucosyl asialo-GM1) that provide a nutritional source specific for this particular organism (8). This represents an example of a nonpathogen manipulating host biochemical pathways for its own benefit. This group also monocolonized gnotobiotic mice with *B. thetaiotaomicron* and analyzed the colonized ileal tissue by high-density microarray analysis. These studies revealed a spectrum of significantly up- and downregulated genes involved in such diverse roles as nutrient absorption, angiogenesis, and barrier function. Immunoinflammatory genes were not affected (37). Thus, commensal bacteria clearly are capable of influencing host cell biology in a manner not normally considered pathogenic (proinflammatory).

A fascinating recent observation is that TTSSs are employed to translocate effector molecules necessary for the establishment of commensal or symbiotic interactions. TTSSs have been characterized in many gramnegative phytopathogenic bacteria. In *Xanthomonas campestris* the TTSS is involved in the elicitation of plant defense mechanisms that lead to host resistance, or "hypersensitive response" (HR). HR is defined as the rapid apoptotic death of plant cells immediately adjacent to the infection site, and serves to restrict the potential systemic spread of an invasive pathogen. In these cases, the translocated proteins act as, and are designated, *avirulence* factors (12, 18). An even more intriguing example is seen among the aforementioned rhizobia. Viprey et al. reported that such symbiotic bacteria elicit the nodulation response in plants by the action of proteins secreted via a type III secretion apparatus. (72). Other examples are seen in the animal kingdom, such as *Sodalis glossindius*, an endosymbiont of tsetse flies. Dale et al. identified *S. glossindius* mutants that were unable to invade insect cells and establish a stable symbiotic state. This approach identified components of a TTSS bearing high homology to the SPI-1 TTSS of *Salmonella enterica* (17). These observations establish that the TTSS is not solely a "virulence" factor, but may be more accurately described as a device employed by the prokaryotic kingdom as a "communication system" with eukaryotic cells. In some cases, as in the traditionally understood enteropathogens, a lineage of bacteria has used the genes of the pathogenicity island (encoding TTSS and contiguous effector genes) to facilitate a lifestyle that is detrimental to the host, thus defining a parasite/pathogenic relationship. As the study of the family *Enterobacteriaceae* illustrates, these organisms have evolved a diverse range of lifestyles within the vertebrate intestinal tract, albeit from our perspective all pathogenic (22). Nonetheless, certain plant- and arthopod-specific bacteria have used a very similar set of genes to establish relationships with their respective hosts that are commensal/symbiotic in nature. Thus, the existence of commensal/symbiotic interactions mediated by these systems may suggest that such relationships are present in the large, complex commensal ecosystem of the human intestine.

Our laboratory group and others have long noted that cultured epithelial cells colonized by several strains of nonpathogenic *Salmonella* fail to induce upregulation of inflammatory effector molecules or activation of NF-κB (29, 51). We made the initial surprising discovery that cells thus colonized for a minimum of 30 min were refractory to activation by known proinflammatory strains or other potent pharmacologic activators of NF-κB. Further work demonstrated that the blockade of proinflammatory gene activation occurred pretranscrip-

tionally by inhibiting the activation of NF-κB and preventing translocation of the DNA binding p50/p65 dimer. Biochemical experiments showed that IκB-α was normally phosphorylated in cells colonized by nonpathogens, but subsequent ubiquitination of the modified IκB-α was totally eliminated. The inability to ubiquitinate IκB thus prevented degradation of IκB and the subsequent translocation of NF-κB. These data were the first reported example of inhibition of the NF-κB pathway at the level of ubiquitination (51). In contrast to the inhibitory mechanisms associated with *Yersinia* infection, nonpathogenic *Salmonella* spp. apparently block the polyubiquitination of IκB without interfering with phosphorylation. It is evident that enteric bacteria have evolved several biochemical mechanisms to influence key regulatory steps of the NF-κB pathway.

INHIBITION OF UBIQUITIN AND RELATED MOLECULES

How could prokaryotic organisms influence the cellular ubiquitination machinery? We have noted that the anti-inflammatory phenomenon mediated by *Salmonella* spp. clearly requires physical contact between living eukaryotic and prokaryotic cells. Therefore, it is unlikely that a protein/toxin secreted into the environment mediates the effect. The anti-inflammatory effect does require an intact TTSS; *S. enterica* serovar Typhimurium mutations that totally block function of this structure (*invA* and *invG*) are not able to repress NF-κB activation. These observations imply that a specific secreted effector molecule may be translocated into the cytoplasm of the colonized cells. Treatment of bacteria with prokaryotic protein synthesis inhibitors does not interfere with anti-inflammatory effects, while heat killing will abolish the phenomenon, suggesting active translocation of a preformed protein (unpublished data). We have shown that the only other known substrate of the β-TrCP SCF complex, phospho-β-catenin, is also prevented from being ubiquitinated in cells colonized with anti-inflammatory organisms. Furthermore, using antibodies to total ubiquitinated protein, we have shown that the anti-inflammatory effects do not obviously affect whole cell levels of ubiquitin-conjugated proteins. These data have led us to suggest that the anti-inflammatory bacteria are translocating a protein that specifically inhibits or reverses the activity of the β-TrCP SCF complex.

Inhibitors of ubiquitination have only recently attracted attention. As mentioned earlier, the Vpu protein of HIV inhibits activation of the NF-κB pathway, by binding to and inactivating the β-TrCP SCF complex (1, 7). A class of endogenous ubiquitin hydrolases has been described that functions in the deubiquitination of modified protein substrates, preventing subsequent degradation (75). Significantly, Orth et al. reported that the *Yersinia* effector YopJ, which is necessary for inhibition of NF-κB in macrophages, bears structural similarity to adenovirus protease (AVP) and yeast Ubl-specific protease 1 (Ulp-1), members of an emerging class of proteins designated ubiquitin-like proteases (54). These enzymes have dual functions: to process the COOH terminus of the ubiquitin-like molecule SUMO-1/Sentrin (Ubl in yeast), which allows the product to be used as a substrate in the convalent modification of the target protein, and to cleave at the COOH terminus of SUMO-1 conjugated to the ε-lysine residue of the modified target protein, effectively desumoylating the protein. These proteases cleave after a Gly-Gly motif, which is found in the isopeptide linkages of both sumoylated and ubiquitinated substrates, suggesting that the Yop protein could also act as a deubiquitinating enzyme. From published data, it appears that YopJ acts to deconjugate SUMO modified proteins, although the effect on proteins conjugated to ubiquitin or related molecules has not been determined. Thus, YopJ is a translocated protein with probable enzymatic activity toward cellular proteins modified by ubiquitin and ubiquitin-like proteins.

Intriguingly, homologs of the YopJ ubiquitin-like protease are found in several organisms with known interactions with eukaryotic hosts. One, AvrBsT, is found in members of phytopathogenic bacteria (*Xanthomonas* spp.) that mediate the "avirulence" function described above (18). Expression of AvrBsT in infected plant cells is required to elicit the defensive "hypersensitivity" response. Mutation of the effector abolishes this response (54). Another homolog present in *Rhizobium* spp., YL4O, may be instrumental in the establishment of a long-term symbiotic state between these bacteria and the cells of root nodules of leguminous plants (72). No clear analog of the NF-κB system has been described in plant immunity, yet these observations may suggest that ubiquitin-dependent signaling, with antiapoptotic end effects, is present in plant responses to infection. Finally, an AvrA homolog is present in most enteropathogenic *Salmonella* spp. (31). In fact, in experiments in our laboratory the AvrA homolog of *S. enterica* serovar Typhimurium displayed potent inhibitory activity toward NF-κB activation (unpublished data).

As discussed, ubiquitin and ubiquitin-like protein modifications are involved at several regulatory points of the NF-κB pathway: (i) the addition of the K63-linked ubiquitin chain on TRAF6 mediated by Ubc13 and Uev1A, (ii) the addition of Nedd8 onto the Cul subunit of the SCF complex by an unknown ligase, and (iii) the addition of K48-linked ubiquitin onto phospho-IκB mediated by the β-TrCP-SCF. Potentially, interference of either of the last two examples is consistent with the observations in *Salmonella* spp. (i.e., blockade of IκB ubiquitination but intact phosphorylation).

INFLAMMATORY REPRESSION IN DISEASE AND HEALTH

Blockade of the inflammatory surveillance (Toll/NF-κB) systems may represent a purely pathogenic mechanism. A disease-causing organism may paralyze the innate (and much of the adaptive) immune system as a mechanism for invasion, systemic spread, and general parasitization. The effects of *Yersinia* spp. may be an example of this strategy. Orth et al. suggest that blockade of the NF-κB pathway serves to "cut the lines of communication" within the macrophage (53). Additionally, blockade of NF-κB is proapoptotic, which in the case of *Yersinia*-infected macrophages would eliminate a key immunomodulatory cell. This has been postulated as a mechanism by which the supremely virulent *Yersinia pestis* is able to disseminate within the host so rapidly. The blockade of proinflammatory pathways by chronic pathogens such as *M. avium* or *B. bronchiseptica* may allow for long-term carriage that is characteristic of these infections. Note that chronic carriage of a pathogen with minimal accompanying tissue injury is close to the definition of commensalism.

Perhaps blockade or attenuation of the NF-κB pathway may be a mechanism of commensalism. Our observations of anti-inflammatory activity in nonpathogenic *Salmonella* spp., which are intestinal commensals in adult birds and reptiles, and the presence of YopJ/AvrA-like molecules in plant and insect symbionts, may be examples of this latter strategy. Furthermore, it could be suggested that microorganisms intimately associated with eukaryotic hosts may have evolved protein (or small molecule) mediators, such as the Avr proteins, to dampen the host proinflammatory and immune responses without provoking apoptotic cell death. This mechanism may contribute to the characteristic tolerance that the vertebrate intestinal epithelium displays toward enteric microflora.

Alternatively, and not necessarily contradictorily, if NF-κB blockade results in accelerated apoptosis of epithelial cells, this plausibly represents an avirulence function by allowing elimination of the infected cells, analogous to the hypersensitivity response in plants. Apoptosis in a rapidly turned over cell type such as epithelia may represent a host response to eliminate invading organisms without escalation to full-scale inflammation and its attendant collateral damage. As epithelial cells are rapidly replaced, one would not necessarily expect massive epithelial loss and exposure of the submucosa, as occurs during *Shigella* infection.

Any given organism in the gut microflora may possess pro- and anti-inflammatory determinants. Proinflammatory determinants may be cell wall components such as LPS, surface appendages such as flagella, and effector proteins secreted from the interior of the bacterial cell. As suggested, translocated components such as the YopJ/AvrA family may serve the opposite function of dampening inflammatory stimuli. Are YopJ/AvrA homologs more widespread among bacteria that interact with eukaryotic cells? Are they present in the normal human flora? If other translocated proteins or secreted small molecules mediate similar functions, then the collective gut ecosystem itself may represent a balance of organisms with pro- and anti-inflammatory potential. Tilting the ecological balance of a healthy flora to a more "proinflammatory" population could conceivably contribute to the initiation and maintenance of idiopathic inflammatory bowel disease (e.g., Crohn's disease and ulcerative colitis). It is also important to remember that similar prokaryotic-eukaryotic interactions are likely to be found along dermal, oral, respiratory, and urogenital epithelia and may contribute to appropriate defensive functions in those tissues as well.

In recent years there has been interest in the use of living organisms as therapeutic agents, or "probiotics." Bacteria employed in this manner are usually members of the human flora, including *Lactobacillus* spp. and *Bifidobacterium* spp. Several controlled clinical trials have shown that administration of such organisms may have beneficial effects in cases of infectious diarrhea (including pseudomembranous colitis) and in inflammatory bowel disease (3). In the laboratory, use of probiotic organisms can prevent or reverse colitis observed in the spontaneous mouse models of inflammatory bowel disease (48). The mechanisms of the observed benefits are totally unknown, but ecologic niche competition and elaboration of bacteriostatic compounds are assumed, while improvement of epithelial barrier function and inhibition of host inflammatory processes have been suggested (3). As discussed, experiments with germ-free mice show that normal flora clearly affect intestinal physiological functions and are capable of directly influencing host cell biochemical regulation. That probiotic organisms possess mechanisms that modulate proinflammatory pathways is certainly an attractive hypothesis.

FUTURE WORK

Among normal tissues, the mammalian intestine is both uniquely colonized by a great diversity and density of microorganisms and also uniquely tolerant of the proinflammatory effects usually elicited by bacteria. This chapter has addressed how bacteria in the gut are capable of modifying host epithelia for their own purposes. Disease-causing bacteria have evolved methods of translocating effector proteins into eukaryotic cells to mediate their parasitic lifestyles, while homologous systems are employed in plant and insect hosts to establish symbiotic states. We have described a biochemical pathway in human cells (NF-κB) by which both nonpathogens and pathogens may be able to attenuate host defense systems and noted specific effector proteins (Avr/Yop) that may mediate these effects.

Work to date indicates that the NF-κB pathway is a critical mediator of immune and inflammatory responses in the intestinal tract, where it acts as a sentry to monitor the presence of potentially pathogenic organisms. Most aspects of the pathway show structural and functional conservation across vast evolutionary time. These observations underscore both the importance of the NF-κB system and the need for eukaryotes to protect themselves from microbial attack. And given the symbiotic and commensal roles many prokaryotes play among and amid eukaryotic hosts, including the human gut flora, how eukaryotes and prokaryotes adjust these responses to establish a mutually beneficial equilibrium is a fascinating question. What is the role of low-level "physiological" inflammation in the gut? How is this elicited and/or modified by the enteric flora? A more complete understanding of the relationship of the intestinal flora with the human host may reveal new understanding of human diseases and suggest novel approaches toward treating them.

REFERENCES

1. **Akari, H., S. Bour, S. Kao, A. Adachi, and K. Strebel.** 2001. The human immunodeficiency virus type 1 accessory protein Vpu induces apoptosis by suppressing the nuclear factor kappa-B dependent expression of anti-apoptotic factors. *J. Exp. Med.* **194:**1299–1312.

2. **Alcamo, E., J. Mizgerd, B. Horwitz, R. Bronson, A. Beg, M. Scott, C. Coerschuk, R. Hynes, and D. Baltimore.** 2001. Targeted mutation of TNF receptor I rescues the RelA-deficient mouse and reveals a critical role for NF-kappa B in leukocyte recruitment. *J. Immunol.* **167:**1592–1560.

3. **Alvarez-Olmos, M., and R. Oberhelman.** 2001. Probiotics and infectious diseases: a modern perspective on a traditional therapy. *Clin. Infect. Dis.* **32:**1567–1576.

4. **Bauerle, P.** 1998. Pro-inflammatory signalling: last pieces in the NF-κB puzzle? *Curr. Biol.* **8:** 19–22.

5. **Baumler, A., R. Tsolis, T. Ficht, and L. Adams.** 1998. Evolution of host adaptation in *Salmonella enterica. Infect. Immun.* **66:**4579–4587.

6. **Beg, A., W. Sha, R. Bronson, S. Ghosh, and D. Baltimore.** 1995. Embryonic lethality and liver degeneration in mice lacking the RelA component of NF-kappaB. *Nature* **376:**167–170.

7. **Bour, S., C. Perrin, H. Akari, and K. Strebel.** 2001. The human immunodeficiency virus type 1 Vpu protein inhibits NF-κB activation by interfering with βTrCP-mediated degradation of IκB. *J. Biol. Chem.* **276:**15920–15928.

8. **Bry, L., P. Falk, T. Midtvedt, and J. Gordon.** 1996. A model of host-microbial interactions in an open intestinal ecosystem. *Science* **273:** 1380–1383.

9. **Butcher, B., L. Kim, P. Johnson, and E. Denkers.** 2001. *Toxoplasma gondii* tachyzoites inhibit proinflammatory cytokine induction in infected macrophages by preventing nuclear translocation of the transcription factor NF-κB. *J. Immunol.* **167:**2193–2201.

10. **Chen, Z., J. Hagler, V. Palombella, F. Melandri, D. Scherer, D. Ballard, and T. Maniatis.** 1995. Signal-induced site-specific phosphorylation targets IκBα to the ubiquitin-proteasome pathway. *Genes Dev.* **9:**1586–1597.

11. **Chen, Z., L. Parent, and T. Maniatis.** 1996. Site-specific phosphorylation of IκBα by a novel

ubiquitination-dependent protein kinase activity. *Cell* **84:**853–862.

12. **Ciesiolka, L., T. Hwin, J. Gearlds, G. Min-savage, R. Saenz, M. Bravo, V. Handley, S. Conover, H. Zhang, J. Caporgno, N. Phen-grasamy, A. Toms, R. Stall, and M. Whalen.** 1999. Regulation of expression of avir-ulence gene avrRxv and identification of a family of host interaction factors by sequence analysis of avrBst. *Mol. Plant Microbe Interact.* **12:**35–44.

13. **Collins, T., M. Read, A. Neish, M. Whitley, D. Thanos, and T. Maniatis.** 1995. Transcrip-tional regulation of endothelial cell adhesion mol-ecules: NF-κB and cytokine-inducible enhancers. *FASEB J.* **9:**899–909.

14. **Cornelis, G., and F. Van Gijsegem.** 2000. As-sembly and function of type III secretion systems. *Annu. Rev. Microbiol.* **54:**735–774.

15. **Cotran, R., V. Kumar, and T. Collins.** 1999. *The Pathologic Basis of Disease*, 6th ed. The W. B. Saunders Co., Philadelphia, Pa.

16. **Cummings, C., and D. Relman.** 2000. Using DNA microarrays to study host-microbe inter-actions. *Emerg. Infect. Dis.* **6:**513–525.

17. **Dale, C., S. Young, D. Haydon, and S. Welburn.** 2001. The insect symbiont *Sodalis glos-sindus* utilizes a type III secretion system for cell invasion. *Proc. Natl. Acad. Sci. USA* **98:**1883–1888.

18. **Dangl, J., and J. Jones.** 2001. Plant pathogens and integrated defense responses to infection. *Na-ture* **411:**826–833.

19. **Day, D., B. Mandall, and B. Morrson.** 1978. The rectal biopsy appearances of *Salmonella colitis*. *Histopathology* **2:**117–131.

20. **Deng, L., C. Wang, E. Spencer, L. Yang, A. Braun, X. You, C. Slaughter, C. Pickart, and Z. Chen.** 2000. Activation of the IκB kinase complex by TRAF6 requires a dimeric ubiquitin-conjugating enzyme complex and a unique polyubiquitin chain. *Cell* **103:**351–361.

21. **DiDonato, J., M. Hayakawa, D. Rothwarf, E. Zandi, and M. Karin.** 1997. A cytokine-responsive IκB kinase that activated the transcrip-tion factor NF-κB. *Nature* **388:**548–554.

22. **Donnenberg, M.** 2000. Pathogenic strategies of enteric bacteria. *Nature* **406:**768–774.

23. **Elewaut, D., J. DiDonato, J. Kim, F. Truong, L. Eckmann, and M. Kagnoff.** 1999. NF-κB is a central regulator of the intes-tinal epithelial cell innate immune response in-duced by infection with enteroinvasive bacteria. *J. Immunol.* **163:**1457–1466.

24. **Falk, P., L. Hooper, T. Midtvedt, and J. Gordon.** 1998. Creating and maintaining the gastrointestinal ecosystem: what we know and

need to know from gnotobiology. *Microbiol. Mol. Biol. Rev.* **62:**1157–1170.

25. **Falkow, S., R. Isberg, and D. Portnoy.** 1992. The interaction of bacteria with mammalian cells. *Annu. Rev. Cell Biol.* **8:**333–363.

26. **Foo, S., and G. Nolan.** 1999. NF-κB to the rescue. Rel's, apoptosis and cellular transforma-tion. *Trends Genet.* **15:**229–235.

27. **Freiberg, C., R. Fellay, A. Bairoch, W. Broughton, A. Rosenthal, and X. Perret.** 1997. Molecular basis of symbiosis between *Rhi-zobium* and legumes. *Nature* **387:**352–353.

28. **Galyov, E., M. Wood, R. Rosqvist, P. Mul-lan, P. Watson, S. Hedges, and T. Wallis.** 1997. A secreted effector protein of *Salmonella dublin* is translocated into eukaryotic cells and mediates inflammation and fluid secretion in in-fected ileal mucosa. *Mol. Microbiol.* **25:**903–912.

29. **Gewirtz, A., A. Rao, P. Simon, D. Merlin, D. Carnes, J. Madara, and A. Neish.** 2000. *Salmonella typhimurium* induces epithelial IL-8 ex-pression via Ca^{+2}-mediated activation of the NF-κB pathway. *J. Clin. Invest.* **105:**79–92.

30. **Hacker, J., and J. Kaper.** 2000. Pathogenicity islands and the evolution of microbes. *Annu. Rev. Microbiol.* **54:**641–679.

31. **Hardt, W.-D., and J. Galan.** 1997. A secreted *Salmonella* protein with homology to an aviru-lence determinant of plant pathogenic bacteria. *Proc. Natl. Acad. Sci. USA* **94:**9887–9892.

32. **Heissmeyer, V., D. Krappmann, E. Hatada, and C. Scheidereit.** 2001. Shared pathways of IκB kinase-induced SCF (beta-TrCP)-mediated ubiquitination and degradation for the NF-κB precursor p105 and IκB alpha. *Mol. Cell. Biol.* **21:**1024–1035.

33. **Hobbie, S., L. Chen, R. Davis, and J. Galan.** 1997. Involvement of mitogen-activated protein kinase pathways in the nuclear responses and cy-tokine production induced by *Salmonella typhi-murium* in cultured intestinal epithelial cells. *J. Immunol.* **159:**5550–5559.

34. **Hoffman, J., F. Kafatos, C. Janeway, and R. Ezekowitz.** 1999. Phylogenetic perspectives in innate immunity. *Science* **284:**1313–1318.

35. **Hooper, L., L. Bry, P. Falk, and J. Gordon.** 1998. Host-microbial symbiosis in the mamma-lian intestine: exploring an internal ecosystem. *BioEssays* **20:**336–343.

36. **Hooper, L., and J. Gordon.** 2001. Commensal host-bacterial relationships in the gut. *Science* **292:**1115–1118.

37. **Hooper, L., M. Wong, A. Thelin, L. Hans-son, P. Falk, and J. Gordon.** 2001. Molecular analysis of commensal host-microbial relation-ships in the intestine. *Science* **291:**881–884.

38. **Jobin, C., and R. Sartor.** 2000. The IκB/NF-κB system; a key determinant for mucosal inflammation and protection. *Am. J. Physiol.* **278:**451–462.

39. **Karin, M.** 1999. The beginning of the end: IκB kinase (IKK) and NF-κB activation. *J. Biol. Chem.* **274:**27339–27342.

40. **Karin, M., and Y. Ben-Neriah.** 2000. Phosphorylation meets ubiquitination: the control of NF-κB activity. *Annu. Rev. Immunol.* **18:**621–663.

41. **Klumpp, D., A. Weiser, S. Sengupta, S. Forrestal, R. Batler, and A. Schaeffer.** 2001. Uropathogenic *Escherichia coli* potentiates type 1 pilus-induced apoptosis by suppressing NF-κB. *Infect. Immun.* **69:**6689–6695.

42. **Kopp, E., and S. Ghosh.** 1995. NF-κB and Rel proteins in innate immunity. *Adv. Immunol.* **58:**1–12.

43. **Kunsch, C., and C. Rosen.** 1993. NF-κB subunit-specific regulation of the interleukin-8 promoter. *Mol. Cell. Biol.* **13:**6137–6146.

44. **Lee, C., M. Silva, A. Siber, A. Kelly, E. Galyov, and B. McCormick.** 2000. A secreted *Salmonella* protein induces a proinflammatory response in epithelial cells, which promotes neutrophil migration. *Proc. Natl. Acad. Sci. USA* **97:**12283–12288.

45. **Lemaitre, B., E. Nicolas, L. Michaut, J.-M. Reichart, and J. Hoffman.** 1996. The dorsoventral regulatory gene cassette spatzle/Toll/cactus controls the potent antifungal response in *Drosophila* adults. *Cell* **86:**973–983.

46. **Looney, R., and R. Steigbigel.** 1986. Role of the Vi antigen of *Salmonella typhi* in resistance to host defense in vitro. *J. Lab. Clin. Med.* **108:**506–516.

47. **Maniatis, T.** 1999. A ubiquitin ligase complex essential for the NF-κB, Wnt/wingless, and hedgehog signalling pathways. *Genes Dev.* **13:**505–510.

48. **Masden, K., J. S. Doyle, L. D. Jewell, M. M. Tavernini, and R. N. Fedorak.** 1999. *Lactobacillus* sp. prevents olitis in interleukin-10 gene deficient mice. *Gastroenterology* **116:**1107–1114.

49. **May, M., and S. Ghosh.** 1999. IκB kinases: kinsmen with different crafts. *Science* **284:**271–273.

50. **Mozaffarian, N., A. Casadevall, and J. Berman.** 2000. Inhibition of human endothelial cell chemokine production by the opportunistic fungal pathogen *Cryptococcus neoformans. J. Immunol.* **165:**1541–1547.

51. **Neish, A., A. Gewirtz, H. Zeng, A. Young, M. Hobert, V. Karmali, A. Rao, and J. Madara.** 2000. Prokaryotic regulation of epithelial responses by inhibition of IκB-α ubiquitination. *Science* **289:**1560–1563.

52. **Oie, K., and D. Pickup.** 2001. Cowpox virus and other members of the orthopoxvirus group interfere with the regulation of NF-κB activation. *Virology* **288:**175–187.

53. **Orth, K., L. Palmer, Z. Bao, S. Stewart, A. Rudolph, J. Bliska, and J. Dixon.** 1999. Inhibition of the mitogen-activated protein kinase kinase superfamily by a *Yersinia* effector. *Science* **285:**1920–1923.

54. **Orth, K., Z. Xu, M. Mudgett, Z. Bao, L. Palmer, J. Bliska, W. Mangel, B. Staskawicz, and J. Dixon.** 2000. Disruption of signaling by *Yersinia* effector YopJ, a ubiquitin-like protein protease. *Science* **290:**1594–1597.

55. **Palmer, L., A. Pancetti, S. Greenberg, and J. Bliska.** 1999. YopJ of *Yersinia* spp. is sufficient to cause downregulation of multiple mitogen-activated protein kinases in eukaryotic cells. *Infect. Immun.* **67:**708–716.

56. **Palombella, V., O. Rando, A. Goldberg, and T. Maniatis.** 1994. The ubiquitin-proteasome pathway is required for processing the NF-κB1 precursor protein and the activation of NF-κB. *Cell* **78:**773–785.

57. **Powell, P., L. Dixon, and R. Parkhouse.** 1996. An IκB homolog encoded by African swine fever virus provides a novel mechanism for downregulation of proinflammatory cytokine responses in host macrophages. *J. Virol.* **70:**8527–8533.

58. **Read, M., J. Brownell, T. Gladysheva, M. Hottelet, L. Parent, M. Coggins, J. Pierce, V. Podust, R.-S. Luo, V. Chau, and J. Palombella.** 2000. Nedd8 modification of Cul-1 activates SCF-β-TrCP-dependent ubiquitination of IκBa. *Mol. Cell. Biol.* **20:**2326–2333.

59. **Read, M., A. Neish, F. Luscinskas, V. Palombella, T. Maniatis, and T. Collins.** 1995. The proteosome pathway is required for cytokine-induced endothelial-leukocyte adhesion molecule expression. *Immunity* **2:**493–505.

60. **Revilla, Y., M. Callejo, J. Rodriguez, E. Culebras, M. Nogal, M. Salas, E. Vinulea, and M. Fresno.** 1998. Inhibition of nuclear factor κB activation by a virus-encoded IκB-like protein. *J. Biol. Chem.* **273:**5405–5411.

61. **Rosenberger, C., A. Pollard, and B. Finlay.** 2001. Gene array technology to determine host responses to *Salmonella. Microbes Infect.* **3:**1353–1360.

62. **Ruckdeschel, K., O. Mannel, K. Richter, C. Jacobi, K. Trulzsch, B. Rouot, and J. Heesemann.** 2001. Yersinia outer protein P of *Yersinia enterocolitica* simultaneously blocks the nuclear factor-κB pathway and exploits lipopolysac-

charide signaling to trigger apoptosis in macrophages. *J. Immunol.* **166:**1823–1831.

63. **Sangari, F., M. Petrofsky, and L. Bermudez.** 1999. *Mycobacterium avium* infection of epithelial cells results in inhibition or delay in the release of interleukin-8 and RANTES. *Infect. Immun.* **67:**5069–5075.

64. **Schesser, K., A.-K. Spiik, J.-M. Dukuzumuremyi, M. Neurath, S. Petterson, and H. Wolf-Watz.** 1998. The yopJ locus is required for *Yersinia*-mediated inhibition of the NF-kappaB activation and cytokine expression: YopJ contains a eukaryotic SH2-like domain that is essential for its repressive activity. *Mol. Microbiol.* **28:**1067–1079.

65. **Schwartz, A., and A. Ciechanover.** 1999. The ubiquitin-proteasome pathway and pathogenesis of human diseases. *Annu. Rev. Med.* **50:** 57–74.

66. **Senfteben, U., Y. Cao, G. Xiao, F. Greten, G. Krahn, G. Bonnizzi, Y. Chen, Y. Hu, A. Fong, S.-C. Sun, and M. Karin.** 2001. Activation by IKKα of a second evolutionary conserved, NF-κB signaling pathway. *Science* **293:** 1495–1499.

67. **Sha, W., H. Liou, E. Tuomanen, and D. Baltimore.** 1995. Targeted disruption of the p50 subunit of NF-kappa B leads to multifocal defects in immune responses. *Cell* **80:**321–330.

68. **Silverman, N., and T. Maniatis.** 2001. NF-κB signaling pathways in mammalian and insect immunity. *Genes Dev.* **15:**2321–2342.

69. **Spencer, E., J. Jiang, and Z. Chen.** 1999. Signal induced ubiquitination of IκBα by the F-box protein slimb/β-TrCP. *Genes Dev.* **13:**284–294.

70. **Thanos, D., and T. Maniatis.** 1995. NF-κB: a lesson in family values. *Cell* **80:**529–532.

71. **Varel, V.** 1987. Activity of fiber degrading microorganisms in the pig large intestine. *J. Anim. Sci.* **65:**488–496.

72. **Viprey, V., A. Del Greco, W. Golinowski, W. Broughton, and X. Perret.** 1998. Symbiotic implications of type III protein secretion machinery in *Rhizobium. Mol. Microbiol.* **28:**1381–1389.

73. **Wang, C., L. Deng, M. Hong, G. Akkaraju, J.-I. Inoue, and Z. Chen.** 2001. Tak1 is a ubiquitin-dependent kinase of MKK and IKK. *Nature* **412:**346–351.

74. **Wang, C.-Y., M. Mayo, R. Korneluk, D. Goeddel, and A. Baldwin.** 1998. NF-κB antiapoptosis: induction of TRAF1 and TRAF2 and c-IAP1 and c-IAP2 to suppress caspase-8 activation. *Science* **281:**1680–1683.

75. **Wilkinson, F.** 1997. Regulation of ubiquitin-dependent processes by deubiquitinating enzymes. *FASEB J.* **11:**1245–1256.

76. **Wilson, K.** 1995. The gastrointestinal microflora, p. 607–615. *In* T. Yamada (ed.), *Textbook of Gastroenterology,* vol. 1. J. P. Lippincott, Philadelphia, Pa.

77. **Wilson, M., R. Seymour, and B. Henderson.** 1998. Bacterial perturbation of cytokine networks. *Infect. Immun.* **66:**2401–2409.

78. **Winston, J., P. Strack, P. Beer-Romero, C. Chu, S. Elledge, and J. Harper.** 1999. The SCF β-TRCP-ubiquitin ligase complex associates specifically with phosphorylated destruction motifs in IκBα and β-catenin and stimulates IκBα ubiquitination *in vitro. Genes Dev.* **13:**270–283.

79. **Yeh, E., L. Gong, and T. Kamitani.** 2000. Ubiquitin-like proteins: new wines in new bottles. *Gene* **248:**1–14.

80. **Yuk, M. H., E. Harvill, P. Cotter, and J. F. Miller.** 2000. Modulation of host immune responses, induction of apoptosis and inhibition of NF-κB activation by the *Bordetella* type III secretion system. *Mol. Microbiol.* **35:**991–1004.

ANTIMICROBIAL PEPTIDE EFFECTORS OF SMALL INTESTINAL INNATE IMMUNITY

Andre J. Ouellette and Michael E. Selsted

12

The lining of the mammalian small intestine consists of a monolayer of epithelial cells that establishes a physical barrier between the contents of the lumen and the circulation. That epithelial sheet forms the largest surface at which any organism is exposed to its external environment. To maximize membrane surface area and facilitate nutrient absorption from the intestinal lumen, the small intestine evolved villus projections and the brush border that characterizes the apical membranes of absorptive enterocytes (chapter 1, this volume). The lumen from which nutrients are absorbed, however, is also occupied by a resident commensal microflora (80), and microorganisms that are ingested represent a continual infectious challenge to the epithelial barrier. In this setting, the small bowel must provide environmental conditions that support nutrient absorption and water and electrolyte homeostasis while preventing most microbes from becoming significant resident populations (68). Although the anatomic features that optimize the absorptive area appear to favor mucosal colonization by the microflora, the number of bacteria in the small intestine is relatively few compared to those in the cecum and colon (231, 232). This fact suggests that there are mechanisms at work in the small intestine that counter microbial colonization of the epithelial lining.

The activities that contribute to the low microbial count of the small intestine are complex and interacting. The varied factors include the digestive, mucous, and immune secretions of the gastrointestinal (GI) tract; acquired immune responses such as secretion of immunoglobulin A (IgA); the release of microbicidal molecules by resident bacteria; the cell dynamics of the continually regenerating gut epithelium; and gene-encoded antimicrobial peptides and proteins that are released by epithelial cells. In this chapter, we consider and review evidence that α-defensins secreted by mucosal Paneth cells contribute to innate immunity against bacteria in the small intestine.

ANTIMICROBIAL PEPTIDES

Growing experimental evidence has led to acceptance of the concept that species produce antimicrobial peptides constitutively or inducibly in response to infection (260). Partly, this evidence has come from the purification of

Andre J. Ouellette and Michael E. Selsted, Department of Pathology and Department of Microbiology and Molecular Genetics, College of Medicine, University of California, Irvine, CA 92697-4800.

peptides with antimicrobial activities from every species investigated, including insects, arachnids, horseshoe crabs and other crustaceans, fish, birds, mollusks, frogs, and many mammalian species, including humans (57, 116–118) (Table 1). Invariably, the isolated molecules exhibit microbicidal peptide activity when assayed in vitro. In species that lack clonal immune mechanisms, microbial infection or antigens stimulate transcriptional activation of target cell-specific proteins and peptides via highly conserved receptor-mediated signaling pathways (94, 234). Once released, those molecules act rapidly to neutralize invading microbes. Genetic studies in mice now confirm that certain of these molecules confer protection against microbial colonization and invasion in mammalian skin and gut (43, 153, 249).

In mammals, antimicrobial proteins and peptide genes are expressed by varied differentiated cell lineages, including epithelial cells and phagocytes (118). In cells of myeloid origin, the peptides are stored in granules and mediate nonoxidative bacterial cell killing after phagocytosis and phagolysosomal fusion (60, 119, 128, 150, 183, 209, 213). In the airway, skin, oropharynx, gingival crevice, urogenital epithelium, and gastrointestinal tract, epithelial cells release peptides to function on those diverse mucosal surfaces (117, 118, 206). Some of these peptides appear to be expressed and released constitutively, and others are induced upon exposure to bacterial antigens for release by apparently similar mechanisms. Still additional peptides may accumulate in secretory granules for later release as components of regulated exocytotic pathways, as occurs in Paneth cells. The general features of antimicrobial peptide biology have been reviewed comprehensively (260).

ANTIMICROBIAL PEPTIDE STRUCTURE

Antimicrobial peptides range from linear, α-helical molecules to dicyclic, β-sheet-containing peptides that contain up to four disulfide bonds and have no α-helical component (Table 1). Because antimicrobial peptides elaborated by different species have conserved structural motifs rather than identical primary structures, this broad class of molecules has generally been categorized according to their biochemical composition or on the basis of secondary structures as (i) linear, random coil peptides that adopt α-helical structure and amphipathicity in hydrophobic environments, (ii) β-sheet-containing peptides stabilized by one or more disulfide bonds, (iii) linear non-α-helical peptides that frequently contain high levels of one or more amino acids, and (iv) peptides that are less amenable to such classifications (Table 1). Despite their diverse primary, secondary, and tertiary structures, most microbicidal peptides are amphipathic (87, 137, 250, 258), and it is their amphipathicity that confers an ability to interact with and selectively disrupt microbial cell membranes (85, 215, 246). It is generally accepted that peptide-mediated membrane disruption creates defects that dissipate the electrochemical gradients of the microbial cell and lead to its eventual death.

DEFENSINS: THREE FAMILIES OF CYSTEINE-RICH ANTIMICROBIAL PEPTIDES

The defensins were among the first antimicrobial peptide families to be described (120, 207). In mammals, the term defensin applies to three families of cationic, cysteine-rich antimicrobial peptides, the α-, β-, and θ-defensins (Fig. 1). α- and β-defensin molecules are cationic peptides of 3 to 4 kDa molecular weight with six cysteine residues that pair invariantly to form distinctive tridisulfide arrays that are characteristic of each peptide subfamily (118). The α-defensins are major constituents of azurophilic granules in mammalian phagocytic leukocytes, and they are released by a limited number of epithelial cell lineages. Accounting for 5 to 18% of total cellular protein in neutrophils, α-defensins are estimated to reach concentrations of $\sim$10 mg/ml as granules dissolve in phagolysosomes following ingestion of microorganisms (60). The

TABLE 1 Representative antimicrobial peptides from plants and animals[a]

Peptide	Primary structure	References
α-Helical		
Cecropin A	KWKLFKKIEKVGQNIRDGIIKAGPAVAVVGQATQIAK*a*	88, 224
Magainin 2	GIGKFLHSAKKFGKAFVGEIMNS	261
Dermaseptin 1	ALWKTMLKKLGTMALHAGKAALGAAADTISQGTQ	144
LL-37	LLGDFFRKSKEKIGKEFKRIVQRIKDFLRNLVPRTES	1, 16
1 Disulfide bond		
Bactenecin 1	RLCRIVVIRVCR	259
Thanatin	GSKKPVPIIYCNRRTGKCQRM	49
Brevinin 1T	VNPIILGVLPKVCLITKKC	110
Ranalexin	FLGGLIKIVPAMICAVTKKC	33
2 Disulfide bonds		
Tachyplesin 1	RWC$_1$FRVC$_2$YRGIC$_2$YRKC$_1$R*a*	148
Androctonin	RSVC$_1$RQIKIC$_2$RRRGGC$_2$YYKC$_1$TNRPY	129
Protegrin 1	RGGRLC$_1$YC$_2$RRRFC$_2$VC$_1$VGR*a*	105
3 Disulfide bonds		
α-Defensin, HNP-2	C$_1$YC$_2$RIPAC$_3$IAGERRYGTC$_2$IYQGRLWAFC$_3$C$_1$	60
β-Defensin, BNBD-4	QRVRNPQSC$_1$RWNMGVC$_2$IPFLC$_3$RVGMRQIGTC$_2$FGPRVPC$_1$C$_3$RR	212
θ-Defensin, RTD-1	GFC$_1$RC$_2$LC$_3$RRGVC$_3$RC$_2$IC$_1$TR[b]	230
Sapecin A	ATC$_1$DLLSGTGINHSAC$_2$AAHC$_3$LLRGNRGGYC$_2$NGKAVC$_3$VC$_1$RN	109, 136
Thionin (crambin)	TTC$_1$C$_2$PSIVARSNFNVC$_3$RIPGTPEAIC$_3$ATYTGC$_2$IIIPGATC$_1$PGDYAN	109
4 Disulfide bonds		
Radish defensin	QKLC$_1$QRPSGTWSGVC$_2$GNNNAC$_3$KNQC$_4$IRLEKARHGSC$_2$NYVFPAHC$_3$IC$_4$YFPC$_1$	235, 236
Drosomycin	DC$_1$LSGRYKGPC$_2$AVWDNETC$_3$RRVC$_4$KEEGRSSGHC$_2$SPSLKC$_3$WC$_4$EGC$_1$	111, 151
Hepcidin	DTHFPIC$_1$IFC$_2$C$_3$GC$_4$C$_1$HRSKC$_2$GMC$_3$C$_4$KT	170
Linear, nonhelical		
Bac5	RFRPPIRRPPIRPPFYPPFRPPIRPPIFPPIRPPFRPPLGRPFP*a*	257, 259
PR-39	RRRPRPPYLPRPRPPPFFPPRLPPRIPPGFPPRFPPRFP*a*	2
Indolicidin	ILPWKPWWPWRR*a*	211
Apidaecin	GNNRPVYIPQPRPPHPRI	30
Pyrrhocoricin	VDKGSYLPRPTPPRPIYNRN	160
Histatin 5	DSHAKRHHGYKRKFHEKHHSHRGY	159

[a] Excerpted from reference 260, with permission. *a*, amide.
[b] Macrocyclic peptide. No free N or C terminus.

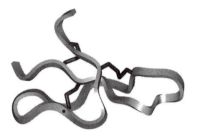

α-defensin monomer
rabbit RK-1

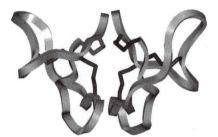

α-defensin dimer
human HNP-3

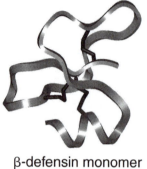

β-defensin monomer
human hBD-1

θ-defensin monomer
rhesus RTD-1

FIGURE 1 Structures of α-, β-, and θ-defensins. The backbone and disulfide structures are shown of RK-1 (upper left), a monomeric rabbit α-defensin (169, 262); HNP-3 (upper right), a dimeric human α-defensin; hBD-1 (lower left), a monomeric human β-defensin; and RTD-1 (lower right), a θ-defensin from rhesus macaque.

β-defensins, discovered in cattle as antimicrobial peptides of neutrophil granules and of airway and lingual epithelial cells (41, 205, 212), exist in several mammalian and avian species and are expressed by a greater variety of epithelial cell types than α-defensins (206). For example, β-defensin peptides or transcripts have been detected in human kidney, skin, pancreas, gingiva, tongue, esophagus, salivary gland, cornea, and airway epithelium and in epithelial cells of a number of species (14, 15, 55, 58, 66, 73, 74, 95, 96, 107, 108, 127, 134, 138, 157, 158, 212, 244, 265). The θ-defensins, RTD-1-3, are macrocyclic peptides of 2-kDa molecular mass that were isolated from neutrophils and monocytes of the rhesus

macaque (122, 230, 240). RTD-1 is a covalently closed circular polypeptide chain of 18 amino acids that is stabilized by three disulfide bonds (Fig. 1). RTD-1 biosynthesis is unusual because the peptide assembles from two distinct precursor molecules, with each precursor contributing a 9-amino-acid moiety to the final RTD-1 peptide. The half-precursors are products of two different genes that contain three exons and resemble all known myeloid α-defensin genes, except that they are truncated by stop codons in exon 3. The homodimeric θ-defensins, RTD-2 and -3, have also been isolated from monkey neutrophils (122, 240), and their presence at 15- to 30-fold lower concentrations than RTD-1 suggests that θ-defensin assembly favors heterodimer formation (240). The mechanisms that catalyze or facilitate θ-defensin assembly in monkeys are not understood (230).

DEFENSIN STRUCTURE

The 3- to 4-kDa α- and β-defensins both contain six cysteine residues that form specific and invariant disulfide bond pairings (208, 229). Although the spacing of the cysteine residues and Cys-Cys pairings of disulfide bonds in α- and β-defensins differs, the peptides have remarkably similar folded conformations (169, 222, 264). The folded conformation of the α-defensins consists of three β-strands and no α-helical content. This highly constrained tertiary structure is required for antimicrobial activity (77, 115, 209). The crystal structure of the human neutrophil α-defensin HNP-3 is a noncovalent, amphipathic dimer in which arginine side chains lie equatorially above a hydrophobic surface consisting of apolar monomer side chains (77). The amino and carboxyl termini of the monomers are clustered on the pole of the dimer opposite the hydrophobic face. Evidence for dimeric (or multimeric) structure of HNP-1 in solution was provided by nuclear magnetic resonance (NMR) experiments (169, 262) and by the immunoreactivity of HNP-1 in a sandwich immunoassay in which the capture and detecting monoclonal antibodies were directed toward similar or identical epitopes (167). The solution structures of α-defensins from rabbit neutrophils and kidney are monomeric (168, 222). As described below, these structural differences are associated with major differences in the mechanisms by which these peptides interact with reconstituted model membranes.

Solution and crystallographic analyses of β-defensins have disclosed the similarity of the α- and β-defensin folds, as well as the amphipathic structures produced by the spatial partitioning of polar and hydrophilic side chains on the peptide surfaces. The folds of human β-defension 1 (hBD-1) and -2 are similar to each other and to bovine β-defensin

12 (82, 83, 202, 264); all three consist predominantly of a triple-stranded β-sheet. Both hBD-1 and -2 possess short α-helical segments. The crystal structure of hBD-2 is dimeric, though the interfacial contacts are dissimilar to those of the α-defensin HNP-3 (77). Moreover, certain hBD-2 crystal forms are oligomeric, as octamers organized through interactions of the amino termini of monomers (83). However, solution structural studies demonstrated that hBD-2 is monomeric at acidic and near-neutral pH (202). Similarly, no hBD-1 quaternary structure was observed in crystals of this peptide. To date, other than the finding that β-defensins possess microbicidal rather than microbistatic properties in vitro, there are few experimental data regarding the mechanism(s) of β-defensin antimicrobial action, and the role of oligomerization in the action of these peptides is unresolved. To date, no tertiary structural information has been reported for human β-defensins 3 and 4.

The solution structure of RTD-1, predicted by Tang et al. to be a double-hairpin β-sheet (230), was confirmed by NMR spectroscopy experiments (239) to exist as an elongated macrocycle (239). The solution structure demonstrates the flexibility of the peptide center, and the overall lack of amphiphilicity distinguishes θ-defensin structures from those of α- and β-defensins. Of note, unlike most α- and β-defensins, RTD-1 is potently bactericidal in the presence of increasing ionic strength, whereas the activity of (synthetic) acyclic RTD-1 was completely inhibited by physiologic NaCl (230, 240). Thus, peptide circularization in vitro confers salt insensitivity to the peptides in a manner that superficially resembles the salt-insensitivity of natural, circularized θ-defensin family peptides from rhesus macaque neutrophils. When the normally salt-sensitive rabbit neutrophil α-defensins were chemically converted to circularized structures, certain analogs retained defensin-like architecture and were active against *Escherichia coli* and *Salmonella enterica* serovar Typhimurium at NaCl concentrations that inhibit the parent NP-1 molecule (256). It will be of interest to learn whether chemical circularization will become a widely applicable means of improving the activities of peptides for applications under physiologic conditions.

MECHANISMS OF MICROBIAL CELL KILLING BY α-DEFENSINS

α-Defensins are generally microbicidal against gram-positive and gram-negative bacteria, certain fungi, spirochetes, protozoa, and enveloped viruses, although it is important to recognize that single amino acid substitutions may alter the target cell specificity of individual peptides (6). Human neutrophil peptides permeabilize the outer and inner membranes of *E. coli* sequentially, and these peptides induce the formation of ion channels in lipid bilayers (115). Both of these peptide-elicited effects are influenced by membrane energetics (60).

The α-defensins from human and rabbit neutrophils achieve bacterial cell killing by distinctive membrane disruptive mechanisms. As noted above, the higher-ordered structures of human and rabbit-human neutrophil α-defensins differ in that human HNP-2 is a noncovalent dimer and rabbit NP-1 is monomeric (77, 169). The dimeric HNP-2 forms stable, 20-Å multimeric pores after insertion into model membranes (250), and a pore model in which six HNP-2 dimers intercalate in the bilayer to form the pore annulus has been proposed based on leakage studies with large unilamellar vesicles (246). In contrast to this stable pore, monomeric NP-1 does not induce stable multimeric pores but permeabilizes the membrane by creating large, short-lived defects in model phospholipid bilayers (86). These findings show that a detailed understanding of the mechanisms by which the mouse and human Paneth cell α-defensins achieve microbial cell killing cannot be extrapolated from other systems and that specific peptides need to be investigated directly.

THE BIOLOGY OF THE INTESTINAL EPITHELIUM

In mammals, the intestinal epithelium is renewed continually throughout the lifetime of the individual (31). Four primary epithelial cell lineages—absorptive enterocytes, goblet cells, enteroendocrine cells, and Paneth cells—are generated daily from stem cell populations that occupy every small intestinal crypt (67, 221). Over a life cycle of 2 to 5 days, depending on the species, the progeny of crypt epithelial stem cells emerge from the proliferative zone, migrate to the villus tip, apoptose, and exfoliate into the lumen (31). In contrast to those upwardly mobile enterocyte lineages, Paneth cell progenitors differentiate as they descend from the stem cell zone toward the base of the crypt (20). In contrast to the short-lived enterocytes that populate the villi, Paneth cells have lifetimes of 20 days or more (31). The epithelial lining, therefore, is a dynamic structure characterized by continually differentiating cell populations that migrate along the crypt-villus axis, and innate immune mechanisms that protect the epithelium from microbial colonization must be viewed within that context.

Lesions in the intestinal epithelial cell monolayer induced by toxic insults, infections, or episodes of inflammation must be repaired, or the disrupted barrier may provide portals of entry for pathogens or opportunistic microbes. Acquired immune responses of intraepithelial T lymphocytes, B cells, gut-associated lymphoid tissue, M cells, and myeloid and lymphoid cells in the lamina propria as well as barriers to paracellular trafficking formed by physical connections between enterocytes all contribute to maintaining mucosal integrity. Increasing evidence shows that activated lymphocytes communicate with epithelial cells to influence phenotype and modify epithelial differentiation programs (7, 101), showing that the cellular components of acquired and innate immunity interact rather than function as separate compartments (4). The polypeptide mediators of intestinal host defense that derive from intestinal epithelial cells will now be described, and the role of those gene products in mucosal immunity will be considered.

The mammalian gut commits extensive energy to clonal immune responses to microbial and dietary antigens. For example, B-cell-mediated humoral immunity via secretory IgA transport across enterocytes to the gut lumen is considered to be vital to small intestinal host defense. This is evident from the protective effects of specific IgA introduced into mice, particularly against enteric viruses (76, 106, 141, 185, 220). Induction of anticommensal secretory IgA by this pathway is antigen driven, requires an intestinal microflora and B-cell-containing lymphoid aggregates, and represents a specific T-cell-independent response of the normal mucosa to commensals (126). Although specific IgA deficiency is the most common immune deficiency in humans, the defect is not usually associated with illness, suggesting that other mechanisms compensate or that additional challenges to the immune system are required to establish disease (36). Intraepithelial T lymphocytes also reside in the villi interspersed among enterocytes and function in cell-mediated immunity (61). Acquired immune responses to infectious agents mediated by T cells and B cells are initiated by specific antigens and are selective, but lymphocytic responses may not be rapid enough to contain acute infections by rapidly growing microorganisms or by pathogens that infect a naïve host (23, 24).

Activities or conditions that are associated with digestion and the normal physiology of the gastrointestinal tract are likely to inhibit the growth of bacteria in the small intestine. Gastric acidity, digestive enzymes and pancreatic secretions, bile salts, peristalsis and the migrating motor complex, mucus, the resident commensal flora, and exfoliation of enterocytes during epithelial renewal are general and nonspecific factors that deter the growth of microbial populations in the small intestine (89, 161). However, the varied intestinal epithelial cell lineages also contribute to innate enteric host defenses by forming physical and biochemical barriers to colonization.

Absorptive enterocytes, goblet cells, and Paneth cells of the small intestine elaborate lineage-specific gene products or exhibit activities that contribute to enteric host defense.

For example, intestinal goblet cells secrete mucins that help to establish a mucopolysaccharide complex that forms a physical polymeric barrier to microbial attachment and colonization (130, 146). Goblet cells also secrete intestinal trefoil factor (mTFF3), a peptide with three intramolecular disulfide bonds that form a trefoil-like motif (103, 178, 225, 237). Secretion of mTFF3 is implicated in colonic barrier function, because mTFF3-deficient mice develop inflammatory bowel disease and megacolon, and they become immunocompromised when challenged with irritants to the bowel lining such as dextran sodium sulfate (132, 133, 238). In addition to transcytosis of secretory IgA, absorptive enterocytes are also capable of contributing to mucosal immunity by producing antimicrobial peptides. In vitro studies show that cultured human intestinal epithelial cell lines produce the human β-defensin hBD-1 constitutively and selectively upregulate production of hBD-2 in response to specific bacterial species (157, 158). Studies of intact villi ex vivo, though, have shown that villus enterocytes do not release detectable bactericidal peptide activity in response to bacterial cell exposure (11).

ANTIMICROBIAL PROTEINS AND PEPTIDES IN THE GASTROINTESTINAL TRACT

Evidence shows that expression of antimicrobial peptides in the gastrointestinal tract has been conserved in evolution. In mosquitos and flesh flies, blood meals upregulate insect defensin gene expression in the midgut (42, 78, 114). Magainin, the major endogenous antimicrobial peptide of Xenopus skin, is also found in specialized cells in the stomach and in glandular cells at the base of folds in the frog intestine (182). In goats, expression of β-defensin precursors preproGBD-1 and -2 has specific patterns of mucosal tissue distribution, with the former expressed principally in the tongue and respiratory tract, and the latter occurring mainly in the intestine (263). Expression of GI tract β-defensins has been reported in ruminants (90, 91). Human colonic epithelial cell lines HT-29 and Caco-2 express hBD-1 mRNA constitutively and induce hBD-2 expression when exposed to interleukin-1 alpha (IL-1α) or when infected with enteroinvasive bacteria (158). Human fetal intestinal xenografts express hBD-1 constitutively but not hBD-2, and intraluminal infection of xenografts with *Salmonella* spp. activates hBD-2 mRNA accumulation, but hBD-1 mRNA levels are not affected (158). In the colonic and gastric epithelium, hBD-2 expression is induced in response to inflammation and *Helicobacter pylori* infection, respectively (157, 158). Also, the colonic, but not small intestinal, epithelium expresses the human cathelicidin family peptide LL-37, and levels of the peptide were markedly higher in biopsies of patients with colonic inflammation (75). The colonic mucosa also upregulates β-defensin synthesis in cattle that are acutely infected with *Cryptococcus neoformans* (233). These findings show that the enteric epithelium elaborates some form of microbicidal peptide in every species investigated, even though the species may differ with respect to the particular antimicrobial peptide that is produced. In the small intestine, α-defensins secreted by Paneth cells constitute a major source of antimicrobial peptide activity.

PANETH CELLS

Paneth cells occupy the base of the crypts of Lieberkühn in the small intestine of most mammals, and the high concentrations of α-defensins in the apically directed secretory granules of these cells implicate them in mucosal immunity (174). A small number of Paneth cells populate every crypt in the small intestine of most mammals, and their abundant and characteristic secretory products accumulate as they descend to the base of the crypt (19). Paneth cell distribution is restricted to the small intestine except in carcinoma or during inflammation such as Barrett's esophagus, Crohn's disease, gastritis, autism, and ulcerative colitis (5, 51, 84, 135, 188, 189, 226). Differentiation does not require the presence of luminal bacteria or dietary components, be-

cause histologically normal Paneth cells develop under germfree conditions and also from fetal intestinal xenografts in isogenic or nude mice (186, 187, 201, 219, 251). Although Paneth cells in germfree and normally reared mice and rats show morphological differences and administration of fecal enema to germfree mice stimulated Paneth cell degranulation (196, 198, 199), Paneth cells do not require contact with bacteria or bacterial antigens to initiate or complete their lineage differentiation program (10, 27, 46, 143). The discovery of Paneth cell lysozyme (172), a muraminidase that hydrolyzes the peptidoglycan of bacterial cell walls, suggested that these epithelial cells and their products might function in host defense (Table 2). The identification of Paneth cell α-defensins provided further evidence of Paneth cell involvement in innate immunity (44, 210).

ANTIMICROBIAL PROTEINS AND PEPTIDES IN PANETH CELLS

Paneth cell granules are rich in antibiotic proteins and peptides, and release of these granules contributes to mucosal defense (174, 195). For example, the granules of Paneth cells contain lysozyme, secretory phospholipase A$_2$ (sPLA$_2$), α-defensins, xanthine oxidase, DNase, CD15, AE2 anion exchanger, the Lim protein CRIP, and tumor necrosis factor alpha (TNF-α) as components of apically oriented secretory granules (8, 9, 50, 65, 142, 145, 154, 165, 175, 216). Many of these components, as well as those listed in Table 2, have direct antimicrobial activities in vitro, or they are associated with host defense or immune regulation. The knowledge that this complex of granule constituents is released into the lumen of the small intestine suggested that Paneth cells are effectors of innate immunity. Evidence continues to build in support of that hypothesis (174).

α-DEFENSINS IN PANETH CELLS

α-Defensins are abundant granule constituents in neutrophils and Paneth cells (35, 60, 175, 183, 209, 210). In human, rat, and mouse small intestine (Fig. 2), enteric α-defensin

TABLE 2 Paneth cell gene products[a]

Gene product	Subcellular localization	References
Lysozyme	Secretory granules	63, 65
Secretory phospholipase A$_2$	Secretory granules	149, 154, 214, 255
α-Defensins	Secretory granules	10, 165, 175
Immunoglobulin A	Secretory granules	45, 184
Cysteine-rich intestinal peptide	Secretory granules	50
TNF-α	Secretory granules	102, 204, 228
AE2 Cl$^-$/HCO$_3^-$ exchanger	Secretory granules	8
Xanthine dehydrogenase/oxidase	Secretory granules	145
Prostaglandin E2	Secretory granules	203
Trypsin/trypsinogen	Granule associated	21, 22
Laminin receptor	Granule associated	218
Rab3D	Granule associated	156
Phospholipase B/lipase	Granule associated	227
Carboxylic ester hydrolase	Granule associated	3
DNase I	Granule associated	216
CRHSP28	Cytoplasm	71
NADPase	Golgi	171
Glutathione-S-transferase	Cytoplasm	40
Multidrug resistance-associated protein	Basolateral membrane	173
Osteopontin	Granule associated	180
C-type lectin, HIH/PAP, 16-kDa stress protein		32, 112, 131, 191
Protein disulfide isomerase	Endoplasmic reticulum	93, 247
Matrilysin, MMP-7	Secretory granules	248
CD15, Lewis X antigen		9
Fas ligand, CD95 ligand	Secretory granules	113
Metallothionein	Granules	147, 152
α1 E voltage-gated Ca^{2+} channel		69
cAMP-activated Cl$^-$ conductance		241

[a] Excerpted from reference 174, with permission.

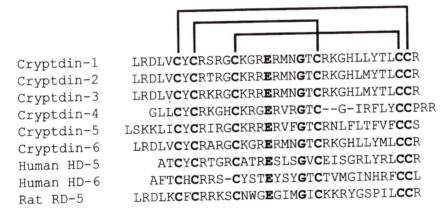

```
Cryptdin-1    LRDLVCYCRSRGCKGRERMNGTCRKGHLLYTLCCR
Cryptdin-2    LRDLVCYCRTRGCKRRERMNGTCRKGHLMYTLCCR
Cryptdin-3    LRDLVCYCRKRGCKRRERMNGTCRKGHLMYTLCCR
Cryptdin-4     GLLCYCRKGHCKRGERVRGTC--G-IRFLYCCPRR
Cryptdin-5    LSKKLICYCRIRGCKRRERVFGTCRNLFLTFVFCCS
Cryptdin-6    LRDLVCYCRARGCKGRERMNGTCRKGHLLYMLCCR
Human HD-5     ATCYCRTGRCATRESLSGVCEISGRLYRLCCR
Human HD-6    AFTCHCRRS-CYSTEYSYGTCTVMGINHRFCCL
Rat RD-5      LRDLKCFCRRKSCNWGEGIMGICKKRYGSPILCCR
```

FIGURE 2 Primary structures of Paneth cell α-defensins. The single letter notation amino acid sequences of mouse cryptdins 1 to 6, human Paneth cell α-defensins HD-5 and HD-6, and rat Paneth cell α-defensin RD-5 were positioned manually to align conserved Cys, Glu, and Gly residues. Dash characters denote spaces introduced to maintain the alignment of conserved amino acids (bolded typeface) that are conserved in all known α-defensin peptides. The cysteine connectivities that characterize the α-defensin tridisulfide array are shown. The HD-5 and HD-6 peptides have been purified from ileal neobladder urine (176), and the RD-5 peptide sequence was deduced from the cDNA sequence and by homology with mouse cryptdin N termini (34).

transcripts and peptides have been localized exclusively to Paneth cells or Paneth cell secretory granules (34, 35, 162, 165, 175, 210). Antibodies to α-defensins HD-5, cryptdin-1, and cryptdin-4 are highly peptide specific, and they react with Paneth cells with specificity (162, 165, 175, 210). In mice, six mouse α-defensin peptides are prevalent in small intestinal Paneth cells, and there are two α-defensins in human Paneth cells (97, 98, 161, 163) (Fig. 2). Levels of individual mouse cryptdins differ, with cryptdins 1, 2, 5, and 6 present at approximately equivalent levels and cryptdins 3 and 4 occurring at lower overall levels (163, 210).

Paneth cell α-defensins have been recovered from luminal rinses of mouse jejunum and ileum (165). Characterized luminal cryptdins include peptides that are identical to the tissue forms of cryptdins 2, 4, and 6, but variants of cryptdins 1, 4, and 6 with amino termini truncated by one or two residues were also purified. In assays of antimicrobial activity against *Staphylococcus aureus*, *E. coli*, and the defensin-sensitive *S. enterica* serovar Typhimurium *phoP*-mutant, the in vitro antibacterial activities of tissue or luminal full-length cryptdins were the same. In general, the N-terminally truncated (des-Leu)-, (des-Leu-Arg)-cryptdin-6, and (des-Gly)-cryptdin-4 peptides had lower overall antimicrobial activities than the corresponding full-length molecules under the conditions of the assays (165). It appears that the N-terminally truncated cryptdin peptides may be generated in the lumen after secretion, and innate enteric immunity may be influenced or modulated by an as yet unknown luminal aminopeptidase(s).

REGULATION OF α-DEFENSIN BIOSYNTHESIS IN PANETH CELLS

Paneth cell defensin genes are closely linked at chromosomal loci with myeloid α-defensin genes. The two human Paneth cell α-defensin genes map to 8p21-8pter, and the mouse genes are syntenic and located on the proximal region of chromosome 8 (164, 223). Charac-

teristically, α-defensin genes have tissue-specific expression patterns, with predominant expression occurring in myeloid cells or in Paneth cells. α-Defensin genes expressed in cells of myeloid origin have three exons, and those genes expressed in Paneth cells have two; examples of α-defensin genes expressed by both cell lineages have not been reported (18, 53, 92, 97, 98, 124). In Paneth cell α-defensin genes, the 5′-untranslated region and the preprosegment are coded by exon 1, but all known myeloid α-defensin and θ-defensin genes contain an additional intron that interrupts the 5′-untranslated region of the transcript (166). In all cases, the most distal exon of α-defensin genes codes for the functional peptide (18, 54, 92, 98, 118, 124). A model for a possible evolutionary history of the human defensin gene family has been proposed (18).

In humans and mice, Paneth cell α-defensin genes are also expressed in reproductive epithelium. Mouse cryptdins have been localized to Sertoli cells and Leydig cells of the testis by immunoperoxidase staining with an anti-cryptdin-1 antibody (70), and cryptdin mRNAs and peptides are also reported to be present in mouse skin (217). Paneth cell α-defensins have been detected in human oropharyngeal and urogenital mucosa (52, 181). Genetic and immunohistochemical experiments have detected the HD-5 peptide in endocervical and vaginal epithelium (181). In rabbit, α-defensins that do not resemble the known rabbit myeloid α-defensins have been purified from kidney (17, 253). Although those findings suggest that the renal epithelium expresses a specific set of α-defensin genes, the rabbit enteric defensins have not been characterized as yet. In the small intestine, α-defensins are specific to Paneth cells (10, 162, 175, 210).

Cryptdin genes are differentially expressed in mouse small intestine. For example, cryptdin-4 is not found in proximal small bowel but occurs at maximal levels in ileal Paneth cells (39, 162). In contrast, the levels of the other known cryptdins are similar throughout the length of the small intestine (39). This differential pattern of cryptdin-4 expression is independent of live bacteria, because the positional specificity is retained in gnotobiotic mice (unpublished). α-Defensin mRNAs accumulate during intestinal development, and their appearance coincides with Paneth cell differentiation during intestinal crypt ontogeny (26, 38). A subset of cryptdin genes are also differentially expressed before Paneth cells are apparent during early postnatal crypt ontogeny in mice (38). The peptides are found in goblet-like cells that are dispersed in the maturing epithelial cell monolayer of the fetal and newborn small intestine (38). The human *HD-5* and *HD-6* genes are expressed in the developing fetus as early as 13.5 weeks of gestation, as detected by reverse transcriptase (RT)-PCR, and their appearance coincides with Paneth cell ontogeny during gestation (127). As in mice (26), the expression of *HD-5* and *HD-6* genes in utero shows that human Paneth cell α-defensin gene activation is independent of infectious stimuli.

ANTIMICROBIAL ACTIVITIES OF PANETH CELL α-DEFENSINS
In vitro, Paneth cell α-defensins display microbicidal activities against a range of microorganisms, including *E. coli, S. enterica* serovar Typhimurium, *Listeria monocytogenes, S. aureus,* and *Giardia lamblia* (6, 44, 163, 177, 210). The bactericidal activity of cryptdin-4 is the most potent of the mouse cryptdins (163). Human Paneth cell HD-5 is active against several bacterial species and also against the fungus *Candida albicans*, and the recombinant HD-5 peptide retains activity even after partial proteolysis, evidence that this peptide could function within the hostile environment of the intestinal lumen (177).

Differential microbicidal activities exhibited by structurally similar mouse cryptdins have suggested structure-activity relationships among these peptides. For example, trophozoites of *G. lamblia* are sensitive to cryptdin-2 and -3 exposure in vitro, but cryptdins 1 and 6 have little to no effect on trophozoite sur-

vival (6). The apparent determinant of that activity is an Arg at residue position 15 in the active cryptdins, in contrast to Gly at residue 15 in the inactive peptides (6). The ability of apically administered cryptdins 2 or 3, but not cryptdin-1 or cryptdins 4 to 6, to elicit reversible, dose-dependent Cl⁻ secretory responses from T84 cell monolayers is another instance of differential cryptdin peptide activities (121, 139). These examples of selective cryptdin isoform activities seem to result from side chain substitutions on surface-accessible residues (166). Structural models of cryptdins 1 to 3 and 6 based on the crystallographic backbone of homologous HNP-3 predict that the side chain at residue position 15 is surface exposed and positioned near a turn in the polypeptide backbone (166). Because membrane phospholipids and cell envelope glycolipids strongly affect peptide:membrane interactions and defensin sensitivity (85), these substitutions may induce topologic differences or otherwise modulate the peptide-membrane interactions and thus effects on target cell envelopes or membrane components.

PANETH CELL DIFFERENTIATION AND ONTOGENY
Mechanisms that regulate Paneth cell maturation and function are essential to understanding the function of α-defensins in innate immunity. The most highly differentiated Paneth cells reside below the stem cell zone at the base of the crypt (26, 68, 252), but cells termed "intermediate," "granulomucous," or "transitional" cells that produce both mucins and contain small electron-dense inclusions in their cytoplasm are also found in crypts (29). Those inclusions are larger than the dense granules of goblet cells but smaller than the apical granules of differentiated Paneth cells (62, 101). In rodents, Paneth cells emerge during cytodifferentiation of the fetal small intestinal endoderm from an intervillous epithelium that leads to crypt ontogeny (26). Paneth cell markers appear in cells in the developing mouse intestinal epithelium early in the differentiation process, including fucosy-

lated and sialylated glycoconjugates, sPLA$_2$, lysozyme, and the matrix metalloproteinase-7 (matrilysin, or MMP-7) (26, 27, 38, 127, 190). With minor differences, the appearance of Paneth cells and their products is the same in germfree and conventionally reared mice, although MMP-7 levels are substantially lower in the germfree state (125). Glycoconjugates that contain terminal α-fucose and are recognized by lectin AAA from *Anguilla anguilla* (27, 79) are more abundant in adult germfree mice than in conventional mice, as shown by levels of AAA staining (27, 68, 81). Colonization of germfree mice with conventional microflora results in a normal AAA staining pattern within 2 weeks. Thus, even though Paneth cell differentiation is independent of the gut microflora, the levels of certain Paneth cell-specific granule components may vary under germfree conditions (81).

PROCESSING AND ACTIVATION OF PANETH CELL α-DEFENSINS

α-Defensin precursors from Paneth cells and neutrophils have similar general features, and they are processed from inactive proforms by specific proteolytic cleavage steps. Both neutrophil and Paneth cell α-defensins derive from ~10-kDa prepropeptides that contain canonical signal sequences, acidic proregions, and an ~3.5-kDa mature α-defensin peptide in the C-terminal portion of the precursor. In cells of myeloid origin, processing of α-defensin precursors occurs within 4 to 24 h after synthesis by sequential events that produce intermediates of 75 and 56 amino acids (59, 140, 242). In mature phagocytic leukocytes, most α-defensins are completely processed (59, 242). Deletions in the prosegment adjacent to the proregion-defensin junction impair posttranslational processing of a human neutrophil pro-α-defensin heterologously expressed in mouse 32DCL3 cells (59). The anionic propeptide segments may also be important for neutralization or folding of the cationic C-terminal defensin peptides, as suggested by the inhibition of α-defensin bactericidal activity in vitro by the addition of intact proregions in *trans* (10, 140, 243). In

humans, several processed forms of HD-5 with varied amino termini have been isolated from postsurgical ileal neobladder urine and from ileal tissue. In ileal neobladder urine, three HD-5 peptides and HD-6 were identified, representing prepro-HD-5 residues 36 to 94 (HD-5$_{36-94}$), HD-5$_{56-94}$, HD-5$_{63-94}$, and HD-6$_{69-100}$ (181). The HD-5$_{63-94}$ peptide is similar to the recombinant HD-5$_{64-94}$ peptide, which has broad-spectrum antimicrobial activity (177). Extracts from washed human ileum contain a major peptide that is immunoreactive with anti-HD5 antiserum, and that ~8-kDa molecule corresponds to HD-5$_{20-94}$, as confirmed by N-terminal protein sequence analysis (35). The same pro-HD-5 molecule was also extracted from isolated human crypts, but HD-5$_{36-94}$, not HD-5$_{20-94}$, was recovered from secretions collected from human crypts. These findings are taken as evidence that human Paneth cells store HD-5 in precursor form that is converted to the mature HD-5 peptide during or after secretion (35, 176). In mice, on the other hand, extensive procryptdin processing takes place intracellularly and prior to secretion.

In mouse Paneth cells, MMP-7 mediates the processing and activation of α-defensins from 8.4-kDa proforms (249). In mouse small intestinal epithelium, MMP-7 is only expressed by Paneth cells where the enzyme is an abundant secretory granule constituent (248). MMP-7 is essential for posttranslational processing of mouse cryptdin precursors to form microbicidal, mature α-defensins (249), and MMP-7-catalyzed cleavage of procryptdins in vitro produces active 3.5-kDa α-defensins by cleaving precursors at conserved sites in the proregion and at the junction of the propeptide and the N terminus of the mature cryptdin peptide (Fig. 3). Conserved internal cleavage sites occur between Ser43 and Val44 in the prosegment and between Ser58 and Leu59, the consensus N terminus for all cryptdin peptides except cryptdins 4 and 5 (10). An additional procryptdin processing site exists between Ser54 and Leu55, as shown by the isolation of corresponding processing intermediates from mouse small intestine (179)

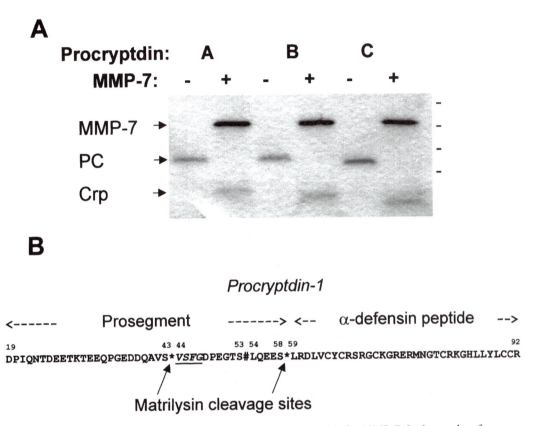

FIGURE 3 Recognition and cleavage of mouse procryptdins by MMP-7. In A, samples of procryptdins A, B, and C were incubated overnight with (+) or without (−) MMP-7, and samples of those digests were resolved electrophoretically and stained. Electrophoretic mobilities of individual components are noted at left in descending order as follows: MMP-7, matrilysin; PC, purified procryptdins; Crp, MMP-7-activated cryptdin peptides. As described in the text, MMP-7 is the activating metalloproteinase for all mouse Paneth cell α-defensins. Dashes at right denote, in descending order, the position of 28-, 18-, 15.6-, and 7.6-kDa molecular size markers. In B, the consensus cleavage sites disclosed by protein sequencing of MMP-7 digests of procryptdins A to C are noted by asterisks (★) that interrupt the procryptdin-1 sequence, and the pound character (#) shows the N terminus of procryptdin intermediates purified from mouse small bowel by Putsep et al. (179) that were not evident in the procryptdin A to C digests. Numerals above the primary structure refer to residue positions, with the initiating Met residue in preprocryptdin-1 as residue #1. Reprinted from reference 10 with permission.

and from in vitro digestion of recombinant procryptdin-4 with MMP-7 (217a). Thus, the mouse procryptdins contain conserved MMP-7-catalyzed processing sites within the precursor prosegment (Fig. 3).

Targeted disruption of the MMP-7 gene results in a measurable impairment in enteric host defense. First, Paneth cells in the small bowel of MMP-7-null mice express cryptdin genes normally and accumulate procryptdins, but the precursors are not processed to mature, bactericidal cryptdin peptides (10, 249). MMP-7-null mice are less effective at clearing noninvasive *E. coli* administered orally, and the mice succumb more rapidly and to lower doses of virulent *S. enterica* serovar Typhimurium (249). Thus, the cryptdin deficiency resulting from a lack of the essential procryptdin processing enzyme is associated with a deficit in mucosal immunity and with an increased risk of systemic disease in vivo.

In mouse small intestine, extensive procryptdin activation occurs in Paneth cells and before secretion into the lumen. Electrophoretic and Western blot analyses of proteins extracted from partially purified Paneth cell granules show that 60 to 70% of the procryptdin pool in the granules have been activated by MMP-7-dependent proteolytic cleavage (10). By immunolocalization, both prosegments and cryptdins occur in secretory granules, and biochemical analyses revealed that Paneth cell granule preparations contain abundant activated cryptdins at levels equivalent to those in intact crypts and extracts of whole intestine (10). As noted previously, human ileum and human crypts contain predominantly proHD-5$_{20-94}$ forms, evidence that pro-α-defensins are processed to functional peptides during or after secretion (35, 176). An alternative and uncharacterized mechanism must convert α-defensin precursors to active peptides in the human small intestine. Although the details of the processing steps have not been elucidated, it seems clear that mouse and human Paneth cells have evolved distinctly different mechanisms for delivering functional α-defensins to the small intestinal lumen.

Procryptdin activation in mice is not sensitive to the presence of the gut microflora. Germfree mice contain less Paneth cell MMP-7 than conventional mice, and colonization of germfree mice with *Bacteroides thetaiotaomicron* stimulates MMP-7 accumulation in Paneth cells to levels found in mice with conventional microflora (125). Because MMP-7 is required for activation of cryptdin precursors (249), it may be reasonable to expect that the extent of procryptdin processing would be modulated as MMP-7 levels change in response to the microflora. However, intestinal protein extracts from conventional and germfree mice contain similar levels of activated cryptdins, and Paneth cells that differentiate in fetal mouse intestinal implants grown subcutaneously also appear to activate cryptdins normally (10). Thus, Paneth cells growing under germfree conditions or free from luminal exposure to bacterial antigens contain sufficient MMP-7 to initiate and complete the conversion of procryptdins to functional peptides. Furthermore, Paneth cell differentiation in mice provides functional cryptdins for secretion, regardless of the luminal microflora.

REGULATION OF PANETH CELL SECRETION

Studies in mice have shown that Paneth cells are responsive to their environment, releasing their secretory granules in response to bacteria and bacterial antigens (Fig. 4). Paneth cell secretion may be stimulated by live or dead gram-negative and gram-positive bacteria and by antigens such as lipopolysaccharide (LPS), lipoteichoic acid, lipid A, and muramyl dipeptide (11). The secretory response to bacteria and LPS is rapid and dose dependent, and it is selective for bacteria, in that crypts do not release peptides when incubated with live fungi or protozoa. The stimulated secretions contain microbicidal peptide activity, and 70% of the bactericidal peptide activity that is released can be neutralized by a polyclonal anti-cryptdin-1 antibody that reacts with cryptdins 1, 2, 3, and 6. In response to the bacterial stimuli, Paneth cells in a single mouse crypt secrete ~360 pg of cryptdin in a discharge consisting of ~100 ng of total protein. That material is released into the crypt lumen, a space calculated to have a volume of ~3 pl per 100 μm of crypt height, to produce a local cryptdin concentration of ~100 mg/ml at secretion (11). Because individual cryptdins have extensive antimicrobial activity in vitro at low μg/ml concentrations, that is, 1 μM or less (44, 162, 163, 165), the release of elicited secretions provides microbicidal peptides to the crypt lumen in vast excess of their minimal bactericidal concentrations. Thus, innate immunity in crypts is an active process and responsive to environmental cues of infection. The receptors for pattern recognition and the signaling pathway(s) associated with the vesicular fusion events that lead to apical secretion remain unknown. These aspects of Paneth cell biology are likely to be relevant to mucosal

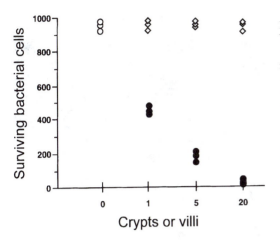

FIGURE 4 Release of microbicidal peptide activity by crypt Paneth cells in response to live bacteria. Crypts (solid circles) or villi (shaded diamonds) were isolated from adult mice and incubated in numbers shown with 10^3 of *S. enterica* serovar Typhimurium CFU for 1 h at 37°C in 50 μl of isotonic buffer. Viable CFU were quantitated by plating the entire mixtures on semisolid nutrient media overnight. Data points show surviving bacteria from individual replicate mixtures. Open circles represent surviving bacteria after incubation of 10^3 CFU for 1 h at 37°C in 50 μl of isotonic buffer in the absence of crypts or villi. As noted in the text, bacteria exposed to crypts die in response to Paneth cell secretions (11), but equivalent exposure to villus epithelium does not affect *S. enterica* serovar Typhimurium viability. Reprinted from reference 11 with permission.

immunity and also to an understanding of regulated secretory pathways that operate in epithelial cells.

Paneth cell secretion is mediated by cytosolic Ca^{2+} levels (197). Pilocarpine, bethanechol, and nonspecific G-protein activation by NaF and $AlCl_3$ induce massive Paneth cell secretion (172, 194, 195), and muscarinic receptor antagonists block Paneth cell degranulation (194). In vitro, carbamyl choline administration to isolated mouse ileal crypts stimulates increased cytosolic Ca^{2+} by mobilizing intracellular Ca^{2+} stores and activating an influx of extracellular Ca^{2+}, and the Ca^{2+} dynamics occur in Paneth cells but not in other cells in the crypt (197). The pattern of the increase in Paneth cell cytosolic Ca^{2+} is biphasic (197, 200), suggestive of an initial cytosolic $[Ca^{2+}]$ rise that depends on Ca^{2+} release from intracellular stores, followed by a second sustaining Ca^{2+} signal that requires the influx of extracellular Ca^{2+}. These observations led to the finding that mouse Paneth cell secretion in response to bacterial stimuli is modulated by a cation selective channel that regulates the influx of extracellular Ca^{2+} (12).

A Ca^{2+}-ACTIVATED, INTERMEDIATE-CONDUCTANCE K^+ CHANNEL MODULATES MOUSE PANETH CELL SECRETION

Paneth cell secretion in response to bacterial stimuli is modulated in part by mIKCa1, a Ca^{2+}-gated K^+ channel that controls the influx of extracellular Ca^{2+}. IK_{Ca} channels have intermediate single channel conductances, are voltage independent, and open in response to changes in intracellular Ca^{2+} (28, 48, 245). The human IKCa1 protein has six transmembrane segments and internal N and C termini; the hIKCa1 C terminus is complexed to calmodulin, the Ca^{2+} sensor for the channel (47). In mouse small intestinal epithelium, mIKCa1 is detected only in Paneth cells and not in isolated villi, in villus enterocytes, or in other crypt epithelial cells (12), a finding that suggests a Paneth cell-specific role for mIKCa1 in mouse small bowel (12). When expressed heterologously, the Paneth cell mIKCa1 channel is Ca^{2+} activated and blocked by specific IKCa1 inhibitors. Charybdotoxin, the IKCa1-selective charybdotoxin analogue ChTx-Glu^{32}, clotrimazole, and the highly selective triarylmethane inhibitors of human (254) and mouse IKCa1 channels, blocked Paneth cell secretion by 50 to 60% following stimulation with bacteria or LPS (12). The involvement of mIKCa1 in Paneth cell secretion does not exclude the possibility that other Ca^{2+}-activated K^+ channel subtypes participate in granule release. mIKCa1 modulates the extent of α-defensin delivery to the intestinal lumen.

The involvement of the Ca^{2+}-activated mIKCa1 channel in Paneth cell secretory responses to bacteria and LPS suggests that the control of cytosolic $[Ca^{2+}]$ regulates the Pa-

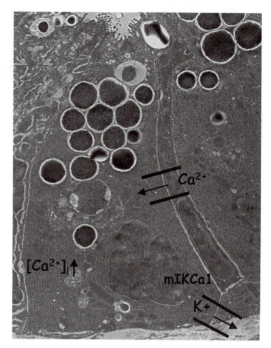

FIGURE 5 Role of mIKCa1 in Paneth cell secretion. Exposure of Paneth cells to pharmacologic agents (197) or bacterial antigens results in an initial increase in cytosolic Ca^{2+} ([Ca^{2+}i]) by mobilization of intracellular stores. mIKCa1 channels in the Paneth cell membrane would be predicted to open as cytosolic [Ca^{2+}i] approaches 300 nM, providing the counterbalancing K^+ efflux necessary to sustain Ca^{2+} entry from the external milieu (12). As noted in detail in the text, blockade of mIKCa1 would depolarize the membrane and attenuate the calcium-signaling response required to generate a complete Paneth cell secretory response. Electron micrograph was generously provided by Susan J. Hagen, Beth Israel Deaconess Medical Center, Boston, Mass.

neth cell pathway. By analogy to events in human T lymphocytes during the specific immune response, mIKCa1 channels in the Paneth cell membrane are predicted to open at cytosolic [Ca^{2+}] of ~300 nM to provide the necessary counterbalancing cation efflux needed to maintain electronegativity of the cell and sustain Ca^{2+} entry from the external milieu (28, 47, 64). By blockade or mutational impairment of mIKCa1, the electrochemical Ca^{2+} gradient would dissipate without K^+ efflux, and the Ca^{2+} signal needed to complete the initiated Paneth cell secretory response would be attenuated (Fig. 5). Of course, the validity of this hypothesis must be tested by electrophysiologic measurements.

DYNAMICS OF PANETH CELL BIOLOGY IN MICE

Conditions that disrupt crypt cell biology induce crypt intermediate or granulomucous cells to accumulate Paneth cell markers and to exhibit an apparent Paneth cell phenotype (Fig. 6). For example, mice that express attenuated diphtheria toxin A fragment or simian

virus 40 large T-antigen transgenes under the control of a mouse cryptdin-2 gene promoter experience a transient Paneth cell deficiency (62). Up to 4 to 5 weeks of age, the majority of small intestinal crypts of these transgenic mice lack apparent Paneth cells. Coincident with the Paneth cell-deficient period, intermediate cells and granule-containing goblet cells increase in number and accumulate electron-dense, secretory granules that contain cryptdins and sPLA$_2$ (62). Thus, transient, genetically induced Paneth cell deficiency alters lineage determination in crypt intermediate cells to increase the production of Paneth cell antimicrobial peptides for secretion.

Paneth cells or other crypt epithelial cells also appear to respond to proinflammatory mediators released by T lymphocytes, neighboring epithelial cells, or cells in the stroma. For example, *Trichinella spiralis* helminth infection of mouse small intestine stimulates a 5- to 10-fold increase in Paneth cell numbers and the accumulation of cryptdins in dense granules of intermediate cells (101) (Fig. 6). These

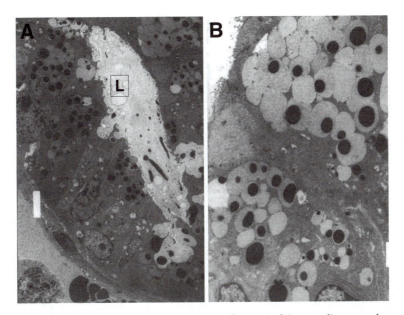

FIGURE 6 Dense granules in mouse small intestinal intermediate granulomucous cells during *T. spiralis* infection. (A) This transmission electron micrograph shows evidence of extensive Paneth cell degranulation into the crypt lumen (L). Cells at the top of the field display large electron dense granules within electron-lucent mucus-containing granules, the hallmark of intermediate granulomucous cells. (B) Two representative intermediate cells that were detected above the crypt villus junction. Such cells are immunopositive for mouse Paneth cell α-defensins and are not found after clearance of the infection (101). Reprinted from reference 101, with permission.

events are mediated by T lymphocytes that are thymic independent (100, 101). Paneth cell numbers also increase rapidly in mice undergoing systemic T-cell activation caused by CD3 ligation (7). Anti-CD3-induced T-cell activation induces dramatic crypt cell apoptosis within 4 to 6 h followed by a three- to fourfold increase in the number of Paneth cells after 36 h. Perhaps, proinflammatory cytokines modulate or redirect lineage determination programs of the gastrointestinal epithelium during such inflammatory episodes. The increase in Paneth cell numbers or the recruitment of granulomucous intermediate cells to secrete active α-defensins are changes that are consistent with the augmentation of small bowel innate immunity in response to local immune stimulation. Collectively, the Paneth cell modifications associated with transgene-mediated Paneth cell deficiency, helminth infection, and T-cell activation disclose a certain plasticity that modifies lineage differentiation programs of crypt cell populations in response to environmental stimuli.

PANETH CELL DEFECTS IN DISEASE
By releasing α-defensins at high local concentrations in response to cholinergic stimulation and microbial antigens, Paneth cells contribute actively to mucosal immunity (Fig. 7). These secretions may protect the crypt epithelium from the potentially lethal effects of acute microbial infection, they may influence the composition of the resident commensal microflora by exerting selective bactericidal effects on different bacterial species, or both. To date, recognized Paneth cell dysfunction is not

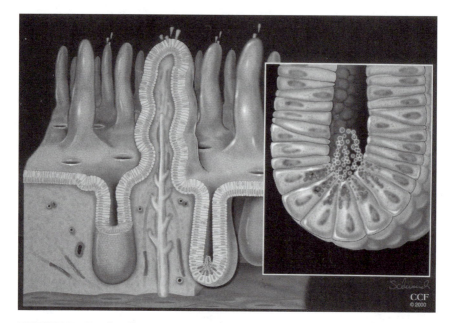

FIGURE 7 Paneth cells in the context of the small intestinal villus–crypt axis (56). Stem cells in small intestinal crypts divide, and their progeny migrate upward toward the villi or descend toward the base of the crypt. Migration toward the villus tips is accompanied by cellular differentiation into absorptive enterocytes, goblet cells, or enteroendocrine cells. The life span of these villus cells from their origin in the crypt, through migration and differentiation, until apoptotic death and exfoliation into the lumen is approximately 2 to 5 days. Stem cell progeny that migrate to the crypt base differentiate into Paneth cells that live for several weeks. (Inset) Paneth cells release secretory vesicles into the narrow lumen of the crypt (56). The secretory responses are mediated by Ca^{2+}, and the secretions contain α-defensins, lysozyme, and secretory phospholipase A_2. Illustration by D. Schumick, Department of Medical Illustration, Cleveland Clinic Foundation, ©2000, Cleveland Clinic Foundation. Reprinted from reference 56, with permission.

identified with predisposition to enteric immunopathology, but the concept may merit consideration. First, Paneth cell products may affect the species distribution and numbers of bacterial species that can reside in the small intestine (19). Changes in the microbial flora secondary to altered Paneth cell function could influence the ability of individuals to control luminal bacteria, resulting in increased susceptibility to inflammatory bowel disease or enteric infection. Also, the integrity of the intestinal epithelial monolayer depends on preserving stem cell viability, and aberrant stem cell function may have adverse consequences for normal barrier maintenance by the intestinal epithelium (56, 174). Because α-defensins and other Paneth cell antimicrobial polypeptides are likely to protect crypts against bacterial overgrowth and infection, defects in Paneth cell physiology may predispose individuals to the adverse effects of insults that disrupt crypt cell biology and impair epithelial cell renewal.

The inflammatory bowel diseases, Crohn's disease and ulcerative colitis, have provided links between altered mucosal barrier function and the intestinal microflora (192, 193). Necrotizing enterocolitis (NEC) is a disease that usually involves the terminal ileum and results in necrosis with hemorrhage, mucosal edema, and limited inflammation (25), and the incidence of NEC in premature newborns suggests that delayed local innate immune development may contribute to the disease (13, 104). The levels of HD-5 and HD-6 α-defensin mRNAs are elevated in NEC relative to controls (190). Also, the number of Paneth cells is twice normal in NEC, suggesting that the disease process may promote the differentiation of greater numbers of Paneth cells (190). Although functional studies of α-defensin biosynthesis and secretion by Paneth cells from NEC patients are needed to test these possibilities, the literature is consistent with a possible involvement of enteric α-defensins in NEC pathophysiology. For example, the relatively low fetal levels of HD-5 and HD-6 expression compared to those of term newborns and adults are a characteristic of normal human intestinal development. The immature innate defenses of premature neonates may predispose them to NEC (190).

Enteric immunity in vivo is impaired in mice that are cryptdin deficient secondary to genetic deletion of procryptdin activation (249), but the Paneth cells of those mice are morphologically normal. It seems reasonable to consider, therefore, that certain individuals may harbor mutations with potentially adverse effects on the pathways for defensin synthesis and secretion and that the defects would escape notice by histological or immunohistochemical evaluation. Furthermore, given the complexity of the immune system in the small intestine, a decrement in Paneth cell output, akin to the loss of secretory IgA (36), may not be sufficient to initiate disease, because alternative innate or adaptive immune mechanisms may compensate to maintain homeostasis and prevent overgrowth by resident or transient microflora. However, under the added stress of inflammation, infectious challenge, or immune stimulation, these hypothetical defects could become manifest as increased susceptibility to disease. As high throughput microarray and alternative approaches to scanning for mutations in target genes improve and achieve widespread use, these issues will be subjected to experimental analysis. Those results should further our understanding of the extent to which impaired innate immunity affects susceptibility to infectious agents or the development of enteric immunopathologies (37, 72, 99, 123, 155).

ACKNOWLEDGMENTS

Supported by NIH grants DK44632 (A.J.O.) and AI22931 (M.E.S.). We thank Charles L. Bevins, Tomas Ganz, Yashwant R. Mahida, Edith Porter, and Michael Zasloff for permission to duplicate published data or to excerpt material from their publications. We thank Klara Osapay for the preparation of Fig. 1.

REFERENCES

1. **Agerberth, B., H. Gunne, J. Odeberg, P. Kogner, H. G. Boman, and G. H. Gudmundsson.** 1995. FALL-39, a putative human peptide antibiotic, is cysteine-free and expressed in bone marrow and testis. *Proc. Natl. Acad. Sci. USA* **92:**195–199.
2. **Agerberth, B., J. Y. Lee, T. Bergman, M. Carlquist, H. G. Boman, V. Mutt, and H. Jornvall.** 1991. Amino acid sequence of PR-39. Isolation from pig intestine of a new member of the family of proline-arginine-rich antibacterial peptides. *Eur. J. Biochem.* **202:**849–854.
3. **Aho, H. J., B. Sternby, M. Kallajoki, and T. J. Nevalainen.** 1989. Carboxyl ester lipase in human tissues and in acute pancreatitis. *Int. J. Pancreatol.* **5:**123–134.
4. **Akira, S., K. Takeda, and T. Kaisho.** 2001. Toll-like receptors: critical proteins linking innate and acquired immunity. *Nat. Immunol.* **2:**675–680.
5. **Albedi, F. M., E. Lorenzetti, M. Contini, and F. Nardi.** 1984. Immature Paneth cells in intestinal metaplasia of gastric mucosa. *Appl. Pathol.* **2:**43–48.
6. **Aley, S. B., M. Zimmerman, M. Hetsko, M. E. Selsted, and F. D. Gillin.** 1994. Killing of *Giardia lamblia* by cryptdins and cationic neutrophil peptides. *Infect. Immun.* **62:**5397–5403.
7. **Alnadjim, Z., S. M. Cohn, T. Ayabe, S. Biafora, A. J. Ouellette, and T. A. Barrett.** 2001. T cell activation instructs epithelial lineage development by inducing Paneth cell expansion and cryptdin production in intestinal crypts. *Gastroenterology* **120:**A21 (Abstract).
8. **Alper, S. L., H. Rossmann, S. Wilhelm, A. K. Stuart-Tilley, B. E. Shmukler, and U. Seidler.** 1999. Expression of AE2 anion exchanger in mouse intestine. *Am. J. Physiol.* **277:** G321–G332.
9. **Ariza, A., D. Lopez, E. M. Castella, C. Munoz, M. J. Zujar, and J. L. Mate.** 1996. Ex-

pression of CD15 in normal and metaplastic Paneth cells of the digestive tract. *J. Clin. Pathol.* **49:**474–477.

10. **Ayabe, T., D. P. Satchell, P. Pesendorfer, H. Tanabe, C. L. Wilson, S. J. Hagen, and A. J. Ouellette.** 2002. Activation of Paneth cell alpha-defensins in mouse small intestine. *J. Biol. Chem.* **277:**5219–5228.

11. **Ayabe, T., D. P. Satchell, C. L. Wilson, W. C. Parks, M. E. Selsted, and A. J. Ouellette.** 2000. Secretion of microbicidal alpha-defensins by intestinal Paneth cells in response to bacteria. *Nat. Immunol.* **1:**113–118.

12. **Ayabe, T., H. Wulff, D. Darmoul, M. D. Cahalan, K. G. Chandy, and A. J. Ouellette.** 2002. Modulation of mouse Paneth cell alpha-defensin secretion by mIKCa1, a Ca^{2+}-activated, intermediate conductance potassium channel. *J. Biol. Chem.* **277:**3793–3800.

13. **Ballance, W. A., B. B. Dahms, N. Shenker, and R. M. Kliegman.** 1990. Pathology of neonatal necrotizing enterocolitis: a ten-year experience. *J. Pediatr.* **117:**S6–S13.

14. **Bals, R., X. Wang, R. L. Meegalla, S. Wattler, D. J. Weiner, M. C. Nehls, and J. M. Wilson.** 1999. Mouse beta-defensin 3 is an inducible antimicrobial peptide expressed in the epithelia of multiple organs. *Infect. Immun.* **67:**3542–3547.

15. **Bals, R., X. Wang, Z. Wu, T. Freeman, V. Bafna, M. Zasloff, and J. M. Wilson.** 1998. Human beta-defensin 2 is a salt-sensitive peptide antibiotic expressed in human lung. *J. Clin. Invest.* **102:**874–880.

16. **Bals, R., X. Wang, M. Zasloff, and J. M. Wilson.** 1998. The peptide antibiotic LL-37/hCAP-18 is expressed in epithelia of the human lung where it has broad antimicrobial activity at the airway surface. *Proc. Natl. Acad. Sci. USA* **95:**9541–9546.

17. **Bateman, A., R. J. MacLeod, P. Lembessis, J. Hu, F. Esch, and S. Solomon.** 1996. The isolation and characterization of a novel corticostatin/defensin-like peptide from the kidney. *J. Biol. Chem.* **271:**10654–10659.

18. **Bevins, C. L., D. E. Jones, A. Dutra, J. Schaffzin, and M. Muenke.** 1996. Human enteric defensin genes: chromosomal map position and a model for possible evolutionary relationships. *Genomics* **31:**95–106.

19. **Bevins, C. L., E. Martin-Porter, and T. Ganz.** 1999. Defensins and innate host defence of the gastrointestinal tract. *Gut* **45:**911–915.

20. **Bjerknes, M., and H. Cheng.** 1981. The stem-cell zone of the small intestinal epithelium. I. Evidence from Paneth cells in the adult mouse. *Am. J. Anat.* **160:**51–63.

21. **Bohe, M., A. Borgstrom, C. Lindstrom, and K. Ohlsson.** 1984. Trypsin-like immunoreactivity in human Paneth cells. *Digestion* **30:**271–275.

22. **Bohe, M., C. Lindstrom, and K. Ohlsson.** 1986. Immunohistochemical demonstration of pancreatic secretory proteins in human paneth cells. *Scand. J. Gastroenterol. Suppl.* **126:**65–68.

23. **Boman, H. G.** 1991. Antibacterial peptides: key components needed in immunity. *Cell* **65:**205–207.

24. **Boman, H. G.** 1995. Peptide antibiotics and their role in innate immunity. *Annu. Rev. Immunol.* **13:**61–92.

25. **Brown, E. G., and A. Y. Sweet.** 1982. Neonatal necrotizing enterocolitis. *Pediatr. Clin. North Am.* **29:**1149–1170.

26. **Bry, L., P. Falk, K. Huttner, A. Ouellette, T. Midtvedt, and J. I. Gordon.** 1994. Paneth cell differentiation in the developing intestine of normal and transgenic mice. *Proc. Natl. Acad. Sci. USA* **91:**10335–10339.

27. **Bry, L., P. G. Falk, T. Midtvedt, and J. I. Gordon.** 1996. A model of host-microbial interactions in an open mammalian ecosystem. *Science* **273:**1380–1383.

28. **Cahalan, M. D., and K. G. Chandy.** 1997. Ion channels in the immune system as targets for immunosuppression. *Curr. Opin. Biotechnol.* **8:**749–756.

29. **Calvert, R., G. Bordeleau, G. Grondin, A. Vezina, and J. Ferrari.** 1988. On the presence of intermediate cells in the small intestine. *Anat. Rec.* **220:**291–295.

30. **Casteels, P., C. Ampe, F. Jacobs, and P. Tempst.** 1993. Functional and chemical characterization of Hymenoptaecin, an antibacterial polypeptide that is infection-inducible in the honeybee (*Apis mellifera*). *J. Biol. Chem.* **268:**7044–7054.

31. **Cheng, H.** 1974. Origin, differentiation and renewal of the four main epithelial cell types in the mouse small intestine. IV. Paneth cells. *Am. J. Anat.* **141:**521–535.

32. **Christa, L., F. Carnot, M. T. Simon, F. Levavasseur, M. G. Stinnakre, C. Lasserre, D. Thepot, B. Clement, E. Devinoy, and C. Brechot.** 1996. HIP/PAP is an adhesive protein expressed in hepatocarcinoma, normal Paneth, and pancreatic cells. *Am. J. Physiol.* **271:**G993–G1002.

33. **Clark, D. P., S. Durell, W. L. Maloy, and M. Zasloff.** 1994. Ranalexin. A novel antimicrobial peptide from bullfrog (*Rana catesbeiana*) skin, structurally related to the bacterial antibiotic, polymyxin. *J. Biol. Chem.* **269:**10849–10855.

34. **Condon, M. R., A. Viera, M. D'Alessio, and G. Diamond.** 1999. Induction of a rat enteric

defensin gene by hemorrhagic shock. *Infect. Immun.* **67:**4787–4793.

35. **Cunliffe, R. N., F. R. Rose, J. Keyte, L. Abberley, W. C. Chan, and Y. R. Mahida.** 2001. Human defensin 5 is stored in precursor form in normal Paneth cells and is expressed by some villous epithelial cells and by metaplastic Paneth cells in the colon in inflammatory bowel disease. *Gut* **48:**176–185.

36. **Cunningham-Rundles, C.** 2001. Physiology of IgA and IgA deficiency. *J. Clin. Immunol.* **21:**303–309.

37. **Cuthbert, A. P., S. A. Fisher, M. M. Mirza, K. King, J. Hampe, P. J. Croucher, S. Mascheretti, J. Sanderson, A. Forbes, J. Mansfield, S. Schreiber, C. M. Lewis, and C. G. Mathew.** 2002. The contribution of NOD2 gene mutations to the risk and site of disease in inflammatory bowel disease. *Gastroenterology* **122:**867–874.

38. **Darmoul, D., D. Brown, M. E. Selsted, and A. J. Ouellette.** 1997. Cryptdin gene expression in developing mouse small intestine. *Am. J. Physiol.* **272:**G197–G206.

39. **Darmoul, D., and A. J. Ouellette.** 1996. Positional specificity of defensin gene expression reveals Paneth cell heterogeneity in mouse small intestine. *Am. J. Physiol.* **271:**G68–G74.

40. **de Bruin, W. C., M. J. Wagenmans, and W. H. Peters.** 2000. Expression of glutathione S-transferase alpha, P1-1 and T1-1 in the human gastrointestinal tract. *Jpn. J. Cancer Res.* **91:**310–316.

41. **Diamond, G., M. Zasloff, H. Eck, M. Brasseur, W. L. Maloy, and C. L. Bevins.** 1991. Tracheal antimicrobial peptide, a cysteine-rich peptide from mammalian tracheal mucosa: peptide isolation and cloning of a cDNA. *Proc. Natl. Acad. Sci. USA* **88:**3952–3956.

42. **Dimopoulos, G., A. Richman, H. M. Muller, and F. C. Kafatos.** 1997. Molecular immune responses of the mosquito *Anopheles gambiae* to bacteria and malaria parasites. *Proc. Natl. Acad. Sci. USA* **94:**11508–11513.

43. **Dorschner, R. A., V. K. Pestonjamasp, S. Tamakuwala, T. Ohtake, J. Rudisill, V. Nizet, B. Agerberth, G. H. Gudmundsson, and R. L. Gallo.** 2001. Cutaneous injury induces the release of cathelicidin anti-microbial peptides active against group A *Streptococcus*. *J. Invest. Dermatol.* **117:**91–97.

44. **Eisenhauer, P. B., S. S. Harwig, and R. I. Lehrer.** 1992. Cryptdins: antimicrobial defensins of the murine small intestine. *Infect. Immun.* **60:**3556–3565.

45. **Erlandsen, S. L., C. B. Rodning, C. Montero, J. A. Parsons, E. A. Lewis, and I. D.** Wilson. 1976. Immunocytochemical identification and localization of immunoglobulin A within Paneth cells of the rat small intestine. *J. Histochem. Cytochem.* **24:**1085–1092.

46. **Falk, P. G., L. V. Hooper, T. Midtvedt, and J. I. Gordon.** 1998. Creating and maintaining the gastrointestinal ecosystem: what we know and need to know from gnotobiology. *Microbiol. Mol. Biol. Rev.* **62:**1157–1170.

47. **Fanger, C. M., S. Ghanshani, N. J. Logsdon, H. Rauer, K. Kalman, J. Zhou, K. Beckingham, K. G. Chandy, M. D. Cahalan, and J. Aiyar.** 1999. Calmodulin mediates calcium-dependent activation of the intermediate conductance KCa channel, IKCa1. *J. Biol. Chem.* **274:**5746–5754.

48. **Fanger, C. M., H. Rauer, A. L. Neben, M. J. Miller, H. Wulff, J. C. Rosa, C. R. Ganellin, K. G. Chandy, and M. D. Cahalan.** 2001. Calcium-activated potassium channels sustain calcium signaling in T lymphocytes. Selective blockers and manipulated channel expression levels. *J. Biol. Chem.* **276:**12249–12256.

49. **Fehlbaum, P., P. Bulet, S. Chernysh, J. P. Briand, J. P. Roussel, L. Letellier, C. Hetru, and J. A. Hoffmann.** 1996. Structure-activity analysis of thanatin, a 21-residue inducible insect defense peptide with sequence homology to frog skin antimicrobial peptides. *Proc. Natl. Acad. Sci. USA* **93:**1221–1225.

50. **Fernandes, P. R., D. A. Samuelson, W. R. Clark, and R. J. Cousins.** 1997. Immunohistochemical localization of cysteine-rich intestinal protein in rat small intestine. *Am. J. Physiol.* **272:**G751–G759.

51. **Frydman, C. P., I. J. Bleiweiss, P. D. Unger, R. E. Gordon, and N. V. Brazenas.** 1992. Paneth cell-like metaplasia of the prostate gland. *Arch. Pathol. Lab. Med.* **116:**274–276.

52. **Frye, M., J. Bargon, N. Dauletbaev, A. Weber, T. O. Wagner, and R. Gropp.** 2000. Expression of human alpha-defensin 5 (HD5) mRNA in nasal and bronchial epithelial cells. *J. Clin. Pathol.* **53:**770–773.

53. **Ganz, T.** 1994. Biosynthesis of defensins and other antimicrobial peptides. *CIBA Found. Symp.* **186:**62–71; discussion, p. 71–76.

54. **Ganz, T.** 1999. Defensins and host defense. *Science* **286:**420–421.

55. **Ganz, T.** 2001. Defensins in the urinary tract and other tissues. *J. Infect. Dis.* **183**(Suppl. 1):S41–S42.

56. **Ganz, T.** 2000. Paneth cells—guardians of the gut cell hatchery. *Nat. Immunol.* **1:**99–100.

57. **Ganz, T., and R. I. Lehrer.** 1999. Antibiotic peptides from higher eukaryotes: biology and applications. *Mol. Med. Today* **5:**292–297.

58. **Ganz, T., and R. I. Lehrer.** 1998. Antimicrobial peptides of vertebrates. *Curr. Opin. Immunol.* **10:**41–44.

59. **Ganz, T., L. Liu, E. V. Valore, and A. Oren.** 1993. Posttranslational processing and targeting of transgenic human defensin in murine granulocyte, macrophage, fibroblast, and pituitary adenoma cell lines. *Blood* **82:**641–650.

60. **Ganz, T., M. E. Selsted, D. Szklarek, S. S. Harwig, K. Daher, D. F. Bainton, and R. I. Lehrer.** 1985. Defensins. Natural peptide antibiotics of human neutrophils. *J. Clin. Invest.* **76:**1427–1435.

61. **Gapin, L., H. Cheroutre, and M. Kronenberg.** 1999. Cutting edge: TCR alpha beta$^+$ CD8 alpha alpha$^+$ T cells are found in intestinal intraepithelial lymphocytes of mice that lack classical MHC class I molecules. *J. Immunol.* **163:**4100–4104.

62. **Garabedian, E. M., L. J. Roberts, M. S. McNevin, and J. I. Gordon.** 1997. Examining the role of Paneth cells in the small intestine by lineage ablation in transgenic mice. *J. Biol. Chem.* **272:**23729–23740.

63. **Geyer, G.** 1973. Lysozyme in Paneth cell secretions. *Acta Histochem.* **45:**126–132.

64. **Ghanshani, S., H. Wulff, M. J. Miller, H. Rohm, A. Neben, G. A. Gutman, M. D. Cahalan, and K. G. Chandy.** 2000. Upregulation of the IKCa1 potassium channel during T-cell activation. Molecular mechanism and functional consequences. *J. Biol. Chem.* **275:**37137–37149.

65. **Ghoos, Y., and G. Vantrappen.** 1971. The cytochemical localization of lysozyme in Paneth cell granules. *Histochem. J.* **3:**175–178.

66. **Goldman, M. J., G. M. Anderson, E. D. Stolzenberg, U. P. Kari, M. Zasloff, and J. M. Wilson.** 1997. Human beta-defensin-1 is a salt-sensitive antibiotic in lung that is inactivated in cystic fibrosis. *Cell* **88:**553–560.

67. **Gordon, J. I., and M. L. Hermiston.** 1994. Differentiation and self-renewal in the mouse gastrointestinal epithelium. *Curr. Opin. Cell. Biol.* **6:**795–803.

68. **Gordon, J. I., L. V. Hooper, M. S. McNevin, M. Wong, and L. Bry.** 1997. Epithelial cell growth and differentiation. III. Promoting diversity in the intestine: conversations between the microflora, epithelium, and diffuse GALT. *Am. J. Physiol.* **273:**G565–G570.

69. **Grabsch, H., A. Pereverzev, M. Weiergraber, M. Schramm, M. Henry, R. Vajna, R. E. Beattie, S. G. Volsen, U. Klockner, J. Hescheler, and T. Schneider.** 1999. Immunohistochemical detection of alpha1E voltage-gated Ca(2$^+$) channel isoforms in cerebellum, INS-1 cells, and neuroendocrine cells of the digestive system. *J. Histochem. Cytochem.* **47:**981–994.

70. **Grandjean, V., S. Vincent, L. Martin, M. Rassoulzadegan, and F. Cuzin.** 1997. Antimicrobial protection of the mouse testis: synthesis of defensins of the cryptdin family. *Biol. Reprod.* **57:**1115–1122.

71. **Groblewski, G. E., M. Yoshida, H. Yao, J. A. Williams, and S. A. Ernst.** 1999. Immunolocalization of CRHSP28 in exocrine digestive glands and gastrointestinal tissues of the rat. *Am. J. Physiol.* **276:**G219–G226.

72. **Hampe, J., H. Frenzel, M. M. Mirza, P. J. Croucher, A. Cuthbert, S. Mascheretti, K. Huse, M. Platzer, S. Bridger, B. Meyer, P. Nurnberg, P. Stokkers, M. Krawczak, C. G. Mathew, M. Curran, and S. Schreiber.** 2002. Evidence for a NOD2-independent susceptibility locus for inflammatory bowel disease on chromosome 16p. *Proc. Natl. Acad. Sci. USA* **99:**321–326.

73. **Harder, J., J. Bartels, E. Christophers, and J. M. Schroder.** 2001. Isolation and characterization of human beta-defensin-3, a novel human inducible peptide antibiotic. *J. Biol. Chem.* **276:**5707–5713.

74. **Harder, J., J. Bartels, E. Christophers, and J. M. Schroder.** 1997. A peptide antibiotic from human skin. *Nature* **387:**861.

75. **Hase, K., L. Eckmann, J. D. Leopard, N. Varki, and M. F. Kagnoff.** 2002. Cell differentiation is a key determinant of cathelicidin LL-37/human cationic antimicrobial protein 18 expression by human colon epithelium. *Infect. Immun.* **70:**953–963.

76. **Herrmann, J. E., S. C. Chen, D. H. Jones, A. Tinsley-Bown, E. F. Fynan, H. B. Greenberg, and G. H. Farrar.** 1999. Immune responses and protection obtained by oral immunization with rotavirus VP4 and VP7 DNA vaccines encapsulated in microparticles. *Virology* **259:**148–153.

77. **Hill, C. P., J. Yee, M. E. Selsted, and D. Eisenberg.** 1991. Crystal structure of defensin HNP-3, an amphiphilic dimer: mechanisms of membrane permeabilization. *Science* **251:**1481–1485.

78. **Hoffmann, J. A., F. C. Kafatos, C. A. Janeway, and R. A. Ezekowitz.** 1999. Phylogenetic perspectives in innate immunity. *Science* **284:**1313–1318.

79. **Hooper, L. V., L. Bry, P. G. Falk, and J. I. Gordon.** 1998. Host-microbial symbiosis in the mammalian intestine: exploring an internal ecosystem. *Bioessays* **20:**336–343.

80. **Hooper, L. V., and J. I. Gordon.** 2001. Commensal host-bacterial relationships in the gut. *Science* **292:**1115–1118.

81. **Hooper, L. V., M. H. Wong, A. Thelin, L. Hansson, P. G. Falk, and J. I. Gordon.** 2001. Molecular analysis of commensal host-microbial relationships in the intestine. *Science* **291:**881–884.

82. **Hoover, D. M., O. Chertov, and J. Lubkowski.** 2001. The structure of human beta-defensin-1. New insights into structural properties of beta-defensins. *J. Biol. Chem.* **276:**39021–39026.

83. **Hoover, D. M., K. R. Rajashankar, R. Blumenthal, A. Puri, J. J. Oppenheim, O. Chertov, and J. Lubkowski.** 2000. The structure of human beta-defensin-2 shows evidence of higher order oligomerization. *J. Biol. Chem.* **275:**32911–32918.

84. **Horvath, K., J. C. Papadimitriou, A. Rabsztyn, C. Drachenberg, and J. T. Tildon.** 1999. Gastrointestinal abnormalities in children with autistic disorder. *J. Pediatr.* **135:**559–563.

85. **Hristova, K., M. E. Selsted, and S. H. White.** 1997. Critical role of lipid composition in membrane permeabilization by rabbit neutrophil defensins. *J. Biol. Chem.* **272:**24224–24233.

86. **Hristova, K., M. E. Selsted, and S. H. White.** 1996. Interactions of monomeric rabbit neutrophil defensins with bilayers: comparison with dimeric human defensin HNP-2. *Biochemistry* **35:**11888–11894.

87. **Huang, H. W.** 1999. Peptide-lipid interactions and mechanisms of antimicrobial peptides. *Novartis Found. Symp.* **225:**188–200; discussion, p. 200–206.

88. **Hultmark, D., H. Steiner, T. Rasmuson, and H. G. Boman.** 1980. Insect immunity. Purification and properties of three inducible bactericidal proteins from hemolymph of immunized pupae of *Hyalophora cecropia. Eur. J. Biochem.* **106:**7–16.

89. **Huttner, K. M., and C. L. Bevins.** 1999. Antimicrobial peptides as mediators of epithelial host defense. *Pediatr. Res.* **45:**785–794.

90. **Huttner, K. M., D. J. Brezinski-Caliguri, M. M. Mahoney, and G. Diamond.** 1998. Antimicrobial peptide expression is developmentally regulated in the ovine gastrointestinal tract. *J. Nutr.* **128:**297S–299S.

91. **Huttner, K. M., M. R. Lambeth, H. R. Burkin, D. J. Burkin, and T. E. Broad.** 1998. Localization and genomic organization of sheep antimicrobial peptide genes. *Gene* **206:**85–91.

92. **Huttner, K. M., M. E. Selsted, and A. J. Ouellette.** 1994. Structure and diversity of the murine cryptdin gene family. *Genomics* **19:**448–453.

93. **Iida, K. I., O. Miyaishi, Y. Iwata, K. I. Kozaki, M. Matsuyama, and S. Saga.** 1996. Distinct distribution of protein disulfide isomerase family proteins in rat tissues. *J. Histochem. Cytochem.* **44:**751–759.

94. **Imler, J. L., and J. A. Hoffmann.** 2000. Toll and Toll-like proteins: an ancient family of receptors signaling infection. *Rev. Immunogenet.* **2:**294–304.

95. **Jia, H. P., T. Starner, M. Ackermann, P. Kirby, B. F. Tack, and P. B. McCray, Jr.** 2001. Abundant human beta-defensin-1 expression in milk and mammary gland epithelium. *J. Pediatr.* **138:**109–112.

96. **Jia, H. P., S. A. Wowk, B. C. Schutte, S. K. Lee, A. Vivado, B. F. Tack, C. L. Bevins, and P. B. McCray, Jr.** 2000. A novel murine beta-defensin expressed in tongue, esophagus, and trachea. *J. Biol. Chem.* **275:**33314–33320.

97. **Jones, D. E., and C. L. Bevins.** 1993. Defensin-6 mRNA in human Paneth cells: implications for antimicrobial peptides in host defense of the human bowel. *FEBS Lett.* **315:**187–192.

98. **Jones, D. E., and C. L. Bevins.** 1992. Paneth cells of the human small intestine express an antimicrobial peptide gene. *J. Biol. Chem.* **267:**23216–23225.

99. **Judge, T., and G. R. Lichtenstein.** 2002. The NOD2 gene and Crohn's disease: another triumph for molecular genetics. *Gastroenterology* **122:**826–828.

100. **Kamal, M., D. Wakelin, and Y. Mahida.** 2001. Mucosal responses to infection with *Trichinella spiralis* in mice. *Parasite* **8:**S110–S113.

101. **Kamal, M., D. Wakelin, A. J. Ouellette, A. Smith, D. K. Podolsky, and Y. R. Mahida.** 2001. Mucosal T cells regulate Paneth and intermediate cell numbers in the small intestine of *T. spiralis*-infected mice. *Clin. Exp. Immunol.* **126:**117–125.

102. **Keshav, S., L. Lawson, L. P. Chung, M. Stein, V. H. Perry, and S. Gordon.** 1990. Tumor necrosis factor mRNA localized to Paneth cells of normal murine intestinal epithelium by in situ hybridization. *J. Exp. Med.* **171:**327–332.

103. **Kindon, H., C. Pothoulakis, L. Thim, K. Lynch-Devaney, and D. K. Podolsky.** 1995. Trefoil peptide protection of intestinal epithelial barrier function: cooperative interaction with mucin glycoprotein. *Gastroenterology* **109:**516–523.

104. **Kliegman, R. M.** 1990. Models of the pathogenesis of necrotizing enterocolitis. *J. Pediatr.* **117:**S2–S5.

105. **Kokryakov, V. N., S. S. Harwig, E. A. Panyutich, A. A. Shevchenko, G. M. Aleshina, O. V. Shamova, H. A. Korneva, and R. I. Lehrer.** 1993. Protegrins: leukocyte antimicrobial peptides that combine features of corticostatic defensins and tachyplesins. *FEBS Lett.* **327:**231–236.

106. **Kraehenbuhl, J. P., E. Pringault, and M. R. Neutra.** 1997. Review article: Intestinal epithelia and barrier functions. *Aliment. Pharmacol. Ther.* **11**(Suppl. 3):3–8; discussion, p. 8–9.

107. **Krisanaprakornkit, S., J. R. Kimball, and B. A. Dale.** 2002. Regulation of human beta-defensin-2 in gingival epithelial cells: the involvement of mitogen-activated protein kinase pathways, but not the NF-kappaB transcription factor family. *J. Immunol.* **168:**316–324.

108. **Krisanaprakornkit, S., A. Weinberg, C. N. Perez, and B. A. Dale.** 1998. Expression of the peptide antibiotic human beta-defensin 1 in cultured gingival epithelial cells and gingival tissue. *Infect. Immun.* **66:**4222–4228.

109. **Kuzuhara, T., Y. Nakajima, K. Matsuyama, and S. Natori.** 1990. Determination of the disulfide array in sapecin, an antibacterial peptide of *Sarcophaga peregrina* (flesh fly). *J. Biochem.* (Tokyo) **107:**514–518.

110. **Kwon, M. Y., S. Y. Hong, and K. H. Lee.** 1998. Structure-activity analysis of brevinin 1E amide, an antimicrobial peptide from *Rana esculenta*. *Biochim. Biophys. Acta* **1387:**239–248.

111. **Landon, C., P. Sodano, C. Hetru, J. Hoffmann, and M. Ptak.** 1997. Solution structure of drosomycin, the first inducible antifungal protein from insects. *Protein Sci.* **6:**1878–1884.

112. **Lasserre, C., C. Colnot, C. Brechot, and F. Poirier.** 1999. HIP/PAP gene, encoding a C-type lectin overexpressed in primary liver cancer, is expressed in nervous system as well as in intestine and pancreas of the postimplantation mouse embryo. *Am. J. Pathol.* **154:**1601–1610.

113. **Lee, S. H., M. S. Shin, W. S. Park, S. Y. Kim, S. M. Dong, H. K. Lee, J. Y. Park, R. R. Oh, J. J. Jang, J. Y. Lee, and N. J. Yoo.** 1999. Immunohistochemical analysis of Fas ligand expression in normal human tissues. *APMIS* **107:**1013–1019.

114. **Lehane, M. J., D. Wu, and S. M. Lehane.** 1997. Midgut-specific immune molecules are produced by the blood-sucking insect *Stomoxys calcitrans*. *Proc. Natl. Acad. Sci. USA* **94:**11502–11507.

115. **Lehrer, R. I., A. Barton, K. A. Daher, S. S. Harwig, T. Ganz, and M. E. Selsted.** 1989. Interaction of human defensins with *Escherichia coli*. Mechanism of bactericidal activity. *J. Clin. Invest.* **84:**553–561.

116. **Lehrer, R. I., and T. Ganz.** 1999. Antimicrobial peptides in mammalian and insect host defence. *Curr. Opin. Immunol.* **11:**23–27.

117. **Lehrer, R. I., and T. Ganz.** 2002. Cathelicidins: a family of endogenous antimicrobial peptides. *Curr. Opin. Hematol.* **9:**18–22.

118. **Lehrer, R. I., and T. Ganz.** 2002. Defensins of vertebrate animals. *Curr. Opin. Immunol.* **14:**96–102.

119. **Lehrer, R. I., T. Ganz, and M. E. Selsted.** 1988. Oxygen-independent bactericidal systems. Mechanisms and disorders. *Hematol. Oncol. Clin. North Am.* **2:**159–169.

120. **Lehrer, R. I., M. E. Selsted, D. Szklarek, and J. Fleischmann.** 1983. Antibacterial activity of microbicidal cationic proteins 1 and 2, natural peptide antibiotics of rabbit lung macrophages. *Infect. Immun.* **42:**10–14.

121. **Lencer, W. I., G. Cheung, G. R. Strohmeier, M. G. Currie, A. J. Ouellette, M. E. Selsted, and J. L. Madara.** 1997. Induction of epithelial chloride secretion by channel-forming cryptdins 2 and 3. *Proc. Natl. Acad. Sci. USA* **94:**8585–8589.

122. **Leonova, L., V. N. Kokryakov, G. Aleshina, T. Hong, T. Nguyen, C. Zhao, A. J. Waring, and R. I. Lehrer.** 2001. Circular minidefensins and posttranslational generation of molecular diversity. *J. Leukoc. Biol.* **70:**461–464.

123. **Lesage, S., H. Zouali, J. P. Cezard, J. F. Colombel, J. Belaiche, S. Almer, C. Tysk, C. O'Morain, M. Gassull, V. Binder, Y. Finkel, R. Modigliani, C. Gower-Rousseau, J. Macry, F. Merlin, M. Chamaillard, A. S. Jannot, G. Thomas, and J. P. Hugot.** 2002. CARD15/NOD2 mutational analysis and genotype-phenotype correlation in 612 patients with inflammatory bowel disease. *Am. J. Hum. Genet.* **70:**845–857.

124. **Linzmeier, R., D. Michaelson, L. Liu, and T. Ganz.** 1993. The structure of neutrophil defensin genes. *FEBS Lett.* **321:**267–273.

125. **Lopez-Boado, Y. S., C. L. Wilson, L. V. Hooper, J. I. Gordon, S. J. Hultgren, and W. C. Parks.** 2000. Bacterial exposure induces and activates matrilysin in mucosal epithelial cells. *J. Cell. Biol.* **148:**1305–1315.

126. **Macpherson, A. J., D. Gatto, E. Sainsbury, G. R. Harriman, H. Hengartner, and**

R. M. Zinkernagel. 2000. A primitive T cell-independent mechanism of intestinal mucosal IgA responses to commensal bacteria. *Science* **288:**2222–2226.

127. Mallow, E. B., A. Harris, N. Salzman, J. P. Russell, R. J. DeBerardinis, E. Ruchelli, and C. L. Bevins. 1996. Human enteric defensins. Gene structure and developmental expression. *J. Biol. Chem.* **271:**4038–4045.

128. Mambula, S. S., E. R. Simons, R. Hastey, M. E. Selsted, and S. M. Levitz. 2000. Human neutrophil-mediated nonoxidative antifungal activity against *Cryptococcus neoformans. Infect. Immun.* **68:**6257–6264.

129. Mandard, N., D. Sy, C. Maufrais, J. M. Bonmatin, P. Bulet, C. Hetru, and F. Vovelle. 1999. Androctonin, a novel antimicrobial peptide from scorpion *Androctonus australis:* solution structure and molecular dynamics simulations in the presence of a lipid monolayer. *J. Biomol. Struct. Dyn.* **17:**367–380.

130. Mantle, M., G. G. Forstner, and J. F. Forstner. 1984. Antigenic and structural features of goblet-cell mucin of human small intestine. *Biochem. J.* **217:**159–167.

131. Masciotra, L., P. Lechene de la Porte, J. M. Frigerio, N. J. Dusetti, J. C. Dagorn, and J. L. Iovanna. 1995. Immunocytochemical localization of pancreatitis-associated protein in human small intestine. *Dig. Dis. Sci.* **40:**519–524.

132. Mashimo, H., D. K. Podolsky, and M. C. Fishman. 1995. Structure and expression of murine intestinal trefoil factor: high evolutionary conservation and postnatal expression. *Biochem. Biophys. Res. Commun.* **210:**31–37.

133. Mashimo, H., D. C. Wu, D. K. Podolsky, and M. C. Fishman. 1996. Impaired defense of intestinal mucosa in mice lacking intestinal trefoil factor. *Science* **274:**262–265.

134. Mathews, M., H. P. Jia, J. M. Guthmiller, G. Losh, S. Graham, G. K. Johnson, B. F. Tack, and P. B. McCray, Jr. 1999. Production of beta-defensin antimicrobial peptides by the oral mucosa and salivary glands. *Infect. Immun.* **67:**2740–2745.

135. Matsubara, F. 1977. Morphological study of the Paneth cell. Paneth cells in intestinal metaplasia of the stomach and duodenum of man. *Acta Pathol. Jpn.* **27:**677–695.

136. Matsuyama, K., and S. Natori. 1988. Molecular cloning of cDNA for sapecin and unique expression of the sapecin gene during the development of *Sarcophaga peregrina. J. Biol. Chem.* **263:**17117–17121.

137. Matsuzaki, K., Y. Mitani, K. Y. Akada, O. Murase, S. Yoneyama, M. Zasloff, and K. Miyajima. 1998. Mechanism of synergism between antimicrobial peptides magainin 2 and PGLa. *Biochemistry* **37:**15144–15153.

138. McNamara, N. A., R. Van, O. S. Tuchin, and S. M. Fleiszig. 1999. Ocular surface epithelia express mRNA for human beta defensin-2. *Exp. Eye Res.* **69:**483–490.

139. Merlin, D., G. Yue, W. I. Lencer, M. E. Selsted, and J. L. Madara. 2001. Cryptdin-3 induces novel apical conductance(s) in Cl-secretory, including cystic fibrosis, epithelia. *Am. J. Physiol. Cell Physiol.* **280:**C296–C302.

140. Michaelson, D., J. Rayner, M. Couto, and T. Ganz. 1992. Cationic defensins arise from charge-neutralized propeptides: a mechanism for avoiding leukocyte autocytotoxicity? *J. Leukoc. Biol.* **51:**634–639.

141. Michetti, P., N. Porta, M. J. Mahan, J. M. Slauch, J. J. Mekalanos, A. L. Blum, J. P. Kraehenbuhl, and M. R. Neutra. 1994. Monoclonal immunoglobulin A prevents adherence and invasion of polarized epithelial cell monolayers by *Salmonella typhimurium. Gastroenterology* **107:**915–923.

142. Moller, P., H. Walczak, S. Reidl, J. Strater, and P. H. Krammer. 1996. Paneth cells express high levels of CD95 ligand transcripts: a unique property among gastrointestinal epithelia. *Am. J. Pathol.* **149:**9–13.

143. Molmenti, E. P., D. H. Perlmutter, and D. C. Rubin. 1993. Cell-specific expression of alpha 1-antitrypsin in human intestinal epithelium. *J. Clin. Invest.* **92:**2022–2034.

144. Mor, A., V. H. Nguyen, A. Delfour, D. Migliore-Samour, and P. Nicolas. 1991. Isolation, amino acid sequence, and synthesis of dermaseptin, a novel antimicrobial peptide of amphibian skin. *Biochemistry* **30:**8824–8830.

145. Morita, Y., M. Sawada, H. Seno, S. Takaishi, H. Fukuzawa, N. Miyake, H. Hiai, and T. Chiba. 2001. Identification of xanthine dehydrogenase/xanthine oxidase as a rat Paneth cell zinc-binding protein. *Biochim. Biophys. Acta* **1540:**43–49.

146. Morrissey, S. M., and M. C. Tymvios. 1978. Acid mucins in human intestinal goblet cells. *J. Pathol.* **126:**197–208.

147. Mullins, J. E., and I. C. Fuentealba. 1998. Immunohistochemical detection of metallothionein in liver, duodenum and kidney after dietary copper-overload in rats. *Histol. Histopathol.* **13:**627–633.

148. Nakamura, T., H. Furunaka, T. Miyata, F. Tokunaga, T. Muta, S. Iwanaga, M. Niwa,

T. Takao, and Y. Shimonishi. 1988. Tachy-plesin, a class of antimicrobial peptide from the hemocytes of the horseshoe crab (*Tachypleus tridentatus*). Isolation and chemical structure. *J. Biol. Chem.* **263:**16709–16713.

149. Nevalainen, T. J., J. M. Gronroos, and M. Kallajoki. 1995. Expression of group II phospholipase A2 in the human gastrointestinal tract. *Lab. Invest.* **72:**201–208.

150. Newman, S. L., L. Gootee, J. E. Gabay, and M. E. Selsted. 2000. Identification of constituents of human neutrophil azurophil granules that mediate fungistasis against *Histoplasma capsulatum. Infect. Immun.* **68:**5668–5672.

151. Nicolas, E., A. J. Nappi, and B. Lemaitre. 1996. Expression of antimicrobial peptide genes after infection by parasitoid wasps in *Drosophila. Dev. Comp. Immunol.* **20:**175–181.

152. Nishimura, H., N. Nishimura, and C. Tohyama. 1989. Immunohistochemical localization of metallothionein in developing rat tissues. *J. Histochem. Cytochem.* **37:**715–722.

153. Nizet, V., T. Ohtake, X. Lauth, J. Trowbridge, J. Rudisill, R. A. Dorschner, V. Pestonjamasp, J. Piraino, K. Huttner, and R. L. Gallo. 2001. Innate antimicrobial peptide protects the skin from invasive bacterial infection. *Nature* **414:**454–457.

154. Nyman, K. M., P. Ojala, V. J. Laine, and T. J. Nevalainen. 2000. Distribution of group II phospholipase A2 protein and mRNA in rat tissues. *J. Histochem. Cytochem.* **48:**1469–1478.

155. Ogura, Y., D. K. Bonen, N. Inohara, D. L. Nicolae, F. F. Chen, R. Ramos, H. Britton, T. Moran, R. Karaliuskas, R. H. Duerr, J. P. Achkar, S. R. Brant, T. M. Bayless, B. S. Kirschner, S. B. Hanauer, G. Nunez, and J. H. Cho. 2001. A frameshift mutation in NOD2 associated with susceptibility to Crohn's disease. *Nature* **411:**603–606.

156. Ohnishi, H., S. A. Ernst, N. Wys, M. McNiven, and J. A. Williams. 1996. Rab3D localizes to zymogen granules in rat pancreatic acini and other exocrine glands. *Am. J. Physiol.* **271:**G531–G538.

157. O'Neil, D. A., S. P. Cole, E. Martin-Porter, M. P. Housley, L. Liu, T. Ganz, and M. F. Kagnoff. 2000. Regulation of human beta-defensins by gastric epithelial cells in response to infection with *Helicobacter pylori* or stimulation with interleukin-1. *Infect. Immun.* **68:**5412–5415.

158. O'Neil, D. A., E. M. Porter, D. Elewaut, G. M. Anderson, L. Eckmann, T. Ganz, and M. F. Kagnoff. 1999. Expression and regulation of the human beta-defensins hBD-1 and hBD-2 in intestinal epithelium. *J. Immunol.* **163:**6718–6724.

159. Oppenheim, F. G., T. Xu, F. M. McMillian, S. M. Levitz, R. D. Diamond, G. D. Offner, and R. F. Troxler. 1988. Histatins, a novel family of histidine-rich proteins in human parotid secretion. Isolation, characterization, primary structure, and fungistatic effects on *Candida albicans. J. Biol. Chem.* **263:**7472–7477.

160. Otvos, L., Jr. 2000. Antibacterial peptides isolated from insects. *J. Pept. Sci.* **6:**497–511.

161. Ouellette, A. J., and C. L. Bevins. 2001. Paneth cell defensins and innate immunity of the small bowel. *Inflamm. Bowel Dis.* **7:**43–50.

162. Ouellette, A. J., D. Darmoul, D. Tran, K. M. Huttner, J. Yuan, and M. E. Selsted. 1999. Peptide localization and gene structure of cryptdin 4, a differentially expressed mouse Paneth cell alpha-defensin. *Infect. Immun.* **67:**6643–6651.

163. Ouellette, A. J., M. M. Hsieh, M. T. Nosek, D. F. Cano-Gauci, K. M. Huttner, R. N. Buick, and M. E. Selsted. 1994. Mouse Paneth cell defensins: primary structures and antibacterial activities of numerous cryptdin isoforms. *Infect. Immun.* **62:**5040–5047.

164. Ouellette, A. J., D. Pravtcheva, F. H. Ruddle, and M. James. 1989. Localization of the cryptdin locus on mouse chromosome 8. *Genomics* **5:**233–239.

165. Ouellette, A. J., D. P. Satchell, M. M. Hsieh, S. J. Hagen, and M. E. Selsted. 2000. Characterization of luminal Paneth cell alpha-defensins in mouse small intestine. Attenuated antimicrobial activities of peptides with truncated amino termini. *J. Biol. Chem.* **275:**33969–33973.

166. Ouellette, A. J., and M. E. Selsted. 1996. Paneth cell defensins: endogenous peptide components of intestinal host defense. *FASEB J.* **10:**1280–1289.

167. Panyutich, A. V., N. N. Voitenok, R. I. Lehrer, and T. Ganz. 1991. An enzyme immunoassay for human defensins. *J. Immunol. Methods* **141:**149–155.

168. Pardi, A., D. R. Hare, M. E. Selsted, R. D. Morrison, D. A. Bassolino, and A. C. Bach 2nd. 1988. Solution structures of the rabbit neutrophil defensin NP-5. *J. Mol. Biol.* **201:**625–636.

169. Pardi, A., X. L. Zhang, M. E. Selsted, J. J. Skalicky, and P. F. Yip. 1992. NMR studies of defensin antimicrobial peptides. 2. Three-dimensional structures of rabbit NP-2 and human HNP-1. *Biochemistry* **31:**11357–11364.

170. **Park, C. H., E. V. Valore, A. J. Waring, and T. Ganz.** 2001. Hepcidin, a urinary antimicrobial peptide synthesized in the liver. *J. Biol. Chem.* **276:**7806–7810.

171. **Parsons, S. M., and C. E. Smith.** 1984. Ultrastructural localization of nicotinamide adenine dinucleotide phosphatase (NADPase) activity within columnar, goblet, and Paneth cells of rat small intestine. *J. Histochem. Cytochem.* **32:**989–997.

172. **Peeters, T., and G. Vantrappen.** 1975. The Paneth cell: a source of intestinal lysozyme. *Gut* **16:**553–558.

173. **Peng, K. C., F. Cluzeaud, M. Bens, J. P. Van Huyen, M. A. Wioland, R. Lacave, and A. Vandewalle.** 1999. Tissue and cell distribution of the multidrug resistance-associated protein (MRP) in mouse intestine and kidney. *J. Histochem. Cytochem.* **47:**757–768.

174. **Porter, E. M., C. L. Bevins, D. Ghosh, and T. Ganz.** 2002. The multifaceted Paneth cell. *Cell Mol. Life Sci.* **59:**156–170.

175. **Porter, E. M., L. Liu, A. Oren, P. A. Anton, and T. Ganz.** 1997. Localization of human intestinal defensin 5 in Paneth cell granules. *Infect. Immun.* **65:**2389–2395.

176. **Porter, E. M., M. A. Poles, J. S. Lee, J. Naitoh, C. L. Bevins, and T. Ganz.** 1998. Isolation of human intestinal defensins from ileal neobladder urine. *FEBS Lett.* **434:**272–276.

177. **Porter, E. M., E. van Dam, E. V. Valore, and T. Ganz.** 1997. Broad-spectrum antimicrobial activity of human intestinal defensin 5. *Infect. Immun.* **65:**2396–2401.

178. **Poulsom, R., R. Chinery, C. Sarraf, E. N. Lalani, G. Stamp, G. Elia, and N. Wright.** 1992. Trefoil peptide expression in intestinal adaptation and renewal. *Scand. J. Gastroenterol.* **192**(Suppl.)**:**17–28.

179. **Putsep, K., L. G. Axelsson, A. Boman, T. Midtvedt, S. Normark, H. G. Boman, and M. Andersson.** 2000. Germ-free and colonized mice generate the same products from enteric prodefensins. *J. Biol. Chem.* **275:**40478–40482.

180. **Qu, H., and A. M. Dvorak.** 1997. Ultrastructural localization of osteopontin immunoreactivity in phagolysosomes and secretory granules of cells in human intestine. *Histochem. J.* **29:**801–812.

181. **Quayle, A. J., E. M. Porter, A. A. Nussbaum, Y. M. Wang, C. Brabec, K. P. Yip, and S. C. Mok.** 1998. Gene expression, immunolocalization, and secretion of human defensin-5 in human female reproductive tract. *Am. J. Pathol.* **152:**1247–1258.

182. **Reilly, D. S., N. Tomassini, C. L. Bevins, and M. Zasloff.** 1994. A Paneth cell analogue in *Xenopus* small intestine expresses antimicrobial peptide genes: conservation of an intestinal host-defense system. *J. Histochem. Cytochem.* **42:**697–704.

183. **Rice, W. G., T. Ganz, J. M. Kinkade, Jr., M. E. Selsted, R. I. Lehrer, and R. T. Parmley.** 1987. Defensin-rich dense granules of human neutrophils. *Blood* **70:**757–765.

184. **Rodning, C. B., I. D. Wilson, and S. L. Erlandsen.** 1976. Immunoglobulins within human small-intestinal Paneth cells. *Lancet* **i:**984–987.

185. **Rose, J., M. Franco, and H. Greenberg.** 1998. The immunology of rotavirus infection in the mouse. *Adv. Virus. Res.* **51:**203–235.

186. **Rubin, D. C., K. A. Roth, E. H. Birkenmeier, and J. I. Gordon.** 1991. Epithelial cell differentiation in normal and transgenic mouse intestinal isografts. *J. Cell Biol.* **113:**1183–1192.

187. **Rubin, D. C., E. Swietlicki, K. A. Roth, and J. I. Gordon.** 1992. Use of fetal intestinal isografts from normal and transgenic mice to study the programming of positional information along the duodenal-to-colonic axis. *J. Biol. Chem.* **267:**15122–15133.

188. **Rubio, C. A.** 1989. Paneth cell adenoma of the stomach. *Am. J. Surg. Pathol.* **13:**325–328.

189. **Rubio, C. A., L. Kanter, J. Bjork, B. Poppen, and L. Bry.** 1996. Paneth cell-rich flat adenoma of the rectum: report of a case. *Jpn. J. Cancer Res.* **87:**109–112.

190. **Salzman, N. H., R. A. Polin, M. C. Harris, E. Ruchelli, A. Hebra, S. Zirin-Butler, A. Jawad, E. Martin Porter, and C. L. Bevins.** 1998. Enteric defensin expression in necrotizing enterocolitis. *Pediatr. Res.* **44:**20–26.

191. **Sansonetti, A., H. Romeo, P. Berthezene, P. Scacchi, N. Dusetti, V. Keim, J. C. Dagorn, and J. L. Iovanna.** 1995. Developmental, nutritional, and hormonal regulation of the pancreatitis-associated protein I and III gene expression in the rat small intestine. *Scand. J. Gastroenterol.* **30:**664–669.

192. **Sartor, R. B.** 1997. Pathogenesis and immune mechanisms of chronic inflammatory bowel diseases. *Am. J. Gastroenterol.* **92:**5S–11S.

193. **Sartor, R. B.** 1997. Review article: Role of the enteric microflora in the pathogenesis of intestinal inflammation and arthritis. *Aliment. Pharmacol. Ther.* **11**(Suppl. 3)**:**17–22; discussion, p. 22–23.

194. **Satoh, Y.** 1988. Atropine inhibits the degranulation of Paneth cells in ex-germ-free mice. *Cell Tissue Res.* **253:**397–402.

195. **Satoh, Y.** 1988. Effect of live and heat-killed bacteria on the secretory activity of Paneth cells in germ-free mice. *Cell Tissue Res.* **251:**87–93.

196. **Satoh, Y.** 1984. Ultrastructure of Paneth cells in germ-free rats, with special reference to the secretory granules and lysosomes. *Arch. Histol. Jpn.* **47:**293–301.

197. **Satoh, Y., Y. Habara, K. Ono, and T. Kanno.** 1995. Carbamylcholine- and catecholamine-induced intracellular calcium dynamics of epithelial cells in mouse ileal crypts. *Gastroenterology* **108:**1345–1356.

198. **Satoh, Y., K. Ishikawa, K. Ono, and L. Vollrath.** 1986. Quantitative light microscopic observations on Paneth cells of germ-free and ex-germ-free Wistar rats. *Digestion* **34:**115–121.

199. **Satoh, Y., K. Ishikawa, H. Tanaka, Y. Oomori, and K. Ono.** 1988. Immunohistochemical observations of lysozyme in the Paneth cells of specific pathogen-free and germ-free mice. *Acta Histochem.* **83:**185–188.

200. **Satoh, Y., M. R. Williams, and Y. Habara.** 1999. Effects of AIF4⁻ and ATP on intracellular calcium dynamics of crypt epithelial cells in mouse small intestine. *Cell Tissue Res.* **298:**295–305.

201. **Savidge, T. C., A. L. Morey, D. J. Ferguson, K. A. Fleming, A. N. Shmakov, and A. D. Phillips.** 1995. Human intestinal development in a severe-combined immunodeficient xenograft model. *Differentiation* **58:**361–371.

202. **Sawai, M. V., H. P. Jia, L. Liu, V. Aseyev, J. M. Wiencek, P. B. McCray, Jr., T. Ganz, W. R. Kearney, and B. F. Tack.** 2001. The NMR structure of human beta-defensin-2 reveals a novel alpha-helical segment. *Biochemistry* **40:**3810–3816.

203. **Schmauder-Chock, E. A., and S. P. Chock.** 1992. Prostaglandin E2 localization in the rat ileum. *Histochem. J.* **24:**663–672.

204. **Schmauder-Chock, E. A., S. P. Chock, and M. L. Patchen.** 1994. Ultrastructural localization of tumour necrosis factor-alpha. *Histochem. J.* **26:**142–151.

205. **Schonwetter, B. S., E. D. Stolzenberg, and M. A. Zasloff.** 1995. Epithelial antibiotics induced at sites of inflammation. *Science* **267:**1645–1648.

206. **Schutte, B. C., and P. B. McCray, Jr.** 2002. β-Defensins in lung host defense. *Annu. Rev. Physiol.* **64:**709–748.

207. **Selsted, M. E., D. M. Brown, R. J. DeLange, and R. I. Lehrer.** 1983. Primary structures of MCP-1 and MCP-2, natural peptide antibiotics of rabbit lung macrophages. *J. Biol. Chem.* **258:**14485–14489.

208. **Selsted, M. E., and S. S. Harwig.** 1989. Determination of the disulfide array in the human defensin HNP-2. A covalently cyclized peptide. *J. Biol. Chem.* **264:**4003–4007.

209. **Selsted, M. E., S. S. Harwig, T. Ganz, J. W. Schilling, and R. I. Lehrer.** 1985. Primary structures of three human neutrophil defensins. *J. Clin. Invest.* **76:**1436–1439.

210. **Selsted, M. E., S. I. Miller, A. H. Henschen, and A. J. Ouellette.** 1992. Enteric defensins: antibiotic peptide components of intestinal host defense. *J. Cell Biol.* **118:**929–936.

211. **Selsted, M. E., M. J. Novotny, W. L. Morris, Y. Q. Tang, W. Smith, and J. S. Cullor.** 1992. Indolicidin, a novel bactericidal tridecapeptide amide from neutrophils. *J. Biol. Chem.* **267:**4292–4295.

212. **Selsted, M. E., Y. Q. Tang, W. L. Morris, P. A. McGuire, M. J. Novotny, W. Smith, A. H. Henschen, and J. S. Cullor.** 1993. Purification, primary structures, and antibacterial activities of beta-defensins, a new family of antimicrobial peptides from bovine neutrophils. *J. Biol. Chem.* **268:**6641–6648.

213. **Selsted, M. E., Y. Q. Tang, W. L. Morris, P. A. McGuire, M. J. Novotny, W. Smith, A. H. Henschen, and J. S. Cullor.** 1996. Purification, primary structures, and antibacterial activities of beta-defensins, a new family of antimicrobial peptides from bovine neutrophils. *J. Biol. Chem.* **271:**16430.

214. **Senegas-Balas, F., D. Balas, R. Verger, A. de Caro, C. Figarella, F. Ferrato, P. Lechene, C. Bertrand, and A. Ribet.** 1984. Immunohistochemical localization of intestinal phospholipase A2 in rat Paneth cells. *Histochemistry* **81:**581–584.

215. **Shai, Y.** 1999. Mechanism of the binding, insertion and destabilization of phospholipid bilayer membranes by alpha-helical antimicrobial and cell non-selective membrane-lytic peptides. *Biochim. Biophys. Acta* **1462:**55–70.

216. **Shimada, O., H. Ishikawa, H. Tosaka-Shimada, T. Yasuda, K. Kishi, and S. Suzuki.** 1998. Detection of deoxyribonuclease I along the secretory pathway in Paneth cells of human small intestine. *J. Histochem. Cytochem.* **46:**833–840.

217. **Shirafuji, Y., T. Oono, H. Kanzaki, S. Hirakawa, and J. Arata.** 1999. Detection of cryptdin in mouse skin. *Clin. Diagn. Lab. Immunol.* **6:**336–340.

217a.**Shirafuji, Y., H. Tanabe, D. P. Satchell, A. Henschen-Edman, C. L. Wilson, and A. J. Ouellette.** 2003. Structural determinants of procryptdin recognition and cleavage by matric metalloproteinase-7. *J. Biol. Chem.* **278:**7910-7919.

218. **Shmakov, A. N., J. Bode, P. J. Kilshaw, and S. Ghosh.** 2000. Diverse patterns of expression of the 67-kD laminin receptor in hu-

man small intestinal mucosa: potential binding sites for prion proteins? *J. Pathol.* **191**:318–322.

219. **Shmakov, A. N., and T. C. Savidge.** 1995. Cellular proliferation in the crypt epithelium of human small intestinal xenografts. *Epithel. Cell Biol.* **4**:104–112.

220. **Silvey, K. J., A. B. Hutchings, M. Vajdy, M. M. Petzke, and M. R. Neutra.** 2001. Role of immunoglobulin A in protection against reovirus entry into murine Peyer's patches. *J. Virol.* **75**:10870–10879.

221. **Simon, T. C., and J. I. Gordon.** 1995. Intestinal epithelial cell differentiation: new insights from mice, flies and nematodes. *Curr. Opin. Genet. Dev.* **5**:577–586.

222. **Skalicky, J. J., M. E. Selsted, and A. Pardi.** 1994. Structure and dynamics of the neutrophil defensins NP-2, NP-5, and HNP-1: NMR studies of amide hydrogen exchange kinetics. *Proteins* **20**:52–67.

223. **Sparkes, R. S., M. Kronenberg, C. Heinzmann, K. A. Daher, I. Klisak, T. Ganz, and T. Mohandas.** 1989. Assignment of defensin gene(s) to human chromosome 8p23. *Genomics* **5**:240–244.

224. **Steiner, H., D. Hultmark, A. Engstrom, H. Bennich, and H. G. Boman.** 1981. Sequence and specificity of two antibacterial proteins involved in insect immunity. *Nature* **292**:246–248.

225. **Suemori, S., K. Lynch-Devaney, and D. K. Podolsky.** 1991. Identification and characterization of rat intestinal trefoil factor: tissue- and cell-specific member of the trefoil protein family. *Proc. Natl. Acad. Sci. USA* **88**:11017–11021.

226. **Symonds, D. A.** 1974. Paneth cell metaplasia in diseases of the colon and rectum. *Arch. Pathol.* **97**:343–347.

227. **Takemori, H., F. N. Zolotaryov, L. Ting, T. Urbain, T. Komatsubara, O. Hatano, M. Okamoto, and H. Tojo.** 1998. Identification of functional domains of rat intestinal phospholipase B/lipase. Its cDNA cloning, expression, and tissue distribution. *J. Biol. Chem.* **273**:2222–2231.

228. **Tan, X., W. Hsueh, and F. Gonzalez-Crussi.** 1993. Cellular localization of tumor necrosis factor (TNF)-alpha transcripts in normal bowel and in necrotizing enterocolitis. TNF gene expression by Paneth cells, intestinal eosinophils, and macrophages. *Am. J. Pathol.* **142**:1858–1865.

229. **Tang, Y. Q., and M. E. Selsted.** 1993. Characterization of the disulfide motif in BNBD-12, an antimicrobial beta-defensin peptide from bovine neutrophils. *J. Biol. Chem.* **268**:6649–6653.

230. **Tang, Y. Q., J. Yuan, G. Osapay, K. Osapay, D. Tran, C. J. Miller, A. J. Ouellette, and M. E. Selsted.** 1999. A cyclic antimicrobial peptide produced in primate leukocytes by the ligation of two truncated alpha-defensins. *Science* **286**:498–502.

231. **Tannock, G. W.** 2000. The intestinal microflora: potentially fertile ground for microbial physiologists. *Adv. Microb. Physiol.* **42**:25–46.

232. **Tannock, G. W.** 2001. Molecular assessment of intestinal microflora. *Am. J. Clin. Nutr.* **73**:410S–414S.

233. **Tarver, A. P., D. P. Clark, G. Diamond, J. P. Russell, H. Erdjument-Bromage, P. Tempst, K. S. Cohen, D. E. Jones, R. W. Sweeney, M. Wines, S. Hwang, and C. L. Bevins.** 1998. Enteric beta-defensin: molecular cloning and characterization of a gene with inducible intestinal epithelial cell expression associated with *Cryptosporidium parvum* infection. *Infect. Immun.* **66**:1045–1056.

234. **Tauszig, S., E. Jouanguy, J. A. Hoffmann, and J. L. Imler.** 2000. Toll-related receptors and the control of antimicrobial peptide expression in *Drosophila. Proc. Natl. Acad. Sci. USA* **97**:10520–10525.

235. **Terras, F. R., I. A. Penninckx, I. J. Goderis, and W. F. Broekaert.** 1998. Evidence that the role of plant defensins in radish defense responses is independent of salicylic acid. *Planta* **206**:117–124.

236. **Thevissen, K., A. Ghazi, G. W. De Samblanx, C. Brownlee, R. W. Osborn, and W. F. Broekaert.** 1996. Fungal membrane responses induced by plant defensins and thionins. *J. Biol. Chem.* **271**:15018–15025.

237. **Thim, L.** 1994. Trefoil peptides: a new family of gastrointestinal molecules. *Digestion* **55**:353–360.

238. **Thim, L.** 1997. Trefoil peptides: from structure to function. *Cell Mol. Life Sci.* **53**:888–903.

239. **Trabi, M., H. J. Schirra, and D. J. Craik.** 2001. Three-dimensional structure of RTD-1, a cyclic antimicrobial defensin from rhesus macaque leukocytes. *Biochemistry* **40**:4211–4221.

240. **Tran, D., P. A. Tran, Y. Q. Tang, J. Yuan, T. Cole, and M. E. Selsted.** 2002. Homodimeric theta-defensins from rhesus macaque leukocytes: isolation, synthesis, antimicrobial activities, and bacterial binding properties of the cyclic peptides. *J. Biol. Chem.* **277**:3079–3084.

241. **Tsumura, T., A. Hazama, T. Miyoshi, S. Ueda, and Y. Okada.** 1998. Activation of cAMP-dependent Cl⁻ currents in guinea-pig Paneth cells without relevant evidence for CFTR expression. *J. Physiol.* **512**(Pt. 3):765–777.

242. **Valore, E. V., and T. Ganz.** 1992. Posttranslational processing of defensins in immature human myeloid cells. *Blood* **79:**1538–1544.

243. **Valore, E. V., E. Martin, S. S. Harwig, and T. Ganz.** 1996. Intramolecular inhibition of human defensin HNP-1 by its propiece. *J. Clin. Invest.* **97:**1624–1629.

244. **Valore, E. V., C. H. Park, A. J. Quayle, K. R. Wiles, P. B. McCray, Jr., and T. Ganz.** 1998. Human beta-defensin-1: an antimicrobial peptide of urogenital tissues. *J. Clin. Invest.* **101:**1633–1642.

245. **Vandorpe, D. H., B. E. Shmukler, L. Jiang, B. Lim, J. Maylie, J. P. Adelman, L. de Franceschi, M. D. Cappellini, C. Brugnara, and S. L. Alper.** 1998. cDNA cloning and functional characterization of the mouse $Ca2^+$-gated K^+ channel, mIK1. Roles in regulatory volume decrease and erythroid differentiation. *J. Biol. Chem.* **273:**21542–21553.

246. **White, S. H., W. C. Wimley, and M. E. Selsted.** 1995. Structure, function, and membrane integration of defensins. *Curr. Opin. Struct. Biol.* **5:**521–527.

247. **Willingham, M. C., A. V. Rutherford, and S. Y. Cheng.** 1987. Immunohistochemical localization of a thyroid hormone-binding protein (p55) in human tissues. *J. Histochem. Cytochem.* **35:**1043–1046.

248. **Wilson, C. L., K. J. Heppner, L. A. Rudolph, and L. M. Matrisian.** 1995. The metalloproteinase matrilysin is preferentially expressed by epithelial cells in a tissue-restricted pattern in the mouse. *Mol. Biol. Cell.* **6:**851–869.

249. **Wilson, C. L., A. J. Ouellette, D. P. Satchell, T. Ayabe, Y. S. Lopez-Boado, J. L. Stratman, S. J. Hultgren, L. M. Matrisian, and W. C. Parks.** 1999. Regulation of intestinal alpha-defensin activation by the metalloproteinase matrilysin in innate host defense. *Science* **286:**113–117.

250. **Wimley, W. C., M. E. Selsted, and S. H. White.** 1994. Interactions between human defensins and lipid bilayers: evidence for formation of multimeric pores. *Protein Sci.* **3:**1362–1373.

251. **Winter, H. S., R. B. Hendren, C. H. Fox, G. J. Russell, A. Perez-Atayde, A. K. Bhan, and J. Folkman.** 1991. Human intestine matures as nude mouse xenograft. *Gastroenterology* **100:**89–98.

252. **Wong, M. H., T. S. Stappenbeck, and J. I. Gordon.** 1999. Living and commuting in intestinal crypts. *Gastroenterology* **116:**208–210.

253. **Wu, E. R., R. Daniel, and A. Bateman.** 1998. RK-2: a novel rabbit kidney defensin and its implications for renal host defense. *Peptides* **19:**793–799.

254. **Wulff, H., M. J. Miller, W. Hansel, S. Grissmer, M. D. Cahalan, and K. G. Chandy.** 2000. Design of a potent and selective inhibitor of the intermediate-conductance $Ca2^+$-activated K^+ channel, IKCa1: a potential immunosuppressant. *Proc. Natl. Acad. Sci. USA* **97:**8151–8156.

255. **Yoshikawa, T., S. Naruse, M. Kitagawa, H. Ishiguro, M. Nagahama, E. Yasuda, R. Semba, M. Tanaka, K. Nomura, and T. Hayakawa.** 2001. Cellular localization of group IIA phospholipase A2 in rats. *J. Histochem. Cytochem.* **49:**777–782.

256. **Yu, Q., R. I. Lehrer, and J. P. Tam.** 2000. Engineered salt-insensitive alpha-defensins with end-to-end circularized structures. *J. Biol. Chem.* **275:**3943–3949.

257. **Zanetti, M., G. Del Sal, P. Storici, C. Schneider, and D. Romeo.** 1993. The cDNA of the neutrophil antibiotic Bac5 predicts a pro-sequence homologous to a cysteine proteinase inhibitor that is common to other neutrophil antibiotics. *J. Biol. Chem.* **268:**522–526.

258. **Zanetti, M., R. Gennaro, and D. Romeo.** 1997. The cathelicidin family of antimicrobial peptide precursors: a component of the oxygen-independent defense mechanisms of neutrophils. *Ann. N. Y. Acad. Sci.* **832:**147–162.

259. **Zanetti, M., L. Litteri, R. Gennaro, H. Horstmann, and D. Romeo.** 1990. Bactenecins, defense polypeptides of bovine neutrophils, are generated from precursor molecules stored in the large granules. *J. Cell. Biol.* **111:**1363–1371.

260. **Zasloff, M.** 2002. Antimicrobial peptides of multicellular organisms. *Nature* **415:**389–395.

261. **Zasloff, M.** 1987. Magainins, a class of antimicrobial peptides from *Xenopus* skin: isolation, characterization of two active forms, and partial cDNA sequence of a precursor. *Proc. Natl. Acad. Sci. USA* **84:**5449–5453.

262. **Zhang, X. L., M. E. Selsted, and A. Pardi.** 1992. NMR studies of defensin antimicrobial peptides. 1. Resonance assignment and secondary structure determination of rabbit NP-2 and human HNP-1. *Biochemistry* **31:**11348–11356.

263. **Zhao, C., T. Nguyen, L. Liu, O. Shamova, K. Brogden, and R. I. Lehrer.** 1999. Differential expression of caprine beta-defensins in digestive and respiratory tissues. *Infect. Immun.* **67:**6221–6224.

264. **Zimmermann, G. R., P. Legault, M. E. Selsted, and A. Pardi.** 1995. Solution structure of bovine neutrophil beta-defensin-12: the peptide fold of the beta-defensins is identical to

that of the classical defensins. *Biochemistry* **34:** 13663–13671.

265. **Zucht, H. D., J. Grabowsky, M. Schrader, C. Liepke, M. Jurgens, P. Schulz-Knappe,** **and W. G. Forssmann.** 1998. Human beta-defensin-1: a urinary peptide present in variant molecular forms and its putative functional implication. *Eur. J. Med. Res.* **3:**315–323.

ROLE OF COMMENSAL ENTERIC BACTERIA IN INTESTINAL INFLAMMATION: LESSONS FROM ANIMAL MODELS

R. Balfour Sartor

13

Ulcerative colitis and Crohn's disease, collectively referred to as inflammatory bowel diseases (IBD), are chronic, spontaneously relapsing diseases of uncertain etiology that preferentially involve the distal intestine (32, 100). These disorders appear to be immune mediated based on global activation of the innate and acquired immune systems and clinical responses to nonspecific and selective immunosuppressive therapies, including corticosteroids, cyclosporin, 6-mercaptopurine/azathioprine, and antibodies to tumor necrosis factor (TNF). Rodent models of colitis and ileitis have been extremely useful in developing insights into the pathogenesis of chronic immune-mediated intestinal inflammation (30, 114). Recent data have firmly implicated the commensal microbiota as the primary antigenic stimulus of pathogenic T-lymphocyte responses in these animal models (101). Experimental colitis and IBD occur in regions of highest bacterial stimulation; the ileum contains approximately 10^8 bacteria per g of luminal content and the cecum contains 10^{11} to 10^{12} CFU/g. This chapter outlines evidence

supporting the hypothesis that chronic immune-mediated intestinal inflammation in genetically susceptible hosts is a consequence of overly aggressive cell-mediated immune responses to a subset of commensal luminal bacteria. Mechanisms of genetic susceptibility include dysregulated immune responses leading to loss of immunologic tolerance to endogenous bacteria and altered mucosal barrier function, resulting in uptake of luminal antigens and adjuvants that overwhelm the intrinsic immunologic protective mechanisms (Color Plate 3). Environmental factors, such as diet, episodic antibiotic exposure, and public health measures, can alter the balance between protective (probiotic) and antigenic bacterial species, thereby profoundly influencing the antigenic stimulation of the mucosal immune system resulting in pathogenic responses.

EVIDENCE THAT NORMAL ENTERIC BACTERIA INDUCE COLITIS

Animal Models

The most compelling evidence that normal luminal bacteria induce colitis is the fact that in at least 11 separate models of induced or spontaneous intestinal inflammation, no disease occurs in the absence of bacteria (germ-

R. Balfour Sartor, Departments of Medicine, Microbiology and Immunology, University of North Carolina School of Medicine, Chapel Hill, NC 25799-7038.

Microbial Pathogenesis and the Intestinal Epithelial Cell, ed. by G. Hecht
© 2003 ASM Press, Washington, D.C.

free or sterile state) (Table 1). However, as early as 1 week after colonization with specific-pathogen-free (SPF) bacteria, susceptible mice or rats develop colitis which progresses to aggressive disease (89, 111). Moreover, the activity of intestinal inflammation correlates closely with the degree of bacterial stimulation. For example, interleukin-10 (IL-10)-deficient mice raised in a conventional rodent facility with parasites and bacterial pathogens, including *Helicobacter pylori*, develop lethal small intestinal and colonic inflammation, but in SPF conditions these mice exhibit isolated colitis with no mortality or small intestinal disease (55). Germfree IL-10 knockout mice have no intestinal inflammation by clinical, histologic, and immunologic criteria, but develop cecal-predominant colitis within 1 week of colonization with SPF fecal bacteria, which progresses to aggressive, transmural inflammation with mucosal ulcers and crypt abscesses by 5 weeks after bacterial colonization (111). Treatment of SPF IL-10$^{-/-}$ mice with broad-spectrum antibiotics (a combination of imipenem and vancomycin) can both prevent and treat colitis in this model (24). Of considerable importance, inflammation is confined to the colon, which is the site of highest bacterial concentrations, despite a generalized defect in immunosuppressive IL-10. Similar results are seen in human leukocyte antigen (HLA)/human β_2-microglobulin transgenic

(TG) rats (103). In conventional housing conditions, HLA B$_{27}$ TG rats develop lethal colitis, gastroduodenitis, and clinically evident arthritis, dermatitis, and orchitis (40, 81). Both gastrointestinal inflammation and arthritis are attenuated in an SPF facility and are absent in a sterile environment; the dermatitis and orchitis persist even in the absence of bacterial colonization (89, 120). Imipenem and vancomycin prevent the onset of disease and treat established colitis in SPF B$_{27}$ TG rats, consistent with a 2-log decrease in fecal bacterial concentrations (91). Moreover, cecal inflammation is potentiated by the creation of a cecal self-filling blind loop (SFBL), which results in a 3-log increase in cecal luminal bacterial concentrations, and is dramatically attenuated by surgical bypass of the cecum, which decreases local bacterial concentrations (90). Together, these results in two independent, genetically engineered models graphically illustrate the close correlation of luminal bacterial concentrations with colonic inflammation.

Similar observations in a number of other widely divergent models of small intestinal and colonic inflammation in knockout mice (21, 108); inbred mouse and nonhuman primate strains with spontaneous disease; T-cell transfer models; and induced disease in rats, mice, and guinea pigs in a germfree or reduced bacterial microenvironment (Table 2) and with antibiotic treatment indicate that the ability of endogenous normal enteric bacteria to induce intestinal inflammation in susceptible hosts is a universal phenomenon that is likely to be relevant to human IBD. The only exceptions to this rule are the mild, highly attenuated colitis, gastritis, and hepatitis that develop in germfree IL-2$^{-/-}$ mice and one report of potentiated colitis in germfree mice fed dextran sodium sulfate (DSS) (7). This latter publication is balanced by a conflicting one by Tlaskalova et al., reporting the absence of disease in germfree mice receiving DSS (122), which is consistent with the observation of Onderdonk et al. in germfree guinea pigs fed carrageenan, a related highly sulfated polysaccharide (80). Bacterial metabolism of

TABLE 1. Animal models that do not develop intestinal inflammation in a germfree (sterile) environment

Animal	Model
Mice	IL-2$^{-/-}$, IL-10$^{-/-}$, T-cell receptor $\alpha^{-/-}$, CD$_3\varepsilon$ transgenic, SAMP-1/Yit, DSS, CD$_{45}$RB^{high} → SCID
Rats	HLA B$_{27}$ transgenic, indomethacin
Guinea pigs	Carrageenan
Nonhuman primates	Cotton top tamarin (Thiry-Vella loop)

TABLE 2 Specificity of induction of colitis in gnotobiotic rodent models by defined bacterial species

Model	Bacterial strains inducing colitis	Bacterial strains *not* inducing colitis
IL-10$^{-/-}$ mice (8, 51, 109, 118)	*Enterococcus faecalis, Escherichia coli*	*Bacteroides vulgatus, Helicobacter hepaticus, Candida albicans, Lactococcus lactis, Bifidobacterium* sp., *Lactobacillus* sp., *Bacillus* sp., *Streptococcus viridans, Clostridium sordellii, Enterococcus faecium, Peptostreptococcus productus, Eubacterium contortium, Streptococcus avium*
CD$_{45}$RB^{high} CD$_4^+$ T cells → SCID mice (49)	*Helicobacter muridarum*	Segmented filamentous bacteria, *Listeria monocytogenes* (actA$^-$), *Morganella morganii, Ochrobactrum anthropi*
HLA B$_{27}$ transgenic rat (89, 92)	*Bacteroides vulgatus*	*Escherichia coli, Enterococcus faecalis, Enterococcus faecium, Streptococcus avium, Peptostreptococcus productus, Eubacterium contortium*

DSS may attenuate its inflammatory potential, although this explanation is inconsistent with decreased DSS-induced colitis by antibiotics (91). Despite the lower concentration of luminal bacteria in the small intestine relative to the colon, at least two models of small intestinal inflammation display similar responses to germfree conditions and antibiotic treatment. The Samp-1/Yit strain of mice does not develop ileitis in a sterile environment, whereas antibiotics attenuate ileal inflammation (71). Likewise, susceptible inbred Lewis rats injected twice with indomethacin develop chronic mid-small intestinal ulcers in an SPF environment. However, disease is attenuated by metronidazole (128) and absent in sterile conditions (104). Mid-small intestinal ulceration is associated with local proliferation of luminal enteric bacteria and translocation of viable bacteria into regional lymph nodes (128). Bacteria also contribute to experimental pouchitis in Lewis rats, based on the association of increased luminal bacterial concentrations in the presence of inflammation and response to treatment with antibiotics active against anaerobic bacteria (61).

Extraintestinal inflammation associated with enterocolitis is also dependent on commensal enteric bacteria. Peripheral arthritis that develops in conventional HLA B$_{27}$ TG rats is attenuated under SPF conditions and absent in a sterile environment (89, 120). Susceptible Lewis and Wistar rats with proliferation of predominantly anaerobic bacteria within jejunal SFBL develop hepatobiliary inflammation resembling some features of sclerosing cholangitis and reactivation of experimental peripheral arthritis (60, 62). These lesions are almost totally prevented by metronidazole and tetracycline, which decrease total and anaerobic luminal bacterial concentrations and eliminate *Bacteroides* species (58).

Results in these models indicate that nonviable components of the indigenous bacterial flora can induce and perpetuate intestinal and extraintestinal inflammation. Purified sterile peptidoglycan-polysaccharide (PG-PS) polymers, the primary structural component of the bacterial cell wall, can induce chronic, spontaneously relapsing T-lymphocyte-dependent, granulomatous ileocolitis with erosive, deforming peripheral arthritis, hepatic granulomas, leukocytosis, and anemia of chronic disease in inbred Lewis rats (72, 107). Luminal PG-PS can potentiate acetic acid-induced colitis and is absorbed in greater amounts as detected by cardiac blood, hepatic, and splenic tissue concentrations (106). Furthermore, PG-PS from endogenous enteric bacteria can induce intestinal and systemic inflammation in susceptible Lewis rats, as demonstrated by the ability of mutanolysin, which degrades PG-PS, to prevent and treat experimental pouchitis (61) as well as hepatobiliary inflammation (59) and arthritis (62) induced by small intestinal bacterial overgrowth in the SFBL Lewis rat model. Mutanolysin splits the β_{1-4} linkage between N-acetylglucosamine and N-acetylmuramic acid of the peptidoglycan polymer backbone, which is the same target specificity as mammalian lysozysome. In our hands, lipopolysaccharide (LPS) does not seem to contribute to intestinal and systemic inflammation in these models. Polymyxin B, which complexes and inactivates LPS, had no beneficial effects on arthritis or hepatobiliary inflammation induced by experimental small intestinal bacterial overgrowth in Lewis rats with SFBL or with ileal pouches postcolectomy (58, 61). In vitro, LPS appears to mediate the ability of *Bacteroides vulgatus* to activate NF-κB-dependent intercellular adhesion molecule-1 (ICAM-1) expression in epithelial cell lines (39). LPS and PG-PS stimulate NF-κB through Toll-like receptors (TLR) 4 and 2, respectively (1); both luminal bacterial cell wall polymers can stimulate intracellular NOD-2 (79) and have important adjuvant activities on innate immune cells (110). Thus, these bacterial components, which are present in high concentrations in the lumen of the distal intestine and whose absorption is enhanced with intestinal inflammation (35, 106), may be critically important in inducing and perpetuating chronic, immune-mediated intestinal and extraintestinal inflammation.

Genetic susceptibility is a key determinant of pathogenic versus homeostatic responses to commensal bacteria. In all the genetically engineered rodent models discussed, wild-type (normal) littermates or controls colonized with identical luminal bacteria fail to display any evidence of gastrointestinal or systemic inflammation. For example, nontransgenic littermate control rats housed in the same cages with HLA B_{27} TG rats had no colitis, gastritis, or arthritis (40, 89). Similarly, germfree, wild-type, genetically matched mice colonized with identical cecal or fecal flora as ex-germfree IL-$10^{-/-}$ mice had no clinical, histologic, or immunologic evidence of immune activation (111). Finally, inbred Fischer F_{344} rats, which are major histocompatibility complex (MHC) matched with Lewis rats, and Buffalo rats injected with intramural PG-PS or which develop small bowel bacterial overgrowth as a result of a jejunal SFBL, have only transient intestinal inflammation with no chronicity and no extraintestinal inflammation (60, 72, 107). However, genetic factors alone are not sufficient to induce disease, as illustrated by the lack of colitis or extraintestinal inflammation in susceptible inbred rodent strains or genetically engineered rats and mice raised in germfree conditions. Chronic intestinal inflammation and extraintestinal disease require the interaction of both genetic susceptibility and environmental (microbial) stimulation.

Relevance to IBD

Observations in human IBD, although less controlled, validate the previously outlined results in animal models. Colonic and distal ileal involvement coincides with regions of highest luminal bacterial concentrations, and postoperative recurrent Crohn's disease in the neoterminal ileum immediately proximal to the ileocolonic anastomosis corresponds with exposure to refluxed colonic bacteria. A number of antibiotics (102), most notably metronidazole (115), ciprofloxacin (14), or the combination of both antibiotics (38), treat Crohn's disease. Of key importance, colonic Crohn's disease responds better to antibiotics than isolated ileal disease (38, 112, 115), and ulcerative colitis responds poorly to most antibiotics (102), although Finnish investigators documented a small additive effect of ciprofloxacin and steroids in ulcerative colitis patients (123).

Multiple investigators have documented a decrease in the activity or rate of postoperative recurrence of Crohn's disease after diversion of the fecal stream, either with a diverting ileostomy for active Crohn's colitis (42) or with proximal ileal diversion after segmental resection and primary anastomosis (98). Reanastomosis with restoration of luminal flow leads to a prompt recurrence of disease. Infusion of ostomy contents also results in rapid reactivation of clinical symptoms or histologic and immunohistochemical evidence of inflammation (20, 41). These results suggest that luminal contents contain factors that induce and perpetuate IBD. The association of three single nucleotide polymorphisms in the LPS-binding region of NOD-2 with Crohn's disease provides indirect evidence of a microbial influence in this disease (48, 78). NOD-2 binds intracellular LPS and PG-PS in innate immune cells activating NF-κB (79).

INDUCTION OF CHRONIC INTESTINAL INFLAMMATION BY SELECTED COMPONENTS OF THE ENDOGENOUS BACTERIAL FLORA

Animal Models

Recent results in several independent gnotobiotic models demonstrate that commensal enteric bacterial species differ in their capacity to induce chronic intestinal inflammation (Table 2). We demonstrated that *B. vulgatus* preferentially induces colitis but not gastritis in monoassociated HLA B$_{27}$ TG rats (92), consistent with Onderdonk's observations in guinea pigs with carrageenan-induced colitis (80). Germfree HLA B$_{27}$ TG rats selectively colonized for 1 month with a group of five bacterial species (*Escherichia coli, Enterococcus faecium, Peptostreptococcus productus, Eubacterium contortium,* and *Streptococcus avium*) isolated from Crohn's disease patients did not develop colitis relative to germfree controls (89). However, B$_{27}$ TG rats selectively colonized with the same group of five IBD bacterial strains plus *B. vulgatus* had almost as much colitis and gastritis as SPF TG rats. The specific role of *B. vulgatus* in this model was confirmed by selective colonization (monoassociation) studies. Monoassociation with *B. vulgatus*

induced moderate colitis but no gastritis, whereas selective colonization with *E. coli* had no effect (92). Of considerable importance, however, this *B. vulgatus* strain, either alone or in combination with the five previously studied human IBD-related bacterial strains, stimulated only minimal inflammation in IL-10$^{-/-}$ mice (111), indicating selectivity of responses in different host genetic backgrounds. Similarly, *Enterococcus faecalis* induces colitis in monoassociated IL-10$^{-/-}$ mice (8, 51), yet a related group D streptococcal (enterococcal) species, *Enterococcus faecium,* has no effect in B$_{27}$ TG rats (89). These bacterial species are not pathogens, since *Enterococcus faecalis* and *B. vulgatus* do not induce inflammation in wild-type mice and rats. In unpublished data, we have demonstrated that murine *E. coli* induces aggressive colitis in monoassociated IL-10$^{-/-}$ mice. As stated earlier, a human *E. coli* strain had no effect in B$_{27}$ TG rats (89). Similarly, the effects of *Helicobacter* species are variable in different models and host genetic backgrounds. *Helicobacter hepaticus* colonization had no inflammatory effects in monoassociated IL-10$^{-/-}$ mice or potentiation of colitis in SPF IL-10$^{-/-}$ mice on a mixed 129/C57/Bl6 background (22), but potentiated disease in inbred C57/Bl6 IL-10$^{-/-}$ mice (57). In contrast, *Helicobacter muridarum* monoassociated severe combined immunodeficient (SCID) mice, but not *H. hepaticus* monoassociated mice, developed colitis following transfer of CD$_{45}$RB^{hi} T cells (49). Of potential relevance to the concept of heterogeneous bacterial antigen stimulation in subsets of IBD patients, the kinetics and location of intestinal inflammation in IL-10$^{-/-}$ mice selectively colonized with *Enterococcus faecalis* and *E. coli* are substantially different. *E. faecalis* monoassociated mice develop a slow onset of predominantly distal colitis that is evident by 12 weeks after the bacterial colonization; after 30 weeks some IL-10$^{-/-}$ mice develop duodenal inflammation with obstruction (51). In contrast, *E. coli* monoassociated IL-10$^{-/-}$ mice have a rapid onset of predominantly right-sided (cecal) colonic inflammation that is clinically apparent after 6 weeks of colonization. In both of these models (IL-10$^{-/-}$ mouse and HLA B$_{27}$ TG rat), colitis is more aggressive in SPF rodents than in monoassociated animals, indicating additive and perhaps synergistic activities of the complex cecal bacterial milieu. This concept is further supported by more potent therapeutic activity of the broad-spectrum antibiotic combination of imipenem and vancomycin in B$_{27}$ TG rats or IL-10$^{-/-}$ mice compared with the effects of selective metronidazole and ciprofloxacin (24, 91). Yet many common enteric bacterial species are unable to induce disease (Table 2), suggesting that a relatively small number of commensal bacterial species induce inflammation, with evidence of host-specific responses to microbial stimulation.

Beneficial Effects

The evolving concept that a subset of commensal bacteria with beneficial effects (probiotic species) can prevent experimental colitis or even reverse established disease has important clinical implications. Madsen et al. (66) attenuated the onset and progression of colitis in IL-10$^{-/-}$ mice by administering commensal *Lactobacillus reuteri* or feeding lactulose, a prebiotic agent that enhances the growth of luminal *Lactobacillus* species. Similarly, we reported that daily administration of *Lactobacillus plantarum* could reverse established colitis in SPF IL-10$^{-/-}$ mice (109). In these models, specificity of both bacterial species and host genetic background are important variables, since *Lactobacillus* sp. strain GG had no benefit in IL-10$^{-/-}$ murine colitis (126). In contrast, *Lactobacillus* sp. strain GG, but not *L. plantarum*, could prevent relapse of colitis in HLA B$_{27}$ TG rats following induction of remission by broad-spectrum antibiotics (vancomycin and imipenem) (23). Recent observations indicate that nonviable components of probiotic bacteria, including nonmethylated DNA, can mediate these protective responses. Rachmilewitz et al. prevented colitis in three separate rodent models with synthetic DNA (88) as well as DNA isolated from VSL3, a combination of eight individual probiotic bacterial species (87).

EVIDENCE OF MUCOSAL AND SYSTEMIC IMMUNE ACTIVATION INDUCED BY COMMENSAL ENTERIC BACTERIA

Pathogenic Immune Responses in Susceptible Hosts

Chronic intestinal inflammation is mediated by T lymphocytes, based on the absence of experimental colitis in T-cell-deficient hosts (19, 63), induction of disease by transfer of CD$_4^+$ T lymphocytes (15, 86, 125), and prevention and reversal of chronic inflammation by blockade of products of T$_{H1}$ cytokines (77, 84). Not only are B lymphocytes not required for induction of experimental colitis (19, 63), but these cells also appear to downregulate disease activity (74). In a variety of rodent models, T lymphocytes are selectively responsive to autochthonous luminal bacteria. For example, CD$_4^+$ T cells from the mesenteric lymph nodes (MLN) of CD$_3\varepsilon$ TG mice produce high amounts of gamma interferon (IFN-γ) when incubated with antigen-presenting cells pulsed with cecal bacterial lysates but not with autologous colonic epithelial cells or cecal lysates from germfree mice (125). Similarly, MLN CD$_4^+$ T cells from *Enterococcus faecalis* monoassociated IL-10$^{-/-}$ mice produce high amounts of IFN-γ in response to *Enterococcus faecalis*, but not to *E. coli* or *B. vulgatus* (51), and CD$_4^+$ lymphocytes from HLA B$_{27}$ TG rats secrete abundant IFN-γ when incubated with cecal bacterial lysates (25). Cong et al. demonstrated that bacterial antigen-specific T lymphocytes can induce disease in SPF T-cell-deficient (SCID) recipients (15); activation of these CD$_4^+$ lymphocytes requires CD$_{40}$/CD$_{40}$ ligand interactions (16). Luminal bacterial antigen needs to be continuously present for development of chronic immune-mediated colitis, as demonstrated in the CD$_3\varepsilon$ TG mouse model (125). T lymphocytes from SPF CD$_3\varepsilon$ TG mice with active colitis can transfer disease to SPF T-cell-deficient recipients, although no disease occurs after a similar transfer to germfree recipients. However, the transfer of CD$_4^+$ lymphocytes from the MLN of germfree mice to SPF recipients induced colitis. These studies indicate that activated mucosal T cells require constant antigenic stimulation to induce and perpetuate colonic inflammation, with no evidence of autoimmune activity.

A key factor in the induction of chronic immune-mediated intestinal inflammation is the loss of tolerance to luminal bacterial antigens in genetically susceptible hosts. Normal (genetically resistant) hosts exhibit downregulated mucosal T-cell responses to commensal autologous luminal bacteria; this protective response is lost in susceptible hosts (25, 29).

Innate immune responses in macrophages, dendritic cells, epithelial cells, and neutrophils are integral components in the inflammatory response, mediating activities via stimulation of proinflammatory cytokines and antigen-presenting cells that activate T lymphocytes. Components of commensal bacteria, including cell wall polymers (LPS and PG-PS) and DNA (methylated DNA [CPG]), activate innate immune cells through pattern-recognition receptors, including TLR2 (binding PG-PS), TLR4 (LPS), TLR9 (DNA), and NOD 1 and 2 (LPS and PG-PS) (Color Plate 4) (1). Binding of these products to TLR and NOD molecules activates NF-κB and other key signaling pathways. These bacterial products function as adjuvants that upregulate costimulatory molecules on antigen-presenting cells and stimulate secreted proinflammatory cytokines such as IL-12, which together activate T_{H1} lymphocytes. For example, autologous cecal bacterial lysates and LPS stimulate IL-12 and TNF secretion by T-lymphocyte-depleted MLN cells from HLA B_{27} TG rats and IL-$10^{-/-}$ mice (25, 50). These same stimulants upregulate costimulatory molecules and enhance IL-12 secretion by cultured dendritic cells or isolated antigen-presenting cells from IL-$10^{-/-}$ mice (2). Recent observations indicate that LPS from *B. vulgatus* and nonpathogenic *E. coli* can stimulate NF-κB and upregulate ICAM-1 mRNA and protein expression in intestinal epithelial cells through TLR4 binding (39).

Induction of Protective Immune Responses in Normal Hosts

Germfree rodents have underdeveloped immune responses which are activated following bacterial colonization (64). In normal hosts, commensal luminal bacteria induce protective innate and acquired mucosal responses that regulate barrier function and homeostatic immune mechanisms. Hooper et al. (47) reported that colonization of germfree mice with *Bacteroides thetaiotaomicron* upregulated a characteristic profile of genes contributing to mucosal barrier function, nutrient absorption, epithelial maturation, and xenobiotic metabolism. In a more complex system, colonization of germfree mice with SPF bacteria stimulated mucin (MUC-2) gene expression and sulfation (68). In a murine radiation mucosal damage model, LPS prevented injury and stimulated cyclooxygenase-2 (COX-2) expression and protective prostaglandins in subepithelial myofibroblasts and villous, but not crypt, epithelial cells (94). Antibiotic treatment of neonatal mice enhanced in vitro IL-4 secretion and diminished IL-12 and IFN-γ expression (82), providing a mechanism for T_{H2} responses associated with atopy in children treated with antibiotics during infancy. Bacterial specificity of immune activation is suggested by reports of selective activation of IL-12 by gram-positive bacteria, but stimulation of IL-4 by LPS and gram-negative organisms (44). Of considerable relevance to mechanisms of immunologic tolerance and the pathogenesis of intestinal inflammation, developing evidence suggests that commensal luminal bacteria induce homeostatic mucosal immune responses. Michalek et al. (73, 127) demonstrated lack of oral tolerance to sheep red blood cells, measured by systemic antibody responses, in germfree mice. Normal protective responses could be restored by colonization with gram-negative bacteria and feeding LPS, but not by monoassociation with gram-positive organisms. These results further support the selective induction of regulatory mucosal immune responses by gram-negative commensal enteric bacteria. More recent results indicate that tolerance to dietary oval-bumin is more easily broken in germfree mice and more rapidly restored following colonization with normal bacteria (34, 75) and that $CD_{45}RB^{low}$ CD_4^+ T cells from germfree mice are less effective in preventing colitis induced by cotransferred $CD_{45}RB^{high}$ lymphocytes than are regulatory cells from SPF mice (95). Direct evidence of this concept is provided by prevention of T-cell-induced colitis by co-transferred cecal bacterial expanded CD_4^+ T cells (17).

Relevance to Human IBD

Loss of tolerance to commensal luminal bacteria by the humoral and cellular immune systems has been documented by multiple investigators (101). Circulating and mucosally secreted antibodies to a variety of enteric commensal bacteria are increased in patients with Crohn's disease (6, 65, 119). More recently, serologic responses to discrete epitopes of *B. vulgatus, Pseudomonas fluorescens*, and mycobacterial species have been proposed as noninvasive diagnostic markers of Crohn's disease (12, 70, 116). Although increased serum humoral responses to luminal bacteria are less evident in ulcerative colitis, perinuclear antineutrophilic autoantibodies (pANCA), which are present in 60 to 80% of ulcerative patients, cross-react with several bacterial species, including *Bacteroides caccae, E. coli*, and mycobacteria (11, 12). Duchmann et al. report enhanced proliferation of CD_4^+ T lymphocytes of IBD patients to ubiquitous enteric bacteria (26). T-cell clones from mucosal biopsies showed specific responses to selected common resident bacterial species, including *Bacteroides, Bifidobacteria*, and *E. coli* (27, 28). These results suggest that commensal luminal bacteria provide a constant antigenic stimulus capable of driving pathogenic immune responses in Crohn's disease and ulcerative colitis patients. Furthermore, selective bacterial responses lay the foundation for possible differential immunologic responses to discrete components of the complex luminal microbial milieu in subsets of IBD patients. As is the case with rodent models, combinations of pro-

biotic bacteria (VSL 3) administered to patients with pouchitis prevent recurrent inflammation (37) and stimulate mucosal IL-10 production while reducing TNF levels (124).

MECHANISMS OF IMMUNE-MEDIATED INFLAMMATION IN RESPONSE TO COMMENSAL BACTERIA IN GENETICALLY SUSCEPTIBLE HOSTS

The data discussed above clearly indicate that chronic inflammation in genetically susceptible hosts is due to an overly aggressive cell-mediated immune response to commensal bacteria. However, exact mechanisms of genetic susceptibility and immune activation remain unclear. Rodent models of colitis indicate that genetic susceptibility to inflammation can result from at least three general pathways: (i) dysregulated host immune responses, (ii) defective mucosal barrier function/healing, or (iii) dysbiosis (abnormal balance of aggressive/protective bacteria).

Dysregulated Host Immune Responses

Intestinal homeostasis depends on a delicate balance between pro- and anti-inflammatory cytokines and cellular activities that downregulate pathogenic immunologic responses to resident microflora, dietary, and host antigens, yet allow effective clearance of enteric pathogens. Tolerogenic immune responses appear to be dependent on transforming growth factor β (TGF-β) and IL-10, which are selectively secreted by activated regulatory T cells (T_{H3} and T_{R1}) as well as antigen-presenting cells (84, 113). The best evidence for prevention of inflammation by regulatory T cells is provided by cotransfer studies. Colitis can be induced in T-cell-deficient mice (SCID or RAG-2$^{-/-}$) by injection of $CD_{45}RB^{high}$ CD_4^+ T cells derived from the spleens of normal SPF mice (86). In contrast, $CD_{45}RB^{low}$ cells from the same source do not induce colitis. A regulatory function of the $CD_{45}RB^{low}$ cell population is evident by prevention of colitis when $CD_{45}RB^{high}$ and RB^{low} T cells are cotransferred. As mentioned earlier, colitis is absent in SCID mice raised in a simplified microflora environment, demonstrating the importance of normal bacteria in inducing pathogenic responses (4). Blockade of either IL-10 or TGF-β by neutralizing antibodies reverses protection by CD$_{45}$RB^{low} T cells (5, 85). Preliminary results indicate the CD$_{45}$RB^{low} cells from germ-free donors have attenuated abilities to prevent colitis in this cotransfer model (95), suggesting that normal bacteria activate protective regulatory T cells. Consistent with this observation, Cong et al. demonstrated that bacterial responsive T$_{R1}$ CD$_4^+$ T cells prevent disease in a cotransfer model (17). Recent results indicate that regulatory T cells have high membrane expression of the IL-2 receptor (CD$_{25}$) (93), perhaps explaining the onset of colitis in SPF IL-2$^{-/-}$ mice (99). Spontaneous intestinal inflammation occurs in genetically engineered mice with targeted deletion of either of the key immunosuppressive molecules IL-10 or TGF-β (9, 55, 56). Inflammation is generalized in multiple organs in TGF-β knockout mice (9, 56), but is selectively localized to the colon in SPF IL-10$^{-/-}$ mice (55, 111). Unfractionated MLN or splenic cells from IL-10$^{-/-}$ mice produce dramatically higher concentrations of IL-1β, IL-12, and TNF when stimulated by LPS or cecal bacterial lysates compared with cells from wild-type mice (50). Similarly, antigen-presenting cells or cultured dendritic cells from IL-10$^{-/-}$ mice produce more IL-12 in response to LPS or cecal bacterial lysates, and cecal bacterial lysate-pulsed antigen-presenting or dendritic cells stimulate more IFN-γ by cultured MLN CD$_4^+$ T cells than do similarly stimulated cells from wild-type mice (2). These results illustrate the key role of endogenous IL-10 in preventing pathogenic immune responses to bacterial stimuli.

Although knockout mice are extremely valuable tools to test hypotheses, the complete absence of intrinsic regulatory molecules in genetically engineered rodents is not physiologic. A role for IL-10 in the suppression of pathogenic immune responses to commensal bacteria in genetically susceptible hosts is suggested by increased IL-12 and IFN-γ responses in unfractionated MLN cells from

HLA B$_{27}$ TG rats compared with wild-type rats in response to cecal bacterial lysate stimulation, but increased IL-10 in stimulated cells from wild-type rats (25). Surprisingly, in selective depletion studies IL-10 appeared to be produced primarily by B lymphocytes. These in vitro results conflict with results of cotransfer studies, which suggest that IL-10-secreting regulatory T cells mediate protection in the CD$_{45}$RB$^{high/low}$ cotransfer model (5, 84). In vivo and in vitro results using probiotic bacterial species show that beneficial bacteria can selectively induce IL-10. Oral Lactobacillus sp. strain GG administration after short-term antibiotic treatment stimulated mucosal IL-10 secretion (23) and the VSL 3 combination of Lactobacillus, Bifidobacteria, and Streptococcus species stimulated IL-10 in unfractionated rat splenocytes (10).

Relevance to IBD. As stated earlier, IBD patients display loss of tolerance to resident luminal bacteria (26) with induction of humoral and cellular immune responses to commensal bacteria (101). Whether defective NF-κB activation by LPS in the innate immune cells of Crohn's disease patients with NOD-2 polymorphisms (78) leads to defective antigen-presenting activities remains to be determined.

Defective Mucosal Barrier Function

A defective mucosal barrier could lead to enhanced uptake of luminal bacterial adjuvants and antigens that overwhelm protective mucosal immune responses. The intestinal barrier is composed of a mucus layer, which prevents epithelial attachment of bacteria; secreted IgA and IgM, which complex luminal antigens; and epithelial tight junctions, which limit uptake of luminal macromolecules. If mucosal injury occurs, epithelial restitution rapidly restores integrity and the proliferation of epithelial cells heals microscopic ulcers. Results in knockout and transgenic mice graphically illustrate the importance of an intact epithelial barrier and effective healing in preventing intestinal inflammation. Targeted deletion of intestinal trefoil factor (ITF), which promotes epithelial restitution and increases viscosity of mucus, increases mortality and delays healing in mice with colitis induced by DSS (69). The protective role of ITF is further demonstrated by enhanced healing by rectally administered ITF. Another major stimulant of epithelial restitution is TGF-β (83), which provides another mechanism in addition to immunosuppression to explain the spontaneous colitis that develops in TGF-$\beta^{-/-}$ mice (9). Likewise, Madsen et al. reported that enhanced mucosal permeability and mucosal adherence/invasion of bacteria occur in IL-10$^{-/-}$ mice before the onset of histologic evidence of colitis (66) and that IL-10 enhances epithelial resistance in vitro (67), suggesting that another immunosuppressive molecule also has protective effects on the mucosal barrier. We have demonstrated that IL-10$^{-/-}$ mice have decreased Muc-2 expression even in the germfree state with no inflammation (68). Direct evidence that defective mucosal barrier function can induce intestinal inflammation is provided by the observation that transgenic mice with a dominant negative N-cadherin gene develop intestinal inflammation (43). N-cadherin is a component of the epithelial junctional complex. Finally, prostaglandins stimulate mucus secretion, enhance mucosal blood flow, and accelerate healing after radiation or DSS-induced injury (13, 121). COX-2$^{-/-}$ mice treated with DSS have increased mortality rates and inflammatory scores relative to wild-type mice; COX-1 mice have intermediate inflammation that is also significantly greater than wild-type mice (76). Together, these results in genetically engineered mice demonstrate that genetically determined defects in different mucosal barrier components can lead to chronic, immune-mediated intestinal inflammation.

In addition, environmental factors affect the mucosal barrier, leading to transient breaks that can induce chronic, self-perpetuating intestinal inflammation due to enhanced uptake of luminal bacterial antigens and adjuvants in genetically susceptible hosts. For example, two subcutaneous injections of indomethacin induce chronic mid-small bowel ulceration in susceptible Lewis rats under SPF conditions, but self-limited, transient ulcers in MHC-matched Fischer F$_{344}$ rats (105). Luminal bacteria are essential for the development of chronic inflammation in this model (104).

Relevance to IBD. Mucosal permeability is clearly increased during active Crohn's disease and ulcerative colitis, with enhanced uptake of LPS and translocation of viable bacteria to serosal surfaces and MLN (3, 36). However, developing evidence points to a primary mucosal barrier defect in IBD patients, particularly in patients with Crohn's disease. Hollander et al. suggested that mucosal permeability is enhanced in asymptomatic relatives of Crohn's disease patients (46), which is supported by the observations of Hilsden et al. (45) indicating that a subset of Crohn's disease families display enhanced mucosal permeability with aspirin challenge. Swidsinski et al. reported increased mucosal adherence of luminal bacteria in IBD patients with evidence of intraepithelial bacterial invasion (117). Similarly, Sutton et al. demonstrated increased P. fluorescens DNA in the lamina propria in the colon of Crohn's disease patients (116). A novel mechanism of decreased mucosal protection is suggested by Korzenik et al., who hypothesize that Crohn's disease patients exhibit defective clearance of bacteria by innate immune cells (53). This hypothesis is supported by a preliminary report of beneficial responses to granulocyte colony-stimulating factor (G-CSF) in Crohn's disease patients (52); this molecule increases production and activity of monocytes, macrophages, and neutrophils. This novel hypothesis may also be relevant to mechanisms of inflammation in Crohn's disease patients with NOD-2 polymorphisms (48, 78). NOD-2 is primarily expressed in innate immune cells, particularly monocytes, macrophages, and dendritic cells; binds intracellular LPS and PG-PS; and transduces signals to NF-κB (79). An unanticipated effect of the polymorphisms in the leucine-rich repeat region of NOD-2, which binds LPS and PG-PS, is *defective* induction of NFκB (78), which could possibly lead to decreased clearance of invading enteric bacteria by innate immune cells.

Dysbiosis (Altered Ratio of Beneficial and Aggressive Luminal Bacteria)

A developing concept in IBD is that the *balance* of beneficial and aggressive luminal bacteria affects mucosal homeostasis and regulates immune responses (Table 3). An altered composition of resident enteric bacteria could adversely affect mucosal barrier and immune function. For example, butyrate and other short-chain fatty acids produced by fermentation of nonabsorbed dietary carbohydrates by enteric commensal bacteria are the primary metabolic fuels of colonic epithelial cells; they both stimulate epithelial differentiation and block NF-κB activity. Conversely, hydrogen sulfide, which is produced by sulfate-reducing bacteria, can block short-chain fatty acid metabolism by colonic epithelial cells (97). Roediger has postulated that ulcerative colitis is the result of epithelial starvation due to defective epithelial short-chain fatty acid metabolism (96). However, almost complete elimination of luminal hydrogen sulfide by bismuth subsalicylate had no effect on acute DSS-included colitis (33). In a careful analysis of sequential microbial colonization, Madsen et al. (66) showed that neonatal IL-10$^{-/-}$ mice were preferentially colonized by streptococci and clostridial species rather than lactobacilli, which are the principal species colonizing wild-type mice of equivalent age. Similarly, in unpublished observations, we have noted expansion of certain commensal bacterial species

and contraction of other bacteria in ex-germfree IL-10$^{-/-}$ mice colonized with feces or cecal contents from wild-type mice (K. Wilson, G. Tannock, and R. B. Sartor, unpublished observations). Whether these results are a consequence or a cause of inflammation and whether they are related to the absence of IL-10 remain to be determined. Observations by Fabia et al. (31) suggest a secondary effect, that *Lactobacillus* species are decreased in nonspecific colitis. However, a role for altered luminal composition in the induction of pathogenic immune responses is suggested by increased IFN-γ secretion by MLN of SPF IL-10$^{-/-}$ mice when stimulated with cecal bacterial lysates from IL-10$^{-/-}$ mice with colitis compared with similarly prepared cecal lysates from wild-type mice (C. Albright, S. Kim, and R. B. Sartor, unpublished observations). Therapeutic manipulation of luminal bacterial products by administering *Lactobacillus* species (109) or lactulose, a prebiotic substance that fosters growth of enteric *Lactobacillus* species (66), indicates that changing the luminal microenvironment can have beneficial outcomes.

Relevance to IBD. Ulcerative colitis patients have decreased luminal concentrations of butyrate and increased hydrogen sulfide (96, 97), although these patients do not routinely respond to butyrate or short-chain fatty acid enemas. IBD patients have altered luminal concentrations of probiotic bacteria relative to potentially aggressive bacterial species (31) and respond clinically to supplemental probiotic species, including *E. coli* Nissle for ulcerative colitis patients (54) and VSL 3 in pouchitis (37). An example of subtle changes in bacterial composition is the increased presence of mucosally adherent/invasive *E. coli* strains in ileal biopsy samples in patients with Crohn's disease relative to noninflamed controls and ulcerative colitis patients (18).

CONCLUSIONS

Many studies discussed here support the hypothesis that chronic intestinal inflammation is a consequence of an overly aggressive cell-

TABLE 3 Relative balance of protective versus detrimental commensal enteric bacterial species determines intestinal inflammation versus mucosal homeostasis

Beneficial species	Aggressive species
Lactobacillus spp.	*Bacteroides vulgatus*
Bifidobacter spp.	*Bacteroides thetaiotaomicron*
Streptococcus salivarius	*Enterococcus faecalis*
Selected *Escherichia coli*	Enteroadherent/toxigenic *Escherichia coli*

mediated immune response to a subset of the complex resident enteric bacterial population in genetically susceptible hosts. Host genetic susceptibility is a key determinant of homeostasis versus pathogenic immune responses to ubiquitous luminal bacterial antigens and adjuvants—susceptible hosts develop injurious responses, while normal resistant hosts exhibit protective, regulatory immune responses. Both pathogenic and homeostatic immune responses are initiated and sustained by luminal bacterial adjuvants such as LPS, PG-PS, and DNA fragments and defined bacterial antigens. Several mechanisms of genetic susceptibility are involved in this loss of immunologic tolerance to commensal bacterial antigens: dysregulated host immune responses, defective mucosal barrier function or repair, and an altered balance of beneficial versus aggressive enteric bacteria (dysbiosis).

Environmental factors prominently influence the induction and reactivation of inflammation. Transient infections, use of nonsteroidal anti-inflammatory drugs, exposure to toxins, and smoking can break the mucosal barrier, leading to increased mucosal uptake of luminal bacterial products and inflammation. Similarly, antibiotics, dietary modification, and public health measures can alter the composition of commensal bacteria. Transient mucosal injury or alteration of the microbial milieu is self-limited in normal, resistant hosts, but becomes self-sustaining and chronic in genetically susceptible hosts that have loss of immunologic tolerance caused by dysregulated mucosal immune responses or defective mucosal repair mechanisms (Color Plate 5). Chronic inflammation is sustained by the constant antigenic drive of commensal bacterial antigens and adjuvants.

These observations in rodent models have important implications for the pathogenesis, diagnosis, and treatment of human IBD. The development of histologically and immunologically similar colitis in knockout mice following deletion of any of a number of regulatory or barrier function genes strongly supports the presence of genetic heterogeneity in Crohn's disease and ulcerative colitis. Each individual genetic defect may have a discrete bacterial antigenic drive, defined clinical phenotype, different natural history, and a selective response to therapeutic agents. Therefore, detection of selective antibody and cellular immune responses to discrete bacterial antigens may identify subsets of IBD patients that have a high response rate to individualized therapeutic regimens. Moreover, it is likely that different dominant bacterial antigens stimulate disease in different regions of the intestinal tract. Results in animal models indicate that manipulation of the luminal microflora by antibiotics, probiotics, and prebiotics can treat established disease and prevent recurrent inflammation. These physiologic bacterial manipulations may have additive and perhaps synergistic activities with more widely used immunosuppressive therapies and emerging growth factor treatments.

ACKNOWLEDGMENTS

I thank Susie May for expert secretarial assistance. Original results described in this chapter were supported by NIH grants DK 40249, DK 53347, and DK 34987 and by the Crohn's and Colitis Foundation of America.

REFERENCES

1. **Aderem, A., and R. J. Ulevitch.** 2000. Toll-like receptors in the induction of the innate immune response. *Nature* **406:**782–787.
2. **Albright, C., S. L. Tonkonogy, and R. B. Sartor.** 2002. Endogenous IL-10 inhibits APC stimulation of T lymphocyte responses to luminal bacteria. *Gastroenterology* **122:**A270.
3. **Ambrose N. S., M. Johnson, D. W. Burdon, and M. R. Keighley.** 1984. Incidence of pathogenic bacteria from mesenteric lymph nodes and ileal serosa during Crohn's disease surgery. *Br. J. Surg.* **71:**623–625.
4. **Aranda, R., B. C. Sydora, P. L. McAllister, S. W. Binder, H. Y. Yang, S. R. Targan, and M. Kronenberg.** 1997. Analysis of intestinal lymphocytes in mouse colitis mediated by transfer of CD4$^+$, CD45RB^{high} T cells to SCID recipients. *J. Immunol.* **158:**3464–3473.
5. **Asseman, C., S. Mauze, M. W. Leach, R. L. Coffman, and F. Powrie.** 1999. An essential role for interleukin 10 in the function of regu-

latory T cells that inhibit intestinal inflammation. *J. Exp. Med.* **190:**995–1004.

6. **Auer, I. O., A. Roder, F. Wensinck, J. P. van de Merwe, and H. Schmidt.** 1983. Selected bacterial antibodies in Crohn's disease and ulcerative colitis. *Scand. J. Gastroenterol.* **18:**217–223.

7. **Axelsson, L. G., T. Midtvedt, and A. C. Bylund-Fellenius.** 1996. The role of intestinal bacteria, bacterial translocation and endotoxin in dextran sodium sulphate-induced colitis in the mouse. *Microb. Ecol. Health Dis.* **9:**225–237.

8. **Balish, E., and T. Warner.** 2002. *Enterococcus faecalis* induces inflammatory bowel disease in interleukin-10 knockout mice. *Am. J. Pathol.* **160:**2253–2257.

9. **Boivin, G. P., B. A. O'Toole, I. E. Orsmby, R. J. Diebold, M. J. Eis, T. Doetschman, and A. B. Kier.** 1995. Onset and progression of pathological lesions in transforming growth factor-beta-1-deficient mice. *Am. J. Pathol.* **146:**276–288.

10. **Cender, C. J., D. Haller, C. Walters, and R. B. Sartor.** 2002. VSL #3 alters cytokine production of unfractionated splenocytes upon stimulation with cecal bacterial lysate: immunomodulation by this probiotic combination. *Gastroenterology* **122:**A145.

11. **Cohavy, O., D. Bruckner, L. K. Gordon, R. Misra, B. Wei, M. E. Eggena, S. R. Targan, and J. Braun.** 2000. Colonic bacteria express an ulcerative colitis pANCA-related protein epitope. *Infect. Immun.* **68:**1542–1548.

12. **Cohavy, O., G. Harth, M. Horwitz, M. Eggena, C. Landers, C. Sutton, S. R. Targan, and J. Braun.** 1999. Identification of a novel mycobacterial histone H1 homologue (HupB) as an antigenic target of pANCA monoclonal antibody and serum immunoglobulin A from patients with Crohn's disease. *Infect. Immun.* **67:**6510–6517.

13. **Cohn, S. M., S. Schloemann, T. Tessner, K. Seibert, and W. F. Stenson.** 1997. Crypt stem cell survival in the mouse intestinal epithelium is regulated by prostaglandins synthesized through cyclooxygenase-1. *J. Clin. Invest.* **99:**1367–1379.

14. **Colombel, J. F., M. Lemann, M. Cassagnou, Y. Bouhnik, B. Duclos, J. L. Dupas, B. Notteghem, and J. Y. Mary.** 1999. A controlled trial comparing ciprofloxacin with mesalazine for the treatment of active Crohn's disease. Groupe d'Etudes Therapeutiques des Affections Inflammatoires Digestives (GETAID). *Am. J. Gastroenterol.* **94:**674–678.

15. **Cong, Y., S. L. Brandwein, R. P. McCabe, A. Lazenby, E. H. Birkenmeier, J. P. Sundberg, and C. O. Elson.** 1998. CD4+ T cells reactive to enteric bacterial antigens in spontaneously colitic C3H/HeJBir mice: increased T helper cell type 1 response and ability to transfer disease. *J. Exp. Med.* **187:**855–864.

16. **Cong, Y., C. T. Weaver, A. Lazenby, and C. O. Elson.** 2000. Colitis induced by enteric bacterial antigen-specific CD4+ T cells requires CD40-CD40 ligand interactions for a sustained increase in mucosal IL-12. *J. Immunol.* **165:**2173–2182.

17. **Cong, Y., C. T. Weaver, A. Lazenby, J. P. Sundberg, and C. O. Elson.** 2000. T-regulatory-1 (TR1) cells prevent colitis induced by enteric bacterial antigen-reactive pathogenic TH1 cells. *Gastroenterology* **118:**A683.

18. **Darfeuille-Michaud, A., C. Neut, N. Barnich, E. Lederman, P. Di Martino, P. Desreumaux, L. Gambiez, B. Joly, A. Cortot, and J. F. Colombel.** 1998. Presence of adherent *Escherichia coli* strains in ileal mucosa of patients with Crohn's disease. *Gastroenterology* **115:**1405–1413.

19. **Davidson, N. J., M. W. Leach, M. M. Fort, L. Thompson-Snipes, R. Kuhn, W. Muller, D. J. Berg, and D. M. Rennick.** 1996. T helper cell 1-type CD4+ T cells, but not B cells, mediate colitis in interleukin 10-deficient mice. *J. Exp. Med.* **184:**241–251.

20. **D'Haens, G. R., K. Geboes, M. Peeters, F. Baert, F. Penninckx, and P. Rutgeerts.** 1998. Early lesions of recurrent Crohn's disease caused by infusion of intestinal contents in excluded ileum. *Gastroenterology* **114:**262–267.

21. **Dianda, L., A. M. Hanby, N. A. Wright, A. Sebesteny, A. C. Hayday, and M. J. Owen.** 1997. T cell receptor-alpha beta-deficient mice fail to develop colitis in the absence of a microbial environment. *Am. J. Pathol.* **150:**91–97.

22. **Dieleman, L. A., A. Arends, S. L. Tonkonogy, M. S. Goerres, D. W. Craft, W. Grenther, R. K. Sellon, E. Balish, and R. B. Sartor.** 2000. *Helicobacter hepaticus* does not induce or potentiate colitis in interleukin-10-deficient mice. *Infect. Immun.* **68:**5107–5113.

23. **Dieleman, L. A., M. Goerres, A. Arends, T. A. Springer, and R. B. Sartor.** 2000. *Lactobacillus* GG prevents recurrence of colitis in HLA B$_{27}$ transgenic rats after antibiotic treatment. *Gastroenterology* **118:**A814.

24. **Dieleman, L. A., F. Hoentjen, C. Ehre, B. A. Mann, and D. Sprengers.** 2001. Antibiotics with a selective aerobic and anaerobic spectrum have different therapeutic activities in various regions of the colon in IL-10 knockout mice. *Gastroenterology* **120:**A687.

25. **Dieleman, L. A., F. Hoentjen, R. Williams, C. Torrice, R. B. Sartor, and S. L. Tonkon-**

ogy. 2002. B cells from mesenteric lymph nodes of resistant rats produce more interleukin-10 than those from B27 transgenic rats following in vitro stimulation with cecal bacterial lysate. *Gastroenterology* **122**:A261.

26. **Duchmann, R., I. Kaiser, E. Hermann, W. Mayet, K. Ewe, and K. H. Meyer zum Buschenfelde.** 1995. Tolerance exists towards resident intestinal flora but is broken in active inflammatory bowel disease (IBD). *Clin. Exp. Immunol.* **102**:448–455.

27. **Duchmann, R., E. Marker-Hermann, and K. H. Meyer zum Buschenfelde.** 1996. Bacteria-specific T-cell clones are selective in their reactivity towards different enterobacteria or *H. pylori* and increased in inflammatory bowel disease. *Scand. J. Immunol.* **44**:71–79.

28. **Duchmann, R., E. May, M. Heike, P. Knolle, M. Neurath, and K. H. Meyer zum Buschenfelde.** 1999. T cell specificity and cross reactivity towards *Enterobacteria, Bacteroides, Bifidobacterium*, and antigens from resident intestinal flora in humans. *Gut* **44**:812–818.

29. **Duchmann, R., E. Schmitt, P. Knolle, K. H. Meyer zum Buschenfelde, and M. Neurath.** 1996. Tolerance towards resident intestinal flora in mice is abrogated in experimental colitis and restored by treatment with interleukin-10 or antibodies to interleukin-12. *Eur. J. Immunol.* **26**:934–938.

30. **Elson, C. O., Y. Cong, S. Brandwein, C. T. Weaver, R. P. McCabe, M. Mahler, J. P. Sundberg, and E. H. Leiter.** 1998. Experimental models to study molecular mechanisms underlying intestinal inflammation. *Ann. N.Y. Acad. Sci.* **859**:85–95.

31. **Fabia, R., A. Ar'Rajab, M. L. Johansson, R. Andersson, R. Willen, B. Jeppsson, G. Molin, and S. Bengmark.** 1993. Impairment of bacterial flora in human ulcerative colitis and experimental colitis in the rat. *Digestion* **54**:248–255.

32. **Fiocchi, C.** 1998. Inflammatory bowel disease: etiology and pathogenesis. *Gastroenterology* **115**:182–205.

33. **Furne, J. K., F. L. Suarez, S. L. Ewing, J. Springfield, and M. D. Levitt.** 2000. Binding of hydrogen sulfide by bismuth does not prevent dextran sulfate-induced colitis in rats. *Dig. Dis. Sci.* **45**:1439–1443.

34. **Gaboriau-Routhiau, V., and M. C. Moreau.** 1996. Gut flora allows recovery of oral tolerance to ovalbumin in mice after transient breakdown mediated by cholera toxin or *Escherichia coli* heat-labile enterotoxin. *Pediatr. Res.* **39**:625–629.

35. **Gardiner, K. R., N. H. Anderson, M. D. McCaigue, P. J. Erwin, M. I. Halliday, and B. J. Rowlands.** 1993. Adsorbents as antiendotoxin agents in experimental colitis. *Gut* **34**:51–55.

36. **Gardiner, K. R., M. I. Halliday, G. R. Barclay, L. Milne, D. Brown, S. Stephens, R. J. Maxwell, and B. J. Rowlands.** 1995. Significance of systemic endotoxaemia in inflammatory bowel disease. *Gut* **36**:897–901.

37. **Gionchetti, P., F. Rizzello, A. Venturi, P. Brigidi, D. Matteuzzi, G. Bazzocchi, G. Poggioli, M. Miglioli, and M. Campieri.** 2000. Oral bacteriotherapy as maintenance treatment in patients with chronic pouchitis: a double-blind, placebo-controlled trial. *Gastroenterology* **119**:305–309.

38. **Greenbloom, S. L., A. H. Steinhart, and G. R. Greenberg.** 1998. Combination ciprofloxacin and metronidazole for active Crohn's disease. *Can. J. Gastroenterol.* **12**:53–56.

39. **Haller, D., M. P. Russo, R. B. Sartor, and C. Jobin.** 2002. IKKβ and phosphatidylinositol 3-kinase/Akt participate in non-pathogenic Gram-negative enteric bacteria-induced RelA phosphorylation and NFκB activation in both primary and intestinal epithelial cell lines. *J. Biol. Chem.* **277**:38168–38178.

40. **Hammer, R. E., S. D. Maika, J. A. Richardson, J. P. Tang, and J. D. Taurog.** 1990. Spontaneous inflammatory disease in transgenic rats expressing HLA-B27 and human beta 2m: an animal model of HLA-B27-associated human disorders. *Cell* **63**:1099–1112.

41. **Harper, P. H., E. C. Lee, M. G. Kettlewell, M. K. Bennett, and D. P. Jewell.** 1985. Role of the faecal stream in the maintenance of Crohn's colitis. *Gut* **26**:279–284.

42. **Harper, P. H., S. C. Truelove, E. C. Lee, M. G. Kettlewell, and D. P. Jewell.** 1983. Split ileostomy and ileocolostomy for Crohn's disease of the colon and ulcerative colitis: a 20 year survey. *Gut* **24**:106–113.

43. **Hermiston, M. L., and J. I. Gordon.** 1995. Inflammatory bowel disease and adenomas in mice expressing a dominant negative N-cadherin. *Science* **270**:1203–1207.

44. **Hessle, C., B. Andersson, and A. E. Wold.** 2000. Gram-positive bacteria are potent inducers of monocytic interleukin-12 (IL-12) while gram-negative bacteria preferentially stimulate IL-10 production. *Infect. Immun.* **68**:3581–3586.

45. **Hilsden, R. J., J. B. Meddings, and L. R. Sutherland.** 1996. Intestinal permeability changes in response to acetylsalicylic acid in relatives of patients with Crohn's disease. *Gastroenterology* **110**:1395–1403.

46. **Hollander, D., C. M. Vadheim, E. Brettholz, G. M. Petersen, T. Delahunty, and**

J. I. Rotter. 1986. Increased intestinal permeability in patients with Crohn's disease and their relatives. A possible etiologic factor. *Ann. Intern. Med.* **105:**883–885.

47. Hooper, L. V., M. H. Wong, A. Thelin, L. Hansson, P. G. Falk, and J. I. Gordon. 2001. Molecular analysis of commensal host-microbial relationships in the intestine. *Science* **291:**881–884.

48. Hugot, J. P., M. Chamaillard, H. Zouali, S. Lesage, J. P. Cezard, J. Belaiche, and S. Almer. 2001. Association of NOD2 leucine-rich repeat variants with susceptibility to Crohn's disease. *Nature* **411:**599–603.

49. Jiang, H. Q., N. Kushnir, M. C. Thurnheer, N. A. Bos, and J. J. Cebra. 2002. Monoassociation of SCID mice with *Helicobacter muridarum,* but not four other enterics, provokes IBD upon receipt of T cells. *Gastroenterology* **122:**1346–1354.

50. Kim, S. C., S. L. Tonkonogy, and R. B. Sartor. 2001. Role of endogenous IL-10 in downregulating proinflammatory cytokine expression. *Gastroenterology* **120:**A183.

51. Kim, S. C., S. L. Tonkonogy, E. Balish, and R. B. Sartor. 2002. Bacterial antigen specific T cell activation precedes intestinal inflammation in *E. faecalis* monoassociated IL-10 deficient mice. *Gastroenterology* **122:**A85.

52. Korzenik, J. R., and B. K. Dieckgraefe. 2000. Immunostimulation in Crohn's disease: results of a pilot study of G-CSF (R-Methug-CSF) in mucosal and fistulizing Crohn's disease. *Gastroenterology* **118:**A874.

53. Korzenik, J. R., and B. K. Dieckgraefe. 2000. Is Crohn's disease an immunodeficiency? A hypothesis suggesting possible early events in the pathogenesis of Crohn's disease. *Dig. Dis. Sci.* **45:**1121–1129.

54. Kruis, W., E. Schutz, P. Fric, B. Fixa, G. Judmaier, and M. Stolte. 1997. Double-blind comparison of an oral *Escherichia coli* preparation and mesalazine in maintaining remission of ulcerative colitis. *Aliment. Pharmacol. Ther.* **11:**853–858.

55. Kuhn, R., J. Lohler, D. Rennick, K. Rajewsky, and W. Muller. 1993. Interleukin-10-deficient mice develop chronic enterocolitis. *Cell* **75:**263–274.

56. Kulkarni, A. B., J. M. Ward, L. Yaswen, C. L. Mackall, S. R. Bauer, C. G. Huh, R. E. Gress, and S. Karlsson. 1995. Transforming growth factor-beta 1 null mice. An animal model for inflammatory disorders. *Am. J. Pathol.* **146:**264–275.

57. Kullberg, M. C., J. M. Ward, P. Gorelick, P. Caspar, S. Hieny, A. Cheever, D. Jan-

kovic, and A. Sher. 1998. *Helicobacter hepaticus* triggers colitis in specific-pathogen-free interleukin-10 (IL-10)-deficient mice through an IL-12 and gamma interferon-dependent mechanism. *Infect. Immun.* **66:**5157–5166.

58. Lichtman, S. N., J. Keku, J. H. Schwab, and R. B. Sartor. 1991. Hepatic injury associated with small bowel bacterial overgrowth in rats is prevented by metronidazole and tetracycline. *Gastroenterology* **100:**513–519.

59. Lichtman, S. N., E. E. Okoruwa, J. Keku, J. H. Schwab, and R. B. Sartor. 1992. Degradation of endogenous bacterial cell wall polymers by the muralytic enzyme mutanolysin prevents hepatobiliary injury in genetically susceptible rats with experimental intestinal bacterial overgrowth. *J. Clin. Invest.* **90:**1313–1322.

60. Lichtman, S. N., R. B. Sartor, J. Keku, and J. H. Schwab. 1990. Hepatic inflammation in rats with experimental small intestinal bacterial overgrowth. *Gastroenterology* **98:**414–423.

61. Lichtman, S. N., J. Wang, B. Hummel, S. Lacey, and R. B. Sartor. 1998. A rat model of ileal pouch-rectal anastomosis. *Inflam. Bowel Dis.* **4:**187–195.

62. Lichtman, S. N., J. Wang, R. B. Sartor, C. Zhang, D. Bender, F. G. Dalldorf, and J. H. Schwab. 1995. Reactivation of arthritis induced by small bowel bacterial overgrowth in rats: role of cytokines, bacteria, and bacterial polymers. *Infect. Immun.* **63:**2295–2301.

63. Ma, A., M. Datta, E. Margosian, J. Chen, and I. Horak. 1995. T cells, but not B cells, are required for bowel inflammation in interleukin 2-deficient mice. *J. Exp. Med.* **182:**1567–1572.

64. MacDonald, T. T., and P. B. Carter. 1979. Requirement for a bacterial flora before mice generate cells capable of mediating the delayed hypersensitivity reaction to sheep red blood cells. *J. Immunol.* **122:**2624–2629.

65. Macpherson, A., U. Y. Khoo, I. Forgacs, J. Philpott-Howard, and I. Bjarnason. 1996. Mucosal antibodies in inflammatory bowel disease are directed against intestinal bacteria. *Gut* **38:**365–375.

66. Madsen, K. L., J. S. Doyle, L. D. Jewell, M. M. Tavernini, and R. N. Fedorak. 1999. *Lactobacillus* species prevents colitis in interleukin 10 gene-deficient mice. *Gastroenterology* **116:**1107–1114.

67. Madsen, K. L., S. A. Lewis, M. M. Tavernini, J. Hibbard, and R. N. Fedorak. 1997. Interleukin 10 prevents cytokine-induced disruption of T84 monolayer barrier integrity and limits chloride secretion. *Gastroenterology* **113:**151–159.

68. Makkink, M. K., N. J. Schwerbrock, M. van der Sluis, H. A. Buller, R. B. Sartor, A. W.

Einerhand, and J. Dekker. 2002. Interleukin 10 deficient mice are defective in colonic MUC2 synthesis both before and after induction of colitis by commensal bacteria. *Gastroenterology* **122:**A30.

69. **Mashimo, H., D. C. Wu, D. K. Podolsky, and M. C. Fishman.** 1996. Impaired defense of intestinal mucosa in mice lacking intestinal trefoil factor. *Science* **274:**262–265.

70. **Matsuda, H., Y. Fujiyama, A. Andoh, T. Ushijima, T. Kajinami, and T. Bamba.** 2000. Characterization of antibody responses against rectal mucosa-associated bacterial flora in patients with ulcerative colitis. *J. Gastroenterol. Hepatol.* **15:**61–68.

71. **Matsumoto, S., Y. Okabe, H. Setoyama, K. Takayama, J. Ohtsuka, H. Funahashi, A. Imaoka, Y. Okada, and Y. Umesaki.** 1998. Inflammatory bowel disease-like enteritis and caecitis in a senescence accelerated mouse P1/Yit strain. *Gut* **43:**71–78.

72. **McCall, R. D., S. Haskill, E. M. Zimmermann, P. K. Lund, R. C. Thompson, and R. B. Sartor.** 1994. Tissue interleukin 1 and interleukin-1 receptor antagonist expression in enterocolitis in resistant and susceptible rats. *Gastroenterology* **106:**960–972.

73. **Michalek, S. M., H. Kiyono, M. J. Wannemuehler, L. M. Mosteller, and J. R. McGhee.** 1982. Lipopolysaccharide (LPS) regulation of the immune response: LPS influence on oral tolerance induction. *J. Immunol.* **128:**1992–1998.

74. **Mizoguchi, A., E. Mizoguchi, R. N. Smith, F. I. Preffer, and A. K. Bhan.** 1997. Suppressive role of B cells in chronic colitis of T cell receptor alpha mutant mice. *J. Exp. Med.* **186:**1749–1756.

75. **Moreau, M. C., and V. Gaboriau-Routhiau.** 1996. The absence of gut flora, the doses of antigen ingested and aging affect the long-term peripheral tolerance induced by ovalbumin feeding in mice. *Res. Immunol.* **147:**49–59.

76. **Morteau, O., S. G. Morham, R. Sellon, L. A. Dieleman, R. Langenbach, O. Smithies, and R. B. Sartor.** 2000. Impaired mucosal defense to acute colonic injury in mice lacking cyclooxygenase-1 or cyclooxygenase-2. *J. Clin. Invest.* **105:**469–478.

77. **Neurath, M. F., I. Fuss, B. L. Kelsall, E. Stuber, and W. Strober.** 1995. Antibodies to interleukin 12 abrogate established experimental colitis in mice. *J. Exp. Med.* **182:**1281–1290.

78. **Ogura, Y., D. K. Bonen, N. Inohara, D. L. Nicolae, F. Chen, R. Ramos, H. Britton, T. Moran, R. Karaliuskas, R. H. Duerr, J. P. Achkar, S. R. Brant, T. M. Bayless, B. S. Kirschner, S. B. Hanauer, G. Nunez, and J. H. Cho.** 2001. A frameshift mutation in NOD2 associated with susceptibility to Crohn's disease. *Nature* **411:**603–606.

79. **Ogura, Y., N. Inohara, A. Benito, F. F. Chen, S. Yamaoka, and G. Nunez.** 2001. Nod2, a Nod1/Apaf-1 family member that is restricted to monocytes and activates NF-kappaB. *J. Biol. Chem.* **276:**4812–4818.

80. **Onderdonk, A. B., M. L. Franklin, and R. L. Cisneros.** 1981. Production of experimental ulcerative colitis in gnotobiotic guinea pigs with simplified microflora. *Infect. Immun.* **32:**225–231.

81. **Onderdonk, A. B., J. A. Richardson, R. E. Hammer, and J. D. Taurog.** 1998. Correlation of cecal microflora of HLA-B27 transgenic rats with inflammatory bowel disease. *Infect. Immun.* **66:**6022–6023.

82. **Oyama, N., N. Sudo, H. Sogawa, and C. Kubo.** 2001. Antibiotic use during infancy promotes a shift in the T(H)1/T(H)2 balance toward T(H)2-dominant immunity in mice. *J. Allergy Clin. Immunol.* **107:**153–159.

83. **Podolsky, D. K.** 1999. Mucosal immunity and inflammation. V. Innate mechanisms of mucosal defense and repair: the best offense is a good defense. *Am. J. Physiol.* **277:**G495–G499.

84. **Powrie, F.** 1995. T cells in inflammatory bowel disease: protective and pathogenic roles. *Immunity* **3:**171–174.

85. **Powrie, F., J. Carlino, M. W. Leach, S. Mauze, and R. L. Coffman.** 1996. A critical role for transforming growth factor-beta but not interleukin 4 in the suppression of T helper type 1-mediated colitis by CD45RB(low) CD4+ T cells. *J. Exp. Med.* **183:**2669–2674.

86. **Powrie, F., M. W. Leach, S. Mauze, L. B. Caddle, and R. L. Coffman.** 1993. Phenotypically distinct subsets of CD4+ T cells induce or protect from chronic intestinal inflammation in C. B-17 SCID mice. *Int. Immunol.* **5:**1461–1471.

87. **Rachmilewitz, D., F. Karmeli, J. Lee, and E. Raz.** 2002. Immunostimulatory DNA sequences decrease the enhanced colonic TNFα and IL-1β generation in IBD. *Gastroenterology* **122:**A148.

88. **Rachmilewitz, D., F. Karmeli, K. Takabayashi, T. Hayashi, L. Leider-Trejo, J. Lee, L. M. Leoni, and E. Raz.** 2002. Immunostimulatory DNA ameliorates experimental and spontaneous murine colitis. *Gastroenterology* **122:**1428–1441.

89. **Rath, H. C., H. H. Herfarth, J. S. Ikeda, W. B. Grenther, T. E. J. Hamm, E. Balish, J. D. Taurog, R. E. Hammer, K. H. Wilson, and R. B. Sartor.** 1996. Normal luminal bacteria, especially *Bacteroides* species, mediate chronic colitis, gastritis, and arthritis in HLA-

B27/human beta2 microglobulin transgenic rats. *J. Clin. Invest.* **98:**945–953.

90. **Rath, H. C., J. S. Ikeda, H. J. Linde, J. Scholmerich, K. H. Wilson, and R. B. Sartor.** 1999. Varying cecal bacterial loads influences colitis and gastritis in HLA-B27 transgenic rats. *Gastroenterology* **116:**310–319.

91. **Rath, H. C., M. Schultz, R. Freitag, L. A. Dieleman, F. Li, H. J. Linde, J. Scholmerich, and R. B. Sartor.** 2001. Different subsets of enteric bacteria induce and perpetuate experimental colitis in rats and mice. *Infect. Immun.* **69:**2277–2285.

92. **Rath, H. C., K. H. Wilson, and R. B. Sartor.** 1999. Differential induction of colitis and gastritis in HLA-B27 transgenic rats selectively colonized with *Bacteroides vulgatus* and *Escherichia coli. Infect. Immun.* **67:**2969–2974.

93. **Read, S., V. Malmstrom, and F. Powrie.** 2000. Cytotoxic T lymphocyte-associated antigen 4 plays an essential role in the function of CD25(+)CD4(+) regulatory cells that control intestinal inflammation. *J. Exp. Med.* **192:**295–302.

94. **Riehl, T., S. Cohn, T. Tessner, S. Schloemann, and W. F. Stenson.** 2000. Lipopolysaccharide is radioprotective in the mouse intestine through a prostaglandin-mediated mechanism. *Gastroenterology* **118:**1106–1166.

95. **Rietdijk, S. T., W. Faubion, C. Albright, Y. P. de Jong, A. Abadia, K. Clarke, R. B. Sartor, and C. Terhorst.** 2002. CD4$^+$ CD25$^+$ regulatory T cells originating from germ free mice have impaired suppressive abilities. *Gastroenterology* **122:**A387.

96. **Roediger, W. E.** 1980. The colonic epithelium in ulcerative colitis: an energy-deficiency disease? *Lancet* **ii:**712–715.

97. **Roediger, W. E., A. Duncan, O. Kapaniris, and S. Millard.** 1993. Reducing sulfur compounds of the colon impair colonocyte nutrition: implications for ulcerative colitis. *Gastroenterology* **104:**802–809.

98. **Rutgeerts, P., K. Goboes, M. Peeters, M. Hiele, F. Penninckx, R. Aerts, R. Kerremans, and G. Vantrappen.** 1991. Effect of faecal stream diversion on recurrence of Crohn's disease in the neoterminal ileum. *Lancet* **338:**771–774.

99. **Sadlack, B., H. Merz, H. Schorle, A. Schimpl, A. C. Feller, and I. Horak.** 1993. Ulcerative colitis-like disease in mice with a disrupted interleukin-2 gene. *Cell* **75:**253–261.

100. **Sartor, R. B.** 1997. Pathogenesis and immune mechanisms of chronic inflammatory bowel diseases. *Am. J. Gastroenterol.* **92:**5S–11S.

101. **Sartor, R. B.** 1999. Microbial factors in the pathogenesis of Crohn's disease, ulcerative colitis and experimental intestinal inflammation, p. 153–178. *In* J. B. Kirsner (ed.), *Inflammatory Bowel Diseases*, 5th ed. The W. B. Saunders Co., Philadelphia, Pa.

102. **Sartor, R. B.** 2000. Antibiotics as therapeutic agents in Crohn's disease, p. 359–362. *In* T. M. Bayless and S. Hanauer (ed.), *Current Advanced Therapy of Inflammatory Bowel Disease.* BC Decker, Inc., Hamilton, Ontario, Canada.

103. **Sartor, R. B.** 2000. Colitis in HLA-B27/beta 2 microglobulin transgenic rats. *Int. Rev. Immunol.* **19:**39–50.

104. **Sartor, R. B., D. E. Bender, W. B. Grenther, and L. C. Holt.** 1994. Absolute requirement for ubiquitous luminal bacteria in the pathogenesis of chronic intestinal inflammation. *Gastroenterology* **106:**A767.

105. **Sartor, R. B., D. E. Bender, and L. C. Holt.** 1992. Susceptibility of inbred rat strains to intestinal and extraintestinal inflammation induced by indomethacin. *Gastroenterology* **102:**A690.

106. **Sartor, R. B., T. M. Bond, and J. H. Schwab.** 1988. Systemic uptake and intestinal inflammatory effects of luminal bacterial cell wall polymers in rats with acute colonic injury. *Infect. Immun.* **56:**2101–2108.

107. **Sartor, R. B., R. A. De La Cadena, K. D. Green, S. W. Davis, A. A. Adam, B. Raymond, F. Legris, and R. W. Colman.** 1996. Selective kallikrein-kinin system activation in inbred rats differentially susceptible to granulomatous enterocolitis. *Gastroenterology* **110:**1467–1481.

108. **Schultz, M., S. L. Tonkonogy, R. K. Sellon, C. Veltkamp, V. L. Godfrey, J. Kwon, W. B. Grenther, E. Balish, I. Horak, and R. B. Sartor.** 1999. IL-2-deficient mice raised under germfree conditions develop delayed mild focal intestinal inflammation. *Am. J. Physiol.* **276:**G1461–G1472.

109. **Schultz, M., C. Veltkamp, L. A. Dieleman, W. B. Grenther, P. B. Wyrick, S. L. Tonkonogy, and R. B. Sartor.** 2002. *Lactobacillus plantarum* 299V in the treatment and prevention of spontaneous colitis in interleukin-10 deficient mice. *Inflamm. Bowel Dis.* **8:**71–80.

110. **Schwab, J. H.** 1993. Phlogistic properties of peptidoglycan-polysaccharide polymers from cell walls of pathogenic and normal-flora bacteria which colonize humans. *Infect. Immun.* **61:**4535–4539.

111. **Sellon, R. K., S. Tonkonogy, M. Schultz, L. A. Dieleman, W. Grenther, E. Balish,**

D. M. Rennick, and R. B. Sartor. 1998. Resident enteric bacteria are necessary for development of spontaneous colitis and immune system activation in interleukin-10-deficient mice. *Infect. Immun.* **66:**5224–5231.

112. Steinhart, A. H., B. G. Feagan, C. J. Wong, M. Vandervoort, S. Mikolainis, K. Croitoru, E. Seidman, D. J. Leddin, A. Bitton, E. Drouin, A. Cohen, and G. R. Greenberg. 2002. Combined budesonide and antibiotic therapy for active Crohn's disease: a randomized controlled trial. *Gastroenterology* **123:**33–40.

113. Strober, W., B. Kelsall, I. Fuss, T. Marth, B. Ludviksson, R. Ehrhardt, and M. Neurath. 1997. Reciprocal IFN-gamma and TGF-beta responses regulate the occurrence of mucosal inflammation. *Immunol. Today* **18:**61–64.

114. Strober, W., B. R. Ludviksson, and I. J. Fuss. 1998. The pathogenesis of mucosal inflammation in murine models of inflammatory bowel disease and Crohn's disease. *Ann. Intern. Med.* **128:**848–856.

115. Sutherland, L., J. Singleton, J. Sessions, S. Hanauer, E. Krawitt, G. Rankin, R. Summers, H. Mekhjian, N. Greenberger, and M. Kelly. 1991. Double blind, placebo controlled trial of metronidazole in Crohn's disease. *Gut* **32:**1071–1075.

116. Sutton, C. L., J. Kim, A. Yamane, H. Dalwadi, B. Wei, C. Landers, S. R. Targan, and J. Braun. 2000. Identification of a novel bacterial sequence associated with Crohn's disease. *Gastroenterology* **119:**23–31.

117. Swidsinski, A., A. Ladhoff, A. Pernthaler, S. Swidsinski, V. Loening-Baucke, M. Ortner, J. Weber, U. Hoffmann, S. Schreiber, M. Dietel, and H. Lochs. 2002. Mucosal flora in inflammatory bowel disease. *Gastroenterology* **122:**44–54.

118. Sydora, B. C., M. M. Tavernini, L. D. Jewell, A. Wessler, R. P. Rennie, and R. N. Fedorak. 2001. Effect of bacterial monoassociation on tolerance and intestinal inflammation in IL-10 gene-deficient mice. *Gastroenterology* **120:**A517.

119. Tabaqchali, S., D. P. O'Donoghue, and K. A. Bettelheim. 1978. *Escherichia coli* antibodies in patients with inflammatory bowel disease. *Gut* **19:**108–113.

120. Taurog, J. D., J. A. Richardson, J. T. Croft, W. A. Simmons, M. Zhou, J. L.
Fernandez-Sueiro, E. Balish, and R. E. Hammer. 1994. The germfree state prevents development of gut and joint inflammatory disease in HLA-B27 transgenic rats. *J. Exp. Med.* **180:**2359–2364.

121. Tessner, T. G., S. M. Cohn, S. Schloemann, and W. F. Stenson. 1998. Prostaglandins prevent decreased epithelial cell proliferation associated with dextran sodium sulfate injury in mice. *Gastroenterology* **115:**874–882.

122. Tlaskalova, H., R. Stepankova, T. Hudcovic, B. Cukrowska, E. Verdu, L. Tuckova, L. Jelinkova, F. Bend-Jelloul, Z. Rehakova, J. Sinkora, D. Sokol, P. Bercik, D. Funda, P. Michetti, and J. Cebra. 1999. The role of bacterial microflora in development of dextran sodium sulphate (DSS) induced colitis in immunocompetent and immunodeficient mice. *Microbial. Ecol. Health Dis.* **11:**115–116.

123. Turunen, U., M. A. Farkkila, and V. Valtonen. 1999. Long-term treatment of ulcerative colitis with ciprofloxacin. *Gastroenterology* **117:**282–283.

124. Ulisse, S., P. Gionchetti, S. D'Alo, F. P. Russo, I. Pesce, G. Ricci, F. Rizzello, U. Helwig, M. G. Cifone, M. Campieri, and C. De Simone. 2001. Expression of cytokines, inducible nitric oxide synthase, and matrix metalloproteinases in pouchitis: effects of probiotic treatment. *Am. J. Gastroenterol.* **96:**2691–2699.

125. Veltkamp, C., S. L. Tonkonogy, Y. P. de Jong, C. Albright, W. B. Grenther, E. Balish, C. Terhorst, and R. B. Sartor. 2001. Continuous stimulation by normal luminal bacteria is essential for the development and perpetuation of colitis in Tg(epsilon26) mice. *Gastroenterology* **120:**900–913.

126. Veltkamp, C., S. L. Tonkonogy, M. Schultz, and R. B. Sartor. 1999. *Lactobacillus plantarum* is superior to *Lactobacillus GG* in preventing colitis in IL-10 deficient mice. *Gastroenterology* **116:**A838.

127. Wannemuehler, M. J., H. Kiyono, J. L. Babb, S. M. Michalek, and J. R. McGhee. 1982. Lipopolysaccharide (LPS) regulation of the immune response: LPS converts germfree mice to sensitivity to oral tolerance induction. *J. Immunol.* **129:**959–965.

128. Yamada, T., E. Deitch, R. D. Specian, M. A. Perry, R. B. Sartor, and M. B. Grisham. 1993. Mechanisms of acute and chronic intestinal inflammation induced by indomethacin. *Inflammation* **17:**641–662.

PHYSIOLOGICAL REGULATION OF GASTROINTESTINAL ION TRANSPORT

Kim E. Barrett and Lone S. Bertelsen

14

The gastrointestinal tract deals with large volumes of fluid on a daily basis to subserve its physiological functions (97). Fluid is both secreted, to provide an environment that promotes the digestion and absorption of ingested nutrients, and absorbed, to avoid excessive fluid loss to the stool and resulting dehydration. On average, the daily fluid balance sheet includes a total of 8 to 9 liters presented to the intestine as oral intake or secreted by the intestine itself or the organs that drain into it (such as the pancreas and biliary system). Of this volume, the majority is absorbed, leaving only about 200 ml to be excreted in the stool in health. Thus, the intestine has a large capacity for both secretory and absorptive fluid fluxes, with net absorption markedly predominating under normal circumstances (97).

The situation can be very different in disease, when imbalances in fluid homeostasis arise as a consequence of altered function of the epithelial cells that line the length of the gastrointestinal tract and serve as the site where fluid transport is controlled (14). Notoriously, many enteropathogens cause derangements in intestinal fluid fluxes, ultimately leading clinically to the symptom of diarrhea. In some cases, the mechanisms underlying such diarrhea are well understood. For example, *Vibrio cholerae* elaborates a toxin that is capable of simultaneously increasing fluid secretion while decreasing absorption, thereby overwhelming the normal capacity to handle fluid in the intestinal lumen and producing a profuse, watery diarrhea (14). For other microorganisms also discussed in this volume, the precise mechanisms leading to the induction of diarrheal illness are less clear and are still the subject of active investigation. Nevertheless, it is clear that an understanding of diarrheal disease associated with intestinal infections must rest first on an appreciation of the normal control of intestinal fluid handling. The goal of this chapter, therefore, is to describe the normal mechanisms whereby fluid is secreted and absorbed along the length of the gastrointestinal tract, and the regulatory pathways that govern these processes.

THE INTESTINAL EPITHELIUM

As alluded to above, the control of fluid transport in the intestine resides in the continuous layer of columnar epithelial cells that line the gastrointestinal tract (97). The epithelium has

Kim E. Barrett and Lone S. Bertelsen, Department of Medicine, School of Medicine, University of California, San Diego, UCSD Medical Center 8414, 200 West Arbor Drive, San Diego, CA 92103-8414.

Microbial Pathogenesis and the Intestinal Epithelial Cell, ed. by G. Hecht
© 2003 ASM Press, Washington, D.C.

evolved a number of specialized properties that allow it to participate in the vectorial flux of fluid across the intestinal wall. In fact, fluid is not transported actively in the intestine (or indeed in other epithelial tissues). Instead, the movement of fluid between compartments is driven secondarily in response to osmotic gradients. These are established by virtue of the active transport of electrolytes and other solutes, mediated by epithelial cells. Thus, epithelial cells are polarized and engage in the asymmetric sorting of specific ion transport proteins to either their apical or basolateral poles, thereby allowing for directed movement of specific ionic species either from the bloodstream to the lumen (termed secretion) or from the lumen to the bloodstream (termed absorption) (97). Other epithelial properties that are relevant to a discussion of transport physiology include their ability to form tight junctions (5) and the development of heterogeneous epithelial phenotypes along the crypt-villus and cephalocaudal axes (33, 115). Each of these critical epithelial properties will be addressed in more detail below.

Epithelial Polarity

Significant information has emerged in recent years regarding the mechanisms employed by epithelial cells to establish and maintain their functional polarity (100). Following synthesis, proteins reside briefly in the trans-Golgi network, where their appropriate destination is analyzed. Some of the membrane proteins involved in translocating solutes across epithelial membrane barriers contain sorting information in their primary sequences that permit for accurate trafficking of the protein only to a single membrane domain (i.e., apical or basolateral). These signals, or sorting motifs, in turn permit the packaging of the respective protein into specific vesicles destined to traffic to the appropriate membrane for fusion and delivery of their cargo. The first sorting motifs to be described, somewhat surprisingly, directed traffic of proteins to the basolateral membrane. This was surprising in that basolateral sorting had hitherto been considered to

represent a constitutive or "default" pathway, while it was presumed that specialized information would be needed to direct proteins to the apical membrane because this domain is not a feature of nonpolarized cells (100). Examples of basolateral signals include the amino acid sequences NPXY or YXXϕ (where X is any amino acid and ϕ is an amino acid with a bulky hydrophobic group) (7). In other cases a dihydrophobic sequence may specify basolateral targeting (89), although an increasing number of basolateral sequences are being identified that fail to conform to any of these patterns and may instead act by specifying a particular tertiary structure (7, 83). In each case, nevertheless, the mechanics of sorting likely involve specific interactions of these sequence motifs with clathrin adaptor protein complexes, which are then targeted to the basolateral pole of the cell (100).

Other proteins may traffic specifically to the apical domain by virtue of their ability to partition into specialized membrane structures known as glycosphingolipid rafts, which self-assemble in the plane of the Golgi membrane (126). These structures, in turn, serve to nucleate vesicles that will ultimately travel to the apical pole of the cell. This mechanism has been shown for several proteins that link to the membrane via glycosylphosphatidylinositol anchors, but may be a more general property shared by a number of apical transmembrane proteins, such as ion transporters (100). In other cases, apical sorting may be dependent on protein glycosylation, or short sequences in one or more transmembrane domains, as has been shown for the gastric H,K-ATPase (46, 117). The machinery that, in turn, mediates the trafficking of these apically marked proteins is still the subject of much research. In some cases, caveolin or specific lectins may bind to the target proteins, but it is also clear that some apical proteins can be trafficked independent of these adaptors.

A final level of protein sorting occurs at the plasma membrane. There is continual turnover of membrane proteins via a regulated process of endocytosis and redelivery of proteins in exocytic vesicles (100). To retain a given protein in a specific membrane domain once it has been delivered there in a polarized fashion, the protein either must not participate in this endocytic/exocytic recycling or must undergo re-sorting so that it is returned to the correct location (100). For example, there is evidence that internalization of the basolateral Na,K-ATPase is restricted by virtue of its close association with the fodrin-based cytoskeleton at points of cell-cell contact (109). On the other hand, if a membrane protein is internalized, a number of molecular events appear to differentiate between those proteins destined for ligand decoupling and/or lysosomal degradation, and those that simply recycle back to the membrane of origin, with or without a period spent "in waiting" in a reserve supply of exocytic vesicles (144). In fact, there is substantial evidence that many of the proteins involved in electrolyte transport mechanisms in intestinal epithelial cells may be recruited from a juxtamembrane vesicular storage pool when the cell is called upon to increase its transport rate. For example, the basolateral pool of NKCC1 protein involved in the chloride secretory mechanism (see below) likely is supplemented with additional transporters in cells stimulated with agonists to sustain high rates of ongoing chloride transport (36). Similarly, there is evidence in at least some cell types, and more recently in intact intestinal tissues, that additional cystic fibrosis transmembrane regulator (CFTR) chloride channels are inserted into the apical membrane of stimulated cells in a cyclic AMP (cAMP)-dependent fashion (107).

Tight Junctions

Another feature of the epithelium that is critical to its ability to perform vectorial transport of electrolytes and other solutes is the property of forming an electrically resistive or "tight" barrier (5). Intestinal epithelial cells are linked to each other in a manner reminiscent of the way in which the plastic holder stabilizes a six-pack—junctional structures near the apical pole of columnar intestinal epithelial cells segregate the apical and basolateral poles and restrict the passive permeation of solutes around the cells. This limits the back-diffusion of substances actively transported via the transcellular pathway. Intercellular junctions that link adjacent epithelial cells include the lateral adherens junction (or zonula adherens), followed by the tight junction (or zonula occludens), which is located close to the apical pole (106). The adherens junction appears to be important in the initial assembly of the epithelium, but it is not designed to resist the passage of solutes significantly (98). On the other hand, the tight junctions provide the majority of the transepithelial resistance barrier, as well as allowing for selective and regulatable permeability of the epithelium on the basis of solute size and/or electrical charge (34, 95, 138).

There has been an explosion of molecular information regarding the specific proteins that both make up and regulate the tight junctions of epithelial cells (95). This information is particularly pertinent in the current volume, since many pathogenic microorganisms may act on the proteinaceous components of the tight junction to breach the epithelial barrier in the intestine and thereby cause both local and disseminated disease. Thus, it is useful to briefly review the constituents of this structure (125).

The actual sealing elements of the tight junction are accomplished by two classes of transmembrane proteins that form both homodimeric and heterodimeric associations at "kiss sites" with partners on adjacent cells. The first of these proteins to be identified was occludin, which was assumed to be the only mediator of junctional integrity until it was shown that a mouse constructed to lack this protein entirely had no discernible defect in intestinal barrier function (53, 116). This led to a search for additional junction proteins and the discovery of the claudins, which is a rapidly growing family of related transmembrane proteins that likewise can interact with partners on adjacent cells (129). The claudins are particularly interesting in terms of their diversity and the fact that they can partner promiscuously with other family members, thereby providing for a large diversity of possible junctional structures (129). Functionally, this appears to lead to junctions with varying degrees of permeability, which, in turn, may underlie the observation that the transepithelial resistance of the epithelium increases along the cephalocaudal axis in the intestine, and may also differ between crypt and villus epithelial cells (112). Finally, there is intense interest in the likelihood that different claudin molecules, or heterodimeric pairs of claudins, may confer tight junctional specificity in terms of the types of molecules (particularly in terms of charge) that can permeate through the junctional complex (34, 95, 112, 124, 138).

There are also large and growing numbers of proteins that localize to the cytoplasmic face of the tight junction, and which are involved in the dynamic regulation of tight junctional properties in response to endogenous and exogenous stimuli (95). Some of these proteins have been established as regulators of the constitutive properties of tight junctions at various sites. For example, the protein zonula occludens-1, or ZO-1, exists as at least two isoforms, and the relative abundance of these determines whether a given junction is "tight" or "leaky" (143). Other perijunctional proteins may be involved in posttranslational modification of junctional elements, such as tyrosine and/or serine threonine phosphorylation. There is evidence that the abundance and stability of several junctional elements, including occludin and ZO-1, are determined by their phosphorylation status (94). Dephosphorylated proteins may no longer be retained at the junctional area, and this dissociation therefore leads to a reduction in junction effectiveness (6, 94).

Finally, it should be emphasized that the tight junctional barrier is not a static structure, but is subject to minute-to-minute regulation to subserve physiological needs. Much of the acute regulation of the tight junction appears to derive from its linkages to the cellular cytoskeleton, mediated by perijunctional proteins, and the actin-myosin ring that encircles the apical pole of intestinal epithelial cells. In response to appropriate physiological stimuli (or when inappropriately altered by toxins or other products of pathogens), this junctional ring can contract, thereby exerting a physical force on the tight junction that may increase its permeability (17, 67, 125). Moreover, some data exist to suggest that the permeability of tight junctions is also linked functionally to the transporting status of the adjacent epithelial cells. Critically, an increase in permeability may accompany the active sodium-linked absorption of glucose, allowing for a passive flux of this nutrient as well as bystander low-molecular-weight molecules, such as oligopeptides, that amplify the overall absorptive mechanism (17, 132). At a biochemical level, the contraction of the actin-myosin ring appears to be secondary to the stimulation of myosin light chain kinase activity, in turn promoting the formation of junctional dilatations (133). While there continues to be some controversy as to the precise contribution of this nutrient-driven increase in permeability to nutrient absorption in vivo, it remains the case that such acute regulation clearly occurs and stands as an excellent example of the mechanisms that potentially can also be exploited by microorganisms to alter the permeability of tight junctions under pathological circumstances.

Epithelial Heterogeneity

The epithelium is subject to continuous turnover and renewal. Anchored stem cells are located toward the base of the intestinal crypts and give rise to the four major cell lineages that form the lining of the mature intestine—enterocytes (or colonocytes), Paneth cells, goblet cells, and enteroendocrine cells (110). Paneth cells migrate downward into the base of the crypt, whereas the other lineages migrate upward toward the villus tip (or surface in the colon) (33, 104). However, in addition to these clear lineage decisions, even enterocytes themselves may display divergent functional properties depending on their position along the crypt-villus axis, as well as in the cephalocaudal dimension. Cells derived from the anchored stem cells initially retain some proliferative potential and undergo cell division as they emerge from the crypts (104). These immature cells largely display a secretory phenotype, expressing the membrane transporters and other regulatory machinery that permit them to conduct chloride secretion (139). However, as the cells move out onto the villus (or surface), they stop dividing and begin to express the transporters required for an absorptive phenotype, as well as the brush border hydrolases and other enzymes required for solute digestion and absorption (139). At the same time, these cells appear to suppress the expression of secretory transporters, and they may also express a new complement of receptors for relevant hormones and neurotransmitters. Some recent evidence implies that the paradigm of secretory crypts coupled with absorptive villi may be something of an oversimplification (80). Some cells in the crypts may be capable of absorption, whereas scattered cells on the villus continue to express the transporters needed for secretion, sometimes at very high levels (2, 80). However, the simple paradigm still largely applies and also provides a functional basis for therapies (such as oral rehydration solution) designed to selectively promote absorption without affecting secretory function, which may be amplified in disease.

Epithelial properties also evolve as one moves from stomach to small intestine to colon. For example, the segmental heterogeneity exists for epithelial permeability, with the colonic epithelium being relatively "tight" compared to the leaky small intestinal epithelium. This may reflect the differing physiological roles of these segments, with the small intestine required to absorb large quantities of ingested nutrients compared to the primary role in fluid conservation and dehydration of the stool seen in the distal intestine. Likewise, transport expression evolves to match the luminal environment (97). Thus, colonocytes express few, if any, apical transporters for glu-

cose or other nutrients, given the efficacy of the absorptive process and the fact that the colonic lumen is essentially devoid of such nutrients in health (97). On the other hand, colonocytes upregulate transporters that are not present, or are present only at low levels, in the small intestine, such as transporters for short-chain fatty acids (SCFA) and sodium channels (97). These are relevant for epithelial function in the specialized environment of the colon. Overall, therefore, epithelial cells in the different segments of the intestine express varied ion and solute transport mechanisms consistent with their location and contributions to gastrointestinal function. More details of these specific transport mechanisms are provided below. Information is emerging as to the nature of transcription factors and other spatial cues that trigger the up- or downregulation of specific gene products along both horizontal and vertical axes in the intestine (128).

INTESTINAL TRANSPORT MECHANISMS

We turn now to a discussion of the precise transport mechanisms that mediate the flux of electrolytes and other solutes in the small and large intestines. In general, a given transport mechanism requires the coordinated participation of at least three membrane transport proteins: one that mediates the uptake of the solute of interest, one that mediates its efflux across the contralateral membrane domain to allow for net vectorial transport, and one that energizes the process overall at the expense of consumption of cellular ATP. All the transport mechanisms discussed here are active, in that they result in the transepithelial transport of the solute of interest against existing electrochemical gradients. However, a transport mechanism may be made up of both active and passive transport pathways at the level of the membrane. Transepithelial transport mechanisms are also characterized as either electrogenic or electroneutral. In the latter case, ions of equal and opposite charge are transported in tandem across the epithelial cell, resulting in no net transfer of charge across the tissue. The resulting osmotic gradient then drives the movement of water via the paracellular pathway. In contrast, an electrogenic mechanism sets up both an electrical and a chemical gradient across the epithelium, mandating that, in this case, both the appropriate counterion and water are driven to move paracellularly. Overall, the distinction of electrogenic and electroneutral mechanisms is most relevant in the experimental setting, where the former type of transport can be detected by monitoring changes in potential difference across the epithelium whereas the latter cannot, and instead can be monitored only by using some type of tracer for the substance(s) being transported.

As mentioned previously, the small intestine and colon differ in the precise complement of transport mechanisms they express consistent with their divergent physiological functions (97). Table 1 lists the major transport mechanisms seen in each segment of the intestine. It is likely that all these mechanisms could be subject to dysregulation by enteric pathogens, depending on the site of colonization.

Intestinal Absorptive Mechanisms

Many intestinal absorptive mechanisms center around the sodium ion. This provides a useful driving force for the absorptive vector, given the low level of intracellular sodium established by the activity of the basolateral Na,K-ATPase.

Nutrient-Coupled Sodium Absorption. Many nutrients are absorbed in the small intestine by coupling their movement across the apical membrane of enterocytes with that of sodium. The absorptive mechanism for glucose is the prototype of this class of transport and is depicted diagrammatically in Fig. 1. An essentially analogous mechanism is shared by many amino acids, certain B vitamins, and conjugated bile acids, with the only variations being the molecular identity of the transporters capable of sodium-coupled uptake of the solute in question and the exit pathway for that solute across the basolateral membrane. Transport mechanisms of this type are expressed throughout the small intestine in the case of nutrients, and selectively in the terminal ileum in the case of bile acids, but they are not seen in the colon, consistent with the relative absence of conventional nutrients from the colonic lumen (97). The nutrient-sodium cotransporter (SGLT1 in the case of glucose) mediates the uphill accumulation of the nutrient in question by coupling its movement across the apical membrane to the sodium gradient established by the basolateral Na,K-ATPase. The stoichiometry of this process may vary depending on the precise solute of interest and has not been established for all substrates using this mechanism. In the case of SGLT1, however, two sodium ions accompany the movement of each glucose molecule (78, 79). This allows the efficient accumula-

TABLE 1 Active transport mechanisms in the mammalian small intestine and colon

Mechanisms	Small intestine[a]	Colon[a]
Absorptive	Nutrient-coupled sodium absorption (E)	Sodium absorption (E)
	Coupled sodium chloride absorption (N)	Coupled sodium chloride absorption (N)
	Proton-coupled peptide absorption (E)	SCFA absorption (N)
	Conjugated bile acid absorption (E)	Potassium absorption (N)
Secretory	Chloride secretion (E)	Chloride secretion (E)
	Bicarbonate secretion (E)	Bicarbonate secretion (E)
		Potassium secretion (E)

[a] Transport mechanisms are characterized as either electrogenic (E) or electroneutral (N).

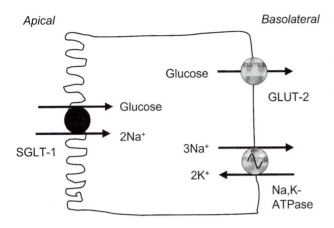

Apical   **Basolateral**

SGLT-1

GLUT-2

Glucose

Glucose

2Na⁺

3Na⁺

2K⁺

Na,K-
ATPase

FIGURE 1 Sodium-coupled glucose absorption. This electrogenic transport process provides for the uphill transport of glucose across the apical membrane of villus epithelial cells in the small intestine by coupling glucose movement to that of sodium via SGLT1. Sodium movement is energized by the low intracellular sodium concentration established by the basolateral Na,K-ATPase. Glucose exits the basolateral membrane via the facilitated diffusion pathway, GLUT-2. Similar mechanisms exist for a variety of other nutrients, such as amino acids. Conjugated bile acids are also reabsorbed in the terminal ileum via a comparable transport mechanism.

tion of glucose, which can then exit the cell via a facilitated diffusion pathway, GLUT-2. Water and chloride ions then follow paracellularly to maintain osmotic and electrical balance. Interestingly, however, recent work by Wright and coworkers has revealed that a large number of water molecules may also traverse the apical membrane in conjunction with the transported sodium and glucose. These scientists have estimated that such water uptake may perhaps be more important than the paracellular route in providing for water reabsorption in the period after eating a meal (85). In either scenario, it is clear that the uptake of sodium in conjunction with various nutrients is the major driving force for overall fluid recovery in the small intestine in the postprandial period. This process also underlies the efficacy of oral rehydration therapy in diseases such as cholera. Likewise, the importance of the sodium/glucose transport mechanism is revealed in children suffering from a rare genetic disorder, glucose-galactose malabsorption, where any one of a number of mutations in the SGLT1 molecule results in profuse diarrhea if glucose, galactose, or more complex carbohydrates containing these residues are provided in the diet (130).

Electrogenic Sodium Absorption. In the colon, where nutrients are absent, sodium

can also be absorbed electrogenically via the participation of sodium channels of the ENaC class. This process accounts for approximately 50% of sodium absorption in the human distal colon, but is apparently largely absent from the small intestine (with the possible exception of the cecum) (97). Luminal sodium enters across the apical membrane via ENaC channels that are identical to those in the distal nephron, in response to gradients established by the basolateral Na,K-ATPase (Fig. 2). Potassium channels, most likely situated in the basolateral membrane, are also required to recycle potassium and provide for the sustained transport of sodium across the epithelium. Chloride and water then follow passively via the paracellular route to restore electroneutrality and osmotic balance between the luminal and basolateral compartments.

In common with the kidney, electrogenic sodium transport in the colon is subject to chronic regulation by the hormone aldosterone. The induction of secondary hyperaldosteronism by feeding a low-salt diet results in upregulated expression of ENaC in both the kidney and colon, enhancing whole-body sodium retention (113). At the level of the colon, this also serves to increase the proportion of sodium that is absorbed via the electrogenic mechanism, as opposed to the electroneutral mechanism discussed below.

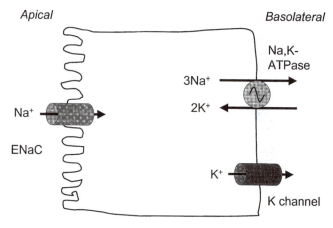

FIGURE 2 Electrogenic sodium absorption. This transport mechanism is found in the colon, and provides sodium uptake via apical ENaC sodium channels in response to gradients established by the basolateral Na,K-ATPase. Basolateral potassium channels provide for potassium recycling as needed. Water and chloride ions are absorbed paracellularly to balance electrical and osmotic forces.

Electroneutral Sodium Chloride Absorption. In the period between meals, when nutrients are largely absent from the small intestinal lumen, the intestine nevertheless needs to maintain an ability to absorb fluid since secretory processes continue, in part to support the motility and cleansing functions of the gut. Absorption during this period is accomplished by the coupled absorption of sodium and chloride (88). This is an electroneutral process, so only water is stimulated to move paracellularly. The details of this absorptive mechanism, which is also expressed to varying degrees in the colon, are depicted in Fig. 3. The mechanism consists of the coupled activity of two exchangers located on the apical membrane—an epithelial isoform of the sodium-hydrogen exchanger (NHE3) and a chloride-bicarbonate exchanger whose molecular identity is still a matter of some controversy, as indicated in the figure (70, 141). The protons and bicarbonate ions required for exchange are assumed to be generated intracellularly via the action of carbonic anhydrase. Sodium exits the cell via the basolateral Na,K-ATPase, whereas chloride as well as potassium taken up by the ATPase can be recycled basolaterally by a protein hypothesized to act in a manner identical to a potassium/chloride cotransporter described in other systems (58).

Peptide Absorption. The intestine has the capability to absorb the products of protein digestion, unlike other nutrients, not only as monomers but also as short peptides. In fact, some amino acids are taken up more efficiently in this form. Peptide uptake is mediated by a process that is electrogenic and linked to the simultaneous uptake of protons

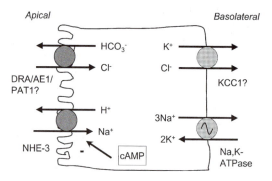

FIGURE 3 Electroneutral sodium chloride absorption. This process is expressed in both the small and large intestine and contributes to water absorption when nutrients are absent. Sodium and chloride are taken up across the apical membrane via the coupled activity of two exchangers. The identity of the chloride/bicarbonate exchanger involved in this process is still controversial, as is the involvement of a basolateral potassium/chloride cotransporter. The apical sodium/hydrogen exhanger, NHE3, can be negatively regulated by increases in cAMP. For additional details, see text.

(and thus likely to be controlled secondarily by the activity of sodium-hydrogen exchangers, which are a major determinant of intracellular pH) (97). The apical transporter involved in this mechanism is designated as PEPT1; it can transport a broad array of different di-, tri-, and even tetrapeptides, which can be positively or negatively charged, or neutral (48). As such, PEPT1 represents something of an enigma for transport physiologists, since the basis for its extremely broad substrate specificity is not yet understood at the molecular level. Once peptides have entered the enterocyte, they are cleaved into their constituent amino acids by intracellular peptidases, and these amino acids can be either used locally or transported to the bloodstream via an array of basolateral amino acid transporters. Overall, the process adds to the electrochemical gradient created across the small intestinal mucosa by nutrient absorption, and thus is predicted to contribute to net water absorption.

Potassium Absorption. The majority of uptake of dietary potassium occurs via passive mechanisms in the small intestine (1). On the other hand, a small proportion of the daily potassium load is absorbed electrogenically in the colon, which implicates this site as a contributor to whole-body potassium homeostasis (particularly since potassium secretion also occurs in this site and can be upregulated by a low-salt diet—see below) (1). However, there is little consensus at present as to the precise mechanism that provides for active potassium absorption in the colon, and several alternative mechanisms have been proposed. The fact that mice lacking the colonic isoform of H,K-ATPase show excessive losses of potassium to the stool may well implicate at least this apical transporter in the process (92).

SCFA Absorption. SCFA are produced during the fermentation of unabsorbed dietary fiber by the colonic flora. They serve as an important energy source for colonocytes, and

are also a major component of the anions and osmolytes in the colonic lumen with a combined concentration of 100 to 150 mM under normal circumstances (27). Absorption of these solutes probably occurs by both passive and active mechanisms. Passive diffusion can contribute significantly to the uptake of SCFA that are protonated, a process that is likely enhanced by the acidic microclimate that has been found to exist immediately adjacent to the colonic epithelium (32). This mode of SCFA uptake has been shown to lead to acidification of the apical pole of colonocytes, leading in turn to the activation of apical sodium/hydrogen exchangers and the accompanying uptake of sodium, which can later be effluxed across the basolateral membrane via the activity of the Na,K-ATPase (31). Transport of ionized SCFA has also been proposed, although the carrier that mediates this process (presumed to be an anion exchanger that exchanges an SCFA anion for intracellular bicarbonate) has yet to be established. In either case, SCFA are either used intracellularly or exit the epithelial cell across the basolateral membrane in ionized form, perhaps by being cotransported with a proton via the monocarboxylate transporter, MCT1 (56).

Secretory Mechanisms

Secretory mechanisms are present in both the small intestine and colon to provide for the regulation of the fluidity of intestinal contents as needed for digestion and absorption, or to subserve specialized roles such as mucosal protection or whole-body potassium homeostasis. Three active secretory mechanisms are recognized: for chloride, bicarbonate, and potassium. Chloride secretion is likely the largest quantitative contributor to net secretory fluxes of fluid in the intestine; chloride also plays an important role in driving the secretion of bicarbonate. Bicarbonate secretion, on the other hand, plays a critical role in protecting the mucosa of the proximal duodenum from acid-peptic damage and is highly expressed in that segment of the small intestine. Lower levels of bicarbonate secretion are observed throughout the small intestine and colon, however, and may play an important role in maintaining an appropriate pH of luminal contents.

Chloride Secretion. For many years, active secretion by intestinal epithelial cells was not well recognized. Classical studies of intestinal transport probably overlooked secretion, since it was masked by the greater magnitude of absorptive flux occurring simultaneously in intact intestinal segments. However, the advent of intestinal epithelial cell lines drew attention to the fact that the intestine constantly secretes as well as absorbs, and, as mentioned above, the primary driving force for secretory fluxes of fluid is provided by the movement of chloride from the bloodstream to the lumen.

The chloride secretory mechanism of intestinal epithelial cells is shown in Fig. 4. As is the case with the other transport mechanisms discussed in this section, the basolateral Na,K-ATPase provides the electromotive force for the overall transport process. The low intracellular sodium concentration established by

this pump drives the secondary active uptake of chloride in association with sodium as well as potassium via a cotransporter protein identified as NKCC1, the Na/K/2Cl cotransporter. Chloride can thus accumulate in the cytosol above its electrochemical equilibrium, and exits across the apical membrane when chloride channels at that site open in response to changes in second messengers. Quantitatively, the most important of these chloride channels is the cystic fibrosis transmembrane conductance regulator, or CFTR, the gene product that is mutated in the setting of cystic fibrosis (14). However, recent studies have also provided evidence of the existence of alternative chloride conductances in the apical membrane of intestinal epithelial cells, most notably those of the CLCA family of channels that are activated by calcium (14, 52). In either case, potassium must be effluxed from the cell to avoid depolarization and to allow for sustained chloride secretion. This likely occurs via one of two presumed classes of basolateral potassium channels sensitive to either calcium or cAMP (39, 57). There is also evidence that additional NKCC1 cotransporters must be in-

FIGURE 4 Electrogenic chloride secretion. This transport mechanism occurs throughout the gastrointestinal tract and drives water and sodium secretion via the paracellular route. Chloride is taken up across the basolateral membrane via the sodium/potassium/chloride cotransporter, NKCC1, in response to the sodium concentration gradient established by the basolateral Na,K-ATPase. Potassium can be recycled by various channels for this cation on the basolateral membrane; one class of channels involved is regulated by calcium and appears to belong to the IK1 family, whereas the existence of cAMP-regulated channels is still hypothetical at present. Chloride exits across the apical membrane predominantly via cAMP-regulated CFTR chloride channels, although there is emerging evidence for additional involvement of calcium-activated CLCA channels.

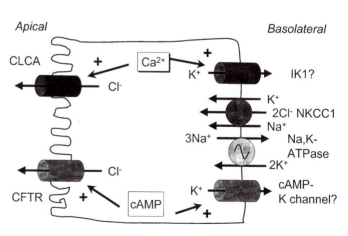

serted into the basolateral membrane and/or otherwise activated if sustained secretion is to take place. In all cases, however, sodium and water are driven to move paracellularly in response to the net transport of chloride ions.

Chloride secretion is clearly a process that can be exploited by specific enteropathogens and/or their toxins, as discussed in detail elsewhere in this volume. The classical example is cholera, which causes a massive and irreversible stimulation of the secretory response (14). The ability of infectious pathogens to activate chloride secretion has led some authors to speculate that partial protection from diseases caused by such organisms may have provided a selective pressure to retain CFTR mutants in the gene pool, with heterozygotes likely to experience fewer diarrheal symptoms (54, 62, 63). While it remains controversial, this is at least an attractive hypothesis for the relatively high prevalence of cystic fibrosis in many populations, despite the devastating nature of the homozygous state.

Bicarbonate Secretion. Large amounts of bicarbonate are secreted by the proximal duodenum and diffuse into an overlying mucus layer to provide protection against acid-peptic damage (69). The physiological role of bicarbonate secretion in other intestinal segments is less well understood. The finding that congenital chloride diarrhea, a disease that arises from a mutation in one of the candidates for the apical chloride/bicarbonate exchanger involved in bicarbonate secretion, downregulated in adenoma (DRA), leads to a profound systemic alkalosis, may imply that intestinal bicarbonate secretion plays a role in whole-body acid-base homeostasis, at least under certain circumstances (38, 99).

Two mechanisms for the net secretion of bicarbonate are recognized (Fig. 5 and 6), which differ both in the pathway used by bicarbonate ions to exit across the apical membrane and on whether the transport mechanism is electrogenic or electroneutral. In the best-studied model, bicarbonate can be generated intracellularly via the action of car-

bonic anhydrase (where a basolateral sodium/hydrogen exchanger serves to efflux liberated protons) or can enter across the basolateral membrane in conjunction with sodium via the NBC sodium/bicarbonate cotransporter (119). The latter process is, once again, driven secondarily by the activity of the Na,K-ATPase. In the electroneutral secretory mechanism (Fig. 5), bicarbonate exits across the apical membrane via a chloride/bicarbonate exchanger, which may be DRA, or perhaps an anion exchanger of the AE family (70, 99). There is also recent evidence of the involvement of a novel anion exchanger known as PAT1 in this process, particularly in the small intestine where expression of DRA is relatively low compared to the colon (141). No matter what its precise molecular identity, this transporter's activity may be driven via the stimulated release of chloride across the apical membrane via CFTR channels, which is then recycled back into the cell by the exchanger. In a second, electrogenic mechanism (Fig. 6), bicarbonate exits the cell through apical channels. There is some evidence that CFTR plays this role, although the rates of permeation of bicarbonate ions through the channel are much lower than those of chloride (111). Alternatively, there may be a specific bicarbonate channel (or channels) that has yet to be identified.

Potassium Secretion. All portions of the mammalian colon are capable of conducting the active secretion of potassium ions. It is likely that this occurs chronically in response to alterations in whole-body electrolyte status, but the physiological significance of acute changes in potassium transport in the colon is unknown at present (131). The model for potassium secretion is depicted in Fig. 7 and is quite analogous to the chloride secretory mechanism shown in Fig. 4 except that apical chloride channels are replaced by those for potassium (64–66). Experimentally, the two processes can be distinguished by the sidedness of their sensitivity to potassium channel blockers; potassium secretion can be blocked by the ad-

FIGURE 5   Electroneutral bicarbonate secretion. Bicarbonate is generated intracellularly via the action of carbonic anhydrase (not shown), or enters across the basolateral membrane via secondary active transport mediated by the sodium/bicarbonate cotransporter, and energized by the sodium gradient established by the Na,K-ATPase. In response to increases in cAMP, apical CFTR chloride channels allow the outflow of chloride across the apical membrane, which is in turn exchanged for intracellular bicarbonate, via an anion exchanger whose identity is still controversial, as shown. A housekeeping basolateral sodium/hydrogen exchanger (NHE-1) is involved in intracellular pH homeostasis during the process. For further details, see text.

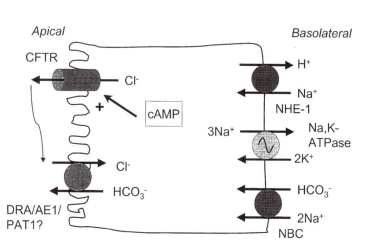

dition of such inhibitors to the apical side of the tissue, whereas these agents are effective in reducing chloride secretion only when added basolaterally.

REGULATION OF EPITHELIAL ION TRANSPORT

Intestinal epithelial ion transport is regulated via complex pathways that are still not fully understood. Regulation can be divided into two complementary mechanisms: (i) an inter-cellular mechanism consisting of stimulation of the epithelium by mediators released from nerves, endocrine cells, and other effector cells and (ii) an intracellular mechanism where second messengers initiate signal transduction pathways within the epithelial cells themselves. The primary ion secreted by the epithelium is chloride, and chloride secretion is increased by neural, humoral, and immune-related mechanisms (11). Conversely, absorptive transport mechanisms are often inhibited

FIGURE 6   Electrogenic bicarbonate secretion. The major features of this model are identical to the transport mechanism depicted in Fig. 5, except that bicarbonate exits the cell across the apical membrane via a conductive pathway, which may be CFTR. For additional details, see text.

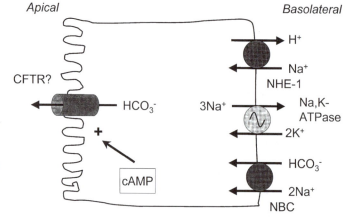

Apical   Basolateral

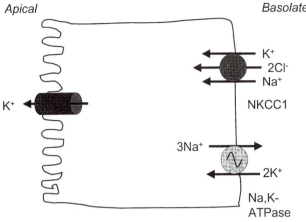

FIGURE 7 Electrogenic potassium secretion. This transport mechanism is expressed in the colon and contributes to whole-body potassium homeostasis. Potassium is taken up across the basolateral membrane by the NKCC1 cotransporter in response to the sodium gradient established by the Na,K-ATPase. Potassium then exits the cell across apical potassium channels that have not yet been identified at the molecular level. Water and chloride follow paracellularly to maintain osmotic and electrical balance between compartments.

by similar events. In either case, the two predominant intracellular pathways use cyclic nucleotides or ionized calcium as second messengers (11). Overall, inappropriate regulation, whether by endogenous factors or in response to bacterial components, may change the gut from a state of net water absorption to one of secretion and thereby lead to the excessive luminal water flow underlying diarrhea.

Targets of Regulation

Ultimately, regulatory mechanisms impinge on the membrane transporters discussed in the preceding sections. To review, ion movement across membranes can be accomplished by three distinct classes of transport mechanisms: carriers, pumps, and channels. Carriers bind and translocate combinations of solutes in tandem, or exchange one ion for another, and are characterized by their dependence on transmembrane ion concentration gradients. On the other hand, pumps are a class of carriers that require the energy of ATP hydrolysis to transport ions against transmembrane electrical and concentration gradients. Finally, channels permit large numbers of ions to move in a conductive fashion when open, but are also dependent on transmembrane ion concentration gradients. Table 2 summarizes the diverse intestinal carriers, pumps, and channels that serve as targets for the regulation

of ion transport in this tissue. Their behavior can be modified by four basic mechanisms: (i) direct interactions between transport proteins and regulatory factors; (ii) covalent modification such as phosphorylation/dephosphorylation; (iii) vesicle transport to and from the membrane, regulating the numbers of transporters located in the membrane; and finally, (iv) alterations in the expression levels of specific transport proteins.

Intercellular Regulation

The epithelium is continuously influenced by cell types resident in the lamina propria including nerves, enteroendocrine cells, mast cells, and myofibroblasts. Blood-borne and autocrine regulation also controls epithelial function. Finally, in disease states, infiltrating inflammatory cells may also contribute to the regulation of intestinal transport. Figure 8 illustrates intercellular regulation.

Neural Regulation. Enteric nerve endings release peptides and other neurotransmitters that are capable of regulating both the epithelium and muscle layers. Many transmitters, including neurotensin, neuropeptide Y, acetylcholine, and 5-hydroxytryptamine (23, 25), have been shown to regulate ion transport mainly by binding directly to epithelial receptors, thereby inducing second messengers. In general, neural regulation probably provides

TABLE 2 Carriers, pumps, and channels expressed in intestinal epithelial cells

Carriers	Pumps	Channels
Na$^+$-solute cotransporters, e.g., SGLT-1	Na$^+$,K$^+$-ATPase	Chloride channels: CFTR, CLCA
H$^+$-solute cotransporters, e.g., PEPT1	H$^+$,K$^+$-ATPase	Sodium channels: ENaC
Na$^+$,K$^+$,2Cl$^-$ cotransporter: NKCC1		Potassium channels
HCO$_3^-$,Na$^+$ cotransporter: NBC		
Na$^+$/H$^+$ exchangers: NHE		
Cl$^-$/HCO$_3^-$ exchangers: DRA, AE1, PAT1		

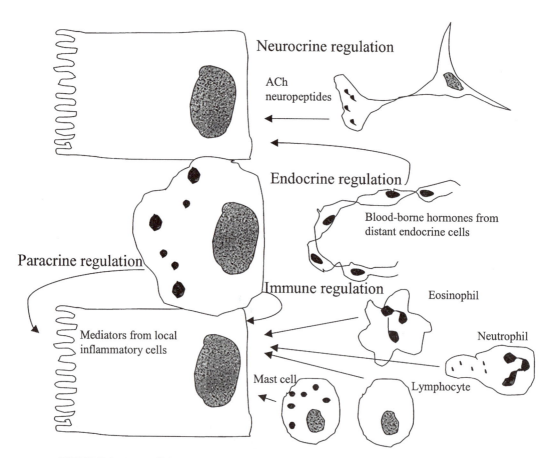

FIGURE 8 Intercellular regulation of gastrointestinal transport. Enteric nerves release neurotransmitters and peptides, which interact largely with the epithelial cells themselves to alter transport. Regulatory peptides from endocrine cells are released both apically and basolaterally, and local diffusion of these peptides to nearby epithelial cells (paracrine regulation) can regulate ion transport. Blood-borne peptides from distant endocrine cells can also induce regulatory actions in a similar fashion. Finally, resident or infiltrating immune/inflammatory cells can be stimulated to release mediators, which in turn act on the epithelium. There is also substantial evidence for cross talk among these various regulatory mechanisms (not shown). For further details, see text.

minute-to-minute control of ion transport as required for handling the meal. For example, physical stroking of the mucosa, a maneuver thought to model the physical passage of contents through the intestine, evokes a cholinergic reflex that induces secretion of both fluid and mucus (59, 123). This likely serves to lubricate the mucosa and protect it from damage. However, neurotransmitters may also exert indirect and sometimes more chronic effects on ion transport through their ability to release secondary hormones and mediators from endocrine and immune cells.

Endocrine Regulation. In keeping with neural regulation, ion transport is also affected by enteroendocrine cells located among the epithelial cells themselves, which release peptides and other mediators capable of influencing ion transport. Blood-borne hormones from distant endocrine cells likely also contribute to epithelial regulation, although the precise participants have not been fully elucidated. Enteroendocrine cells can register the nature and composition of the luminal contents and alter ion transport responses via direct effects on epithelial cells. Well-known hormones and related factors that can influence ion transport include secretin, insulin, gastrin, and epidermal growth factor (EGF) (24, 29, 51, 103). Another recently identified endocrine regulator is pituitary adenylate cyclase-activating polypeptide, PACAP, a novel hypothalamic peptide that has been shown to evoke anion secretion in the intestine. It has been suggested that the regulation of anion secretion by intestinal epithelial cells in vivo may be mediated by locally formed PACAP in an autocrine or paracrine fashion (84).

Immune Regulation. If stimulated, immunologic effector cells release substances that can also regulate epithelial function. For example, resident immune cells in the gastrointestinal mucosa, such as mast cells, are now recognized not only to react to antigens but also to modulate epithelial transport and bar-

rier functions. Upon stimulation by antigen or other agonists such as neuropeptides, mast cells release bioactive mediators via a process of regulated exocytosis into the adjoining tissue. This in turn induces physiological responses (146), which can include ion transport abnormalities, especially during inflammation (35, 105). Mast cell mediators known to induce Cl^- secretion include histamine and adenosine (9). Similarly, phagocytic leukocytes (macrophages, neutrophils, eosinophils) that may infiltrate the lamina propria in disease states possess the enzymatic machinery necessary to form large amounts of reactive oxygen metabolites (ROS) (61), many of which have been demonstrated to contribute to secretory responses (55). Neutrophils may additionally migrate into the lumen, forming crypt abscesses where bacterial factors evoke release of the ion transport modulator $5'AMP$, a precursor for adenosine (87). Other effects of immune cells may be indirect. For example, the myofibroblast sheath underlying the epithelium is thought to act as a site where signals from the lamina propria are "translated." This function may be due to the ability of these fibroblasts to release prosecretory mediators such as prostaglandin E_2 (PGE_2) in response to neurohumoral or inflammatory agents (19). In general, activation of immune cells results in net secretion and could therefore be considered deleterious. On the other hand, this secretory response, resulting from the cooperation of immune cells, myofibroblasts, and the epithelium, may represent a primitive host-defense response intended to rid the lumen of invading pathogens.

Intracellular Ion Transport Regulation
The intestinal epithelium has evolved a complex network of pathways that can regulate its function in a largely autonomous fashion, once an initial signal has been received. For example, when extracellular agents, such as hormones or toxins, bind to specific receptors on epithelial cells, intracellular signaling cascades are initiated. Important constituents of these cascades are the small signaling mole-

cules that act within the cell as second messengers. The levels of these second messengers regulate the activity of various protein kinases and other effectors within the cell. Thus, changes in these messengers will alter, directly or indirectly, the activity and/or abundance in the membrane of the various transport proteins that make up epithelial transport mechanisms. However, the process is not strictly linear, since cross talk between receptors and divergent signaling cascades occurs concomitantly. Thus, while cyclic nucleotides and free cytosolic Ca^{2+} are the predominant intracellular signals that regulate intestinal epithelial ion transport, the generation and/or activity of these messengers may be amplified, antagonized, or secondarily mediated by a host of additional signaling molecules (13).

Cyclic Nucleotides. It has long been documented that cAMP and cyclic guanosine phosphate (cGMP) play important roles in the control of intestinal epithelial ion transport (45, 114). cAMP is generated from ATP through the action of adenylate cyclase, a membrane-bound enzyme that is coupled through stimulatory (Gs) and inhibitory (Gi) G proteins to a number of hormone and neurotransmitter receptors (49). Gs-dependent activation of adenylate cyclase and increases in cAMP production are associated with the induction of ion transport by a variety of endogenous hormonal regulators including prostaglandins and vasoactive intestinal polypeptide (47). Many exogenous substances, e.g., a diversity of bacteria, may also stimulate epithelial transport by activation of the cAMP-dependent pathway. cGMP, on the other hand, is generated by guanylate cyclase. This enzyme is found in two forms in the colon, particulate and soluble, while the small intestine contains only the former (49).

cAMP-dependent chloride secretion is induced through protein kinase A (PKA) (16, 121) whereas cGMP-induced Cl^- secretion has recently been documented to occur via a protein kinase GII (PKGII) pathway (120). The kinetics of either cyclic nucleotide-induced secretory response are sustained in the continued presence of agonist and quantitatively proportional to cyclic nucleotide levels (11). Both PKA and PKGII appear to be capable of phosphorylating and thereby activating CFTR in the presence of appropriate levels of intracellular ATP. In addition, some authors have shown that a pool of CFTR resides in subapical vesicular compartments, which rapidly redistribute from the cytoplasm to the apical surface upon cAMP stimulation (3, 4). This cAMP-regulated CFTR trafficking is assumed to contribute to the regulation of CFTR-mediated anion transport (102, 108). In fact, regulation of transporters by insertion into, or retrieval from, the plasma membrane is now known to be a common mechanism whereby the regulation of a number of different transporters can be achieved, such as for NKCC1 (36), SGLT1 (68), Na,K-ATPase (140), Na^+ channels (50), and NHE3 (76).

Absorptive mechanisms may also be affected by changes in cyclic nucleotides, although in this case the influence can be inhibitory. NHE3 is the third of six cloned Na^+/H^+ exchangers. It is the predominant epithelial isoform and is mainly expressed on the villus in the intestine (147). Like CFTR, NHE3 is regulated by phosphorylation events via cAMP-induced PKA action, although this phosphorylation induces inhibition of NHE3 activity (28, 96). Therefore, activation of PKA leads concomitantly to inhibition of NHE3 and activation of CFTR.

CFTR, while functioning as a Cl^- channel, may also act as a regulator of other ion transporters, (Fig. 9). For example, cAMP-dependent activation of CFTR results in a reciprocal inhibition of ENaC Na^+ channels (60, 81). It has been suggested that this regulation is due to the fact that Cl^- ions control ENaC activity (81). Another emerging regulatory role for CFTR is in the control of K^+ transport. This may depend on the type of K^+ channel considered (22). Thus, while cAMP appears to exert an inhibitory influence on apical K^+ transport (42), CFTR stimulates the

Apical

Basolateral

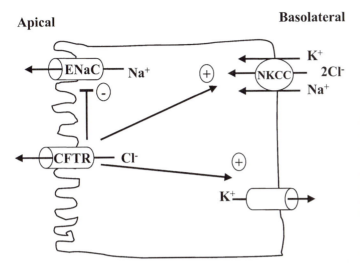

FIGURE 9 The regulatory action of CFTR on other ion channels and transporters. In addition to its role as a chloride channel, CFTR exerts modulatory influences over a variety of other transport proteins and processes as shown. These include inhibition of the epithelial Na^+ channel, ENaC, induction of increased expression of NKCC1, and activation of basolateral K^+ channels.

activity of basolaterally located K^+ channels (60), as well as upregulates the expression of NKCC1 (122).

Intracellular cAMP also stimulates basolateral K^+ uptake via NKCC1 and decreases the ratio of basolateral versus apical K^+ conductances, leading to increased luminal and reduced serosal K^+ efflux (42). This is important for maintaining the membrane potential and thereby Cl^- secretion (42, 93). Thus, as depicted in Fig. 4, an increase in the levels of either cAMP or cGMP within the epithelium through PKA activates apical chloride channels and thereby stimulates Cl^- secretion, stimulates activation of basolateral potassium channels, and inhibits neutral Na^+,Cl^- absorption (26, 145).

Intracellular Calcium. Ionized calcium plays a central role as a second messenger in cellular functions (45), and intracellular levels are accordingly tightly regulated. Increases in Ca^{2+} have been shown to stimulate both Cl^- and HCO_3^- secretion while inhibiting electroneutral NaCl absorption (12). In contrast to the sustained secretory responses induced by cyclic nucleotides, the Ca^{2+}-dependent chloride secretory response, at least, is transient, even in the continued presence of agonist or elevated intracellular Ca^{2+} (11, 41). Many

neuroimmune mediators, including acetylcholine, serotonin, and histamine, regulate epithelial ion transport by activation of Ca^{2+} signaling. The mechanisms by which increases in intracellular Ca^{2+} regulate ion transport processes appear to be more complex and are less well understood than for cAMP.

Taking the example of chloride secretion, the initiation of the Ca^{2+}-mediated transport process involves receptor-mediated activation of phospholipase C (PLC), which cleaves membrane phosphatidylinositides to yield inositol(1,4,5)triphosphate (InsP3) and diacylglycerol (101). InsP3 stimulates the release of Ca^{2+} from intracellular stores (18), which appears also to initiate Ca^{2+} influx from the extracellular milieu (18). Diacylglycerol, on the other hand, activates and translocates protein kinase C (PKC) to the plasma membrane (101). This enzyme, in turn, reduces the Ca^{2+} sensitivity of large conductance Ca^{2+}-activated K^+ channels (15), thereby reducing the coupling strength between localized Ca^{2+} transients and the channel. This possibly functions as a negative feedback mechanism. In fact, PKC appears to have a dual role in regulation of epithelial ion transport (43), since activation of this enzyme can initially be shown to induce active Cl^- secretion, but over longer periods reduces secretory responses induced by both cAMP and Ca^{2+} mobilizing agents (72). This discrepancy may well be accounted for by the divergent effects of different PKC isozymes (30, 127). On the other hand, increases in Ca^{2+} within the epithelial cytosol can activate Ca^{2+}-calmodulin-dependent protein kinase, CaMK, which has been implicated in the regulation of the putative calcium-activated apical Cl^- channel in secretory epithelia (8).

Finally, increases in intracellular Ca^{2+} may alter ion transport by a direct effect on basolateral, calcium-activated K^+ channels (77). Activation of these channels results in K^+ exit from the cell, which, in turn, increases the driving force for Cl^- exit across the apical membrane (40). Also, volume increases will activate K^+ channels through CaMK-mediated phosphorylation, although there is some evidence that this occurs secondary to an increase in cytosolic acidification rather than an increase in $[Ca^{2+}]_{(i)}$ (86).

Interactions between cAMP and Calcium.　Viewing Ca^{2+}- or cAMP-regulated ion transport as separate events may not provide a full understanding of their physiological impact, due to overlap and synergy between the signaling events initiated by each second messenger. Thus, potassium recycling through basolateral K^+ channels is essential for cAMP-activated chloride secretion (91), but basolateral K^+ conductance is under the dominant control of intracellular Ca^{2+}. In fact, the predominant effect of cAMP on basolateral K^+ conductance may be an inhibitory one, perhaps due to a decrease in intracellular Ca^{2+} (118). An increase in cytosolic Ca^{2+} results in the opening of basolateral K^+ channels, which causes a hyperpolarization of the cell membrane, indirectly supporting Cl^- secretion by increasing the driving force for Cl^- exit. On the other hand, apical chloride exit is likely the rate-limiting step for calcium-mediated chloride secretion. Thus, when secretory epithelial cells are exposed simultaneously to agonists that increase cAMP and calcium, the secretory response overall is amplified. These synergistic effects reflect cooperative interactions between basolateral potassium channels and apical chloride channels. This cross talk between second messenger generation provides for an enhanced secretory response to a given level of agonist (e.g., hormones or neurotransmitters) or in response to pathogens. At the same time, Ca^{2+}-induced secretion is limited, unless coordinated with a cAMP-dependent response. This therefore indirectly prevents excessive secretion to Ca^{2+}-dependent secretagogues alone (20, 142).

Effects of Tyrosine Kinases on Ion Transport.　The downstream effects mediated by calcium and cyclic nucleotides are, as mentioned above, in general thought to be mediated through actions of protein kinases and phosphatases (121). In addition to the serine/threonine kinases discussed above, however, tyrosine kinases are known to play a variety of roles in signal transduction, and in recent years their involvement in the regulation of ion transport has emerged. The activation of these kinases often results in a complex cascade of events modulating numerous functions, and recently the EGF receptor tyrosine kinase, in particular, has been shown to play a key role in regulation of ion transport.

Calcium-Stimulated Activation of Tyrosine Kinase Activity.　Recent studies indicate that, in addition to stimulating chloride secretion, calcium-dependent agonists such as the muscarinic agonist carbachol (CCh) also evoke signaling pathways that play a role in inhibiting ion transport (75). Two such mechanisms appear to exist. One, which is involved in the long-term inhibition of chloride secretion, is mediated by elevations in inositol tetrakisphosphate (71). The other mechanism participates in limiting ongoing Ca^{2+}-dependent secretory responses and is mediated by the agonist-stimulated influx of extracellular calcium (21, 137). Epithelial tyrosine kinases are now known to play important roles in these inhibitory effects on Ca^{2+}-dependent chloride secretion. In addition to stimulating chloride secretion, CCh induces tyrosine phosphorylation of the EGF receptor, EGFr. This response appears to involve the calcium-dependent soluble tyrosine kinase, Pyk-2, another soluble kinase, Src (73), and perhaps the release of an EGFr ligand, transforming growth factor α (TGF-α) (90). In turn, EGFr transactivation activates mitogen–activated protein kinases (MAPK) (ERK1/2 and p38), which, through mechanisms yet to be elucidated, inhibit chloride secretion. Since pharmacological inhibition of either EGFr phosphorylation or MAPK activation results in a potentiation and increased duration of CCh-stimulated secretory responses, it appears that these events represent a mechanism by which chloride secretion in response to CCh may be self-limited (74); the mechanisms are depicted in Fig. 10.

EGF itself may also activate the EGFr, thereby initiating a separate cascade of events (134). First among these is activation of the receptor kinase activity, which also leads to autophosphorylation of the receptor (135) and to tyrosine phosphorylation of additional substrates. EGF thereby also activates various enzymes that are involved in inositol phosphate and phospholipid metabolism (134). While EGF does not itself stimulate chloride secretion, the growth factor inhibits calcium-dependent chloride secretion by "uncoupling" the rise in intracellular calcium from downstream effector responses (135). At least part of this inhibitory effect on chloride secretion is exerted through the activation of phosphatidylinositol 3-kinase (PI 3-K) and an inhibitory effect on basolateral K^+ channels (136). Interestingly, similar signaling pathways are involved in regulating other modes of ion transport. For example, EGF has been shown to increase NaCl absorption via basolateral membrane receptors (44) through a mechanism involving PI 3-K (76). The downstream effect of PI 3-K on chloride secretion is to inhibit K^+ channels via PKC, whereas EGF stimulation of PI 3-K in regard to NHE3 ac-

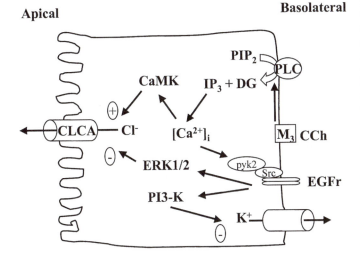

Apical

Basolateral

FIGURE 10 Pathways for the stimulation and inhibition of Ca^{2+}-dependent chloride secretory responses. Agonists that evoke increases in intracellular Ca^{2+} (here exemplified by the muscarinic agonist, CCh, binding to an M_3-muscarinic receptor) are capable of inducing CaMK-stimulated chloride secretory responses via activation of calcium-activated chloride channel (CLCA). At the same time, increases in intracellular Ca^{2+} will transactivate the EGF receptor and subsequently recruit the ERK1/2 isoforms of MAPK, which by as yet unknown mechanisms reduces the secretory responses. In a divergent mechanism, activation of EGFr by EGF itself results in stimulation of PI 3-K, which inhibits but does not also stimulate chloride secretion. This action is mediated by inhibition of a basolateral potassium channel, reducing the driving force for apical chloride secretion. For further details, see text.

tivation appears to induce trafficking of NHE3 to the plasma membrane (82). In sum, these complementary actions ensure that the net effect of EGF is to increase overall intestinal fluid absorption.

These mechanisms whereby similar intracellular signaling pathways have reciprocal effects on secretory and absorptive processes illustrate the complexity of the intestinal secretory apparatus. The physiological relevance of the induced inhibitory pathways on chloride secretion is still unclear, but it is thought that they may act as a "braking" mechanism to prevent excessive ion and fluid loss from the body in response to calcium-dependent hormones and neurotransmitters, particularly in the setting of mucosal injury (10).

SUMMARY AND CONCLUSIONS

The mammalian intestine actively transports a wide range of solutes to fulfill its physiological roles of nutrient digestion and absorption. In addition to the uptake of digested products of the meal, electrolytes are secreted and absorbed to regulate the fluidity of the intestinal contents appropriately. These functions are undertaken by intestinal epithelial cells, which are subject to a plethora of inter- and intracellular regulatory mechanisms that impinge ultimately on membrane transport proteins, thereby altering their activity, location, and/ or expression. Increased knowledge of the molecular nature of both signaling and transport proteins has enhanced our understanding of intestinal transport and offers the opportunity to intervene when transport is dysregulated.

In health, net absorption of fluid and solutes predominates in the intestine overall, preventing dehydration. However, as is discussed elsewhere in this volume, bacterial pathogens may cause disease by subverting this balance, resulting in net secretion and thus the clinical symptom of diarrhea. An understanding of the normal molecular physiology of intestinal transport should thus provide a complementary appreciation of these pathophysiological events, particularly since many bacteria can di-

rectly influence the transporters and signal transduction proteins discussed here. Ultimately, such knowledge may allow the development of highly targeted therapies that will be useful in reducing the scourge of infectious diarrhea.

ACKNOWLEDGMENTS

Studies from our laboratory have been supported by grants from the National Institutes of Health (DK28305, DK35108 [Project5]) and from the Crohn's and Colitis Foundation of America. We thank our colleagues for helpful discussions and Glenda Wheeler for assistance with manuscript submission.

REFERENCES

1. **Agarwal, R., R. Afzalpurkar, and J. S. Fordtran.** 1994. Pathophysiology of potassium absorption and secretion by the human intestine. *Gastroenterology* **107:**548–571.
2. **Ameen, N. A., T. Ardito, M. Kashgarian, and C. R. Marino.** 1995. A unique subset of rat and human villus cells express the cystic fibrosis transmembrane conductance regulator. *Gastroenterology* **108:**1016.
3. **Ameen, N. A., B. Martensson, L. Bourguinon, C. Marino, J. Isenberg, and G. E. McLaughlin.** 1999. CFTR channel insertion to the apical surface in rat duodenal villus epithelial cells is upregulated by VIP in vivo. *J. Cell Sci.* **112:**887–894.
4. **Ameen, N. A., E. van Donselaar, G. Posthuma, H. de Jonge, G. McLaughlin, H. J. Geuze, C. Marino, and P. J. Peters.** 2000. Subcellular distribution of CFTR in rat intestine supports a physiologic role for CFTR regulation by vesicle traffic. *Histochem. Cell Biol.* **114:**219–228.
5. **Anderson, J. M.** 2001. Molecular structure of tight junctions and their role in epithelial transport. *News Physiol. Sci.* **16:**126–130.
6. **Andreeva, A. Y., E. Krause, E. C. Muller, I. E. Blasig, and D. I. Utepbergenov.** 2001. Protein kinase C regulates the phosphorylation and cellular localization of occludin. *J. Biol. Chem.* **276:**38480–38486.
7. **Aroeti, B., P. A. Kosen, I. D. Kuntz, F. E. Cohen, and K. E. Mostov.** 1993. Mutational and secondary structural analysis of the basolateral sorting signal of the polymeric immunoglobulin receptor. *J. Cell Biol.* **123:**1149–1160.
8. **Arreola, J., J. E. Melvin, and T. Begenisich.** 1998. Differences in regulation of Ca^{2+}-activated Cl^- channels in colonic and parotid secretory

cells. *Am. J. Physiol. Cell Physiol.* **274:**C161–C166.

9. **Barrett, K. E.** 1991. Immune regulation of intestinal ion transport: implications for inflammatory diarrhea. *Progr. Inflamm. Bowel Dis.* **12:**8–11.

10. **Barrett, K. E.** 1993. Chloride secretion by the colonic epithelial cell line, T₈₄: mechanisms and regulation, p. 215–235. *In* W. Clauss (ed.), *Ion Transport in Vertebrate Colon.* Springer-Verlag, Berlin, Germany.

11. **Barrett, K. E.** 1993. Positive and negative regulation of chloride secretion in T₈₄ cells. *Am. J. Physiol.* **265:**C859–C868.

12. **Barrett, K. E.** 1997. Integrated regulation of intestinal epithelial transport: intercellular and intracellular pathways. 1996 Bowditch Lecture. *Am. J. Physiol.* **272:**C1069–C1076.

13. **Barrett, K. E., and K. Dharmsathaphorn.** 1991. Secretion and absorption: small intestine and colon, p. 265–294. *In* T. Yamada (ed.), *Textbook of Gastroenterology.* J. B. Lippincott Company, Philadelphia, Pa.

14. **Barrett, K. E., and S. J. Keely.** 2000. Chloride secretion by the intestinal epithelium: molecular basis and regulatory aspects. *Annu. Rev. Physiol.* **62:**535–572.

15. **Bayguinov, O., B. Hagen, J. L. Kenyon, and K. M. Sanders.** 2001. Coupling strength between localized Ca²⁺ transients and K⁺ channels is regulated by protein kinase C. *Am. J. Physiol. Cell Physiol.* **281:**C1512–C1523.

16. **Berger, H. A., S. M. Travis, and M. J. Welsh.** 1993. Regulation of the cystic fibrosis transmembrane conductance regulator Cl⁻ channel by specific protein kinases and protein phosphatases. *J. Biol. Chem.* **268:**2037–2047.

17. **Berglund, J. J., M. Riegler, Y. Zolotarevsky, E. Wenzl, and J. R. Turner.** 2001. Regulation of human jejunal transmucosal resistance and MLC phosphorylation by Na⁺-glucose cotransport. *Am. J. Physiol. Gastrointest. Liver Physiol.* **281:**G1487–G1493.

18. **Berridge, M. J.** 1993. Inositol trisphosphate and calcium signalling. *Nature* **361:**315–324.

19. **Berschneider, H. M., and D. W. Powell.** 1992. Fibroblasts modulate intestinal secretory responses to inflammatory mediators. *J. Clin. Invest.* **89:**484–489.

20. **Binder, H. J., and G. I. Sandle.** 1994. Electrolyte transport in the mammalian colon, p. 2133–2171. *In* L. R. Johnson (ed.), *Physiology of the Gastrointestinal Tract,* 3rd ed. Raven Press, New York, N.Y.

21. **Bischof, G., B. Illek, W. W. Reenstra, and T. E. Machen.** 1995. Role for tyrosine kinases in carbachol-regulated Ca entry into colonic epithelial cells. *Am. J. Physiol.* **268:**C154–C161.

22. **Boucherot, A., R. Schreiber, and K. Kunzelmann.** 2001. Regulation and properties of KCNQ1 (K(V)LQT1) and impact of the cystic fibrosis transmembrane conductance regulator. *J. Membr. Biol.* **182:**39–47.

23. **Brown, D. R., S. L. Boster, M. F. Overend, A. M. Parsons, and B. G. Treder.** 1990. Actions of neuropeptide Y on basal, cyclic AMP-induced and neurally evoked ion transport in porcine distal jejunum. *Regul. Pept.* **29:**31–47.

24. **Brown, D. R., and S. M. O'Grady.** 1997. Regulation of ion transport in the porcine intestinal tract by enteric neurotransmitters and hormones. *Comp. Biochem. Physiol. A Physiol.* **118:**309–317.

25. **Brown, D. R., and B. G. Treder.** 1989. Neurohormonal regulation of ion transport in the porcine distal jejunum. Actions of neurotensin and its natural homologs. *J. Pharmacol. Exp. Ther.* **249:**348–357.

26. **Brzuszczak, I. M., J. Zhao, C. Bell, D. Stiel, I. Fielding, J. Percy, R. Smith, and E. V. O'Loughlin.** 1996. Cyclic AMP-dependent anion secretion in human small and large intestine. *J. Gastroenterol. Hepatol.* **11:**804–810.

27. **Burgaut, M.** 1987. Occurrence, absorption and metabolism of short chain fatty acids in the digestive tract of mammals. *Comp. Biochem. Physiol.* **86B:**439–472.

28. **Cabado, A. G., F. H. Yu, A. Kapus, G. Lukacs, S. Grinstein, and J. Orlowski.** 1996. Distinct structural domains confer cAMP sensitivity and ATP dependence to the Na⁺/H⁺ exchanger NHE3 isoform. *J. Biol. Chem.* **271:**3590–3599.

29. **Canani, R. B., M. Bisceglia, E. Bruzzese, G. Mallardo, and A. Guarino.** 1999. Growth hormone stimulates, through tyrosine kinase, ion transport and proliferation in human intestinal cells. *J. Pediatr. Gastroenterol. Nutr.* **28:**315–320.

30. **Chow, J. Y. C., J. M. Uribe, and K. E. Barrett.** 2000. A role for protein kinase Cε in the inhibitory effect of epidermal growth factor on calcium-stimulated chloride secretion in human colonic epithelial cells. *J. Biol. Chem.* **275:**21169–21176.

31. **Chu, S., and M. H. Montrose.** 1996. Nonionic diffusion and carrier-mediated transport drive extracellular pH regulation of mouse colonic crypts. *J. Gen. Physiol.* **494:**783–793.

32. **Chu, S., and M. H. Montrose.** 1999. The glow of the colonic pH microclimate kindled by short-chain fatty acids, chloride and bicarbonate. *J. Physiol.* **517:**315.

33. **Clatworthy, J. P., and V. Subramanian.** 2001. Stem cells and the regulation of proliferation, differentiation and patterning in the intes-

tinal epithelium: emerging insights from gene expression patterns, transgenic and gene ablation studies. *Mech. Devel.* **101**:3–9.

34. **Colegio, O. R., C. M. Van Itallie, H. J. McCrea, C. Rahner, and J. M. Anderson.** 2002. Claudins create charge-selective channels in the paracellular pathway between epithelial cells. *Am. J. Physiol. Cell Physiol.* **283**:C142–C147.

35. **Crowe, S. E., G. K. Luthra, and M. H. Perdue.** 1997. Mast cell mediated ion transport in intestine from patients with and without inflammatory bowel disease. *Gut* **41**:785–792.

36. **D'Andrea, L., C. Lytle, J. B. Matthews, P. Hofman, B. Forbush III, and J. L. Madara.** 1996. Na:K:2Cl cotransporter (NKCC) of human intestinal epithelial cells. Surface expression in response to cAMP. *J. Biol. Chem.* **271**:28969–28976.

37. Reference deleted.

38. **Darrow, D. C.** 1945. Congenital alkalosis with diarrhea. *J. Pediatr.* **26**:519.

39. **Devor, D. C., and M. E. Duffey.** 1992. Carbachol induces K^+, Cl^-, and nonselective cation conductances in T84 cells: a perforated patch-clamp study. *Am. J. Physiol.* **263**:C780–C787.

40. **Devor, D. C., S. M. Simasko, and M. E. Duffey.** 1990. Carbachol induces oscillations of membrane potassium conductance in a colonic cell line, T84. *Am. J. Physiol.* **258**:G318–G326.

41. **Dharmsathaphorn, K., and S. J. Pandol.** 1986. Mechanisms of chloride secretion induced by carbachol in a colonic epithelial cell line. *J. Clin. Invest.* **77**:348–354.

42. **Diener, M., F. Hug, D. Strabel, and E. Scharrer.** 1996. Cyclic AMP-dependent regulation of K^+ transport in the rat distal colon. *Br. J. Pharmacol.* **118**:1477–1487.

43. **Donowitz, M., M. E. Cohen, M. Gould, and G. W. Sharp.** 1989. Elevated intracellular Ca^{2+} acts through protein kinase C to regulate rabbit ileal NaCl absorption. Evidence for sequential control by Ca^{2+}/calmodulin and protein kinase C. *J. Clin. Invest.* **83**:1953–1962.

44. **Donowitz, M., J. L. Montgomery, M. S. Walker, and M. E. Cohen.** 1994. Brush-border tyrosine phosphorylation stimulates ileal neutral NaCl absorption and brush-border Na^+/H^+ exchange. *Am. J. Physiol.* **266**:G647–G656.

45. **Donowitz, M., and M. J. Welsh.** 1986. Ca^{++} and cyclic AMP in regulation of intestinal Na, K, and Cl transport. *Annu. Rev. Physiol.* **48**:135–150.

46. **Dunbar, L. A., and M. J. Caplan.** 2001. Ion pumps in polarized cells: sorting and regulation of the Na^+, K^+- and H^+, K^+-ATPases. *J. Biol. Chem.* **276**:29617–29620.

47. **Eberhart, C., and R. Dubois.** 1995. Eicosanoids and the gastrointestinal tract. *Gastroenterology* **109**:285–301.

48. **Fei, Y. J., V. Ganapathy, and F. H. Leibach.** 1998. Molecular and structural features of the proton-coupled oligopeptide transporter superfamily. *Prog. Nucleic Acid Res. Mol. Biol.* **58**:239–261.

49. **Field, M., M. C. Rao, and E. B. Chang.** 1989. Intestinal electrolyte transport and diarrheal disease. (First of two parts.) *N. Engl. J. Med.* **321**:800–806.

50. **Fisher, R. S., F. G. Grillo, and S. Sariban-Sohraby.** 1996. Brefeldin A inhibition of apical Na^+ channels in epithelia. *Am. J. Physiol.* **270**:C138–C147.

51. **Fukuda, M., A. Ohara, T. Bamba, and Y. Saek.** 2000. Activation of transepithelial ion transport by secretin in human intestinal Caco-2 cells. *Jpn. J. Physiol.* **50**:215–225.

52. **Fuller, C. M., and D. J. Benos.** 2000. Ca^{2+}-activated Cl^- channels: a newly emerging anion transport family. *News Physiol. Sci.* **15**:165–171.

53. **Furuse, M., T. Hirase, M. Itoh, A. Nagafuchi, S. Yonemura, S. Tsukita, and S. Tsukita.** 1993. Occludin: a novel integral membrane protein localizing at tight junctions. *J. Cell Biol.* **123**:1777.

54. **Gabriel, S. E., K. N. Brigman, B. H. Koller, R. C. Boucher, and M. J. Stutts.** 1994. Cystic fibrosis heterozygote resistance to cholera toxin in the cystic fibrosis mouse model. *Science* **266**:107–109.

55. **Gaginella, T. S., J. F. Kachur, H. Tamai, and A. Keshavarzian.** 1995. Reactive oxygen and nitrogen metabolites as mediators of secretory diarrhea. *Gastroenterology* **109**:2019–2028.

56. **Garcia, C. K., J. L. Goldstein, R. K. Pathak, R. G. W. Anderson, and M. S. Brown.** 1994. Molecular characterization of a membrane transporter for lactate, pyruvate, and other monocarboxylates: implications for the Cori cycle. *Cell* **76**:865–873.

57. **Gerlach, A. C., N. N. Gangopadhyay, and D. C. Devor.** 2000. Kinase-dependent regulation of the intermediate conductance, calcium-dependent potassium channel, hIK1. *J. Biol. Chem.* **275**:585–598.

58. **Gillen, C. M., S. Brill, J. A. Payne, and B. Forbush III.** 1996. Molecular cloning and functional expression of the K-Cl cotransporter from rabbit, rat, and human. *J. Biol. Chem.* **271**:16237–16244.

59. **Goyal, R. K., and I. Hirano.** 1996. The enteric nervous system. *N. Engl. J. Med.* **334**:1106–1115.

60. **Greger, R.** 2000. Role of CFTR in the colon. *Annu. Rev. Physiol.* **62**:467–491.

61. **Grisham, M. B., and D. N. Granger.** 1988. Neutrophil-mediated mucosal injury. Role of reactive oxygen metabolites. *Dig. Dis. Sci.* **33**:6S–15S.

62. **Grout, M., T. Zaidi, G. Meluleni, S. S. Mueschenborn, G. Banting, R. Ratcliff, M. J. Evans, W. H. Colledge, and G. B. Pier.** 1998. *Salmonella typhi* uses CFTR to enter intestinal epithelial cells. *Nature* **393**:79–82.

63. **Grubb, B. R., and S. E. Gabriel.** 1997. Intestinal physiology and pathology in gene-targeted mouse models of cystic fibrosis. *Am. J. Physiol.* **273**:G258–G266.

64. **Halm, D. R., and R. A. Frizzell.** 1986. Active K transport across rabbit distal colon: relation to Na absorption and Cl secretion. *Am. J. Physiol.* **251**:C252.

65. **Halm, D. R., and S. T. Halm.** 1994. Aldosterone stimulates K secretion prior to onset of Na absorption in guinea pig distal colon. *Am. J. Physiol.* **266**:C552–C558.

66. **Halm, D. R., and R. Rick.** 1992. Secretion of K and Cl across colonic epithelium: cellular localization using electron microprobe analysis. *Am. J. Physiol.* **262**:C1392–C1402.

67. **Hecht, G., C. Pothoulakis, J. T. LaMont, and J. L. Madara.** 1988. *Clostridium difficile* toxin A perturbs cytoskeletal structure and tight junction permeability of cultured human intestinal epithelial monolayers. *J. Clin. Invest.* **82**:1516–1524.

68. **Hirsch, J. R., D. D. F. Loo, and E. M. Wright.** 1996. Regulation of Na$^+$/glucose cotransporter expression by protein kinases in *Xenopus laevis* oocytes. *J. Biol. Chem.* **271**:14740–14746.

69. **Hogan, D. L., and J. I. Isenberg.** 1988. Gastroduodenal bicarbonate production, p. 385–408. *In* G. Stollerman (ed.), *Advances in Internal Medicine.* Year Book Medical, Chicago, Ill.

70. **Jacob, P., H. Rossmann, G. Lamprecht, A. Kretz, C. Neff, E. Lin-Wu, M. Gregor, D. A. Groneberg, J. Kere, and U. Seidler.** 2002. Down-regulated in adenoma mediates apical Cl$^-$/HCO$_3^-$ exchange in rabbit, rat and human duodenum. *Gastroenterology* **122**:709–724.

71. **Kachintorn, U., M. Vajanaphanich, K. E. Barrett, and A. E. Traynor-Kaplan.** 1993. Elevation of inositol tetrakisphosphate parallels inhibition of calcium-dependent chloride secretion in T$_{84}$ colonic epithelial cells. *Am. J. Physiol.* **264**:C671–C676.

72. **Kachintorn, U., P. Vongkovit, M. Vajanaphanich, S. Dinh, K. E. Barrett, and K. Dharmsathaphorn.** 1992. Dual effects of a phorbol ester on calcium-dependent chloride secretion by T$_{84}$ human colonic epithelial cells. *Am. J. Physiol.* **262**:C15–C22.

73. **Keely, S. J., S. O. Calandrella, and K. E. Barrett.** 2000. Carbachol-stimulated transactivation of epidermal growth factor receptor and MAP kinase in T$_{84}$ cells is mediated by intracellular Ca^{2+}, PYK-2, and p60^{src}. *J. Biol. Chem.* **275**:12619–12625.

74. **Keely, S. J., J. M. Uribe, and K. E. Barrett.** 1997. Carbachol stimulates transactivation of the EGF receptor and MAP kinase in T$_{84}$ epithelial cells: implications for calcium-dependent chloride secretion. *Gastroenterology* **112**:A375.

75. **Keely, S. J., J. M. Uribe, and K. E. Barrett.** 1998. Carbachol stimulates transactivation of epidermal growth factor receptor and MAP kinase in T$_{84}$ cells: implications for carbachol-stimulated chloride secretion. *J. Biol. Chem.* **273**:27111–27117.

76. **Khurana, S., S. K. Nath, S. A. Levine, J. M. Bowser, C. M. Tse, M. E. Cohen, and M. Donowitz.** 1996. Brush border phosphatidylinositol 3-kinase mediates epidermal growth factor stimulation of intestinal NaCl absorption and Na$^+$/H$^+$ exchange. *J. Biol. Chem.* **271**:9919–9927.

77. **Kidd, J. F., and P. Thorn.** 2000. Intracellular Ca^{2+} and Cl$^-$ channel activation in secretory cells. *Annu. Rev. Physiol.* **62**:493–513.

78. **Kimmich, G. A.** 1981. Gradient coupling in isolated intestinal cells. *Fed. Proc.* **40**:2474–2479.

79. **Kimmich, G. A.** 1984. Sodium-sugar coupling stoichiometry in chick intestinal cells. *Am. J. Physiol.* **247**:C74–C82.

80. **Kockerling, A., and M. Fromm.** 1993. Origin of cAMP-dependent Cl$^-$ secretion from both crypts and surface epithelia of rat intestine. *Am. J. Physiol.* **264**:C1294–C1301.

81. **Kunzelmann, K., R. Schreiber, and A. Boucherot.** 2001. Mechanisms of the inhibition of epithelial Na$^+$ channels by CFTR and purinergic stimulation. *Kidney Int.* **60**:455–461.

82. **Kurashima, K., E. Z. Szabo, G. Lukacs, J. Orlowski, and S. Grinstein.** 1998. Endosomal recycling of the Na$^+$/H$^+$ exchanger NHE3 isoform is regulated by the phophatidylinositol 3-kinase pathway. *J. Biol. Chem.* **273**:20828–20836.

83. **Le Gall, A. H., S. K. Powell, C. A. Yeaman, and E. Rodriguez-Boulan.** 1997. The neural cell adhesion molecule expresses a tyrosine-independent basolateral sorting signal. *J. Biol. Chem.* **272**:4559–4567.

84. **Leung, P. S., S. C. So, S. Y. Lam, L. L. Tsang, Y. W. Chung, and H. C. Chan.** 2001. Local regulation of anion secretion by pituitary

adenylate cyclase-activating polypeptide in human colonic T84 cells. *Cell Biol. Int.* **25:**123–129.

85. **Loo, D. D., B. A. Hirayama, A. K. Meinild, G. Chandy, T. Zeuthen, and E. M. Wright.** 1999. Passive water and ion transport by cotransporters. *J. Physiol.* **518:**195–202.

86. **MacLeod, R. J., and J. R. Hamilton.** 1999. Ca^{2+}/Calmodolin kinase II and decreases in intracellular pH are required to activate K^+ channels after substantial swelling in villus epithelial cells. *J. Membr. Biol.* **172:**59–66.

87. **Madara, J. L., T. W. Patapoff, B. Gillece-Castro, S. Colgan, C. Parkos, C. Delp, and R. J. Mrsny.** 1993. 5′-AMP is the neutrophil derived paracrine factor that elicits chloride secretion from T_{84} intestinal epithelial cell monolayers. *J. Clin. Invest.* **91:**2320–2325.

88. **Maher, M. M., J. D. Gontarek, R. S. Bess, M. Donowitz, and C. J. Yeo.** 1997. The Na/H exchange isoform NHE3 regulates basal canine ileal Na^+ absorption in vivo. *Gastroenterology* **112:**174–183.

89. **Matter, K., E. M. Yamamoto, and I. Mellman.** 1994. Structural requirements and sequence motifs for polarized sorting and endocytosis of LDL and Fc receptors in MDCK cells. *J. Cell Biol.* **126:**991–1004.

90. **McCole, D. F., S. J. Keely, and K. E. Barrett.** 2001. Carbachol transactivation of the EGF receptor in T84 cells requires TGF-α release. *Gastroenterology* **120:**A526–A527.

91. **McNamara, B., D. C. Winter, J. E. Cuffe, G. C. O'Sullivan, and B. J. Harvey.** 1999. Basolateral K^+ channel involvement in forskolin-activated chloride secretion in human colon. *J. Physiol.* **519:**251–260.

92. **Meneton, P., P. J. Schultheis, J. Greeb, M. L. Nieman, L. H. Liu, L. L. Clarke, J. J. Duffy, T. Doetschman, J. N. Lorenz, and G. E. Shull.** 1998. Increased sensitivity to K^+ deprivation in colonic H,K-ATPase-deficient mice. *J. Clin. Invest.* **101:**536–542.

93. **Merlin, D., X. Guo, C. L. Laboisse, and U. Hopfer.** 1995. Ca^{2+} and cAMP activate different K^+ conductances in the human intestinal goblet cell line HT29-Cl.16E. *Am. J. Physiol. Cell Physiol.* **268:**C1503–C1511.

94. **Meyer, T. N., C. Schweisinger, J. Ye, B. M. Denker, and S. K. Nigam.** 2001. Reassembly of the tight junction after oxidative stress depends on tyrosine kinase activity. *J. Biol. Chem.* **276:**22048–22055.

95. **Mitic, L. L., C. M. Van Itallie, and J. M. Anderson.** 2000. Molecular physiology and pathophysiology of tight junctions. I. Tight junc-

tion structure and function: lessons from mutant animals and proteins. *Am. J. Physiol.* **279:**G250.

96. **Moe, O. W., M. Amemiya, and Y. Yamaji.** 1995. Activation of protein kinase A acutely inhibits and phosphorylates Na/H exchanger NHE-3. *J. Clin. Invest.* **96:**2187–2194.

97. **Montrose, M. H., S. J. Keely, and K. E. Barrett.** 1999. Secretion and absorption: small intestine and colon, p. 320–355. *In* T. Yamada, D. H. Alpers, L. Laine, C. Owyang, and D. W. Powell (ed.), *Textbook of Gastroenterology*, 3rd ed. Lippincott, Williams and Wilkins, Philadelphia, Pa.

98. **Morgado-Diaz, J. A., and W. de Souza.** 2001. Evidence that increased tyrosine phosphorylation causes disassembly of adherens junctions but does not perturb paracellular permeability in Caco-2 cells. *Tissue Cell* **33:**500–513.

99. **Moseley, R. H., P. Hoglund, G. D. Wu, D. G. Silberg, S. Haila, A. de la Chapelle, C. Holmberg, and J. Kere.** 1999. Downregulated in adenoma gene encodes a chloride transporter defective in congenital chloride diarrhea. *Am. J. Physiol.* **276:**G185–G192.

100. **Nelson, W. J., and C. Yeaman.** 2001. Protein trafficking in the exocytic pathway of polarized epithelial cells. *Trends Cell Biol.* **11:**483–486.

101. **Nishizuka, Y.** 1984. Turnover of inositol phospholipids and signal transduction. *Science* **225:**1365.

102. **Nusrat, A., C. Delp, and J. L. Madara.** 1992. Intestinal epithelial restitution. Characterization of a cell culture model and mapping of cytoskeletal elements in migrating cells. *J. Clin. Invest.* **89:**1501–1511.

103. **Olsen, P. S., D. M. Preben, P. Kirkegaard, S. S. Poulsen, and E. Nexo.** 1994. Effect of secretin and somatostatin on secretion of epidermal growth factor from Brunner's glands in the rat. *Dig. Dis. Sci.* **39:**2186–2190.

104. **Ouellette, A.** 1997. Paneth cells and innate immunity in the crypt microenvironment. *Gastroenterology* **113:**1779–1784.

105. **Perdue, M. H., J. Marshall, and S. Masson.** 1990. Ion transport abnormalities in inflamed rat jejunum. Involvement of mast cells and nerves. *Gastroenterology* **98:**561–567.

106. **Perreault, N., and J. F. Beaulieu.** 1998. Primary cultures of fully differentiated and pure human intestinal epithelial cells. *Exp. Cell Res.* **25:**34–42.

107. **Peters, K. W., J. Qi, J. P. Johnson, S. C. Watkins, and R. A. Frizzell.** 2001. Role of snare proteins in CFTR and ENaC trafficking. *Pflugers Arch.* **443**(Suppl. 1)**:**S65–S69.

108. **Peters, K. W., J. Qi, S. C. Watkins, and R. A. Frizzell.** 2000. Mechanisms underlying regulated CFTR trafficking. *Med. Clin. North Am.* **84:**633–640.

109. **Piepenhagen, P. A., and W. J. Nelson.** 1998. Biogenesis of polarized epithelial cells during kidney development in situ: roles of E-cadherin-mediated cell-cell adhesion and membrane cytoskeleton organization. *Mol. Biol. Cell* **9:**3161–3177.

110. **Potten, C. S.** 1998. Stem cells in gastrointestinal epithelium: numbers, characteristics, and death. *Phil. Trans. R. Soc. London* **353:**821.

111. **Poulsen, J. H., H. Fischer, B. Illek, and T. E. Machen.** 1994. Bicarbonate conductance and pH regulatory capability of cystic fibrosis transmembrane conductance regulator. *Proc. Natl. Acad. Sci. USA* **91:**5340–5344.

112. **Rahner, C., L. L. Mitic, and J. M. Anderson.** 2001. Heterogeneity in expression and subcellular localization of claudins 2, 3, 4, and 5 in the rat liver, pancreas, and gut. *Gastroenterology* **120:**411.

113. **Rajendran, V. M., M. Kashgarian, and H. J. Binder.** 1989. Aldosterone induction of electrogenic sodium transport in the apical membrane vesicles of rat distal colon. *J. Biol. Chem.* **264:**18638–18644.

114. **Rao, M. C., S. A. Orellana, M. Field, D. C. Robertson, and R. A. Giannella.** 1981. Comparison of the biological actions of three purified heat-stable enterotoxins: effects on ion transport and guanylate cyclase activity in rabbit ileum in vitro. *Infect. Immun.* **33:**167.

115. **Rubin, D. C., E. Sweitlicki, K. A. Roth, and J. I. Gordon.** 1992. Use of fetal intestinal isografts from normal and transgenic mice to study the programming of positional information along the duodenal-to-colonic axis. *J. Biol. Chem.* **267:**15122–15133.

116. **Saitou, M., M. Furuse, H. Sasaki, J. D. Schulzke, M. Fromm, H. Takano, T. Noda, and S. Tsukita.** 2000. Complex phenotype of mice lacking occludin, a component of tight junction strands. *Mol. Biol. Cell* **11:**4131–4142.

117. **Scheiffele, P., J. Peranen, and K. Simons.** 1997. N-glycans as apical sorting signals in epithelial cells. *Nature* **378:**96–98.

118. **Schultheiss, G., and M. Diener.** 1998. K^+ and Cl^- conductances in the distal colon of the rat. *Gen. Pharmacol.* **31:**337–342.

119. **Seidler, U., O. Bachmann, P. Jacob, S. Christiani, I. Blumenstein, and H. Rossmann.** 2001. Na+/HCO3- cotransport in normal and cystic fibrosis intestine. *J. Pancreas* (On line) **2**(Suppl. 4)**:**247–256.

120. **Selveraj, N. G., R. Prasad, J. L. Goldstein, and M. C. Rao.** 2000. Evidence for the presence of cGMP-dependent pretin kinase-II in human distal colon and in T84, the colonic cell line. *Biochim. Biophys. Acta* **1498:**32–43.

121. **Shlatz, L. J., D. V. Kimberg, and K. A. Cattieu.** 1979. Phosphorylation of specific rat intestinal microvillus and basal-lateral membrane proteins by cyclic nucleotides. *Gastroenterology* **76:**293.

122. **Shumaker, H., and M. Soleimani.** 1999. CFTR upregulates the expression of the basolateral Na^+-K^+-$2Cl^-$ cotransporter in cultured pancreatic duct cells. *Am. J. Physiol. Cell Physiol.* **277:**C1100–C1110.

123. **Sidhu, M., and H. J. Cooke.** 1995. Role for 5-HT and ACh in submucosal reflexes mediating colonic secretion. *Am. J. Physiol.* **269:**G346–G351.

124. **Simon, D. B., Y. Lu, K. A. Choate, H. Velazquez, E. Al-Sabban, M. Praga, G. Casari, A. Bettinelli, G. Colussi, J. Rodriguez-Soriano, D. McCredie, D. Milford, S. Sanjad, and R. P. Lifton.** 1999. Paracellin-1, a renal tight junction protein required for paracellular Mg^{2+} resorption. *Science* **285:**103–106.

125. **Simonovic, I., M. Arpin, A. Koutsouris, H. J. Falk-Krzesinski, and G. Hecht.** 2001. Enteropathogenic *Escherichia coli* activates ezrin, which participates in disruption of tight junction barrier function. *Infect. Immun.* **69:**5679–5688.

126. **Simons, K., and E. Ikonen.** 1997. Functional rafts in cell membranes. *Nature* **387:**569–572.

127. **Toker, A., M. Meyer, K. K. Reddy, J. R. Falck, R. Aneja, S. Aneja, A. Parra, D. J. Burns, L. M. Ballas, and L. C. Cantley.** 1994. Activation of protein kinase C family members by the novel polyphosphoinositides PtdIns-3,4-P2 and PtdIns-3,4,5-P3. *J. Biol. Chem.* **269:**32358–32367.

128. **Traber, P. G.** 1997. Epithelial cell growth and differentiation. V. Transcriptional regulation, development, and neoplasia of the intestinal epithelium. *Am. J. Physiol. Gastrointest. Liver Physiol.* **273:**G979–G981.

129. **Tsukita, S., M. Furuse, and M. Itoh.** 2001. Multifunctional strands in tight junctions. *Nat. Rev. Mol. Cell Biol.* **2:**285–293.

130. **Turk, E., B. Zabel, S. Mundlos, J. Dyer, and E. M. Wright.** 1991. Glucose/galactose malabsorption caused by a defect in the Na^+/glucose cotransporter. *Nature* **350:**354–356.

131. **Turnamian, S. G., and H. J. Binder.** 1989. Regulation of active sodium and potassium transport in the distal colon of the rat. Role of

the aldosterone and glucocorticoid receptors. *J. Clin. Invest.* **84**:1924–1929.

132. **Turner, J. R., and J. L. Madara.** 1995. Physiological regulation of intestinal epithelial tight junctions as a consequence of Na+-coupled nutrient transport. *Gastroenterology* **109**:1391–1396.

133. **Turner, J. R., B. K. Rill, S. L. Carlson, D. Carnes, R. Kerner, R. J. Mrsny, and J. L. Madara.** 1997. Physiological regulation of epithelial tight junctions is associated with myosin light-chain phosphorylation. *Am. J. Physiol. Cell Physiol.* **273**:C1378–C1385.

134. **Ullrich, A., and J. Schlessinger.** 1990. Signal transduction by receptors with tyrosine kinase activity. *Cell* **61**:203–212.

135. **Uribe, J. M., C. M. Gelbmann, A. E. Traynor-Kaplan, and K. E. Barrett.** 1996. Epidermal growth factor inhibits calcium-dependent chloride secretion in T_{84} human colonic epithelial cells. *Am. J. Physiol.* **271**:C914–C922.

136. **Uribe, J. M., S. J. Keely, A. E. Traynor-Kaplan, and K. E. Barrett.** 1996. Phosphatidylinositol 3-kinase mediates the inhibitory effect of epidermal growth factor on calcium-dependent chloride secretion. *J. Biol. Chem.* **271**:26588–26595.

137. **Vajanaphanich, M., C. Schultz, R. Y. Tsien, A. E. Traynor-Kaplan, S. J. Pandol, and K. E. Barrett.** 1993. Crosstalk between epithelial calcium and cAMP signalling pathways: implications for secretion. *Gastroenterology* **104**:A286.

138. **Van Itallie, C., C. Rahner, and J. M. Anderson.** 2001. Regulated expression of claudin-4 decreases paracellular conductance through a selective decrease in sodium permeability. *J. Clin. Invest.* **107**:1319–1327.

139. **Venkatasubramanian, J., J. Sahi, and M. C. Rao.** 2000. Ion transport during growth and differentiation. *Ann. N.Y. Acad. Sci.* **915**:357–372.

140. **Verrey, F., J. Beron, and B. Spindler.** 1996. Corticosteroid regulation of renal Na,K-ATPase. *Mineral Electrolyte Metab.* **22**:279–292.

141. **Wang, Z., S. Petrovic, E. Mann, and M. Soleimani.** 2002. Identification of an apical Cl^-/HCO_3^- exchanger in the small intestine. *Am. J. Physiol. Gastrointest. Liver Physiol.* **282**:G573–G579.

142. **Warhurst, G., K. Fogg, N. Higgs, A. Tonge, and J. Grundy.** 1994. Ca^{2+}-mobilising agonists potentiate forskolin- and VIP-stimulated cAMP production in human colonic cell line, HT29-cl.19A: role of $[Ca^{2+}]_i$ and protein kinase C. *Cell Calcium* **15**:162–174.

143. **Willott, E., M. S. Balda, M. Heintzelman, B. Jameson, and J. M. Anderson.** 1992. Localization and differential expression of two isoforms of the tight junction protein ZO-1. *Am. J. Physiol.* **262**:C1119–C1124.

144. **Woodman, P. G.** 2000. Biogenesis of the sorting endosome: the role of Rab5. *Traffic* **1**:695–701.

145. **Yao, B., D. L. Hogan, K. Bukhave, M. A. Koss, and J. I. Isenberg.** 1993. Bicarbonate transport by rabbit duodenum in vitro: effect of vasoactive intestinal polypeptide, prostaglandin E_2, and cyclic adenosine monophosphate. *Gastroenterology* **104**:732–740.

146. **Yu, L. C., and M. H. Perdue.** 2001. Role of mast cells in intestinal mucosal function: studies in models of hypersensitivity and stress. *Immunol. Rev.* **179**:61–73.

147. **Yun, C. H. C., C. M. Tse, S. K. Nath, S. A. Levine, S. R. Brant, and M. Donowitz.** 1995. Mammalian Na^+/H^+ exchanger gene family: structure and function studies. *Am. J. Physiol.* **269**:G1–G11.

EPITHELIAL RESPONSE TO ENTERIC PATHOGENS: ACTIVATION OF CHLORIDE SECRETORY PATHWAYS

V. K. Viswanathan and Gail Hecht

15

INTRODUCTION: INTESTINAL SECRETION OF WATER AND ELECTROLYTES

The closely regulated secretion of water and electrolytes is a key physiological process of the gastrointestinal tract. The intestine handles approximately 8 to 9 liters of fluid per day, most of which is resorbed under healthy conditions. Physiologic levels of fluid secretion are important for diffusion and activity of digestive enzymes, as well as for the transport of water-soluble digestion products across the absorptive surface of intestinal cells. Additionally, high levels of bicarbonate secretion in the proximal duodenum protect it from the potentially damaging effects of gastric acid and pepsin. Transient fluid secretion in response to mechanical stimulation of the mucosa by a passing food bolus provides lubrication and protects the mucosa from physical damage. In contrast, dysregulation of intestinal secretion has pathological consequences. Indeed, fluid loss is the predominant reason for the high

mortality and morbidity associated with intestinal bacterial infections.

With some exceptions, crypt cells are usually secretory while villus cells are absorptive. This spatial segregation of fluid secretory function is correlated with the polarized distribution of various transporters such as the cystic fibrosis transmembrane conductance regulator (CFTR) and the $Na^+/K^+/2Cl^-$ cotransporter (NKCC). Water moves paracellularly along a standing gradient established in the lateral spaces of absorptive enterocytes. Tight junctions between the epithelial cell act as a regulatable barrier for paracellular movement, and also play an important role in maintaining the polarity of the epithelial cell, referred to as fence function, by restricting the movement of various membrane-bound molecules, including ion transporters (65). The gradient that drives fluid secretion results from active transport of electrolytes and other solutes. The predominant electrolyte driving transcellular fluid secretion into the lumen is chloride. Paracellular movement of sodium accompanies chloride secretion, and the resulting luminal accumulation of sodium chloride generates the osmotic gradient responsible for water movement (4). The focus of this review is the disruption of transcellular chloride secretion by

V. K. Viswanathan and Gail Hecht, Division of Digestive Diseases and Nutrition, Department of Medicine, University of Illinois at Chicago, Room 714, Clinical Sciences Building (M/C 716), 840 S. Wood Street, Chicago, IL 60612-7323.

Microbial Pathogenesis and the Intestinal Epithelial Cell, ed. by G. Hecht
© 2003 ASM Press, Washington, D.C.

microbial pathogens, with emphasis on recent advances in this field. Only a brief review of normal chloride secretion is outlined herein. For a recent and comprehensive overview of this topic, the reader is referred to chapter 14 of this volume.

GENERAL ASPECTS OF TRANSCELLULAR FLUID SECRETION: AN OVERVIEW

Chloride accumulates within intestinal epithelial cells by entering across the basolateral membrane along with sodium and potassium via NKCC1 in an electroneutral manner ($1Na^+:1K^+;2Cl^-$) (Fig. 1). Accumulation of

intracellular chloride above its electrochemical equilibrium is due to the activity of the Na^+ K^+-ATPase, which lowers the sodium concentration and increases the K^+ concentration within the cell. Potassium channels at the basolateral surface prevent cellular depolarization, preserving the electrical driving force for chloride exit from the cell. Thus, the driving force for chloride can be generated by a direct effect on the chloride transporters on the apical surface or by modulation of the Na^+/K^+ levels within the cell. A net decrease in the Na^+/K^+ levels within the cells results in intracellular chloride levels beyond its electrochemical equilibrium such that when apical

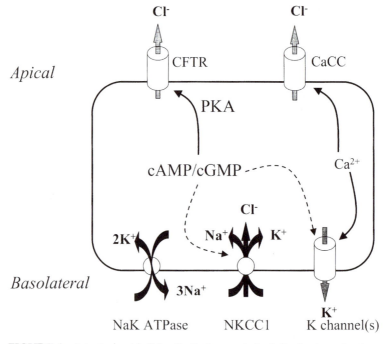

FIGURE 1 Intestinal epithelial cells display a polarized distribution of various ion transporters. Electroneutral transport of chloride across the basolateral surface is primarily driven by the sodium concentration gradient established by the Na^+K^+ ATPase. Potassium channels on the basolateral surface are involved in potassium recycling, thereby preventing cellular depolarization. Accumulation of chloride within the cell beyond its electrochemical equilibrium is the electrical driving force for chloride movement across apical chloride channels. While the bulk of this transport occurs via the CFTR, the CaCC also contribute, especially toward acute secretory responses. The intermediate messengers cAMP and cGMP potentiate chloride secretion by acting primarily on CFTR and NKCC1. Figure adapted from Barrett and Keely (4).

chloride channels open, chloride flows out of the cell and into the lumen.

Chloride exits into the lumen via chloride-specific channels in the apical membrane. Transcellular Cl⁻ secretion is electrogenic, since this anion exits without the active transport of an accompanying cation or the exchange of another anion. Most of the chloride secretion across the apical membrane occurs via CFTR (14). The two mandatory steps required for activation of CFTR are the ordered phosphorylation of various sites by the cyclic AMP (cAMP)-dependent protein kinase A (PKA) and nucleotide binding and hydrolysis (8). This channel may also be regulated by the cAMP-dependent delivery of preformed CFTR from subapical membrane vesicles, thereby increasing channel density on the apical surface (30). Alternatively, downregulation of this receptor can be achieved by reduction of its levels in the membrane by endocytosis, driven by a tyrosine-based motif, as well as other motifs in the C terminus of the molecule (26). CFTR is also activated by increases in cyclic guanosine monophosphate (cGMP) in intestinal epithelial cells (IEC). This may be due to the cross-activation of PKA by high levels of cGMP, and/or a direct effect of a type II cGMP-dependent protein kinase (PKGII) on the CFTR molecule. Table 1 lists the various molecules that affect chloride secretion by modulating the cAMP or cGMP levels within the cell. Also listed are the various bacterial products that affect cAMP/cGMP levels within the cells, thereby dysregulating chloride secretion.

Mutations in the CFTR gene that lead to mislocalization, altered function, or expression of this protein have serious pathophysiological consequences. CFTR knockout mice exhibit severe intestinal pathophysiology, leading to both neonatal and adult mortality (10, 57). The high rate of mortality appears to result from the inability of the intestinal tract to secrete either Cl⁻ or HCO_3^- in both basal and stimulated states (9, 17, 23, 55). The primary defect in cystic fibrosis is the inadequate hydration of mucosal surfaces due to reduced chloride secretion.

A second class of channels, the calcium-activated chloride channels (CaCC), are also involved in chloride secretion across the apical membrane of IEC (28). As the name suggests, these channels mediate chloride secretion in response to agonists that alter cytosolic calcium levels. The intermediary signaling molecules in these processes are various phosphorylated phosphoinositides. Agonists and antagonists of these channels, and the microbial products that dysregulate them, are listed in Table 1. While the cAMP/cGMP-mediated stimulation of chloride secretion by CFTR is a sustained response, calcium activation of chloride channels results only in a transient increase in chloride secretion. Activation of these channels requires the integration of several signals, possibly including phosphorylation of the receptor by calmodulin-dependent protein kinase type II (CaMKII). The controversy regarding the role of these channels in chloride secretion may at least in part be due to the complexity of their regulation (28). Since negative signaling mechanisms rapidly downregulate CaCC, even in the continued presence of the agonist, Ca^{2+}-induced chloride secretion is transient in nature.

cAMP SIGNALING AND CHLORIDE SECRETION

Introduction

cAMP is synthesized in cells by the action of adenylate cyclase. The engagement of receptors linked to this enzyme leads to the modulation of intracellular cAMP levels. Receptors coupled to inhibitory GTP-binding proteins (G_i) attenuate adenylate cyclase activity and decrease cAMP levels. Alternatively, receptors coupled to stimulatory GTP-binding proteins (G_s) increase cAMP levels by activating adenylate cyclase (58). An increase in cytoplasmic cAMP leads to activation of cAMP-dependent protein kinases and the phosphorylation of various intracellular pro-

TABLE 1 Modulators of chloride secretion pathways

Pathway	Physiological	Microbial
cAMP dependent	Vasoactive intestinal peptide Adenosine[a] Porcine intestinal peptide Secretin Bradykinin Cyclooxygenase pathway products[a]	Cholera toxin[a] Heat-stable *E. coli* enterotoxin[a] *Salmonella* enterotoxin *Campylobacter jejuni* enterotoxin *Pseudomonas aeruginosa* enterotoxin *Shigella dysenteriae* enterotoxin
cGMP dependent	Guanylin[a] Uroguanylin[a] Nitric oxide Atrial natriuretic peptide	Heat-stable *E. coli* enterotoxin[a] *Yersinia enterocolitica* enterotoxin *Klebsiella pneumoniae* enterotoxin Heat-stable *Vibrio cholerae* enterotoxin EAST-1[a]
Phosphorylated phosphoinositides dependent	Bombesin Vasopressin Vasotocin Bradykinin Polyamines	*Salmonella* SopB[a] *C. difficile* toxin A[a]
Ca^{2+} dependent	Carbachol[a] ATP Serotonin Substance P Bradykinin Neurotensin Histamine	*C. difficile* enterotoxin[a] *Cryptosporidium* enterotoxin *Vibrio parahemolyticus* TDH[a] Rotavirus NSP4[a]

[a] Discussed in the text.

teins. Prostaglandins and vasoactive intestinal polypeptide (VIP) are two endogenous regulators of ion transport that activate adenylate cyclase and increase intracellular cAMP levels in a G-protein-dependent fashion (29, 54). cAMP regulates the Cl$^-$ secretory response by a PKA-dependent opening of apical channels, and the secretory response is proportional to the elevation of cAMP levels (8, 37).

Pathogenic Mechanisms Involving cAMP

Direct Stimulation: CT and the *E. coli* Heat-Labile Enterotoxins LTI and LTII. Cholera toxin (CT) from *Vibrio cholerae* and the type I and type II heat-labile enterotoxins (LTI and LTII) from *Escherichia coli* are the primary agents that mediate the diarrhea caused by these organisms. These toxins be-

long to the AB5 enterotoxin family (31), wherein each member has an A polypeptide noncovalently linked to five identical B polypeptides (Fig. 2). The A subunit is composed of two structural domains, termed A1 and A2 peptides, that are linked by an exposed loop containing a serine protease-sensitive "nick" site and a single disulfide bond. Proteolytic cleavage of the A subunit and reduction of the linking disulfide bond release the enzymatically active N-terminal A1 fragment from the C-terminal A2 fragment.

The two serogroups of heat-labile enterotoxins, I and II, have structurally and functionally similar A polypeptides, but distinct B polypeptides. CT and LTI belong to serogroup I, while serogroup II includes the LTII variants LTIIa and LTIIb. Antiserum against CT or LTI can neutralize all serogroup I enterotoxins but not those in serogroup II, and

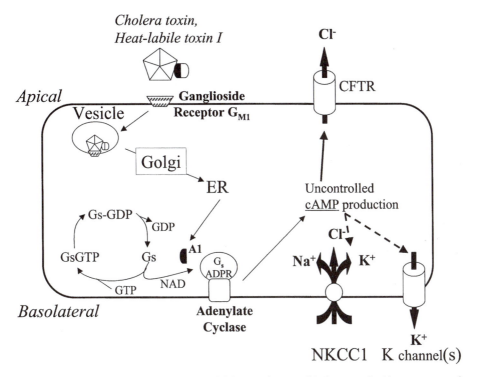

FIGURE 2 Cholera toxin and the heat-labile *E. coli* toxins bind to ganglioside receptors and enter epithelial cells as an AB5 complex by retrograde membrane trafficking through the Golgi and ER. Dissociation and cleavage of the A subunit result in the A1-peptide-mediated ADP-ribosylation of $G_s\alpha$. This results in a sustained activation of adenylate cyclase and elevation of cAMP, which in turn increases electrogenic chloride secretion.

vice versa. The pentameric B subunit exhibits lectin-like activity and binds specifically and avidly to the oligosaccharide domain of ganglioside receptors, thereby tethering the toxin to the host cell. The two serogroups show distinct receptor-binding specificities. CT and LTI bind to ganglioside G_{M1} on intestinal epithelial cells, resulting in chloride secretion. LTIIa binds to ganglioside G_{D1b}, while LTIIb binds with high affinity to G_{D1a} (68). Toxicity, in general, is determined primarily by the origin and receptor-binding specificity of the B subunit and not by the origin of the A1 polypeptide. Thus, a chimeric toxin created by combining the A subunit of CT with the B subunit of LTIIb failed to induce a Cl⁻ secretory response, although it bound avidly to G_{D1b} gangliosides.

It was recently demonstrated that toxin binding to G_{M1} on T84 cells was necessary and sufficient for targeting CT into intracellular compartments and eliciting a cellular response. CT binding to G_{M1} concentrates the toxin in detergent-insoluble, glycolipid-rich apical membrane microdomains (lipid rafts), an event that correlates with toxicity. Binding of one pentameric subunit cross-links five ganglioside receptors at the cell surface. Small changes in the binding affinity of CT could abolish toxicity. Thus, mutation of the B subunit His-57 to Ala in the conserved exposed peptide loop (Glu-51–Ile-58) resulted in a failure to induce toxicity. CT-H57A bound to only a fraction of the cell-surface receptors available to wild-type CT. The bulk of cell-surface receptors inaccessible to CT-H57A localized to detergent-insoluble apical membrane micro-domains (lipid rafts) (53). These studies demonstrate that CT action depends on stable high-affinity binding to G_{M1} and emphasize the importance of lipid trafficking in CT action.

The lag phase between toxin binding and detectable signs of toxicity is thought to represent the time required for various intracellular events. CT, unlike pore-forming toxins, enters epithelial cells by a complex pathway involving apical endocytosis and retrograde membrane trafficking through the Golgi to the endoplasmic reticulum (ER). For a detailed description of toxin trafficking, the reader is referred to chapter 4 of this volume. CT can be endocytosed by clathrin-dependent as well as by caveolae- and clathrin-independent endocytosis in various cell types (63). Following endocytosis, CT enters the ER wherein the A1 peptide unfolds and translocates into the cytosol. Subsequent movement of A1 to the adenylate cyclase may be by diffusion or by vesicular transport via the secretory pathway. The A2 peptide also contains the KDEL motif, a sorting signal that increases the efficiency of toxin function, presumably by facilitating toxin entry into the ER. CT variants lacking a functional KDEL motif can intoxicate host epithelial cells, albeit less efficiently.

The A1 subunit of CT is an ADP-ribosyltransferase that catalyzes the transfer of an ADP-ribose from NAD^+ to Arg-187 in the $G_s\alpha$ chain, a member of the G protein family. ADP-ribosylation of $G_s\alpha$ by CT stabilizes the GTP-bound conformation, thereby producing sustained stimulation of adenylate cyclase and elevated intracellular cAMP. The resulting electrogenic Cl^- secretion leads to massive secretory diarrhea. CT has also been reported to have indirect effects on secretion via the enteric nervous system. These effects are mediated by 5-hydroxytryptamine, which induces calcium-dependent chloride secretion (66).

Indirect Involvement of cAMP: *C. difficile* toxin. *Clostridium difficile*, the leading cause of nosocomial enteric infections, is a noninvasive pathogen that causes colitis entirely by the action of two potent exotoxins, toxin A and toxin B. Unlike CT and *E. coli* enterotoxin, which elicit secretion without an acute inflammatory component, *C. difficile* toxin triggers marked intestinal inflammation. Toxin A (2,710 amino acids [aa], 308 kDa), one of the largest known bacterial toxins, elicits chloride secretion and alters permeability in intestinal loops of experimental animals (43). In addition, toxin A induces epithelial cell necrosis and inflammation in the lamina propria. Toxin B (2,366 aa, 270 kDa), though closely related to toxin A (49% aa identity), possesses potent cytotoxic activity against various cultured cells, but has no enterotoxic effects in animal models. Only the secretion effects of these toxins are discussed herein, and the reader is referred to a recent review (49) and chapters 19 and 28 of this volume for details on the inflammatory pathways.

While it is known that the toxins inactivate low-molecular-weight GTPases, the relationship to cAMP-dependent secretion is not very clear. A recent study established one pathway connecting the two events (2). It was demonstrated that toxin A induced the expression of cyclooxygenase-2 (COX-2) in a lamina propria cell population (but not in epithelial cells). COX-2 induction has been observed in various cell types in response to proinflammatory cytokines, lipopolysaccharide, and infectious agents. COX-2 is involved in the conversion of arachidonic acid to prostaglandin E2 (PGE_2). PGE_2 can induce cAMP-mediated chloride secretion, increase salt and water secretion, and inhibit neutral sodium chloride and water absorption in the intestine. While toxin A-induced COX-2 production elevated PGE_2 levels, inhibition of COX-2 blocked not only toxin A-mediated PGE_2 production, but also fluid secretion, mucosal injury, and inflammation. Induction of secretion via elevated PGE_2 levels has also been reported to occur with *Salmonella* infection (see below).

The C-terminal receptor-binding domain consists of repeating units of 20 to 30 aa that bind with high specificity to the trisaccharide Galα1-3Galβ1-4GlcNAc. While this receptor is present in rodents and other animals, it is absent in humans, implying that binding of toxin A to human enterocytes involves a different mechanism. Deletion mutants lacking the C-terminal domain of toxin B have a 10-fold reduced cytotoxicity compared with the holotoxin. Microinjection of such a deletion mutant containing only the first 546 aa of toxin B, however, continued to induce phenotypes such as cell rounding. While the specific receptors for these toxins on human cells have not been identified, they are thought to be present on a wide variety of cells including neutrophils, lymphocytes, and macrophages. The central hydrophobic portion of these toxins (aa 956–1,130) may be involved with cellular uptake and processing. Mutant toxins containing intact catalytic and binding domains, but lacking the central portion, have sharply reduced cytotoxicity (49).

Following binding to the receptor, toxin A is rapidly internalized (Fig. 3). Unlike the retrograde transport described for CT, *C. difficile* toxin appears to enter the cytosol from the low-pH compartment of endosomes (5, 50). Recent data suggest that the acidic conditions of the endosomes aid membrane insertion of the toxin (5, 50). Furthermore, toxin B was also observed to induce the formation of ion-permeable channels.

Within 10 min, the toxin is localized in the mitochondria, an event accompanied by a rapid fall in intracellular ATP levels, release of mitochondrial cytochrome *c*, and the production of free radicals (19). The N-terminal glucosyltransferase activity, expressed in the first 550 aa, acts upon low-molecular-weight GTPases of the Rho family (Rho ABC, Rac, and CDC42), key regulators of cellular actin (1). Transfer of glucose from UDP-glucose to these signaling proteins results in their inactivation. This, in turn, results in dispersion of actin stress fibers, cell detachment, and rounding. In Chinese hamster ovary cells and human colonic cell lines, mitochondrial impairment precedes Rho glucosylation. Additional effects on tight junctions and paracellular permeability have also been observed and are discussed in chapter 16 of this volume (21, 47, 52).

cGMP SIGNALING IN CHLORIDE SECRETION

Introduction
In the normal intestine, increases in cGMP lead to the phosphorylation and activation of the CFTR by the membrane-bound cGMP-dependent protein kinase II (PKGII) or by cross-activation of the cAMP-dependent protein kinase (4). This results in the release of chloride and/or bicarbonate from the cell. Guanylin and uroguanylin are peptides that bind to and activate intestinal guanylate cyclase C (GC-C) receptors in the brush border membrane leading to cGMP production (6) (Fig. 4). The active 15-aa peptide, human guanylin, is generated by proteolytic cleavage of the inactive precursor, pro-guanylin. Guanylin mRNA is abundant in the intestine, although some expression is also observed in the kidney, adrenal gland, uterus, and oviduct. Guanylin peptide is widely distributed from the duodenum to the colon in rats and humans, with the highest concentrations being observed in the ileum and proximal colon.

Uroguanylin, a 16-aa peptide, is released by proteolytic cleavage of the precursor protein pro-uroguanylin. Uroguanylin is more widely distributed, being found in the stomach, kidney, lung, and pancreas, in addition to the intestine. These two peptides are approximately 50% identical at the amino acid level (Table 2). Both molecules are secreted into the intestinal lumen and blood in response to sodium chloride administration. Guanylin and uroguanylin may cooperatively regulate GC activity in a pH-dependent fashion (18). While guanylin was maximally active at an alkaline pH of 8, uroguanylin was found to be 100-fold more active at an acidic mucosal pH of 5 in stimulating cGMP production and transepithelial chloride secretion.

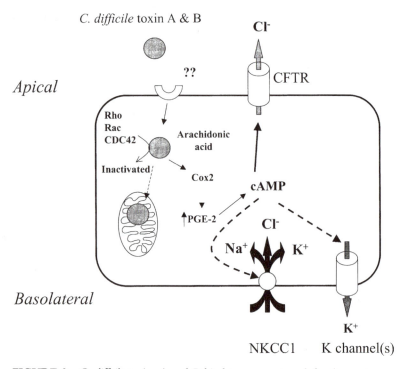

FIGURE 3 *C. difficile* toxins A and B bind to an as yet undefined receptor on human intestinal epithelial cells and enter cells via an endosomal compartment. These toxins inactivate low-molecular-weight GTPases of the Rho family by glucosylation. In addition, the toxins rapidly localize to the mitochondria, leading to cytotoxic effects. The effect of toxin A on secretion may involve the induction of COX-2-mediated elevation of PGE_2 levels. PGE_2, in turn, is known to induce cAMP-mediated chloride secretion in intestinal epithelial cells.

Pathogenic Mechanisms Involving cGMP: Heat-Stable Enterotoxins

Enterotoxigenic *E. coli* (ETEC) is a significant pathogen in developing countries and is often associated with traveler's diarrhea. ETEC and other pathogens such as *Klebsiella pneumoniae* elaborate a family of heat-stable enterotoxins (ST) that mimic the activity of the endogenous agonists of GC-C (45). ST_a of ETEC shares 50% homology with guanylin and binds competitively to GC-C (Table 2). Another heat-stable enterotoxin, EAST-1, produced by enteroaggregative *E. coli*, was shown to be structurally and functionally similar to guanylin (41). The EAST-1 genotype has been detected with notable frequency in enterohemorrhagic *E. coli* (EHEC) (100% in EHEC O157:H7 and 89% in EHEC O26), ETEC (41%, plasmid encoded), and enteropathogenic *E. coli* (EPEC; 21.5%). The potency of GC-C stimulation, in descending order, is ST > uroguanylin > guanylin. St_a, which is 40-fold more active than guanylin, is responsible for the increased fluid secretion associated with ETEC infection. The cysteine disulfide bridges in these peptides are indispensable for optimal activity and may explain the higher potency of ST. While guanylin and uroguanylin have two disulfide bridges linking four cysteine residues, ST have six cysteines linked by three disulfide bridges (Table 2). A functional GC-C receptor is required for ST_a-mediated fluid secretion. This was demonstrated by the finding that GC-C null mice were resistant to ST, while infection with ST_a enterotoxigenic bacteria led to di-

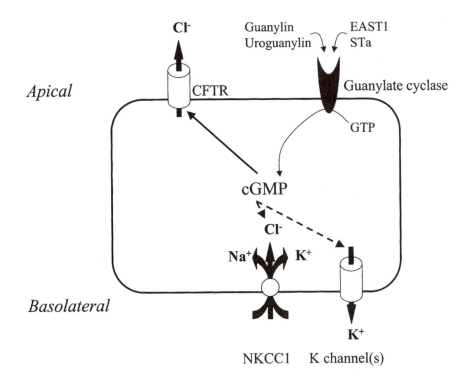

FIGURE 4 Guanylin, uroguanylin, and the homologous peptides from bacteria, EAST-1 and STₐ, bind to the guanylate cyclase C receptor, leading to the production of cGMP. cGMP mediates the phosphorylation and activation of CFTR by either the cGMP- or cAMP-dependent protein kinase.

arrhea and death in wild-type and heterozygous mice (38).

The elevated cGMP concentration resulting from GC activation induces the PKGII-mediated phosphorylation and activation of CFTR (45). PKGII null mice displayed a selective loss of ST_a-mediated chloride secre-

tion, while retaining cAMP-dependent responses (33, 48). CFTR knockout mice had marked reductions of Cl^- and bicarbonate secretion responses to guanylin and uroguanylin. In addition to elevation of chloride secretory responses, ST_a and related peptides inhibit Na^{2+} absorption by an undefined mechanism

TABLE 2 Comparison of the amino acid sequences of guanylin and related peptide ligands of guanylate cyclase C[a]

Ligand	Sequence
Guanylin	P G T C E I C A Y A A C T G C
Uroguanylin	N D D C E L C V N V A C T G C L
EAST-1	.. A S S Y A S C I W C T – T A C A S C H G ..
E. coli STₐ	N T F Y C C E L C C N P A C A G C Y

[a] Intramolecular cysteine–disulfide linkages are indicated. As indicated, *E. coli* STₐ has an extra disulfide bond.

(34). A recent study concluded that ST_a-induced water secretion could not be explained by an isotonic Cl^- fluid exit alone (64). Rather, the additional fluid output in renal cells was correlated with secretion through the water channels, aquaporins. The relevance of these findings to intestinal epithelial cells is presently not clear, since these cells do not appear to express aquaporins (64).

CALCIUM-DEPENDENT CHLORIDE SECRETION

Introduction

Calcium-dependent chloride secretion is a transient response even in the continued presence of the agonist (28). Thus, the CaCC are subject to rapid up- and downregulatory events, suggesting that they may play a role in acute secretion processes. Agents such as the muscarinic agonist carbachol mobilize calcium from intracellular stores by increasing the production of inositol-1,4,5-phosphate [$Ins(1,4,5)P_4$]. Calcium, in turn, activates basolateral potassium channels and apical chloride channels to stimulate chloride secretion. In addition, calcium also activates calmodulin-dependent protein kinase II, triggering a cascade leading to elevated levels of $Ins(3,4,5,6)P_4$ phosphate. $Ins(3,4,5,6)P_4$ appears to target an apical chloride channel to block the effects of a rise in intracellular calcium. Alternatively, peptide factors such as epidermal growth factor (EGF), which do not themselves act as agonists of chloride secretion, can downregulate calcium-dependent secretion by activation of phosphatidyl inositol-3 (PI3) kinase. This, in turn, downregulates a basolateral potassium channel. For a detailed discussion of these pathways, the reader is referred to the recent review by Keely and Barrett (28).

Pathogenic Mechanisms Involving Calcium

TDH. *Vibrio parahemolyticus* is a diarrheagenic pathogen that has been reported in worldwide outbreaks often associated with the consumption of undercooked shellfish. Thermostable direct hemolysin (TDH) produced by *V. parahemolyticus* has been implicated in the pathogenesis of the diarrheal disease caused by this organism. TDH-positive strains cause hemolysis on Wagatsuma agar, referred to as the Kanagawa phenomenon (KP). The addition of TDH to the mucosal side of human colonic tissue in Ussing chambers caused increased short-circuit current (Isc), a measure of net ion transport, that was inhibited by the CaCC-specific inhibitor DIDS (60). Increased intracellular Ca^{2+} concentrations and Isc, inhibitable by protein kinase C inhibitors, were also observed in Caco-2 cells treated apically with TDH (60) (Fig. 5). The details of these processes are currently unknown.

It was recently reported that KP-negative *V. parahemolyticus* strains produce a TDH-related hemolysin (TRH). Although the two proteins are immunologically similar, it is not known if TRH plays a role in diarrhea. TRH may be particularly important in KP-negative strains known to cause gastroenteritis (25). In contrast to TDH, TRH activity is labile to heat treatment for 10 min at 60°C (25). TRH, which stimulates fluid secretion in the rabbit loop model (24), was recently shown to elevate Ca^{2+} levels and induce Cl^- secretion in cultured human epithelial cells (59). Although TRH is a pore-forming toxin, Cl^- secretion does not occur through these pores since it could be inhibited by the CaCC-specific inhibitor DIDS as well as by the depletion of calcium.

Rotavirus NSP4 Enterotoxin. Rotavirus is a common cause of diarrhea in children, particularly between the ages of 6 months and 2 years, and is responsible for nearly 20% of diarrhea-associated deaths in children below the age of 5 years (35). This double-stranded RNA virus establishes a lytic infection of villous enterocytes. The onset of diarrhea occurs prior to alterations in cytopathology, and cytoprotective agents that inhibit histologic changes fail to inhibit diarrhea (44). At later stages, destruction of these cells may contribute to diarrhea by reducing intestinal sodium and water absorption.

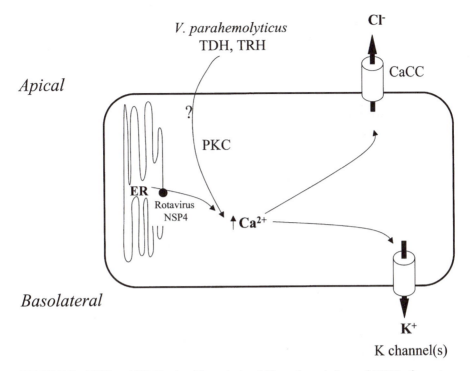

FIGURE 5   TDH and TDH-related hemolysin of *V. parahaemolyticus* and NSP4 of rotavirus elevate intracellular calcium concentrations by a protein kinase C-dependent mechanism. This results in the activation of the CaCC.

One major mechanism is via the Ca^{2+}-dependent enterotoxic activity of the 175-aa nonstructural protein NSP4 (Fig. 5). NSP4 is inserted into the ER membrane and may serve as a receptor for immature rotavirus particles. Sf9 insect cells expressing NSP4 in a baculovirus system, but not the other viral proteins, demonstrated Ca^{2+} mobilization. Interestingly, NSP4 evoked age-dependent diarrhea and Ca^{2+}-dependent chloride secretion in CFTR-deficient mice, unlike carbachol and the cAMP-mobilizing compound forskolin, suggesting that NSP4-induced diarrhea is not mediated by CFTR.

Delivery of the full-length or truncated NSP4 peptide (aa 114–135) into murine ilea induced diarrhea (3). Also, $NSP4_{114-135}$ added to pup small intestinal mucosal sheets caused Ca^{2+}-dependent chloride secretion in Ussing chamber experiments. A unique age dependence, similar to whole-animal diarrheal response, was demonstrated, in that chloride secretion did not occur in adult mucosa. In addition, virus-infected cells secrete a carboxy-terminal 7-kDa peptide of NSP4 containing the active domain (aa 112–175) via a nonclassical, Golgi-dependent secretory pathway (70). This peptide, after binding to an unidentified apical receptor, mobilized $[Ca^{2+}]_i$ through phospholipase C signaling and was able to induce diarrhea in neonatal mice. The importance of NSP4 for human infection remains to be established. Rotavirus infection also attenuates the sodium glucose symporter SGLT1 and disaccharidase activity. These events decrease absorption of water, electrolytes, glucose, and amino acids, all of which contribute to rotavirus-induced diarrhea (35).

PHOSPHOINOSITIDES AND CHLORIDE SECRETION

Introduction

Phosphorylated inositol derivatives play a key role in Ca^{2+}-mediated chloride secretion.

While Ins(1,4,5)P$_4$ is required for Ca^{2+} mobilization (62), other derivatives such as Ins(3,4,5,6)P$_4$ play a key role in downregulating the secretory response by blocking the apical chloride channel.

Pathogenic Mechanisms Involving Phosphoinositides: *S. enterica*

The serovars of *Salmonella enterica* (Typhimurium, Typhi, etc.) cause a range of illnesses in various animals. Infections with this pathogen are a frequent cause of food-borne outbreaks of gastroenteritis in the United States. *Salmonella* sp. encodes two type III secretion systems and various effector molecules that modulate host cellular functions (16). *Salmonella*-induced chloride secretion may be mediated by modulation of the inositol phosphate fluxes in the host cell. Infection of intestinal epithelial cells with *S. enterica* serovar Dublin or Typhi induced nearly a 10-fold increase in Ins(1,4,5,6)P$_4$ levels and was suggested to promote Cl$^-$ flux by antagonizing EGF inhibition mediated through phosphatidyl (PtdIns) 3 kinase and PtdInsP$_3$ (12). It was subsequently shown that the SopB protein of serovar Dublin, which shows homology to mammalian inositol polyphosphate 4-phosphatases, had the corresponding phosphatase activity in vitro (Fig. 6). SopB is one of several proteins secreted into host cells by the type III secretion system. Recombinant SopB hydrolyzed phosphotidylinositol 3,4,5-triphosphate [PtdIns(3,4,5)P$_3$], an inhibitor of Ca^{2+}-dependent chloride secretion. In addition, SopB could also hydrolyze PtdIns(1,3,4,5,6)P to Ins(1,4,5,6)P, a signaling molecule that antagonizes PtdIns(3,4,5), thereby indirectly elevating chloride secretion. A *sopB*$^-$ strain of serovar Dublin was unable to elevate Ins(1,4,5,6) levels and was defective for fluid secretion (46). Overexpression of SopB in embryonic 293 cells was able to alter phosphoinositide levels and induce chloride secretion (15). A recent study demonstrated that SopB also mediates actin cytoskeleton rearrangements in a Cdc42-dependent manner, thereby exhibiting overlapping functions with the other two effectors of bacterial entry, the Rho family GTP exchange factors SopE and SopE2 (71). More interestingly, SopB-independent inositol fluxes were demonstrated to be a consequence of the SopE-dependent activation of an endogenous inositol phosphatase. It is presently unclear if these SopB-independent mechanisms contribute to secretion.

Salmonella spp. may also induce secretion by other mechanisms. For instance, infection of cultured human epithelial cell lines with invasive bacteria such as *S. enterica* serovars Typhi and Dublin, *Yersinia enterocolitica*, *Shigella dysenteriae*, and enteroinvasive *E. coli* mediated an increase in PGE$_2$ levels by elevating the rate-limiting enzymes of prostaglandin formation, PGHS-2 (13). Such an increase was not seen with noninvasive pathogens such as EPEC or EHEC.

OTHER PATHOGENIC CHLORIDE SECRETORY PATHWAYS: EPEC

Infection with EPEC perturbs various intestinal functions including ion secretion. Infection of cultured human intestinal epithelial Caco-2 cells stimulated a rapid and transient increase in Isc, which was partly due to Cl$^-$ secretion (11). In contrast, infection of the T84 IEC line failed to demonstrate a similar response. Instead, stimulation of EPEC-infected monolayers with the classic Ca^{2+}- and cAMP-mediated secretagogues carbachol and forskolin yielded an attenuated response that was not attributable to altered Cl$^-$ secretion (20). Further investigation suggested that perturbation of bicarbonate-dependent transport processes accounted for this paradoxical response. The variability between transport properties of the different cell lines and the different models of infection potentially explains the discrepancy between these studies.

In fact, other studies have demonstrated the difference between Caco-2 and T84 cell lines in their secretory responses (51). Enteroinvasive bacteria, unlike nonpathogenic, noninvasive bacteria, elicited a more robust chloride secretory response in Caco-2 cells than in T84 cells. Similarly, while enteroinvasive bacteria

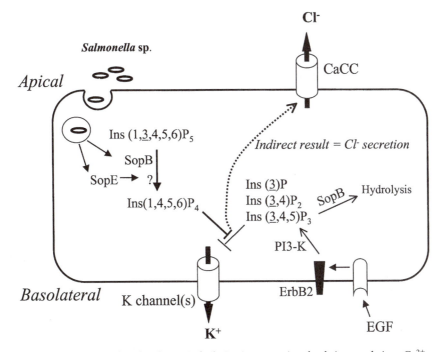

FIGURE 6 Phosphorylated inositol derivatives are involved in regulating Ca^{2+}-mediated chloride secretion and may have stimulatory or inhibitory effects. Derivatives such as $Ins(3,4,5)P_3$ inhibit basolateral potassium channels, thereby elevating the positive charge within the cell, thus favoring the retention of chloride ions within the cell. Proteins injected into epithelial cells by *Salmonella* sp. promote the production of $Ins(1,4,5,6)P_4$, which in turn blocks $Ins(3,4,5)P_3$-mediated K channel inhibition. In addition, the *Salmonella* protein SopB also hydrolyzes $Ins(3,4,5)P_3$. Removal of K^+ channel inhibition results in the export of potassium ions and renders the cell with a net negative charge, thereby favoring the exit of chloride ions through the apical channels.

mediated inducible nitric oxide synthase (iNOS)- and COX-2-dependent alteration of transepithelial resistance in Caco-2 cells, this effect was not observed in T84 cells. Correspondingly, only Caco-2 cells registered an increase in NO and PGE_2 levels upon infection. Interestingly, both cAMP and cGMP analogs could evoke increases in Isc in both HT29/cl.19A and T84 cells. Infection with invasive bacteria potentiated the Isc response in HT29/cl.19A, but dampened the response in T84 cells, underscoring the variable responses in these cell lines. Enteroinvasive bacteria also upregulated the iNOS-dependent expression and/or membrane abundance of CFTR and NKCC1 (51).

INFLAMMATORY RESPONSES AND CHLORIDE SECRETION

In addition to direct elicitation of secretory responses by enteric bacterial pathogens and their products, these infections typically elicit host inflammatory responses. Numerous pathogens trigger the activation of the NF-κB family of transcriptional activators (61). The importance of NF-κB to host resistance to infection is underscored by studies demonstrating that mice deficient in different NF-κB subunits were more susceptible to infections. NF-κB is sequestered in the cytoplasm by the inhibitory-kappa B (IκB) proteins. Infection with various pathogens stimulates signaling pathways leading to phosphorylation and degradation of IκB, exposing a nuclear localization signal on the NF-κB dimer. Translocation of NF-κB to the nucleus results in the expression of numerous genes involved in immune function, including cytokines such as gamma interferon, interleukin-8 (IL-8), and IL-12, receptors such as CD25 and Gal1R, and intercellular adhesion molecules such as ICAM-1. The regulation of IκB gene expression by NF-κB results in a feedback regulation loop.

The upregulation and secretion of IL-8 result in the transmigration of neutrophils across intestinal epithelia. Upon entry into the lumen, neutrophils release 5′-AMP, which is converted to adenosine by an apical membrane 5′-ectonucleotidase, CD73. Of the four adenosine receptor subtypes cloned so far, the A2b receptor appears to be the only one found on intestinal epithelial cells. Interaction of adenosine with A2bR results in the activation of the coupled Gαs and the stimulation of cAMP-mediated electrogenic chloride secretion (36). It was recently demonstrated that A2bR is recruited to the plasma membrane as a microdomain complex with ezrin and NHE-3 kinase regulatory protein (E3KARP) (56).

Galanin

Galanin, a 30-aa neuropeptide, is widely distributed in the central nervous system and enteric nerve terminals lining the human gastrointestinal tract. This peptide interacts with the specific receptors Gal1R, Gal2R, and Gal3R. While all three receptors are expressed in the smooth muscle cells of the gastrointestinal tract, only Gal1R is expressed in intestinal epithelial cells. Galanin modulates intestinal motility by stimulating smooth muscle contraction. Additionally, galanin causes chloride secretion in the colon by binding the intestinal epithelial cell Gal1R (7).

The Gal1R promoter includes several consensus binding sites for binding of the proinflammatory transcription factor NF-κB. Consistent with this, Gal1R expression was shown to be transcriptionally regulated by

NF-κB, resulting in a dose-dependent increase in Cl⁻ secretion in response to the ligand galanin. NF-κB activation resulting from dextran sodium sulfate-induced murine colitis or infection with intestinal pathogens caused a Gal1R-dependent elevation in fluid secretion (22, 39). Consistent with the absence of Gal1R in normal mouse epithelia, galanin had no significant effect on murine colonic tissue ex vivo. Galanin, however, progressively increased Isc and colonic fluid secretion in mice infected with enteric pathogens or treated with dextran sodium sulfate. These events correlated with an increase in Gal1R expression and were attenuated by a galanin-specific antibody.

With respect to infection-induced Gal1R expression, pathogenic E. coli, but not nonpathogenic E. coli, activated NF-κB and thereby elevated Gal1R expression (22). While galanin induced a 5-fold increase in Isc in uninfected T84 cells, infection of cells to pathogenic E. coli increased Isc approximately 20-fold. Disparate pathogens, including S. enterica serovar Typhimurium and S. flexneri, similarly increased colonocyte Gal1R expression, leading to increased fluid secretion (40). Gal1R⁻/⁻ mice were not compromised for survival or basal colonic fluid secretion, yet infection-induced fluid secretion was abrogated in both the heterozygous and homozygous knockout mice. Other studies revealed that HT29/cl.19A, but not T84 cells, responded to galanin under baseline conditions, although this peptide stimulated pathogen-induced Isc increases in both cell lines (51).

Defensins

There are indications that immune mediators may link with secretory processes in additional ways. Cryptdins or intestinal defensins are small peptide molecules produced by mouse Paneth cells. Apart from antibacterial activity, defensins have also been demonstrated to engage the adaptive immune system. It was demonstrated that of the six mouse intestinal defensins, cryptdins 2 and 3 were able to elicit a chloride secretory response in human IEC (32). Although these two peptides differ only at a single residue position, cryptidin 3 was able to elicit a more profound response. Similar observations were noted in human embryonic kidney cells (69). By inserting into the membrane, these peptides form an ion-selective pore, thereby facilitating chloride secretion (42).

NO

NO has been reported to regulate both absorptive and secretory functions (27). NO is a second messenger that modulates various cellular processes including inflammation (67). NF-κB and proinflammatory cytokines can regulate NO levels by upregulating the levels of iNOS. NO stimulates soluble guanylate cyclase, leading to the formation of cGMP. While soluble guanylate cyclase is not abundant in IEC, stimulation of this isoform in enteric neurons could lead to the release of other secretagogues such as acetylcholine, vasoactive intestinal polypeptide, and substance P. As described above, infection with enteroinvasive bacteria elevates NO levels in epithelial cells. Under physiological conditions, however, NO is believed to play a pro-absorptive role by suppressing prostaglandin formation and opening basolateral K$^+$ channels (27).

SUMMARY

Secretion via the transcellular pathway is an exquisitely regulated process. Various pathogens and their toxins can directly disrupt these pathways, frequently by invoking multiple mechanisms. In addition, host cell responses elicited by pathogens can also contribute to the chloride secretory response. Beyond this, immune cells such as neutrophils release products that are ultimately converted into prosecretory molecules. The continued investigation of host-pathogen interactions will undoubtedly result in a deeper understanding of these mechanisms and enhance our knowledge of the regulation of secretion under both physiological and pathophysiological circumstances.

REFERENCES

1. **Aktories, K., G. Schmidt, and I. Just.** 2000. Rho GTPases as targets of bacterial protein toxins. *Biol. Chem.* **381:**421–426.
2. **Alcantara, C., W. F. Stenson, T. S. Steiner, and R. L. Guerrant.** 2001. Role of inducible cyclooxygenase and prostaglandins in *Clostridium difficile* toxin A-induced secretion and inflammation in an animal model. *J. Infect. Dis.* **184:**648–652.
3. **Ball, J. M., P. Tian, C. Q. Zeng, A. P. Morris, and M. K. Estes.** 1996. Age-dependent diarrhea induced by a rotaviral nonstructural glycoprotein. *Science* **272:**101–104.
4. **Barrett, K. E., and S. J. Keely.** 2000. Chloride secretion by the intestinal epithelium: molecular basis and regulatory aspects. *Ann. Rev. Physiol.* **62:**535–572.
5. **Barth, H., G. Pfeifer, F. Hofmann, E. Maier, R. Benz, and K. Aktories.** 2001. Low pH-induced formation of ion channels by *Clostridium difficile* toxin B in target cells. *J. Biol. Chem.* **276:**10670–10676.
6. **Beltowski, J.** 2001. Guanylin and related peptides. *J. Physiol. Pharmacol.* **52:**351–375.
7. **Benya, R. V., K. A. Matkowskyj, A. Danilkovich, and G. Hecht.** 1998. Galanin causes Cl$^-$ secretion in the human colon. Potential significance of inflammation-associated NF-kappa B activation on galanin-1 receptor expression and function. *Ann. N.Y. Acad. Sci.* **863:**64–77.
8. **Bradbury, N.** 2002. cAMP signaling cascades and CFTR: is there more to learn? *Pflugers Arch. Eur. J. Physiol.* **443:**S85–S91.
9. **Clarke, L. L., B. R. Grubb, S. E. Gabriel, O. Smithies, B. H. Koller, and R. C. Boucher.** 1992. Defective epithelial chloride transport in a gene-targeted mouse model of cystic fibrosis. *Science* **257:**1125–1128.
10. **Colledge, W. H., R. Ratcliff, D. Foster, R. Williamson, and M. J. Evans.** 1992. Cystic fibrosis mouse with intestinal obstruction. *Lancet* **340:**680.
11. **Collington, G. K., I. W. Booth, and S. Knutton.** 1998. Rapid modulation of electrolyte transport in Caco-2 cell monolayers by enteropathogenic *Escherichia coli* (EPEC) infection. *Gut* **42:**200–207.
12. **Eckmann, L., M. T. Rudolf, A. Ptasznik, C. Schultz, T. Jiang, N. Wolfson, R. Tsien, J. Fierer, S. B. Shears, M. F. Kagnoff, and A. E. Traynor-Kaplan.** 1997. D-myo-Inositol

1,4,5,6-tetrakisphosphate produced in human intestinal epithelial cells in response to *Salmonella* invasion inhibits phosphoinositide 3-kinase signaling pathways. *Proc. Natl. Acad. Sci. USA* **94:** 14456–14460.

13. **Eckmann, L., W. F. Stenson, T. C. Savidge, D. C. Lowe, K. E. Barrett, J. Fierer, J. R. Smith, and M. F. Kagnoff.** 1997. Role of intestinal epithelial cells in the host secretory response to infection by invasive bacteria. Bacterial entry induces epithelial prostaglandin h synthase-2 expression and prostaglandin E2 and F2alpha production. *J. Clin. Invest.* **100:**296–309.

14. **Eggermont, E.** 1996. Gastrointestinal manifestations in cystic fibrosis. *Eur. J. Gastroenterol. Hepatol.* **8:**731–738.

15. **Feng, Y. C., S. R. Wente, and P. W. Majerus.** 2001. Overexpression of the inositol phosphatase SopB in human 293 cells stimulates cellular chloride influx and inhibits nuclear mRNA export. *Proc. Natl. Acad. Sci. USA* **98:** 875–879.

16. **Galan, J. E.** 2001. *Salmonella* interactions with host cells: type III secretion at work. *Annu. Rev. Cell Dev. Biol.* **17:**53–86.

17. **Grubb, B. R., E. Lee, A. J. Pace, B. H. Koller, and R. C. Boucher.** 2000. Intestinal ion transport in NKCC1-deficient mice. *Am. J. Physiol. Gastrointest. Liver Physiol.* **279:**G707–G718.

18. **Hamra, F. K., S. L. Eber, D. T. Chin, M. G. Currie, and L. R. Forte.** 1997. Regulation of intestinal uroguanylin guanylin receptor-mediated responses by mucosal acidity. *Proc. Natl. Acad. Sci. USA* **94:**2705–2710.

19. **He, D., S. J. Hagen, C. Pothoulakis, M. Chen, N. D. Medina, M. Warny, and J. T. LaMont.** 2000. *Clostridium difficile* toxin A causes early damage to mitochondria in cultured cells. *Gastroenterology* **119:**139–150.

20. **Hecht, G., and A. Koutsouris.** 1999. Enteropathogenic *E. coli* attenuates secretagogue-induced net intestinal ion transport but not Cl⁻ secretion. *Am. J. Physiol.* **276:**G781–G788.

21. **Hecht, G., A. Koutsouris, C. Pothoulakis, J. T. LaMont, and J. L. Madara.** 1992. *Clostridium difficile* toxin B disrupts the barrier function of T84 monolayers. *Gastroenterology* **102:** 416–423.

22. **Hecht, G., J. A. Marrero, A. Danilkovich, K. A. Matkowskyj, S. D. Savkovic, A. Koutsouris, and R. V. Benya.** 1999. Pathogenic *Escherichia coli* increase Cl⁻ secretion from intestinal epithelia by upregulating galanin-1 receptor expression. *J. Clin. Invest.* **104:**253–262.

23. **Hogan, D. L., D. L. Crombie, J. I. Isenberg, P. Svendsen, O. B. Schaffalitzky de**

Muckadell, and M. A. Ainsworth. 1997. Acid-stimulated duodenal bicarbonate secretion involves a CFTR-mediated transport pathway in mice. *Gastroenterology* **113:**533–541.

24. **Honda, T., and T. Iida.** 1993. The pathogenicity of *Vibrio parahaemolyticus* and the role of the thermostable direct haemolysin and related haemolysins. *Rev. Med. Microbiol.* **4:**106–113.

25. **Honda, T., Y. X. Ni, and T. Miwatani.** 1988. Purification and characterization of a hemolysin produced by a clinical isolate of Kanagawa phenomenon-negative *Vibrio parahaemolyticus* and related to the thermostable direct hemolysin. *Infect. Immun.* **56:**961–965.

26. **Hu, W., M. Howard, and G. L. Lukacs.** 2001. Multiple endocytic signals in the C-terminal tail of the cystic fibrosis transmembrane conductance regulator. *Biochem. J.* **354:**561–572.

27. **Izzo, A. A., N. Mascolo, and F. Capasso.** 1998. Nitric oxide as a modulator of intestinal water and electrolyte transport. *Dig. Dis. Sci.* **43:** 1605–1620.

28. **Keely, S. J., and K. E. Barrett.** 2000. Regulation of chloride secretion. Novel pathways and messengers. *Ann. N.Y. Acad. Sci.* **915:**67–76.

29. **Kimberg, D. V., M. Field, J. Johnson, A. Henderson, and E. Gershon.** 1971. Stimulation of intestinal mucosal adenyl cyclase by cholera enterotoxin and prostaglandins. *J. Clin. Invest.* **50:**1218–1230.

30. **Kleizen, B., I. Braakman, and H. R. de Jonge.** 2000. Regulated trafficking of the CFTR chloride channel. *Eur. J. Cell Biol.* **79:**544–556.

31. **Lencer, W. I.** 2001. Microbes and microbial toxins: paradigms for microbial-mucosal interactions: *V. cholera*: invasion of the intestinal epithelial barrier by a stably folded protein toxin. *Am. J. Physiol. Gastroenterol. Liver Physiol.* **280:**G781–G786.

32. **Lencer, W. I., G. Cheung, G. R. Strohmeier, M. G. Currie, A. J. Ouellette, M. E. Selsted, and J. L. Madara.** 1997. Induction of epithelial chloride secretion by channel-forming cryptdins 2 and 3. *Proc. Natl. Acad. Sci. USA* **94:** 8585–8589.

33. **Lohmann, S. M., A. B. Vaandrager, A. Smolenski, U. Walter, and H. R. De Jonge.** 1997. Distinct and specific functions of cGMP-dependent protein kinases. *Trends Biochem. Sci.* **22:**307–312.

34. **Lucas, M. L.** 2001. A reconsideration of the evidence for *Escherichia coli* STa (heat stable) enterotoxin-driven fluid secretion: a new view of STa action and a new paradigm for fluid absorption. *J. Appl. Microbiol.* **90:**7–26.

35. **Lundgren, O., and L. Svensson.** 2001. Pathogenesis of rotavirus diarrhea [Review]. *Microbes Infect.* **3:**1145–1156.

36. **Madara, J. L., T. W. Patapoff, B. Gillece-Castro, S. P. Colgan, C. A. Parkos, C. Delp, and R. J. Mrsny.** 1993. 5′-adenosine monophosphate is the neutrophil-derived paracrine factor that elicits chloride secretion from T84 intestinal epithelial cell monolayers. *J. Clin. Invest.* **91:**2320–2325.

37. **Mandel, K. G., K. Dharmsathaphorn, and J. A. McRoberts.** 1986. Characterization of a cyclic AMP-activated Cl⁻ transport pathway in the apical membrane of a human colonic epithelial cell line. *J. Biol. Chem.* **261:**704–712.

38. **Mann, E. A., M. L. Jump, J. Wu, E. Yee, and R. A. Giannella.** 1997. Mice lacking the guanylyl cyclase C receptor are resistant to STa-induced intestinal secretion. *Biochem. Biophys. Res. Commun.* **239:**463–466.

39. **Marrero, J. A., K. A. Matkowskyj, K. Yung, G. Hecht, and R. V. Benya.** 2000. Dextran sulfate sodium-induced murine colitis activates NF-kappaB and increases galanin-1 receptor expression. *Am. J. Physiol. Gastrointest. Liver Physiol.* **278:**G797–804.

40. **Matkowskyj, K. A., A. Danilkovich, J. Marrero, S. D. Savkovic, G. Hecht, and R. V. Benya.** 2000. Galanin-1 receptor up-regulation mediates the excess colonic fluid production caused by infection with enteric pathogens. *Nat. Med.* **6:**1048–1051.

41. **Menard, L., and J. Dubreuil.** 2002. Enteroaggregative *Escherichia coli* heat-stable enterotoxin 1 (EAST1): a new toxin with an old twist. *Crit. Rev. Microbiol.* **28:**43–60.

42. **Merlin, D., G. Yue, W. I. Lencer, M. E. Selsted, and J. L. Madara.** 2001. Cryptdin-3 induces novel apical conductance(s) in Cl⁻ secretory, including cystic fibrosis, epithelia. *Am. J. Physiol. Cell Physiol.* **280:**C296–C302.

43. **Moore, R., C. Pothoulakis, J. T. LaMont, S. Carlson, and J. L. Madara.** 1990. *C. difficile* toxin A increases intestinal permeability and induces Cl⁻ secretion. *Am. J. Physiol.* **259:**G165–G172.

44. **Morris, A. P., and M. K. Estes.** 2001. Microbes and microbial toxins: paradigms for microbial-mucosal interactions. VIII. Pathological consequences of rotavirus infection and its enterotoxin. *Am. J. Physiol. Gastrointest. Liver Physiol.* **281:**G303–G310.

45. **Nakazato, M.** 2001. Guanylin family: new intestinal peptides regulating electrolyte and water homeostasis. *J. Gastroenterol.* **36:**219–225.

46. **Norris, F. A., M. P. Wilson, T. S. Wallis, E. E. Galyov, and P. W. Majerus.** 1998. SopB, a protein required for virulence of *Salmonella dublin*, is an inositol phosphate phosphatase. *Proc. Natl. Acad. Sci. USA* **95:**14057–14059.

47. **Nusrat, A., C. von Eichel-Streiber, J. R. Turner, P. Verkade, J. L. Madara, and C. A. Parkos.** 2001. *Clostridium difficile* toxins disrupt epithelial barrier function by altering membrane microdomain localization of tight junction proteins. *Infect. Immun.* **69:**1329–1336.

48. **Pfeifer, A., A. Aszodi, U. Seidler, P. Ruth, F. Hofmann, and R. Fassler.** 1996. Intestinal secretory defects and dwarfism in mice lacking cGMP-dependent protein kinase II. *Science* **274:**2082–2086.

49. **Pothoulakis, C., and J. T. Lamont.** 2001. Microbes and microbial toxins: paradigms for microbial-mucosal interactions—II. The integrated response of the intestine to *Clostridium difficile* toxins. *Am. J. Physiol. Gastrointest. Liver Physiol.* **280:**G178–G183.

50. **Qa'Dan, M., L. M. Spyres, and J. D. Ballard.** 2000. pH-induced conformational changes in *Clostridium difficile* toxin B. *Infect. Immun.* **68:**2470–2474.

51. **Resta-Lenert, S., and K. E. Barrett.** 2002. Enteroinvasive bacteria alter barrier and transport properties of human intestinal epithelium: role of iNOS and COX-2. *Gastroenterology* **122:**1070–1087.

52. **Riegler, M., R. Sedivy, C. Pothoulakis, G. Hamilton, J. Zacherl, G. Bischof, E. Cosentini, W. Feil, R. Schiessel, and J. T. LaMont.** 1995. *Clostridium difficile* toxin B is more potent than toxin A in damaging human colonic epithelium in vitro. *J. Clin. Invest.* **95:**2004–2011.

53. **Rodighiero, C., Y. Fujinaga, T. R. Hirst, and W. I. Lencer.** 2001. A cholera toxin B-subunit variant that binds ganglioside G_{M1} but fails to induce toxicity. *J. Biol. Chem.* **276:**36939–36945.

54. **Schwartz, C. J., D. V. Kimberg, H. E. Sheerin, M. Field, and S. I. Said.** 1974. Vasoactive intestinal peptide stimulation of adenylate cyclase and active electrolyte secretion in intestinal mucosa. *J. Clin. Invest.* **54:**536–544.

55. **Seidler, U., I. Blumenstein, A. Kretz, D. Viellard-Baron, H. Rossmann, W. H. Colledge, M. Evans, R. Ratcliff, and M. Gregor.** 1997. A functional CFTR protein is required for mouse intestinal cAMP-, cGMP- and Ca^{2+}-dependent HCO_3^- secretion. *J. Physiol.* **505:**411–423.

56. **Sitaraman, S. V., L. Wang, M. Wong, M. Bruewer, M. Hobert, C.-H. Yun, D. Merlin, and J. L. Madara.** 2002. The adenosine 2b receptor is recruited to the plasma membrane and associates with E3KARP and ezrin upon agonist stimulation. *J. Biol. Chem.* **277:**33188–33195.

57. Snouwaert, J. N., K. K. Brigman, A. M. Latour, N. N. Malouf, R. C. Boucher, O. Smithies, and B. H. Koller. 1992. An animal model for cystic fibrosis made by gene targeting. *Science* **257**:1083–1088.

58. Stryer, L., and H. R. Bourne. 1986. G proteins: a family of signal transducers. *Annu. Rev. Cell Biol.* **2**:391–419.

59. Takahashi, A., N. Kenjyo, K. Imura, Y. Myonsun, and T. Honda. 2000. Cl(-) secretion in colonic epithelial cells induced by the *Vibrio parahaemolyticus* hemolytic toxin related to thermostable direct hemolysin. *Infect. Immun.* **68**: 5435–5438.

60. Takahashi, A., Y. Sato, Y. Shiomi, V. V. Cantarelli, T. Iida, M. Lee, and T. Honda. 2000. Mechanisms of chloride secretion induced by thermostable direct haemolysin of *Vibrio parahaemolyticus* in human colonic tissue and a human intestinal epithelial cell line. *J. Med. Microbiol.* **49**:801–810.

61. Tato, C., and C. Hunter. 2002. Host-pathogen interactions: subversion and utilization of the NF-kappa B pathway during infection. *Infect. Immun.* **70**:3311–3317.

62. Tkachuk, V. A. 1998. Phosphoinositide metabolism and Ca^{2+} oscillation. *Biochem. Russia* **63**: 38–46.

63. Torgenstern, M. L. 2001. Internalization of cholera toxin by different endocytic mechanisms. *J. Cell Sci.* **114**:3737–3747.

64. Toriano, R., A. Kierbel, M. A. Ramirez, G. Malnic, and M. Parisi. 2001. Spontaneous water secretion in T84 cells: effects of STa enterotoxin, bumetanide, VIP, forskolin, and A-23187. *Am. J. Physiol. Gastrointest. Liver Physiol.* **281**: G816–G822.

65. Tsukita, S., M. Furuse, and M. Itoh. 2001. Multifunctional strands in tight junctions. *Nat. Rev. Molec. Cell Biol.* **2**:285–293.

66. Turvill, J. L., F. H. Mourad, and M. J. Farthing. 1998. Crucial role for 5-HT in cholera toxin but not *Escherichia coli* heat-labile enterotoxin-intestinal secretion in rats. *Gastroenterology* **115**:883–890.

67. Wapnir, R., and S. Teichberg. 2002. Regulation mechanisms of intestinal secretion: implications in nutrient absorption. *J. Nutr. Biochem.* **13**:190–199.

68. Wimer-Mackin, S., R. K. Holmes, A. A. Wolf, W. I. Lencer, and M. G. Jobling. 2001. Characterization of receptor-mediated signal transduction by *Escherichia coli* type IIa heat-labile enterotoxin in the polarized human intestinal cell line T84. *Infect. Immun.* **69**:7205–7212.

69. Yue, G., D. Merlin, M. Selsted, W. I. Lencer, J. L. Madara, and D. Eaton. 2002. Cryptidin 3 forms anion selective channels in cytoplasmic membranes of human embryonic kidney cells. *Am. J. Physiol. Gastrointest. Liver Physiol.* **282**:G757–G765.

70. Zhang, M., C. Q. Zeng, A. P. Morris, and M. K. Estes. 2000. A functional NSP4 enterotoxin peptide secreted from rotavirus-infected cells. *J. Virol.* **74**:11663–11670.

71. Zhou, D. G., L. M. Chen, L. Hernandez, S. B. Shears, and J. E. Galan. 2001. A *Salmonella* inositol polyphosphatase acts in conjunction with other bacterial effectors to promote host cell actin cytoskeleton rearrangements and bacterial internalization. *Molec. Microbiol.* **39**:248–259.

ENTERIC PATHOGENS THAT AFFECT INTESTINAL EPITHELIAL TIGHT JUNCTIONS

Gail Hecht

16

An interesting confluence of events has been the recent emergence of vast amounts of information regarding two seemingly disparate areas—host-pathogen interactions and tight junction (TJ) biology. As a result, new mechanisms of TJ regulation and microbial pathogenesis have been recognized. While initial studies centered on bacterial pathogens, new studies have also examined the impact of viruses on this important physiological structure. This review covers the effects of both enteric bacterial and viral pathogens on intestinal epithelial TJs.

TJ STRUCTURE AND FUNCTION

The intercellular TJ is a complex multiprotein structure that serves to provide a barrier to the movement of substances between adjacent cells. It is composed of both intracellular and membrane-spanning proteins. The roles of both categories of proteins in the formation and regulation of TJs are subjects of tremendous attention. As the intent of this review is to discuss the various mechanisms by which

microbes can alter TJs, the reader is referred to recently published reviews regarding TJ structure and function (1, 69, 71). To set the stage, however, a schematic of TJs is depicted in Fig. 1. Briefly, the intracellular complex of TJ-associated proteins includes zonula occludens protein 1 (ZO-1), ZO-2, ZO-3, cingulin, 7H6, symplekin, and ZA-1TJ, in addition to several signaling molecules such as Rab-3B, Rab-13, c-Yes, c-Src, PKCζ, and Gα. To date, four integral TJ membrane proteins have been identified: occludin (23), the family of claudins (46), junctional adhesion molecule (JAM) (39), and the coxsackievirus and adenovirus receptor (CAR) (10). Both occludin and the claudins have four transmembrane-spanning domains that create two extracellular loops within the paracellular space. Homotypic interactions between occludin and homo- or heterotypic interaction between the various claudin isoforms serve to create the paracellular barrier (70). JAM and CAR possess a single transmembrane region.

Occludin, the first TJ transmembrane protein to be identified (23), possesses a long C-terminal cytoplasmic tail that contains numerous phosphorylatable residues. Several investigators using different approaches have shown that phosphorylated forms of occludin associate with the TJ per se while lesser- or

Gail Hecht, Professor of Medicine, Chief, Digestive Diseases and Nutrition, University of Illinois at Chicago, Department of Medicine, Section of Digestive Diseases and Nutrition, 840 S. Wood Street, MC 716, Chicago, IL 60612.

Microbial Pathogenesis and the Intestinal Epithelial Cell, ed. by G. Hecht
© 2003 ASM Press, Washington, D.C.

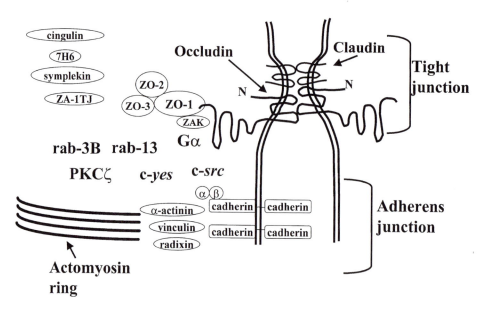

FIGURE 1 Schematic of TJ structure. TJs are macromolecular structures consisting of both transmembrane-spanning proteins, such as occludin, and a number of claudin isoforms. Two additional integral membrane proteins with a single transmembrane domain (not shown) are JAM and CAR. These molecules contribute to the barrier function of TJs. In addition to the transmembrane proteins, a number of other proteins form an intracellular plaque that likely aids in the targeting of transmembrane proteins. A number of signaling molecules also localize to the TJ and likely contribute to the regulation of permeability. The exact roles of these signaling molecules have not been defined. (Modified from L. L. Mitic and J. M. Anderson, *Annu. Rev. Physiol.* **60:**121–142, 1998.)

nonphosphorylated occludin resides in the basolateral membrane or cytosol (78). Many studies have also demonstrated a role for occludin in providing barrier function to the TJs (41, 78). On the other hand, knockout of the occludin gene in mouse embryonic stem cells did not ablate the formation of TJs (57). As such, the family of claudins was discovered (22, 46). Although the topology of claudins is similar to that of occludin, claudin has a much shorter C-terminal cytoplasmic tail and phosphorylation has not been demonstrated. Recent data support a more major role for claudins in providing barrier function (1, 69, 71), than for occludin, although both are likely important. It has been convincingly demonstrated, however, that the variability in ion selectivity and the degree of barrier function can be modulated by the level of expression of certain claudin isoforms (74).

For example, regulated expression of human claudin-4 in Madin-Darby canine kidney (MDCK) cells increased the complexity of TJ strands and transepithelial electrical resistance (TER), an electrophysiological measurement of TJ barrier function. The latter was found to be attributable to a selective decrease in Na^+ permeability, thus providing the first demonstration that claudins create selective ion channels in the TJ. As such, the wide variability in TER reported for many different epithelial tissues (53) can likely be attributed to differences in homotypic or heterotypic interactions between claudin isoforms (24). In fact, expression of certain claudins is tissue specific (16, 47, 55).

Only a few years ago, a third TJ integral membrane protein, called JAM (junctional adhesion molecule), was discovered. JAM contains a single transmembrane domain, two extracellular immunoglobulin domains, and a short cytoplasmic tail (39). JAM is a TJ component of both epithelial and endothelial cells and has recently been found to interact with several other TJ-associated proteins, including ZO-1, occludin, cingulin (4), and AF-6 (14). Through its associations with other TJ proteins as well as with the cytoskeleton, JAM may contribute to the overall organizational process of TJ formation. Another intriguing role for JAM is that of participation in the transepithelial or transendothelial migration of neutrophils during the inflammatory response (12, 39).

CAR (coxsackievirus and adenovirus receptor), like JAM, has a single transmembrane-spanning domain, two extracellular immunoglobulin-like domains, and a 107-amino-acid cytoplasmic tail (10). The potential of CAR as a target for adenoviral vectors used as gene therapy for cystic fibrosis, on the basis of its expression in airway epithelia, was thwarted because of its restricted localization to the basolateral surface (9). Therefore, initial attention was focused on defining the regions within this protein that conferred basolateral sorting. It was also recognized that CAR was capable of homotypic cell adhesion (32) and that it was concentrated at sites of cell-cell interactions (9, 52). These findings set the stage for the recent discovery that CAR is actually a transmembrane component of the TJ and that it confers some degree of barrier function (10).

It is the extracellular portions of the TJ transmembrane proteins that interact, probably in a "ziplock" fashion, to create the paracellular barrier. To some degree, the number of TJ strands correlates with TER (8). However, this relationship is now believed to be much more complex, involving the state (open or closed) of aqueous pores within the TJs. Multiple lines of evidence now suggest that claudins form such aqueous pores and that the variation in the heterotypic interaction may account for the difference in "tightness" of various epithelia (69, 71). The role of occludin in barrier function is somewhat less clear. Published data suggest that occludin

may contribute to the formation of aqueous pores that regulate the paracellular flow of noncharged solutes (2). The contributions of occludin to TJ fence function (cell polarity) and signaling remain to be explored.

Many interactions exist between the intracellular and transmembrane TJ proteins, as well as with proteins primarily localized to the underlying zonula adherens, i.e., actin and myosin (71). Many of these protein-protein interactions occur through PDZ domains. The peripheral membrane proteins ZO-1, -2, and -3 all contain three PDZ domains, one SH3 domain, and a guanylyl kinase-like domain. Many of the interactions between TJ proteins have been mapped to these regions (reviewed in reference 1). The TJ complex, therefore, is a macromolecular structure that is likely involved in intercellular signaling that participates in the regulation of crucial cellular events including proliferation, differentiation, and polarity. The presence of signaling molecules, such as Rab-3b, Rab-13, c-Src, c-Yes, and atypical PKCζ, supports this view.

Perturbation of the TJ barrier by microbial pathogens can likely occur at any of these levels. Beyond this, there are newly published reports that TJ proteins can even serve as receptors for a bacterial toxin and specific viruses (discussed below). This review focuses on the mechanisms by which enteric bacterial and viral pathogens can disrupt this important structure.

MECHANISMS OF TJ DISRUPTION BY MICROBIAL PATHOGENS

Exploitation of Cytoskeletal Contraction by Phosphorylation of MLC

Enteropathogenic *Escherichia coli* (EPEC) and enterohemorrhagic *E. coli* (EHEC) are in many ways similar. Neither invades host cells; instead, both adhere intimately to intestinal epithelial cells, causing characteristic attaching and effacing (A/E) lesions. From this extracellular location, both trigger host cell signal transduction cascades that ultimately disrupt cellular functions including that of the TJ barrier (27). The ability to induce both morphological and functional changes in the host epithelium has a genetic basis. Specifically, both of these pathogens harbor a 35-kb pathogenicity island within the chromosome, called the locus of enterocyte effacement (LEE) (43). Encoded within this locus are proteins required for intimate attachment to host cells and for the formation of a type III secretory apparatus (see chapters 22 and 23 for details). The latter, simplistically stated, is a molecular syringe through which the microbe delivers bacterial proteins directly into host cells (Fig. 2). While some of the EPEC secreted proteins (Esp) have been identified and characterized, the specific mechanisms by

which they affect host cell functions have not been defined. What has been clarified, however, is that targeted host cell signaling molecules are activated by infection. Both EPEC and EHEC markedly enhance the phosphorylation of the 20-kDa myosin light chain (MLC) (38, 82). It is the phosphorylated form of MLC that interacts with actin, thus catalyzing myosin ATPase, which drives cytoskeletal contraction. A ring of cytoskeletal proteins circumscribes intestinal epithelial cells and inserts into the lateral membrane immediately beneath the TJs. Several studies employing a variety of models, including genetic approaches (30, 73), physiological stimulation (6, 72), and pathophysiological models such as infection (51, 82), have demonstrated that

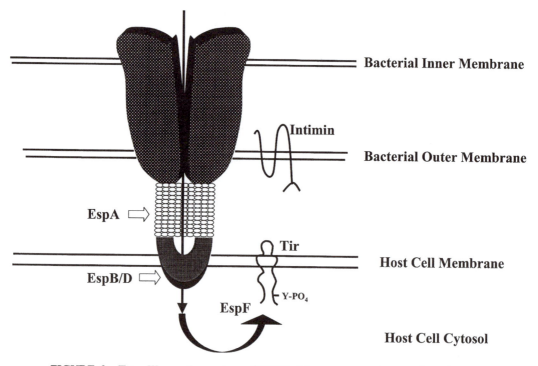

FIGURE 2 Type III secretion system of EPEC. Most gram-negative enteric pathogens, including EPEC, EHEC, and *Salmonella*, *Shigella*, and *Yersinia* spp., express a type III secretory system through which effector molecules can be directly delivered into host cells. Of particular relevance to EPEC is the translocated intimin receptor (Tir), which is tyrosine phosphorylated once inside the host cell and inserted into the host cell membrane where it serves as a receptor for the outer membrane EPEC adhesin, intimin. Effector molecules, such as EspF, are also injected into host cells where they perturb physiologic processes. (Modified from D. L. Goosney, S. Gruenheid, and B. B. Finlay, *Annu. Rev. Cell Dev. Biol.* **16:**173–189, 2000.)

phosphorylated MLC-driven cytoskeletal contraction is one mechanism whereby TJ permeability is enhanced. We have shown that EPEC-induced MLC phosphorylation is one way that this pathogen disrupts the TJ barrier; others have shown the same for EHEC (51, 82). Specifically, infection of model intestinal epithelia by EPEC caused a progressive increase in MLC phosphorylation. Inhibition of MLC kinase (MLCK) activity by buffering calcium, using specific MLCK pharmacologic inhibitors (82), or by cell-permeant inhibitory peptides (83) significantly reduced the EPEC-associated decrease in TER, a functional measurement of TJ permeability.

Others have reported similar findings regarding EHEC (51). EHEC infection, independent of Shiga-like toxin production, of intestinal epithelial cells has been shown to decrease TER, in part by activating MLCK (51). Changes in the distribution of ZO-1 were also described, but the effects on other TJ proteins have not been examined. Whether the effects of MLCK on TJs are a result of displacing TJ proteins that interact with the actomyosin cytoskeleton or triggering key signaling molecules that regulate the TJ barrier is not known.

TJ Disruption by Fragmentation of Actin

Actin has been demonstrated to interact with several TJ proteins including ZO-1, ZO-2, ZO-3, cingulin, occludin, and claudins (reviewed in reference 1). Disruption of the actin cytoskeleton by various methods has been shown to perturb the TJ barrier (29, 31, 48, 49). The best example of pathogen-induced actin fragmentation causing disruption of TJs is *Clostridium difficile*. *C. difficile*, the organism responsible for antibiotic-associated pseudomembranous colitis, produces two structurally similar (45% amino acid identity) exotoxins, toxin A and toxin B, whose targets are Rho GTP binding proteins, Rho, Rac, and Cdc42 (see chapter 27) (13, 34, 35). Both toxins UDP-glucosylate a critical threonine residue of Rho, rendering it inactive. As a result, actin is depolymerized at both the apical and basal

poles of cells (49). Associated with these changes in the actin cytoskeleton was a loss of occludin, ZO-1, and ZO-2 from the TJ (49). Loss of the TJ barrier correlated with these structural changes (29, 31). The impact of toxins A and B on the TJ barrier and structure has been demonstrated in cultured epithelia (29, 31, 49) as well as mammalian, including human, tissues (56). Whether all the effects of *C. difficile* toxins on TJs are mediated by actin depolymerization or whether there are also direct effects on TJ-associated proteins is not clear.

Another clostridial toxin, C3 transferase produced by *Clostridium botulinum*, also inactivates Rho but via ADP-ribosylation. The effect on the actin cytoskeleton, however, is the same as that caused by *C. difficile* toxins, namely, actin fragmentation. The impact of this toxin on polarized intestinal epithelial cells was examined using an efficient delivery system whereby C3 transferase was coupled to the cell binding, but enzymatically inactive, domain of diptheria toxin (48). As was seen in response to *C. difficile* toxins, C3 transferase also induced the dissociation of ZO-1 from TJs and a corresponding disruption of the TJ barrier. That two different bacterial toxins with targeted effects on the actin cytoskeleton also perturb the structure and function of TJs highlights the physiological relevance of the interactions between these two important structures (11, 17, 77).

Disruption of TJs by Bacterial Proteases

Several microbes elaborate proteases. In this era of attention to host-pathogen interactions, the functional impact of some of these bacterial products is becoming apparent. With regard to the intestinal tract, the *Bacteroides fragilis* enterotoxin (BFT) and the haemagglutinin protease (HA/P) of *Vibrio cholerae* are the best-characterized examples of bacterial-derived proteases that disrupt TJs.

B. fragilis enterotoxin (discussed in greater detail in chapter 17), a 20-kDa, zinc-dependent metalloprotease, has been clearly linked to diarrhea. Interestingly, this toxin, which is not internalized by cells, requires contact with the basolateral surface of intestinal epithelial cells to exert its effects, which include the rearrangement of actin, stimulation of chloride secretion, and disruption of TJs (7). Careful and logical studies by Wu et al. (79) showed that BFT cleaves the cell-cell adhesion molecule E-cadherin. The initial cleavage site of this transmembrane protein occurs near the plasma membrane and is ATP independent. The subsequent intracellular degradation, which requires both ATP and cellular proteases, likely triggers the dissociation of ZO-1 and occludin from TJs. The effects of BFT on TJs are believed to be the result of a series of events that include the loss of E-cadherin/β-catenin interactions, disruption of the actin cytoskeleton, and ultimately disassembly of TJ structures.

In contrast, the HA/P of *V. cholerae* has direct proteolytic effects on TJs. Specifically, HA/P degrades the transmembrane TJ protein occludin (81). Unlike the more extensive degradation of E-cadherin by BFT, HA/P appears to leave the cytoplasmic portion of occludin associated with TJs. In fact, others have previously shown that this particular domain of occludin is sufficient for TJ targeting (40). While ZO-1 also redistributed following exposure to HA/P, this event was not attributed to degradation. Rather, the primary effects of HA/P on occludin are believed to disrupt its association with ZO-1, leaving it free to migrate away from the TJ complex. Corresponding with these structural changes in intestinal epithelial TJs was loss of function (45, 80). The strong correlation between HA/P production and effects on the TJ barrier raised questions regarding the role of another *V. cholerae* toxin, zonula occludin toxin (19), in *V. cholerae*-induced TJ effects. Even *zot⁻* strains had a significant impact on TER, while a *hap* mutant strain had only modest effects (45), suggesting that, at least in the cultured human intestinal epithelial T84 cell model, factors other than Zot are responsible for the alteration in TJ barrier. Zot is discussed in detail in

chapter 17 of this volume, and the controversy surrounding this area is discussed in chapter 26.

Pathogens Having Direct Effects on TJ Proteins

As the structural basis of the TJ complex is now more clearly defined, there are increased opportunities to investigate the effects of microbial pathogens on specific TJ proteins. Our laboratory has focused on the effect of EPEC infection, on occludin and found that this protein is dramatically altered. When viewed by immunofluorescent staining, occludin loses its uniform distribution at the level of the TJ early after EPEC infection, taking on a "beaded" appearance. Later, however, at times that correlate with decreasing TER, occludin dissociates from the TJ and redistributes to an intracellular compartment (62). This morphological change corresponds to a decrease in occludin phosphorylation. Others have shown, using a variety of model systems, that occludin phosphorylation is required for its association with TJs (18, 58, 78). The enzyme that dephosphorylates occludin has not been identified. In fact, it is not known whether a host or a bacterial enzyme is responsible. Bacterial proteins that possess phosphatase activity have been described. For example, YopH of *Yersinia* sp. is a tyrosine phosphatase that is delivered into host cells through a type III secretion system and targets eukaryotic proteins (25). Another potential explanation of these data is that EPEC infection could cause the dissociation of kinases from occludin, thus shifting the balance toward phosphatase activity.

Although the specific phosphatase responsible for this effect on occludin has not been identified, we have found that an EPEC-secreted protein (Esp), F, is required for the full effect of EPEC on TJ barrier function (44). EspF is not a structural component of the type III secretion apparatus but is delivered into host cells by this system. The type III secretory system of EPEC is discussed in detail in chapter 23 of this book. Mutation of the *espF* gene significantly diminished the impact of EPEC on the TER of intestinal epithelial monolayers and on the redistribution of occludin (44). A direct relationship between the amount of EspF produced and the extent of the decrease in TER was demonstrated using an isopropyl-β-D-thiogalactopyranoside (IPTG)-inducible system for EspF expression. Furthermore, mutation of any of the type III secretion genes essentially abrogated the impact of EPEC on TJs. Whether EspF is the only EPEC effector molecule that alters TJ proteins and permeability is unclear. In addition, the mechanisms by which EspF exerts such dramatic effects on host cell function are not known. However, EspF contains three proline-rich repeats, suggesting that there is high potential for interacting with host cell protein(s). Identification of such interacters will further our understanding of how the TJ barrier is regulated as well as enhance our knowledge of EPEC pathogenesis.

Interestingly, one protein that redistributes to the A/E lesions of EPEC and appears to be involved in the cross talk between bacteria and host is ezrin (61). Ezrin is a membrane-cytoskeletal linker protein with signal transducing capability through its interaction with actin. In its dormant state, the N and C termini of ezrin interact in an intramolecular fashion, thereby masking its membrane and cytoskeletal binding domains, respectively. Activation of ezrin by phosphorylation of key threonine and tyrosine residues breaks the interaction, thus exposing the critical binding sites. The author's laboratory has shown that EPEC infection induces threonine and tyrosine phosphorylation of ezrin and enhances its cytoskeletal binding. The latter event is considered synonymous with ezrin activation. A functional type III secretion system is required for full activation of ezrin. Expression of a dominant-negative ezrin molecule, consisting of the N terminus and specifically lacking the 35-amino-acid C-terminal actin binding domain, reduced EPEC-induced decrease in TER by ca. 50% (61). These data suggest that signaling events initiated by the interaction

between EPEC and host intestinal epithelial cells involve ezrin and that these activated signals have downstream effects on the TJ barrier. Whether other proteins that localize to A/E lesions also participate in this cross talk has yet to be determined.

A functional phenotype similar to that described above for EPEC EspF has been attributed to a *Yersinia* outer membrane protein, YopE. Several groups have demonstrated that infection of intestinal epithelial cells by *Yersinia* spp. perturbs TJ barrier function (60, 66). Tafazoli, et al. recently reported that *Yersinia* infection of MDCK-1 monolayers disrupted F-actin as well as two key TJ proteins, ZO-1 and occludin (66). A *yopE* mutant, however, failed to induce these effects, suggesting a direct role for this bacterial protein in TJ disruption. As for EspF, the mechanism by which YopE perturbs the TJ barrier is unknown.

The combination of molecular microbiological and cell physiological approaches, however, provides a powerful tool for identifying microbial virulence factors. It was this type of "functional screening" of a series of EPEC mutant strains that led to the identification of the role of *rorf10*, a gene also encoded on the EPEC pathogenicity island or LEE. While the *rorf10* mutant was found to exhibit normal adherence, A/E lesion formation, and secretion of EspA, -B, and -D, it was attenuated in its effects on TJ permeability measured as TER and translocation of EspF into host cells. Subsequent studies showed that this intracellular, α-helical protein interacted with EspF, but not the translocated intimin receptor Tir or other EPEC-secreted proteins. Together, these properties suggested that this protein operates as a chaperone for EspF and hence was named chaperone for EPEC-secreted protein F or CesF (15). The more routine application of this type of genetic or physiologic approach to investigating microbial pathogenesis will undoubtedly yield fruitful results.

Although EHEC is genetically similar to EPEC, i.e., both contain a LEE that shares 94% nucleotide homology, their effects on host cell physiology are quite different. For example, nonpathogenic *E. coli* K-12 transformed to express the LEE of EPEC decreased TER and redistributed occludin in a manner similar to that induced by wild-type EPEC (62). In contrast, K-12 transformed with the LEE of EHEC has no effect on TER or occludin localization (75), suggesting that factors outside of the LEE are important for inducing host cell effects. One similar feature in the mechanisms by which EPEC and EHEC increase the permeability of TJs, however, is through the activation of MLCK, as discussed earlier in this chapter.

Perturbation of TJs Allows Microbes Access to Basolateral Membrane Receptors

Intestinal epithelial cell receptors for several enteric bacterial pathogens are, interestingly, restricted to the basolateral membrane of these polarized cells. In addition to providing barrier function to epithelial sheets, TJs also contribute to the maintenance of cell polarity, that is, the segregation of apical and basolateral membrane proteins. There is strong evidence to show that disruption of TJs by several means, including transmigration of inflammatory cells and perturbation of TJ proteins, can either allow microbes to traverse the paracellular pathway or disrupt the polar distribution of membrane proteins (fence function) such that basolaterally restricted molecules relocalize to the apical domain. Either scenario results in access of pathogenic microbes to cognate host receptors.

Yersinia

The best-characterized example of disruption of TJ fence function enhancing the access of a pathogen to a basolaterally restricted receptor relates to *Yersinia* spp. and β_1 integrin. β_1 integrin is the eukaryotic receptor for the outer membrane *Yersinia* protein invasin (33). Under physiological circumstances, β_1 integrin is localized to the basolateral membrane of cells, serving to anchor cells to the extracellular matrix or to each other. Upon disruption of TJs, fence function is perturbed and

membrane proteins can redistribute, gaining access to the apical domain. In the case of *Yersinia* sp. initial invasion is believed to occur through M cells, which apparently harbor β_1 integrin on the apical membrane. An early response to infection is an acute inflammatory response manifested as neutrophil infiltration into the lamina propria followed by transmigration across the intestinal epithelium via TJs. McCormick et al. demonstrated that the transepithelial migration of neutrophils resulted in the disruption of TJ fence function and the appearance of β_1 integrin on the apical cell surface (42). As such, the rate of invasion of *Yersinia* sp. increased as a result of enhanced access of invasin to its cognate receptor, β_1 integrin.

EPEC

A similar scenario has been demonstrated for EPEC (28). Although the best-characterized ligand/receptor pair for EPEC is the outer membrane adhesin, intimin, and the bacterial-produced type III secreted protein Tir, intimin can also bind to β_1 integrin (20). While the contribution of this interaction to EPEC pathogenesis was unclear, we have shown that, following disruption of TJs by EPEC infection, β_1 integrin redistributes to the apical surface of intestinal epithelial cells and potentiates the drop in TER. Blocking antibodies against an extracellular domain of β_1 integrin inhibits this response. The hypothesis is that the initial interaction between intimin and Tir is crucial for the activation of signals that trigger the disruption of TJs, as a *tir* deletion strain has no impact on the TJ barrier. Once perturbed, however, the redistribution of basolateral membrane proteins to the apical surface provides a second binding partner for intimin or potentially other unidentified adhesins. Signals activated by this interaction could then have additional effects on the TJ barrier.

Shigella

Another enteric pathogen lacking the ability to bind to the apical surface of host intestinal epithelial cells, thus initially employing M cells to invade the epithelium, is *Shigella* sp. The subsequent inflammatory response, including the transepithelial migration of neutrophils, enhances the access of *Shigella* sp. to the basolateral aspect of epithelial cells by opening TJs and forging a route for translocation through the paracellular pathway (50, 59). *Shigella*, interestingly, shows little binding to host cells, although it does briefly interact with the basolateral membrane of these cells prior to being engulfed. The Ipa B/C complex secreted by *Shigella* sp. has been shown to bind to $\alpha_5\beta_1$ integrin (76), a component of focal adhesion complexes. This is not an exclusive event, however, in that an interaction between the hyaluronic acid receptor, CD44, and IpaB has been shown to recruit ezrin (64) and to activate Rho (67). It is the disruption of TJs that enhances the access of *Shigella* sp. to these basolateral membrane proteins, thus triggering events that lead to engulfment of the microbe.

TJ PROTEINS AS RECEPTORS FOR ENTERIC PATHOGENS

An interesting paradigm has emerged over the past few years—the exploitation of TJ transmembrane proteins as microbial receptors. First, several claudin isoforms were shown to function as receptors for *Clostridium perfringens* enterotoxin (CPE), the toxin responsible for the diarrhea associated with *C. perfringens* type A food poisoning. Second, three unrelated viruses have now been shown to use TJ transmembrane proteins as receptors. The details of these findings are discussed below.

Claudins are Receptors for CPE

It was recognized only a few years ago that a 22-kDa eukaryotic cell protein served as a receptor for CPE (36). Subsequent studies showed that two human homologues, hCPE-R and hRVP-1, were functional receptors for CPE (37). Functionality was determined by showing that transfection of either of these proteins into mouse L cells conferred the phenotype of CPE cytotoxicity. Abundant expression of these receptors was found to occur in the small intestine. hRVP-1 and hCPE-R were subsequently identified as isoforms of the

family of claudins, claudin-3 and -4, respectively. CPE reportedly binds to the second extracellular loop of claudin-3. To date, more than 20 claudin isoforms have been identified, but only claudins 3, 4, 6, 7, 8, and 14 can bind CPE (21).

More recent data suggest that CPE can also interact with occludin. This is not a result of the interaction between occludin and claudins since occludin could be identified only in the late-forming 200-kDa CPE complex, while claudins were present in CPE complexes of all sizes (63). Furthermore, single point mutations in the N termini of nontoxic CPEs rendered them incapable of forming the larger complexes, suggesting that CPE itself participates in pulling occludin into this complex.

The net effect of CPE on TJ structure has been demonstrated by two independent groups. Exposure of the basolateral surface of MDCK cells to a nontoxic C-terminal fragment of CPE (C-CPE) induced the dissociation of claudin-4 from TJs, the subsequent disintegration of TJ fibrils, and an increase in paracellular permeability (65). Similarly, perfusion of rat liver with CPE, resulting in basolateral exposure of hepatocytes to this toxin, caused fragmentation of TJ strands (54). CPE also induced the ablation of canalicular microvilli and flattening of the membrane surface. The fact that TJ disruption by CPE requires basolateral access of this toxin suggests that this effect is not the initial event. Rather, CPE rapidly induces cytotoxicity of intestinal epithelial cells, probably by pore formation in the apical membranes, and fluid and electrolyte secretion (26). Such damage to the intestinal epithelium is certainly sufficient to allow access of CPE to the basolateral domain of remaining epithelial cells, thus enabling secondary TJ effects to occur. In this scenario, enhanced paracellular permeability would contribute to, although not initiate, the diarrhea caused by CPE.

JAM as a Receptor for Reovirus

Reovirus can infect many animals including humans, primarily children, and cause gastrointestinal or respiratory disease. Viral attachment to host cells is the critical initial step in establishing disease. The reovirus attachment protein $\sigma 1$ binds to cell surface receptors, but the identity of such receptors was not defined until recently. An expression cloning approach was used and identified JAM as a reovirus receptor by screening a human neuronal-precursor cell cDNA library (3). Further, reovirus-resistant murine erythroleukemia (MEL) or chicken embryo fibroblast (CEF) cells were rendered permissive following transfection with human JAM (hJAM). Also, hJAM monoclonal antibodies blocked reovirus binding to competent cells. Beyond these findings, it was demonstrated that reovirus-induced activation of NF-κB and apoptosis were dependent upon interactions between the reovirus attachment protein $\sigma 1$ and JAM, although other molecules, namely, α-linked sialyic acid, could mediate the attachment step. This intriguing realization indicates that viral replication alone is insufficient to stimulate such crucial host responses and highlights the possibility that TJ proteins may serve as environmental sensors and respond to microbial pathogens by inducing the inflammatory response and apoptosis. As for some other microbial pathogens and the above-discussed CPE, reovirus must gain access to the basolateral domain of the cell to access its receptor. In the case of reovirus, transport across microfold (M) cells allows for access to JAM.

CAR Is a TJ Protein

CAR was identified a few years ago (5, 68); however, its cellular function was not known. Recently, Cohen et al. (10) found that CAR is actually a transmembrane TJ protein that assists in the provision of the paracellular barrier. Initial experiments showed that the transfection of Chinese hamster ovary (CHO) cells with CAR resulted in the localization of CAR to areas of cell-cell contact, but only when CAR was present on the membrane of apposing cells. Such localization did not occur upon contact with mock-transfected cells. The localization of ZO-1 in CHO-CAR cells was synonomous with that of CAR but

remained diffusely distributed in mock-transfected cells. Further studies confirmed that CAR, as ZO-1, localizes to the TJs of polarized epithelial cells, including the human colonic epithelial cell line T_{84}, human airway epithelial cells, and MDCK cells. Immuno-gold electron microscopy clearly demonstrated the association of CAR with TJs. Co-immunoprecipitation studies showed that CAR and ZO-1 associate either directly or via interactions with other TJ proteins. To assess the role of CAR in barrier function, the paracellular flux of fluorescein isothiocyanate (FITC)-labeled dextran across CHO-pcDNA and CHO-CAR cells grown on permeable supports was assessed. Expression of CAR significantly decreased the paracellular movement of dextran. Similarly, expression of human CAR in MDCK cells approximately doubled the TER of monolayers. Most significant was the demonstration that the sequestration of CAR within the TJ complex severely limited the degree of infection by both coxsackievirus B3 and adenovirus type 5. This occurred despite the presentation of virus to either the apical or basolateral surface of confluent monolayers. In contrast, disruption of TJs by treatment with EDTA caused a significant increase in infection by these specific viruses, which could be inhibited by polyclonal CAR antibodies. Therefore, for infection by coxsackievirus or adenovirus to ensue, disruption of TJs by some other means is a prerequisite.

Several intriguing conclusions derive from these studies. First, a fourth member of the family of transmembrane TJ proteins has been identified. Second, this is the third reported example of a TJ transmembrane protein serving as a receptor for microbial pathogens or their products. Third, it is clearly demonstrated that sequestration of a microbial receptor within the TJ complex protects the cell from infection by specific pathogens attacking from either the apical or basolateral pole, providing yet another example of the importance of maintaining epithelial integrity.

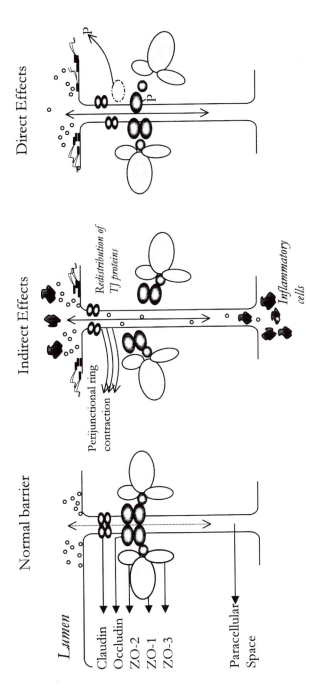

FIGURE 3 Under normal conditions, TJs provide a barrier to the paracellular space, thus preventing free access of bacteria or their products to the underlying compartments. Pathogens, however, can disrupt the TJ barrier by indirect and direct mechanisms. Examples of indirect perturbation of TJs include contraction of the perijunctional actomyosin ring through the activation of MLCK and subsequent phosphorylation of MLC. Redistribution of TJ proteins likely occurs as a consequence of cytoskeletal contraction through the numerous interactions that exist between TJ proteins and actin or myosin. The transepithelial migration of inflammatory cells, in particular neutrophils, occurs across TJs and opens, at least temporarily, these structures. One example of a more direct effect is the dephosphorylation of occludin by EPEC (62). Less- or nonphosphorylated forms of occludin dissociate from the TJ and thereby alter paracellular permeability.

CONCLUDING REMARKS

This is an exciting time to explore host-pathogen interactions, with so many tools readily available. The number of ways that pathogens can disrupt and/or exploit TJ proteins continues to expand (Fig. 3). The most recent studies identifying TJ proteins as receptors for both viruses and a bacterial toxin exemplify exploitation. Similarly, perturbation of TJ fence function and cell polarity is an event that favors the microbe. On the other hand, whether disruption of the TJ barrier is advantageous to the host or pathogen is less clear. Arguments can be made for each case. Since loss of the TJ barrier could render electrolyte and nutrient absorption less efficient, this process may contribute to diarrhea. Diarrhea benefits the host by flushing the organisms from the intestinal lumen. At the same time, diarrhea serves as a means of transmission of the pathogen.

In any event, many questions remain regarding the specific mechanisms by which enteric microbial pathogens disrupt TJs. Future studies exploring interactions between microbial effector molecules and host proteins will undoubtedly yield new information regarding the regulation of TJs and at the same time provide insight into mechanisms of microbial pathogenesis.

REFERENCES

1. Anderson, J. M. 2001. Molecular structure of tight junctions and their role in epithelial transport. News Physiol. Sci. 16:126–130.
2. Balda, M. S., J. A. Witney, C. Flores, S. Gonzalez, M. Cereijido, and K. Matter. 1996. Functional dissociation of paracellular permeability and transepithelial electrical resistance and disruption of the apical-basolateral intramembrane diffusion barrier by expression of a mutant tight junction membrane protein. J. Cell. Biol. 134:1031–1049.
3. Barton, E., J. Forrest, J. Conolly, J. Chappel, Y. Liu, F. Schnell, A. Nusrat, C. A. Parkos, and T. Dermody. 2001. Junction adhesion molecule is a receptor for reovirus. Cell 104:441–451.
4. Bazzoni, G., O. M. Martinez Estrada, F. Orsenigo, M. Cordenonsi, S. Citi, and E. Dejana. 2000. Interaction of junctional adhesion molecule with the tight junction components ZO-1, cingulin, and occludin. J. Biol. Chem. 275:20520–20526.
5. Bergelson, J. M., J. A. Cunningham, G. Droguett, E. A. Kurt-Jones, A. Krithivas, J. S. Hong, M. S. Horwitz, R. L. Crowell, and R. W. Finberg. 1997. Isolation of a common receptor for coxsackie B viruses and adenoviruses 2 and 5. Science 275:1320–1323.
6. Berglund, J. J., M. Riegler, Y. Zolotarevsky, E. Wenzl, and J. R. Turner. 2001. Regulation of human jejunal transmucosal resistance and MLC phosphorylation by Na$^+$-glucose cotransport. Am. J. Physiol. 281:G1487–G1493.
7. Chambers, F., S. Koshy, R. Saidi, D. Clark, R. Moore, and C. Sears. 1997. Bacteroides fragilis toxin exhibits polar activity on monolayers of human intestinal epithelial cells (T84 cells) in vitro. Infect. Immun. 65:3561–3570.
8. Claude, P. 1978. Morphological factors influencing transepithelial permeability: a model for the resistance of the zonula occludens. J. Membr. Biol. 10:219–232.
9. Cohen, C., J. Gaetz, T. Ohman, and J. M. Bergelson. 2001. Multiple regions within the coxsackievirus and adenovirus receptor cytoplasmic domain are required for basolateral sorting. J. Biol. Chem. 276:25392–25398.
10. Cohen, C. J., J. T. Shieh, R. J. Pickles, T. Okegawa, J. T. Hsieh, and J. M. Bergelson. 2001. The coxsackievirus and adenovirus receptor is a transmembrane component of the tight junction. Proc. Natl. Acad. Sci. USA 98:15191–15196.
11. Cordenonsi, M., F. D'Atri, E. Hammar, D. A. D. Parry, J. Kendrick-Jones, D. Shore, and S. Citi. 1999. Cingulin contains globular and coiled-coil domains and interacts with ZO-1, ZO-2, ZO-3, and myosin. J. Cell. Biol. 147:1569–1581.
12. Del Maschio, A., A. De Luigi, I. Martin-Padura, R. Furlan, M. G. De Simoni, and E. Dejana. 1999. Leukocyte recruitment in the cerebrospinal fluid of mice with experimental meningitis is inhibited by an antibody to junctional adhesion molecule (JAM). J. Exp. Med. 190:1351–1356.
13. Dillon, S., E. Rubin, M. Yakubovich, C. Pothoulakis, J. T. LaMont, L. Feig, and R. Gilbert. 1995. Involvement of Ras-related Rho proteins in the mechanisms of action of Clostridium difficile Toxin A and Toxin B. Infect. Immun. 63:1421–1426.
14. Ebnet, K., C. U. Schulz, M. K. Meyer Zu Brickwedded, G. G. Pendl, and D. Vestwe-

ber. 2000. Junctional adhesion molecule interacts with the PDZ domain-containing proteins AF-6 and ZO-1. *J. Biol. Chem.* **275**:27979–27988.

15. **Elliot, S. J., C. B. O'Connell, A. Koutsouris, M. S. Donnenberg, G. Hecht, and J. B. Kaper.** 2002. A novel gene required for EPEC to increase tight junction permeability encodes a chaperone for EspF. *Infect. Immun.* **70**:2271–2277.

16. **Enck, A. H., U. V. Berger, and A. S. Yu.** 2001. Claudin-2 is selectively expressed in proximal nephron in mouse kidney. *Am. J. Physiol.* **281**:F966–F974.

17. **Fanning, A., B. J. Jameson, L. Jesaitis, and J. M. Anderson.** 1998. The tight junction protein ZO-1 establishes a link between the transmembrane protein occludin and the actin cytoskeleton. *J. Biol. Chem.* **273**:29745–29753.

18. **Farshori, P., and B. Kachar.** 1999. Redistribution and phosphorylation of occludin during opening and resealing of tight junctions in cultured epithelial cells. *J. Membr. Biol.* **170**:147–156.

19. **Fasano, A., B. Baudry, D. Pumplin, S. Wasserman, B. Tall, J. Ketley, and J. Kaper.** 1991. *Vibrio cholera* produces a second enterotoxin, which affects intestinal tight junctions. *Proc. Natl. Acad. Sci. USA* **88**:5242–5246.

20. **Frankel, G., O. Lider, R. Hershkoviz, A. P. Mould, S. G. Kachalsky, D. C. A. Candy, L. Cahalon, M. J. Humphries, and G. Dougan.** 1996. The cell-binding domain of intimin from enteropathogenic *Escherichia coli* binds to beta1 integrins. *J. Biol. Chem.* **271**:20359–20364.

21. **Fujita, K., J. Katahira, Y. Horiguchi, N. Sonoda, M. Furuse, and S. Tskuita.** 2000. *Clostridium perfringens* enterotoxin binds to the second extracellular loop of claudin-3, a tight junction membrane protein. *FEBS Lett.* **476**:258.

22. **Furuse, M., K. Fujita, T. Hiiragi, K. Fujimoto, and S. Tsukita.** 1998. Claudin-1 and -2 novel integral membrane proteins localizing at tight junctions with no sequence similarity to occludin. *J. Cell Biol.* **141**:1539–1550.

23. **Furuse, M., T. Hirase, M. Itoh, A. Nagafuchi, S. Yonemura, S. Tsukita, and S. Tsukita.** 1993. Occludin: a novel integral membrane protein localizing at tight junctions. *J. Cell Biol.* **123**:1777–1788.

24. **Furuse, M., H. Sasaki, and S. Tsukita.** 1999. Manner of interaction of heterogeneous claudin species within and between tight junction strands. *J. Cell Biol.* **147**:891–903.

25. **Guan, K., and J. E. Dixon.** 1990. Protein tyrosine phosphatase activity of an essential viru-

lence determinant in *Yersinia*. *Science* **249**:553–556.

26. **Hardy, S., P. Denmead, N. Parekh, and P. E. Granum.** 1999. Cationic currects induced by *Clostridium perfringens* type A enterotoxin in human intestinal Caco-2 cells. *J. Med. Microbiol.* **48**:235.

27. **Hecht, G.** 2001. Microbes and microbial toxins: paradigms for microbial-mucosal interactions. VII. Enteropathogenic *Escherichia coli*: physiological alterations from an extracellular position. *Am. J. Physiol. Gastrointest. Liver Physiol.* **281**:G1–G7.

28. **Hecht, G., A. Koutsouris, and M. M. Muza.** 2001. EPEC infection allows migration of B1 integrin to apical membrane which contributes to functional perturbations. *Gastroenterology* **120**:A325.

29. **Hecht, G., A. Koutsouris, C. Pothoulakis, J. T. LaMont, and J. Madara.** 1992. *Clostridium difficile* toxin B disrupts the barrier function of T$_{84}$ monolayers. *Gastroenterology* **102**:416–423.

30. **Hecht, G., L. Pestic, G. Nikcevic, A. Koutsouris, D. Tripuraneni, D. Lorimer, G. Nowak, J. V. Guerriero, E. L. Elson, and P. de Lanerolle.** 1996. Expression of the catalytic domain of myosin light chain kinase increases paracellular permeability. *Am. J. Physiol.* **271**:C1678–C1684.

31. **Hecht, G., C. Pothoulakis, J. T. LaMont, and J. L. Madara.** 1988. *Clostridium difficile* toxin A perturbs cytoskeletal structure and tight junction permeability of cultured human intestinal epithelial monolayers. *J. Clin. Invest.* **82**:1516–1524.

32. **Honda, T., H. Saitoh, M. Masuko, T. Katagiri-Abe, K. Tominaga, I. Kozakai, K. Kobayashi, T. Kumanishi, Y. G. Watanabe, S. Odani, and R. Kuwano.** 2000. The coxsackievirus-adenovirus receptor protein as a cell adhesion molecule in the developing mouse brain. *Brain Res. Mol. Brain Res.* **77**:19–28.

33. **Isberg, R. R., D. L. Voorhis, and M. Leong.** 1990. Multiple β1 chain integrins are receptors for invasin, a protein that promotes bacterial penetration into mammalian cells. *Cell* **60**:861–871.

34. **Just, I., G. Fritz, K. Aktories, M. Giry, M. Popoff, P. Boquet, S. Hegenberth, and C. von Eichel-Streiber,** 1994. *Clostridium difficile* toxin B acts on the GTP-binding protein Rho. *J. Biol. Chem.* **269**:10706–10712.

35. **Just, I., J. Selzer, M. Wilm, C. von Eichel-Streiber, M. Mann, and K. Aktories.** 1995. Glucosylation of Rho proteins by *Clostridium difficile* toxin B. *Nature* **375**:500–503.

36. **Katahira, J., N. Inoue, Y. Horiguchi, M. Matsuda, and N. Sugimoto.** 1997. Mo-

lecular cloning and functional characterization of the receptor for *Clostridium perfringens* enterotoxin. *J. Cell Biol.* **136:**1239–1247.

37. **Katahira, J., H. Sugiyama, N. Inoue, Y. Horiguchi, M. Matsuda, and N. Sugimoto.** 1997. *Clostridium perfringens* enterotoxin utilizes two structurally related membrane proteins as functional receptors in vivo. *J. Biol. Chem.* **272:**26652–26658.

38. **Manjarrez-Hernandez, H. A., B. Amess, L. Sellers, T. J. Baldwin, S. Knutton, P. H. Williams, and A. Aitken.** 1991. Purification of a 20kDa phosphoprotein from epithelial cells and identification as myosin light chain. *FEBS Lett.* **292:**121–127.

39. **Martin-Padura, I., S. Lostaglio, M. Schneemann, L. Williams, M. Romano, P. Fruscella, C. Panzeri, A. Stoppacciaro, L. Ruco, A. Villa, D. Simmons, and E. Dejana.** 1998. Junctional adhesion molecule, a novel member of the immunoglobulin superfamily that distributes at intercellular junctions and modulates monocyte transmigration. *J. Cell Biol.* **142:**117–127.

40. **Matter, K., and M. S. Balda.** 1998. Biogenesis of tight junctions: the C-terminal domain of occludin mediates basolateral targeting. *J. Cell Sci.* **111:**511–519.

41. **McCarthy, K. M., I. B. Skare, M. C. Stankewich, M. Furuse, S. Tsukita, R. A. Rogers, R. D. Lynch, and E. Schneeberger.** 1996. Occludin is a functional component of the tight junction. *J. Cell Sci.* **109:**2287–2298.

42. **McCormick, B., A. Nusrat, C. Parkos, L. D'Andrea, P. Hofman, D. Carnes, T. Liang, and J. Madara.** 1997. Unmasking of intestinal epithelial lateral membrane β1 integrin consequent to transepithelial neutrophil migration in vitro facilitates *inv*-mediated invasion by *Yersinia pseudotuberculosis*. *Infect. Immun.* **65:**1414–1421.

43. **McDaniel, T. K., K. G. Jarvis, M. S. Donnenberg, and J. B. Kaper.** 1995. A genetic locus of enterocyte effacement conserved among diverse enterobacterial pathogens. *Proc. Natl. Acad. Sci. USA* **92:**1664–1668.

44. **McNamara, B. P., A. Koutsouris, C. B. O'Connell, J. P. Nougayrede, M. S. Donnenberg, and G. Hecht.** 2001. Translocated EspF protein from enteropathogenic *Escherichia coli* disrupts host intestinal barrier function. *J. Clin. Invest.* **107:**1–10.

45. **Mel, S. F., K. J. Fullner, S. Wimer-Mackin, W. I. Lencer, and J. J. Mekalanos.** 2000. Association of protease activity in *Vibrio cholerae* vaccine strains with decreases in transcellular epithelial resistance of polarized T84 intestinal epithelial cells. *Infect. Immun.* **68:**6487–6492.

46. **Morita, K., M. Furuse, K. Fujimoto, and S. Tsukita.** 1999. Claudin multigene family encoding four-transmembrane domain protein components of tight junctions strands. *Proc. Natl. Acad. Sci. USA* **96:**511–516.

47. **Morita, K., H. Sasaki, M. Furuse, and S. Tsukita.** 1999. Endothelial claudin: claudin-5/TMVCF constitutes tight junction strands in endothelial cells. *J. Cell Biol.* **147:**185–194.

48. **Nusrat, A., M. Giry, J. R. Turner, S. P. Colgan, C. A. Parkos, D. Carnes, E. Lemichez, P. Boquet, and J. Madara.** 1995. Rho protein regulates tight junctions and perijunctional actin organization in polarized epithelia. *Proc. Natl. Acad. Sci. USA* **92:**10629–10633.

49. **Nusrat, A., C. von Eichel-Streiber, J. Turner, P. Verkade, J. Madara, and C. Parkos.** 2001. *Clostridium difficile* toxins disrupt epithelial barrier function by altering membrane microdomain localization of tight junction proteins. *Infect. Immun.* **69:**1329–1336.

50. **Perdomo, J. J., P. Gounon, and P. J. Sansonetti.** 1994. Polymorphonuclear leukocyte transmigration promotes invasion of colonic epithelial monolayers by *Shigella flexneri*. *J. Clin. Invest.* **93:**633–643.

51. **Philpott, D., D. McKay, W. Mak, M. Perdue, and P. Sherman.** 1998. Signal transduction pathways involved in enterohemorrhagic *Escherichia coli*-induced alterations in T84 epithelial permeability. *Infect. Immun.* **66:**1680–1687.

52. **Pickles, R. J., D. McCarty, H. Matsui, P. J. Hart, S. H. Randell, and R. C. Boucher.** 1998. Limited entry of adenovirus vectors into well-differentiated airway epithelium is responsible for inefficient gene transfer. *J. Virol.* **72:**6014–6023.

53. **Powell, D. W.** 1981. Barrier function of epithelia. *Am. J. Physiol.* **241:**G275–G288.

54. **Rahner, C., L. Mitic, B. McClane, and J. Anderson.** 1999. *Clostridium perfringens* enterotoxin impairs bile flow in the isolated perfused rat liver and induces fragmentation of tight junction fibrils. *Hepatology* **30:**326A.

55. **Rahner, C., L. L. Mitic, and J. M. Anderson.** 2001. Heterogeneity in expression and subcellular localization of claudins 2, 3, 4, and 5 in the rat liver, pancreas, and gut. *Gastroenterology* **120:**411–422.

56. **Riegler, M., R. Sedivy, C. Pothoulakis, G. Hamilton, J. Zacheri, G. Bischof, E. Consentini, W. Feil, R. Schiessel, J. T. LaMont, and E. Wenzl.** 1995. *Clostridium difficile* toxin B is more potent than toxin A in damaging human colonic epithelium in vitro. *J. Clin. Invest.* **95:**2004–2011.

57. Saitou, M., K. Fujimoto, Y. Doi, M. Itoh, T. Fujimoto, M. Furuse, H. Takano, T. Noda, and S. Tsukita. 1998. Occludin-deficient embryonic stem cells can differentiate into polarized epithelial cells bearing tight junctions. *J. Cell Biol.* **141:**397–408.

58. Sakakibara, A., M. Furuse, M. Saitou, Y. Ando-Akatsuka, and S. Tsukita. 1997. Possible involvement of phosphorylation of occludin in tight junction formation. *J. Cell Biol.* **137:**1393–1401.

59. Sansonetti, P. J., M. Arondel, M. Huerre, A. Harada, and K. Matsushima. 1999. Interleukin-8 controls bacterial transepithelial translocation at the cost of epithelial destruction in experimental shigellosis. *Infect. Immun.* **67:** 1471–1480.

60. Serrander, R., K.-E. Magnusson, E. Kihlstrom, and T. Sundqvist. 1986. Acute *Yersinia* infections in man increase intestinal permeability towards low-molecular weight polyethyleneglycols (PEB 400). *Scand. J. Infect. Dis.* **18:**409–413.

61. Simonovic, I., M. Arpin, A. Koutsouris, H. J. Falk-Krzesinski, and G. Hecht. 2001. Enteropathogenic *Escherichia coli* activates ezrin, which participates in disruption of tight junction barrier function. *Infect. Immun.* **69:**5679–5688.

62. Simonovic, I., J. Rosenberg, A. Koutsouris, and G. Hecht. 2000. Enteropathogenic *E. coli* dephosphorylates and dissociates occludin from intestinal epithelial tight junctions. *Cell Microbiol.* **2:**305–315.

63. Singh, U., C. Van Itallie, L. Mitic, J. Anderson, and B. McClane. 2000. CaCo-2 cells treated with *Clostridium perfringens* enterotoxin form multiple large complex species, one of which contains the tight junction protein occludin. *J. Biol. Chem.* **275:**18407–18417.

64. Skoudy, A., G. T. Nhieu, M. Mantis, J. Arpin, J. Mounier, P. Gounon, and P. J. Sansonetti. 1999. A functional role for ezrin during *Shigella flexneri* entry into epithelial cells. *J. Cell Sci.* **112:**2059–2068.

65. Sonoda, N., M. Furuse, T. Sasaki, S. Yonemura, J. Kathaira, Y. Horiguchi, and S. Tsukita. 1999. *Clostridium perfringens* enterotoxin fragment removes specific claudins from tight junction strands: evidence for direct involvement of claudins in tight junction barrier. *J. Cell Biol.* **147:**195–204.

66. Tafazoli, F., A. Holmstrom, A. Forsberg, and K-E. Magnusson. 2000. Apically exposed, tight junction-associated β1-integrins allow binding and YopE-mediated perturbation of epithelial barriers by wild-type *Yersinia* bacteria. *Infect. Immun.* **68:**5335–5343.

67. Takahashi, K., T. Sasaki, A. Mammoto, K. Takaishi, T. Kameyama, S. Tsukita, and Y. Takai. 1997. Direct interaction of the Rho GDP dissociation inhibitor with ezrin/radixin/moesin initiates the activation of the Rho small G protein. *J. Biol. Chem.* **272:**23371–23375.

68. Tomko, R. P., R. Xu, and L. Philipson. 1997. HCAR and MCAR: the human and mouse cellular receptors for subgroup C adenoviruses and group B coxsackieviruses. *Proc. Natl. Acad. Sci. USA* **94:**3352–3356.

69. Tsukita, S., and M. Furuse. 2002. Claudin-based barrier in simple and stratified cellular sheets. *Curr. Opin. Cell Biol.* **14:**531–536.

70. Tsukita, S., and M. Furuse. 2000. Pores in the wall: claudins constitute tight junction strands containing aqueous pores. *J. Cell Biol.* **149:**13–16.

71. Tsukita, S., M. Furuse, and M. Itoh. 2001. Multifunctional strands in tight junctions. *Nat. Rev.* **2:**285–293.

72. Turner, J. R., E. D. Black, J. Ward, C. M. Tse, F. A. Uchwat, H. A. Alli, M. Donowitz, J. Madara, and J. M. Angle. 2000. Transepithelial resistance can be regulated by the intestinal brush-border Na^+/H^+ exchanger NHE3. *Am. J. Physiol.* **279:**C1918–C1924.

73. Turner, J. R., B. K. Rill, S. L. Carlson, D. Carnes, R. Kerner, R. J. Mrsny, and J. L. Madara. 1997. Physiological regulation of epithelial tight junctions is associated with myosin light-chain phosphorylation. *Am. J. Physiol.* **273:** C1378–C1385.

74. Van Itallie, C., C. Rahner, and J. M. Anderson. 2001. Regulated expression of claudin-4 decreases paracellular conductance through a selective decrease in sodium permeability. *J. Clin. Invest.* **107:**1319–1327.

75. Viswanathan, V. K., S. Lukic, A. Koutsouris, and G. Hecht. 2002. Enteropathogenic and enterohemorrhagic *E. coli* disrupt tight junctions by distinct mechanisms. *Gastroenterology* **122:**A4.

76. Watarai, M., S. Funato, and C. Sasakawa. 1996. Interaction of Ipa proteins of *Shigella flexneri* with alpha5beta1 integrin promotes entry of the bacteria into mammalian cells. *J. Exp. Med.* **183:**991–999.

77. Wittchen, E., J. Haskins, and B. Stevenson. 1999. Protein interactions at the tight junction. *J. Biol. Chem.* **274:**35179–35185.

78. Wong, V. 1997. Phosphorylation of occludin correlates with occludin localization and function at the tight junction. *Am. J. Cell Physiol.* **273:** C1859–C1867.

79. Wu, S., K. Lim, J. Huang, R. Saidi, and C. Sears. 1998. *Bacteroides fragilis* enterotoxin

cleaves the zonula adherens protein, E–cadherin. *Proc. Natl. Acad. Sci. USA* **95:**14979–14984.

80. **Wu, Z., D. Milton, P. Nybom, A. Sjo, and K. E. Magnusson.** 1996. *Vibrio cholerae* hemagglutinin/protease (HA/protease) causes morphological changes in cultured epithelial cells and perturbs their paracellular barrier function. *Microb. Pathogen* **21:**111–123.

81. **Wu, Z., P. Nybom, and K. Magnusson.** 2000. Distinct effects of *Vibrio cholerae* haemagglutinin/protease on the structure and localization of the tight junction-associated proteins occludin and ZO-1. *Cell Microbial.* **2:**11–17.

82. **Yuhan, R., A. Koutsouris, S. D. Savkovic, and G. Hecht.** 1997. Enteropathogenic *Escherichia coli*-induced myosin light chain phosphorylation alters intestinal epithelial permeability. *Gastroenterology* **113:**1873–1882.

83. **Zolotarevsky, Y., G. Hecht, A. Koutsouris, D. E. Gonzalez, C. Quan, J. Tom, R. J. Mrsny, and J. R. Turner.** 2002. A membrane-permeant peptide that inhibits MLC kinase restores barrier function in in vitro models of intestinal disease. *Gastroenterology* **123:**163–172.

ENTERIC MICROBIAL TOXINS AND THE INTESTINAL EPITHELIAL CYTOSKELETON

James P. Nataro, Cynthia Sears, Alessio Fasano, and Robert J. Bloch

17

The cytoskeleton provides structure and organization to the epithelial cell. In addition to providing support and rigidity on demand, the cytoskeleton mediates adhesion of cells to surfaces and to each other, anchoring of proteins into the plasma membrane, and, to a large extent, control of cellular processes.

The cytoskeletal system is composed of three main categories of proteins (Fig. 1; see Table 1). (i) Structural proteins, such as actin and myosin, provide rigidity to the cell. (ii) Accessory proteins modulate the actions of the structural proteins, typically by binding at specialized domains. Accessory proteins may induce structural changes in their target proteins and/or may modify the cytoskeleton by bringing interacting proteins into favorable juxtaposition. Among others, cross-linking,

James P. Nataro, Center for Vaccine Development, Departments of Pediatrics and Medicine, University of Maryland School of Medicine, Baltimore, MD 21201. *Cynthia Sears*, Department of Medicine, The Johns Hopkins School of Medicine, Baltimore, MD 21205. *Alessio Fasano*, Center for Vaccine Development, Departments of Pediatrics and Medicine and Department of Physiology, University of Maryland School of Medicine, Baltimore, MD 21201. *Robert J. Bloch*, Department of Physiology, University of Maryland School of Medicine, Baltimore, MD 21201.

nucleating, and bundling proteins fall into this category. (iii) Cytoskeletal control proteins are responsible for executing the most dynamic changes in the cytoskeleton. These factors include the Rho family GTPases, as well as a plethora of phosphatases and kinases.

In an astonishing feat of evolutionary finesse, many pathogenic bacteria exploit the cytoskeleton to execute their pathogenic strategies. The results include cell death, exfoliation, and the induction of secretory or inflammatory states. Frank invasion of the intestinal epithelium is a common pathogenic strategy of enteric pathogens, but despite intensive and highly sophisticated investigations in a number of systems, the precise evolutionary advantage of this strategy remains a matter of speculation.

Perhaps not unexpectedly, given the elegance of biological systems, bacterial pathogens have coopted to their own purposes nearly every facet of the eukaryotic cytoskeleton. We shall see below that enteric pathogens modify the structural proteins of the cytoskeleton and divert or, more impressively, mimic the effects of cytoskeletal regulators. Themes in both convergent and divergent evolution are dramatically evident among these systems.

Microbial Pathogenesis and the Intestinal Epithelial Cell, ed. by G. Hecht
© 2003 ASM Press, Washington, D.C.

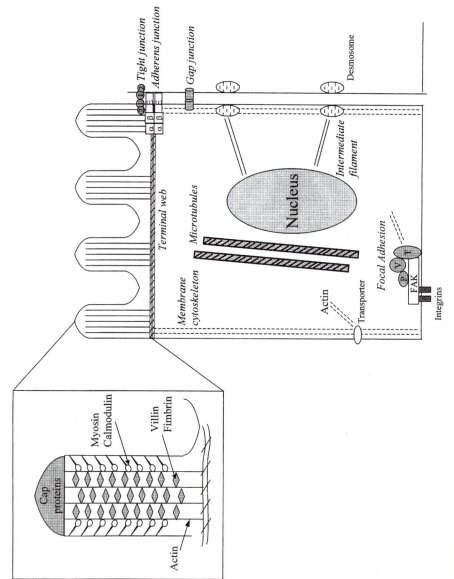

FIGURE 1 The enterocyte cytoskeleton. The enterocyte is supported by three major structural polymers. (i) Actin microfilaments are prominent in the microvilli, the terminal web, and the membrane cytoskeleton. Actin filaments connect to several proteins and protein complexes on the inner face of the cytoplasmic membrane, including adherens junctions, focal adhesions, and transporters in the basolateral membrane. (ii) Intermediate filaments connect to desmosomes on the basolateral membrane, giving rigidity and resistance to shear forces. (iii) Microtubules provide support and serve as tracks for molecular motors. Proteins illustrated at the adherens junction are the α- and β-catenins and the transmembrane protein E-cadherin ('E'). TJs comprise integral membrane proteins ("1" in Fig.), including occludins and claudins, and signaling proteins ("2" in Fig.).

TABLE 1 Major structural proteins of the cytoskeleton

Protein	Mol mass (kDa)	Function	Distribution
Actin	42	Forms filaments that provide structure to cell	Abundant (8 to 14% of total cell protein). Filamentous (F) and soluble (G) forms in dynamic equilibrium
α-Actinin	100	Cross-links actin filaments	Stress fibers, focal adhesions (FA)
Ankyrin	200	Binds and cross-links spectrin, stabilizing membrane cytoskeleton	Membrane cytoskeleton
Catenins	102 (α) 88 (α)	Cross-link actin filaments to adherens junction	Adherens junction
Claudin	Variable	Family of proteins comprising TJ strands; mediates barrier function	TJs
Cofilin	19	Actin-severing protein; regulates actin polymerization	Binds to actin filaments via 13-amino-acid F-actin binding domain
Ezrin	80	Microfilament-bundling protein; links actin filaments to PM	Microvilli; FA
Filamin	250	Actin-cross-linking protein; mediates loose actin gel formation	Cytoplasm
Fimbrin	68	Microfilament-bundling protein; forms tight bundles at core of microvilli	Microvilli
Gelsolin	90	Nucleates actin polymerization; cleaves actin at high concentration	Cytoplasm
Myosin I	111–128	Motor ATPase that interacts with actin filaments	Microvilli; stress fibers; PM; cytoplasm
Occludin	60	Integral membrane protein providing barrier function in TJs	TJ
Paxillin	68	Major component of FA; binds to talin and focal adhesion kinase	FA
Plectin	>500	Major cytoskeletal cross-linker	Hemidesmosomes, intermediate filaments
Profilin	15	Forms complex with G-actin to regulate polymerization	Cytoplasm
Radixin	82	Actin barbed-end capping protein	Adherens junction
Spectrin	220–240	Heterodimeric protein; major constituent of membrane cytoskeleton; stabilizes Golgi	Membrane cytoskeleton, adherens junction; Golgi
Tropomyosin	66	Stabilizes F-actin	Microfilaments
Villin	95	Tight microfilament cross-linking protein; forms actin bundles in microvilli; caps filaments at low calcium concentration, severs at high calcium concentration	Microvilli

STRUCTURAL ELEMENTS OF
THE CYTOSKELETON

The cytoskeleton of transporting epithelia contributes to the polarized structure that is required for directed transport of ions and metabolites. It also reinforces the cell-to-cell junctions that stabilize the epithelial layer and that separate the lumenal and serosal compartments.

The cytoskeleton of epithelial cells, as in most mammalian cells, is composed of three major structures: microtubules, intermediate filaments, and microfilaments. Microtubules, composed of tubulin and its associated proteins, play an important role in maintaining the overall cell shape and in the subcellular trafficking of membrane-bound vesicles destined for the apical or basolateral surfaces (67). Intermediate filaments of the cytokeratin subfamily stabilize the epithelial monolayer by forming a belt within each cell that attaches to the lateral membrane at desmosomes (56). Desmosomes are cell-to-cell junctions that, through their attachments to cytokeratins, create a cytoskeletal superstructure within and between cells that stabilizes and interlinks the entire epithelial monolayer (215). Actin-based microfilaments and the structures they support play an essential role in determining the polarity, compartmentation, and organization of transporting epithelia (47, 48).

Microfilaments are composed largely of actin monomers, termed G-actin, that polymerize to form filaments (F-actin) of variable length (158, 161, 186). Actin polymerization is directional. Under normal physiological conditions, new G subunits tend to be added selectively to the "plus" end of the filament, though growth from the "minus" end is also possible. These ends are also called the "barbed" and "pointed" ends, respectively, because of their arrowhead-like appearance when they are decorated with myosin heads, the globular actin-binding portion of myosin. Actin polymerization is accompanied by the hydrolysis of one ATP molecule for each monomer added. This enhances the directionality of actin filament polymerization and can

result in a process termed "treadmilling," in which monomers of G-actin are selectively added at the plus end and removed from the minus end, with no net growth or reduction in length of the filament. Thus, the formation of actin filaments is a pseudo-equilibrium dependent upon the hydrolysis of ATP.

Several proteins that bind G-actin, such as profilin, and proteins that sever F-actin filaments, such as gelsolin and cofilin/ADF (actin depolymerization factor), influence this pseudo-equilibrium and the average length of F-actin filaments (104, 127, 158, 161, 186). Filament lengths are also affected by "capping" proteins, such as actin-capping protein beta and tropomodulin, which interact selectively with the plus and minus ends, respectively. The initiation of new sites of filament growth is also regulated by actin-binding proteins, including filament-severing proteins, which create new plus ends, and two actin-related proteins, Arp2 and Arp3 (139–141). Arp2 and Arp3 form a complex with members of the Wiskott-Aldrich syndrome protein (WASP) family, which nucleate new filament formation from the sides of existing F-actin filaments. All of these interactions are subject to complex patterns of regulation (see below).

The properties of actin and its ability to interact with a wide variety of cytoplasmic and membrane proteins allow it to form several different structures fulfilling specific roles in epithelial cells. Indeed, the actin-based structures of epithelial cells are as highly specialized as the regions they occupy.

The apical epithelial surface is covered with ca. 1-μm-long microvilli, which are supported by F-actin filaments oriented into tightly packed, parallel bundles (47, 48). These filaments are cross-linked by several proteins, including villin, fimbrin, and espin (15), which bring neighboring filaments so close together that other actin-associated proteins, like myosin and α-actinin, cannot interact with actin in the interior of the bundle. Actin on the surface of the bundle, which is closely apposed to the microvillar membrane, can interact with other proteins, however. In particular, it interacts with an unusual form of myosin termed myosin I (because it has a single myosin head). Myosin I binds to the cytoplasmic surface of the microvillar membrane with its head appropriately positioned to be activated by actin (135). That activation affects the shape and motility of the microvillus and is likely to be essential for microvillar formation. Another class of proteins of the ERM (ezrin, radixin, moesin) family also participates in the formation of microvilli by binding simultaneously to actin and to cytoplasmic domains of integral microvillar membrane proteins (118, 220).

The parallel arrays of actin filaments are anchored at either end of the microvillus. The plus ends of the filaments attach to a dense array of proteins at the microvillar tip that have not yet been identified. The minus ends of the filamentous bundle are anchored within the terminal web, a highly interwoven set of actin and spectrin filaments that also contains myosin II (106), so called because it contains two myosin heads. The spectrin in this structure, termed TW260/240 for its location in the terminal web and the apparent molecular weights of its subunits (68), has not been well characterized. Intermediate filaments are concentrated just below the terminal web, presumably to provide additional stability.

Actin filaments in the cytoplasm of epithelial cells can be organized into thick bundles, or they can assume a looser, netlike organization. The filaments in the latter, which are typically found coursing through the cytoplasm, are composed of individual actin filaments that are loosely cross-linked to each other by large proteins such as filamin or ABP280 (191). In addition, microfilaments in the cytoplasm may be linked to other elements of the cytoskeleton, including intermediate filaments and microtubules, by giant macromolecules such as plectin (189).

By contrast, large bundles of actin filaments tend to concentrate in the cytoplasm near the basolateral membrane (158). These bundles, often termed "stress fibers," are more tightly organized than the cytoplasmic web just mentioned, but they are more loosely organized than the microvillar bundles of actin filaments at the apical surface. Typically, they also contain tropomyosin and α-actinin as well as myosin II. α-Actinin cross-links F-actin and, as it is a rodlike molecule of ca. 30 to 40 nm in length, tends to maintain spaces of about this dimension between neighboring actin filaments (130). These distances are sufficient to accommodate myosin II, which is typically organized into bipolar filaments with multiple heads all of which are capable of interacting with and being activated by actin. These filaments are joined in the middle by the myosin rod domain, which mediates the assembly of myosin II into thick, rodlike elements. Tropomyosin, which is expressed as several distinct isoforms in epithelia (196), lies in the shallow groove of the F-actin filament and regulates its ability to interact with myosin. Although these proteins could in principle distribute almost uniformly along the actin filaments of stress fibers, they tend to segregate into distinct, alternating structures that contain myosin II or α-actinin.

Unlike striated muscle, where the actin-myosin interactions are regulated by the binding of Ca^{2+} to the troponin complex, which in turn binds to tropomyosin, actin-myosin interactions in the cytoplasm of epithelial cells are regulated by phosphorylation and dephosphorylation of a small protein associated with the myosin head, called myosin light chain. This reaction is catalyzed by a Ca^{2+}-calmodulin-dependent myosin light chain kinase in a process that is also subject to regulation by signal transducing pathways (see below). Several additional myosin light chain kinases exist to serve a variety of cellular processes, and they too are subject to multiple regulatory mechanisms (103).

Stress fibers attach to the basolateral membrane in several distinct structures, including focal contacts, adherens junctions, and hemidesmosomes. Surrounding these sites of attachment to the membrane is a tight web of membrane-associated filaments composed of spectrin, which can bind to proteins and phospholipids in the membrane directly (117) or, more commonly, through another peripheral membrane protein called ankyrin (17). The spectrins at the basolateral membrane of epithelial cells are in the spectrin II subfamily, also known as "fodrin" (203). Ankyrin 3, also known as ankyrin G, mediates spectrin's association with a number of integral membrane proteins in epithelial cells, the most prominent of which is the Na/K-ATPase (137, 146), which plays a major role in transepithelial ion transport.

CELL JUNCTION AND ADHERENCE CONTACTS

Focal Contacts and Hemidesmosomes

Epithelial cells adhere to one another at their lateral surfaces through desmosomes, adherens junctions, and tight junctions and to a surrounding basal lamina through hemidesmosomes and focal contacts (65). Focal contacts are specialized adhesion complexes that form in cells grown in tissue culture, where the cells are tightly attached to the culture substrate, and in epithelial cells in vivo, where cells adhere to a basal lamina. Focal contacts are characterized by high concentrations of integrins that mediate attachment to the substrate or the basal lamina and that anchor the plus ends of actin microfilaments in stress fibers to the cytoplasmic surface of the basolateral membrane (174). It should be noted that the term "focal adhesion" (FA) is sometimes used to designate a particularly complex focal contact (65); here the terms will be used synonymously.

Integrins are heterodimeric proteins composed of α and β subunits, both of which span the membrane once. On the extracellular surface, the two subunits combine to form a kidney-shaped domain with affinity for one of a number of extracellular proteins, including vitronectin, fibronectin, collagen, sulfated proteoglycans, and laminin (132). The latter three proteins are key components of the basal lamina of intestinal epithelia and are known to interact preferentially with integrins of the β1 subfamily. The β1 subunit of integrin can associate with different α subunits to form heterodimers with varying specificities for extracellular proteins. Several α subunits, including 1, 2, 3, and 9, are expressed in the intestine.

The cytoplasmic domains of the β1 integrins provide binding sites for at least two proteins that mediate the anchoring of bundles of actin filaments to the membrane at focal contacts. α-Actinin binds with high affinity to the β1 subunit and simultaneously to actin (156). It also binds to tensin, which has actin-binding activity as well. Another cytoskeletal protein, talin, binds with lower affinity to the β1 subunit and simultaneously to vinculin (93), which is also capable of binding actin (98). Thus, the attachment of actin filaments to focal contacts is the result of multiple crosslinked interactions among vinculin, talin, and α-actinin complex and both actin and integrin.

Focal contacts are also sites at which a complex form of signal transduction occurs. As integrins accumulate in focal contacts, or are stimulated to aggregate in the cell membrane by other means, a tyrosine kinase cascade is initiated that results in changes in local morphology and, ultimately, in gene expression (174, 211). This cascade begins with a soluble tyrosine kinase, called focal adhesion kinase or FAK (175), which, like α-actinin and talin, binds to the cytoplasmic sequence of the β1 subunit of integrin (176). As FAK molecules are brought together by their integrin "carriers," transphosphorylation occurs, much as it occurs with receptor tyrosine kinases such as the epidermal growth factor receptors. Phosphorylation of FAK activates its tyrosine kinase activity, which can then act on a number of downstream components, including pp60src and paxillin, a structural protein that is tethered to the cytoplasmic surface of focal contacts by virtue of its ability to bind to vinculin (202). Paxillin, which binds FAK (91) and can also be phosphorylated on serine/threonine residues, is believed to serve as a nexus in the FAK signaling cascade.

Like focal contacts, hemidesmosomes are adhesion complexes on the basolateral membrane that bind via integrins (192). Adhesion is mediated primarily by α_6-β_4 integrin, which is selectively enriched at hemidesmosomes and which appears to interact preferentially with laminin in the extracellular matrix (187). Intracellular links to the cytoskeleton are primarily between the cytoplasmic portion of integrin and intermediate filaments and are mediated by plectin (149). Because plectin is a multipurpose cytoskeletal cross-linker (189), additional links to microfilaments and microtubules may form at these sites as well.

TJs

A key function of the intercellular junction complex between neighboring intestinal epithelial cells is the formation of selective barriers that permit the generation and maintenance of tissue compartments with distinct compositions. Tight junctions (TJs) represent the major barrier within the paracellular space (120). Evidence now exists that TJs, once regarded as static structures, are in fact dynamic and readily adapt to a variety of developmental, physiological, and pathological circumstances (Fig. 2). The adaptive mechanisms and specific regulation of TJs are areas of active investigation, and they remain incompletely understood.

The structure of TJs has been studied extensively. Freeze-fracture electron microscopy reveals that these contacts, which encircle the apical side of the lateral surface of each cell, are continuous strands of transmembrane particles that interact with similar structures of adjacent cells. These interactions define the paracellular permeability characteristics. A number of proteins are associated with TJs.

The first protein found to be associated with the TJ, occludin, was identified in 1993 (60). Occludin is composed of four transmembrane domains, two extracellular domains, and a long cytoplasmic carboxyl-terminal tail. Electrophoretic evidence suggests that the phosphorylated form of oc-

cludin appears to be the major form located within the TJ, whereas the less phosphorylated forms are found in the basolateral membrane and in the cytosol. Knockout experiments using murine embryo stem cells suggest that occludin is not the only component responsible for TJ competency (171).

Another large family of TJ membrane proteins, the claudins, was recently described (59, 136). The functional importance of claudins in forming fibrils was demonstrated by using a claudin-11 knockout mouse model, in which a complete loss of TJ fibrils was observed in Sertoli cells. It is believed that each of the 20 known claudins possesses selective permeability properties. Similar to occludins, some claudins on adjacent cells interact to form intercellular connections, while other claudins do not (61).

A third membrane protein, JAM (junction-associated membrane protein), was identified by raising monoclonal antibodies against endothelial cells (122). JAM has only one putative transmembrane domain, and the extracellular portion of JAM contains two domains with intrachain disulfide bonds, a theme typical of immunoglobulin (Ig)-like loops of the V type. JAM mediates homotypic cell-cell adhesion (122). It remains unknown whether JAM could form a functional barrier to prevent the free flux of ions and small solutes.

Zonula occludens protein 1 (ZO-1), ZO-2, and ZO-3 are proteins associated with the cytoplasmic side of the TJ. ZO-1 is a ~220-kDa peripheral membrane protein that is localized to the TJ in both epithelial and endothelial cells (190). ZO-1 has been demonstrated to interact with the actin cytoskeleton through spectrin (200). Other peripheral proteins, called ZO-2 and ZO-3, with molecular masses of 160 and 100 kDa, respectively, have been identified as ZO-1 binding proteins (73, 81). Sequence analysis shows that ZO-1, ZO-2, and ZO-3 are members of the large family of membrane-associated guanylate kinase (MAGUK) proteins. MAGUK proteins share several structural motifs, including variable numbers of PDZ domains, one *src* ho-

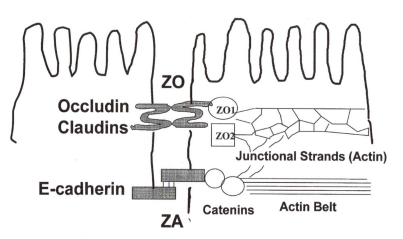

FIGURE 2 The epithelial junctional complex. TJs (zonula occludens or ZO) comprise transmembrane proteins (occludin, claudins, and JAM), which form a tight barrier in the paracellular space. Occludin and the claudins interact with the cytoskeleton via ZO-1, ZO-2, and ZO-3, and a series of downstream adapter and signaling proteins, ultimately interfacing with actin and actin-binding proteins. Basal to the ZO is the zonula adherens (ZA). This complex is attached to the apical actin belt via catenins and also to the junctional actin strands of the ZO. Catenins are involved in cellular signaling reactions (see text).

mology 3 (SH3) region, and one guanylate kinase (GUK) homology region. The PDZ domains of these proteins appear to interact with the C-terminal cytoplasmic tail of transmembrane proteins, and this is believed to be the mechanism of ZO-1-occludin interaction.

Several other peripheral membrane proteins have also been localized to the TJ, including cingulin, 7H6, Rab-13, $G\alpha_{i\text{-}2}$, and PKC (12). Another protein named symplekin has been described that is not only associated with TJs, but can also be localized to the nucleus (110). In cells that do not form TJs, symplekin appears to be localized only in the nucleus. Interestingly, ZO-1 can also be localized to the nucleus, but unlike symplekin, ZO-1 can be found in the nucleus under conditions of cell growth but not in fully differentiated epithelial cells (70). This pattern of dual localization for TJ components suggests that beside regulation of paracellular permeability, TJ structures might also be involved in the regulation of gene expression, cell growth, and differentiation (12).

Adherens Junctions (ZA)

The ~120-kDa intercellular adhesion glycoprotein, E-cadherin, is the key structural protein of the zonula adherens (ZA) in the intestinal epithelial cell (43, 74, 76, 79, 96, 219). This protein has a single transmembrane domain and five repeating extracellular domains (~75% of the protein) responsible for calcium-dependent, homotypic (i.e., cadherin-cadherin) cell adhesion (30). Cell-to-cell adhesion, in part, provides the cell surface with cues directing the development of intestinal epithelial cell polarity, in turn defined by the asymmetric assembly of the cytoskeleton, membrane domains, and vectorial transport properties of these cells (43, 74, 79). The cytoplasmic domain of E-cadherin binds to β-catenin, which is tethered to α-catenin and which connects the cadherin-catenin complex to the F-actin terminal web in the apex of the enterocyte (71) (Fig. 1). The terminal web provides linkages among the ZA, the ZO, and the F-actin core of the microvilli.

Additional catenin proteins, γ-catenin and p120[ctn], associate with the cytoplasmic domain of E-cadherin (8). Formation of this cadherin-catenin-actin complex strengthens cell-to-cell adhesion and provides the framework for association of a rich signaling network at the adherens junction that includes tyrosine kinases and phosphatases, protein kinase C, and small GTP-binding proteins (43, 77, 150). Cadherin-mediated adhesion is a highly dynamic process that not only is a target for signaling pathways (to regulate cell adhesion) but also sends signals (through the catenins) that regulate basic cellular processes (71).

The role and importance of the ZA-associated catenin proteins in signal transduction are incompletely understood and an area of active investigation (43, 75, 77, 78, 150). For example, β-catenin exists in two cellular pools, a cytoplasmic pool (normally complexed with a serine/threonine kinase, glycogen synthase kinase-3β [GSK-3β], the adenomatous polyposis coli [APC] protein and axin) and the membrane pool associated with E-cadherin. Cytoplasmic β-catenin is an essential signaling molecule in the Wnt/Wingless signaling pathway that contributes, upon activation and nuclear translocation, to normal embryonic development and differentiation (32, 50, 142). However, mutation of one or more proteins in this signaling cascade correlates epidemiologically with cancer formation (142). In contrast to the clear-cut role for the cytoplasmic β-catenin pool in nuclear signaling, conflicting data have been reported regarding the capacity for E-cadherin-bound β-catenin to activate nuclear signaling (13, 14, 18, 77, 78). Limited data suggest that γ-catenin may substitute for β-catenin and also participate in nuclear signaling. The p120^{ctn} protein appears to play a central role in defining the adhesive properties of the ZA and has both positive and negative effects on cadherin-mediated adhesion (7–9). However, p120^{ctn} consists of a family of proteins with up to 32 protein isoforms as products of both C- and N-terminal alternative splicing of a single gene. Four major human isoforms exist, but the functional importance of each isoform is, as yet, unknown.

REGULATION OF THE CYTOSKELETON

The organization and assembly of the actin cytoskeleton are influenced by the usual cast of the cell's metabolic regulators, including protein phosphorylation, Ca^{2+}, and small molecules such as phosphoinositides (PIs). Some key examples are the ability of Ca^{2+} to promote not only actomyosin interactions, but also the formation of new actin filaments by stimulating the severing protein, gelsolin (194). Phosphorylation of cofilin by LIM kinase has the opposite effect, inhibiting cofilin activity and its ability to sever filaments (33). PIP2 (phosphatidylinositol 4,5-biphosphate) released into the cytoplasm following activation of G-protein-linked receptors, promotes the dissociation of profilin and gelsolin from G- and F-actin, respectively. The dissociation of G-actin from its complex with profilin increases the pool of cytoplasmic G-actin, while the dissociation of gelsolin from the barbed ends of the filaments it has severed exposes newly formed barbed ends (194). Both reactions promote filament growth. Tyrosine phosphorylation of the cytoplasmic domain of integrin by Src can also affect the state of the actin cytoskeleton by inhibiting its ability to anchor at focal contacts (92). This in turn may weaken the organization of focal contacts and decrease cellular adhesiveness.

Although many other mechanisms that link receptor-induced signaling cascades to the cytoskeleton are still under investigation, results to date have implicated a unique class of small GTPases of the Rho, Rac, and Cdc42 family (163, 164). This family, of which nearly two dozen members have been identified in the human genome, controls the assembly of actin into its three most distinctive structures—stress fibers, lamellipodia, and filopodia—the last resembling microvilli structurally. Of particular interest in epithelial cells are Rac and Cdc42, which drive the assembly of lamellipodia and filopodia, respectively. Both proteins act by stimulating the ability of the ARP2/3 complex to nucleate the formation of new actin filaments (90).

The small GTPases are active when they are bound to GTP, but they are inactive in the GDP-bound state (Fig. 3) (163, 164). Thus, the state of actin polymerization is governed at least in part by proteins that control the form of bound guanine nucleotide. This control is effected by a set of proteins that interact with each of the small GTPases in distinct ways to promote the formation of the GTP- or GDP-bound forms.

The best understood of these are the GDP-GTP exchange factors, or GEFs, which activate the GTPases by promoting the formation of the GTP-bound form. GEFs typically have a "double homology" (DH) domain, which catalyzes GDP-GTP exchange, located just N terminal to a pleckstrin homology (PH) domain (31). Like other PH domains, those found in GEFs can bind PIP3, which increases GEF activity and promotes actin polymerization. Paired DH and PH domains are often found embedded in much larger proteins with structural motifs, like immunoglobulin (Ig) or spectrin-like domains, that presumably help to target the GEF to particular structures in the cytoplasm. Approximately 50 proteins with DH domains have been identified, i.e., more than two for each of the small GTPases. This suggests that several GEFs can act on the same GTPase and, perhaps, that some of the GEFs are active in only particular subcellular environments.

Just as the GEFs can stimulate small GTPases, GAPs, or GTPase-activating proteins, can inhibit their activity by promoting the hydrolysis of bound GTP to GDP (64). The prototypical member of this subfamily is RhoGAP, although several other proteins with GAP activity have also been characterized. Like the GEFs, GAPs can be much larger than the GTPases they regulate. Also like the GEFs, approximately 50 proteins with GAP-like sequences have been identified, but their specificities remain unknown. The mechanisms that regulate their effects on the small GTPases are now under investigation. For example, recent evidence indicates that tyrosine phosphorylation by cytoplasmic tyrosine ki-

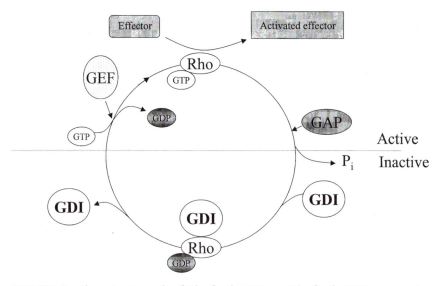

FIGURE 3 The activation cycle of Rho family GTPases. Rho family GTPases are active when bound to GTP and inactive when bound to GDP. They possess intrinsic GTPase activity, which is accelerated by GAP proteins or inhibited by GEF proteins. GDI proteins stabilize the GDP-bound state. Activated GTPases are commonly bound to the plasma membrane, but become detached on inactivation. The effect shown here for Rho is activation of an effector, illustrated with an asterisk. Many effectors exist, including kinases, phosphatases, phospholipases, and adaptor proteins. See text for details.

nases such as Src can increase GAP activity, leading to a decrease in actin polymerization (51).

The third class of proteins that regulate the activity of the small GTPases are the guanine nucleotide dissociation inhibitors, or GDIs, which bind to and stabilize the GDP-bound form, thereby inhibiting actin polymerization (173). While the structure of the GDI-Rho complex has been determined, the factors that govern GDI-Rho interactions are still poorly understood. Among the likely factors are phosphorylation and binding to ERM proteins, but the details remain to be discovered.

Although the small GTPases play an important role in determining the extent, form, and locus of actin polymerization, they control other important cytoskeletal functions as well. For example, Rho in the GTP-bound form activates Rho kinase, or ROCK (25), a cytoplasmic serine/threonine kinase that in turn phosphorylates myosin light chain. This reaction, as well as the parallel phosphorylation of myosin light chain phosphatase, also catalyzed by ROCK, activates the myosin light chain, promoting its ability to stimulate actomyosin activity. This provides an alterative pathway by which the activation of small GTPases can promote the formation and tensile strength of stress fibers (25).

BACTERIAL TOXINS AFFECTING THE CYTOSKELETON OF INTESTINAL EPITHELIAL CELLS

Given the many important roles of the epithelial cytoskeleton, it should come as no surprise that bacterial toxins have evolved to subvert these functions. What is astonishing, however, is the breadth and complexity of instances in which toxins target the cytoskeleton and its regulators. Below we consider many of the best-studied examples of this extraordinary phenomenon.

Toxins Affecting Rho GTPases or Actin

Four toxins produced by *Clostridium* spp. and a toxin produced by select *Escherichia coli* strains have been demonstrated to directly modify either Rho GTPases or actin. These toxins have been reviewed extensively (5, 26, 100, 101, 113, 162, 177–179, 207, 213) and are considered only briefly here. In each case, it is unclear how the precise mechanism of action defined for each protein toxin contributes to disease pathogenesis.

C. difficile **Toxins A and B.** *Clostridium difficile*, the only definitive microbiologic cause of antibiotic-associated diarrhea, produce two toxins often mislabeled as an enterotoxin (toxin A; molecular mass, 308 kDa) and a cytotoxin (toxin B; molecular mass, 270 kDa) (5, 101). In animal experiments, toxin A induces hemorrhagic fluid secretion and an inflammatory response and markedly damages ileal and colonic epithelium, whereas toxin B appears inactive. However, toxin B is a potent cytotoxin when tested in cultured cells in vitro. Recent experiments examining the action of toxins A and B on the human colon in vitro revealed that both toxins stimulated a decrease in intestinal barrier function (decreased epithelial resistance) (159), and, surprisingly, toxin B was more potent than toxin A. Additional studies of polarized intestinal epithelial cells in vitro revealed that both toxins diminished the barrier function of the cells without inducing cytotoxicity. However, the time course of resistance changes and the pattern of F-actin changes in the cells were distinct. This is notable since both toxin A and toxin B have been shown to act identically to monoglucosylate (at Thr-37) members of the Rho family of GTP-binding proteins. These divergent in vitro and in vivo responses to toxin A and toxin B suggest that the toxins bind to distinct receptors, differ in their ability to stimulate intracellular signaling pathways, and/or traffic differently in intestinal epithelial cells. Additional studies of the mechanism of action of toxin A confirm that the cellular response to toxin A is complex (160). For example, toxin A localizes to mitochondria within minutes of cellular application and prior to the onset of Rho glucosylation that requires approximately 15 to 30 min (84). Activation of multiple proinflammatory pathways (e.g., release of reactive oxygen species, activation of primary sensory neurons, stimulation of interleukin-8 [IL-8] production) occurs rapidly, and the pathophysiologic response to toxin A is attenuated by inhibitors directed at suppressing the inflammatory response (6).

***C. botulinum* C2 Toxin.** The C2 toxin stimulates secretion in mouse intestinal loops associated with intestinal damage and is not a neurotoxin like other *Clostridium botulinum* toxins (100, 162). Its role in human disease is unknown. The C2 toxin consists of two components that are not covalently or noncovalently linked. One component (105 kDa) mediates cellular binding, and the second (55 kDa) confers biologic activity. The C2 toxin exhibits substrate specificity by ADP-ribosylating β/γ-nonmuscle cytoplasmic and γ-smooth muscle G (monomeric) actin, but not α-muscle actins, at Arg-177, leading to loss of actin ATPase activity. α-Muscle and γ-smooth muscle actin isoforms differ only in three N-terminal amino acids, suggesting that this region of actin is critical to the substrate specificity of the C2 toxin. ADP-ribosylation of G-actin by the C2 toxin prevents its polymerization into F-actin and, over time, results in depolymerization of cellular F-actin accompanied by cellular rounding and eventually lysis.

***C. botulinum* C3 Toxin.** The C3 toxin ADP-ribosylates RhoA, B, and C (but not Rac or Cdc42) at asparagine 41 within the GTPase effector region (reviewed in reference 213). Inactivation of Rho leads to cell rounding, redistribution of actin, and inhibition of other Rho-dependent processes. While it is now clear that Rho GTPase proteins influence numerous cellular processes, it may be important that inactivation of Rho GTPases by C3 toxin regulates the organization of apical F-actin in polarized intestinal epithelial cells, resulting in enhanced TJ permeability (diminished barrier function) associated with dissociation of the ZO-1 protein from the ZO (TJ) (152).

The C3 toxin has no known role in human disease, and its ability to enter cells is poor (26). However, discovery of its mechanism of action enabled this toxin to be used as an in vitro probe to examine the mechanisms of other toxins altering the function Rho GTPases.

***E. coli* CNF-1 and CNF-2.** In limited studies, strains of *E. coli* producing cytotoxic necrotizing factor 1 (CNF-1) have been associated with human disease including enteritis, urinary tract infections, and prostatitis, whereas *E. coli* strains producing CNF-2 have been associated with enteric disease of farm animals (11, 22, 166). The amino acid content of the two toxins indicates that they are closely related, with 85% identical and 99% conserved sequences. Both toxins are cell associated, and it is hypothesized that they are delivered to host cells by the bacteria, possibly by a type III secretion system. The CNF toxins deamidate glutamine 63 (into glutamic acid) of Rho or glutamine 61 of Rac and Cdc42 (also members of the Rho GTPase protein family). This modification blocks GTPase activity (i.e., preventing the hydrolysis of GTP to GDP), locking the Rho proteins in their GTP-bound activated state and resulting in permanent activation of the proteins (22). Thus, similar to the C3 toxin, these toxins also serve as useful molecular tools to investigate the biologic function of the Rho GTPase proteins in a variety of cell types. The classic cellular phenotype associated with CNF-1 treatment is multinucleation with cellular enlargement and increased filamentous actin bundles. In intestinal epithelial cell monolayers, intoxication with CNF-1 results in diminished barrier function with enhanced F-actin filament formation (66). Specific effects on tight junctional proteins have not been reported. It is intriguing to note that in intestinal epithelial cell monolayers, both inactivation and activation of Rho GTPases result in diminished barrier function.

Type III Secretion Effectors

TTSS Considered. Type III secretion systems (TTSS) are highly conserved clusters of bacterial virulence genes that play multiple roles in the pathogenic schemes of their host bacteria. The secretion apparatae themselves are conserved among the various host organisms and are apparently derived from a common bacterial ancestor (4, 94, 147). Indeed, recent evidence suggests that all TTSS are descended from, or share a common ancestor with, the gram-negative flagellar apparatus (4, 147).

All known TTSS share certain characteristics. Each comprises a multiprotein secretion channel complex that mediates the passage of effector proteins through the inner membrane, periplasm, and outer membrane of the bacterial cell. It is thought that all TTSS also feature a needle complex at the bacterial cell surface through which the effector proteins are secreted (4, 21, 36, 193). In the cases of *Salmonella* spp., *Yersinia* spp., and *E. coli*, these needle complexes serve to directly inject effector and translocator proteins into the cytoplasm of a target eukaryotic cell (see below). The roles of several proteins in the assembly and function of the secretion apparatus are known, whereas other proteins are as yet cryptic in function.

Another notable feature of TTSS is that assembly and function of the systems are tightly regulated. In the cases of *Salmonella* spp. and *Yersinia* spp. (and presumably for other TTSS), the assembly of the apparatus occurs under conditions present in the mammalian intestine. Secretion of the effectors and injection into target cells occur in response to direct contact of the needle complex with the target eukaryotic cell membrane. It is thought as well that synthesis of the effectors is coupled to the secretion process, although this phenomenon may be different among the various systems and even for different effectors within the same system (27, 214). TTSS effectors do not exhibit classical signal sequences, and the precise signals permitting recognition by the secreton are still controversial (10, 116).

Each of the TTSS serves an important, highly specialized function in the pathogenic strategy of its bacterial host. We discuss here only those systems that act primarily on the intestinal epithelial cell. The *Yersinia* TTSS, thought to prevent uptake by professional phagocytic cells, has been reviewed elsewhere (3, 19, 20).

***Salmonella* SPI-1 Effectors.** Pathogenic nontyphoid *Salmonella* serotypes feature two TTSS on their chromosomes, located on *Salmonella* pathogenicity island 1 (SPI-1) and SPI-2. Although the secretion complexes of these two TTSS are homologous, they secrete different effector proteins and respond to different signals mediating their respective synthesis and function.

SPI-1 is activated in the lumen of the small intestine, where it injects its effectors into the cytoplasm of intestinal epithelial cells (62); SPI-1 effectors mediate invasion of the bacterium into the target enterocyte. The *Salmonella* entry process into epithelial cells and macrophages follows a distinctive pathway most similar to macropinocytosis (114). As a result, the invading bacterium becomes encased in a vacuole that is relatively safe from the actions of lysosomal enzymes and other antibacterial defenses. Effectors secreted by the SPI-1 system are responsible for executing this elegant strategy. In contrast to SPI-1, SPI-2 is activated upon entry into intestinal leukocytes and serves to subvert the intestinal immune response, thereby promoting persistence of the infection. The functions of SPI-2 effectors are not as well studied as those of SPI-1 and do not seem to target the intestinal epithelial cells. Therefore, only SPI-1 effectors will be considered here.

Nontyphoid salmonellae induce phagocytosis by normally nonphagocytic epithelial cells lining the small intestine. This uptake process begins with binding of the bacterium to the apical plasma membrane; the bacterium then stimulates the cell to form long filopodia, which wrap around the bacterium, ultimately leading to internalization. Remarkably, the plasma membrane re-forms behind the engulfed bacterium (the so-called "splash" phenotype). Importantly, the endosome in which the bacterium resides does not follow the typical phagosomal pathway and therefore represents an intracellular sanctuary for the bacterium.

Uptake of *Salmonella* spp. by epithelial cells is mediated by at least 13 secreted products of the SPI-1 TTSS. These products include SipA, SipB, SipC, SipD, SopA, SopB, SopD, SopE, SopE2, AvrA, SptP, SlrP, and SspH1. Together, these proteins effect the intricate and finely tuned cytoskeletal modifications that characterize the *Salmonella* entry process (221). Not unexpectedly, this process coopts the normal processes for cytoskeletal control, but remarkably, the bacterial proteins that interdict the cell's regulatory cascades often have little identifiable homology to their eukaryotic counterparts. Nevertheless, certain telltale signatures required for their actions, e.g., SH2 and SH3 domains, have been found among SPI-1 effectors.

In this context, it is not surprising that *Salmonella* sp. exploits the Rho family GTPase Cdc42 for its uptake: cells with dominant negative Cdc42 mutations are reduced in their ability to engulf salmonellae by more than fivefold (30a). The effect of *Salmonella* spp. on the GTPases is an example of the fine balance that pathogenic bacteria effect to induce disease, while eliciting only as much damage to the host as this mission necessitates (62).

SopE, SopE2, and SptP. Rac-dependent uptake of *Salmonella* spp. is induced predominantly by the balanced effects of GAP and GEF-like factors. Using a γgt11 library, Hardt et al. (80) implicated Rac and Cdc42 as SopE-binding partners and demonstrated intrinsic GEF activity. Rudolph et al. confirmed these findings and suggested that the kinetics of the SopE-Cdc42 complex formation and GTPase activation were similar to those of natural GEFs, even though SopE has no apparent structural similarity to GEFs (168).

The remarkable mimicry of GEF activity by SopE left an unanswered question. If the SPI-1 TTSS induced activation of Rac-1- and Cdc42-induced cytoskeletal rearrangements, how did the cell recover from this effect, knowing that normal cycling of Rho GTPases is finely tuned by competing GEFs, GDIs, and GAPs (see above)? SptP provided the answer: *Salmonella* sp. also employs a balancing act of GEF and GAP-like SPI-1 effectors. Fu and Galan (54) showed that SptP mutants of *Salmonella enterica* serovar Typhimurium induced ruffles and entered Ref52 epithelial cells, but that the plasma membrane did not re-form after bacterial internalization. They further microinjected Ref52 cells with purified GST-SopE, GST-SptP, or a mixture of both proteins. Microinjection of SopE induced membrane ruffling and actin microfilament reorganization; SptP microinjected alone induced a more general cytoskeletal disruption. However, when the two proteins were injected together, cells remained normal in appearance. The authors went on to show that SptP bound to Rac1 in vitro and that the effector stimulated in vitro GTPase activity of Rac and Cdc42, but not Ras or Rho. Importantly, despite no overall homology with mammalian GAPs, the authors demonstrated that SptP GAP activity was abolished by mutagenesis of an arginine finger motif, known to be required for activity of mammalian GAPs. In addition, these authors had previously noted that SptP is apparently bifunctional in its ability to modulate the cytoskeleton: whereas the N terminus confers GAP activity, the C-terminal domain of SptP encodes tyrosine phosphatase activity that is able to independently alter the cytoskeleton when microinjected (55).

SipA. Although the SopE/SptP system is clearly important, it does not wholly account for *Salmonella* invasiveness. Encoded within the SPI-1 TTSS is a set of effector proteins (the *Salmonella* invasion proteins, or Sips) with homology to the IpaABCD proteins of *Shi-*

gella spp. (95) (see below). Whereas there is some overlap of function and mechanism between Sips and Ipas, there is also significant divergence.

SipA (also called SspA) is an 87-kDa protein with homology to the *Shigella* IpaA protein (133, 223, 224). Mutations in SipA result in a decrease in *S. enterica* serovar Typhimurium invasion in the very early stage (5 min), although invasion returns to near wild-type levels by 15 min. Zhou et al. reported that SipA binds F-actin in vitro and in vivo (224). This binding activity greatly increased the stability of F-actin, decreased the critical concentration for F-actin polymerization, and inhibited actin depolymerization. These workers also showed that SipA forms a complex with the actin-bundling protein T-plastin; this interaction may be mediated via F-actin, perhaps by the induction of a conformational change in actin that promotes its binding to T-plastin. T-plastin was shown to localize to the site of *Salmonella* invasion, and T-plastin dominant-negative mutants did not take up *Salmonella* spp. at wild-type levels. These workers also observed that SipA mutants were less effective in inducing actin cytoskeletal reorganization and that the rearrangements were diffuse rather than localized to the site of ruffle formation and bacterial uptake. Their conclusion was that SipA promoted bacterial uptake by focusing F-actin filament formation in the vicinity of ruffles, thus increasing the stability and competence of the ruffles and filopodia.

Using MDCK cells, however, Jepson et al. (97) found that an *S. enterica* serovar Typhimurium *sipA* mutant was indeed deficient in early entry, but that ruffle formation and actin filament organization appeared unchanged compared with the wild type. These authors found that the bacteria appeared to remain within the ruffle for longer periods prior to uptake and that they did not remain localized to the center of the ruffle. Reconciling the observations of Zhou et al. and Jepson et al. is challenging, but both groups agree on a role for SipA in facilitating uptake; both also agree

that SipA does not bind vinculin, as does its *Shigella* homolog IpaA. The full effect of SipA on the cytoskeleton and ruffle formation remains unclear.

SipB. The SipB effector is homologous to the IpaB protein of *Shigella* spp. Like IpaB, SipB has been shown to induce macrophage apoptosis by binding to caspase 1 (89). Hayward et al. (83) have found that SipB localizes to the bacterial outer membrane and that purified SipB mediates the fusion of lipid bilayers. It is unclear whether or not this fusion process occurs in the setting of *Salmonella* invasion or even how such an effect could contribute to the invasion mechanism. Further work is required to determine the role of SipB in *Salmonella* pathogenesis.

SipC. SipC is essential for the invasion of epithelial cells by *Salmonella* spp. (82, 126, 155). Purified SipC directly bundles actin filaments via its N-terminal domain, while the SipC C-terminal domain nucleates actin polymerization. Both of these effects occur in the absence of additional eukaryotic cell proteins. McGhie et al. have shown that SipA potentiates the effects of SipC (126), lending support to the suggestions of Zhou et al. (224) that SipA acts via its interactions with actin and T-plastin.

SopB and SigD. SopB is a secreted effector protein, initially found in isolates of *S. enterica* serovar Dublin, which has been shown to be required for induction of fluid secretion in a bovine loop model (63). A SopB homolog (initially called SigD) is now known to be present in other *Salmonella* strains as well. Notably, although SopB is secreted by the SPI-1 TTSS, it is not encoded within SPI-1 (but rather within the SPI-5 island).

SopB mutants were initially reported to be deficient in fluid secretion and neutrophil infiltration in calf ileal loops, but the gene was not thought to contribute to invasiveness. Norris et al. (151) found that SopB possesses two motifs found in inositol polyphosphate 4-phosphatase enzymes. Recombinant GST-SopB was shown to possess broad-spectrum inositol phosphate phosphatase activity, which was abolished by site-directed mutation of the predicted active site cysteine residue. In *Salmonella*-infected cells, however, the authors of this work detected accumulation only of Ins $(1,4,5,6)P_4$, which was abolished by mutagenesis of SopB. This Ins $(1,4,5,6)P_4$ could have been derived from Ins $(1,3,4,5,6)P_5$, which antagonizes the effect of PtdIns $(3,4,5)P3$ in closing chloride channels. A specific effect of SopB on the function of chloride channels was demonstrated by intracellular expression of SopB in a tetracycline-inducible mammalian expression vector (49). Induction of inflammation by SopB may occur via activation of the proto-oncogene Akt, which is an activator of NF-κB (188).

Subsequently, Zhou et al. found that SopB did indeed play a role in *Salmonella* internalization, but in a manner at least partially redundant with SopE and SopE2: mutants in any one of these three SPI-1 effectors entered cells normally, whereas mutants in all three were deficient in internalization (222). SopB mutated at the proposed catalytic cysteine behaved like a null mutant, suggesting that inositol polyphosphate phosphatase activity interfaced with Rac/Cdc42 GTPase activity. The precise mechanism whereby this effect occurs is not yet known.

Other Salmonella *effectors.* A number of other secreted effectors of SPI-1 apparently play roles in virulence. SspH1 is a leucine-rich protein that is encoded by a minority of *Salmonella* strains (131) but may play a role in diarrheagenicity. SopA is a secreted protein that may also contribute to fluid secretion and inflammation in an as yet unknown manner (216).

Shigella Mxi-Spa Effectors. *Shigella* spp. are pathogens of the human colon. Data from animal models suggest that these pathogens interact with the intestinal mucosa at M cells overlying the colonic Peyer's patches; thereupon *Shigella* spp. enter and pass through the cells to enter the gut-associated lymphoid follicle. Here, the bacteria encounter and are engulfed by macrophages. However, instead of being killed by the host macrophage, *Shigella* spp. lyse the phagosome and, once in the cytoplasm, induce apoptosis and inflammation. This sequence results in the familiar inflammatory enteritis manifested most dramatically as dysentery.

Binding of *Shigella* spp. to the epithelial plasma membrane, a process most efficient at the basolateral surface, is followed by the induction of cellular extensions, rising several microns from the cell surface (1). These extensions then wrap around the bacterium, engulfing the organism in a phagosome. The formation of cellular extensions is induced by the rearrangement of cytoskeletal proteins. Vinculin is recruited to the plasma membrane in close apposition to the adherent bacteria. In addition, a dense network of actin, α-actinin, and cortactin assembles within the cellular extensions, whereas ezrin is specifically recruited to the tips of the processes and presumably links the actin network to the plasma membrane.

The GTPases Rho, Rac, and Cdc42 have all been shown to be involved in *Shigella* spp. uptake: treatment of cells with the clostridial exoenzyme C3 (which ADP-ribosylates RhoA) inhibits *Shigella* entry (2), while dominant-negative mutants of Rac and Cdc42 also display decreased uptake (138).

Like *Salmonella* spp., *Shigella* sp. requires the secreted effectors of a TTSS to invade epithelial cells. The *Shigella* TTSS is encoded within a ca. 31-kb region residing on the *Shigella* virulence plasmid. A large number of proteins could be secreted by the *Shigella* TTSS (24), but only a few of these have been studied in any significant detail, and in general less is known about *Shigella* entry than about that of *Salmonella* spp. The Ipa proteins, IpaA, -B, -C, and -D, are homologous to the Sip effectors of the *Salmonella* SPI-1. Remarkably, however, although the uptake mechanisms are comparable, the details of Ipa- and Sip-induced uptake differ significantly.

In concert, the Ipa proteins induce the formation of a membrane protein complex most reminiscent of the FA complex (see above) (129, 148). Although signficant details remain to be elucidated, it has been shown convincingly that IpaB and IpaC form a complex in the extracellular environment and that this complex is sufficient to mediate the internalization of latex beads into epithelial cells in culture (129). The IpaB-IpaC complex binds to both $\alpha_5\beta_1$ integrin and CD44, the hyaluronan receptor. CHO cells overexpressing $\alpha_5\beta_1$ integrin displayed increased internalization of *Shigella* spp. (210). Likewise, pretreatment of cells with anti-CD44 antibodies may also decrease uptake (184, 199).

Purified IpaB-IpaC complexes bind to cells and trigger actin polymerization and the formation of filopodia and lamellipodia (199). Notably, however, the IpaB-IpaC complex alone does not trigger all the cytoskeletal rearrangements induced by wild-type *Shigella* spp. The IpaA protein has been shown to bind vinculin (23, 198), which, as noted above, is recruited to the immediate vicinity of adherent bacteria. It has been suggested that IpaA and the IpaB-IpaC complex work in concert, therefore, to promote efficient internalization of *Shigella* spp. and by analogous mechanisms. Both vinculin and ezrin are multidomain proteins that comprise binding domains for actin in one domain and the membrane or membrane-associated proteins in the other. In the inactive conformation, both vinculin (34, 98, 99) and ezrin (201) are folded, thereby concealing the respective binding domains. Upon activation, these proteins unfold to reveal and activate their binding domains and thereby serve to establish a link between actin microfilaments and the plasma membrane, typically as part of the FA complex. Thus, expression of IpaA is thought to activate the actin-binding ability of vinculin, whereas

binding of IpaB-IpaC to the CD44 receptor provides a similar signal to ezrin. The secretion of these three effectors may be sufficient to effect cytoskeletal rearrangements that act via Rho GTPases to trigger bacterial engulfment. However, significant questions remain. It has not been established with certainty that the Ipa proteins work exclusively at the level of the plasma membrane, or whether they are actively injected into the cytoplasm like the *Salmonella* effectors. Clearly the *Shigella* TTSS is capable of injecting proteins into the eukaryotic cell upon contact (197), but the relative contributions of cytoplasmic and membrane-bound effectors are not clearly established. In addition, it is likely that there are other effectors that may play additional roles in the invasion process.

***E. coli* LEE effectors.** Enteropathogenic *E. coli* (EPEC) and enterohemorrhagic *E. coli* (EHEC) induce striking rearrangements of the host cell cytoskeleton by virtue of their related chromosomally encoded TTSS. The TTSS of each is encoded on an island called the locus of enterocyte effacement (LEE) island (105, 125, 212). When expressed in *E. coli* K-12, the 35-kb LEE island is sufficient to mediate bacterial attachment and induction of the characteristic attaching and effacing (A/E) phenotype (125). Proteins known to be secreted by the LEE TTSS include EspA, EspB, EspD, EspF, EspG, Tir, and Map.

EspABD. EspB and D are secreted LEE proteins that are thought to be part of the translocation apparatus, most likely serving as the pore through which other effector proteins enter the eukaryotic cell. However, when expressed within cultured HeLa cells via a mammalian expression vector, EspB was shown to induce cytoskeletal rearrangements (195). Thus, this protein may serve more than one function, including serving as a cytoskeletal toxin in addition to facilitating delivery of other effectors. EspA assembles into a filamentous surface organelle that serves as an accessory bacterial adhesin (111).

EspF. EspF is a 206-amino-acid protein encoded within the EPEC and EHEC LEE regions. Although the protein has been shown to be a secreted TTSS effector, and indeed to be injected into eukaryotic cells, it is not required for induction of the A/E lesion (128). EspF features several (two to five) 19-amino-acid proline-rich repeat regions, which resemble the eukaryotic proline-rich repeats known to interact with the SH-3 domains implicated in signal transduction. Crane et al. expressed EspF in Cos and HeLa cells using mammalian expression vectors and demonstrated that EspF induced cellular apoptosis (35). McNamara et al. demonstrated that EspF is required for EPEC-induced loss of transepithelial electric resistance, increased monolayer permeability, and redistribution of TJ-associated occludin in T84 monolayers (128). By complementing an *espF* mutant with *espF* under the control of an inducible promoter, the investigators showed that the drop in transepithelial resistance exhibited a dose-response effect with increasing *espF* expression. EspF may be a multifunctional effector whose full mode of action is as yet uncharacterized.

Tir. The identification of Tir marked the first time a bacterial pathogen was found to adhere to eukaryotic cells by virtue of a receptor that was of bacterial origin (107). Finlay and colleagues had initially suggested that intimin mediated binding to host membranes by virtue of a ca. 90-kDa protein (so-called Hp90), which was shown to be tyrosine-phosphorylated during formation of the A/E lesion (167). Surprisingly, however, further experiments showed that Hp90 actually originated as a 78-kDa EPEC protein which was injected into the cell by the LEE TTSS and which spuriously migrates as the larger species after several phosphorylation events (107). We now know that mature phosphorylated Tir assumes a hairpin-like transmembrane structure: the N and C termini are anchored within the

eukaryotic cell, and the central portion, to which the C terminus of intimin binds, protrudes to the cell exterior (37, 119).

In addition to serving as the anchor for bacterial adherence to the cell, Tir serves as the catalyst for the cytoskeletal rearrangements that form the A/E lesion. A series of reports have described the direct binding of purified Tir to FA proteins, including α-actinin, talin, and vinculin (28, 53, 69). Finlay and coworkers have shown recently that phosphorylated Tir tyrosine residue 474 binds directly to the adapter protein Nck, which is required for the recruitment of N-WASP and the Arp2/3 complex to the site of bacterial attachment, giving rise, in turn, to the characteristic pedestal complex (72, 102). Moreover, these investigators showed that cells with mutant Nck alleles did not form A/E lesions when infected with EPEC. This report may provide the vital link between phosphorylation of Tir and the molecular interactions that constitute the nucleation of actin beneath the bacterium and the abundant polymerization of actin microfilaments. This series of cytoskeletal rearrangements gives rise to the characteristic A/E pedestal. Interestingly, EHEC Tir does not feature a tyrosine at residue 474. Instead, an unmodified phenylalanine residue apparently serves a similar function to Y474 of EPEC Tir (40).

Intimin represents the ligand of Tir and, as such, promotes the cytoskeletal effects associated with the latter. However, intimin apparently also binds other receptors endogenous to the eukaryotic cell. β_1-Integrin (52) and nucleolin (183) have each been suggested as receptors for intimin binding. Binding to each of these molecules could result in signal transduction; indeed, intimin expressed on latex beads induced elongation of microvilli in the absence of Tir (157).

Map. Kenny and Jepson found that so-called *orf19*, located immediately upstream of the *tir* gene, encoded a ca. 20-kDa protein that was secreted via the LEE TTSS (109). Interestingly, the Orf19 predicted protein was found to feature a putative mitochondrial pre-sequence cleavage site. These authors demonstrated that the Orf19 protein was localized by cellular fractionation to the detergent-insoluble fraction and that the Orf19 protein colocalized with mitochondria by immunofluorescence microscopy. Moreover, the authors found that mitochondria of EPEC-infected cells failed to label with the cationic mitochondrion-specific fluoroprobe tetramethyl-rhodamine, which labels mitochondria only in the presence of native mitochondrial membrane potential. Orf19 null mutants did not induce abnormalities of mitochondrial staining with this probe. Thus, the authors conclude that Orf19, renamed Map for mitochondrial-associated protein, is a TTSS effector that specifically poisons cellular mitochondria. Although a role for this protein in pathogenesis is not yet apparent, the authors speculate that it could either induce activation of ATP-sensitive ion channels or perhaps play a role in modulating apoptotic pathways.

More recently, Kenny et al. have suggested that Map may have GAP-like activity and that it may counterbalance the effects of Tir on the cytoskeleton (108). This strategy is reminiscent of the finely tuned actions of the *Salmonella* TTSS effectors.

EspG. EspG is a 44-kDa effector of the LEE TTSS that has significant similarity to the VirA protein of *Shigella* spp. EspG has been shown to be injected into epithelials cells, although an EPEC EspG mutant did not reveal any differences compared with the wild type in in vitro interaction with epithelial cells. The precise role of EspG in EPEC infection is as yet undefined.

Protease Toxins

BFT, a Zinc-Dependent Metalloprotease Toxin. *Bacteroides fragilis* toxin (BFT) is encoded by a gene, *bft*, consisting of one open reading frame of 1,191 nucleotides that predicts a protein of 397 amino acid residues (181, 217). A comparison of the N-terminal

sequence determined from purified BFT with the predicted protein from the nucleotide sequence suggests that BFT is synthesized with three consecutive peptide domains: pre (signal) sequence (18 amino acid residues), propeptide (193 amino acid residues), and the mature protein (186 amino acid residues). This structure suggests that BFT belongs to the intramolecular chaperone protease family (181). Covalently linked propeptides in this family (serving as the intramolecular chaperone) are essential to both proper protein folding for biologic activity and secretion of the biologically active protein. Currently, no details are available on the intracellular synthesis, processing, and secretion of the BFT protein by enterotoxigenic *B. fragilis* (ETBF) strains. Three distinct chromosomal *bft* sequences (termed *bft-1*, *bft-2*, and *bft-3*) have been reported that are 92 to 96% identical in their predicted amino acid sequences, with the majority (>90%) of the amino acid differences identified in the mature toxin protein (217). BFT proteins purified from culture supernatants of ETBF strains secreting these distinct BFT isotypes exhibit biochemical differences but only modest changes in biologic activity to date.

BFT exhibits two major biologic activities: stimulation of secretion in ligated ileal and colonic segments (lambs, calves, rabbits, and rats) and alteration of the morphology of epithelial cells (e.g., HT29/Cl, T84, Caco-2, MDCK) capable of forming TJ complexes (i.e., ZO and ZA) (29, 112, 154, 169, 170, 180, 181, 218). BFT does not exhibit biologic activity on epithelial cell lines (such as HeLa or Hep-2) that do not polarize. The cloned HT29/C1 cell line, human colonic carcinoma cells, has been studied most extensively as a model for investigating the mechanism of action of BFT. These cells exhibit a rapid and striking change in morphology when exposed to BFT without a loss of viability (170). Available data using inhibitors of endosomal function and intracellular vesicular trafficking suggest that BFT is not internalized and, thus, is thought to modify cell structure and function from an extracellular location (218). The half-maximal concentration of BFT-2 altering HT29/C1 cell morphology is ~12.5 pM, whereas it is ~1 nM in polarized T84 monolayers. Only 0.5 pM (0.01 ng/ml) BFT is required to alter HT29/C1 cell morphology after an 18-h incubation. The potency of BFT in modifying intestinal epithelial cell structure and function is consistent with the hypothesis that ETBF strains (presumably with release of small amounts of BFT) stimulate acute and possibly chronic intestinal pathology.

Intestinal tissues exhibit a submucosal inflammatory response when infected with ETBF or treated with purified BFT (181, 182). Higher doses of BFT lead to secretion of mildly hemorrhagic fluid with patchy mucosal wall hemorrhage. Consistent with these observations, BFT stimulates intestinal epithelial cells in vitro to secrete the polymorphonuclear cell chemoattractant IL-8, in a dose-dependent manner. It is unknown if BFT stimulates proinflammatory chemokine secretion in vivo in animals or humans. No pathology from human disease or studies to evaluate intestinal inflammation in human ETBF disease is yet available.

To date, all of the pathophysiologic outcomes following BFT treatment of intestinal epithelial cells have been linked to coincident morphologic changes in these cells. When polarized monolayers of epithelial cells (T84, MDCK, HT29, HT29/C1, Caco-2) are treated with BFT in vitro, BFT decreases the resistance of the epithelial monolayers in a dose- and time-dependent manner (29, 153, and C. L. Sears, unpublished observations). Electron microscopic analysis of T84 monolayers after BFT treatment reveals swollen cells in which apical F-actin staining is diminished and the microvilli are unraveled. Between some cells there is complete effacement of the ZO (TJ) and the ZA (29). However, increased F-actin is detected at the basolateral pole of the intestinal epithelial cells, suggesting that BFT stimulates a dynamic restructuring of cellular F-actin via as yet unknown mechanisms. Consistent with this hypothesis, total F-actin content of BFT-treated cells is unchanged. Similar structural and pathophysio-

logic changes are observed in human colon examined in vitro (165).

Recent data indicate that BFT acts as a protease, consistent with the predictions of its gene structure (134, 218). Of the cellular structural proteins examined, only E-cadherin, the major structural protein of the ZA, is cleaved by BFT in a time- and concentration-dependent manner (218). Onset of E-cadherin cleavage is detected within 1 min in HT29/C1 cells, preceding the first detected morphology changes (detected at ca. 10 min); similarly, resynthesis of E-cadherin correlates with recovery of HT29/C1 cell morphology. Additional studies suggest that cleavage of E-cadherin by BFT is a two-step process in which the extracellular domain of E-cadherin is first degraded in an ATP-independent manner (potentially directly mediated by BFT), followed by the degradation of the intracellular domain of E-cadherin in an ATP-dependent manner (potentially mediated by one or more cellular proteases). BFT was the first bacterial toxin identified to remodel the intestinal epithelial cytoskeleton and F-actin architecture via cleavage of a cell surface molecule.

Serine Protease Autotransporters of Enterobacteriaceae. A growing number of proteins have been found to be secreted through the gram-negative outer membrane in a mechanism similar to that first described for the IgA protease of *Neisseria* spp. (88). Proteins secreted by this so-called autotransporter mechanism carry a dedicated C-terminal domain, which is thought to fold into a beta-barrel, through which the mature protein exits the bacterium. A family of these secreted proteins possesses a functional serine protease motif at a conserved position. The proteases cleave a variety of substrates and are thought to execute a variety of functions for their respective pathogens (86).

One family of these proteases, called the SPATEs (serine protease autotransporters of *Enterobacteriaceae*), are expressed by diarrheagenic and uropathogenic *E. coli* and *Shigella* strains (86). They are generally the most abundant proteins in the supernatants of their host strains when grown in laboratory conditions. Several have been shown to induce cytopathic effects, but the precise roles in pathogenesis have not been determined for any of these proteins.

Many strains of enteroaggregative *E. coli* (EAEC) carry the gene for a SPATE protein called Pet (plasmid-encoded toxin) (42, 85, 143–145). Navarro-Garcia et al. showed that the Pet protein induced rounding of HEp-2 and HT-29 cells in culture. Although actin microfilaments were dissolved, no cleavage of actin was detected. In vitro organ cultures of pediatric colonic tissue revealed that EAEC strain 042 induced less mucosal damage in the absence of an intact *pet* gene. In addition, Pet was shown to elicit enterotoxic effects on rat jejunal tissue mounted in an Ussing chamber.

Pet appears to act intracellularly. Studies using confocal microscopy reveal internalization and trafficking of the toxin in epithelial cells, and the effects of Pet are blocked by preincubating cells with Brefeldin A (143). Recently, Sui and Nataro have reproduced Pet's cellular effects by expressing the toxin within the cytoplasm using mammalian expression vectors (unpublished observations).

Pet has been shown to cleave spectrin, a component of the membrane cytoskeleton (206), and disruption of spectrin in the membrane cytoskeleton precedes dissolution of actin stress fibers (Color Plate 6) (R. Cappello and J. Nataro, unpublished observations). Spectrin is thought to assist in maintenance of membrane domains, in providing stability and shape to organelles, and in linking the membrane to motors of transport and to the major filament systems (38, 39). Disruption of the spectrin system could induce a myriad of cellular abnormalities, including disorders of barrier function and ion secretion.

Other Toxins

Zot. Several microorganisms have been shown to exert a cytopathic effect on epithelial cells that involves the TJ complex. These bacteria alter the intestinal permeability either directly (i.e., EPEC) or through the elaboration of toxins (e.g., *C. difficile, B. fragilis*) (44). A more direct action on TJ permeability has been proposed for the ZO toxin (Zot) elaborated by *Vibrio cholerae* (16, 45). Zot is a single polypeptide chain of 44.8 kDa encoded by the bacteriophage CTXφ present in toxigenic strains of *V. cholerae* (208). Zot possesses multiple domains that suggest a dual function of the protein as a morphogenetic phage peptide for the *V. cholerae* phage CTXφ and as an enterotoxin that modulates intestinal TJ (204). Zot localizes in the bacterial outer membrane of *V. cholerae*, with subsequent cleavage and secretion of a C-terminal fragment in the host intestinal milieu (204). Structure-function analysis of the toxin suggested that these two fragments have distinctive biological functions (41). Its ~33-kDa N-terminal portion possesses homology with pI proteins of other filamentous bacteriophages (204) and, therefore, is possibly involved in the CTXφ phage assembly, while the ~12-kDa C-terminal fragment of the toxin seems responsible for the permeating action on intestinal TJ (41). Interestingly, the Zot C-terminal fragment shares a putative receptor-binding motif with zonulin, the recently described Zot mammalian analog involved in TJ modulation (209). Amino acid comparison between the Zot active fragment and zonulin, combined with site-directed mutagenesis experiments, confirmed the presence of an octapeptide receptor-binding domain toward the N terminus of the processed Zot (41).

Zot effects on TJ modulation are mediated by a cascade of intracellular events that lead to a PKCα-dependent polymerization of actin microfilaments strategically localized to regulate the paracellular pathway (45). The toxin exerts this effect by interacting with the zonulin surface receptor, whose distribution varies within the intestine. The zonulin receptor is detectable in the jejunum and distal ileum, but not in the colon, and decreases along the villous-crypt axis (46). This receptor distribution coincides with the regional effect of Zot on intestinal permeability (46) and with the preferential F-actin redistribution induced by Zot in the mature cells of the villi (45). These data also suggest that the expression of the zonulin receptor(s) is upregulated during enterocyte differentiation. This hypothesis is supported by the observation that human intestinal epithelial CaCo$_2$ cells (which resemble the mature absorptive enteric cell of the villi), but not cryptlike T84 cells, express this receptor(s) on their surface (205). The paucity of Zot binding in the crypt area may also reflect the fact that this region is already leaky, as compared to the more mature epithelium of the tip of the villi (121), and thus might not need to express a significant amount of the zonulin receptor involved in TJ regulation.

Following binding to the zonulin receptor, Zot induces actin polymerization (45), followed by ZO-1-occludin and ZO-1-claudin disengagement (A. Fasano, unpublished observation) and downregulation of occludin expression. These changes occur as soon as 15 to 30 min following Zot exposure in both enterocyte cell lines and whole intestinal tissues and are temporally coincident with TJ disassembly.

Taken together, these data suggest that Zot regulates TJ in a rapid, reversible, and reproducible fashion and activates intracellular signals involved in zonulin-mediated modulation of the paracellular pathway.

CPE. Native *Clostridium perfringens* enterotoxin (CPE) is a 35-kDa peptide that acts as a potent cytotoxin in in vitro and in vivo studies (reviewed in reference 172). Detailed studies suggest that CPE binds irreversibly with several membrane proteins, yielding a pore-forming complex and resulting in rapid cell death. In rabbits, intestinal secretion is always associated with histopathologic damage. Recently, a carboxy-terminal fragment of CPE has been shown to cleave claudins 3 and 4, key proteins of the ZO, resulting in diminished barrier function without cytotoxicity (123, 124, 185). These data provided the first evidence indicating the physiologic importance of the claudin proteins in the barrier function of the ZO. Whether this mechanism contributes to the in vivo effects of CPE is unknown.

V. cholerae **RTX toxin.** The RTX ("repeats-in-toxin") toxin (encoded by *rtxA*) produced by El Tor and O139, but not by classical *V. cholerae* strains, elicits rounding of both epithelial and nonepithelial cell lines (115). This cellular phenotype occurs by an unknown mechanism that involves depolymerization of F-actin and cross-linking of G-actin into dimers, trimers, and higher multimers (58). Initial experiments examining the effect of mutant El Tor strains on the physiology of human colonic epithelial cell (T84) monolayers revealed that production of the RTX toxin was associated with a loss of barrier function consistent with its described in vitro effects on F- and G-actin (57).

CONCLUSIONS AND DIRECTIONS

Enteric toxins now provide a remarkable set of tools with which to dissect the complex interactions of the epithelial cytoskeleton. The field lies at the nexus of bacteriology, protein chemistry, and cell biology and provides a prominent example of synergistic research among scientific disciplines. The next era of research in this field will likely include pharmacology as clinical applications come to the fore. Such advances will occupy center stage in the field of cellular microbiology.

ACKNOWLEDGMENTS

Work in the authors' laboratories is supported by AI33096 and AI43615 (J.P.N.), DK48373 (A.F.), NS17282 and HL63404 (R.J.B.), and DK45496 (C.L.S.).

REFERENCES

1. **Adam, T., M. Arpin, M. C. Prevost, P. Gounon, and P. J. Sansonetti.** 1995. Cytoskeletal rearrangements and the functional role of T-plastin during entry of *Shigella flexneri* into HeLa cells. *J. Cell. Biol.* **129:**367–381.
2. **Adam, T., M. Giry, P. Boquet, and P. Sansonetti.** 1996. Rho-dependent membrane folding causes *Shigella* entry into epithelial cells. *EMBO J.* **15:**3315–3321.

3. **Aepfelbacher, M., and J. Heesemann.** 2001. Modulation of Rho GTPases and the actin cytoskeleton by *Yersinia* outer proteins (Yops). *Int. J. Med. Microbiol.* **291:**269–276.

4. **Aizawa, S. I.** 2001. Bacterial flagella and type III secretion systems. *FEMS Microbiol. Lett.* **202:** 157–164.

5. **Aktories, K., G. Schmidt, and I. Just.** 2000. Rho GTPases as targets of bacterial protein toxins. *Biol. Chem.* **381:**421–426.

6. **Alcantara, C., W. F. Stenson, T. S. Steiner, and R. L. Guerrant.** 2001. Role of inducible cyclooxygenase and prostaglandins in *Clostridium difficile* toxin A-induced secretion and inflammation in an animal model. *J. Infect. Dis.* **184:**648–652.

7. **Anastasiadis, P. Z., S. Y. Moon, M. A. Thoreson, D. J. Mariner, H. C. Crawford, Y. Zheng, and A. B. Reynolds.** 2000. Inhibition of RhoA by p120 catenin. *Nat. Cell. Biol.* **2:**637–644.

8. **Anastasiadis, P. Z., and A. B. Reynolds.** 2000. The p120 catenin family: complex roles in adhesion, signaling and cancer. *J. Cell. Sci.* **113**(Part 8):1319–1334.

9. **Anastasiadis, P. Z., and A. B. Reynolds.** 2001. Regulation of Rho GTPases by p120-catenin. *Curr. Opin. Cell Biol.* **13:**604–610.

10. **Anderson, D. M., and O. Schneewind.** 1999. *Yersinia enterocolitica* type III secretion: an mRNA signal that couples translation and secretion of YopQ. *Mol. Microbiol.* **31:**1139–1148.

11. **Andreu, A., A. E. Stapleton, C. Fennell, H. A. Lockman, M. Xercavins, F. Fernandez, and W. E. Stamm.** 1997. Urovirulence determinants in *Escherichia coli* strains causing prostatitis. *J. Infect. Dis.* **176:**464–469.

12. **Balda, M. S., and K. Matter.** 1998. Tight junctions. *J. Cell. Sci.* **111:**541–547.

13. **Barker, N., and H. Clevers.** 2000. Catenins, Wnt signaling and cancer. *Bioessays* **22:**961–965.

14. **Barker, N., P. J. Morin, and H. Clevers.** 2000. The Yin-Yang of TCF/beta-catenin signaling. *Adv. Cancer Res.* **77:**1–24.

15. **Bartles, J. R., L. Zheng, A. Li, A. Wierda, and B. Chen.** 1998. Small espin: a third actin-bundling protein and potential forked protein ortholog in brush border microvilli. *J. Cell Biol.* **143:**107–119.

16. **Baudry, B., A. Fasano, J. Ketley, and J. B. Kaper.** 1992. Cloning of a gene (zot) encoding a new toxin produced by *Vibrio cholerae*. *Infect. Immun.* **60:**428–434.

17. **Bennett, V., and L. Chen.** 2001. Ankyrins and cellular targeting of diverse membrane proteins to physiological sites. *Curr. Opin. Cell Biol.* **13:**61–67.

18. **Ben-Ze'ev, A., M. Shtutman, and J. Zhurinsky.** 2000. The integration of cell adhesion with gene expression: the role of beta-catenin. *Exp. Cell Res.* **261:**75–82.

19. **Bleves, S., and G. R. Cornelis.** 2000. How to survive in the host: the *Yersinia* lesson. *Microbes Infect.* **2:**1451–1460.

20. **Bliska, J. B.** 2000. Yop effectors of *Yersinia* spp. and actin rearrangements. *Trends Microbiol.* **8:** 205–208.

21. **Blocker, A., N. Jouihri, E. Larquet, P. Gounon, F. Ebel, C. Parsot, P. Sansonetti, and A. Allaoui.** 2001. Structure and composition of the *Shigella flexneri* "needle complex," a part of its type III secreton. *Mol. Microbiol.* **39:**652–663.

22. **Boquet, P.** 2001. The cytotoxic necrotizing factor 1 (CNF1) from *Escherichia coli*. *Toxicon* **39:** 1673–1680.

23. **Bourdet-Sicard, R., M. Rudiger, B. M. Jockusch, P. Gounon, P. J. Sansonetti, and G. T. Nhieu.** 1999. Binding of the *Shigella* protein IpaA to vinculin induces F-actin depolymerization. *EMBO J.* **18:**5853–5862.

24. **Buchrieser, C., P. Glaser, C. Rusniok, H. Nedjari, H. D'Hauteville, F. Kunst, P. Sansonetti, and C. Parsot.** 2000. The virulence plasmid pWR100 and the repertoire of proteins secreted by the type III secretion apparatus of *Shigella flexneri*. *Mol. Microbiol.* **38:**760–771.

25. **Burridge, K.** 1999. Crosstalk between Rac and Rho. *Science* **283:**2028–2029.

26. **Busch, C., and K. Aktories.** 2000. Microbial toxins and the glycosylation of rho family GTPases. *Curr. Opin. Struct. Biol.* **10:**528–535.

27. **Cambronne, E. D., L. W. Cheng, and O. Schneewind.** 2000. LcrQ/YscM1, regulators of the *Yersinia* yop virulon, are injected into host cells by a chaperone-dependent mechanism. *Mol. Microbiol.* **37:**263–273.

28. **Cantarelli, V. V., A. Takahashi, I. Yanagihara, Y. Akeda, K. Imura, T. Kodama, G. Kono, Y. Sato, and T. Honda.** 2001. Talin, a host cell protein, interacts directly with the translocated intimin receptor, Tir, of enteropathogenic *Escherichia coli*, and is essential for pedestal formation. *Cell Microbiol.* **3:**745–751.

29. **Chambers, F. G., S. S. Koshy, R. F. Saidi, D. P. Clark, R. D. Moore, and C. L. Sears.** 1997. *Bacteroides fragilis* toxin exhibits polar activity on monolayers of human intestinal epithelial cells (T84 cells) in vitro. *Infect. Immun.* **65:**3561–3570.

30. **Chappuis-Flament, S., E. Wong, L. D. Hicks, C. M. Kay, and B. M. Gumbiner.** 2001. Multiple cadherin extracellular repeats mediate homophilic binding and adhesion. *J. Cell Biol.* **154:**231–243.

30a.Chen, L. M., S. Hobbie, and J. E. Galan. 1996. Requirement of CDC42 for *Salmonella*-induced cytoskeletal and nuclear responses. *Science* **274**:2115–2118.

31. Cherfils, J., and P. Chardin. 1999. GEFs: structural basis for their activation of small GTP-binding proteins. *Trends Biochem. Sci.* **24**:306–311.

32. Clements, W. M., J. Wang, A. Sarnaik, O. J. Kim, J. MacDonald, C. Fenoglio-Preiser, J. Groden, and A. M. Lowy. 2002. beta-Catenin mutation is a frequent cause of Wnt pathway activation in gastric cancer. *Cancer Res.* **62**:3503–3506.

33. Condeelis, J. 2001. How is actin polymerization nucleated in vivo? *Trends Cell Biol.* **11**:288–293.

34. Craig, S. W., and R. P. Johnson. 1996. Assembly of focal adhesions: progress, paradigms, and portents. *Curr. Opin. Cell Biol.* **8**:74–85.

35. Crane, J., B. McNamara, and M. Donnenberg. 2001. Role of EspF in host cell death induced by enteropathogenic *Escherichia coli*. *Cell. Microbiol.* **3**:197–211.

36. Daniell, S. J., N. Takahashi, R. Wilson, D. Friedberg, I. Rosenshine, F. P. Booy, R. K. Shaw, S. Knutton, G. Frankel, and S. Aizawa. 2001. The filamentous type III secretion translocon of enteropathogenic *Escherichia coli*. *Cell Microbiol.* **3**:865–871.

37. de Grado, M., A. Abe, A. Gauthier, O. Steele-Mortimer, R. DeVinney, and B. B. Finlay. 1999. Identification of the intimin-binding domain of Tir of enteropathogenic *Escherichia coli*. *Cell. Microbiol.* **1**:7–17.

38. De Matteis, M. A., and J. S. Morrow. 1998. The role of ankyrin and spectrin in membrane transport and domain formation. *Curr. Opin. Cell Biol.* **10**:542–549.

39. De Matteis, M. A., and J. S. Morrow. 2000. Spectrin tethers and mesh in the biosynthetic pathway. *J. Cell Sci.* **113**:2331–2343.

40. DeVinney, R., J. L. Puente, A. Gauthier, D. Goosney, and B. B. Finlay. 2001. Enterohaemorrhagic and enteropathogenic *Escherichia coli* use a different Tir-based mechanism for pedestal formation. *Mol. Microbiol.* **41**:1445–1458.

41. Di Pierro, M., R. Lu, S. Uzzau, W. Wang, K. Margaretten, C. Pazzani, F. Maimone, and A. Fasano. 2001. Zonula occludens toxin structure-function analysis. Identification of the fragment biologically active on tight junctions and of the zonulin receptor binding domain. *J. Biol. Chem.* **276**:19160–19165.

42. Eslava, C., F. Navarro-Garcia, J. R. Czeczulin, I. R. Henderson, A. Cravioto, and J. P. Nataro. 1998. Pet, an autotransporter enterotoxin from enteroaggregative *Escherichia coli*. *Infect. Immun.* **66**:3155–3163.

43. Fagotto, F., and B. M. Gumbiner. 1996. Cell contact-dependent signaling. *Dev. Biol.* **180**:445–454.

44. Fasano, A. 1999. Cellular microbiology: can we learn cell physiology from microorganisms? *Am. J. Physiol.* **276**:C765–C776.

45. Fasano, A., C. Fiorentini, G. Donelli, S. Uzzau, J. B. Kaper, K. Margaretten, X. Ding, S. Guandalini, L. Comstock, and S. E. Goldblum. 1995. Zonula occludens toxin modulates tight junctions through protein kinase C-dependent actin reorganization, in vitro. *J. Clin. Invest.* **96**:710–720.

46. Fasano, A., S. Uzzau, C. Fiore, and K. Margaretten. 1997. The enterotoxic effect of zonula occludens toxin on rabbit small intestine involves the paracellular pathway. *Gastroenterology* **112**:839–846.

47. Fath, K. R., and D. R. Burgess. 1995. Microvillus assembly. Not actin alone. *Curr. Biol.* **5**:591–593.

48. Fath, K. R., S. N. Mamajiwalla, and D. R. Burgess. 1993. The cytoskeleton in development of epithelial cell polarity. *J. Cell Sci. Suppl.* **17**:65–73.

49. Feng, Y., S. R. Wente, and P. W. Majerus. 2001. Overexpression of the inositol phosphatase SopB in human 293 cells stimulates cellular chloride influx and inhibits nuclear mRNA export. *Proc. Natl. Acad. Sci. USA* **98**:875–879.

50. Filali, M., N. Cheng, D. Abbott, V. Leontiev, and J. F. Engelhardt. 2002. Wnt-3A/beta-catenin signaling induces transcription from the LEF-1 promoter. *J. Biol. Chem.* **277**:33398–33410.

51. Fincham, V. J., A. Chudleigh, and M. C. Frame. 1999. Regulation of p190 Rho-GAP by v-Src is linked to cytoskeletal disruption during transformation. *J. Cell Sci.* **112**(Pt. 6):947–956.

52. Frankel, G., O. Lider, R. Hershkoviz, A. Mould, S. Kachalsky, D. Candy, L. Cahalon, M. Humphries, and G. Dougan. 1996. The cell-binding domain of intimin from enteropathogenic *Escherichia coli* binds to beta1 integrins. *J. Biol. Chem.* **23**:20359–20364.

53. Freeman, N. L., D. V. Zurawski, P. Chowrashi, J. C. Ayoob, L. Huang, B. Mittal, J. M. Sanger, and J. W. Sanger. 2000. Interaction of the enteropathogenic *Escherichia coli* protein, translocated intimin receptor (Tir), with focal adhesion proteins. *Cell Motil. Cytoskel.* **47**:307–318.

54. Fu, Y., and J. E. Galan. 1999. A *Salmonella* protein antagonizes Rac-1 and Cdc42 to mediate

host-cell recovery after bacterial invasion. *Nature* **401**:293–297.

55. **Fu, Y., and J. E. Galan.** 1998. The *Salmonella typhimurium* tyrosine phosphatase SptP is translocated into host cells and disrupts the actin cytoskeleton. *Mol. Microbiol.* **27**:359–368.

56. **Fuchs, E., and K. Weber.** 1994. Intermediate filaments: structure, dynamics, function, and disease. *Annu. Rev. Biochem.* **63**:345–382.

57. **Fullner, K. J., W. I. Lencer, and J. J. Mekalanos.** 2001. *Vibrio cholerae*-induced cellular responses of polarized T84 intestinal epithelial cells are dependent on production of cholera toxin and the RTX toxin. *Infect. Immun.* **69**:6310–6317.

58. **Fullner, K. J., and J. J. Mekalanos.** 2000. In vivo covalent cross-linking of cellular actin by the *Vibrio cholerae* RTX toxin. *EMBO J.* **19**:5315–5323.

59. **Furuse, M., K. Fujita, T. Hiiragi, K. Fujimoto, and S. Tsukita.** 1998. Claudin-1 and -2: novel integral membrane proteins localizing at tight junctions with no sequence similarity to occludin. *J. Cell Biol.* **141**:1539–1550.

60. **Furuse, M., T. Hirase, M. Itoh, A. Nagafuchi, S. Yonemura, and S. Tsukita.** 1993. Occludin: a novel integral membrane protein localizing at tight junctions. *J. Cell Biol.* **123**:1777–1788.

61. **Furuse, M., H. Sasaki, and S. Tsukita.** 1999. Manner of interaction of heterogeneous claudin species within and between tight junction strands. *J. Cell Biol.* **147**:891–903.

62. **Galan, J. E., and D. Zhou.** 2000. Striking a balance: modulation of the actin cytoskeleton by *Salmonella. Proc. Natl. Acad. Sci. USA* **97**:8754–8761.

63. **Galyov, E. E., M. W. Wood, R. Rosqvist, P. B. Mullan, P. R. Watson, S. Hedges, and T. S. Wallis.** 1997. A secreted effector protein of *Salmonella dublin* is translocated into eukaryotic cells and mediates inflammation and fluid secretion in infected ileal mucosa. *Mol. Microbiol.* **25**:903–912.

64. **Gamblin, S. J., and S. J. Smerdon.** 1998. GTPase-activating proteins and their complexes. *Curr. Opin. Struct. Biol.* **8**:195–201.

65. **Geiger, B., A. Bershadsky, R. Pankov, and K. M. Yamada.** 2001. Transmembrane crosstalk between the extracellular matrix—cytoskeleton crosstalk. *Nat. Rev. Mol. Cell Biol.* **2**:793–805.

66. **Gerhard, R., G. Schmidt, F. Hofmann, and K. Aktories.** 1998. Activation of Rho GTPases by *Escherichia coli* cytotoxic necrotizing factor 1 increases intestinal permeability in Caco-2 cells. *Infect. Immun.* **66**:5125–5131.

67. **Gilbert, T., A. Le Bivic, A. Quaroni, and E. Rodriguez-Boulan.** 1991. Microtubular organization and its involvement in the biogenetic pathways of plasma membrane proteins in Caco-2 intestinal epithelial cells. *J. Cell Biol.* **113**:275–288.

68. **Glenney, J. R., Jr., P. Glenney, and K. Weber.** 1983. The spectrin-related molecule, TW-260/240, cross-links the actin bundles of the microvillus rootlets in the brush borders of intestinal epithelial cells. *J. Cell Biol.* **96**:1491–1496.

69. **Goosney, D. L., R. DeVinney, and B. B. Finlay.** 2001. Recruitment of cytoskeletal and signaling proteins to enteropathogenic and enterohemorrhagic *Escherichia coli* pedestals. *Infect. Immun.* **69**:3315–3322.

70. **Gottardi, C. J., M. Arpin, A. S. Fanning, and D. Louvard.** 1996. The junction-associated protein, zonula occludens-1, localizes to the nucleus before the maturation and during the remodeling of cell-cell contacts. *Proc. Natl. Acad. Sci. USA* **93**:10779–10784.

71. **Gottardi, C. J., and B. M. Gumbiner.** 2001. Adhesion signaling: how beta-catenin interacts with its partners. *Curr. Biol.* **11**:R792–R794.

72. **Gruenheid, S., R. DeVinney, F. Bladt, D. Goosney, S. Gelkop, G. D. Gish, T. Pawson, and B. B. Finlay.** 2001. Enteropathogenic *E. coli* Tir binds Nck to initiate actin pedestal formation in host cells. *Nat. Cell Biol.* **3**:856–859.

73. **Gumbiner, B., T. Lowenkopf, and D. Apatira.** 1991. Identification of a 160-kDa polypeptide that binds to the tight junction protein ZO-1. *Proc. Natl. Acad. Sci. USA* **88**:3460–3464.

74. **Gumbiner, B. M.** 1996. Cell adhesion: the molecular basis of tissue architecture and morphogenesis. *Cell* **84**:345–357.

75. **Gumbiner, B. M.** 1993. Proteins associated with the cytoplasmic surface of adhesion molecules. *Neuron* **11**:551–564.

76. **Gumbiner, B. M.** 2000. Regulation of cadherin adhesive activity. *J. Cell Biol.* **148**:399–404.

77. **Gumbiner, B. M.** 1995. Signal transduction of beta-catenin. *Curr. Opin. Cell Biol.* **7**:634–640.

78. **Gumbiner, B. M., and P. D. McCrea.** 1993. Catenins as mediators of the cytoplasmic functions of cadherins. *J. Cell Sci. Suppl.* **17**:155–158.

79. **Gumbiner, B. M., and K. M. Yamada.** 1995. Cell-to-cell contact and extracellular matrix. *Curr. Opin. Cell Biol.* **7**:615–618.

80. **Hardt, W. D., L. M. Chen, K. E. Schuebel, X. R. Bustelo, and J. E. Galan.** 1998. *S. typhimurium* encodes an activator of Rho GTPases that induces membrane ruffling and nuclear responses in host cells. *Cell* **93**:815–826.

81. **Haskins, J., L. Gu, E. S. Wittchen, J. Hibbard, and B. R. Stevenson.** 1998. ZO-3, a

novel member of the MAGUK protein family found at the tight junction, interacts with ZO-1 and occludin. *J. Cell Biol.* **141**:199–208.

82. **Hayward, R. D., and V. Koronakis.** 1999. Direct nucleation and bundling of actin by the SipC protein of invasive *Salmonella. EMBO J.* **18:** 4926–4934.

83. **Hayward, R. D., E. J. McGhie, and V. Koronakis.** 2000. Membrane fusion activity of purified SipB, a *Salmonella* surface protein essential for mammalian cell invasion. *Mol. Microbiol.* **37:** 727–739.

84. **He, D., S. J. Hagen, C. Pothoulakis, M. Chen, N. D. Medina, M. Warny, and J. T. LaMont.** 2000. *Clostridium difficile* toxin A causes early damage to mitochondria in cultured cells. *Gastroenterology* **119**:139–150.

85. **Henderson, I. R., S. Hicks, F. Navarro-Garcia, W. P. Elias, A. D. Philips, and J. P. Nataro.** 1999. Involvement of the enteroaggregative *Escherichia coli* plasmid-encoded toxin in causing human intestinal damage. *Infect. Immun.* **67**:5338–5344.

86. **Henderson, I. R., and J. P. Nataro.** 2001. Virulence functions of autotransporter proteins. *Infect. Immun.* **69**:1231–1243.

87. [Reference deleted.]

88. **Henderson, I. R., F. Navarro-Garcia, and J. P. Nataro.** 1998. The great escape: structure and function of the autotransporter proteins. *Trends Microbiol.* **6**:370–378.

89. **Hersh, D., D. M. Monack, M. R. Smith, N. Ghori, S. Falkow, and A. Zychlinsky.** 1999. The *Salmonella* invasin SipB induces macrophage apoptosis by binding to caspase-1. *Proc. Natl. Acad. Sci. USA* **96**:2396–2401.

90. **Higgs, H. N., and T. D. Pollard.** 2001. Regulation of actin filament network formation through ARP2/3 complex: activation by a diverse array of proteins. *Annu. Rev. Biochem.* **70:** 649–676.

91. **Hildebrand, J. D., M. D. Schaller, and J. T. Parsons.** 1995. Paxillin, a tyrosine phosphorylated focal adhesion-associated protein binds to the carboxyl terminal domain of focal adhesion kinase. *Mol. Biol. Cell* **6**:637–647.

92. **Hirst, R., A. Horwitz, C. Buck, and L. Rohrschneider.** 1986. Phosphorylation of the fibronectin receptor complex in cells transformed by oncogenes that encode tyrosine kinases. *Proc. Natl. Acad. Sci. USA* **83**:6470–6474.

93. **Horwitz, A., K. Duggan, C. Buck, M. C. Beckerle, and K. Burridge.** 1986. Interaction of plasma membrane fibronectin receptor with talin—a transmembrane linkage. *Nature* **320**:531–533.

94. **Hueck, C. J.** 1998. Type III protein secretion systems in bacterial pathogens of animals and plants. *Microbiol. Mol. Biol. Rev.* **62**:379–433.

95. **Hueck, C. J., M. J. Hantman, V. Bajaj, C. Johnston, C. A. Lee, and S. I. Miller.** 1995. *Salmonella typhimurium* secreted invasion determinants are homologous to *Shigella* Ipa proteins. *Mol. Microbiol.* **18**:479–490.

96. **Ishii, K., and K. J. Green.** 2001. Cadherin function: breaking the barrier. *Curr. Biol.* **11:** R569–R572.

97. **Jepson, M., B. Kenny, and A. Leard.** 2001. Role of *sipA* in the early stages of *Salmonella typhimurium* entry into epithelial cells. *Cell. Microbiol.* **3**:417–426.

98. **Johnson, R. P., and S. W. Craig.** 1995. F-actin binding site masked by the intramolecular association of vinculin head and tail domains. *Nature* **373**:261–264.

99. **Johnson, R. P., and S. W. Craig.** 1994. An intramolecular association between the head and tail domains of vinculin modulates talin binding. *J. Biol. Chem.* **269**:12611–12619.

100. **Just, I., F. Hofmann, and K. Aktories.** 2000. Molecular mode of action of the large clostridial cytotoxins. *Curr. Top. Microbiol. Immunol.* **250**:55–83.

101. **Just, I., F. Hofmann, H. Genth, and R. Gerhard.** 2001. Bacterial protein toxins inhibiting low-molecular-mass GTP-binding proteins. *Int. J. Med. Microbiol.* **291**:243–250.

102. **Kalman, D., O. D. Weiner, D. L. Goosney, J. W. Sedat, B. B. Finlay, A. Abo, and J. M. Bishop.** 1999. Enteropathogenic *E. coli* acts through WASP and Arp2/3 complex to form actin pedestals. *Nat. Cell Biol.* **1**:389–391.

103. **Kamm, K. E., and J. T. Stull.** 2001. Dedicated myosin light chain kinases with diverse cellular functions. *J. Biol. Chem.* **276**:4527–4530.

104. **Kang, F., D. L. Purich, and F. S. Southwick.** 1999. Profilin promotes barbed-end actin filament assembly without lowering the critical concentration. *J. Biol. Chem.* **274**:36963–36972.

105. **Kaper, J. B., T. K. McDaniel, K. G. Jarvis, and O. Gomez-Duarte.** 1997. Genetics of virulence of enteropathogenic *E. coli. Adv. Exp. Med. Biol.* **412**:279–287.

106. **Keller, T. C., 3rd, K. A. Conzelman, R. Chasan, and M. S. Mooseker.** 1985. Role of myosin in terminal web contraction in isolated intestinal epithelial brush borders. *J. Cell Biol.* **100**:1647–1655.

107. **Kenny, B., R. DeVinney, M. Stein, D. J. Reinscheid, E. A. Frey, and B. B. Finlay.** 1997. Enteropathogenic *E. coli* (EPEC) transfers

its receptor for intimate adherence into mammalian cells. *Cell* **91:**511–520.

108. **Kenny, B., S. Ellis, A. D. Leard, J. Warawa, H. Mellor, and M. A. Jepson.** 2002. Co-ordinate regulation of distinct host cell signalling pathways by multifunctional enteropathogenic *Escherichia coli* effector molecules. *Mol. Microbiol.* **44:**1095–1107.

109. **Kenny, B., and M. Jepson.** 2000. Targeting of an enteropathogenic *Escherichia coli* (EPEC) effector protein to host mitochondria. *Cell Microbiol.* **2:**579–590.

110. **Keon, B. H., S. Schafer, C. Kuhn, C. Grund, and W. W. Franke.** 1996. Symplekin, a novel type of tight junction plaque protein. *J. Cell Biol.* **134:**1003–1018.

111. **Knutton, S., I. Rosenshine, M. J. Pallen, I. Nisan, B. C. Neves, C. Bain, C. Wolff, G. Dougan, and G. Frankel.** 1998. A novel EspA-associated surface organelle of enteropathogenic *Escherichia coli* involved in protein translocation into epithelial cells. *EMBO J* **17:**2166–2176.

112. **Koshy, S. S., M. H. Montrose, and C. L. Sears.** 1996. Human intestinal epithelial cells swell and demonstrate actin rearrangement in response to the metalloprotease toxin of *Bacteroides fragilis. Infect. Immun.* **64:**5022–5028.

113. **Lerm, M., G. Schmidt, and K. Aktories.** 2000. Bacterial protein toxins targeting rho GTPases. *FEMS Microbiol. Lett.* **188:**1–6.

114. **Lesser, C. F., C. A. Scherer, and S. I. Miller.** 2000. Rac, ruffle and rho: orchestration of *Salmonella* invasion. *Trends Microbiol.* **8:**151–152.

115. **Lin, W., K. J. Fullner, R. Clayton, J. A. Sexton, M. B. Rogers, K. E. Calia, S. B. Calderwood, C. Fraser, and J. J. Mekalanos.** 1999. Identification of a *Vibrio cholerae* RTX toxin gene cluster that is tightly linked to the cholera toxin prophage. *Proc. Natl. Acad. Sci. USA* **96:**1071–1076.

116. **Lloyd, S. A., A. Forsberg, H. Wolf-Watz, and M. S. Francis.** 2001. Targeting exported substrates to the *Yersinia* TTSS: different functions for different signals? *Trends Microbiol.* **9:**367–371.

117. **Lombardo, C. R., S. A. Weed, S. P. Kennedy, B. G. Forget, and J. S. Morrow.** 1994. Beta II-spectrin (fodrin) and beta I epsilon 2-spectrin (muscle) contain NH2- and COOH-terminal membrane association domains (MAD1 and MAD2). *J. Biol. Chem.* **269:**29212–29219.

118. **Louvet-Vallee, S.** 2000. ERM proteins: from cellular architecture to cell signaling. *Biol. Cell* **92:**305–316.

119. **Luo, Y., E. A. Frey, R. A. Pfuetzner, A. L. Creagh, D. G. Knoechel, C. A. Haynes,** B. B. Finlay, and N. C. Strynadka. 2000. Crystal structure of enteropathogenic *Escherichia coli* intimin-receptor complex. *Nature* **405:**1073–1077.

120. **Madara, J. L., and K. Dharmsathaphorn.** 1985. Occluding junction structure-function relationships in a cultured epithelial monolayer. *J. Cell Biol.* **101:**2124–2133.

121. **Marcial, M. A., S. L. Carlson, and J. L. Madara.** 1984. Partitioning of paracellular conductance along the ileal crypt-villus axis: a hypothesis based on structural analysis with detailed consideration of tight junction structure-function relationships. *J. Membr. Biol.* **80:**59–70.

122. **Martin-Padura, I., S. Lostaglio, M. Schneemann, L. Williams, M. Romano, P. Fruscella, C. Panzeri, A. Stoppacciaro, L. Ruco, A. Villa, D. Simmons, and E. Dejana.** 1998. Junctional adhesion molecule, a novel member of the immunoglobulin superfamily that distributes at intercellular junctions and modulates monocyte transmigration. *J. Cell Biol.* **142:**117–127.

123. **McClane, B. A.** 2000. *Clostridium perfringens* enterotoxin and intestinal tight junctions. *Trends Microbiol.* **8:**145–146.

124. **McClane, B. A.** 2001. The complex interactions between *Clostridium perfringens* enterotoxin and epithelial tight junctions. *Toxicon* **39:**1781–1791.

125. **McDaniel, T. K., and J. B. Kaper.** 1997. A cloned pathogenicity island from enteropathogenic *Escherichia coli* confers the attaching and effacing phenotype on *E. coli* K-12. *Mol. Microbiol.* **23:**399–407.

126. **McGhie, E. J., R. D. Hayward, and V. Koronakis.** 2001. Cooperation between actin-binding proteins of invasive *Salmonella*: SipA potentiates SipC nucleation and bundling of actin. *EMBO J.* **20:**2131–2139.

127. **McGrath, J. L., E. A. Osborn, Y. S. Tardy, C. F. Dewey, Jr., and J. H. Hartwig.** 2000. Regulation of the actin cycle in vivo by actin filament severing. *Proc. Natl. Acad. Sci. USA* **97:**6532–6537.

128. **McNamara, B., A. Koutsouris, C. O'Connell, J.-P. Nougayrede, M. Donnenberg, and G. Hecht.** 2001. Translocated EspF protein from enteropathogenic *Escherichia coli* disrupts host intestinal barrier function. *J. Clin. Invest.* **107:**621–629.

129. **Menard, R., M. C. Prevost, P. Gounon, P. Sansonetti, and C. Dehio.** 1996. The secreted Ipa complex of *Shigella flexneri* promotes entry into mammalian cells. *Proc. Natl. Acad. Sci. USA* **93:**1254–1258.

130. **Meyer, R. K., and U. Aebi.** 1990. Bundling of actin filaments by alpha-actinin depends on its molecular length. *J. Cell Biol.* **110:**2013–2024.

131. **Miao, E. A., C. A. Scherer, R. M. Tsolis, R. A. Kingsley, L. G. Adams, A. J. Baumler, and S. I. Miller.** 1999. *Salmonella typhimurium* leucine-rich repeat proteins are targeted to the SPI1 and SPI2 type III secretion systems. *Mol. Microbiol.* **34:**850–864.

132. **Miner, J. H.** 1999. Renal basement membrane components. *Kidney Int.* **56:**2016–2024.

133. **Mitra, K., D. Zhou, and J. E. Galan.** 2000. Biophysical characterization of SipA, an actin-binding protein from *Salmonella enterica*. *FEBS Lett.* **482:**81–84.

134. **Moncrief, J. S., R. Obiso, Jr., L. A. Barroso, J. J. Kling, R. L. Wright, R. L. Van Tassell, D. M. Lyerly, and T. D. Wilkins.** 1995. The enterotoxin of *Bacteroides fragilis* is a metalloprotease. *Infect. Immun.* **63:**175–181.

135. **Mooseker, M. S., K. A. Conzelman, T. R. Coleman, J. E. Heuser, and M. P. Sheetz.** 1989. Characterization of intestinal microvillar membrane disks: detergent-resistant membrane sheets enriched in associated brush border myosin I (110K-calmodulin). *J. Cell Biol.* **109:**1153–1161.

136. **Morita, K., M. Furuse, K. Fujimoto, and S. Tsukita.** 1999. Claudin multigene family encoding four-transmembrane domain protein components of tight junction strands. *Proc. Natl. Acad. Sci. USA* **96:**511–516.

137. **Morrow, J. S., C. D. Cianci, T. Ardito, A. S. Mann, and M. Kashgarian.** 1989. Ankyrin links fodrin to the alpha subunit of Na,K-ATPase in Madin-Darby canine kidney cells and in intact renal tubule cells. *J. Cell Biol.* **108:**455–465.

138. **Mounier, J., V. Laurent, A. Hall, P. Fort, M. F. Carlier, P. J. Sansonetti, and C. Egile.** 1999. Rho family GTPases control entry of *Shigella flexneri* into epithelial cells but not intracellular motility. *J. Cell Sci.* **112:**2069–2080.

139. **Mullins, R. D., J. A. Heuser, and T. D. Pollard.** 1998. The interaction of Arp2/3 complex with actin: nucleation, high affinity pointed end capping, and formation of branching networks of filaments. *Proc. Natl. Acad. Sci. USA* **95:**6181–6186.

140. **Mullins, R. D., J. F. Kelleher, J. Xu, and T. D. Pollard.** 1998. Arp2/3 complex from Acanthamoeba binds profilin and cross-links actin filaments. *Mol. Biol. Cell.* **9:**841–852.

141. **Mullins, R. D., and T. D. Pollard.** 1999. Structure and function of the Arp2/3 complex. *Curr. Opin. Struct. Biol.* **9:**244–249.

142. **Nakatani, Y., K. Masudo, Y. Miyagi, Y. Inayama, N. Kawano, Y. Tanaka, K. Kato, T. Ito, H. Kitamura, Y. Nagashima, S. Yamanaka, N. Nakamura, J. Sano, N. Ogawa, N. Ishiwa, K. Notohara, M. Resl, and E. J. Mark.** 2002. Aberrant nuclear localization and gene mutation of beta-catenin in low-grade adenocarcinoma of fetal lung type: up-regulation of the Wnt signaling pathway may be a common denominator for the development of tumors that form morules. *Mod. Pathol.* **15:**617–624.

143. **Navarro-Garcia, F., A. Canizalez-Roman, J. Luna, C. Sears, and J. P. Nataro.** 2001. Plasmid-encoded toxin of enteroaggregative *Escherichia coli* is internalized by epithelial cells. *Infect. Immun.* **69:**1053–1060.

144. **Navarro-Garcia, F., C. Eslava, J. M. Villaseca, R. Lopez-Revilla, J. R. Czeczulin, S. Srinivas, J. P. Nataro, and A. Cravioto.** 1998. In vitro effects of a high-molecular-weight heat-labile enterotoxin from enteroaggregative *Escherichia coli*. *Infect. Immun.* **66:**3149–3154.

145. **Navarro-Garcia, F., C. Sears, C. Eslava, A. Cravioto, and J. P. Nataro.** 1999. Cytoskeletal effects induced by pet, the serine protease enterotoxin of enteroaggregative *Escherichia coli*. *Infect. Immun.* **67:**2184–2192.

146. **Nelson, W. J., and P. J. Veshnock.** 1987. Ankyrin binding to (Na^{++} K$^+$)ATPase and implications for the organization of membrane domains in polarized cells. *Nature* **328:**533–536.

147. **Nguyen, L., I. T. Paulsen, J. Tchieu, C. J. Hueck, and M. H. Saier, Jr.** 2000. Phylogenetic analyses of the constituents of Type III protein secretion systems. *J. Mol. Microbiol. Biotechnol.* **2:**125–144.

148. **Nhieu, G. T., and P. J. Sansonetti.** 1999. Mechanism of *Shigella* entry into epithelial cells. *Curr. Opin. Microbiol.* **2:**51–55.

149. **Nievers, M. G., I. Kuikman, D. Geerts, I. M. Leigh, and A. Sonnenberg.** 2000. Formation of hemidesmosome-like structures in the absence of ligand binding by the (alpha)6(beta)4 integrin requires binding of HD1/plectin to the cytoplasmic domain of the (beta)4 integrin subunit. *J. Cell Sci.* **113**(Part 6):963–973.

150. **Noren, N. K., C. M. Niessen, B. M. Gumbiner, and K. Burridge.** 2001. Cadherin engagement regulates Rho family GTPases. *J. Biol. Chem.* **276:**33305–33308.

151. **Norris, F. A., M. P. Wilson, T. S. Wallis, E. E. Galyov, and P. W. Majerus.** 1998. SopB, a protein required for virulence of *Salmonella dublin*, is an inositol phosphate phosphatase. *Proc. Natl. Acad. Sci. USA* **95:**14057–14059.

152. **Nusrat, A., M. Giry, J. R. Turner, S. P. Colgan, C. A. Parkos, D. Carnes, E. Lemichez, P. Boquet, and J. L. Madara.** 1995. Rho protein regulates tight junctions and perijunctional actin organization in polarized epithelia. *Proc. Natl. Acad. Sci. USA* **92:**10629–10633.

153. **Obiso, R. J., Jr., A. O. Azghani, and T. D. Wilkins.** 1997. The *Bacteroides fragilis* toxin fragilysin disrupts the paracellular barrier of epithelial cells. *Infect. Immun.* **65:**1431–1439.

154. **Obiso, R. J., Jr., D. M. Lyerly, R. L. Van Tassell, and T. D. Wilkins.** 1995. Proteolytic activity of the *Bacteroides fragilis* enterotoxin causes fluid secretion and intestinal damage in vivo. *Infect. Immun.* **63:**3820–3826.

155. **Osiecki, J. C., J. Barker, W. L. Picking, A. B. Serfis, E. Berring, S. Shah, A. Harrington, and W. D. Picking.** 2001. IpaC from *Shigella* and SipC from *Salmonella* possess similar biochemical properties but are functionally distinct. *Mol. Microbiol.* **42:**469–481.

156. **Otey, C. A., F. M. Pavalko, and K. Burridge.** 1990. An interaction between alpha-actinin and the beta 1 integrin subunit in vitro. *J. Cell Biol.* **111:**721–729.

157. **Phillips, A., J. Giron, S. Hicks, G. Dougan, and G. Frankel.** 2000. Intimin from enteropathogenic *Escherichia coli* mediates remodelling of the eukaryotic cell surface. *Microbiology* **146:**1333–1344.

158. **Pollard, T. D., L. Blanchoin, and R. D. Mullins.** 2001. Actin dynamics. *J. Cell Sci.* **114:**3–4.

159. **Pothoulakis, C.** 2000. Effects of *Clostridium difficile* toxins on epithelial cell barrier. *Ann. N.Y. Acad. Sci.* **915:**347–356.

160. **Pothoulakis, C., and J. T. Lamont.** 2001. Microbes and microbial toxins: paradigms for microbial-mucosal interactions. II. The integrated response of the intestine to *Clostridium difficile* toxins. *Am. J. Physiol. Gastrointest. Liver Physiol.* **280:**G178–G183.

161. **Ressad, F., D. Didry, C. Egile, D. Pantaloni, and M. F. Carlier.** 1999. Control of actin filament length and turnover by actin depolymerizing factor (ADF/cofilin) in the presence of capping proteins and ARP2/3 complex. *J. Biol. Chem.* **274:**20970–20976.

162. **Richard, J. F., L. Petit, M. Gibert, J. C. Marvaud, C. Bouchaud, and M. R. Popoff.** 1999. Bacterial toxins modifying the actin cytoskeleton. *Int. Microbiol.* **2:**185–194.

163. **Ridley, A. J.** 2001. Rho family proteins: coordinating cell responses. *Trends Cell Biol.* **11:**471–477.

164. **Ridley, A. J.** 2001. Rho GTPases and cell migration. *J. Cell Sci.* **114:**2713–2722.

165. **Riegler, M., M. Lotz, C. Sears, C. Pothoulakis, I. Castagliuolo, C. C. Wang, R. Sedivy, T. Sogukoglu, E. Cosentini, G. Bischof, W. Feil, B. Teleky, G. Hamilton, J. T. LaMont, and E. Wenzl.** 1999. *Bacteroides fragilis* toxin 2 damages human colonic mucosa in vitro. *Gut* **44:**504–510.

166. **Rippere-Lampe, K. E., A. D. O'Brien, R. Conran, and H. A. Lockman.** 2001. Mutation of the gene encoding cytotoxic necrotizing factor type 1 (cnf[1]) attenuates the virulence of uropathogenic *Escherichia coli*. *Infect. Immun.* **69:**3954–3964.

167. **Rosenshine, I., S. Ruschkowski, M. Stein, D. J. Reinscheid, S. D. Mills, and B. B. Finlay.** 1996. A pathogenic bacterium triggers epithelial signals to form a functional bacterial receptor that mediates actin pseudopod formation. *EMBO J.* **15:**2613–2624.

168. **Rudolph, M. G., C. Weise, S. Mirold, B. Hillenbrand, B. Bader, A. Wittinghofer, and W. D. Hardt.** 1999. Biochemical analysis of SopE from *Salmonella typhimurium*, a highly efficient guanosine nucleotide exchange factor for Rho GTPases. *J. Biol. Chem.* **274:**30501–30509.

169. **Saidi, R. F., K. Jaeger, M. H. Montrose, S. Wu, and C. L. Sears.** 1997. *Bacteroides fragilis* toxin rearranges the actin cytoskeleton of HT29/C1 cells without direct proteolysis of actin or decrease in F-actin content. *Cell Motil. Cytoskel.* **37:**159–165.

170. **Saidi, R. F., and C. L. Sears.** 1996. *Bacteroides fragilis* toxin rapidly intoxicates human intestinal epithelial cells (HT29/C1) in vitro. *Infect. Immun.* **64:**5029–5034.

171. **Saitou, M., Y. Ando-Akatsuka, M. Itoh, M. Furuse, J. Inazawa, K. Fujimoto, and S. Tsukita.** 1997. Mammalian occludin in epithelial cells: its expression and subcellular distribution. *Eur. J. Cell Biol.* **73:**222–231.

172. **Sarker, M. R., U. Singh, and B. A. McClane.** 2000. An update on *Clostridium perfringens* enterotoxin. *J. Nat. Toxins* **9:**251–266.

173. **Sasaki, T., and Y. Takai.** 1998. The Rho small G protein family-Rho GDI system as a temporal and spatial determinant for cytoskeletal

control. *Biochem. Biophys. Res. Commun.* **245:** 641–645.

174. **Sastry, S. K., M. Lakonishok, S. Wu, T. Q. Truong, A. Huttenlocher, C. E. Turner, and A. F. Horwitz.** 1999. Quantitative changes in integrin and focal adhesion signaling regulate myoblast cell cycle withdrawal. *J. Cell Biol.* **144:**1295–1309.

175. **Schaller, M. D., C. A. Borgman, B. S. Cobb, R. R. Vines, A. B. Reynolds, and J. T. Parsons.** 1992. pp125FAK, a structurally distinctive protein-tyrosine kinase associated with focal adhesions. *Proc. Natl. Acad. Sci. USA* **89:**5192–5196.

176. **Schaller, M. D., C. A. Otey, J. D. Hildebrand, and J. T. Parsons.** 1995. Focal adhesion kinase and paxillin bind to peptides mimicking beta integrin cytoplasmic domains. *J. Cell Biol.* **130:**1181–1187.

177. **Schmidt, G., and K. Aktories.** 1998. Bacterial cytotoxins target Rho GTPases. *Naturwissenschaften* **85:**253–261.

178. **Schmidt, G., and K. Aktories.** 2000. Rho GTPase-activating toxins: cytotoxic necrotizing factors and dermonecrotic toxin. *Methods Enzymol.* **325:**125–136.

179. **Schnittler, H. J., S. W. Schneider, H. Raifer, F. Luo, P. Dieterich, I. Just, and K. Aktories.** 2001. Role of actin filaments in endothelial cell-cell adhesion and membrane stability under fluid shear stress. *Pflugers Arch.* **442:** 675–687.

180. **Sears, C. L.** 2000. Molecular physiology and pathophysiology of tight junctions V. Assault of the tight junction by enteric pathogens. *Am. J. Physiol. Gastrointest. Liver Physiol.* **279:**G1129–G1134.

181. **Sears, C. L.** 2001. The toxins of *Bacteroides fragilis. Toxicon* **39:**1737–1746.

182. **Sears, C. L., L. L. Myers, A. Lazenby, and R. L. Van Tassell.** 1995. Enterotoxigenic *Bacteroides fragilis. Clin. Infect. Dis.* **20**(Suppl. 2): S142–S148.

183. **Sinclair, J. F., and A. D. O'Brien.** 2002. Cell-surface localized nucleolin is a eucaryotic receptor for the adhesin intimin-γ of enterohemorrhagic *Escherichia coli* O157:H7. *J. Biol. Chem.* **277:**2876–2885.

184. **Skoudy, A., J. Mounier, A. Aruffo, H. Ohayon, P. Gounon, P. Sansonetti, and G. Tran Van Nhieu.** 2000. CD44 binds to the *Shigella* IpaB protein and participates in bacterial invasion of epithelial cells. *Cell Microbiol.* **2:**19–33.

185. **Sonoda, N., M. Furuse, H. Sasaki, S. Yonemura, J. Katahira, Y. Horiguchi, and S. Tsukita.** 1999. *Clostridium perfringens* enter-

otoxin fragment removes specific claudins from tight junction strands: evidence for direct involvement of claudins in tight junction barrier. *J. Cell Biol.* **147:**195–204.

186. **Southwick, F. S.** 2000. Gelsolin and ADF/cofilin enhance the actin dynamics of motile cells. *Proc. Natl. Acad. Sci. USA* **97:**6936–6938.

187. **Spinardi, L., S. Einheber, T. Cullen, T. A. Milner, and F. G. Giancotti.** 1995. A recombinant tail-less integrin beta 4 subunit disrupts hemidesmosomes, but does not suppress alpha 6 beta 4-mediated cell adhesion to laminins. *J. Cell Biol.* **129:**473–487.

188. **Steele-Mortimer, O., L. A. Knodler, S. L. Marcus, M. P. Scheid, B. Goh, C. G. Pfeifer, V. Duronio, and B. B. Finlay.** 2000. Activation of Akt/protein kinase B in epithelial cells by the *Salmonella typhimurium* effector sigD. *J. Biol. Chem.* **275:**37718–37724.

189. **Steinbock, F. A., and G. Wiche.** 1999. Plectin: a cytolinker by design. *Biol. Chem.* **380:** 151–158.

190. **Stevenson, B. R., J. D. Siliciano, M. S. Mooseker, and D. A. Goodenough.** 1986. Identification of ZO-1: a high molecular weight polypeptide associated with the tight junction (zonula occludens) in a variety of epithelia. *J. Cell Biol.* **103:**755–766.

191. **Stossel, T. P., J. Condeelis, L. Cooley, J. H. Hartwig, A. Noegel, M. Schleicher, and S. S. Shapiro.** 2001. Filamins as integrators of cell mechanics and signalling. *Nat. Rev. Mol. Cell. Biol.* **2:**138–145.

192. **Stutzmann, J., A. Bellissent-Waydelich, L. Fontao, J. F. Launay, and P. Simon-Assmann.** 2000. Adhesion complexes implicated in intestinal epithelial cell-matrix interactions. *Microsc. Res. Tech.* **51:**179–190.

193. **Sukhan, A., T. Kubori, J. Wilson, and J. E. Galan.** 2001. Genetic analysis of assembly of the *Salmonella enterica* serovar Typhimurium type III secretion-associated needle complex. *J. Bacteriol.* **183:**1159–1167.

194. **Sun, H. Q., M. Yamamoto, M. Mejillano, and H. L. Yin.** 1999. Gelsolin, a multifunctional actin regulatory protein. *J. Biol. Chem.* **274:**33179–33182.

195. **Taylor, K. A., P. W. Luther, and M. S. Donnenberg.** 1999. Expression of the EspB protein of enteropathogenic *Escherichia coli* within HeLa cells affects stress fibers and cellular morphology. *Infect. Immun.* **67:**120–125.

196. **Temm-Grove, C. J., B. M. Jockusch, R. P. Weinberger, G. Schevzov, and D. M. Helfman.** 1998. Distinct localizations of tropomyosin isoforms in LLC-PK1 epithelial cells

suggests specialized function at cell-cell adhesions. *Cell Motil. Cytoskeleton* **40:**393–407.

197. **Toyotome, T., T. Suzuki, A. Kuwae, T. Nonaka, H. Fukuda, S. Imajoh-Ohmi, T. Toyofuku, M. Hori, and C. Sasakawa.** 2001. *Shigella* protein IpaH(9.8) is secreted from bacteria within mammalian cells and transported to the nucleus. *J. Biol. Chem.* **276:**32071–32079.

198. **Tran Van Nhieu, G., A. Ben-Ze'ev, and P. J. Sansonetti.** 1997. Modulation of bacterial entry into epithelial cells by association between vinculin and the *Shigella* IpaA invasin. *EMBO J.* **16:**2717–2729.

199. **Tran Van Nhieu, G., E. Caron, A. Hall, and P. J. Sansonetti.** 1999. IpaC induces actin polymerization and filopodia formation during *Shigella* entry into epithelial cells. *EMBO J.* **18:**3249–3262.

200. **Tsukamoto, T., and S. K. Nigam.** 1997. Tight junction proteins form large complexes and associate with the cytoskeleton in an ATP depletion model for reversible junction assembly. *J. Biol. Chem.* **272:**16133–16139.

201. **Tsukita, S., K. Oishi, N. Sato, J. Sagara, and A. Kawai.** 1994. ERM family members as molecular linkers between the cell surface glycoprotein CD44 and actin-based cytoskeletons. *J. Cell Biol.* **126:**391–401.

202. **Turner, C. E., J. R. Glenney, Jr., and K. Burridge.** 1990. Paxillin: a new vinculin-binding protein present in focal adhesions. *J. Cell Biol.* **111:**1059–1068.

203. **Ursitti, J., and R. Bloch.** 2001. Spectrin, p. 2965–2971. *In* T. Creighton (ed.), *Encyclopedia of Molecular Medicine*, vol. 5. John Wiley & Sons, New York. N.Y.

204. **Uzzau, S., P. Cappuccinelli, and A. Fasano.** 1999. Expression of *Vibrio cholerae* zonula occludens toxin and analysis of its subcellular localization. *Microb. Pathog.* **27:**377–385.

205. **Uzzau, S., R. Lu, W. Wang, C. Fiore, and A. Fasano.** 2001. Purification and preliminary characterization of the zonula occludens toxin receptor from human (CaCo2) and murine (IEC6) intestinal cell lines. *FEMS Microbiol. Lett.* **194:**1–5.

206. **Villaseca, J. M., F. Navarro-Garcia, G. Mendoza-Hernandez, J. P. Nataro, A. Cravioto, and C. Eslava.** 2000. Pet toxin from enteroaggregative *Escherichia coli* produces cellular damage associated with fodrin disruption. *Infect. Immun.* **68:**5920–5927.

207. **Wahl, S., H. Barth, T. Ciossek, K. Aktories, and B. K. Mueller.** 2000. Ephrin-A5 induces collapse of growth cones by activating Rho and Rho kinase. *J. Cell Biol.* **149:**263–270.

208. **Waldor, M. K., and J. J. Mekalanos.** 1996. Lysogenic conversion by a filamentous phage encoding cholera toxin. *Science* **272:**1910–1914.

209. **Wang, W., S. Uzzau, S. E. Goldblum, and A. Fasano.** 2000. Human zonulin, a potential modulator of intestinal tight junctions. *J. Cell Sci.* **113**(Part 24):4435–4440.

210. **Watarai, M., S. Funato, and C. Sasakawa.** 1996. Interaction of Ipa proteins of *Shigella flexneri* with alpha5beta1 integrin promotes entry of the bacteria into mammalian cells. *J. Exp. Med.* **183:**991–999.

211. **Werb, Z., P. M. Tremble, O. Behrendtsen, E. Crowley, and C. H. Damsky.** 1989. Signal transduction through the fibronectin receptor induces collagenase and stromelysin gene expression. *J. Cell Biol.* **109:**877–889.

212. **Wieler, L. H., T. K. McDaniel, T. S. Whittam, and J. B. Kaper.** 1997. Insertion site of the locus of enterocyte effacement in enteropathogenic and enterohemorrhagic *Escherichia coli* differs in relation to the clonal phylogeny of the strains. *FEMS Microbiol. Lett.* **156:**49–53.

213. **Wilde, C., and K. Aktories.** 2001. The Rho-ADP-ribosylating C3 exoenzyme from *Clostridium botulinum* and related C3-like transferases. *Toxicon* **39:**1647–1660.

214. **Williams, A. W., and S. C. Straley.** 1998. YopD of *Yersinia pestis* plays a role in negative regulation of the low-calcium response in addition to its role in translocation of Yops. *J. Bacteriol.* **180:**350–358.

215. **Windoffer, R., M. Borchert-Stuhltrager, and R. E. Leube.** 2002. Desmosomes: interconnected calcium-dependent structures of remarkable stability with significant integral membrane protein turnover. *J. Cell Sci.* **115:**1717–1732.

216. **Wood, M. W., M. A. Jones, P. R. Watson, A. M. Siber, B. A. McCormick, S. Hedges, R. Rosqvist, T. S. Wallis, and E. E. Galyov.** 2000. The secreted effector protein of *Salmonella dublin*, SopA, is translocated into eukaryotic cells and influences the induction of enteritis. *Cell Microbiol.* **2:**293–303.

217. **Wu, S., L. A. Dreyfus, A. O. Tzianabos, C. Hayashi, and C. L. Sears.** 2002. Diversity of the metalloprotease toxin produced by enterotoxigenic *Bacteroides fragilis*. *Infect. Immun.* **70:**2463–2471.

218. **Wu, S., K. C. Lim, J. Huang, R. F. Saidi, and C. L. Sears.** 1998. *Bacteroides fragilis* enterotoxin cleaves the zonula adherens protein, E-cadherin. *Proc. Natl. Acad. Sci. USA* **95:**14979–14984.

219. **Yap, A. S., W. M. Brieher, and B. M. Gumbiner.** 1997. Molecular and functional

analysis of cadherin-based adherens junctions. *Annu. Rev. Cell Dev. Biol.* **13**:119–146.

220. **Yonemura, S., and S. Tsukita.** 1999. Direct involvement of ezrin/radixin/moesin (ERM)-binding membrane proteins in the organization of microvilli in collaboration with activated ERM proteins. *J. Cell Biol.* **145**:1497–1509.

221. **Zhou, D.** 2001. Collective efforts to modulate the host actin cytoskeleton by *Salmonella* type III-secreted effector proteins. *Trends Microbiol.* **9**:567–569.

222. **Zhou, D., L. M. Chen, L. Hernandez, S. B. Shears, and J. E. Galan.** 2001. A *Salmonella* inositol polyphosphatase acts in conjunction with other bacterial effectors to promote host cell actin cytoskeleton rearrangements and bacterial internalization. *Mol. Microbiol.* **39**:248–259.

223. **Zhou, D., M. S. Mooseker, and J. E. Galan.** 1999. An invasion-associated *Salmonella* protein modulates the actin-bundling activity of plastin. *Proc. Natl. Acad. Sci. USA* **96**:10176–10181.

224. **Zhou, D., M. S. Mooseker, and J. E. Galan.** 1999. Role of the *S.* Typhimurium actin-binding protein SipA in bacterial internalization. *Science* **283**:2092–2095.

ONTOGENY OF THE HOST RESPONSE TO ENTERIC MICROBIAL INFECTION

Bobby J. Cherayil and W. Allan Walker

18

The gastrointestinal tract contains, both within the epithelial layer and in the lamina propria, large numbers of cells involved in immune responses. The location of these cells adjacent to the intestinal lumen exposes them constantly to innumerable foreign antigens derived from food and commensal microbial flora. If the intestinal immune system responded vigorously to these antigens, a dangerous state of reactivity would develop, resulting in food intolerance and chronic intestinal inflammation. On the other hand, if the immune cells did not respond to foreign antigens at all, microorganisms could spread from the intestine to wreak havoc throughout the body. Fortunately, neither of these sets of circumstances occurs in most individuals. Soluble food antigens do not provoke an immune response and, in fact, usually lead to a state of systemic nonresponsiveness, a phenomenon known as oral tolerance (87). Commensal microbes are recognized and are confined to the lumen by responses that minimize inflammation and tissue damage. Microbial pathogens, however, activate a full-fledged inflammatory and adaptive immune response that is directed at their elimination, even at the cost of some tissue damage. This ability to distinguish friend (food, commensals) from foe (potential pathogens) is an important characteristic of normal intestinal immune responses and is key to immune homeostasis in this tissue.

How does this property develop? Normal newborn animals, including humans, do not have the discriminatory function of the fully mature form; as a result, they are more likely to have abnormal responses to food and commensal organisms (18). The development of this important function is intimately associated with changes in the intestinal immune system that occur during ontogeny in response to intrinsic genetic programs, exposure to food antigens, and colonization by a normal commensal flora. In this chapter, we review what these changes are, when they take place, what mechanisms drive them, and how they contribute to the function of the mature response to enteric microbes. Before beginning this discussion, we briefly describe the elements of the mature intestinal immune system.

THE ELEMENTS OF THE INTESTINAL IMMUNE SYSTEM

Illustrated in Fig. 1 are the components that play an important role in normal immune re-

Bobby J. Cherayil and W. Allan Walker, Combined Program in Pediatric Gastroenterology and Nutrition, Massachusetts General Hospital and Harvard Medical School, Boston, MA 02114.

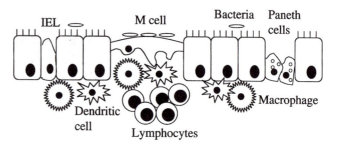

FIGURE 1 Elements of the mucosal immune system. The various cellular components that contribute to immune defense of the intestine are depicted.

sponses in the mature intestine. A key element is the polarized monolayer of epithelial cells that lines the lumen. The tight intercellular junctions formed by these cells, together with the secretions they produce and the surface glycoconjugates they express, limit the movement of molecules across the monolayer. Interspersed within the monolayer, particularly in the follicle-associated epithelium that lies over Peyer's patches, are specialized epithelial cells known as M (for microfold) cells, which actively take up antigens from the lumen and transport them to underlying antigen-presenting cells (92). Sampling of lumenal antigens and organisms can also be carried out by macrophages and dendritic cells that extend processes between the epithelial cells (64, 104). Distributed throughout the lamina propria, often in close apposition to the basal surface of the epithelial cells, are macrophages that are poised to phagocytose any microorganisms that might get across the epithelium. Interestingly, the lamina propria macrophages, unlike similar cells at other sites in the body, are devoid of the surface molecule CD14, making them less responsive to lipopolysaccharide (LPS) (112). This property would allow these cells to eliminate small numbers of bacteria without unnecessarily inciting an inflammatory response. Paneth cells, another component of innate defense, are located in the crypt epithelium, where they are able to release antimicrobial peptides in response to contact with bacteria (33, 96). In addition to macrophages, the lamina propria also contains mast cells and large numbers of lymphocytes, particularly immunoglobulin A (IgA)-producing B cells. Mast cells contribute to in-

nate and adaptive immune responses (71, 130). Dimeric IgA produced by B cells is transcytosed across the epithelial monolayer via the polymeric immunoglobulin receptor (pIgR) and acts on lumenal bacteria to prevent their adherence. In addition to lymphocytes within the lamina propria, specialized T cells, known as intraepithelial lymphocytes (IEL), are located within the epithelial layer itself. The IEL have a repertoire of antigen receptors designed especially to recognize either bacterial antigens or surface molecules expressed by stressed epithelial cells. They are in a constitutively active state, ready to respond quickly when the appropriate stimulus is perceived.

The intestinal epithelium, together with the associated phagocytic and lymphoid cells, constitutes a physical and functional barrier that separates lumenal contents from the rest of the body, including the rest of the immune system. This barrier ensures that microorganisms either do not cross over from the lumen or do so in numbers that can be handled without inflammatory tissue damage. At the same time, this barrier allows absorption of soluble nutrients and continuous sampling of lumenal contents. Furthermore, as will be discussed in more detail below, the epithelial cells that form part of the barrier are capable of sensing potential dangers in the lumenal environment, such as the presence of invasive bacteria, and responding with the expression of inflammatory mediators. These mediators initiate an acute inflammatory reaction, recruiting neutrophils, monocytes, and lymphocytes into the lamina propria to deal with the offending agent by means of innate and adaptive immune mechanisms. We will now discuss the normal ontogeny of the various components described above.

EPITHELIAL CELLS

Barrier Functions

In the context of defense against microbial infection, an important function of intestinal epithelial cells is to act as a physical barrier. Morphologically normal intercellular tight junctions have been observed even in the early human fetus, although these structures may be more dynamic than those in the adult (100). However, it has been noted that the barrier function of the epithelium is not fully developed at birth. In newborn animals and humans, the permeability of the intestine to various proteins is abnormally high compared with that in the adult state (5, 122). This increased epithelial permeability in the neonatal period is attributable to several factors, including quantitative and qualitative differences in the mucus of newborn and adult animals (109), lower gastric acid and pancreatic enzyme secretion (56, 68), and reduced gut motility (82). Mucus composition may be particularly relevant to the present discussion since it has been shown that competition between mucus glycoproteins and receptors on epithelial cells can influence interactions with bacteria (27, 127).

Antigen Sampling and M Cells

Somewhat at odds with its role as a physical barrier, the epithelial layer must also have some means of sampling the contents of the lumen so that lumenal antigens can tolerize or activate the cells of the adaptive immune system depending on the microenvironmental circumstances. This function is carried out by M cells (reviewed in reference 92). These morphologically distinct, specialized enterocytes are first seen at about 17 weeks of gestation in the human fetus, shortly after the appearance of intestinal lymphoid aggregates (85). This temporal sequence of events is significant, since in vitro tissue culture experiments have suggested that B lymphocytes are involved in inducing the differentiation of M cells from enterocytes (62). The finding that mice lacking B cells have impaired development of Peyer's patches, follicle-associated epithelium, and M cells provides in vivo support for this idea (38). More recent work with recombinase activating gene knockout (Rag1$^{-/-}$) mice, which lack T and B cells, indicates that although B lymphocytes are required for the formation of full-sized follicle-associated epithelium, nonlymphocytes can also support M-cell differentiation (26). Various viruses, bacteria, and parasites have been shown to interact specifically with M cells (61).

Sensing and Responding to the Lumenal Microbial Environment

Enterocytes are among the first cells to come into contact with lumenal microorganisms and have the important function of sensing and responding to the intestinal microbial population. Several enterocyte surface molecules and some intracellular proteins are involved in the sensing function via binding to microorganisms or their products. When abnormalities in the local environment are detected, the epithelial cells respond with changes in their own functions, as well as the expression of various secreted and surface molecules that influence the behavior of cells of the immune system. The latter response often results in the activation of a local inflammatory cascade. Epithelial cells thus serve as an active interface that monitors the microbial environment of the lumen and communicates the information to the intestinal immune system. Developmentally regulated changes in enterocyte sensing or response mechanisms can give rise to age-specific differences in susceptibility to the consequences of enteric infection. Some of the important factors involved in the interactions between enterocytes and microorganisms are considered below.

Surface Glycosylation Patterns. The surface of epithelial cells, including the apical surface facing the intestinal lumen, is covered with oligosaccharides attached to membrane proteins and lipids. Depending on their exact structure, these sugar moieties can facilitate adhesion by different kinds of microorganisms. Therefore, there has been considerable interest in elucidating the details of enterocyte surface glycosylation. In the rat small intestine, most surface oligosaccharides on intestinal epithelial cells demonstrate terminal sialylation prior to weaning, whereas terminal fucosylation becomes the predominant pattern after weaning (119). This corresponds with an alteration in sialyl- and fucosyltransferases (17). A recent study has documented a steady postnatal decline in surface sialylation and α-2,6-sialyltransferase activity in the mouse small intestine (but not the colon), and showed further that this alteration occurred predominantly in goblet cells (24). Cortisone was found to accelerate this decline. Similar changes occur in intestinal glycosylation patterns during human ontogeny; that is, a fetal pattern of predominant sialylation followed by an adult pattern of predominant fucosylation and galactosylation (23). These changes may alter the susceptibility of the intestine to colonization by specific commensal or pathogenic organisms. Indeed, it has been shown that attachment of *Helicobacter pylori* to fucosylated versus sialylated glycans influences pathogenicity, while colonization with the commensal *Bacteroides thetaiotaomicron*, which uses terminal L-fucose residues as a nutrient source, is facilitated by a glycosylation pattern rich in this sugar (51). Some of these weaning-related changes in glycosylation are genetically programmed, whereas others are caused by the introduction of specific nutrients or their breakdown products (40). The commensal bacteria have also been shown to contribute to these changes by the induction of specific glycosyltransferases (11), the most interesting example of which is the induction of the relevant fucosyltransferase by *B. thetaiotaomicron* as a means of providing its own nutrient source (11, 53). *B. thetaiotaomicron* thus modifies the gut microenvironment to favor its own nutritional needs, a process that probably gives it a distinct survival advantage over other bacteria. Recent studies have shown that the

introduction of commensal microflora into germfree mice is required for the normal maturation of intestinal glycosyltransferase activities (N. N. Nanthakumar, D. Dai, D. S. Newburg, and W. A. Walker, submitted for publication).

Receptors for Bacterial Toxins. Several enteric bacterial pathogens produce their clinical effects on the intestine through the release of exotoxins. These toxins then bind to specific receptors on the plasma membrane to initiate signaling cascades that lead ultimately to derangements in enterocyte function. The effects of some of these toxins have been found to be developmentally regulated. Newborn animals are more susceptible than older animals to the effects of cholera toxin and *Escherichia coli* heat-stable toxin. The former effect involves postreceptor mechanisms (16), while the latter involves a postweaning decrease in receptor number (3, 19, 20, 59). In contrast, newborn animals are less susceptible than their older counterparts to *Clostridium difficile* toxin and Shiga toxin. Newborn rabbits lack high-affinity receptors for *C. difficile* toxin A, whereas the receptor is present in adult animals (29). These findings in animals may correlate with the well-known clinical observation that 10 to 50% of normal human neonates and infants carry toxin-producing *C. difficile* in their gastrointestinal tracts without exhibiting evidence of disease, whereas very few older children are asymptomatic carriers of the organism (58). Similarly, there is an age-dependent increase in expression of the receptor for Shiga toxin (83, 84).

TLRs. Enterocytes are constantly exposed to large quantities of LPS and other bacterial products derived from the commensal flora in the lumen of the intestine. It is relevant to ask, therefore, whether these cells are capable of responding to these common bacterial determinants. Interest in this issue was sparked recently by the identification of a family of receptor proteins, known as the Toll-like receptors (TLRs), that have been implicated in the recognition of, and in the triggering of an inflammatory response to, LPS and other microbial molecules (reviewed in reference 80). The expression of the TLRs in intestinal epithelial cells has been examined, with conflicting results in some cases (1, 12, 13, 88). These various studies suggest that enterocytes are not very responsive to LPS, in part because of insufficient expression of the relevant TLR or an essential coreceptor. However, this issue, which is discussed in more detail in chapter 5, will undoubtedly benefit from further investigation. In relation to the ontogeny of intestinal immune responses, it is pertinent to note that TLR2 and TLR4 mRNA and protein have been found to be expressed in a fetal intestinal epithelial cell line and in primary fetal enterocytes, suggesting that if the intestinal epithelium does indeed respond to LPS, this ability may already be present from a very early stage of development (32).

TLR5, the receptor for bacterial flagellin, is noteworthy in the context of the intestine's ability to discriminate between commensal and pathogenic bacteria. This receptor has been found to be expressed selectively on the basolateral surface of T84 cells (34). If it is assumed that this characteristic applies to primary enterocytes, bacteria in the lumen of the intestine would not have access to basolaterally expressed TLR5 and would not activate TLR5-dependent inflammatory signals. On the other hand, invasive bacteria that cross the epithelial monolayer in significant numbers would be able to activate the receptor. In keeping with this idea, a commensal *E. coli* strain applied to the apical surface of a polarized T84 monolayer did not stimulate TLR5, whereas a pathogenic *Salmonella* strain did (35). Interestingly, this differential behavior was shown to be related to the ability of *Salmonella*, but not *E. coli*, to induce the transcytosis of flagellin in the apical to basolateral direction. Flagellin has been shown recently to stimulate production of the dendritic cell-recruiting chemokine CCL20 from human intestinal epithelial cell lines (110), a factor that

may be relevant to the initiation of adaptive immune responses. To our knowledge, TLR5 expression has not been examined at different stages of intestinal development, although this would clearly be an interesting area of investigation.

NOD Proteins. In addition to surface receptors for LPS, intracellular, cytosolic proteins also interact with this bacterial component. These proteins (reviewed in reference 7), including the NOD1 and NOD2 proteins, respond to LPS with the activation of NF-κB, a transcription factor crucial for turning on the genetic program involved in inflammation. Invasive strains of *Shigella* spp., which escape from the phagosome to the cytosol of cells that they infect, have been shown to activate NF-κB in epithelial cells in a NOD1-dependent manner (36). Furthermore, mutations in NOD2 have recently been implicated in human Crohn's disease (44, 55, 94), tying together abnormalities in innate immune responses to bacteria and bowel inflammation (124). No information on developmental regulation of NOD1 or NOD2 expression or function is yet available.

Production of Cytokines and Other Mediators Involved in Inflammation. Interactions between lumenal microorganisms and enterocytes (involving the sensing molecules described above) can induce the latter to produce cytokines, chemokines, and other inflammatory mediators (reviewed in reference 79). Commensal bacteria do not activate these responses, whereas pathogenic ones do, either because of peculiarities in the interactions with enterocyte surface molecules or because the pathogenic bacteria express specific virulence factors that activate proinflammatory signaling pathways (125). For example, effector proteins that are translocated into the host cytosol by virulent strains of *Salmonella* turn on the mitogen-activated protein (MAP) kinase pathway, leading to cytokine production (50). Other factors produced by enterocytes in response to infection include tumor necrosis factor alpha (TNF-α), macrophage chemotactic protein 1 (MCP-1), granulocyte-macrophage colony-stimulating factor (GM-CSF), and interleukin 6 (IL-6), as well as an as yet unidentified, *Salmonella*-induced, apically secreted chemotactic agent (78). Recently, the T-cell chemoattractants IP-10, Mig, and I-TAC, acting preferentially on Th1 cells, have been shown to be produced by human enterocytes in response to *Salmonella* and invasive *E. coli* (28). These secreted molecules serve to recruit inflammatory cells from the circulation to the site of epithelial infection and, in some cases, to induce the transmigration of the inflammatory cells across the epithelium so that they can deal with the infecting organism. Protozoan and helminth intestinal parasites and viruses have also been shown to elicit similar epithelial inflammatory responses (79).

The ability to produce cytokines in response to inflammatory stimuli may be developmentally regulated. A recent study has demonstrated that a human fetal intestinal epithelial cell line, as well as fetal intestinal explants, produces relatively more IL-8 in response to inflammatory stimuli than mature intestinal epithelial cells (89). This difference may be relevant to the pathogenesis of age-specific inflammatory disorders of the intestine, such as necrotizing enterocolitis (discussed further below).

Expression of Stress-Associated Molecules. In addition to producing secreted inflammatory mediators, enterocytes can also respond to changes in the local environment by expressing specific surface molecules that act as "danger signals." Two such molecules are the MICA and MICB proteins, nonclassical relatives of the major histocompatibility complex (MHC) class I proteins (reviewed in reference 117). MICA and MICB are expressed in a patchy distribution on the intestinal epithelium, and their levels are significantly increased by stressful conditions such as heat shock (41) and infection (25, 42). These proteins function as ligands for the NKG2D receptor, which is expressed on nat-

ural killer (NK) cells, γδ IEL (43), peripheral blood γδ T cells (25), and CD8 αβ T cells (42), and provide a costimulus for antigen-specific responses. The upregulation of MICA and MICB on enterocytes by infection could thus increase the responsiveness of lymphocyte populations to microbial antigens. Another nonclassical MHC molecule, TL, which is also expressed prominently in the gut, has been shown to interact with CD8αα and thereby inhibit IEL proliferation while enhancing cytokine production (70). Although developmental regulation of these nonclassical MHC molecules has not been determined, this issue is probably worth examining, especially in view of the postulated importance of γδ IEL in controlling infection in the neonatal period (48).

CELLS OF THE INNATE IMMUNE SYSTEM

The intestinal epithelium is closely associated with several cell types involved in innate immunity (the rapidly deployed, antigen-nonspecific arm of the immune response). Included are phagocytic and antigen-presenting cells, such as macrophages and dendritic cells, Paneth cells, and mast cells, which are involved in the production and release of various antimicrobial molecules.

Macrophages

Macrophages are the major resident phagocytic population in the gut. They can be found diffusely in the lamina propria, mainly in a subepithelial distribution (86, 98), as well as clustered in the Peyer's patches. In human fetal intestine, macrophages can be detected from about 12 weeks of gestation onward, although specific subpopulations (based on surface marker phenotype) differ with gestational age and location (lamina propria versus Peyer's patches) (46, 116). A peculiarity of lamina propria macrophages is that they lack CD14, an essential coreceptor for TLR4, and therefore are LPS hyporesponsive (112). This regional specialization may be important in preventing inappropriate activation of inflammatory signals in response to the LPS normally present in the intestinal lumen and/or carried over by the small numbers of commensal organisms that may penetrate the epithelial barrier. Since the expression of CD14 on lamina propria macrophages has not been examined during intestinal ontogeny, it is not clear whether levels of this molecule are developmentally regulated, or whether a CD14-negative subset of macrophages is specifically recruited into the developing organ.

Dendritic Cells

Dendritic cells are antigen-processing cells that function at the interface between innate and adaptive immunity (reviewed in reference 81). Immature dendritic cells are avidly phagocytic and endocytotic and can take up and process antigens, including those derived from various microorganisms. In the presence of the appropriate microbial signals (such as LPS), they become activated and migrate out of the tissue to regional lymph nodes, where they present the processed antigen to T cells, along with costimulatory signals and immunoregulatory cytokines. Dendritic cells are thus key elements involved in the initiation and regulation of adaptive immune responses to infectious organisms (103). They may also be involved in the discrimination between commensal and pathogenic bacteria in the gut. Recent work has shown that intestinal lamina propria dendritic cells can extend cytoplasmic processes between enterocytes without disrupting the integrity of the epithelial barrier. They use these processes to take up both commensal and pathogenic bacteria from the lumen, but the subsequent behavior of the cells varies with the kind of organism phagocytosed. Pathogenic bacteria such as *Salmonella* spp. activate the dendritic cells to leave the intestine and (presumably) migrate to the regional lymph node. Commensal bacteria, on the other hand, do not induce this migration (104). This differential migratory behavior could contribute to the difference in immune response to the two kinds of organisms. The ontogeny of dendritic cells in the intestine has not been examined in detail. They appear at about the same time as macrophages and have a similar distribution. Interestingly, a recent report has indicated that dendritic cells derived from umbilical cord monocytes of newborn humans are impaired in the LPS-induced production of IL-12 (39), suggesting that these cells may be in an immature state in the neonatal period.

Paneth Cells

A cluster of Paneth cells, derived from the same stem cells that give rise to enterocytes, is located at the bottom of each crypt. These specialized secretory cells release broad-spectrum, antimicrobial peptides, known as defensins, in response to contact with bacteria (reviewed in references 33 and 96). The function of these cells in mucosal immunity is discussed in detail in chapter 11. They are first seen in the human fetus at about 17 weeks of gestation (120).

Mast Cells

Mast cells, which are present in significant numbers in the lamina propria, are traditionally considered to be effector cells in IgE-mediated allergic responses (reviewed in references 71 and 130). Besides their involvement in food allergies, intestinal mast cells can also play a role in defense against intestinal parasites and enteric bacterial pathogens (30, 77). The latter function involves neutrophil recruitment in response to TNF-α released by bacterially activated mast cells (77). Precise information on the ontogeny of mast cells in the intestine is not available, other than data indicating that these cells are present in approximately equivalent numbers and distribution in the fetal and adult stages, both in humans and in rodents (54).

CELLS OF THE ADAPTIVE IMMUNE SYSTEM

Adaptive immune responses take longer to develop than innate responses, are exquisitely antigen specific, and are characterized by the development of immunological memory. The lymphocyte is the signature cell type that mediates adaptive immunity. During gut ontogeny, lymphocyte populations develop in the human fetal intestine from about 11 weeks of gestation onward. An initial appearance of aggregates of MHC class II$^+$ cells in the lamina propria is followed by the appearance of T and B cells in these aggregates by about 16 weeks, separation into distinct T and B zones by 19 weeks, and an adult-type pattern by about mid-gestation (73, 107). Most of the B cells in the aggregates of fetal intestine are IgM$^+$, with only rare IgA$^+$ or IgG$^+$ cells (114, 115). IgA-expressing B cells and plasma cells are seen in the lamina propria in significant numbers only after birth, especially from the second postnatal week onward (106, 107). IEL appear at around 16 weeks of gestation and are predominantly of the $\gamma\delta$ variety (113). pIgR, necessary for the transcytosis of secretory IgA across the epithelial monolayer, appears in the intestinal epithelium between 16 and 29 weeks of gestation (9, 93). Significant changes occur in intestinal B- and T-cell populations in the postnatal period in response to feeding and colonization with commensal flora. These changes are discussed in more detail in a subsequent section.

The fetus appears to have the ability to mount an adaptive immune response against foreign antigens. A recent clinical study found evidence of both T-cell and B-cell immunoreactivity to *Plasmodium* antigens in the cord blood of infants born in an area of high malaria endemicity (65). However, there are likely to be differences between the immune responsiveness of neonatal and adult lymphocytes, suggesting a gradual maturation from the fetal, through the newborn, and into the adult stages. The immune system of neonatal mice and humans appears to have an intrinsic Th2 bias (2, 6, 101). This skew toward Th2 differentiation normally declines over the first 2 years of life (102), a change that has been attributed to exposure to environmental microorganisms, including intestinal pathogens and commensal bacteria (97, 128). In addition to the tendency toward Th2 differentiation, T cells from newborn humans and mice differ in

their requirement for costimulatory signals, such that it is often more difficult to activate them in vitro, and perhaps in vivo, when compared to their more mature counterparts (2).

The microenvironment of the intestine is traditionally considered to favor suppression of local immune responses. This has been attributed to local production of IL-10, transforming growth factor beta (TGF-β) and other immunoregulatory molecules by T cells, macrophages, dendritic cells, and epithelial cells (4, 10, 57, 91). The precise ontogeny of these features has not been examined, but it is likely that some, if not all, of them may be related to interactions with commensal bacteria or their products (63, 118).

FACTORS THAT INFLUENCE IMMUNE ONTOGENY IN THE GUT

Commensal Bacteria

Commensal bacteria have an important influence on the postnatal development of epithelial and lymphocyte function in the gut (14). Most observations in this area have been made with rodents, but it is likely that they have broad applicability, since clinical studies indicate that commensal bacteria have an important influence on human immune responses.

Epithelial Cells. An earlier section discussed changes in surface glycosylation patterns of enterocytes induced by commensal bacteria (11, 52). In addition, recent microarray analysis has indicated that *B. thetaiotaomicron*, a major component of the commensal flora in mice and humans, has significant global effects on gene expression in intestinal epithelial cells, with the potential to influence multiple intestinal functions, including barrier function (52). Epithelial expression of matrilysin, an enzyme involved in the processing of pro-defensins, has also been shown to be activated by this organism (72). Experiments with a noninvasive *Salmonella* strain, mimicking commensal bacteria, suggest that such organisms may have an inhibitory effect on epithelial NF-κB activation and inflammatory gene expression (90), perhaps helping to explain why the intestine is not in a chronically inflamed state. The developing human intestine appears to overrespond to inflammatory stimuli (89) and requires anti-inflammatory agents that are present in breast milk to modulate inflammation until maturation occurs (37).

B Lymphocytes. The postnatal increase in IgA-producing B cells, alluded to above, is probably related to the antigenic stimulation associated with feeding and the introduction of a commensal bacterial flora (22). Prior to bacterial colonization of the gut, the predominant circulating immunoglobulin is IgM, with a repertoire that is largely independent of external antigen (47). There is no intestinal secretory IgA against commensal organisms (74). When bacterial flora is introduced to formerly germfree mice, Peyer's patch hypertrophy associated with the appearance of germinal centers is seen. A transient bacteremia occurs, leading to a systemic immune response to the bacteria. Simultaneously, secretory IgA to bacterial components develops in the intestine, which limits bacterial translocation across the epithelial barrier and reduces the systemic immune response and the Peyer's patch germinal center reaction (108). Once the secretory IgA response to the commensal flora has been established, it can influence subsequent reactivity to antigens expressed by intestinal bacteria, confining the response to the mucosa without evidence of systemic T-cell priming (74). At least some of the anticommensal secretory IgA production is independent of both T cells and organized lymphoid tissue, but is dependent on a novel pathway of B-cell development involving switching to IgA in the intestine (75). Conventional IgM to IgA switching can also occur in situ in the intestinal lamina propria (31).

T Lymphocytes. Commensal organisms can influence the activation state of CD4$^+$ T cells in the Peyer's patches, leading to an increase in the number of cells with an activated phenotype (15). The effect of commensal bacteria is particularly apparent in the IEL population. Neonatal mice, like fetal humans (113), have a high proportion of $\gamma\delta$ IEL. Germfree animals maintain this characteristic, but colonization with gut flora results in a progressive increase in $\alpha\beta$ IEL (123) and an increase in the constitutive cytolytic activity of $\gamma\delta$ IEL (69). Studies in the rat have indicated similar changes and further showed that the commensal flora influenced the Vβ repertoire of the IEL (49). Developmentally regulated changes in the T-cell receptor repertoire of $\gamma\delta$ IEL in the human gut have also been noted (60), but the relationship to the commensal flora has not been worked out.

Do the changes in the intestinal immune system induced by commensal flora have a role in determining the outcome of subsequent infection with enteric pathogens? A number of studies indicate that precolonization of germfree animals with commensal organisms protects against a subsequent challenge with enteric pathogens (14). The mechanisms underlying this protection have not yet been completely elucidated, but at least in some cases it was independent of the pathogen's effects on intestinal colonization (76, 111). Studies also indicate that the gut commensal flora is important in initiating or maintaining normal systemic Th1/Th2 balance (97, 128) and the normal local immunosuppressive microenvironment (63, 118).

Feeding

The antigenic stimulation and bacterial colonization that result from oral feeding are required for the development of IgM- and IgA-producing plasma cells in the intestinal lamina propria (66). Breast milk deserves special mention because it has a number of positive effects on the intestine and mucosal immune system. Besides providing passive protection with antibacterial components such as IgA, lysozyme, and lactoferrin, it promotes development of a commensal flora rich in bifidobacteria and decreases colonization with potential pathogens (45, 129). It also provides growth factors, such as epidermal growth factor (EGF), insulin-like growth factor (IGF), and TGF-β, that influence enterocyte growth, migration, and maturation (67), all of which may help to decrease the permeability of the epithelial barrier to proteins (105, 121). Indeed, it has been shown that colostrum deprivation delays closure of mucosal membranes (8). Breast milk also provides immunomodulatory molecules, including various cytokines and chemokines, that have the potential to influence the development and function of the mucosal immune system (67) and to modulate inflammation (37).

CLINICAL IMPLICATIONS

Allergies

An increase in atopic diseases worldwide has been associated with declining exposure to environmental microorganisms (21). Antibiotic use in the neonatal period and infancy, which has significant effects on the intestinal flora and therefore on the maturation of the intestinal immune system, has also been associated with the subsequent development of allergic disease (126). Similar observations have been made in experimental animals, indicating that oral kanamycin administration to young mice resulted in an increase in serum IgE and the development of Th2-skewed responses (97). The association between decreased microbial exposure and increased incidence of atopy has been linked to the fact that many bacteria, including the intestinal flora, induce the release of anti-inflammatory cytokines such as IL-10 and TGF-β at some point in their interactions with cells of the immune system. These molecules have important inhibitory effects on the inflammation and Th2-dominated responses seen in allergy, so exposure to lower levels of environmental microorganisms could lead to more exuberant Th2 responses (128). Accordingly, one approach to managing this problem is to deliberately increase contact with harmless microbial flora. Support for this strategy has been provided by the observation that the oral administration of bacteria (*Lactobacillus*) inhibits Th2 responses, in part by stimulating IL-10 production (99).

Necrotizing Enterocolitis

Necrotizing enterocolitis is an inflammatory condition of the bowel that is seen almost exclusively in premature infants. Although the exact pathogenesis of this disease is still unclear, the immature state of the intestine and mucosal immune system is very likely to play a role in the generation of an abnormal inflammatory response to enteric bacteria (18). The decreased barrier function of the immature intestine, coupled with delayed and abnormal bacterial colonization (95), and the paucity of secretory IgA-producing plasma cells are likely to contribute to increased bacterial translocation across the epithelium. The result is activation of a mucosal immune system that has not yet reached its mature state of dampened responsiveness. The enhanced inflammatory responses of immature epithelial cells may also contribute to an exaggerated local inflammatory state.

SUMMARY AND CONCLUSIONS

The developmental changes taking place in the intestinal epithelium and associated immune system are summarized in the time line depicted in Fig. 2. It can be seen that the important cellular elements involved in innate and adaptive immune defense are in place by around mid-gestation, and it would be reasonable to assume that the ability to mount an effective response exists from this point onward. Indeed, the ability of the fetus to mount immune responses to microbial antigens supports this idea (65). This initial phase of ontogeny is probably controlled to a large extent by inherent genetic programs, although environmental stimuli, such as those provided by swallowed amniotic fluid and maternal antibodies, are also likely to contribute. The major changes after this period occur in the epithelial and lymphocyte populations. The epithelial monolayer undergoes alterations in its surface characteristics and permeability, while T and B cells are subjected to a refinement of their repertoire and function. The bulk of this latter phase takes place after birth, largely under the influence of environmental

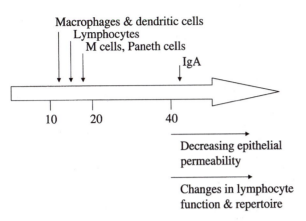

FIGURE 2 Changes in the mucosal immune system during ontogeny. The appearance of various cell types, molecules, and functional changes associated with immune defense of the intestine are depicted along a time line representing the fetal and early neonatal periods. The numbers refer to weeks of gestation.

stimuli provided by feeding and microbial colonization.

To return to the issue raised at the beginning of this review, how do the developmental processes we have described culminate in a mature intestine that has the ability to distinguish between harmful and harmless microorganisms? It is tempting to speculate that this discriminatory function arises as a result of the initial contact with the commensal flora. The changes induced by this contact constitute a molding or "educational" process by which the intestinal epithelium and associated immune system become uniquely adapted to the presence of the commensal microorganisms. A state of détente is thus established in which the organisms are kept from crossing the epithelial barrier in large numbers by mechanisms that have developed to provide defense without inflammation. Any organism that evades or defeats these mechanisms because of special invasive or other properties, and succeeds in multiplying on the lamina propria side of the epithelium, is interpreted by the body as potentially pathogenic. Sensors for such organisms (e.g., TLR5 expressed on the basolateral aspect of the epithelium, or signaling cascades that are activated by bacterial virulence factors [125]) then come into play to activate a full-scale inflammatory reaction. Further study of the role of commensal-host interactions in guiding the maturation of intestinal immune function will provide added insight, not only into the responses that protect against enteric infections, but also into more general mechanisms involved in immunoregulation.

ACKNOWLEDGMENTS

Work in our laboratories is supported by grants from the National Institutes of Health, R01AI48815 (B.J.C.) and R01HD31852, P01DK33506, P30DK40561, and R37HD12437 (W.A.W.). We are grateful to our colleagues Cathryn Nagler-Anderson, Tor Savidge, and Hai Ning Shi for their helpful review of this manuscript.

REFERENCES

1. **Abreu, M. T., P. Vora, E. Faure, L. S. Thomas, E. T. Arnold, and M. Arditi.** 2001. Decreased expression of Toll-like receptor-4 and MD-2 correlates with intestinal epithelial cell protection against dysregulated proinflammatory gene expression in response to bacterial lipopolysaccharide. *J. Immunol.* **167:**1609–1616.
2. **Adkins, B.** 1999. T cell function in newborn mice and humans. *Immunol. Today* **20:**330–335.
3. **al-Majali, A. M., J. P. Robinson, E. K. Asem, C. Lamar, M. J. Freeman, and A. M. Saeed.** 1999. Age-dependent variation in the density and affinity of *Escherichia coli* heat-stable enterotoxin in mice. *Adv. Exp. Med. Biol.* **473:**137–145.
4. **Autschbach, F., J. Braunstein, B. Helmke, I. Zuna, G. Schurmann, Z. I. Niemir, R. Wallich, H. F. Otto, and S. C. Meuer.** 1998. In situ expression of interleukin-10 in noninflamed human gut and in inflammatory bowel disease. *Am. J. Pathol.* **153:**121–130.
5. **Axelsson, I., I. Jakobsson, T. Lindberg, S. Poleberger, B. Benediktsson, and N. Raiha.**

1989. Macromolecular absorption in pre-term and term infants. *Act. Paed. Scand.* **78:**532–537.

6. **Barrios, C., P. Brawand, M. Berney, C. Brandt, P. H. Lambert, and C. A. Siegrist.** 1996. Neonatal and early life immune responses to various forms of vaccine antigens differ from adult responses: predominance of a Th2-biased pattern which persists after adult boosting. *Eur. J. Immunol.* **26:**1489–1496.

7. **Beutler, B.** 2001. Autoimmunity and apoptosis: the Crohn's connection. *Immunity* **15:**5–14.

8. **Bines, J. E., and W. A. Walker.** 1991. Growth factors and the development of neonatal host defence. *Adv. Exp. Med. Biol.* **30:**31–39.

9. **Brandtzaeg, P., D. E. Nilssen, T. O. Rognum, and P. S. Thrane.** 1991. Ontogeny of the mucosal immune system and IgA deficiency. *Gastroenterol. Clin. North Am.* **20:**397–439.

10. **Braunstein, J., L. Qiao, F. Autschbach, G. Schumann, and S. Meuer.** 1997. T cells of the human intestinal lamina propria are high producers of interleukin-10. *Gut* **41:**215–220.

11. **Bry, L., P. G. Falk, T. Midtvedt, and J. I. Gordon.** 1996. A model of host-microbial interactions in an open mammalian ecosystem. *Science* **273:**1380–1383.

12. **Cario, E., and D. K. Podolsky.** 2000. Differential alteration in intestinal epithelial cell expression of TLR3 and TLR4 in inflammatory bowel disease. *Infect. Immun.* **68:**7010–7017.

13. **Cario, E., I. M. Rosenberg, S. L. Brandwein, P. L. Beck, H. C. Reinecker, and D. K. Podolsky.** 2000. Lipopolysaccharide activates distinct signaling pathways in intestinal epithelial cell lines expressing Toll-like receptors. *J. Immunol.* **164:**966–972.

14. **Cebra, J. J.** 1999. Influences of microbiota on intestinal immune system development. *Am. J. Clin. Nutr.* **69:**1046S–1051S.

15. **Cebra, J. J., S. B. Periwal, G. Lee, F. Lee, and K. E. Shroff.** 1998. Development and maintenance of the gut-associated lymphoid tissue (GALT): the roles of enteric bacteria and viruses. *Dev. Immunol.* **6:**13–18.

16. **Chu, S. H., I. G. Ely, and W. A. Walker.** 1989. Age and cortisone alter host responsiveness to cholera toxin in the developing gut. *Am. J. Physiol.* **256:**G220–G225.

17. **Chu, S. H., and W. A. Walker.** 1986. Developmental changes in the activities of sialyl- and fucosyltransferases in rat small intestine. *Biochim. Biophys. Acta* **883:**496–500.

18. **Claud, E. C., and W. A. Walker.** 2001. Hypothesis: inappropriate colonization of the premature intestine can cause neonatal necrotizing enterocolitis. *FASEB J.* **15:**1398–1403.

19. **Cohen, M. B., A. Guarino, R. Shukla, and R. A. Giannella.** 1988. Age-related differences in receptors for *E. coli* heat-stable enterotoxin in the small and large intestine of children. *Gastroenterology* **94:**367–373.

20. **Cohen, M. B., M. S. Moyer, M. Luttrell, and R. A. Giannella.** 1986. The immature rat small intestine exhibits an increased sensitivity and response to *Escherichia coli* heat-stable enterotoxin. *Pediatr. Res.* **20:**555–560.

21. **Committee, I. S.** 1998. World variation in prevalence of symptoms of asthma, allergic rhinoconjunctivitis, and atopic eczema. *Lancet* **351:**1225–1232.

22. **Crabbe, P. A., H. Bazin, H. Eyssen, and J. F. Heremans.** 1968. The normal microbial flora as a major stimulus for proliferation of plasma cells synthesizing IgA in the gut. *Int. Arch. Allerg.* **34:**362–375.

23. **Dai, D., N. N. Nanthakumar, D. S. Newburg, and W. A. Walker.** 2000. Role of oligosaccharides and glycoconjugates in intestinal host defense. *J. Ped. Gastroenterol. Nutr.* **30:**S23–S33.

24. **Dai, D., N. N. Nanthakumar, T. C. Savidge, D. S. Newburg, and W. A. Walker.** 2002. Region-specific ontogeny of α-2,6-sialyltransferase during normal and cortisone-induced maturation in mouse intestine. *Am. J. Physiol. Gastrointest. Liver Physiol.* **282:**G480–G490.

25. **Das, H., V. Groh, C. Kuijl, M. Sugita, C. T. Morita, T. Spies, and J. F. Bukowski.** 2001. MICA engagement by human Vγ2Vδ2 T cells enhances their antigen-dependent effector function. *Immunity* **15:**83–93.

26. **Debard, N., F. Sierro, J. Browning, and J. P. Kraehenbuhl.** 2001. Effect of mature lymphocytes and lymphotoxin on the development of follicle-associated epithelium and M cells in mouse Peyer's patches. *Gastroenterology* **120:**1173–1182.

27. **Denari, G., T. L. Hale, and O. Washington.** 1986. Effect of guinea pig or monkey colonic mucus on *Shigella* aggregation and invasion of HeLa cells by *Shigella flexneri* 1b and 2a. *Infect. Immun.* **51:**975–978.

28. **Dwinell, M. B., N. Lugering, L. Eckmann, and M. F. Kagnoff.** 2001. Regulated production of interferon-inducible T cell chemoattractants by human intestinal epithelial cells. *Gastroenterology* **120:**49–59.

29. **Eglow, R., C. Pothoulakis, S. Itzkowitz, E. J. Israel, C. J. O'Keane, D. Gong, N. Gao, Y. L. Xu, W. A. Walker, and J. T. LaMont.** 1992. Diminished *Clostridium difficile* toxin A sensitivity in newborn rabbit ileum is associated with decreased toxin A receptor. *J. Clin. Invest.* **90:**822–829.

30. **Else, K. J., and F. D. Finkelman.** 1998. Intestinal nematode parasites, cytokines, and effector mechanisms. *Int. J. Parasitol.* **28:**1145–1158.

31. **Fagarasan, S., K. Kinoshita, M. Muramatsu, K. Ikuta, and T. Honjo.** 2001. In situ class switching and differentiation to IgA-producing cells in the gut lamina propria. *Nature* **413:**639–643.

32. **Fusunyan, R. D., N. N. Nanthakumar, M. E. Baldeon, and W. A. Walker.** 2001. Evidence for an innate immune response in the immature human intestine: Toll-like receptors on fetal enterocytes. *Pediatr. Res.* **49:**589–593.

33. **Ganz, T.** 2000. Paneth cells—guardians of the gut cell hatchery. *Nature Immunol.* **1:**99–100.

34. **Gewirtz, A. T., T. A. Navas, S. Lyons, P. J. Godowski, and J. L. Madara.** 2001. Cutting edge: bacterial flagellin activates basolaterally expressed TLR5 to induce epithelial proinflammatory gene expression. *J. Immunol.* **167:**1882–1885.

35. **Gewirtz, A. T., P. O. Simon, C. K. Schmitt, L. J. Taylor, C. H. Hagedorn, A. D. O'Brien, A. S. Neish, and J. L. Madara.** 2001. *Salmonella typhimurium* translocates flagellin across intestinal epithelia, inducing a proinflammatory response. *J. Clin. Investig.* **107:**99–109.

36. **Girardin, S. E., R. Tournebize, M. Mavris, A.-L. Page, X. Li, G. R. Stark, J. Bertin, P. S. DiStefano, M. Yaniv, P. J. Sansonetti, and D. J. Philpott.** 2001. CARD4/Nod1 mediates NF-κB and JNK activation by invasive *Shigella flexneri*. *EMBO Rep.* **2:**736–742.

37. **Goldman, A. S.** 1993. The immune system of human milk: anti-microbial, anti-inflammatory and immunomodulating properties. *Pediatr. Infect. Dis. J.* **12:**664–671.

38. **Golovkina, T. V., M. Shlomchik, L. Hannum, and A. Chervonsky.** 1999. Organogenic role of B lymphocytes in mucosal immunity. *Science* **286:**1965–1968.

39. **Goriely, S., B. Vincart, P. Stordeur, J. Vekemans, F. Willems, M. Goldman, and D. De Wit.** 2001. Deficient IL-12 (p35) gene expression by dendritic cells derived from neonatal monocytes. *J. Immunol.* **166:**2141–2146.

40. **Greco, S., I. Hugueny, P. George, P. Perrin, P. Louisot, and M. C. Biol.** 2000. Influence of spermine on intestinal maturation of the glycoprotein glycosylation process in neonatal rats. *Biochem. J.* **345:**69–75.

41. **Groh, V., S. Bahram, S. Bauer, A. Herman, M. Beauchamp, and T. Spies.** 1996. Cell stress-related human major histocompatibility complex class I gene expressed in gastrointestinal epithelium. *Proc. Natl. Acad. Sci. USA* **93:**12445–12450.

42. **Groh, V., R. Rhinehart, J. Randolph-Habecker, M. S. Topp, S. R. Riddell, and T. Spies.** 2001. Costimulation of CD8αβ T cells by NKG2D via engagement by MIC induced on virus-infected cells. *Nature Immunol.* **2:**198–200.

43. **Groh, V., A. Steinle, S. Bauer, and T. Spies.** 1998. Recognition of stress-induced MHC molecules by intestinal epithelial γδ T cells. *Science* **279:**1737–1740.

44. **Hampe, J., A. Cuthbert, P. J. Croucher, M. M. Mirza, S. Mascheretti, S. Fisher, H. Frenzel, K. King, A. Hasselmeyer, A. J. MacPherson, S. Bridger, S. van Deventer, A. Forbes, S. Nikolaus, J. E. Lennard-Jones, U. R. Foelsch, M. Krawczak, C. Lewis, S. Schreiber, and C. G. Mathew.** 2001. Association between insertion mutation in NOD2 gene and Crohn's disease in German and British populations. *Lancet* **357:**1902–1904.

45. **Harmsen, H. J., A. C. Wildeboer-Veloo, G. C. Raangs, A. A. Wagendorp, N. Klijn, J. G. Bindels, and G. W. Welling.** 2000. Analysis of intestinal flora development in breast-fed and formula-fed infants by using molecular identification and detection methods. *J. Pediatr. Gastroenterol. Nutr.* **30:**61–67.

46. **Harvey, J., D. B. Jones, and D. H. Wright.** 1990. Differential expression of MHC- and macrophage-associated antigens in human fetal and postnatal small intestine. *Immunology* **69:**409–415.

47. **Haury, M., A. Sundblad, A. Grandien, C. Barreau, A. Coutinho, and A. Nobrega.** 1997. The repertoire of serum IgM in normal mice is largely independent of external antigenic contact. *Eur. J. Immunol.* **27:**1557–1563.

48. **Hayday, A., E. Theodoridis, E. Ramsburg, and J. Shires.** 2001. Intraepithelial lymphocytes: exploring the third way in immunology. *Nature Immunol.* **2:**997–1003.

49. **Helgeland, L., J. T. Vaage, B. Rolstad, T. Midtvedt, and P. Brandtzaeg.** 1996. Microbial colonization influences composition and T cell receptor V beta repertoire of intraepithelial lymphocytes in rat intestine. *Immunology* **89:**494–501.

50. **Hobbie, S., L. M. Chen, R. J. Davis, and J. E. Galan.** 1997. Involvement of mitogen-activated protein kinase pathways in the nuclear responses and cytokine production induced by *Salmonella typhimurium* in cultured intestinal epithelial cells. *J. Immunol.* **159:**5550–5559.

51. **Hooper, L. V., and J. I. Gordon.** 2001. Glycans as legislators of host-microbial interactions: spanning the spectrum from symbiosis to pathogenicity. *Glycobiology* **11:**1R–10R.

52. **Hooper, L. V., M. H. Wong, A. Thelin, L. Hansson, P. G. Falk, and J. L. Gordon.** 2001. Molecular analysis of commensal host-microbial relationships in the intestine. *Science* **291**:881–884.

53. **Hooper, L. V., J. Xu, P. G. Falk, T. Midtvedt, and J. I. Gordon.** 1999. A molecular sensor that allows a gut commensal to control its nutrient foundation in a competitive ecosystem. *Proc. Natl. Acad. Sci. USA* **96**:9833–9838.

54. **Horie, K., J. Fujita, K. Takakura, H. Kanzaki, H. Suginami, M. Iwai, H. Nakayama, and T. Mori.** 1993. The expression of c-kit protein in human adult and fetal tissues. *Hum. Repr.* **8**:1955–1962.

55. **Hugot, J. P., M. Chamaillard, H. Zouali, S. Lesage, J. P. Cezard, J. Belaiche, S. Almer, C. Tysk, C. A. O'Morain, M. Gassull, V. Binder, Y. Finkel, A. Cortot, R. Modigliani, P. Laurent-Puig, C. Gower-Rousseau, J. Macry, J. F. Colombel, M. Sahbatou, and G. Thomas.** 2001. Association of NOD2 leucine-rich repeat variants with susceptibility to Crohn's disease. *Nature* **411**:537–539.

56. **Hyman, P. E., D. D. Clarke, S. L. Everett, B. Sonne, D. Steward, T. Harada, J. H. Walsh, and I. L. Taylor.** 1985. Gastric acid secretory function in pre-term infants. *J. Pediatr.* **106**:467–471.

57. **Iwasaki, A., and B. L. Kelsall.** 2001. Unique functions of CD11b⁻ CD8α⁺ and double negative Peyer's patch dendritic cells. *J. Immunol.* **166**:4884–4890.

58. **Jarvis, W. B., and R. A. Feldman.** 1984. *Clostridium difficile* and gastroenteritis: how strong is the association in children? *Pediatr. Infect. Dis. J.* **3**:4.

59. **Jaso-Friedmann, L., L. A. Dreyfus, S. C. Whipp, and D. C. Robertson.** 1992. Effect of age on activation of porcine intestinal guanylate cyclase and binding of *Escherichia coli* heat-stable enterotoxin (STα) to porcine intestinal cells and brush border membranes. *Am. J. Vet. Res.* **53**:2251–2258.

60. **Kagnoff, M. F.** 1998. Current concepts in mucosal immunity. III. Ontogeny and function of γδ T cells in the intestine. *Am. J. Physiol.* **274**:G455–G458.

61. **Kato, T., and R. L. Owen.** 1999. Structure and function of intestinal mucosal epithelium, p. 115–132. *In* P. L. Ogra, J. Mestecky, M. E. Lamm, W. Strober, J. Bienenstock, and J. R. McGhee (ed.), *Mucosal Immunology*, 2nd ed. Academic Press Inc., San Diego, Calif.

62. **Kerneis, S., A. Bogdanova, J. P. Kraehenbuhl, and E. Pringault.** 1997. Conversion by Peyer's patch lymphocytes of human enterocytes into M cells that transport bacteria. *Science* **277**:910–911.

63. **Kim, J. H., and M. Ohsawa.** 1995. Oral tolerance to ovalbumin in mice as a model for detecting modulation of the immunologic tolerance to a specific antigen. *Biol. Pharmacol. Bull.* **18**:854–858.

64. **Kimura, A.** 1977. The epithelial-macrophage relationship in Peyer's patches: an immunopathological study. *Bull. Osaka Med. Sch.* **23**:67–91.

65. **King, C. L., I. Malhotra, A. Wamachi, J. Kioko, P. Mungai, S. A. Wahab, D. Koech, P. Zimmerman, J. Ouma, and J. W. Kazura.** 2002. Acquired immune responses to *Plasmodium falciparum* merozoite surface protein-1 in the human fetus. *J. Immunol.* **168**:356–364.

66. **Knox, W. F.** 1986. Restricted feeding and human intestinal plasma cell development. *Arch. Dis. Child.* **61**:744–749.

67. **Koldovsky, O., and A. S. Goldman.** 1999. Growth factors and cytokines in milk, p. 1523–1530. *In* P. L. Ogra, J. Mestecky, M. E. Lamm, W. Strober, J. Bienenstock, and J. R. McGhee (ed.), *Mucosal Immunology*, 2nd ed. Academic Press Inc., San Diego, Calif.

68. **Lebenthal, E., and P. C. Lee.** 1982. Alternate pathways of digestion and absorption in early infancy. *J. Pediatr. Gastroenterol. Nutr.* **3**:1–3.

69. **Lefrancois, L., and T. Goodman.** 1989. In vivo modulation of cytolytic activity and Thy-1 expression in TCR-γδ+ intraepithelial lymphocytes. *Science* **243**:1716–1718.

70. **Leishman, A. J., O. V. Naidenko, A. Attinger, F. Koning, C. J. Lena, Y. Xiong, H.-C. Chang, E. Reinherz, M. Kronenberg, and H. Cheroutre.** 2001. T cell responses modulated through interaction between CDαα and the nonclassical MHC class I molecule TL. *Science* **294**:1936–1939.

71. **Lin, T.-J., and A. D. Befus.** 1999. Mast cells and eosinophils in mucosal defenses and pathogenesis, p. 469–482. *In* P. L. Ogra, J. Mestecky, M. E. Lamm, W. Strober, J. Bienenstock, and J. R. McGhee (ed.), *Mucosal Immunology*, 2nd ed. Academic Press Inc., San Diego, Calif.

72. **Lopez-Boado, Y. S., C. L. Wilson, L. V. Hooper, J. I. Gordon, S. J. Hultgren, and W. C. Parks.** 2000. Bacterial exposure induces and activates matrilysin in mucosal epithelial cells. *J. Cell Biol.* **148**:1305–1315.

73. **MacDonald, T. T., and J. Spencer.** 1994. Ontogeny of the gut-associated lymphoid system in man. *Acta Paed. Suppl.* **83**:3–5.

74. **Macpherson, A. J., D. Gatto, E. Sainsbury, G. R. Harriman, H. Hengartner, and R. M. Zinkernagel.** 2000. A primitive T cell-independent mechanism of intestinal mucosal IgA

responses to commensal bacteria. *Science* **288:** 2222–2226.

75. **Macpherson, A. J. S., A. Lamarre, K. McCoy, G. R. Harriman, B. Odermatt, G. Dougan, H. Hengartner, and R. M. Zinkernagel.** 2001. IgA production without μ or ∂ chain expression in developing B cells. *Nature Immunol.* **2:**625–631.

76. **Maia, O. B., R. Duarte, A. M. Silva, D. C. Cara, and J. R. Nicoli.** 2001. Evaluation of the components of a commercial probiotic in gnotobiotic mice experimentally challenged with *Salmonella enterica* subsp. *enterica* ser. *typhimurium. Vet. Microbiol.* **79:**183–189.

77. **Malaviya, R., T. Ikeda, E. Ross, and S. N. Abraham.** 1996. Mast cell modulation of neutrophil influx and bacterial clearance at sites of infection through TNFα. *Nature* **381:**77–80.

78. **McCormick, B. A., C. A. Parkos, S. P. Colgan, D. K. Carnes, and J. L. Madara.** 1998. Apical secretion of a pathogen-elicited epithelial chemoattractant activity in response to surface colonization of intestinal epithelia by *Salmonella typhimurium. J. Immunol.* **160:**455–466.

79. **McGee, D. W.** 1999. Inflammation and mucosal cytokine production, p. 559–573. *In* P. L. Ogra, J. Mestecky, M. E. Lamm, W. Strober, J. Bienenstock, and J. R. McGhee (ed.), *Mucosal Immunology*, 2nd ed. Academic Press Inc., San Diego, Calif.

80. **Medzhitov, R.** 2001. Toll-like receptors and innate immunity. *Nature Rev. Immunol.* **1:**135–145.

81. **Mellman, I., and R. M. Steinman.** 2001. Dendritic cells: specialized and regulated antigen processing machines. *Cell* **106:**255–258.

82. **Milla, P. J.** 1996. Intestinal motility during ontogeny and intestinal pseudo-obstruction in children. *Pediatr. Clin. North Am.* **43:**511–532.

83. **Mobassaleh, M., A. Donohue-Rolfe, M. Jacewicz, R. J. Grand, and G. T. Keusch.** 1988. Pathogenesis of *Shigella* diarrhea: evidence for a developmentally-regulated glycolipid receptor for *Shigella* toxin involved in the fluid secretory response of rabbit small intestine. *J. Infect. Dis.* **157:**1023–1031.

84. **Mobassaleh, M., S. K. Gross, R. H. McCluer, A. Donohue-Rolfe, and G. T. Keusch.** 1989. Quantitation of the rabbit intestinal glycolipid receptor for Shiga toxin. Further evidence for the developmental regulation of globotriaosylceramide in microvillus membranes. *Gastroenterology* **97:**384–391.

85. **Moxey, P. C., and J. S. Trier.** 1978. Specialized cell types in the human fetal small intestine. *Anat. Rec.* **191:**269–286.

86. **Nagashima, R., K. Maeda, Y. Imai, and T. Takahashi.** 1996. Lamina propria macrophages in the human gastrointestinal mucosa: their distribution, immunohistological phenotype, and function. *J. Histochem. Cytochem.* **44:**721–731.

87. **Nagler-Anderson, C., and H. N. Shi.** 2001. Peripheral nonresponsiveness to orally administered soluble protein antigens. *Crit. Rev. Immunol.* **21:**121–132.

88. **Naik, S., E. J. Kelly, L. Meijer, S. Pettersson, and I. R. Sanderson.** 2001. Absence of Toll-like receptor 4 explains endotoxin hyporesponsiveness in human intestinal epithelium. *J. Pediatr. Gastroenterol. Nutr.* **32:**449–453.

89. **Nanthakumar, N. N., R. D. Fusunyan, I. Sanderson, and W. A. Walker.** 2000. Inflammation in the developing human intestine: a possible pathophysiologic contribution to necrotizing enterocolitis. *Proc. Natl. Acad. Sci. USA* **97:**6043–6048.

90. **Neish, A. S., A. T. Gewirtz, H. Zeng, A. N. Young, M. E. Hobert, V. Karmali, A. S. Rao, and J. L. Madara.** 2000. Prokaryotic regulation of epithelial responses by inhibition of IκBα degradation. *Science* **289:**1560–1563.

91. **Newberry, R. D., W. F. Stenson, and R. G. Lorenz.** 1999. Cyclooxygenase-2-dependent arachidonic acid metabolites are essential modulators of the intestinal immune response to dietary antigen. *Nature Med.* **5:**900–906.

92. **Niedergang, F., and J.-P. Kraehenbuhl.** 2000. Much ado about M cells. *Tr. Cell Biol.* **10:** 137–141.

93. **Ogra, S. S., P. L. Ogra, J. Lippes, and T. B. J. Tomasi.** 1972. Immunohistologic localization of immunoglobulins, secretory component, and lactoferrin in the developing human fetus. *Proc. Soc. Exp. Biol. Med.* **139:**570–574.

94. **Ogura, Y., D. K. Bonen, N. Inohara, D. L. Nicolae, F. F. Chen, R. Ramos, H. Britton, T. Moran, R. Karaliuskas, R. H. Duerr, J. P. Achkar, S. R. Brant, T. M. Bayless, B. S. Kirschner, S. B. Hanauer, G. Nunez, and J. H. Cho.** 2001. A frameshift mutation in NOD2 associated with susceptibility to Crohn's disease. *Nature* **31:**603–606.

95. **Orrahge, K., and C. E. Nord.** 1999. Factors controlling the bacterial colonization of the intestine in breast-fed infants. *Act. Paed. Suppl.* **88:** 47–57.

96. **Ouellette, A. J., and C. L. Bevins.** 2001. Paneth cell defensins and innate immunity of the small bowel. *Inflamm. Bowel Dis.* **7:**43–50.

97. **Oyama, N., N. Sudo, H. Sogawa, and C. Kubo.** 2001. Antibiotic use during infancy promotes a shift in the Th1/Th2 balance toward Th2-dominated immunity in mice. *J. Allerg. Clin. Immunol.* **107:**153–159.

98. **Pavli, P., L. Maxwell, E. Van de Pol, and F. Doe.** 1996. Distribution of human colonic dendritic cells and macrophages. *Clin. Exp. Immunol.* **104:**124–132.

99. **Pessi, T., Y. Sutas, M. Hurme, and E. Isolauri.** 2000. IL-10 generation in atopic children following oral *Lactobacillus rhamnosus GG*. *Clin. Exp. Allerg.* **30:**1804–1808.

100. **Polak-Charcon, S., J. Shoham, and Y. Ben-Shaul.** 1980. Tight junctions in epithelial cells of human fetal hindgut, normal colon and adenocarcinoma. *JNCI* **65:**53–62.

101. **Prescott, S. L., C. Macaubas, B. J. Holt, T. B. Smallacombe, R. Loh, P. D. Sly, and P. G. Holt.** 1998. Transplacental priming of the human immune system to environmental allergens: universal skewing of initial T cell responses toward the Th2 cytokine profile. *J. Immunol.* **160:**4730–4737.

102. **Prescott, S. L., C. Macaubas, T. Smallacombe, B. J. Holt, P. D. Sly, R. Loh, and P. G. Holt.** 1998. Reciprocal age-related patterns of allergen-specific T-cell immunity in normal vs atopic infants. *Clin. Exp. Allerg.* **28:** 38–44.

103. **Rescigno, M., and P. Borrow.** 2001. The host-pathogen interaction: new themes from dendritic cell biology. *Cell* **106:**267–270.

104. **Rescigno, M., M. Urbano, B. Valzasina, M. Francolini, G. Rotta, R. Bonasio, F. Graucci, J.-P. Kraehenbuhl, and P. Ricciardi-Castagnoli.** 2001. Dendritic cells express tight junction proteins and penetrate gut epithelial monolayers to sample bacteria. *Nature Immunol.* **2:**361–367.

105. **Roberton, D. M., R. Paganelli, R. Dinwiddie, and R. J. Levinsky.** 1982. Milk antigen absorption in the preterm and term neonate. *Arch. Dis. Child.* **57:**369–372.

106. **Rognum, T. O., S. Thrane, L. Stoltenberg, A. Vege, and P. Brandtzaeg.** 1992. Development of intestinal mucosal immunity in fetal life and the first postnatal months. *Pediatr. Res.* **32:**145–149.

107. **Russell, G. J., A. K. Bhan, and H. S. Winter.** 1990. The distribution of T and B lymphocyte populations and MHC class II expression in human fetal and postnatal intestine. *Pediatr. Res.* **27:**239–244.

108. **Shroff, K. E., K. Meslin, and J. J. Cebra.** 1995. Commensal enteric bacteria engender a self-limiting humoral mucosal immune response while permanently colonizing the gut. *Infect. Immun.* **63:**3904–3913.

109. **Shub, M. D., K. Y. Pang, D. A. Swann, and W. A. Walker.** 1983. Age-related changes in chemical composition and physical properties of mucus glycoproteins from rat small intestine. *Biochem. J.* **215:**405–411.

110. **Sierro, F., B. Dubois, A. Coste, D. Kaiserlian, J. P. Kraehenbuhl, and J. C. Sirard.** 2001. Flagellin stimulation of intestinal epithelial cells triggers CCL20-mediated migration of dendritic cells. *Proc. Natl. Acad. Sci. USA* **98:** 13722–13727.

111. **Silva, A. M., E. A. Bambirra, A. L. Oliveira, P. P. Souza, D. A. Gomes, E. C. Vieira, and J. R. Nicoli.** 1999. Protective effect of bifidus milk on the experimental infection with *Salmonella enteritidis* subsp. *typhimurium* in conventional and gnotobiotic mice. *J. Appl. Microbiol.* **86:**331–336.

112. **Smith, P. D., L. E. Smythies, M. Mosteller-Barnum, D. A. Sibley, M. W. Russell, M. Merger, M. T. Sellers, J. M. Orenstein, T. Shimada, M. F. Graham, and H. Kubagawa.** 2001. Intestinal macrophages lack CD14 and CD89 and consequently are down-regulated for LPS- and IgA-mediated activities. *J. Immunol.* **167:**2651–2656.

113. **Spencer, J., P. G. Isaacson, T. C. Diss, and T. T. MacDonald.** 1989. Expression of disulphide-linked and non-disulphide-linked forms of T cell receptor gamma/delta heterodimer in human intestinal intraepithelial lymphocytes. *Eur. J. Immunol.* **19:**1335–1338.

114. **Spencer, J., T. T. MacDonald, T. Finn, and P. G. Isaacson.** 1986. The development of the gut-associated lymphoid tissue in the terminal ileum of fetal human intestine. *Clin. Exp. Immunol.* **64:**536–543.

115. **Spencer, J., T. T. MacDonald, and P. G. Isaacson.** 1987. Development of human gut-associated lymphoid tissue. *Adv. Exp. Med. Biol.* **216B:**1421–1430.

116. **Spencer, J., T. T. MacDonald, and P. G. Isaacson.** 1987. Heterogeneity of non-lymphoid cells expressing HLA-DR region antigens in human fetal gut. *Clin. Exp. Immunol.* **67:**415–424.

117. **Stephens, H. A. F.** 2001. MICA and MICB genes: can the enigma of their polymorphism be resolved? *Tr. Immunol.* **22:**378–385.

118. **Sudo, N., S. Sawamura, K. Tanaka, Y. Aiba, C. Kubo, and Y. Koga.** 1997. The requirement of intestinal bacterial flora for the development of an IgE production system fully susceptible to oral tolerance induction. *J. Immunol.* **159:**1739–1745.

119. **Torres-Pinedo, R., and A. Mahmood.** 1984. Postnatal changes in biosynthesis of microvillus membrane glycans of rat small intestine. I. Evidence of developmental shift from

terminal sialylation to fucosylation. *Biochem. Biophys. Res. Commun.* **125:**546–553.

120. **Trier, J. S., and P. C. Moxey.** 1979. Morphogenesis of the small intestine during fetal development. *CIBA Found. Symp.* **70:**3–29.

121. **Udall, J. N., P. Colony, L. Fritze, K. Pang, J. S. Trier, and W. A. Walker.** 1981. Development of gastrointestinal mucosal barrier. II. The effect of natural versus artificial feeding on intestinal permeability to macromolecules. *Pediatr. Res.* **15:**245–249.

122. **Udall, J. N., K. Pang, L. Fritze, R. Kleinman, and W. A. Walker.** 1981. Development of gastrointestinal mucosal barrier. I. The effect of age on intestinal permeability to macromolecules. *Pediatr. Res.* **15:**241–244.

123. **Umesaki, Y., H. Setoyama, S. Matsumoto, and Y. Okada.** 1993. Expansion of $\alpha\beta$ T cell receptor bearing intestinal intraepithelial lymphocytes after microbial colonization in germfree mice and its independence from thymus. *Immunol.* **79:**32–37.

124. **Van Heel, D. A., D. P. McGovern, and D. P. Jewell.** 2001. Crohn's disease: genetic susceptibility, bacteria and innate immunity. *Lancet* **357:**1925–1928.

125. **Wallis, T. S., and E. E. Galyov.** 2000. Molecular basis of *Salmonella*-induced enteritis. *Mol. Microbiol.* **36:**997–1005.

126. **Wickens, K., N. Pearce, J. Crane, and R. Beasley.** 1999. Antibiotic use in early childhood and the development of asthma. *Clin. Exp. Allergy* **29:**766–771.

127. **Williams, R. C., and R. J. Gibbons.** 1975. Inhibition of streptococcal attachment of receptors on human buccal epithelial cells by antigenically similar salivary glycoproteins. *Infect. Immun.* **11:**711–715.

128. **Wills-Karp, M., J. Santeliz, and C. L. Karp.** 2001. The germless theory of allergic disease: revisiting the hygiene hypothesis. *Nature Rev. Immunol.* **1:**69–75.

129. **Wold, A. E., and I. Adlerberth.** 2000. Breast feeding and the intestinal microflora of the infant—implications for protection against infectious diseases. *Adv. Exp. Med. Biol.* **478:**77–93.

130. **Yu, L. L., and M. H. Perdue.** 2001. Role of mast cells in intestinal mucosal function: studies in models of hypersensitivity and stress. *Immunol. Rev.* **179:**61–73.

NEUROIMMUNE INTERACTIONS AND PATHOGENESIS OF INTESTINAL INFLAMMATION IN INFECTIOUS DISEASES

Charalabos Pothoulakis

19

THE NEUROPEPTIDE GALANIN MODULATES *E. COLI*–MEDIATED DIARRHEA

The attachment of bacteria to mucosal surfaces is the initial event in the pathogenesis of several bacterial infections in the gastrointestinal tract. The best-studied examples of diarrhea and inflammation caused by enterobacterial pathogens are infection due to *Salmonella* spp. and pathogenic *Escherichia coli*, including enteropathogenic *E. coli* (EPEC) and enterohemorrhagic *E. coli* (EHEC). Although it is well recognized that enteric pathogens can stimulate several secretory and proinflammatory responses following contact with intestinal epithelial cells (30, 42, 94), the mechanism by which these responses are generated is not entirely clear. A series of elegant studies demonstrated that the peptide-hormone galanin and galanin receptors localized in the intestinal mucosa may be involved in the pathophysiology of infectious diarrhea. Galanin is a 29-amino-acid peptide with brain-gut distribution that regulates several intestinal functions, including gastrointestinal motility, acid secretion, and hormone release (3). Galanin is localized in the myenteric and the submucosal plexus in close proximity to the epithelium, and galanin type 1 (Gal1) receptors have been identified in the human intestine (57).

In colonic adenocarcinoma T84 cells expressing endogenous Gal1 receptors, galanin exposure causes Cl^- secretion that is mediated via increased calcium (4). Interestingly, the addition of EHEC, EPEC, and enterotoxigenic *E. coli* (ETEC), but not normal commensal *E. coli*, to T84 cell monolayers results in increased expression of Gal1 receptors at the mRNA and protein levels (39) (Color Plate 7). Moreover, colonic tissues from infected mice placed in Ussing chambers demonstrated substantial Cl^- secretion in response to galanin (39), indicating that upregulation of galanin receptors in response to enteric pathogens represents a pivotal mechanism for fluid secretion during infection. The importance of Gal1 receptors in infectious diarrhea was directly confirmed in animals genetically deficient in these receptors, which demonstrated a substantial reduction in fluid secretion following infection (67). Interestingly, *Salmonella enterica* serovar Typhimurium and *Shigella flexneri* also lead to upregulation of Gal1 receptors in the colonic epithelium, and the absence of these receptors results in reduced colonic fluid secretion in

Charalabos Pothoulakis, Division of Gastroenterology, Beth Israel Deaconess Medical Center, Harvard Medical School, 330 Brookline Avenue, Boston, MA 02215.

response to these pathogens (67). Together, these findings suggest that epithelial-neuronal interactions during infection with enteric pathogenic microbes represent a major functional component of secretory responses to these organisms (Color Plate 7). It is noteworthy that the enteric nervous system also plays a pivotal role in the intestinal secretory responses to toxins released from ETEC (58). An intriguing aspect of the Gal1 receptor-mediated gut secretion and inflammation is the mechanism of its upregulation during bacterial infections. Exposure of mice to an array of bacterial pathogens causes increased NF-κB immunoreactivity as well as increased expression of Gal1 receptors at the colonocyte level (39) (Color Plate 7). Increased NF-κB activation and Gal1 expression were dramatically reduced by the general NF-κB inhibitor dexamethazone, suggesting that Gal1 receptor expression is linked to NF-κB (Color Plate 7). In support of this hypothesis, Lorimer et al. identified two NF-κB binding sites in the promoter region of the Gal1 receptor gene that appear to be important for the regulation of this promoter (57). These findings are consistent with increased expression of these receptors not only during infection with pathogenic organisms (39, 67), but also during dextran sodium sulfate (DSS)-induced colitis, a condition where NF-κB activation is also evident (63).

ROLE OF SP IN SALMONELLA INFECTION

Substance P (SP) and its receptors have been implicated in the mediation of inflammation in many organs, including the gastrointestinal tract. Several pieces of evidence also indicate that this neuropeptide participates in the pathophysiology of Salmonella infection. For example, oral administration of Salmonella to mice resulted in a rapid and substantial upregulation of mRNAs for the high-affinity SP and neurokinin-1 (NK-1) receptor in the Peyer's patches and mesenteric lymph nodes (46). Pretreatment of mice with a peptide SP antagonist prior to Salmonella infection resulted in an earlier appearance of infection, in-

creased lethality, and reduced mucosal levels of interleukin 12 (IL-12) and gamma interferon (IFN-γ) mRNAs in infected mice (46). Interestingly, endogenous IL-12 enhances the immune response and protects mice from Salmonella infection (48), and SP via its NK-1 receptor stimulates IL-12 release from macrophages (47). Macrophages also express SP mRNA, which can be upregulated, leading to the release of SP when exposed to bacterial lipopolysaccharide (LPS) in vitro or during intestinal inflammation in vivo (10, 14). Salmonella enters the host and survives in macrophages and neutrophils. Furthermore, immunity against this bacterium is based on the capacity of these cells to kill ingested bacteria (40). Thus, SP and the NK-1 receptor may play an important role in the host's protective immune responses to Salmonella and possibly other pathogens. The cellular mechanism(s) of proinflammatory effects of SP in the gut may be directly related to its capacity to induce cellular activation of NF-κB (55), a transcription factor related to upregulation of genes for several proinflammatory cytokines linked to intestinal inflammation.

Neuroimmune interactions and the enteric nervous system also play a major role in the pathogenesis of intestinal secretion due to Salmonella infection. Ileal and duodenal fluid secretion following intragastric inoculation of S. enterica serovar Typhimurium to rats was diminished by administration of the nerve blocking agents hexamethonium and lidocaine, as well as by intravenous administration of the prostaglandin inhibitor indomethacin (11). Thus, S. enterica serovar Typhimurium invades the intestinal mucosa and stimulates an inflammatory response leading to the release of prostaglandins and activation of nerve reflexes within the enteric nervous system (ENS) that regulate fluid secretion in response to this pathogen. In agreement with these observations, exposure of porcine small intestine to S. enterica serovar Typhimurium resulted in increased fluid secretion and elevated serotonin (5-HT) and prostaglandin E2 (PGE2) levels (35). Moreover, the 5-HT receptor antagonist ondansetron reduced fluid accumulation to serovar Typhimurium. Thus, serovar Typhimurium triggers the release of 5-HT and PGE2, which mediate a large part of small intestinal fluid secretion in response to this pathogen.

NEUROIMMUNE INTERACTIONS AND PATHOGENESIS OF *C. DIFFICILE* TOXIN-INDUCED INFLAMMATION

Clostridium difficile toxin-mediated diarrhea and enterocolitis represent one of the best disease models, demonstrating how neuro-immune interactions modulate intestinal enterotoxin responses. *C. difficile* is the primary etiologic agent of antibiotic-associated colitis in animals and humans and a major health problem in hospitalized patients worldwide (54). Diarrhea and colitis in response to this pathogen are mediated by the release of two large exotoxins, toxin A and toxin B, with potent cytotoxic and enterotoxic properties (82). The cellular mechanism of toxins A and B involves binding to surface receptors and, following endocytosis, disruption of the actin cytoskeletal network mediated by modification of the Rho family of GTPases (1, 82). Application of toxin A, but not toxin B, into animal intestine causes fluid secretion, increases mucosal permeability, and stimulates intestinal inflammation characterized by the release of several inflammatory mediators and extravasation and transmigration of neutrophils into the mucosa (15, 45, 71, 81, 97).

Mast Cells and Macrophages in Toxin A Responses

Several different cell types of the intestinal lamina propria appear to play a major role in the mediation of toxin A's inflammatory signaling in the intestine. Mucosal mast cells are activated and degranulated early during toxin A enteritis and release several mast cell mediators, including rat mast cell protease II, which play an important role in fluid secretion and inflammation in response to this toxin (17, 81).

Administration of the mast cell inhibitor ketotifen, a drug used in bronchial asthma and eosinophilic gastroenteritis, inhibits toxin-A-mediated enterotoxicity and reduces the levels of the mast cell mediators leukotriene B4 and C4, platelet-activating factor, and rat mast cell protease II (81). Moreover, the mast cell stabilizer lodoxamide or the histamine 1 receptor antagonist hydroxyzine substantially reduces albumin permeability in rat mesenteric venules in response to toxin A (53). Interestingly, mast cell-deficient mice have reduced toxin-A-associated ileal secretion and mucosal neutrophil infiltration (107), providing direct evidence of the importance of these multifunctional cells in the pathogenesis of enterotoxin-induced inflammatory diarrhea. Isolated peritoneal mast cells also respond to toxin A in vitro by releasing tumor necrosis factor alpha (TNF-α) (13). Thus, mediators released from mast cells in response to toxin A directly or indirectly signal leukocyte-endothelial cell interactions, leading to neutrophil transmigration, gut inflammation, and epithelial cell damage (75, 78).

Nitric oxide (NO) may represent an important molecule in the signaling pathway of toxin A-induced mast cell activation. It is well established that NO-mast cell interactions modulate several intestinal responses linked to inflammation, including gut permeability (43), vasodilation (66), and epithelial cell damage and ulceration (52). Studies with the toxin A model in rats demonstrated that administration of a neuronal NO synthase inhibitor worsened while an NO donor substantially inhibited toxin A-induced intestinal secretion, inflammation, and mast cell degranulation (83). These results suggest that an NO–mast-cell-dependent pathway is involved in the modulation of intestinal secretion and neutrophil transmigration following ileal toxin A exposure.

Lamina propria macrophages are important in both acute and chronic intestinal inflammatory reactions. Evidence also suggests that these cells participate in the intestinal inflammatory responses to toxin A. Thus, lamina propria macrophages isolated from toxin A-injected ileal loops release substantial amounts of TNF-α and macrophage inflammatory protein-2 (MIP-2) (14–16). Moreover, pretreatment of rats with the potent anti-inflammatory cytokine IL-11 reduced toxin A-mediated enterotoxic responses, and this effect was accompanied by reduced TNF-α and MIP-2 levels released from purified intestinal lamina propria macrophages (16). Interestingly, both *C. difficile* toxins can directly stimulate human peripheral monocytes and macrophages to release a large array of proinflammatory cytokines (56, 88, 103). Based on these considerations, macrophage-dependent mechanisms participate in the pathogenesis of toxin A-mediated enterocolitis.

Activation of Sensory Neurons and the Inflammatory Response

Several pieces of evidence indicate that the mechanism of these enterotoxic responses involves interactions between epithelial, endothelial, and mucosal immune and inflammatory cells with neuropeptides released in the intestine in response to toxin A. In vivo experiments in anesthetized rats suggested that sensory neurons and enteric nerves might play a significant role in the in vivo mechanisms of toxin A. Early observations in the *C. difficile* toxin A model of acute enteritis demonstrated that application of the local anesthetic lidocaine or administration of the ganglionic blocker hexamethonium abrogated toxin A-induced ileal fluid secretion, mucosal permeability to mannitol, and neutrophil activation in the rat ileum (17). Primary sensory afferent neurons, with their cell bodies localized in the dorsal root ganglia of the spinal cord, represent an important system in the mediation of pain and inflammation in peripheral organs. Experiments using animals chronically pretreated with the neurotoxin capsaicin, which desensitizes sensory neurons by depleting their nerve endings from sensory neuropeptides, demonstrated almost complete inhibition of the enterotoxic responses to toxin A (17, 62). The importance of sensory neurons in the pathophysiology of toxin A-mediated gut inflammation was further underscored by experiments demonstrating that surgical extrinsic

denervation diminishes toxin A-associated responses in rat ileum (61). Moreover, pretreatment with the capsaicin vanilloid receptor subtype 1 (VR1) antagonist, capsazepine, also significantly inhibited toxin A-induced intestinal inflammation (69).

Since SP and calcitonin gene-related peptide (CGRP) represent the major peptide transmitters of sensory neurons in the gut and elsewhere, experiments with peptide antagonists examined their possible involvement in the toxin A model. Early important studies demonstrated increased SP, NK-1 receptor expression in colonic sections from patients with inflammatory bowel disease (IBD) (59), suggesting its possible involvement in bowel inflammation. Administration of SP or CGRP antagonists dramatically reduced intestinal secretion and neutrophil infiltration in response to toxin A (44, 62, 79), suggesting participation of these peptides in toxin A-induced inflammation. SP and CGRP levels were also elevated in the cell bodies of the dorsal root ganglia in the spinal cord soon after intraluminal toxin administration, followed by increased peptide expression in the intestinal mucosa (14, 44). The high affinity SP, NK-1 receptor was also upregulated at the mRNA and protein level shortly after ileal toxin A exposure, and before epithelial cell damage and inflammation in response to toxin A were established (62, 80). Interestingly, NK-1 receptors during toxin A inflammation were localized in the intestinal mucosa, including on epithelial cells (80), cells of the intestinal lamina propria such as macrophages (14), and enteric nerves (62). Using quantitative autoradiography, Mantyh et al. reported a dramatic increase in NK-1 receptors in tissue from a patient with *C. difficile*-associated colitis (60), indicating that these receptors may be related to *C. difficile* infection in humans.

Studies with Gene Knockout Animals

Direct evidence for the pathophysiologic significance of SP and its NK-1 receptors and the mechanism of their involvement in *C. difficile*-induced enteritis was generated from studies using genetically deficient animals. Animals deficient in NK-1 receptors were protected from all enterotoxic effects of toxin A and showed dramatically reduced mucosal TNF-α expression compared with that in wild type, despite the similar increases in SP levels in response to toxin A in both genotypes (19) (Fig. 1). The cell-surface enzyme neutral endopeptidase (NEP) degrades SP and represents a major pathway for termination of its biologic responses, including SP's participation in colonic inflammation in an IBD-related model (95). Studies with mice genetically lacking this enzyme showed enhanced toxin A-mediated ileal inflammation (50). Moreover, increased toxin A-mediated inflammation in these mice was prevented by administration of recombi-

nant NEP, while pretreatment of wild-type mice with the NEP inhibitor phosphoramidon exacerbated toxin A-mediated inflammation (50), providing further evidence of SP's importance in enterotoxin-mediated secretion and inflammation.

Several anatomical observations and experiments with animal models suggest that communication between mucosal mast cells and nerves plays an important role in the pathophysiology of intestinal inflammation (5, 76, 92). Interactions between SP, released from intestinal nerves, and mast cells modulate secretory and inflammatory responses in the gastrointestinal (GI) tract (72, 84, 86). Mast cell degranulation in response to toxin A was also diminished either by chronic capsaicin pre-

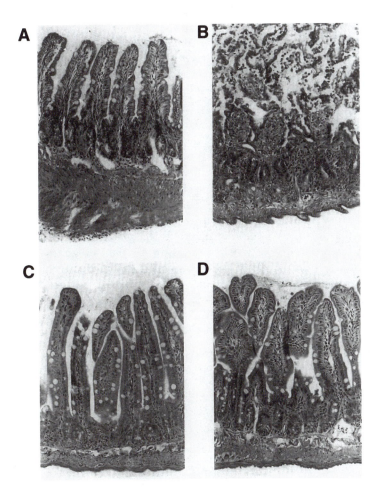

FIGURE 1 Reduced epithelia cell damage in NK-1 receptor-deficient (NK-1R$^{-/-}$) mice in response to *C. difficile* toxin A. Histologic evaluation of toxin A-induced enteritis in wild-type and NK-1R$^{-/-}$ mice. Injection of toxin A to mouse ileum of normal +/+ mice causes acute necroinflammatory damage with epithelial cell destruction and infiltration of the lamina propria with neutrophils (B), compared to buffer injection (A). Buffer-injected ileum of NK-1R$^{-/-}$ shows normal epithelial architecture (C) compared to +/+ mice (A). Toxin A administration to NK-1R$^{-/-}$ mouse ileum shows a dramatic diminution of toxin A-associated histopathologic changes (D) compared to a histopathology section from toxin A-exposed ileum of +/+ mice (B). Original magnification, ×160. (From reference 19, with permission.)

treatment (17) or by administration of NK-1 receptor antagonists (79). Together, these results indicate a sensory, SP-mediated neuronal control of mast cell activation during gut inflammation in response to *C. difficile* toxin A. Studies with mice deficient in mast cells have further contributed to our understanding of mast cell-nerve interactions in the modulation of enterotoxin-induced inflammatory responses in the gut. Thus, experiments using NK-1 receptor antagonists in mast cell-deficient versus normal mice demonstrated the functional importance of mast cell-SP-mediated pathways in the modulation of toxin A-induced intestinal secretion and neutrophil infiltration (107).

NT as a Proinflammatory Mediator

Neurotensin (NT) is a 13-amino-acid peptide synthesized primarily in the brain and gut. The primary cellular sources of this peptide in the intestine are specialized neuroendocrine cells, called N cells (2), while the enteric neurons represent another source. NT can be released from the intestine in response to several secretagogues, including cholera toxin (25), and exerts several diverse effects linked to gut inflammation such as chloride secretion (87), motility changes (73), colonic prostaglandin and mucin secretion (18), proliferation of T lymphocytes (28), and mast cell activation (70). Novel evidence also indicates that NT is a proinflammatory peptide in enterotoxin-induced inflammation. Toxin A administration into rat colon results in increased expression of NT and its type 1 receptor in the colonic mucosa (20) (Fig. 2). Moreover, blockade of these receptors with a newly synthesized NT type 1 receptor antagonist inhibits toxin A-associated colonic secretion, mucosa permeability, and neutrophil transmigration, as well as mast cell degranulation in response to toxin A (20). A large part of the effect of NT in mast cell activation in the toxin A model involves release of SP from the colonic mucosa (20), indicating communication between SP and NT in toxin A-induced colitis.

An interesting question evolving from these results is related to the cellular mechanism of action of NT leading to gut inflammation. In a recent report, Zhao and colleagues identified the presence of NT type 1 receptor (NTR1) mRNA on normal, nontransformed colonocytes (110). Binding of NT to colonocytes overexpressing this receptor caused increased IL-8 synthesis and release mediated by both NF-κB- and extracellular signal-regulated kinase (ERK)-dependent pathways (110), suggesting the capacity of this peptide to initiate a potent proinflammatory response at the colonocyte level. Another important question is related to the mechanism of the rapid increase of NT and its receptors 15 to 30 min after colonic administration of toxin A. Yeh et al. recently reported that ischemia-reperfusion in rat jejunum leads to significant proinflammatory changes in the jejunal mucosa, including increased activity of the transcription factors NF-κB and AP-1, which was accompanied by increased NT mRNA expression after reperfusion (109). Since AP-1 and AP-1/CRE binding sites in the promoter region of the NT gene have been shown to regulate expression of this peptide (12, 29), it was suggested that these and possibly other factors may be involved in the regulation of NT expression in ischemia-reperfusion-induced injury (109). The presence of putative binding sites for transcription factors on the promoter region of the NTR1 gene (96) may implicate a similar mechanism for the upregulation of this receptor during toxin A-mediated colonic inflammation (20), since toxin A stimulates expression of transcription factors in vitro (103).

MAST CELL-NERVE COMMUNICATION IN THE PATHOGENESIS OF PARASITIC INFECTIONS

Parasitic infections of the intestine represent a major health problem primarily in underdeveloped countries throughout the world. Studies using the *Trichinella spiralis* and *Nippostrongylus brasiliensis* animal models of

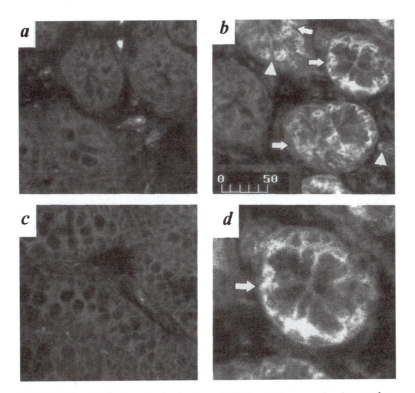

FIGURE 2 *C. difficile* toxin A stimulates NTR1 protein expression in rat colon. Rat colonic loops were injected with purified toxin A or buffer and after 2 h colonic tissues were processed for immunohistochemistry using an antibody directed against two N-terminal peptides of NTR1. Toxin A injection resulted in increased NTR1 expression (b) compared to control colon (a). (c) Toxin A-exposed colon incubated with NTR1 antiserum preabsorbed with an excess of the receptor peptides used to generate the antibody shows the complete disappearance of signal. Higher magnification of (d) demonstrates the presence of intense signal on epithelial cells (arrows in b and d) as well as on cells of the lamina propria (arrowhead). Bar, 50 μm. (From reference 39, with permission.)

parasitic infections provided important information not only on the pathophysiology of these diseases, but also on the outcome of immune cell-nerve interactions in the pathogenesis of diarrhea and intestinal inflammation. Valuable information from use of these models has had wide application in studies involving neuroimmune interactions in other forms of infectious diarrhea and inflammation. Studies in humans and animal models of *T. spiralis* infection demonstrated a marked increase in the number, activation, and differentiation of intestinal mast cells (32, 36, 108). Moreover, mastocytosis in this model is func-

tionally related to the development of infection and expulsion of the nematode (37, 51, 108). Substantial interactions between mast cells and intestinal nerves also play a major role in the regulation of electrolyte transport in the *T. spiralis* model. Thus, challenge of jejunal and colonic tissue from nematode-infected animals with *T. spiralis* antigens caused ion transport changes that are mediated by mast cells and cholinergic nerves (89, 102), as well as histamine and prostaglandins (22, 90). Signaling between mast cells via histamine and submucosal neurons is also involved in colonic anaphylactic responses to *T. spiralis* sensitizing antigens (31). Motility changes evident during *T. spiralis* infection may also involve mast cell-nerve communication in the GI tract. For example, studies with wild-type and IL-5-deficient mice suggested that IL-5 plays a major role in intestinal eosinophilia and muscle hypercontractility in *T. spiralis* infection (98).

N. BRASILIENSIS

Infection with *N. brasiliensis* has been widely used as a model to study intestinal pathophysiology. It is well established that infection with this parasite causes acute pathological and biochemical changes in the small intestine, including villus atrophy, crypt hyperplasia, and inflammation (85); motility changes (24, 101); and alterations in intestinal permeability (85) (Table 1). Mast cells have also been recognized as an important cell population associated with the pathophysiology of inflammation and colonic motility changes during *N. brasiliensis* infection (49, 64, 108). Immunologically activated rat intestinal mast cells obtained from *N. brasiliensis*-infected animals release more prostaglandins and leukotrienes (38). Moreover, intestinal mucosal injury in response to the nematode was temporally associated with mast cell activation and increased levels of leukotrienes in the jejunum (77). In *N. brasiliensis*-sensitized rats, mucosal mast cell degranulation is associated with jejunal paracellular permeability changes (91). As well, intestinal hypersensitivity and motility changes following infection with *N. brasiliensis* in rats depend on mast cell activation (33, 68).

TABLE 1 Intestinal responses regulated by neuroimmune interactions during inflammatory parasitic infection

Fluid accumulation
Cl⁻ secretion
Motility
Paracellular permeability
Mucosal blood flow
Parasitic granuloma formation
Release of immune mediators

Several reports provided evidence for the pathophysiologic importance of intestinal nerves in the development of *N. brasiliensis* infection (Table 1). Using Ussing chambers, Masson et al. demonstrated that neuronally mediated ion secretion was diminished in rat jejunum 10 and 35 days after *N. brasiliensis* infection, and this effect was associated with increased SP levels in nerve fibers of infected rats (65). Consistent with this observation, Jodal et al. reported that net fluid transport changes during *N. brasiliensis* infection are mediated in large part by the enteric nervous system (41). Infection with this nematode also resulted in early activation of brain Fos expression (a parameter of nerve cell activation) that was associated with intestinal inflammatory and motility changes (21). Thus, during intestinal inflammation, activation of intestinal neuronal afferents may communicate signals to the brain.

Important anatomical observations also underscored the existence of mast cell-nerve interactions in the intestinal lamina propria and opened the field for further studies to identify the functional significance of this interaction. In the *N. brasiliensis* nematode animal model, 67% of intestinal mucosal mast cells were found to be in contact with nerves in the small intestinal subepithelium (5, 93). Nerve endings associated with mast cells in these studies contained the neuropeptides SP and CGRP. Electron microscopy experiments identified a population of mast cells having membrane-to-membrane contact with unmyelinated axons, while another mast cell population embraced nerve bundles through lamellopodia formation (93). Substantial remodeling of intestinal nerves also takes place during the different phases of *N. brasiliensis* infection (92). These results provided substantial evidence for possible cross talk between the immune and nervous systems in the gut. Mast cell-nerve interactions play a functional role in the intestinal responses to *N. brasiliensis*. Perdue et al. demonstrated activation of mucosal mast cells during *N. brasiliensis*-induced inflammation and implicated mast cell-nerve interactions in the modulation of ion secretion from the intestinal epithelium (76). Along these lines, mast cell stabilization with ketotifen decreases jejunal inflammation in the acute stage of the infection, but it results in prolonged intestinal inflammation (34). Ablation of extrinsic sensory neurons with capsaicin worsened intestinal inflammation in *N. brasiliensis*-infected rats, but it did not affect the duration of the infection (34). These results suggest that sensory neurons may play a protective role in this model via a pathway that does not involve mast cells.

NEUROIMMUNE CIRCUITS IN *S. MANSONI* INFECTION

Role of SP

The parasite *Schistosoma mansoni* causes several acute and chronic clinical conditions involving the intestine, the liver, and the spleen. Schistosomiasis, a serious cause of morbidity and mortality in endemic regions, is characterized by the formation of granulomas in the liver and intestinal tract. Although the pathophysiology of this disease is not entirely clear, several pieces of evidence demonstrate that interactions between neuropeptides with immune cells in the affected organs play a major role in the development of schistosomiasis. Early observations demonstrated that schistosome granulomas isolated from the livers of mice infected with the parasite contained nerve growth factor (99). Moreover, microscopy studies showed substantial nerve cell destruction in the myenteric plexus and the submucus and mucosal plexi of the ileum and colon of infected mice in close proximity to schistosoma granulomas (100), suggesting involvement of enteric nerves in the inflammatory response to this parasite. Several neuropeptides and neuropeptide receptors were also localized within granulomas during schistosoma infection from several target tissues. For example, eosinophils from liver schistosoma granulomas express SP and its mRNA (104), and an authentic SP, NK-1 receptor has been shown to be expressed in *S. mansoni* granuloma T lymphocytes (23).

Other tachykinins, such as substance K and neuropeptide K, were also identified in these granulomas (105), albeit at lower levels. Moreover, SP modulates immunoglobulin secretion in spleen and granuloma cell preparations obtained from infected mice (74), and stimulates IFN-γ secretion from spleen or granuloma inflammatory cells primed in vitro by antigen (7). Studies using mice deficient in NK-1 receptors also showed that SP via its NK-1 receptor participates in the formation of granulomas and IFN-γ production in schistosoma-infected mice (8). Taken together, these findings indicate that SP and the NK-1 receptor represent important components of the immune response and granuloma formation during *S. mansoni* infection.

Somatostatin-SP Interactions

Somatostatin (SOM) is a 14-amino-acid cyclic peptide that is released from nerve endings and from endocrine-like cells in the intestinal and colonic mucosa. SOM acting through specific G protein-coupled receptors exerts inhibitory effects in many GI functions, including motility and blood flow. SOM, via its interactions with immune cells, also plays an important role in the neuroimmune response and granuloma formation during *S. mansoni* infection. Thus, macrophages from granulomas isolated from *S. mansoni*-infected animals secrete SOM (106). Furthermore, expression of preprosomatostatin mRNA expression correlates well with granuloma formation during S. *mansoni* infection, and its expression can be stimulated in normal splenocytes in vitro by several proinflammatory mediators (26). Interestingly, SP, acting through NK-1 receptors, downregulates SOM gene and protein expression from schistosoma granulomas (6). Granuloma T lymphocytes in murine schistosomiasis have SOM receptors, and exposure to SOM leads to diminished IFN-γ secretion (9, 27). In conclusion, communication between SP and SOM represents an important system that controls the generation of inflammatory and immune responses in granulomatous schisto-somiasis.

CONCLUSIONS

The pathogenic mechanism of infectious inflammatory diarrhea of multiple etiologies involves extensive interactions between intestinal nerves and mucosal immune cells and epithelial cells. Activation of nerves, neuroendocrine cells, and immune cells of the intestinal lamina propria following mucosal exposure to infectious agents leads to the release of several important neuropeptides with brain-gut distribution. Increased expression of neuropeptide receptors during infectious or enterotoxin-mediated diarrhea and inflammation is also evident in many in vivo studies and represents a key component in the initiation and development of intestinal inflammation, since receptors for neuropeptides are expressed at very low levels under normal conditions. Signaling of neuropeptide receptors (NK-1, NT-1, and Gal1) following ligand exposure in many cell types appears to be related to activation and nuclear translocation of transcription factors such as NF-κB, leading to upregulation of proinflammatory genes and release of proinflammatory cytokines. Evidence also indicates that pathways linked to transcription factors may also be involved in the expression of some neuropeptides and possibly neuropeptide receptors following exposure of the intestinal mucosa to bacteria, bacterial enterotoxins, and parasites. The successful inhibition of several types of infectious diarrhea and inflammation by neuropeptide and neuropeptide receptor antagonists in animal models opens the possibility that these or similar antagonists may be beneficial in the amelioration of the intestinal inflammation in human infection. Further studies examining the mechanism of action of these peptides and elucidation of signaling of their receptors on intestinal epithelial and lamina propria immune cells are required, however, before embarking on clinical studies.

REFERENCES

1. **Aktories, K., G. Schmidt, and I. Just.** 2000. Rho GTPases as targets of bacterial protein toxins. *Biol. Chem.* **381:**421–426.
2. **Barber, D. L., A. M. Buchan, J. H. Walsh, and A. H. Soll.** 1986. Isolated canine ileal mucosal cells in short-term culture: a model for study of neurotensin release. *Am. J. Physiol.* **250:**G374–G384.
3. **Bauer, F. E., A. Zintel, M. J. Kenny, D. Calder, M. A. Ghatei, and S. R. Bloom.** 1989. Inhibitory effect of galanin on postprandial gastrointestinal motility and gut hormone release in humans. *Gastroenterology* **97:**260–264.
4. **Benya, R. V., J. A. Marrero, D. A. Ostrovskiy, A. Koutsouris, and G. Hecht.** 1999. Human colonic epithelial cells express galanin-1 receptors, which when activated cause Cl⁻ secretion. *Am. J. Physiol.* **276:**G64–G72.
5. **Bienenstock, J., M. Tomioka, H. Matsuda, R. H. Stead, G. Quinonez, G. T. Simon, M. D. Coughlin, and J. A. Denburg.** 1987. The role of mast cells in inflammatory processes: evidence for nerve/mast cell interactions. *Int. Arch. Allergy Appl. Immunol.* **82:**238–243.
6. **Blum, A. M., D. E. Elliott, A. Metwali, J. Li, K. Qadir, and J. V. Weinstock.** 1998. Substance P regulates somatostatin expression in inflammation. *J. Immunol.* **161:**6316–6322.
7. **Blum, A. M., A. Metwali, G. Cook, R. C. Mathew, D. Elliott, and J. V. Weinstock.** 1993. Substance P modulates antigen-induced, IFN-gamma production in murine *Schistosomiasis mansoni. J. Immunol.* **151:**225–233.
8. **Blum, A. M., A. Metwali, M. Kim-Miller, J. Li, K. Qadir, D. E. Elliott, B. Lu, Z. Fabry, N. Gerard, and J. V. Weinstock.** 1999. The substance P receptor is necessary for a normal granulomatous response in murine schistosomiasis mansoni *J. Immunol.* **162:**6080–6085.
9. **Blum, A. M., A. Metwali, R. C. Mathew, G. Cook, D. Elliott, and J. V. Weinstock.** 1992. Granuloma T lymphocytes in murine schistosomiasis mansoni have somatostatin receptors and respond to somatostatin with decreased IFN-gamma secretion *J. Immunol.* **149:**3621–3626.
10. **Bost, K. L., S. A. Breeding, and D. W. Pascual.** 1992. Modulation of the mRNAs encoding substance P and its receptor in rat macrophages by LPS. *Reg. Immunol.* **4:**105–112.
11. **Brunsson, I.** 1987. Enteric nerves mediate the fluid secretory response due to *Salmonella typhimurium* R5 infection in the rat small intestine. *Acta Physiol. Scand.* **131:**609–617.
12. **Bullock, B. P., G. P. McNeil, and P. R. Dobner.** 1994. Synergistic induction of neurotensin gene transcription in PC12 cells parallels

changes in AP-1 activity. *Brain Res. Mol. Brain Res.* **27**:232–242.

13. Calderon, G. M., J. Torres-Lopez, T. J. Lin, B. Chavez, M. Hernandez, O. Munoz, A. D. Befus, and J. A. Enciso. 1998. Effects of toxin A from *Clostridium difficile* on mast cell activation and survival. *Infect. Immun.* **66**:2755–2761.

14. Castagliuolo, I., A. C. Keates, B. Qiu, C. P. Kelly, S. Nikulasson, S. E. Leeman, and C. Pothoulakis. 1997. Increased substance P responses in dorsal root ganglia and intestinal macrophages during *Clostridium difficile* toxin A enteritis in rats. *Proc. Natl. Acad. Sci. USA* **94:** 4788–4793.

15. Castagliuolo, I., A. C. Keates, C. C. Wang, A. Pasha, L. Valenick, C. P. Kelly, S. T. Nikulasson, J. T. LaMont, and C. Pothoulakis. 1998. *Clostridium difficile* toxin A stimulates macrophage-inflammatory protein-2 production in rat intestinal epithelial cells. *J. Immunol.* **160:** 6039–6045.

16. Castagliuolo, I., C. P. Kelly, B. S. Qiu, S. T. Nikulasson, J. T. LaMont, and C. Pothoulakis. 1997. IL-11 inhibits *Clostridium difficile* toxin A enterotoxicity in rat ileum. *Am. J. Physiol.* **273**:G333–G341.

17. Castagliuolo, I., J. T. LaMont, R. Letourneau, C. Kelly, J. C. O'Keane, A. Jaffer, T. C. Theoharides, and C. Pothoulakis. 1994. Neuronal involvement in the intestinal effects of *Clostridium difficile* toxin A and *Vibrio cholerae* enterotoxin in rat ileum. *Gastroenterology* **107**:657–665.

18. Castagliuolo, I., S. E. Leeman, E. Bartolak-Suki, S. Nikulasson, B. Qiu, R. E. Carraway, and C. Pothoulakis. 1996. A neurotensin antagonist, SR 48692, inhibits colonic responses to immobilization stress in rats. *Proc. Natl. Acad. Sci. USA* **93**:12611–12615.

19. Castagliuolo, I., M. Riegler, A. Pasha, S. Nikulasson, B. Lu, C. Gerard, N. P. Gerard, and C. Pothoulakis. 1998. Neurokinin-1 (NK-1) receptor is required in *Clostridium difficile*-induced enteritis. *J. Clin. Invest.* **101**:1547–1550.

20. Castagliuolo, I., C. C. Wang, L. Valenick, A. Pasha, S. Nikulasson, R. E. Carraway, and C. Pothoulakis. 1999. Neurotensin is a proinflammatory neuropeptide in colonic inflammation. *J. Clin. Invest.* **103**:843–849.

21. Castex, N., J. Fioramonti, J. Ducos de Lahitte, G. Luffau, J. More, and L. Bueno. 1998. Brain Fos expression and intestinal motor alterations during nematode-induced inflammation in the rat. *Am. J. Physiol.* **274**:G210–G216.

22. Castro, G. A., and Y. Harari. 1991. Immunoregulation of endometrial and jejunal epithelia

sensitized by infection. *Int. Arch. Allergy Appl. Immunol.* **95**:184–190.

23. Cook, G. A., D. Elliott, A. Metwali, A. M. Blum, M. Sandor, R. Lynch, and J. V. Weinstock. 1994. Molecular evidence that granuloma T lymphocytes in murine schistosomiasis mansoni express an authentic substance P (NK-1) receptor. *J. Immunol.* **152**:1830–1835.

24. Crosthwaite, A. I., J. D. Huizinga, and J. A. Fox. 1990. Jejunal circular muscle motility is decreased in nematode-infected rat. *Gastroenterology* **98**:59–65.

25. Eklund, S., L. Karlstrom, A. Rokaeus, E. Theodorsson, M. Jodal, and O. Lundgren. 1989. Effects of cholera toxin, *Escherichia coli* heat stable toxin and sodium deoxycholate on neurotensin release from the ileum in vivo. *Regul. Pept.* **26**:241–252.

26. Elliott, D. E., A. M. Blum, J. Li, A. Metwali, and J. V. Weinstock. 1998. Preprosomatostatin messenger RNA is expressed by inflammatory cells and induced by inflammatory mediators and cytokines. *J. Immunol.* **160**:3997–4003.

27. Elliott, D. E., A. Metwali, A. M. Blum, M. Sandor, R. Lynch, and J. V. Weinstock. 1994. T lymphocytes isolated from the hepatic granulomas of schistosome-infected mice express somatostatin receptor subtype II (SSTR2) messenger RNA. *J. Immunol.* **153**:1180–1186.

28. Evers, B. M., R. J. Bold, J. A. Ehrenfried, J. Li, C. M. Townsend, Jr., and G. R. Klimpel. 1994. Characterization of functional neurotensin receptors on human lymphocytes. *Surgery* **116:** 134–139; discussion, **116**:139–140.

29. Evers, B. M., X. Wang, Z. Zhou, C. M. Townsend, Jr., G. P. McNeil, and P. R. Dobner. 1995. Characterization of promoter elements required for cell-specific expression of the neurotensin/neuromedin N gene in a human endocrine cell line. *Mol. Cell Biol.* **15**:3870–3881.

30. Fleckenstein, J. M., and D. J. Kopecko. 2001. Breaching the mucosal barrier by stealth: an emerging pathogenic mechanism for enteroadherent bacterial pathogens. *J. Clin. Invest.* **107:** 27–30.

31. Frieling, T., J. M. Palmer, H. J. Cooke, and J. D. Wood. 1994. Neuroimmune communication in the submucous plexus of guinea pig colon after infection with *Trichinella spiralis*. *Gastroenterology* **107**:1602–1609.

32. Friend, D. S., N. Ghildyal, K. F. Austen, M. F. Gurish, R. Matsumoto, and R. L. Stevens. 1996. Mast cells that reside at different locations in the jejunum of mice infected with *Trichinella spiralis* exhibit sequential changes in their granule ultrastructure and chymase phenotype. *J. Cell Biol.* **135**:279–290.

33. Gay, J., J. Fioramonti, R. Garcia-Villar, and L. Bueno. 2000. Alterations of intestinal motor responses to various stimuli after *Nippostrongylus brasiliensis* infection in rats: role of mast cells. *Neurogastroenterol. Motil.* **12:**207–214.

34. Gay, J., J. Fioramonti, R. Garcia-Villar, and L. Bueno. 2000. Development and sequels of intestinal inflammation in nematode-infected rats: role of mast cells and capsaicin-sensitive afferents. *Neuroimmunomodulation* **8:**171–178.

35. Grondahl, M. L., G. M. Jensen, C. G. Nielsen, E. Skadhauge, J. E. Olsen, and M. B. Hansen. 1998. Secretory pathways in *Salmonella typhimurium*-induced fluid accumulation in the porcine small intestine. *J. Med. Microbiol.* **47:**151–157.

36. Gustowska, L., E. J. Ruitenberg, A. Elgersma, and W. Kociecka. 1983. Increase of mucosal mast cells in the jejunum of patients infected with *Trichinella spiralis*. *Int. Arch. Allergy Appl. Immunol.* **71:**304–308.

37. Ha, T. Y., N. D. Reed, and P. K. Crowle. 1983. Delayed expulsion of adult *Trichinella spiralis* by mast cell-deficient W/Wv mice. *Infect. Immun.* **41:**445–447.

38. Heavey, D. J., P. B. Ernst, R. L. Stevens, A. D. Befus, J. Bienenstock, and K. F. Austen. 1988. Generation of leukotriene C4, leukotriene B4, and prostaglandin D2 by immunologically activated rat intestinal mucosa mast cells. *J. Immunol.* **140:**1953–1957.

39. Hecht, G., J. A. Marrero, A. Danilkovich, K. A. Matkowskyj, S. D. Savkovic, A. Koutsouris, and R. V. Benya. 1999. Pathogenic *Escherichia coli* increase Cl⁻ secretion from intestinal epithelia by upregulating galanin-1 receptor expression. *J. Clin. Invest.* **104:**253–262.

40. Hsu, H. S. 1989. Pathogenesis and immunity in murine salmonellosis. *Microbiol. Rev.* **53:**390–409.

41. Jodal, M., U. Wingren, M. Jansson, M. Heidemann, and O. Lundgren. 1993. Nerve involvement in fluid transport in the inflamed rat jejunum. *Gut* **34:**1526–1530.

42. Kagnoff, M. F., and L. Eckmann. 1997. Epithelial cells as sensors for microbial infection. *J. Clin. Invest.* **100:**6–10.

43. Kanwar, S., J. L. Wallace, D. Befus, and P. Kubes. 1994. Nitric oxide synthesis inhibition increases epithelial permeability via mast cells. *Am. J. Physiol.* **266:**G222–G229.

44. Keates, A. C., I. Castagliuolo, B. Qiu, S. Nikulasson, A. Sengupta, and C. Pothoulakis. 1998. CGRP upregulation in dorsal root ganglia and ileal mucosa during *Clostridium difficile* toxin A-induced enteritis. *Am. J. Physiol.* **274:**G196–G202.

45. Kelly, C. P., S. Becker, J. K. Linevsky, M. A. Joshi, J. C. O'Keane, B. F. Dickey, J. T. LaMont, and C. Pothoulakis. 1994. Neutrophil recruitment in *Clostridium difficile* toxin A enteritis in the rabbit. *J. Clin. Invest.* **93:**1257–1265.

46. Kincy-Cain, T., and K. L. Bost. 1996. Increased susceptibility of mice to *Salmonella* infection following in vivo treatment with the substance P antagonist, spantide II. *J. Immunol.* **157:**255–264.

47. Kincy-Cain, T., and K. L. Bost. 1997. Substance P-induced IL-12 production by murine macrophages. *J. Immunol.* **158:**2334–2339.

48. Kincy-Cain, T., J. D. Clements, and K. L. Bost. 1996. Endogenous and exogenous interleukin-12 augment the protective immune response in mice orally challenged with *Salmonella dublin. Infect. Immun.* **64:**1437–1440.

49. King, S. J., H. R. Miller, G. F. Newlands, and R. G. Woodbury. 1985. Depletion of mucosal mast cell protease by corticosteroids: effect on intestinal anaphylaxis in the rat. *Proc. Natl. Acad. Sci. USA* **82:**1214–1218.

50. Kirkwood, K. S., N. W. Bunnett, J. Maa, I. Castagliolo, B. Liu, N. Gerard, J. Zacks, C. Pothoulakis, and E. F. Grady. 2001. Deletion of neutral endopeptidase exacerbates intestinal inflammation induced by *Clostridium difficile* toxin A. *Am. J. Physiol. Gastrointest. Liver Physiol.* **281:**G544–G551.

51. Knight, P. A., S. H. Wright, C. E. Lawrence, Y. Y. Paterson, and H. R. Miller. 2000. Delayed expulsion of the nematode *Trichinella spiralis* in mice lacking the mucosal mast cell-specific granule chymase, mouse mast cell protease-1. *J. Exp. Med.* **192:**1849–1856.

52. Konaka, A., M. Nishijima, A. Tanaka, T. Kunikata, S. Kato, and K. Takeuchi. 1999. Nitric oxide, superoxide radicals and mast cells in pathogenesis of indomethacin-induced small intestinal lesions in rats. *J. Physiol. Pharmacol.* **50:**25–38.

53. Kurose, I., C. Pothoulakis, J. T. LaMont, D. C. Anderson, J. C. Paulson, M. Miyasaka, R. Wolf, and D. N. Granger. 1994. *Clostridium difficile* toxin A-induced microvascular dysfunction. Role of histamine. *J. Clin. Invest.* **94:**1919–1926.

54. Kyne, L., R. J. Farrell, and C. P. Kelly. 2001. *Clostridium difficile. Gastroenterol. Clin. N. Am.* **30:**753–777; ix–x.

55. Lieb, K., B. L. Fiebich, M. Berger, J. Bauer, and K. Schulze-Osthoff. 1997. The neuropeptide substance P activates transcription factor NF-kappa B and kappa B-dependent gene expression

in human astrocytoma cells. *J. Immunol.* **159:** 4952–4958.

56. **Linevsky, J. K., C. Pothoulakis, S. Keates, M. Warny, A. C. Keates, J. T. LaMont, and C. P. Kelly.** 1997. IL-8 release and neutrophil activation by *Clostridium difficile* toxin-exposed human monocytes. *Am. J. Physiol.* **273:**G1333–G1340.

57. **Lorimer, D. D., K. Matkowskj, and R. V. Benya.** 1997. Cloning, chromosomal location, and transcriptional regulation of the human galanin-1 receptor gene (GALN1R). *Biochem. Biophys. Res. Commun.* **241:**558–564.

58. **Lundgren, O.** 1998. 5-Hydroxytryptamine, enterotoxins, and intestinal fluid secretion. *Gastroenterology* **115:**1009–1012.

59. **Mantyh, C. R., T. S. Gates, R. P. Zimmerman, M. L. Welton, E. P. Passaro, Jr., S. R. Vigna, J. E. Maggio, L. Kruger, and P. W. Mantyh.** 1988. Receptor binding sites for substance P, but not substance K or neuromedin K, are expressed in high concentrations by arterioles, venules, and lymph nodules in surgical specimens obtained from patients with ulcerative colitis and Crohn's disease. *Proc. Natl. Acad. Sci. USA* **85:** 3235–3239.

60. **Mantyh, C. R., J. E. Maggio, P. W. Mantyh, S. R. Vigna, and T. N. Pappas.** 1996. Increased substance P receptor expression by blood vessels and lymphoid aggregates in *Clostridium difficile*-induced pseudomembranous colitis. *Dig. Dis. Sci.* **41:**614–620.

61. **Mantyh, C. R., D. C. McVey, and S. R. Vigna.** 2000. Extrinsic surgical denervation inhibits *Clostridium difficile* toxin A- induced enteritis in rats. *Neurosci. Lett.* **292:**95–98.

62. **Mantyh, C. R., T. N. Pappas, J. A. Lapp, M. K. Washington, L. M. Neville, J. R. Ghilardi, S. D. Rogers, P. W. Mantyh, and S. R. Vigna.** 1996. Substance P activation of enteric neurons in response to intraluminal *Clostridium difficile* toxin A in the rat ileum. *Gastroenterology* **111:**1272–1280.

63. **Marrero, J. A., K. A. Matkowskyj, K. Yung, G. Hecht, and R. V. Benya.** 2000. Dextran sulfate sodium-induced murine colitis activates NF-kappa B and increases galanin-1 receptor expression. *Am. J. Physiol. Gastrointest. Liver Physiol.* **278:**G797–G804.

64. **Marzio, L., P. Blennerhassett, D. Vermillion, S. Chiverton, and S. Collins.** 1992. Distribution of mast cells in intestinal muscle of nematode-sensitized rats. *Am. J. Physiol.* **262:** G477–G482.

65. **Masson, S. D., D. M. McKay, R. H. Stead, A. Agro, A. Stanisz, and M. H. Perdue.** 1996. *Nippostrongylus brasiliensis* infection evokes neuronal abnormalities and alterations in neurally regulated electrolyte transport in rat jejunum. *Parasitology* **113:**173–182.

66. **Mathison, R., and J. S. Davison.** 1995. Regulation of jejunal arterioles by capsaicin-sensitive nerves in *Nippostrongylus brasiliensis*-sensitized rats. *J. Pharmacol. Exp. Ther.* **273:**337–343.

67. **Matkowskyj, K. A., A. Danilkovich, J. Marrero, S. D. Savkovic, G. Hecht, and R. V. Benya.** 2000. Galanin-1 receptor up-regulation mediates the excess colonic fluid production caused by infection with enteric pathogens. *Nat. Med.* **6:**1048–1051.

68. **McLean, P. G., C. Picard, R. Garcia-Villar, R. Ducos de Lahitte, J. More, J. Fioramonti, and L. Bueno.** 1998. Role of kinin B1 and B2 receptors and mast cells in post intestinal infection-induced hypersensitivity to distension. *Neurogastroenterol. Motil.* **10:**499–508.

69. **McVey, D. C., and S. R. Vigna.** 2001. The capsaicin VR1 receptor mediates substance P release in toxin A-induced enteritis in rats. *Peptides* **22:**1439–1446.

70. **Miller, L. A., D. E. Cochrane, R. E. Carraway, and R. S. Feldberg.** 1995. Blockade of mast cell histamine secretion in response to neurotensin by SR 48692, a nonpeptide antagonist of the neurotensin brain receptor. *Br. J. Pharmacol.* **114:**1466–1470.

71. **Mitchell, T. J., J. M. Ketley, S. C. Haslam, J. Stephen, D. W. Burdon, D. C. Candy, and R. Daniel.** 1986. Effect of toxin A and B of *Clostridium difficile* on rabbit ileum and colon. *Gut* **27:**78–85.

72. **Moriarty, D., N. Selve, A. W. Baird, and J. Goldhill.** 2001. Potent NK1 antagonism by SR-140333 reduces rat colonic secretory response to immunocyte activation. *Am. J. Physiol. Cell Physiol.* **280:**C852–C858.

73. **Mule, F., R. Serio, and A. Postorino.** 1995. Motility pattern of isolated rat proximal colon and excitatory action of neurotensin. *Eur. J. Pharmacol.* **275:**131–137.

74. **Neil, G. A., A. Blum, and J. V. Weinstock.** 1991. Substance P but not vasoactive intestinal peptide modulates immunoglobulin secretion in murine schistosomiasis. *Cell Immunol.* **135:**394–401.

75. **Panes, J., and D. N. Granger.** 1998. Leukocyte-endothelial cell interactions: molecular mechanisms and implications in gastrointestinal disease. *Gastroenterology* **114:**1066–1090.

76. **Perdue, M. H., J. Marshall, and S. Masson.** 1990. Ion transport abnormalities in inflamed rat jejunum. Involvement of mast cells and nerves. *Gastroenterology.* **98:**561–567.

77. Perdue, M. H., J. K. Ramage, D. Burget, J. Marshall, and S. Masson. 1989. Intestinal mucosal injury is associated with mast cell activation and leukotriene generation during *Nippostrongylus*-induced inflammation in the rat. *Dig. Dis. Sci.* **34**:724–731.

78. Pothoulakis, C., I. Castagliuolo, and J. T. LaMont. 1998. Nerves and intestinal mast cells modulate responses to enterotoxins. *News Physiol. Sci.* **13**:58–63.

79. Pothoulakis, C., I. Castagliuolo, J. T. LaMont, A. Jaffer, J. C. O'Keane, R. M. Snider, and S. E. Leeman. 1994. CP-96,345, a substance P antagonist, inhibits rat intestinal responses to *Clostridium difficile* toxin A but not cholera toxin. *Proc. Natl. Acad. Sci. USA* **91**:947–951.

80. Pothoulakis, C., I. Castagliuolo, S. E. Leeman, C. C. Wang, H. Li, B. J. Hoffman, and E. Mezey. 1998. Substance P receptor expression in intestinal epithelium in *Clostridium difficile* toxin A enteritis in rats. *Am. J. Physiol.* **275**:G68–G75.

81. Pothoulakis, C., F. Karmeli, C. P. Kelly, R. Eliakim, M. A. Joshi, C. J. O'Keane, I. Castagliuolo, J. T. LaMont, and D. Rachmilewitz. 1993. Ketotifen inhibits *Clostridium difficile* toxin A-induced enteritis in rat ileum. *Gastroenterology* **105**:701–707.

82. Pothoulakis, C., and J. T. LaMont. 2001. Microbes and microbial toxins: paradigms for microbial-mucosal interactions. II. The integrated response of the intestine to *Clostridium difficile* toxins. *Am. J. Physiol. Gastrointest. Liver Physiol.* **280**:G178–G183.

83. Qiu, B., C. Pothoulakis, I. Castagliuolo, Z. Nikulasson, and J. T. LaMont. 1996. Nitric oxide inhibits rat intestinal secretion by *Clostridium difficile* toxin A but not *Vibrio cholerae* enterotoxin. *Gastroenterology* **111**:409–418.

84. Raithel, M., H. T. Schneider, and E. G. Hahn. 1999. Effect of substance P on histamine secretion from gut mucosa in inflammatory bowel disease. *Scand. J. Gastroenterol.* **34**:496–503.

85. Ramage, J. K., R. H. Hunt, and M. H. Perdue. 1988. Changes in intestinal permeability and epithelial differentiation during inflammation in the rat. *Gut* **29**:57–61.

86. Riegler, M., I. Castagliuolo, P. T. So, M. Lotz, C. Wang, M. Wlk, T. Sogukoglu, E. Cosentini, G. Bischof, G. Hamilton, B. Teleky, E. Wenzl, J. B. Matthews, and C. Pothoulakis. 1999. Effects of substance P on human colonic mucosa in vitro. *Am. J. Physiol.* **276**:G1473–G1483.

87. Riegler, M., I. Castagliuolo, C. Wang, M. Wlk, T. Sogukoglu, E. Wenzl, J. B. Matthews, and C. Pothoulakis. 2000. Neurotensin stimulates Cl(−) secretion in human colonic mucosa in vitro: role of adenosine. *Gastroenterology* **119**:348–357.

88. Rocha, M. F., M. E. Maia, L. R. Bezerra, D. M. Lyerly, R. L. Guerrant, R. A. Ribeiro, and A. A. Lima. 1997. *Clostridium difficile* toxin A induces the release of neutrophil chemotactic factors from rat peritoneal macrophages: role of interleukin-1 beta, tumor necrosis factor alpha, and leukotrienes. *Infect. Immun.* **65**:2740–2746.

89. Russell, D. A. 1986. Mast cells in the regulation of intestinal electrolyte transport. *Am. J. Physiol.* **251**:G253–G262.

90. Russell, D. A., and G. A. Castro. 1989. Immunological regulation of colonic ion transport. *Am. J. Physiol.* **256**:G396–G403.

91. Scudamore, C. L., E. M. Thornton, L. McMillan, G. F. Newlands, and H. R. Miller. 1995. Release of the mucosal mast cell granule chymase, rat mast cell protease-II, during anaphylaxis is associated with the rapid development of paracellular permeability to macromolecules in rat jejunum. *J. Exp. Med.* **182**:1871–1881.

92. Stead, R. H., U. Kosecka-Janiszewska, A. B. Oestreicher, M. F. Dixon, and J. Bienenstock. 1991. Remodeling of B-50 (GAP-43)- and NSE-immunoreactive mucosal nerves in the intestines of rats infected with *Nippostrongylus brasiliensis*. *J. Neurosci.* **11**:3809–3821.

93. Stead, R. H., M. Tomioka, G. Quinonez, G. T. Simon, S. Y. Felten, and J. Bienenstock. 1987. Intestinal mucosal mast cells in normal and nematode-infected rat intestines are in intimate contact with peptidergic nerves. *Proc. Natl. Acad. Sci. USA* **84**:2975–2979.

94. Steiner, T. S., J. P. Nataro, C. E. Poteet-Smith, J. A. Smith, and R. L. Guerrant. 2000. Enteroaggregative *Escherichia coli* expresses a novel flagellin that causes IL-8 release from intestinal epithelial cells. *J. Clin. Invest.* **105**:1769–1777.

95. Sturiale, S., G. Barbara, B. Qiu, M. Figini, P. Geppetti, N. Gerard, C. Gerard, E. F. Grady, N. W. Bunnett, and S. M. Collins. 1999. Neutral endopeptidase (EC 3.4.24.11) terminates colitis by degrading substance P. *Proc. Natl. Acad. Sci. USA* **96**:11653–11658.

96. Sun, Y. J., H. Maeno, S. Aoki, and K. Wada. 2001. Mouse neurotensin receptor 2 gene (Ntsr2): genomic organization, transcriptional regulation and genetic mapping on chromosome 12. *Brain Res. Mol. Brain Res.* **95**:167–171.

97. Triadafilopoulos, G., C. Pothoulakis, R. Weiss, C. Giampaolo, and J. T. LaMont. 1989. Comparative study of *Clostridium difficile* toxin A and cholera toxin in rabbit ileum. *Gastroenterology* **97**:1186–1192.

98. **Vallance, B. A., P. A. Blennerhassett, Y. Deng, K. I. Matthaei, I. G. Young, and S. M. Collins.** 1999. IL-5 contributes to worm expulsion and muscle hypercontractility in a primary *T. spiralis* infection. *Am. J. Physiol.* **277:** G400–G408.

99. **Varilek, G. W., J. V. Weinstock, and N. J. Pantazis.** 1991. Isolated hepatic granulomas from mice infected with *Schistosoma mansoni* contain nerve growth factor. *Infect. Immun.* **59:** 4443–4449.

100. **Varilek, G. W., J. V. Weinstock, T. H. Williams, and J. Jew.** 1991. Alterations of the intestinal innervation in mice infected with *Schistosoma mansoni. J. Parasitol.* **77:**472–478.

101. **Vermillion, D. L., P. B. Ernst, R. Scicchitano, and S. M. Collins.** 1988. Antigen-induced contraction of jejunal smooth muscle in the sensitized rat. *Am. J. Physiol.* **255:**G701–G708.

102. **Wang, Y. Z., J. M. Palmer, and H. J. Cooke.** 1991. Neuroimmune regulation of colonic secretion in guinea pigs. *Am. J. Physiol.* **260:**G307–G314.

103. **Warny, M., A. C. Keates, S. Keates, I. Castagliuolo, J. K. Zacks, S. Aboudola, A. Qamar, C. Pothoulakis, J. T. LaMont, and C. P. Kelly.** 2000. p38 MAP kinase activation by *Clostridium difficile* toxin A mediates monocyte necrosis, IL-8 production, and enteritis. *J. Clin. Invest.* **105:**1147–1156.

104. **Weinstock, J. V., A. Blum, J. Walder, and R. Walder.** 1988. Eosinophils from granulomas in murine *Schistosomiasis mansoni* produce substance P. *J. Immunol.* **141:**961–966.

105. **Weinstock, J. V., and A. M. Blum.** 1989. Tachykinin production in granulomas of murine *Schistosomiasis mansoni. J. Immunol.* **142:**3256–3261.

106. **Weinstock, J. V., A. M. Blum, and T. Malloy.** 1990. Macrophages within the granulomas of murine *Schistosoma mansoni* are a source of a somatostatin 1-14-like molecule. *Cell Immunol.* **131:**381–390.

107. **Wershil, B. K., I. Castagliuolo, and C. Pothoulakis.** 1998. Direct evidence of mast cell involvement in *Clostridium difficile* toxin A-induced enteritis in mice. *Gastroenterology* **114:** 956–964.

108. **Woodbury, R. G., H. R. Miller, J. F. Huntley, G. F. Newlands, A. C. Palliser, and D. Wakelin.** 1984. Mucosal mast cells are functionally active during spontaneous expulsion of intestinal nematode infections in rat. *Nature* **312:** 450–452.

109. **Yeh, K. Y., M. Yeh, J. Glass, and D. N. Granger.** 2000. Rapid activation of NF-kappaB and AP-1 and target gene expression in postischemic rat intestine. *Gastroenterology.* **118:** 525–534.

110. **Zhao, D., A. C. Keates, S. Kuhnt-Moore, M. P. Moyer, C. P. Kelly, and C. Pothoulakis.** 2001. Signal transduction pathways mediating neurotensin-stimulated interleukin-8 expression in human colonocytes. *J. Biol. Chem.* **276:**44464–44471.

APOPTOSIS AND ENTERIC BACTERIAL INFECTIONS

Bärbel Raupach and Arturo Zychlinsky

20

Apoptosis (programmed cell death) is an innate host mechanism whereby controlled cell suicide occurs to maintain homeostasis within multicellular organisms. Induction or prevention of cell death can be a decisive factor in the course of an infection. In some cases, apoptosis of host cells contributes to the mammalian defense against invading pathogens. However, the contrary scenario also occurs. Many bacteria can trigger apoptosis in the host cell and thereby promote the infection. Bacterial virulence factors interfere with the host cell integrity by various mechanisms. Pathogenic strategies to induce cell death can include production of pore-forming toxins, secretion of protein synthesis inhibitors, type-III-secretion-dependent delivery of effector proteins as activators of the endogenous death machinery, stimulation of Toll-like receptors (TLR) by pathogen-associated molecular patterns (PAMPs), and targeting of immune cells by superantigens. In this chapter, we summarize the numerous mechanisms that enteropathogenic bacteria use to induce apoptosis in

host cells. We will focus on bacterium-induced cell death by three enteric pathogens: *Shigella, Salmonella,* and *Yersinia.* Despite the many mechanistic commonalities shared by these enteric bacteria, the outcome of infection differs considerably. Our aim is to illustrate how each of the three microbes manages to manipulate the relationship between apoptotic events and pathogenesis according to its individual needs.

APOPTOSIS

Cell death is crucial for the development and homeostasis of multicellular organisms, and it can also play a role in infections. Based on histological observations, cell death can be classified as either necrosis or apoptosis. These two forms of cell death have distinct morphological characteristics; necrosis is distinguished by swelling of the whole cell as well as the organelles within it. The integrity of the cell membrane is compromised, resulting in leakage of intracellular contents. In contrast, apoptosis is characterized by cell shrinkage, chromatin condensation, and often loss of contact with adjacent cells. This distinctive morphology is transient, and eventually apoptotic cells undergo "secondary necrosis,"

Bärbel Raupach and Arturo Zychlinsky, Department of Cellular Microbiology, Max Planck Institute for Infection Biology, Schumannstrasse 21/22, D-10117 Berlin, Germany.

Microbial Pathogenesis and the Intestinal Epithelial Cell, ed. by G. Hecht
© 2003 ASM Press, Washington, D.C.

which is indistinguishable from necrosis. However, an exclusive characteristic of apoptotic, but not necrotic, cells is that the DNA is fragmented to multimers of 200 bp, reflecting the size of nucleosomes.

Cell death can also be classified depending on whether the molecules that kill the cell were made by the cell itself (programmed cell death) or not. Mostly, cells that activate their program for cell death acquire apoptotic morphology. In contrast, necrotic cells are often killed by external agents or molecules made by other cells (31).

The last 10 years have witnessed an impressive accumulation of information regarding the molecular mechanisms leading to apoptosis. Here, we briefly describe the sequence of signaling events in apoptosis, including the activation of death receptors, the role of mitochondria in cell death, and the eventual clearance of apoptotic material.

Death Receptors

The term "death receptors" applies to proteins in the cell surface that, upon binding of a ligand, initiate a signal sequence cascade that culminates in cell death. Two of the best-characterized cell death receptors are the tumor necrosis factor alpha (TNF-α) receptor (TNF-R) and Fas. These two receptors need to be trimerized in order to signal. They recruit different adaptor molecules that directly or indirectly mobilize caspase-8. Caspases are cysteine proteases that cleave after an aspartate. Every member of this family activates apoptosis when overexpressed in vitro. The caspases have different substrate specificity and are classified into regulatory or effector caspases depending on their role in cell death. Caspase-8 (Casp8), a regulatory caspase, is recruited to a complex formed in response to a death receptor binding its ligand. This recruitment is crucial for the progression of apoptosis. Interestingly, some death receptors, like TNF-R, can also activate a pathway to inhibit cell death via the transactivator NF-κB. However, it is still unclear how the decision is

made that receptor activation leads to either apoptosis or NF-κB activation (4).

The TLR family of cell death receptors is directly involved in the response to bacterial infections. These receptors are activated by factors that are unique to microorganisms, for example, lipopolysaccharide (LPS), bacterial lipopeptides (BLP), or methylated DNA (CpG). The innate immune system has evolved to recognize these molecules, collectively called PAMPs, because they are essential for microbial viability and therefore bacteria cannot modify them. The innate immune system uses the TLR recognition of PAMPs as a signal to mount an inflammatory response. In a system reminiscent of the TNF-R function, TLR can activate two pathways: NF-κB-dependent transcription or apoptosis (Fig. 1). In addition, both NF-κB activation and the induction of apoptosis can lead to the release of proinflammatory cytokines. As in the case of TNF-R activation, it is still not known how the coordination of these two distinct programs is achieved (2, 57).

The Mitochondria and Beyond

The activation of an apoptotic cascade results in a transient permeability change across the mitochondrial membrane. This change causes the release of cytochrome C and of a protein called apoptotic protease activating factor (APAF). When these molecules are released into the cytoplasm, they complex with caspases and together form a complex called the "apoptosome." Effector caspases such as caspase-3, which are part of the apoptosome, are different from the regulatory caspases and are also referred to as "executioner" caspases. Formation of the apoptosome indicates that the cell is past the "point of no return" and is targeted for death. It is still not clear which substrates the executioner caspases need to cleave to kill a cell (78).

Apoptosis is a highly regulated event. Additional regulatory mechanisms within the cascade include (i) a number of serpins that act as caspase inhibitors and (ii) the Bcl-2 family

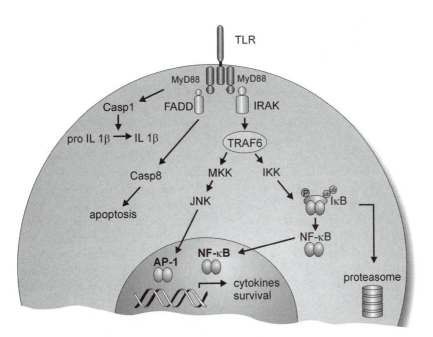

FIGURE 1 TLR signaling cascades. Upon activation, TLR recruit the adaptor molecule MyD88, which can initiate two independent outcomes: apoptosis and transcriptional activation. Apoptosis is activated by the initial recruitment of the FADD protein, which recruits the regulatory Casp8. Recruitment of FADD also provokes the maturation of Casp1, which in turns cleaves pro-IL-1β to its active form. Alternatively, MyD88 can recruit IRAK, which through TRAF6 activates MKK and IKK. MKK can phosphorylate JNK, which activates the transcription factor AP-1. Alternatively, IKK phosphorylates and targets I-κB (inhibitor of κB) to the proteasome, allowing NF-κB to migrate to the nucleus and initiate transcription.

of both pro- and antiapoptotic proteins that control mitochondrial integrity (1).

Clearing of Apoptotic Cells

It is important that the content of apoptotic cells be prevented from spilling out to avoid presentation of endogenous antigens, which would lead to the induction of acquired immune responses and ultimately to autoimmunity. Apoptotic cells achieve this effect by displaying specific markers on their surface, such as phosphatidylserine. These molecules are recognized by professional phagocytes such as neutrophils and macrophages, which can clear apoptotic bodies with high efficiency (73).

APOPTOSIS AND ENTERIC BACTERIAL INFECTIONS

Before entering the fascinating field of how type III-secreted bacterial effectors manipulate endogenous signaling pathways within the infected host cell to mediate apoptosis, we would like to point out that certain enteropathogens also employ toxins as a parallel strategy to induce host cell death. Enteric pathogens are generally classified based on the distinct pathogenic mechanism by which they cause disease, i.e., either toxin production or epithelial cell penetration. Thus, it is remarkable that certain microorganisms have developed both an invasive and a toxigenic strategy to induce apoptosis, a property that in our opinion can only reflect the view that the contribution of bacterium-induced cell death to disease is largely underestimated.

Shigella dysenteriae and enterohemorrhagic *Escherichia coli* (EHEC), which cause severe diarrheal diseases and hemolytic uremic syndrome (HUS), produce A-B type toxins, called Shiga toxin and Shiga-like toxins or verotoxins, respectively (59, 68). Shiga-like toxin 1 (Stx1 or VT1) is almost identical to Shiga toxin, while Stx2 or VT2 contains significant differences in sequence, yet remains structurally similar. The pentameric B subunit of the toxins mediates binding to the host cell via its glycolipid receptor globotriaosylceramide Gb3 (CD77). Subsequently, the toxin is endocytosed and transported all the way from the cell surface to the Golgi and the endoplasmic reticulum (ER) (68). Via retrograde transport, the enzymatically active A subunit of the molecule gains access to the cytosol. Once there, it efficiently inhibits protein synthesis by removing a single adenine residue from the 28S RNA of the 60S ribosomal subunit.

Shiga toxins do not only disrupt ribosome function. The toxin-induced synthesis of proinflammatory cytokines has been reported in epithelial cells of both intestine and kidney (25, 84). In addition, results from two independent groups support the hypothesis (69) that Shiga toxins can induce cell death independent of their effect on protein synthesis. Toxin-mediated apoptosis might involve members of the Bcl-2 family (29, 75). Although the apoptogenic activity of the holotoxin by far exceeds that of the B subunit, additional data suggest that Gb3-dependent endocytosis of the pentameric B subunit is sufficient to induce apoptosis in the absence of inhibition of protein biosynthesis (40, 41).

Shiga toxins induce apoptosis at various epithelial sites, thereby helping the bacteria to break this barrier and reach the submucosa. Compared to many other broad-spectrum protein toxins, Shiga toxins act on a limited number of cell types. Selective targeting of certain epithelial cell subsets may be based on the availability of toxin binding sites, i.e., Gb3

receptors. Enterocytes of the villi may be preferentially killed because they contain more Gb3 receptors compared to crypt cells, which are unaffected by the toxins (30). Moreover, the renal complications associated with *S. dysenteriae* and EHEC infections may directly result from the relative abundance of Gb3 receptors in the kidney epithelium.

Since the discovery that *S. dysenteriae* type 1 produces an exotoxin, many attempts have been made to correlate the unique clinical and epidemiological features of this strain with toxin production. However, experimental evidence from studies in monkeys and human volunteers suggests that invasion and epithelial penetration are the virulence properties central to the pathogenesis of shigellosis in humans (19, 34). Invasive, nontoxigenic strains are still capable of causing dysentery, although the severity and duration of the disease are milder and more closely resemble the clinical symptoms caused by *Shigella flexneri*. Furthermore, Shiga toxin itself cannot function as an enterotoxin and cause diarrhea in humans, implying that its pathogenic role in disease may lie in its cytotoxic activities. Potential targets of the cytotoxin include epithelial cells of the intestine as well as the kidney and possibly also endothelial cells. Thus, Shiga toxin is responsible for the particularly severe colitis and renal sequelae, such as HUS, associated with *S. dysenteriae* infections. However, the precise role of Shiga toxin in human infections remains to be defined.

In enteric infections, toxin-mediated apoptosis preferentially targets epithelial cells, while the bacterial effector proteins interfering with the endogenous death machinery of the cell appear to selectively affect macrophages. Induction of apoptosis in phagocytes may have several advantages for the bacteria. Bacterium-induced cell death can protect the microorganisms against phagocytosis and/or killing. Apoptotic macrophage death, triggered by bacteria, can either result in an impressive localized infiltration of inflammatory cells or occur silently without any signs of inflammation, as has been described for *Shigella* and *Yersinia* infections, respectively. Induction of apoptosis in macrophages can also promote infection. At mucosal sites such as the M cells of Peyer's patches, phagocytes control bacterial entry. Bacterium-induced cell death, in macrophages underlying the M cells, permits access to the submucosa or even the bloodstream and peripheral organs. *Salmonella* sp. employs this strategy in two sequential steps to successfully establish systemic infection.

SHIGELLA-INDUCED MACROPHAGE DEATH

The paradigm for bacteria–induced cell death is that employed by *S. flexneri*. *Shigella* sp. is the etiologic agent of bacillary dysentery or shigellosis, a severe form of bloody diarrhea that significantly contributes to infant mortality in the underdeveloped regions of the world. While the Shiga toxin-producing species *S. dysenteriae* type 1 represents the cause of dysentery epidemics, its nontoxigenic relative, *S. flexneri*, accounts for most of the worldwide endemic form of disease. After oral ingestion, these gram–negative enteropathogens invade the colonic epithelium, where they cause a localized infection by inducing a severe inflammatory response characterized by a massive influx of neutrophils. Inflammation serves a dual purpose in the pathogenesis of disease, since it contributes to both establishment and control of infection. Initially, tissue damage caused by the inflammatory response helps the bacteria to gain access to deeper tissues and promotes further bacterial colonization. However, at the same time inflammation is also the prerequisite for eventual eradication of the microorganisms (89). The key event in all of these processes is the *Shigella*-mediated activation of Casp1 in macrophages, which causes cell death and induces inflammation (72).

Shigella spp. and Macrophage Death

The first encounter between bacteria and phagocytes occurs subsequent to *Shigella*'s traversing the colonic barrier through specialized epithelial cells, called M cells (60, 82). These cells are located within the follicle-associated epithelium as part of the GALT (gut-associated lymphoid tissue). M cells constitutively sample intestinal antigens, including enteropathogens, and transport them from the gut lumen to underlying lymphoid tissues. Resident macrophages are positioned underneath the M cells, ready to deal with intruding microorganisms. Ideally, phagosomal processing will destroy the bacteria and produce the microbial antigens required to initiate specific immunity (32). Many pathogens not only use M cells as their port of entry to the intestinal mucosa, but also have designed strategies to evade elimination by professional phagocytes. In the case of *Shigella* spp., the microorganisms actively invade host cells and then escape from the endosome to the cytoplasm. Inside epithelial cells, the bacteria multiply and employ actin-based motility to move intracellularly and spread from cell to cell, while inside macrophages, *Shigella* sp. induces apoptosis and interleukin (IL)-1 and IL-18 release (86, 88). *Shigella*-induced macrophage killing has been demonstrated not only in vitro, but also in animal models of infection (Fig. 2) (72, 90) and in biopsies from patients with shigellosis (26).

The genes for *Shigella* invasion and cytotoxicity are located on a large virulence plasmid, and strains lacking this plasmid are avirulent (71). The invasion plasmid antigen (*ipa*) operon encodes for the respective effector molecules, which are secreted by a type III secretion system also present on the plasmid. IpaB alone is necessary (87) and sufficient to induce cell death in macrophages (Fig. 3); it activates an apoptotic cascade by binding to Casp1 (11, 77). *Shigella* appears to trigger a specialized cell death pathway, since Casp1-deficient macrophages are resistant to *Shigella*-induced cell death, yet respond to classical apoptotic stimuli (24, 35). Furthermore, *Shigella*-induced apoptosis does not require caspase-3 or -11, occurs independently of p53, and is not regulated by the antiapoptotic proteins of the Bcl-2 family (24). The role of Casp1 in programmed cell death in develop-

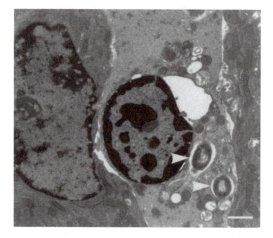

FIGURE 2 Transmission electron micrograph of lymphoid follicles infected with *S. flexneri*. Virulence of the wild-type *S. flexneri* strain M90T was assessed in the rabbit ligated ileal loop model. At 8 h post-infection, tissue samples were fixed and processed for transmission electron microscopy. Cells with apoptotic morphology were detected and contain intracellular bacteria (arrowhead). Bar, 1 μm. (Reprinted from reference 90.)

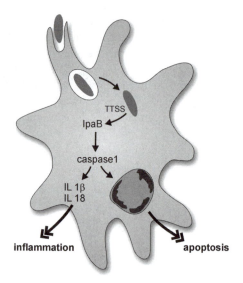

FIGURE 3 Casp1 activation by *Shigella* results in inflammation and cell death. After internalization by macrophages, *Shigella* escapes from the phagosome into the cytoplasm of the host cell where it secretes the virulence factor IpaB via a type III secretion system. As a consequence of the direct interaction between IpaB and Casp1, this cysteine protease initiates both an apoptotic cascade leading to cell death and processing and release of the proinflammatory cytokines IL-1β and IL-18, resulting in inflammation.

ment and homeostasis is unclear, since Casp1-deficient mice do not display the same developmental defects seen in other caspase-deficient animals (39). Casp1 is unique in that it not only plays a role in cell death pathways, but is also essential for the processing of proinflammatory cytokines, as its original name—IL-1β converting enzyme (ICE)—indicates (79). Both IL-1β and IL-18 are produced as zymogens that are proteolytically converted to their mature form by Casp1 (18). Neither of these two cytokines is required for Casp1-dependent *Shigella*-induced macrophage apoptosis, since phagocytes from IL-1β- and IL-18-deficient mice are efficiently killed upon infection. However, it remains unclear whether *Shigella*-induced Casp1 activation and subsequent cell death may mediate release of the processed cytokines, which are synthesized without a conventional leader peptide for secretion.

Shigella and Inflammation

The role of Casp1 activation in macrophage apoptosis and inflammation during *Shigella* in-

fections has recently been analyzed in the murine lung model of shigellosis (72). During experimental pulmonary infections, where bacteria are administered intranasally to mice, *Shigella* sp. elicits an acute inflammatory response in the lung tissue comparable to the inflammation that occurs in the intestinal mucosa of dysenteric patients (61). In immunocompetent mice, severe tracheobronchitis and alveolitis combined with massive infiltration of polymorphonuclear cells (PMN) are observed as early as 6 h postinfection. At 48 h, similar to most cases of human dysentery, both bacterial load and inflammation decrease and the infection starts to resolve. In contrast, Casp1-deficient mice develop a delayed inflammatory response. Inflammation is more severe and dominated by monocytes rather than neutrophils. These animals are incapable of restricting bacterial replication and rapidly succumb to *Shigella* infection.

Results from experimental *Shigella* infections in Casp1-deficient mice reconstituted with either recombinant IL-1β or IL-18, as well as animals defective in these cytokines, suggest that IL-1β and IL-18 display their function at different stages of infection. IL-1β appears to be required for the initial inflammatory response to *Shigella* sp. and for the establishment of infection. Early after infection, very few infectious foci are found in both IL-1β- and Casp1-deficient animals compared with wild-type and IL-18-deficient mice, a phenotype that could be compensated for by the exogenous administration of recombinant IL-1β (72). These data suggest that the initial IL-1β-dependent inflammatory response and associated tissue disruption enable the non-motile *Shigella* sp. to more efficiently spread within the epithelium. This hypothesis is in accordance with earlier reports demonstrating that IL-1β is induced and activated rapidly after *Shigella* infection and that administration of the IL-1 receptor agonist (IL-1ra) reduces inflammation in the rabbit ileal loop model (3, 70).

Functional IL-18, however, is required during a later phase of infection, when the inflammatory response eradicates the bacteria. Similar to Casp1-deficient animals, mice lacking IL-18 do not generate an effective inflammation and thus succumb to uncontrolled microbial replication. A normal inflammatory response during *Shigella* infection was observed in Casp1-deficient mice reconstituted with recombinant IL-18, thus supporting the important role of IL-18 in the control of shigellosis (72). Although gamma interferon (IFN-γ)-deficient mice have been reported to be highly susceptible to *Shigella* infections (83), the functional contribution of IL-18 to control of disease remains to be elucidated. In addition to its role as an IFN-γ-inducing factor, IFN-γ-independent functions in innate and acquired immunity have recently been described (53, 76).

Taken together, Casp1 activation by the *Shigella* virulence factor IpaB represents a prime example of how coordination of both apoptotic and inflammatory pathways ultimately determines the outcome of infection. Casp1 activation is a key step in both microbial pathogenesis of and innate immunity to *Shigella* infections. Protease activation in infected macrophages connects two cellular signaling pathways that lead to cell death and inflammation. Whether a causative link between apoptosis and cytokine release exists remains to be determined. However, Casp1 is essential in coordinating the inflammatory responses required for establishing and controlling infection.

SALMONELLA-INDUCED MACROPHAGE DEATH

In contrast to *Shigella*, which causes a severe but localized and usually self-limiting inflammation in dysenteric patients, *Salmonella* serovars can infect a broad range of hosts including humans, causing diseases ranging from mild enteritis to severe systemic salmonellosis. *Salmonella enterica* serovar Typhimurium is a common cause of gastroenteritis in humans. However, in mice it elicits a systemic disease similar to *S. enterica* serovar Typhi infections in humans and thus represents a suitable animal model to study the pathogenesis of typhoid fever. The bacteria enter the host by the oral route, invade M cells, colonize the Peyer's patches of the small intestine, and gain access to GALT. Infection is characterized by inflammation at the site of bacterial invasion and in underlying tissues. Both *Salmonella*-induced tissue alterations and infiltration of PMN and monocytes contribute to damage of the intestinal mucosa (15, 28). Once *Salmonella* has successfully crossed the epithelial barrier, it selects phagocytes as its preferred host cells. These cells serve as vehicles to the mesenteric lymph nodes, allowing *Salmonella* to disseminate to the liver and spleen (63). Following replication at systemic sites, the bacteria recirculate to their initial port of entry. *Salmonella* infections result in either fatal bacteremia, when unrestricted, or the formation of microabscesses that lead to bacterial clearance, when successfully controlled. Occasionally, the bacteria can persist in asymptomatic carriers, who contribute substantially to dissemination of disease by shedding pathogens via the gallbladder into the environment.

The fact that *Salmonella* preferentially infects macrophages appears counterintuitive, since these phagocytic cells are designed by the host as an early antimicrobial response mechanism. To be successful within this habitat and use it to establish systemic infection, *Salmonella* has evolved a multitude of survival strategies, which enable resistance to antimicrobial effector mechanisms of the host and allow nutrient acquisition for intracellular proliferation (9).

Salmonella-induced macrophage death has been the subject of much attention lately. Macrophage killing mediated by *Salmonella* has been demonstrated both in vitro (10, 20, 38, 50) and in vivo (47, 63). Although initially described as programmed cell death, *Salmonella*-induced macrophage killing does not strictly conform to either classical apoptosis or necrosis (13). In contrast to *Shigella*, two signaling pathways ultimately resulting in macrophage death have been identified for *Salmonella*. These two pathways are different in their kinetics and the virulence factors and caspases involved. *Salmonella* pathogenicity island 1 (SPI1) and SPI2 encode different effectors as well as independent type III secretion systems. SPI1 is responsible for intestinal infection and early macrophage death, while SPI2 encodes genes important for systemic infection and delayed macrophage death.

Early SPI1-Dependent Macrophage Death

Rapid killing of macrophages by *S. enterica* serovar Typhimurium is mechanistically very similar to *Shigella*-induced apoptosis (Fig. 4A). The bacteria inject an effector protein, called SipB, via a type III secretion system into the host cell. SipB is both structurally and functionally homologous to IpaB and also binds to and activates Casp1 to trigger cell death and inflammation (23). Like IpaB, SipB is not only involved in macrophage killing but also plays an essential role in host cell invasion. The 40-kb region of DNA at centisome 63 of the *Salmonella* chromosome, referred to as SPI1, encodes a set of genes required for regulation

and secretion of the virulence factors mediating epithelial cell invasion. Gene expression is tightly regulated by environmental conditions and the bacterial growth state (7). Only invasive bacteria that actively induce their own uptake are cytotoxic to macrophages (20, 50). However, not only the physiological state of the bacteria, but also the activation status of the macrophage can affect the magnitude of *Salmonella*-induced cell death. Activated macrophages stimulated with LPS and IFN-γ are even more rapidly killed by invasive *Salmonella* sp. than nonactivated cells.

The crucial role of *Salmonella*-mediated early macrophage death has been demonstrated both in vitro and in vivo. Casp1 activation by invasive *Salmonella* strains in infected macrophages leads to proteolytic processing of pro–IL-1β and pro–IL-18 to their mature forms as well as to cell death (23, 27). The most striking evidence illustrating the key role of Casp1 activation in salmonellosis arises from the finding that Casp1-deficient mice are resistant to *S. enterica* serovar Typhimurium infection via the natural route. The oral 50% lethal dose (LD_{50}) is increased 1,000-fold in Casp1 knockout animals compared to control mice (47). Interestingly, when mice were challenged intraperitoneally, no difference in susceptibility between Casp1-deficient and wild-type animals was observed. These results indicate that Casp1 is crucial for *Salmonella* pathogenesis in the gastrointestinal, but not the systemic, phase of infection. In the absence of this protease, progression to the systemic phase of *Salmonella* infection is inhibited. Although invasion of M cells and Peyer's patches still occurs, the lack of bacteria-induced cell death and the failure to induce an inflammatory response restrict the infection to the GALT.

Even though *Salmonella* and *Shigella* pursue very similar virulence strategies to initially establish local infection in the gastrointestinal tract, the outcome of infection in Casp1-deficient animals is surprisingly different. In the absence of active Casp1, animals are more susceptible to *Shigella* and ultimately succumb to infection, while they are more resistant to

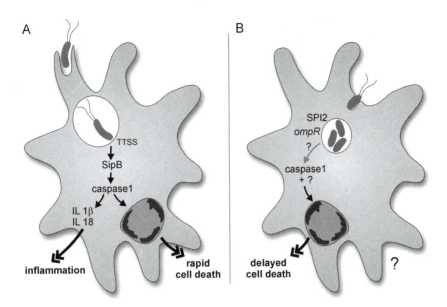

FIGURE 4 Pathways of *Salmonella*-induced cell death in macrophages. (A) SPI1-dependent cell death occurs rapidly after infection with invasive *Salmonella* strains and depends on the interaction between Casp1 and the bacterial effector SipB. As for *Shigella*, SipB-mediated activation of Casp1 leads to the processing of proinflammatory cytokines and cell death. (B) An SPI1-independent mechanism of *Salmonella*-induced cell death is observed later after infection. The exact sequence of events leading to macrophage killing is still unclear; however, delayed cell death depends on the *ompR*-regulated pathogenicity island SPI2 and in part on Casp1.

Salmonella and prevent progression to fatal disease. Within Casp1-deficient mice, invading *Shigella* are able to infect and multiply in individual cells within the follicle-associated epithelium. From there, they gradually spread and generate a fulminate infection that cannot be controlled. In contrast, we assume that invading *Salmonella* are eliminated by resident macrophages within the Peyer's patches of Casp1-deficient animals, since rapid cell death as an evasion strategy of host effector functions is not an option. Thus, the difference in susceptibility to shigellosis and salmonellosis observed in Casp1-deficient mice is a direct reflection of the pathogenesis of these two distinct diseases.

Delayed SPI2-Dependent Macrophage Death

Noninvasive *Salmonella* strains are not capable of inducing early macrophage death, yet they mediate killing of macrophages at later time points postinfection (Fig. 4B). Interestingly, both types of *Salmonella*-induced cell death were described simultaneously (10, 38, 50); however, the mechanistic differences underlying either the rapid or delayed killing of macrophages by *Salmonella* have only recently been dissected (46, 80). As initially described by Lindgren et al. (38), late activation of macrophage death is dependent on a functional *ompR* gene and its regulation of SPI2 genes (33, 80). In addition, the *Salmonella* virulence plasmid *spv* genes have been linked to delayed killing of macrophages (37). However, at this stage it cannot be excluded that cytotoxicity is not a direct result of *spv*-mediated virulence functions, but rather occurs as an indirect consequence of bacterial multiplication, since *S. enterica* serovar Typhimurium *spv* mutants did not proliferate inside the human monocyte-derived macrophages used in this study. Furthermore, SPI1-dependent delayed cell death mediated by Casp2 has been proposed to occur in the absence of Casp1 (27).

The mechanistic basis for SPI2-dependent delayed macrophage killing by *S. enterica* serovar Typhimurium has been recently investigated. SPI2 encodes a type III secretion system and effectors essential for intraphagocyte survival during the systemic phase of salmonellosis (22). Infections of macrophages derived from Casp1-deficient mice with isogenic *S. enterica* serovar Typhimurium strains revealed that delayed SPI2-dependent macrophage death is in part mediated by Casp1. Similar to rapid SPI1-induced macrophage death, SPI2-dependent Casp1 activation leads to the release of mature IL-1β. However, as for *Shigella*-mediated apoptosis, neither IL-1β nor IL-18 is required for rapid or delayed macrophage killing (46). To date, the specific effector molecules within SPI2 that trigger the delayed death cascade macrophages infected with *Salmonella* remain to be identified.

The role of SPI2-dependent delayed macrophage death in the pathogenesis of infection is unclear. Both local and systemic dissemination of disease appears to directly depend on the processing and secretion of proinflammatory cytokines in a Casp1-dependent process. Why would *Salmonella* require multiple distinct mechanisms for activation of Casp1? One plausible explanation could be that rapid and delayed macrophage deaths are alternative strategies for Casp1 activation that occur under different in vivo conditions at distinct locations and time points during infections. SPI2-dependent macrophage death may replace SPI1-mediated Casp1 activation at stages subsequent to invasion of host cells, when *Salmonella* downregulates expression of SPI1 genes. Future studies are required to clarify whether seemingly overlapping mechanisms of bacterium-induced cell death and cytokine processing are designed for purposes of backup or amplification or serve separate functions.

YERSINIA-INDUCED CELL DEATH

In addition to *Yersinia pestis*, the etiological agent of the plague, the genus *Yersinia* contains two enteric pathogens, *Yersinia enterocolitica* and *Yersinia pseudotuberculosis*, which cause gastrointestinal syndromes, lymphadenitis, and septicemia. Like *Shigella* and *Salmonella*, *Yersinia* uses a type III secretion system to deliver bacterial effector molecules to the host cell cytosol to adapt cellular processes according to its pathogenic lifestyle. So far, six *Yersinia* outer protein (Yop) effectors have been identified for *Y. pseudotuberculosis*: YopE, YopH, YopM, YopJ, YpkA, and YopT. Their genes are located on the 70-kb virulence plasmid pYV and encode for virulence factors that interfere with host effector functions at different levels (14). As an immediate effect of these Yops, *Yersinia* blocks phagocytosis and resists killing by macrophages. Moreover, *Yersinia* suppresses the production of proinflammatory cytokines (8, 58) and induces apoptosis in macrophages (45, 49, 67). Both effects are advantageous for the extracellular lifestyle of *Yersinia*.

The effector molecule responsible for the anti-inflammatory and proapoptotic properties of *Yersinia* is YopJ in *Y. pseudotuberculosis*, or its homologue YopP in *Y. enterocolitica*. YopJ is an essential virulence factor, since a *Y. pseudotuberculosis* mutant strain carrying a deletion of *yopJ* is significantly attenuated in mice (48). YopJ-mediated apoptosis of macrophages and inhibition of TNF-α production are important steps in establishing the systemic phase of *Yersinia* infection.

The Anti-Inflammatory Aspects of *Yersinia* Infection

The proinflammatory cytokines, TNF-α, IFN-γ, and IL-8 play a crucial role in control of bacterial infections, including *Yersinia*. *Yersinia* is able to suppress the expression of these cytokines in vivo, a capacity that is required for its proliferation in the host (5, 52). Inhibition of cytokine production during *Yersinia* infection correlates with YopJ-dependent downregulation of mitogen-activated protein kinase (MAPK) signaling pathways, including extracellular signal-regulated kinases (ERK), p38 and Jun amino-terminal kinase (JNK) (8, 58, 65). However, the inhibitory effects of

YopJ on signaling pathways are not restricted to MAPK activities; they also extend to the NF-κB pathway, a signaling system that is central to innate immunity (44, 64, 74).

A recent report by Orth et al. (56) has solved the mystery of how a single effector molecule can function as a universal inhibitor of multiple signaling pathways. YopJ was shown to directly bind to members of the MAPK kinase superfamily, blocking both phosphorylation and activation of these signaling molecules (Fig. 5). Affected kinases include both the MAPK kinases (MKKs) essential for signaling via the MAPK pathways (ERK, P38, JNK) and the I-κB kinase complex (IKKβ) required for NF-κB activation.

The Apoptotic Aspects of *Yersinia* Infection: Anti- or Proapoptosis?

The link between the abilities of *Yersinia* to induce apoptosis in macrophages and to sup-

press cytokine production has been appointed to the transcription factor NF-κB (64). NF-κB not only stimulates expression of cytokines, acute-phase proteins, and adhesion molecules, but also controls cellular survival pathways through the activation of antiapoptotic factors such as inhibitor of apoptosis protein (IAP), TNF receptor activating factor (TRAF), and Bcl-2 (6, 21). Following *Yersinia* infection, NF-κB activity is rapidly downregulated after initial stimulation (64). As NF-κB mediates survival by upregulation of proteins that counteract proapoptotic pathways, YopJ-mediated inhibition of NF-κB activity will result in macrophage cell death. As several studies indicate, however, prevention of NF-κB activation alone is not sufficient to trigger apoptosis in eukaryotic cells, but rather a secondary proapoptotic signal is required for cell death. Activation of TLRs by BLP or LPS appears to be the prime candidate for this secondary stimulus. Stimulation of TLRs with their respective PAMPs not only activates NF-κB by the classical cascade dependent on the IKK complex, in which I-κB is phosphorylated, ubiquitinated, and degraded (42, 43), but also triggers apoptotic pathways through activation of caspases (2). Recent studies in which YopP- and *Yersinia*-mediated apoptosis was specifically prevented by transient overexpression of NF-κB p65 provide evidence that YopP achieves macrophage death by subverting the NF-κB signaling pathway (66). This report also shows that LPS-induced signaling strongly enhances the apoptosis-inducing properties of YopP. Thus, during *Yersinia* infection the action of Yop effectors reverses LPS-mediated signals, since proapoptotic signaling pathways leading to macrophage apoptosis will predominate upon inhibition of NF-κB activation.

YopJ-mediated cell death can be inhibited by the broad-spectrum caspase inhibitor zVAD, but does not involve Casp1 (16, 49). Activation of this, yet to be identified, caspase leads to the cleavage of Bid, a proapoptotic Bcl-2-like protein. Truncated Bid is translocated to the mitochondria, where it induces cytochrome C release and formation

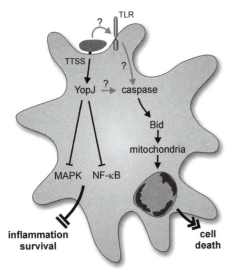

FIGURE 5 *Yersinia* induces cell death by inhibition of survival pathways and by inducing apoptosis. *Yersinia* delivers the effector molecule YopJ into the host cell via type III secretion. YopJ blocks activation of the superfamily of MAPK kinases, thus inactivating both MAPK signaling and NF-κB activity. Inhibition of these pathways prevents the cell from producing cytokines and antiapoptotic factors. In addition, *Yersinia* can activate the cell death machinery. Whether this process directly involves YopJ is unclear.

of the apoptosome complex. Activation of procaspases-9, -3, and -7 mediates the execution of death. Results from Denecker et al. suggest that YopP-dependent cell death is initiated by caspases upstream of Bid, most likely Casp8 (16). However, no clear evidence for a direct physical interaction between YopP and Casp8 could be obtained (74). The mechanistic basis of caspase activation during *Yersinia* infection remains elusive. Future studies on the targets of YopJ/P will help to clarify the issue of whether YopJ/P-mediated macrophage death results from a manipulation of LPS-induced pro- and antiapoptotic signals or from a direct activation of the death machinery.

YopJ/P Functions and Targets

YopJ/P, a global inhibitor of signaling pathways, is a 33-kDa protein that belongs to a family of effector proteins found in various animal and plant pathogens. However, amino acid sequence alignments of these effectors do not reveal any insight into their function. In contrast, the comparison of the predicted secondary structure of YopJ with known crystallographic data provided valuable information about its molecular mechanism of action (57). YopJ resembles adenovirus protease (AVP), which in turn was described to be similar to ubiquitin-like protein protease 1 (Ulp1) from yeast (36). Based on this observation, YopJ was identified as a cysteine protease that cleaves the small ubiquitin-related modifier (SUMO). Ulp activity leads to proteolytic processing of SUMO molecules with two carboxy-terminal glycine residues, which are required for subsequent formation of an isopeptide bond to the ε-amine of lysines on target proteins. Alternatively, SUMO can be removed from modified target proteins by proteolytic cleavage. Both SUMO-1 and its protein conjugates appear to be substrates for YopJ (57). In addition, overexpression of YopJ was reported to result in a decrease of proteins modified by SUMO and ubiquitin (55).

Although ubiquitination of target proteins is classically linked to marking these molecules for proteasomal degradation, increasing evidence exists that correlates this modification with signaling events (62). Thus, the addition of ubiquitin and ubiquitin-like proteins to target molecules can be regarded as a post-translational protein modification comparable to phosphorylation. In both cases, post-translational modifications are reversible and energy dependent and result in a change of activation state or location within the cell (55). Various regulatory proteins, including c-Jun and p53, have been reported to be modified by ubiquitin-like proteins (51). Consequently, it is tempting to speculate that YopJ-dependent removal of SUMO-1 from target proteins may influence the posttranslational modification profile of key elements involved in the inhibition of the signaling pathways central to *Yersinia* infection.

While previous studies have convincingly demonstrated that YopJ directly binds to the superfamily of MKK to block their activation, no supporting evidence exists to show that MKK are modified by SUMO. In contrast, the NF-κB signaling pathways are regulated by ubiquitination at multiple levels. The most prominent modification step is the targeting of I-κB to the ubiquitin-proteasome pathway following IKK-dependent phosphorylation (12). Other ubiquitin-related posttranslational modifications within the NF-κB pathway are linked to TRAF6-mediated ubiquitination events involved in IKK activation in response to proinflammatory mediators. IKK activation by TRAF6 relies on two intermediary factors, TRAF6-regulated IKK activator 1 (TRIKA1) and TRIKA2. TRIKA1 is a dimeric ubiquitin-conjugating enzyme complex (17), while TRIKA2 represents a trimeric protein kinase complex comprising TAK1, TAB1, and TAB2 (81). Together with TRAF6, TRIKA1 was shown to catalyze the synthesis of K63-linked poly-ubiquitin chains that lead to the activation of TAK1. TAK1 then phosphorylates and activates IKK directly without any involvement of the intermediary kinase NIK. In contrast to earlier findings, NIK acts in an extremely receptor-restricted manner instead of representing the universal kinase upstream of

IKK that mediates NF-κB activation in response to many different stimuli (85). Interestingly, ubiquitin-dependent activation of TAK1 has also been associated with activation of the MAPK signaling. TAK1 can phosphorylate MKK6, which in turn activates the JNK-p38 kinase pathway (54). That TRAF6 is essential for both IKK and JNK activation suggests that TAK1 acts as the central kinase (both IKKK and MKKK) that may link MAPK and NF-κB signaling pathways. How ubiquinated TRAF6 mediates activation of the endogenous TAK1 complex and whether transient ubiquitination of TAK1 itself occurs remain unclear.

If we now recall that a signaling step upstream of IKK and MKK was postulated as the potentially common YopJ target, abrogated TAK1 signaling would simultaneously inhibit both antiapoptotic and proinflammatory pathways during *Yersinia* infection. Mechanistically, this profound inhibition could result from the interference of YopJ with the signaling complex required for TAK1 activation. In summary, identification of *Yersinia* effector protein YopJ as a Ulp not only promotes the relevance of ubiquitin and ubiquitin-like protein modifications as a regulatory element, but also explains how a single virulence factor can manipulate diverse signaling pathways.

CONCLUSIONS

Apoptotic cell death in the pathogenesis of infectious diseases was initially studied with regard to viruses. However, bacteria also use modulation of host cell death pathways to enhance pathogenicity. Depending on its individual lifestyle, the microbe makes a clear decision whether to let the host cell live or die. Obligate intracellular pathogens such as *Rickettsia* and *Chlamydia* will—like viruses—inhibit host cell death to preserve their habitat for proliferation. In contrast, facultative intracellular bacteria and extracellular pathogens generally trigger apoptosis within the host to facilitate their infections. As in the case of the enteropathogenic bacteria, reviewed here, bacteria-induced cell death serves the prime function of eliminating or modulating host

defense mechanisms of the innate immune system. Destruction of phagocytes occurs before these effector cells can eradicate the intruding microorganism and is crucial for systemic infections such as salmonellosis. Stimulation of a strong inflammatory response represents a key feature of locally restricted infections such as shigellosis. Interestingly, the pathological alterations observed at the level of the intestinal epithelium as a result of *Shigella*-induced apoptosis share conceptual similarities with the hypersensitivity response occurring in plants. Here, an infection by microbial pathogens is accompanied by rapid cell death at the initial site of infection. Recent studies have provided functional evidence that the basic mechanisms of pathogen-mediated activation of programmed cell death are conserved in the animal and plant system. Astonishing parallels exist on the level of both the signaling components of the host defense and the bacterial effectors. Homologues of YopJ/P are present not only in viral or bacterial pathogens of mammals but also in phytopathogenic bacteria, such as the *Xanthomonas campestris* AvrRxv protein, which was shown to trigger the plant immune system by inducing Black Spot on tobacco leaves (57).

Thus, pathogen-induced programmed cell death is a concept prevalent both in the animal and the plant kingdoms. Bacteria have evolved such that each effector is perfectly tailored to suit the needs of the individual pathogen. As our understanding of the role of apoptosis in response to infection progresses, more surprising similarities may be revealed.

ACKNOWLEDGMENTS

We thank Juana de Diego, Molly Ingersoll, Peter Aichele, and Antoine Galmiche for helpful comments. Diane Schad is gratefully acknowledged for expert graphical assistance.

REFERENCES

1. **Adams, J. M., and S. Cory.** 1998. The Bcl-2 protein family: arbiters of cell survival. *Science* **281:**1322–1326.
2. **Aliprantis, A. O., R. B. Yang, D. S. Weiss, P. Godowski, and A. Zychlinsky.** 2000. The

apoptotic signaling pathway activated by Toll-like receptor-2. *EMBO J.* **19**:3325–3336.

3. **Arondel, J., M. Singer, A. Matsukawa, A. Zychlinsky, and P. J. Sansonetti.** 1999. Increased interleukin-1 (IL-1) and imbalance between IL-1 and IL-1 receptor antagonist during acute inflammation in experimental shigellosis. *Infect. Immun.* **67**:6056–6066.

4. **Ashkenazi, A., and V. M. Dixit.** 1998. Death receptors: signaling and modulation. *Science* **281**:1305–1308.

5. **Autenrieth, I. B., and J. Heesemann.** 1992. In vivo neutralization of tumor necrosis factor alpha and interferon-gamma abrogates resistance to *Yersinia enterocolitica* infection in mice. *Med. Microbiol. Immunol.* **181**:333–338.

6. **Baichwal, V. R., and P. A. Baeuerle.** 1997. Activate NF-κB or die? *Curr. Biol.* **7**:94–96.

7. **Bajaj, V., R. L. Lucas, C. Hwang, and C. A. Lee.** 1996. Co-ordinate regulation of *Salmonella typhimurium* invasion genes by environmental and regulatory factors is mediated by control of hilA expression. *Mol. Microbiol.* **22**:703–714.

8. **Boland, A., and G. R. Cornelis.** 1998. Role of YopP in suppression of tumor necrosis factor alpha release by macrophages during *Yersinia* infection. *Infect. Immun.* **66**:1878–1884.

9. **Buchmeier, N., A. Blanc-Potard, S. Ehrt, D. Piddington, L. Riley, and E. A. Groisman.** 2000. A parallel intraphagosomal survival strategy shared by *Mycobacterium tuberculosis* and *Salmonella enterica*. *Mol. Microbiol.* **35**:1375–1382.

10. **Chen, L. M., K. Kaniga, and J. E. Galan.** 1996. *Salmonella* spp. are cytotoxic for cultured macrophages. *Mol. Microbiol.* **21**:1101–1115.

11. **Chen, Y., M. R. Smith, K. Thirumalai, and A. Zychlinsky.** 1996. A bacterial invasin induces macrophage apoptosis by directly binding ICE. *EMBO J.* **15**:3853–3860.

12. **Chen, Z., J. Hagler, V. J. Palombella, F. Melandri, D. Scherer, D. Ballard, and T. Maniatis.** 1995. Signal-induced site-specific phosphorylation targets I kappa B alpha to the ubiquitin-proteasome pathway. *Genes Dev.* **9**:1586–1597.

13. **Cookson, B. T., and M. A. Brennan.** 2001. Pro-inflammatory programmed cell death. *Trends Microbiol.* **9**:113–114.

14. **Cornelis, G. R., A. Boland, A. P. Boyd, C. Geuijen, M. Iriarte, C. Neyt, M. P. Sory, and I. Stainier.** 1998. The virulence plasmid of *Yersinia*, an antihost genome. *Microbiol. Mol. Biol. Rev.* **62**:1315–1352.

15. **Darwin, K. H., and V. L. Miller.** 1999. Molecular basis of the interaction of *Salmonella* with the intestinal mucosa. *Clin. Microbiol. Rev.* **12**:405–428.

16. **Denecker, G., W. Declercq, C. A. Geuijen, A. Boland, R. Benabdillah, M. van Gurp, M. P. Sory, P. Vandenabeele, and G. R. Cornelis.** 2001. *Yersinia enterocolitica* YopP-induced apoptosis of macrophages involves the apoptotic signaling cascade upstream of bid. *J. Biol. Chem.* **276**:19706–19714.

17. **Deng, L., C. Wang, E. Spencer, L. Yang, A. Braun, J. You, C. Slaughter, C. Pickart, and Z. J. Chen.** 2000. Activation of the IkappaB kinase complex by TRAF6 requires a dimeric ubiquitin-conjugating enzyme complex and a unique polyubiquitin chain. *Cell* **103**:351–361.

18. **Fantuzzi, G., and C. A. Dinarello.** 1999. Interleukin-18 and interleukin-1 beta: two cytokine substrates for ICE (caspase-1). *J. Clin. Immunol.* **19**:1–11.

19. **Fontaine, A., J. Arondel, and P. J. Sansonetti.** 1988. Role of Shiga toxin in the pathogenesis of bacillary dysentery, studied by using a Tox-mutant of *Shigella dysenteriae* 1. *Infect. Immun.* **56**:3099–3109.

20. **Guilloteau, L. A., T. S. Wallis, A. V. Gautier, S. MacIntyre, D. J. Platt, and A. J. Lax.** 1996. The *Salmonella* virulence plasmid enhances *Salmonella*-induced lysis of macrophages and influences inflammatory responses. *Infect. Immun.* **64**:3385–3393.

21. **Hatada, E. N., D. Krappmann, and C. Scheidereit.** 2000. NF-kappaB and the innate immune response. *Curr. Opin. Immunol.* **12**:52–58.

22. **Hensel, M., J. E. Shea, C. Gleeson, M. D. Jones, E. Dalton, and D. W. Holden.** 1995. Simultaneous identification of bacterial virulence genes by negative selection. *Science* **269**:400–403.

23. **Hersh, D., D. Monack, M. Smith, N. Ghori, S. Falkow, and A. Zychlinsky.** 1999. The *Salmonella* invasin SipB induces macrophage apoptosis by binding to Caspase-1. *Proc. Natl. Acad. Sci. USA* **96**:2396–2401.

24. **Hilbi, H., J. E. Moss, D. Hersh, Y. Chen, J. Arondel, S. Banerjee, R. A. Flavell, J. Yuan, P. J. Sansonetti, and A. Zychlinsky.** 1998. *Shigella*-induced apoptosis is dependent on caspase-1 which binds to IpaB. *J. Biol. Chem.* **273**:32895–32900.

25. **Hughes, A. K., P. K. Stricklett, D. Schmid, and D. E. Kohan.** 2000. Cytotoxic effect of Shiga toxin-1 on human glomerular epithelial cells. *Kidney Int.* **57**:2350–2359.

26. **Islam, D., B. Veress, P. K. Bardhan, A. A. Lindberg, and B. Christensson.** 1997. In situ characterization of inflammatory responses in the rectal mucosae of patients with shigellosis. *Infect. Immun.* **65**:739–749.

27. Jesenberger, V., K. J. Procyk, J. Yuan, S. Reipert, and M. Baccarini. 2000. *Salmonella*-induced caspase-2 activation in macrophages: a novel mechanism in pathogen-mediated apoptosis. *J. Exp. Med.* **192:**1035–1046.

28. Jones, B. D., and S. Falkow. 1996. Salmonellosis: host immune responses and bacterial virulence determinants. *Annu. Rev. Immunol.* **14:**533–561.

29. Jones, N. L., A. Islur, R. Haq, M. Mascarenhas, M. A. Karmali, M. H. Perdue, B. W. Zanke, and P. M. Sherman. 2000. *Escherichia coli* Shiga toxins induce apoptosis in epithelial cells that is regulated by the Bcl-2 family. *Am. J. Physiol. Gastrointest. Liver Physiol.* **278:**G811–G819.

30. Keenan, K., D. Dharpnack, S. Formal, and A. O'Brien. 1986. Morphologic evaluation of the effects of Shiga toxin and *E. coli* Shiga-like toxin on the rabbit intestine. *Am. J. Pathol.* **125:**69–80.

31. Kerr, J., A. Wyllie, and A. Currie. 1972. Apoptosis: a basic biological phenomenon with wide ranging implications in tissue kinetics. *Br. J. Cancer* **26:**239–257.

32. Kraehenbuhl, J.-P., and M. R. Neutra. 1992. Molecular and cellular basis of immune protection of mucosal surfaces. *Physiol. Rev.* **72:**853–879.

33. Lee, A. K., C. S. Detweiler, and S. Falkow. 2000. OmpR regulates the two-component system SsrA-SsrB in *Salmonella* pathogenicity island 2. *J. Bacteriol.* **182:**771–781.

34. Levine, M. M., H. L. DuPont, S. B. Formal, R. B. Hornick, A. Takeuchi, E. J. Gangarosa, M. J. Snyder, and J. P. Libonati. 1973. Pathogenesis of *Shigella dysenteriae* 1 (Shiga) dysentery. *J. Infect. Dis.* **127:**261–270.

35. Li, P., H. Allen, S. Banerjee, S. Franklin, L. Herzog, C. Johnston, J. McDowell, M. Paskind, L. Rodman, J. Salfeld, E. Towne, D. Tracey, S. Wardwell, F.-Y. Wei, W. Wong, R. Kamen, and T. Seshadri. 1995. Mice deficient in IL-1β-converting enzyme are defective in production of mature IL-1β and resistant to endotoxic shock. *Cell* **80:**401–411.

36. Li, S. J., and M. Hochstrasser. 1999. A new protease required for cell-cycle progression in yeast. *Nature* **398:**246–251.

37. Libby, S. J., M. Lesnick, P. Hasegawa, E. Weidenhammer, and D. G. Guiney. 2000. The *Salmonella* virulence plasmid *spv* genes are required for cytopathology in human monocyte-derived macrophages. *Cell Microbiol.* **2:**49–58.

38. Lindgren, S. W., I. Stojiljkovic, and F. Heffron. 1996. Macrophage killing is an essential

39. Los, M., S. Wesselborg, and K. Schulze-Osthoff. 1999. The role of caspases in development, immunity, and apoptotic signal transduction: lessons from knockout mice. *Immunity* **10:**629–639.

40. Mangeney, M., C. Lingwood, S. Taga, B. Caillou, T. Tursz, and J. Wiels. 1993. Apoptosis induced in Burkitt's lymphoma cells via Gb3/CD77, a glycolipid antigen. *Cancer Res.* **53:**5314–5319.

41. Marcato, P., G. Mulvey, and G. D. Armstrong. 2002. Cloned Shiga toxin 2 B subunit induces apoptosis in Ramos Burkitt's lymphoma B cells. *Infect. Immun.* **70:**1279–1286.

42. Medzhitov, R., P. Preston-Hurlburt, and C. A. Janeway, Jr. 1997. A human homologue of the *Drosophila* Toll protein signals activation of adaptive immunity. *Nature* **388:**394–397.

43. Medzhitov, R., P. Preston-Hurlburt, E. Kopp, A. Stadlen, C. Chen, S. Ghosh, and C. A. Janeway, Jr. 1998. MyD88 is an adaptor protein in the hToll/IL-1 receptor family signaling pathways. *Mol. Cell* **2:**253–258.

44. Meijer, L. K., K. Schesser, H. Wolf-Watz, P. Sassone-Corsi, and S. Pettersson. 2000. The bacterial protein YopJ abrogates multiple signal transduction pathways that converge on the transcription factor CREB. *Cell Microbiol.* **2:**231–238.

45. Mills, S. D., A. Boland, M.-P. Sory, P. van der Smissen, C. Kerbourch, B. B. Finlay, and G. R. Cornelis. 1997. *Yersinia enterocolitica* induces apoptosis in macrophages by a process requiring functional type III secretion and translocation mechanisms and involving YopP, presumably acting as an effector protein. *Proc. Natl. Acad. Sci. USA* **94:**12638–12643.

46. Monack, D. M., C. S. Detweiler, and S. Falkow. 2001. *Salmonella* pathogenicity island 2-dependent macrophage death is mediated in part by the host cysteine protease caspase-1. *Cell Microbiol.* **3:**825–837.

47. Monack, D. M., D. Hersh, N. Ghori, D. Bouley, A. Zychlinsky, and S. Falkow. 2000. *Salmonella* exploits caspase-1 to colonize Peyer's patches in a murine typhoid model. *J. Exp. Med.* **17:**249–258.

48. Monack, D. M., J. Mecsas, D. Bouley, and S. Falkow. 1998. *Yersinia*-induced apoptosis in vivo aids in the establishment of a systemic infection of mice. *J. Exp. Med.* **188:**2127–2137.

49. Monack, D. M., J. Mecsas, N. Ghori, and S. Falkow. 1997. *Yersinia* signals macrophages to undergo apoptosis and YopJ is necessary for this

virulence mechanism of *Salmonella typhimurium*. *Proc. Natl. Acad. Sci. USA* **93:**4197–4201.

cell death. *Proc. Natl. Acad. Sci. USA* **94:**10385–10390.

50. **Monack, D. M., B. Raupach, A. E. Hromockyj, and S. Falkow.** 1996. *Salmonella typhimurium* invasion induces apoptosis in infected macrophages. *Proc. Natl. Acad. Sci. USA* **93:** 9833–9838.

51. **Muller, S., M. Berger, F. Lehembre, J. S. Seeler, Y. Haupt, and A. Dejean.** 2000. c-Jun and p53 activity is modulated by SUMO-1 modification. *J. Biol. Chem.* **275:**13321–13329.

52. **Nakajima, R., and R. R. Brubaker.** 1993. Association between virulence of *Yersinia pestis* and suppression of gamma interferon and tumor necrosis factor alpha. *Infect. Immun.* **61:**23–31.

53. **Neighbors, M., X. Xu, F. J. Barrat, S. R. Ruuls, T. Churakova, R. Debets, J. F. Bazan, R. A. Kastelein, J. S. Abrams, and A. O'Garra.** 2001. A critical role for interleukin 18 in primary and memory effector responses to *Listeria monocytogenes* that extends beyond its effects on interferon gamma production. *J. Exp. Med.* **194:**343–354.

54. **Ninomiya-Tsuji, J., K. Kishimoto, A. Hiyama, J. Inoue, Z. Cao, and K. Matsumoto.** 1999. The kinase TAK1 can activate the NIK-I kappaB as well as the MAP kinase cascade in the IL-1 signalling pathway. *Nature* **398:**252–256.

55. **Orth, K.** 2002. Function of the Yersinia effector YopJ. *Curr. Opin. Microbiol.* **5:**38–43.

56. **Orth, K., L. E. Palmer, Z. Q. Bao, S. Stewart, A. E. Rudolph, J. B. Bliska, and J. E. Dixon.** 1999. Inhibition of the mitogen-activated protein kinase kinase superfamily by a *Yersinia* effector. *Science* **285:**1920–1923.

57. **Orth, K., Z. Xu, M. B. Mudgett, Z. Q. Bao, L. E. Palmer, J. B. Bliska, W. F. Mangel, B. Staskawicz, and J. E. Dixon.** 2000. Disruption of signaling by Yersinia effector YopJ, a ubiquitin-like protein protease. *Science* **290:**1594–1597.

58. **Palmer, L. E., S. Hobbie, J. E. Galan, and J. B. Bliska.** 1998. YopJ of *Yersinia pseudotuberculosis* is required for the inhibition of macrophage TNF-α production and downregulation of the MAP kinases p38 and JNK. *Mol. Microbiol.* **27:**953–965.

59. **Paton, J. C., and A. W. Paton.** 1998. Pathogenesis and diagnosis of Shiga toxin-producing *Escherichia coli* infections. *Clin. Microbiol. Rev.* **11:** 450–479.

60. **Perdomo, O. J., J. M. Cavaillon, M. Huerre, H. Ohayon, P. Gounon, and P. J. Sansonetti.** 1994. Acute inflammation causes epithelial invasion and mucosal destruction in experimental shigellosis. *J. Exp. Med.* **180:**1307–1319.

61. **Phalipon, A., M. Kaufmann, P. Michetti, J. M. Cavaillon, M. Huerre, P. Sansonetti,** **and J. P. Kraehenbuhl.** 1995. Monoclonal immunoglobulin A antibody directed against serotype-specific epitope of *Shigella flexneri* lipopolysaccharide protects against murine experimental shigellosis. *J. Exp. Med.* **182:**769–778.

62. **Pickart, C. M.** 2000. Ubiquitin in chains. *Trends Biochem. Sci.* **25:**544–548.

63. **Richter-Dahlfors, A., A. M. J. Buchan, and B. B. Finlay.** 1997. Murine salmonellosis studied by confocal microscopy: *Salmonella typhimurium* resides intracellularly inside macrophages and exerts a cytotoxic effect on phagocytes in vivo. *J. Exp. Med.* **186:**569–580.

64. **Ruckdeschel, K., S. Harb, A. Roggenkamp, M. Hornef, R. Zumbihl, S. Kohler, J. Heesemann, and B. Rouot.** 1998. *Yersinia enterocolitica* impairs activation of transcription factor NF-κB: involvement in the induction of programmed cell death and in the suppression of the macrophage tumor necrosis factor alpha production. *J. Exp. Med.* **187:**1069–1079.

65. **Ruckdeschel, K., J. Machold, A. Roggenkamp, S. Schubert, J. Pierre, R. Zumbihl, J. P. Liautard, J. Heesemann, and B. Rouot.** 1997. *Yersinia enterocolitica* promotes deactivation of macrophage mitogen-activated protein kinases extracellular signal-regulated kinase-1/2, p38, and c-Jun NH2-terminal kinase. Correlation with its inhibitory effect on tumor necrosis factor-alpha production. *J. Biol. Chem.* **272:**15920–15927.

66. **Ruckdeschel, K., O. Mannel, K. Richter, C. A. Jacobi, K. Trulzsch, B. Rouot, and J. Heesemann.** 2001. *Yersinia* outer protein P of *Yersinia enterocolitica* simultaneously blocks the nuclear factor-kappa B pathway and exploits lipopolysaccharide signaling to trigger apoptosis in macrophages. *J. Immunol.* **166:**1823–1831.

67. **Ruckdeschel, K., A. Roggenkamp, V. Lafont, P. Mangeat, J. Heesemann, and B. Rouot.** 1997. Interaction of *Yersinia enterocolitica* with macrophages leads to macrophage cell death through apoptosis. *Infect. Immun.* **65:**4813–4821.

68. **Sandvig, K.** 2001. Shiga toxins. *Toxicon* **39:** 1629–1635.

69. **Sandvig, K., and B. van Deurs.** 1992. Toxin induced cell lysis: protection by 3-methyladenine and cycloheximide. *Exp. Cell Res.* **200:**253–262.

70. **Sansonetti, P. J., J. Arondel, J. M. Cavaillon, and M. Huerre.** 1995. Role of interleukin-1 in the pathogenesis of experimental shigellosis. *J. Clin. Invest.* **96:**884–892.

71. **Sansonetti, P. J., D. J. Kopecko, and S. B. Formal.** 1982. Involvement of a plasmid in the invasive ability of *Shigella flexneri. Infect. Immun.* **35:**852–860.

72. Sansonetti, P. J., A. Phalipon, J. Arondel, K. Thirumalai, S. Banerjee, S. Akira, K. Takeda, and A. Zychlinsky. 2000. Caspase-1 activation of IL-1b and IL-18 are essential for *Shigella flexneri* induced inflammation. *Immunity* **12:**581–590.

73. Savill, J., and V. Fadok. 2000. Corpse clearance defines the meaning of cell death. *Nature* **407:**784–788.

74. Schesser, K., A. K. Spiik, J. M. Dukuzu-muremyi, M. F. Neurath, S. Pettersson, and H. Wolf-Watz. 1998. The *yopJ* locus is required for *Yersinia*-mediated inhibition of NF-κB activation and cytokine expression: YopJ contains a eukaryotic SH2-like domain that is essential for its repressive activity. *Mol. Microbiol.* **28:**1067–1079.

75. Suzuki, A., H. Doi, F. Matsuzawa, S. Ai-kawa, K. Takiguchi, H. Kawano, M. Haya-shida, and S. Ohno. 2000. Bcl-2 antiapoptotic protein mediates verotoxin II-induced cell death: possible association between bcl-2 and tissue failure by *E. coli* O157:H7. *Genes Dev.* **14:**1734–1740.

76. Swain, S. L. 2001. Interleukin 18: tipping the balance towards a T helper cell 1 response. *J. Exp. Med.* **194:**F11–F14.

77. Thirumalai, K., K. Kim, and A. Zychlinsky. 1997. IpaB, a *Shigella flexneri* invasin, colocalizes with Interleukin-1β converting enzyme (ICE) in the cytoplasm of macrophages. *Infect. Immun.* **65:** 787–793.

78. Thornberry, N. A. 1996. The caspase family of cysteine proteases. *Br. Med. Bull.* **53:**478–490.

79. Thornberry, N. A., H. G. Bull, J. R. Calay-cay, K. T. Chapman, A. D. Howard , M. J. Kostura, D. K. Miller, S. M. Molineaux, J. R. Weidner, J. Aunins, K. O. Elliston, J. M. Ayala, F. J. Casano, J. Chin, J.-F. Ding, L. A. Egger, E. P. Gaffney, G. Limjuco, O. C. Palyha, S. M. Raju, A. M. Rolando, J. P. Salley, T. T. Yamin, T. D. Lee, J. E. Shively, M. MacCross, R. A. Mumford, J. A. Schmidt, and M. J. Tocci. 1992. A novel heterodimeric cysteine protease is required for interleukin-1β processing in monocytes. *Nature* **356:**768–774.

80. van der Velden, A. W., S. W. Lindgren, M. J. Worley, and F. Heffron. 2000. *Salmonella* pathogenicity island 1-independent induction of apoptosis in infected macrophages by *Salmonella enterica* serotype Typhimurium. *Infect. Immun.* **68:**5702–5709.

81. Wang, C., L. Deng, M. Hong, G. R. Ak-karaju, J. Inoue, and Z. J. Chen. 2001. TAK1 is a ubiquitin-dependent kinase of MKK and IKK. *Nature* **412:**346–351.

82. Wassef, J. S., D. F. Keren, and J. L. Mail-loux. 1989. Role of M cells in initial antigen uptake and in ulcer formation in rabbit intestinal loop model of shigellosis. *Infect. Immun.* **57:**858–863.

83. Way, S. S., A. C. Borczuk, R. Dominitz, and M. B. Goldberg. 1998. An essential role for gamma interferon in innate resistance to *Shigella flexneri* infection. *Infect. Immun.* **66:**1342–1348.

84. Yamasaki, C., Y. Natori, X. T. Zeng, M. Ohmura, S. Yamasaki, Y. Takeda, and Y. Natori. 1999. Induction of cytokines in a human colon epithelial cell line by Shiga toxin 1 (Stx1) and Stx2 but not by non-toxic mutant Stx1 which lacks N-glycosidase activity. *FEBS Lett.* **442:**231–234.

85. Yin, L., L. Wu, H. Wesche, C. D. Arthur, J. M. White, D. V. Goeddel, and R. D. Schreiber. 2001. Defective lymphotoxin-beta receptor-induced NF-kappaB transcriptional activity in NIK-deficient mice. *Science* **291:**2162–2165.

86. Zychlinsky, A., C. Fitting, J. M. Cavaillon, and P. J. Sansonetti. 1994. Interleukin-1 is released by murine macrophages during apoptosis induced by *Shigella flexneri*. *J. Clin. Invest.* **94:** 1328–1332.

87. Zychlinsky, A., B. Kenny, R. Ménard, M. C. Prévost, I. B. Holland, and P. J. San-sonetti. 1994. IpaB mediates macrophage apoptosis induced by *Shigella flexneri*. *Mol. Microbiol.* **11:**619–627.

88. Zychlinsky, A., M. C. Prévost, and P. J. Sansonetti. 1992. *Shigella flexneri* induces apoptosis in infected macrophages. *Nature* **358:**167–168.

89. Zychlinsky, A., and P. J. Sansonetti. 1997. Apoptosis as a proinflammatory event or, what we can learn from bacterial induced cell death. *Trends Microbiol.* **5:**201–204.

90. Zychlinsky, A., K. Thirumalai, J. Arondel, J. R. Cantey, A. Aliprantis, and P. J. San-sonetti. 1996. In vivo apoptosis in *Shigella flexneri* infections. *Infect. Immun.* **64:**5357–5365.

TRAFFICKING OF CHOLERA TOXIN AND RELATED BACTERIAL ENTEROTOXINS: PATHWAYS AND ENDPOINTS

Chiara Rodighiero and Wayne I. Lencer

21

Pathogenic enteric bacteria have evolved by natural selection to elaborate molecular devices that take advantage of the human host. Protein toxins represent elegant examples of such agents. Because of their potency, bacterial toxins can kill or severely alter the physiology of mammalian cells. The enteric bacterial toxins discussed in this chapter, cholera toxin (CT) and the related *Escherichia coli* heat-labile and Shiga or Vero toxins, represent some of the most potent pathogenic factors causing diseases that have affected the course of human history and continue to affect current public health policy.

The enterotoxins of the cholera and Shiga families are produced by noninvasive bacteria. To cause disease, these enterotoxins must breech the barrier of the intestinal epithelium as fully folded proteins and perform their activity in the host cell cytosol. As such, the structure of these protein toxins encodes for all determinants that drive entry, trafficking, and intoxication of the host. Studies on the structure and function of cholera and Shiga toxins, in particular, have elucidated critical

aspects of the epithelial cell biology that affect intestinal physiology in both health and disease.

In this chapter, we focus on toxins of the cholera family as a paradigm for the opportunistic invasion of the mammalian intestine by exploitation of eukaryotic mechanisms of membrane trafficking, protein transport, and signal transduction. CT enters epithelial cells of the human intestine after binding specific lipids on the host cell apical membrane. These lipid receptors dictate trafficking of the toxin retrograde through apical endosomes, the Golgi apparatus, and into the endoplasmic reticulum (ER), where the toxin unfolds and has been proposed to dislocate into the cytosol, using the protein-conducting channel sec61. The mechanism of toxin entry is a near mirror image of protein biosynthesis in eukaryotic cells.

CT AND RELATED ENTEROTOXINS

CT represents one of the best-characterized virulence factors produced by pathogenic microorganisms, and its mode of action will be discussed here in detail. We will also discuss heat-labile toxins (LT) produced by enterotoxigenic strains of *E. coli* (ETEC) and Shiga-like toxins produced by enterohemorrhagic strains of *E. coli* (EHEC) and *Shigella dysenter-*

Chiara Rodighiero and Wayne I. Lencer, GI Cell Biology, Children's Hospital/Harvard Medical School, 300 Longwood Avenue, Boston, MA 02115.

Microbial Pathogenesis and the Intestinal Epithelial Cell, ed. by G. Hecht
© 2003 ASM Press, Washington, D.C.

iae. E. coli heat-labile and Shiga toxins exhibit a similar structure and function to CT, and both are pathogenic in humans (see Table 1).

In 1884, Koch identified the etiologic agent responsible for cholera by reporting the isolation from the stool of patients with acute diarrhea of a "comma shaped" bacillus. The bacillus was later designated *Vibrio cholerae*. Koch described the severe cramps and the production of copious quantities of "rice-water" diarrhea that characterized the disease (42, 95), and postulated that a "poison" produced by the microorganism was responsible (33). More than 70 years of research elapsed before CT was isolated and identified (9, 14).

In 1956, De demonstrated that culture filtrates of *V. cholerae* elicited fluid secretion in rabbit intestines and that certain *E. coli* strains caused a similar cholera-like diarrheal illness (10). Finkelstein and LoSpalluto isolated and purified CT from sterile culture filtrates of *V. cholerae* (17, 18). We now know that CT is a multimeric protein actively secreted by *V. cholerae* in response to the gut environment (48) and that CT primarily accounts for the life-threatening watery diarrhea induced by *V. cholerae* infection.

Toxigenic strains of ETEC produce a similar but less potent toxin. In 1969 Gyles and Barnum described an enterotoxin produced by *E. coli* similar to that of CT (28). The factor was named heat-labile toxin (LT) to define its instability upon heating and to distinguish it from heat-stable toxin (ST), also produced by some *E. coli* strains. Unlike CT, LTs exist in a number of isoforms. All LTs produced by *E. coli* and CT produced by *V. cholerae* are structurally and functionally related (95). Labile toxins from *E. coli* that are antigenically similar to CT are classified as type I toxins (35). An LT-type II enterotoxin family consisting of LTIIa and LTIIb has been designated by Holmes and colleagues as antigenically distinct from the LT I toxins (35). LT type II toxins have been isolated from *E. coli* obtained from cattle and humans, but their role in the pathogenesis of clinical disease remains to be established (26, 27, 34).

S. dysenteriae and certain strains of *E. coli* produce Shiga toxin, which can induce a variety of clinical diseases including bloody diarrhea and hemolytic-uremic syndrome (HUS) (69, 90). Certain strains of EHEC also produce a similar toxin, structurally and functionally related to Shiga toxin, termed Shiga-like toxin or Vero toxin.

STRUCTURE OF CT AND *E. COLI* ENTEROTOXINS: HOMOLOGY WITH RELATED AB TOXINS

CT belongs to a family of so-called AB-type toxins (see Table 1 and Fig. 1) in which the B component (or B-subunit) functions in membrane binding required for entry into host cells. The A component (or A-subunit) exhibits enzymatic activity that activates or modulates a specific intracellular target. The AB toxins may be subdivided into groups on the basis of structural homology or catalytic activity. The enterotoxins CT, LTI, LTIIa, LTIIb, and ST are composed of a single A-subunit and five identical "binding" B-subunits. The plant toxin ricin, *Pseudomonas* exotoxin A (PEA), and diphtheria toxin, on the other hand, are examples of AB toxins that are expressed as single-chain polypeptides made up of two distinct A and B domains that function in enzymatic and membrane binding activities, respectively (Fig. 1).

The A-subunits of CT, LTI, and LTII exhibit ADP-ribosyltransferase activity and ribosylate a specific Arg residue on the alpha-subunit of the heterotrimeric GTPase, Gs. ADP-ribosylation irreversibly inhibits the intrinsic GTPase activity of Gs, and this activates adenylyl cyclase (67) (Table 1). The A-subunit of Shiga toxin or Vero toxin exhibits *N*-glycosidase activity that removes a specific adenine residue from a highly conserved loop present in 28S rRNA (Table 1). This function inhibits protein synthesis (15).

CT and LT exhibit high amino acid sequence homology, with more than 80% identity for both A- and B-subunits. The A-subunits of CT and LT (human, type I) con-

TABLE 1 Selection of AB enterotoxins[a]

Toxin (source)	Abbreviation; structure	Receptor	Cleavage site	S-S bound	ER retrieval sequence	Intracellular target	Enzymatic activity	Clinical effects
CT (*V. cholerae*)	CT; heterohexamer, AB$_5$	Ganglioside G$_{M1}$	CT A-subunit 192, 193	CT A-subunit Cys-187, 199	KDEL	Gsα	ADP-ribosyltransferase	Elevated cAMP, severe watery diarrhea
LTI (*E. coli*, ETEC)	LT; heterohexamer, AB$_5$	Ganglioside G$_{M1}$	LT A-subunit 192, 193	LT A-subunit Cys-187, 199	RDEL	Gsα	ADP-ribosyltransferase	Elevated cAMP, watery diarrhea
LTIIa (*E. coli*)	LTIIa; heterohexamer, AB$_5$	Ganglioside G$_{D1b}$	LTIIa A-subunit 192, 193	LTIIa A-subunit Cys-187, 199	RDEL	Gsα	ADP-ribosyltransferase	Elevated cAMP, diarrhea in animals
LTIIb (*E. coli*)	LTIIb; heterohexamer, AB$_5$	Ganglioside G$_{D1a}$	LTIIb A-subunit 192, 193	LTIIb A-subunit Cys-187, 199	KDEL	Gsα	ADP-ribosyltransferase	Elevated cAMP, diarrhea in animals
Shiga toxin (*S. dysenteriae*)	Shiga toxin; heterohexamer, AB$_5$	Globotriaosylceramide G$_{b3}$	Shiga toxin A-subunit 251, 252	Shiga toxin A-subunit Cys-240, 259	Not present	rRNA 28S	N-Glycosidase	Watery diarrhea, dysentery
Shiga-like or Vero toxin (*E. coli*, EHEC)	Shiga toxin; heterohexamer, AB$_5$	Globotriaosylceramide G$_{b3}$	Shiga toxin A-subunit 251, 252	Shiga toxin A-subunit Cys-240, 259	Not present	rRNA 28S	N-Glycosidase	Watery diarrhea, renal disease HUS
RT (*Ricinus communis*)	RT; polypeptide, AB	Any glycolipid and/or glycoprotein with terminal galactose	Cotranslation modifications remove a 12-residue linker	RT A-subunit Cys-259; RT B-subunit Cys-4	Not present	rRNA 28S	N-Glycosidase	Cell death, lethal
PEA (*Pseudomonas*)	PEA, polypeptide A, T, B domains	Low-density lipoprotein receptor LRP	PEA Arg-279	PEA A domain Cys-287; T domain Cys-265	REDLK	Elongation factor 2	ADP-ribosyltransferase	Cell death, lethal

[a] cAMP, cyclic AMP; RT, ricin toxin.

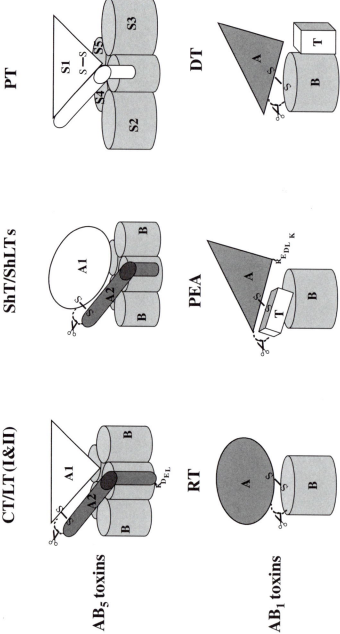

FIGURE 1 Schematic representation of the structural organization of some AB toxins. (Top, from left) CT together with *E. coli* heat-labile enterotoxins type I and II (LT); Shiga toxin (ShT) together with Shiga-like toxins (ShLTs); pertussis toxin (PT). (Bottom, from left) Ricin toxin (RT), PEA, and diphtheria toxin (DT). Identical shapes indicate conserved functional domains, where receptor-binding subunits are cylinders, ADP-ribosyltransferase catalytic subunits are triangles, *N*-glycosidase catalytic subunits are ovals, and translocation domains are cubes. The A domain of C/LT and Shiga and Shiga-like toxins can also be divided into an N-terminal domain (A1) and a C-terminal domain (A2) that anchor domain A1 to the pentameric binding component. The pair of scissors indicates a proteolysis-sensitive loop, and disulfide bonds are also represented (S-S). The ER retention sequence at the C terminus of the A2 fragment of Ctx is KDEL (represented) and RDEL for LT (omitted), while for PEA the signal is REDLK (represented).

tain two distinct structural domains linked by a disulfide bridge at cysteine residues 187 and 199 that defines a loop region where the homology drops to less than 40% (Fig.1). Proteolytic cleavage or "nicking" of the A-subunit in this loop, at Arg 192, gives rise to two fragments, termed A1 and A2, that remain linked via the disulfide bridge (95). The A1 fragment exhibits ADP-ribosyltransferase activity, a property essential for toxicity (6, 24, 61, 79). The A2 fragment comprises 47 residues, amino acids 193 through 240, and tethers the A1 fragment to the pentameric ring of the B-subunit via noncovalent but otherwise stable interactions (81, 92, 93, 111). The C-terminal segment of A2 protrudes through the pore of the doughnut-shaped B pentamer to emerge on the opposite side of the B-subunit cavity, where the last four residues of the CT and LTI A2 fragment are Lys/Arg-Asp-Glu-Leu-COOH (K/RDEL). KDEL defines a protein-sorting motif that functions to localize ER lumenal proteins to the ER. A similar sequence (REDLK) has been found in another AB-type toxin, PEA, that also requires transport to the ER for bioactivity (7) (Table 1). LT type II toxins share high levels of homology in structure and function with A-subunits of CT and LT type I (47). Both LTIIa and LTIIb toxins are organized into A1 and A2 domains and also contain a C-terminal K/RDEL motif.

The B-subunits of CT, LTI, LTII, and Shiga toxins function to bind specific receptors on the host cell membrane. The B-subunits of CT and LT differ minimally in primary amino acid sequence (81) and exhibit almost identical function, with only mild variations in their binding specificities (57) and in pH and thermal stability (25, 83). The B-subunits of LT type II toxins and Shiga-like toxins, however, differ more dramatically in primary structure and function. Nonetheless, they still display a high degree of three-dimensional structural homology with the B-subunits of CT and LT type I toxin (62). As such, LTII and Shiga toxins bind distinct receptors at the cell surface of epithelial cells.

TOXIN SORTING BY STABLE BINDING TO LIPID RECEPTORS AT THE CELL SURFACE OF EUKARYOTIC CELLS

To induce toxicity, CT, *E. coli* LT types I and II, and Shiga and Shiga-like toxins must traffic via a retrograde pathway to the ER from where they translocate into the cytosol (Fig. 2). We have proposed that trafficking into this pathway depends on the biology of the membrane receptor to which the toxin binds at the cell surface, a function of the B-subunit. The evidence for this hypothesis will be discussed below.

Ganglioside G_{M1}: the Functional Receptor for the Toxins of the Cholera Family

Following bacterial expression and release of CT and LT type I into the small intestine of the host, the fully folded holotoxins bind to ganglioside G_{M1} on the apical membrane of intestinal epithelial cells. As described above, the B-subunit dictates specificity for binding. Ganglioside G_{M1} is a glycosphingolipid composed of a ceramide moiety anchored in the outer leaflet of the plasma membrane and a hydrophilic pentasaccharide that extends extracellularly. In the broadest sense, gangliosides include all sialic acid-containing glycosphingolipids. In the specific case of G_{M1}, the sialic acid is indicated by the subscribed capital letter M, which stands for monosialo, and the number 1 refers to the five neutral sugars that form the basic oligosaccharide structure of all gangliosides (110). Mammalian cells ubiquitously express G_{M1}, which may function in regulation of cell growth (29). The binding pocket for G_{M1} was defined by site-directed mutagenesis and by solution of the crystal structure of the B pentamer complexed to the G_{M1} pentasaccharide or galactose alone (38, 63, 68, 94, 100). These studies show that the B pentamer contains five G_{M1}-oligosaccharide binding sites. Although the majority of the oligosaccharide/toxin association occurs through residues contained within a single B monomer, the functional binding pocket

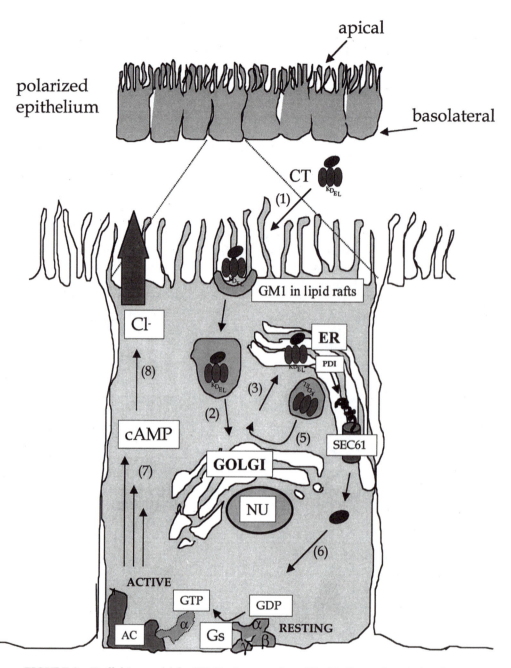

FIGURE 2 Trafficking model for CT. Toxin enters the cell by binding to the apical surface of the polarized epithelium via G_{M1} and association with lipid rafts (1). Toxin moves via endosomes to the Golgi network (2), where the C-terminal KDEL motif facilitates retrograde movement of the CT-G_{M1} complex to the ER (3). Release and translocation of the A-subunit occur in the ER and is a process mediated by PDI (4), while the B-subunit undergoes Golgi/ER recycling prior to degradation (5). Once in the cytosol, the A-subunit is transported to the basolateral membrane where the Gs/adenylate cyclase complex is located (6). ADP-ribosylation of the heterotrimeric GTPase Gsα by the toxin, produces an increase of intracellular cyclic AMP (cAMP) (7) that causes an active secretion of chloride (8).

depends critically on residues from the adjacent B monomer. As a consequence, the B monomer, derived from the disassembled pentamer, can no longer bind to G_{M1}. The orientation of the membrane-associated holotoxin has also been well defined. The position of the A-subunit, relative to the B-subunit bound to its receptor, faces away from the membrane (94).

As the amino acids that contribute to the formation of the G_{M1} binding pockets in CT and LT are conserved, the receptor-binding properties of CT and LTI were thought to be identical. Whereas it is generally accepted that both CT and LT bind to G_{M1} with a very high affinity ($K_d \approx 6 \times 10^{-10}$) (22, 45), it has been proposed that these toxins may also bind to other functional receptors. Indeed, both toxins have been found to bind to the glycosphingolipid G_{D1b} with an affinity approximately 10-fold lower than that of G_{M1} as measured by surface plasmon resonance and solid-phase radioimmunoassay (22, 57). Nonetheless, we have recently found that a loss of only three- to fourfold in binding affinity for G_{M1} is associated with an almost complete loss of toxicity (1, 82). This and another study using a CT mutant that lacked the ability to bind G_{M1} but not G_{D1b}, and was nonfunctional, indicate that G_{D1b} is not likely to serve as a functional trafficking receptor for CT or LTI (106).

Some studies indicate that LT may bind cell surface components that CT cannot bind. This is based on the observation that LT holotoxin induces toxicity in rabbit intestine previously treated with an excess of CT B-subunit. In contrast, pretreatment of rabbit intestines with excess LT B-subunit (type I) completely inhibits CT action (36; T. R. Hirst and W. I. Lencer, personal communication). LT has been found to bind significantly to glycoprotein receptors present in the intestine of several species (36, 37) and with a low affinity to other glycosphingolipids such as asialo-G_{M1} and G_{M2} (22, 57). On the other hand, LTI exhibits a higher apparent binding affinity for G_{M1} when compared with CT as measured by surface plasmon resonance (57). This alone may explain how LT can successfully compete with CT for binding to intestinal receptors and not conversely.

The bioactivity of CT depends on binding to G_{M1} specifically (106, 108). This was ascertained by the use of the LTIIb and LTIIa toxins. CT, LTI, and the LTII toxins share a high degree of homology in A-subunit structure and function. The structures of the B-subunit of these toxins, however, diverge, and the B-subunits of LTIIa and LTIIb bind gangliosides G_{D1b} and G_{D1a}, respectively. LTIIb does not bind G_{M1} at all, and LTIIa binds G_{M1} with low affinity. When tested for toxicity on the polarized human intestinal T84 cell line, both LTIIa and LTIIb bound well to apical membrane receptors but did not induce a functional response. Studies using recombinant chimeras prepared from the A-subunit of CT and the B-subunit of LTIIb and vice versa showed that only toxin chimeras that bound G_{M1} induced toxicity (108). These data indicate specificity for G_{M1} in toxin function. We now hold the view that CT and LTI binding to G_{M1} represents a form of protein acylation that anchors the toxin to the cell membrane and provides the sorting motif for retrograde trafficking into the biosynthetic pathway of host cells. This idea will be developed further below.

Globotriaosylceramide G_{b3}: the Functional Receptor for Shiga and Shiga-Like Toxins

The homopentameric B-subunits of Shiga and Shiga-like toxins also bind to glycolipid receptors on the cell surface of host cells: the glycolipid G_{b3} for Shiga toxin and Shiga-like toxins 1 and 2 (VT1 and VT2); and Gb4 for VT2e (55). The noncovalent interaction has been described to involve as many as 15 receptors per pentameric subunit, with three binding sites per monomer (54).

A Common Feature: Toxin Association with Detergent-Insoluble Membranes

Given that the ceramide domains of G_{M1} and other glycolipids interact directly only with the outer leaflet of the membrane bilayer, how can a lipid-based membrane anchor such as that provided by G_{M1} impart specificity for protein trafficking?

Recent studies indicate that in both the human intestinal T84 and Caco2 cell lines, G_{M1} functions to concentrate CT in detergent-insoluble membrane microdomains (termed "lipid rafts"). This correlates with toxin function (73, 107). Lipid rafts are distinct membrane structures rich in cholesterol, glycolipids, and certain lipid-modified proteins that function in various cell types as membrane-organizing centers for signal transduction, protein and lipid sorting, endocytosis, and transcytosis (described in detail below) (21, 30, 103). Shiga toxin also fractionates with lipid rafts in HeLa cells, but not in monocyte cells, and this correlates with toxin function (80, 96, 102). Similar findings were also obtained with LT type II toxins (106, 108).

Based on these data, we recently hypothesized that toxin-binding glycolipids associate CT, LTI, LTII, and Shiga toxins with lipid rafts and the cellular machinery required for trafficking retrograde into the biosynthetic pathway of host cells. Not all glycolipids in every cell type exhibit this function, and specificity for lipid receptors that use this common trafficking motif has evolved separately for each enterotoxin. Thus, for CT, LTI, and Shiga and Shiga-like toxins, targeting into the retrograde pathway of host cells coopts the machinery for membrane trafficking preprogrammed in the plasma membrane by the structure of the glycolipid receptor itself.

TOXIN ENDOCYTOSIS

CT, LTI, LTII, and Shiga-like toxins enter the host cell by receptor-mediated endocytosis. Non-clathrin-mediated mechanisms are utilized, although Shiga and Shiga-like toxins may enter some cells via clathrin-coated pits. Studies on endocytosis of CT contributed to the characterization of 50- to 80-nm non-coated plasma membrane invaginations, later termed caveolae for "small caves." Caveolae exhibit resistance to solubilization in nonionic

detergents and represent a subset of the membrane microdomains described above as lipid rafts. The biochemistry of caveolae has been greatly facilitated by the characterization of VIP21-caveolin, an integral membrane protein proposed to be part of the "caveolar coat" (74, 76). Caveolae, like lipid rafts, are enriched in glycosphingolipids, sphingomyelin, and cholesterol but lack phospholipids (76). This unique lipid composition confers the biophysical property of insolubility in nonionic detergents at 4°C (thus, the name lipid rafts).

Montesano and coauthors first reported the localization of gold-labeled CT in non-clathrin-coated membrane invaginations of cultured liver cells and proposed the existence of at least two distinct pathways for internalization of surface-bound ligands (65). At present, a total of four pinocytotic pathways in mammalian cells have been described (46). In some cell types, CT and G_{M1} concentrate preferentially in caveolae (75). Human intestinal epithelial cells, however, express low levels of caveolin-1 and -2 and do not exhibit caveolae as assessed morphologically. CT, however, localizes with lipid rafts in this cell type (2).

Despite the evidence that CT and related toxins utilize lipid rafts for entry and sorting into the host cell, CT can also enter cells by clathrin-dependent mechanisms, and the idea that lipid rafts or caveolae, or both, function as distinct structures in endocytosis remains debated in the literature. Evidence supporting this idea includes the discovery that caveolae isolated from lung tissue appear to contain and utilize the same machinery as clathrin-coated pits to pinch off from the plasma membrane and move inside the cell (32, 70, 89). Many questions, however, remain unanswered (44). Mice lacking caveolin-1 and -2, for example, and any structural evidence of caveolae, exhibit an almost normal phenotype, with only subtle defects in cardiopulmonary function (13). Thus, caveolae per se do not appear to be essential for life. On the other hand, caveolin knockout mice exhibit lipid rafts in wild-type concentrations and composition in all cell types examined. Thus, lipid rafts may provide redundant or essential function with respect to caveolae. These data are consistent with our recent observation that lipid rafts that function in trafficking CT in intestinal epithelial cells do not contain caveolin-1 (2).

Sandvig and van Deurs have extensively investigated the intracellular transport of Shiga toxin and reported that this molecule enters the cell in clathrin-coated pits (87). Apparently, the glycolipid G_{b3} becomes fixed in coated pits, possibly interacting with a protein already anchored there (56). Other studies indicate, however, that Shiga toxins may also enter host cells by lipid rafts (16, 43). Ultimately, both the clathrin-dependent and clathrin-independent uptake routes converge in endosomes that can act as a sorting station for subsequent trafficking into the cell.

RETROGRADE TRANSPORT INTO THE GOLGI AND ER

Trafficking of internalized CT and related toxins beyond the early endosome was initially followed by electron microscopy (40, 59, 109). A significant amount of toxin accumulated in the trans-Golgi network at steady state. Initially, these data were interpreted as indicating that the CT A-subunit translocated to the cytosol from the trans-Golgi network. Many lines of evidence now point to the idea that these toxins move first into the Golgi and from there to the ER, where the toxin unfolds and dislocates to the cytosol.

Studies with the fungal metabolite brefeldin A (BFA) provided the first clear evidence that certain bacterial toxins, including CT, LTI, and Shiga toxin, must enter the Golgi apparatus and ER for bioactivity. BFA disrupts membrane traffic in eukaryotic cells such that the Golgi apparatus collapses into the ER (Golgi enzymes rapidly redistribute to the ER after treatment with BFA) and protein transport out of the ER and, in many cell types, retrograde from the plasma membrane into the Golgi are completely blocked. BFA acts by inhibiting the function of the small GTPase ADP-ribosylating factor ARF exchange factor (ARF-GEF), and this blocks the assembly of coat proteins on Golgi membranes necessary for membrane trafficking (8, 11, 97). In all studies, BFA completely and reversibly inhibited CT, LTI, and Shiga toxin action (12, 51, 72, 85, 99). Remarkably, in some cell lines, such as MDCK, BFA does not affect ARF-GEF function and accordingly does not protect against toxin action in this cell type (85).

The existence of the ER-targeting KDEL motif at the C terminus of the A2 peptide in CT, LTI, and LTII provided further evidence that these enterotoxins had to traffic retrograde into the ER for bioactivity (Table 1) (78). The ER retention sequence KDEL was first observed in studies on the ER resident proteins Bip and protein disulfide isomerase (PDI) (77). Pelham and collaborators also noticed that many other luminal ER proteins exhibited a KDEL sequence and discovered that mutants lacking these last four amino acids were no longer retained in the ER but were targeted instead for secretion. The search for the KDEL receptor in yeast produced the identification of two *Saccharomyces cerevisiae* mutants that were unable to retain proteins in the ER. The two mutant proteins were called ERD1 and ERD2, for ER retention defective. It was later established that both mutations were in the *erd2* gene, whose product was an integral membrane protein predicted to have seven transmembrane-spanning domains (98).

Exactly how the ERD2 receptor accomplishes its function of retaining soluble ER proteins in the ER remains to be fully determined. Available data indicate that soluble KDEL proteins that escape the ER bind to the ERD2 receptor resident in the Golgi apparatus that recycles the protein back to the ER. Upon arrival in the ER, the ERD2 receptor releases its cargo and returns to the Golgi apparatus for another cycle of retrieval (53). Ligand binding to ERD2 in vitro appears to require acidic pH (105), and this may account for the vectorial sorting of KDEL proteins backwards to the ER in vivo (87). ERD2 can function in the retrieval of KDEL-containing proteins from the most distal Golgi stack (64).

One of the earliest pieces of evidence that some bacterial toxins may exploit the ERD2 receptor for retrograde transport to the ER came from studies on PEA (7). Deleting the C-terminal REDLK motif on PEA strongly inhibited toxicity, and replacing the C-terminal REDLK sequence with KDEL increased PEA activity.

In later studies, inactivating mutations in the KDEL motif of CT and LTI reduced (but did not ablate) the efficiency by which CT and LT intoxicated human intestinal T84 (49). In CT, the COOH-terminal KDEL sequence was replaced by the unrelated 7-amino-acid sequence LEDERAS, whereas in LT, the COOH-terminal RDEL sequence was altered by a single point mutation, replacing the last leucine (L) with valine (V). In comparison with the wild-type toxins, both CT and LT KDEL mutants elicited a two- to threefold reduced secretory response. This implied a direct and specific interaction of these toxins with endogenous KDEL receptors during signal transduction. Unlike for PEA, however, the KDEL or equivalent RDEL motif was not essential for CT or LT action. These data are consistent with our current view that toxin binding to or clustering G_{M1} represents the dominant sorting motif required for retrograde transport of CT into host cells.

Similar data exist for Shiga toxin. Shiga and Shiga-like toxins do not contain a C-terminal ERD2-binding motif. Nonetheless, electron microscopy studies indicate that horseradish peroxidase conjugates of Shiga toxin move retrograde all the way into the ER and fill the nuclear envelope (84). Incubation of human A431 epithelial cells with butyric acid induced an enhancement of such retrograde transport, which correlated with a marked sensitization of A431 cells to Shiga toxin action. Butyric acid caused a change in the fatty acid structure of the Shiga toxin G_{b3} receptor, suggesting that the ceramide domain of G_{b3} drives retrograde transport (86).

Immunofluorescence and subcellular fractionation experiments with CT provide additional and strong evidence that CT trafficks through the Golgi to the ER (59). In these studies, both the A- and B-subunits of CT were found localized in the Golgi apparatus after an incubation time of about 30 min. However, only the A-subunit was detected in the ER at later time points (3). Fluorescence energy transfer studies by these same investigators provided evidence that CT remains as an AB5 complex during vesicular transport from the plasma membrane to the Golgi complex where the CT A- and B-subunits appeared to separate. The A-subunit was visualized moving into the ER, whereas the B-subunit remained stably localized to the Golgi apparatus.

These data, however, may require reinterpretation in accord with recent findings on the retrograde transport of the pentameric subunits of Shiga toxin and CT (39; Y. Fujinaga, unpublished data). Johannes et al. have investigated the movement of Shiga toxin along the biosynthetic/secretory pathway using recombinant Shiga toxin B-subunits carrying a motif for N-glycosylation. N-Glycosylation occurs only in the ER, and the Shiga toxin B-subunit was glycosylated when applied to Vero cells. This correlated with toxin function. We have obtained similar results with CT (Y. Fujinaga and W. I. Lencer, unpublished studies). The identification of the ER chaperone PDI as the enzyme that unfolds and dissociates the A-subunit from the B-subunit of CT also challenges the idea that the unfolding reaction for CT occurs in the Golgi apparatus (99; described below).

INTRACELLULAR PROCESSING OF CT AND RELATED ENTEROTOXINS: REQUIREMENTS NECESSARY FOR MEMBRANE TRANSLOCATION TO THE CYTOSOL

A single disulfide bond subtends the proteolytic cleavage site on almost all AB toxins (Fig. 1). Like proteolytic cleavage, reduction of this bond also enhances CT, LTI, LTII, and Shiga-like toxin activities in vivo (66). Reduction precedes toxin action in vivo (71). Reduction of the disulfide bond linking the

CT A1- and A2-peptides depends on the enzymatic or chaperone activity of PDI, located primarily in the lumen of the ER (71, 99). PDI acts as a thiol/disulfide isomerase and, depending on the nature of the substrate, will promote disulfide bond formation, isomerization, or reduction to ensure the correct folding of nascent proteins (19, 23). Orlandi first investigated the possible role of PDI in mediating the reduction of the disulfide bond in the A-subunit of CT. These studies showed that a postnuclear supernatant prepared from the human intestinal epithelial cell line Caco-2 was enriched in PDI and reduced CTA in vitro and in vivo. Reduction was dependent on PDI, as evidenced by inhibition with specific anti-PDI neutralizing antibodies (71). Pure PDI was also shown to reduce CTA in vitro (99).

As mentioned above, PDI exists as a soluble protein in the ER, where it is retained by a KDEL C-terminal sequence. PDI, in much lower concentrations, can also be found associated with the plasma membrane of mammalian cells. The cell surface pool of PDI has been shown to facilitate the reduction of diphtheria toxin before it enters the cell by endocytosis. The cell surface pool of PDI, however, does not catalyze reduction of the CT A-subunit. Recently, Tsai et al. identified a factor from crude ER luminal extracts responsible for the reduction and unfolding of CT that was found to be PDI and showed that purified PDI can also act as a chaperone to unfold and dissociate the A1-peptide from the B-pentamer (99; see below). Consistent with these data, the CT A1-peptide and PDI were found to colocalize in the ER of Vero cells, as assessed by confocal microscopy (58).

WHY TRAFFIC TO THE ER: TOXIN UNFOLDING AND TRANSLOCATION TO THE CYTOSOL

During biogenesis, many AB toxins produced by gram-negative bacteria, including CT, LTI, LTII, and Shiga toxins, require translocation across the bacterial inner membrane to fold properly in the bacterial periplasm. Similar to the ER of eukaryotic cells, the pro-karyotic periplasm maintains an oxidizing potential and contains PDIs and other chaperones that assist protein and toxin folding. Thus, CT, LTI, LTII, and Shiga toxins already exhibit the ability to cross biologic membranes (though as nascent peptides) and assemble into stably folded proteins. Entry into the cytosol of host eukaryotic cells requires almost the exact opposite series of events.

In eukaryotic cells, translocation of nascent proteins into the ER occurs via the protein conducting channel Sec61, termed the translocon (60). Recent studies indicate that protein translocation through the translocon and protein folding in the ER are reversible processes. For nascent proteins that do not fold properly during biogenesis, a finely tuned machinery exists to unfold and dislocate aberrant proteins backwards out of the ER through Sec61 to the cytosol, where they are degraded by the proteosome (4). This represents the machinery for protein quality control and has been termed ERAD for ER-associated protein degradation (5). Based on the discovery of this system, and the discovery that certain toxins require trafficking into the ER for bioactivity, several investigators recently proposed the idea that CT, LTI, LTII, and Shiga toxins (among other toxins not discussed in this review) have evolved to exploit ERAD to reach the cytosol of host intestinal epithelial cells (31, 88, 91).

In eukaryotic cells, the Sec61 complex represents the gate for entry of newly synthesized proteins in eukaryotic cells to move from the ribosome/cytosol into the ER and thus the secretory pathway (104). Protein transport into the mammalian ER involves molecular chaperones at various stages. Some act in the cytosol to maintain nascent proteins in a transport-competent state. Others trigger the initial insertion of precursor polypeptides into the Sec61 complex, and another makes transient contact with secretory proteins during later stages of translocation. Inside the ER, the chaperone BiP may make first and critical contact with nascent polypeptides emerging from the pore of Sec61. PDI may also participate in the completion of protein translocation (41) and in catalyzing disulfide bond formation (20). Thus, protein translocation and folding in the ER is an assisted process. This complex system guarantees the delivery of properly folded proteins to their site of action. The ERAD system operates similarly, but in reverse order. Thus, it should be no surprise to find that nature has evolved certain bacterial protein toxins that exploit this very system to invade the cytosol of eukaryotic host cells. Several lines of experimental data are in favor of this hypothesis.

First, it has been shown recently that the CT A-subunit, engineered to carry a eukaryotic signal sequence, will target and translocate into microsomes during in vitro translation (88). Entry into the microsome was assessed by monitoring cleavage of the signal sequence. Remarkably, this form of the CT A-subunit was dislocated back out of the microsome via Sec61, as evidenced by co-immunoprecipitation. These data support the concept, but do not yet prove, that the CT A-subunit may dislocate through Sec61 in vivo. For example, the CT A-subunit used in this study included both the A1- and A2-peptides, which may not fold correctly in the absence of coexpression with the B-subunit. Second, using the A-subunit alone to model the dislocation reaction does not correctly replicate what occurs in vivo, since CT appears to enter the ER as a stably folded holotoxin (99; Fujinaga and Lencer, unpublished data). This represents a major limitation of the experimental approach. Nonetheless, these data provide important evidence in support of the hypothesis.

Tsai et al. recently examined the mechanism for CT unfolding in the ER (99). An in vitro unfolding assay for CT was developed and used in a screen for ER lumenal proteins that catalyzed such activity. PDI was identified and found to unfold and dissociate the A1-peptide from the B-pentamer, but only after the A-subunit was proteolytically nicked. Unlike other chaperones that depend on hydrolysis of ATP, the unfolding of CT by PDI was driven by a redox cycle. PDI appeared to unfold CT variants lacking the single disulfide bond in the A-subunit. These data indicate that the chaperone activity of PDI cannot depend on formation of disulfide adducts between PDI and the CT A-subunit in the unfolding reaction. The results of these studies explain the mechanism and motive force for unfolding CT, localize the reaction to the ER, and explain why CT folds properly in the periplasmic space of *V. cholerae*, but then unfolds in the ER of host cells. As discussed above, the periplasm and ER represent very similar environments organized to assist in protein folding and disulfide bond formation. Here, the single proteolytic nick in the CT A-subunit converts the A-subunit into a substrate for PDI. Nicking of CT occurs after release from *Vibrio* sp. in the lumen of the gastrointestinal tract or when the toxin enters the intestinal epithelial cell. Thus, it seems that proteolytic nicking of the CT A-subunit defines the molecular switch that dictates the vectorial nature of toxin action.

INDIRECT TRANSCYTOSIS ACROSS THE INTESTINAL EPITHELIAL BARRIER

Targeting of these AB5 toxins into the biosynthetic/secretory pathway of host eukaryotic cells positions these toxins for absorption into the systemic circulation by transcytosis across the intestinal cell itself (52). By binding G_{M1}, CT and other bacterial toxins that require entry into the ER for bioactivity have evolved an efficient strategy to exploit an endogenous lipid-based retrograde trafficking pathway from cell surface to Golgi cisternae and ER. The Golgi and ER represent the central organelles in the biosynthetic pathway for intrinsic membrane and secretory proteins, and the Golgi apparatus ultimately feeds nascent proteins to both the apical and basolateral domains of polarized epithelial cells. Sorting to apical and basolateral membrane proteins occurs in the trans-Golgi network. Once CT has arrived inside the Golgi apparatus or ER, the toxin has the opportunity to recycle back to the plasma membrane from an organelle that normally delivers proteins to both sides of the cell. Even a stochastic process of trafficking out of the Golgi would result in redistributing CT to both apical and basolateral membrane domains. The result would be transcytosis. Once across the epithelial barrier, CT would then be in a position to interact with other cells present in the subepithelial space or to redistribute systemically, as may occur for Shiga and Vero toxins that induce disease both locally at the site of infection and systemically, causing hemolytic uremic syndrome.

CONCLUDING REMARKS

To induce disease, CT, LTI, LTII, and Shiga and Shiga-like toxins traverse the entire biosynthetic/secretory pathway of host intestinal epithelial cells in reverse. They do so by exploiting glycolipids in lipid rafts, endogenous mechanisms of lipid and protein traffic, and endogenous mechanisms of protein quality control. The pathway for toxin entry into host cells represents the near mirror image of protein biosynthesis. Thus, nature has finely tuned these protein toxins to infect the host by entering and exploiting the ER, an intracellular compartment that, at first glimpse, would be least accessible to stably folded proteins entering the cell from the plasma membrane.

REFERENCES

1. **Aman, A. T., S. Fraser, E. A. Merritt, C. Rodighiero, M. Kenny, M. Ahn, W. G. Hol, N. A. Williams, W. I. Lencer, and T. R. Hirst.** 2001. A mutant cholera toxin B subunit that binds GM1-ganglioside but lacks immunomodulatory or toxic activity. *Proc. Natl. Acad. Sci. USA* **98:**8536–8541.
2. **Badizadegan, K., B. L. Dickinson, H. E. Wheeler, R. S. Blumberg, R. K. Holmes, and W. I. Lencer.** 2000. Heterogeneity of detergent insoluble membranes from human epithelia containing caveolin-1 and ganglioside G_{M1}. *Am. J. Physiol.* **278:**G895–G904.
3. **Bastiaens, P. I. H., I. V. Majoul, P. J. Verveer, H.-D. Söling, and T. M. Jovin.** 1996. Imaging the intracellular trafficking and state of the AB5 quaternary structure of cholera toxin. *EMBO J.* **15:**4246–4253.
4. **Bonifacino, J. S., and A. M. Weissman.** 1998. Ubiquitin and the control of protein fate in the secretory and endocytic pathways, p. 19–57. *In* J. A. Spudich (ed.), *Annual Review of Cell and Developmental Biology,* vol. 14. Annual Reviews, Palo Alto, Calif.
5. **Brodsky, J. L., and A. A. McCracken.** 1999. ER protein quality control and proteasome-mediated protein degradation. *Semin. Cell Dev. Biol.* **10:**507–513.
6. **Cassel, D., and T. Pfeuffer.** 1978. Mechanism of cholera toxin action: covalent modification of the guanyl nucleotide-binding protein of the adenylate cyclase system. *Proc. Natl. Acad. Sci. USA* **75:**2669–2673.
7. **Chaudry, V. K., Y. Jinno, D. Fitzgerald, and I. Pastan.** 1990. *Pseudomonas* exotoxin contains a specific sequence at the carboxyl terminus that is required for cytotoxicity. *Proc. Natl. Acad. Sci. USA* **87:**308–312.
8. **Chege, N. W., and S. R. Pfeffer.** 1990. Compartmentation of the Golgi complex: brefeldin-A distinguishes trans-Golgi cisternae from the trans-Golgi network. *J. Cell Biol.* **111:**893–899.
9. **De, S. N.** 1959. Enterotoxicity of bacterial-free culture-filtrate of *Vibrio cholerae. Nature* **183:**1533–1534.
10. **De, S. N., K. Bhattacharva, and J. K. Sarkar.** 1956. A study on the pathogenicity of strains of *Bacterium coli* from acute and chronic enteritis. *J. Pathol. Bacteriol.* **71:**201–209.
11. **Donaldson, J. G., J. Lippincott-Schwartz, and R. D. Klausner.** 1991. Guanine nucleotides modulate the effects of brefeldin A in semipermeable cells: regulation of the association of a 110-kD peripheral membrane protein with the Golgi apparatus. *J. Cell Biol.* **112:**579–588.
12. **Donta, S. T., S. Beristain, and T. K. Tomicic.** 1993. Inhibition of heat-labile cholera and *Escherichia coli* enterotoxins by brefeldin A. *Infect. Immun.* **61:**3282–3286.
13. **Drab, M., P. Verkade, M. Elger, M. Kasper, M. Lohn, B. Lauterbach, J. Menne, C. Lindschau, F. Mende, F. C. Luft, A. Schedl, H. Haller, and T. V. Kurzchalia.** 2001. Loss of caveolae, vascular dysfunction, and pulmonary defects in caveolin-1 gene-disrupted mice. *Science* **293:**2449–2452.
14. **Dutta, N. K., M. V. Panse, and D. R. Kulkami.** 1959. Role of cholera toxin in experimental cholera. *J. Bacteriol.* **78:**594–595.
15. **Endo, Y., K. Mitsui, M. Motizuki, and K. Tsurugi.** 1987. The mechanism of action of ricin and related toxic lectins on eukaryotic ribosomes. The site and the characteristics of the modification in 28S ribosomal RNA caused by the toxins. *J. Biol. Chem.* **262:**5908–5912.
16. **Falguieres, T., F. Mallard, C. Baron, D. Hanau, C. Lingwood, B. Goud, J. Salamero,**

and L. Johannes. 2001. Targeting of Shiga toxin b-subunit to retrograde transport route in association with detergent-resistant membranes. *Mol. Biol. Cell* **12**:2453–2468.

17. **Finkelstein, R. A., and J. J. LoSpalluto.** 1969. Pathogenesis of experimental cholera: preparation of choleragen and choleragenoid. *J. Exp. Med.* **130**:185–202.

18. **Finkelstein, R. A., H. T. Norris, and N. K. Dutta.** 1964. Pathogenesis of bacterial cholera in infant rabbits. *J. Infect. Dis.* **114**:203–216.

19. **Freedman, R. B.** 1989. Protein disulfide isomerase: multiple roles in the modification of nascent secretory proteins. *Cell* **57**:1069–1072.

20. **Freedman, R. B., T. R. Hirst, and M. F. Tuite.** 1994. Protein disulphide isomerase: building bridges in protein folding. *Trends Biochem. Sci.* **19**:331–336.

21. **Friedrichson, T., and T. V. Kurzchalia.** 1998. Microdomains of GPI-anchored proteins in living cells revealed by crosslinking. *Nature* **394**: 802–805.

22. **Fukuta, S., J. L. Magnani, E. M. Twiddy, R. K. Holmes, and V. Ginsburg.** 1988. Comparison of the carbohydrate-binding specificities of cholera toxin and *Escherichia coli* heat-labile enterotoxins LTh-I, LT-IIa, and LT-IIb. *Infect. Immun.* **56**:1748–1753.

23. **Gething, M. J., and J. Sambrook.** 1992. Protein folding in the cell. *Nature* **355**:33–45.

24. **Gill, D. M., and R. Meren.** 1978. ADP-ribosylation of membrane proteins catalyzed by cholera toxin: basis of the activation of adenylate cyclase. *Proc. Natl. Acad. Sci. USA* **75**:3050–3054.

25. **Goins, B., and E. Freire.** 1988. Thermal stability and intersubunit interactions of cholera toxin in solution and in association with its cell-surface receptor ganglioside G_{M1}. *Biochemistry* **27**: 2046–2052.

26. **Green, B. A., R. J. Neill, W. T. Ruyechan, and R. K. Holmes.** 1983. Evidence that a new enterotoxin of *Escherichia coli* which activates adenylate cyclase in eucaryotic target cells is not plasmid mediated. *Infect. Immun.* **41**:383–390.

27. **Guth, B. E. C., E. M. Twiddy, L. R. Trabulsi, and R. K. Holmes.** 1986. Variation in chemical properties and antigenic determinants among type II heat-labile enterotoxins of *Escherichia coli*. *Infect. Immun.* **54**:529–536.

28. **Gyles, C. L., and D. A. Barnum.** 1969. A heat-labile enterotoxin form *Escherichia coli* enteropathogenic for pigs. *J. Infect. Dis.* **120**:419–426.

29. **Hakomori, S., and Y. Igarashi.** 1993. Gangliosides and glycosphingolipids as modulators of cell growth, adhesion, and transmembrane signaling. *Adv. Lipid Res.* **25**:147–162.

30. **Harder, T., P. Scheiffele, and K. Simons.** 1998. Lipid domain structure of the plasma membrane revealed by patching of membrane components. *J. Cell Biol.* **141**:929–942.

31. **Hazes, B., and R. J. Read.** 1997. Accumulating evidence suggests that several AB-toxins subvert the endoplasmic reticulum-associated protein degradation pathway to enter target cells. *Biochemistry* **36**:11051–11054.

32. **Henley, J. R., E. W. A. Krueger, B. J. Oswald, and M. A. McNiven.** 1998. Dynamin-mediated internalization of caveolae. *J. Cell Biol.* **141**:85–99.

33. **Hirst, T. R.** 1995. Biogenesis of cholera and related oligomeric enterotoxins, p. 123–184. *In* J. Moss, M. Vaughan, B. Iglewski, and A. T. Tu (ed.), *Bacterial Toxins and Virulence Factors in Disease*, vol. 8. Marcel Dekker, Inc., New York, N.Y.

34. **Holmes, R. K.** 1997. Heat-labile enterotoxins (*Escherichia coli*), p. 30–33. *In* R. Rappuoli and C. Montecucco (ed.), *Guidebook to Protein Toxins and Their Use in Cell Biology*. Oxford University Press, Oxford, United Kingdom.

35. **Holmes, R. K., and E. M. Twiddy.** 1983. Characterization of monoclonal antibodies that react with unique and cross-reacting determinants of cholera enterotoxin and its subunits. *Infect. Immun.* **42**:914–923.

36. **Holmgren, J., P. Fredman, M. Lindblad, A. M. Svennerholm, and L. Svennerholm.** 1982. Rabbit intestinal glycoprotein receptor for *Escherichia coli* heat-labile enterotoxin lacking affinity for cholera toxin. *Infect. Immun.* **38**:424–433.

37. **Holmgren, J., M. Lindblad, P. Fredman, L. Svennerholm, and H. Myrvold.** 1985. Comparison of receptors for cholera toxin and *Escherichia coli* enterotoxins in human intestine. *Gastroenterology* **89**:27–35.

38. **Jobling, M. G., and R. K. Holmes.** 1991. Analysis of structure and function of the B subunit of cholera toxin by the use of site-directed mutagenesis. *Mol. Microbiol.* **5**:1755–1767.

39. **Johannes, L., D. Tenza, C. Antony, and B. Goud.** 1997. Retrograde transport of KDEL-bearing B-fragment of Shiga toxin. *J. Biol. Chem.* **272**:19554–19561.

40. **Joseph, K. C., A. Stieber, and N. K. Gonatas.** 1979. Endocytosis of cholera toxin in GERL-like structures of murine neuroblastoma cells pretreated with GM1 ganglioside. *J. Cell Biol.* **81**:543–554.

41. **Klappa, P., T. Stromer, R. Zimmermann, L. W. Ruddock, and R. B. Freedman.** 1998. A pancreas-specific glycosylated protein disulphide-isomerase binds to misfolded proteins

and peptides with an interaction inhibited by oestrogens. *Eur. J. Biochem.* **254:**63–69.

42. **Koch, R.** 1884. An address on cholera and its bacillus. *Br. Med. J.* **2:**403–407.

43. **Kovbasnjuk, O., M. Edidin, and M. Donowitz.** 2001. Role of lipid rafts in Shiga toxin 1 interaction with the apical surface of Caco-2 cells. *J. Cell Sci.* **114:**4025–4031.

44. **Kurzchalia, T. V., and R. G. Parton.** 1996. And still they are moving.... dynamic properties of caveolae. *FEBS Lett.* **389:**52–54.

45. **Kuziemko, G. M., M. Stroh, and R. C. Stevens.** 1996. Cholera toxin binding affinity and specificity for gangliosides determined by surface plasmon resonance. *Biochemistry* **35:**6375–6384.

46. **Lamaze, C., and S. L. Schmid.** 1995. The emergence of clathrin-independent pinocytotic pathways. *Curr. Opin. Cell Biol.* **7:**573–580.

47. **Lee, C.-M., P. P. Chang, S.-C. Tsai, R. Adamik, S. R. Price, B. C. Kunz, J. Moss, E. M. Twiddy, and R. K. Holmes.** 1991. Activation of *Escherichia coli* heat-labile enterotoxins by native and recombinant adenosine diphosphate-ribosylation factors, 20-kD guanine nucleotide-binding proteins. *J. Clin. Invest.* **87:**1780–1786.

48. **Lee, S. H., D. L. Hava, M. K. Waldor, and A. Camilli.** 1999. Regulation and temporal expression patterns of *Vibrio cholerae* virulence genes during infection. *Cell* **99:**625–634.

49. **Lencer, W. I., C. Constable, S. Moe, M. Jobling, H. M. Webb, S. Ruston, J. L. Madara, T. Hirst, and R. Holmes.** 1995. Targeting of cholera toxin and *E. coli* heat labile toxin in polarized epithelia: role of C-terminal KDEL. *J. Cell Biol.* **131:**951–962.

50. **Lencer, W. I., C. Constable, S. Moe, P. A. Rufo, A. Wolf, M. G. Jobling, S. P. Ruston, J. L. Madara, R. K. Holmes, and T. R. Hirst.** 1997. Proteolytic activation of cholera toxin and *Escherichia coli* labile toxin by entry into host epithelial cells: signal transduction by a protease-resistant toxin variant. *J. Biol. Chem.* **272:**15562–15568.

51. **Lencer, W. I., J. B. de Almeida, S. Moe, J. L. Stow, D. A. Ausiello, and J. L. Madara.** 1993. Entry of cholera toxin into polarized human intestinal epithelial cells: identification of an early brefeldin A sensitive event required for A1-peptide generation. *J. Clin. Invest.* **92:**2941–2951.

52. **Lencer, W. I., S. Moe, P. A. Rufo, and J. L. Madara.** 1995. Transcytosis of cholera toxin subunits across model human intestinal epithelia. *Proc. Natl. Acad. Sci. USA* **92:**10094–10098.

53. **Lewis, M. J., and H. R. B. Pelham.** 1992. Ligand-induced redistribution of a human KDEL receptor from the Golgi complex to the endoplasmic reticulum. *Cell* **68:**353–364.

54. **Ling, H., A. Boodhoo, B. Hazes, M. D. Cummings, G. D. Armstrong, J. L. Brunton, and R. J. Read.** 1998. Structure of the Shiga-like toxin I B-pentamer complexed with an analogue of its receptor Gb₃. *Biochemistry* **37:**1777–1788.

55. **Lingwood, C. A.** 1993. Verotoxins and their glycolipid receptors. *Adv. Lipid Res.* **25:**189–211.

56. **Lord, J. M., and L. M. Roberts.** 1998. Toxin entry: retrograde transport through the secretory pathway. *J. Cell Biol.* **140:**733–736.

57. **MacKenzie, C. R., T. Hirama, K. K. Lee, E. Altman, and N. M. Young.** 1997. Quantitative analysis of bacterial toxin affinity and specificity for glycolipid receptors by surface plasmon resonance. *J. Biol. Chem.* **272:**5533–5538.

58. **Majoul, I., D. Ferrari, and H. D. Soling.** 1997. Reduction of protein disulfide bonds in an oxidizing environment. The disulfide bridge of cholera toxin A-subunit is reduced in the endoplasmic reticulum. *FEBS Lett.* **401:**104–108.

59. **Majoul, I. V., P. I. H. Bastiaens, and H.-D. Söling.** 1996. Transport of an external Lys-Asp-Glu-Leu (KDEL) protein from the plasma membrane to the endoplasmic reticulum: studies with cholera toxin in Vero cells. *J. Cell Biol.* **133:**777–789.

60. **Matlack, K. E., W. Mothes, and T. A. Rapoport.** 1998. Protein translocation: tunnel vision. *Cell* **92:**381–390.

61. **Mekalanos, J. J., R. J. Collier, and W. R. Romig.** 1979. Enzymic activity of cholera toxin. II. Relationships to proteolytic processing, disulfide bond reduction, and subunit composition. *J. Biol. Chem.* **254:**5855–5861.

62. **Merritt, E. A., and W. G. J. Hol.** 1995. AB₅ toxins. *Curr. Opin. Struct. Biol.* **5:**165–171.

63. **Merritt, E. A., S. Sarfaty, M. G. Jobling, T. Chang, R. K. Holmes, T. R. Hirst, and W. G. Hol.** 1997. Structural studies of receptor binding by cholera toxin mutants. *Protein Sci.* **6:**1516–1528.

64. **Miesenbock, G., and J. E. Rothman.** 1995. The capacity to retrieve escaped ER proteins extends to the *trans*-most cisterna of the Golgi stack. *J. Cell Biol.* **129:**309–319.

65. **Montesano, R., J. Roth, A. Robert, and L. Orci.** 1982. Non-coated membrane invaginations are involved in binding and internalization of cholera and tetanus toxins. *Nature* **296:**651–653.

66. **Moss, J., and M. Vaughan.** 1988. ADP-ribosylation of guanyl nucleotide-binding regulatory proteins by bacterial toxins. *Adv. Enzymol. Relat. Areas Mol. Biol.* **61:**303–379.

67. **Moss, J., and M. Vaughan.** 1977. Mechanism of action of choleragen: evidence for ADP-ribosyltransferase activity with arginine as an acceptor. *J. Biol. Chem.* **252**:2455–2457.

68. **Nashar, T. O., H. M. Webb, S. Eaglestone, N. A. Williams, and T. R. Hirst.** 1996. Potent immunogenicity of the B subunits of *Escherichia coli* heat-labile enterotoxin: receptor binding is essential and induces differential modulation of lymphocyte subsets. *Proc. Nat. Acad. Sci. USA* **93**: 226–230.

69. **O'Brien, A. D., V. L. Tesh, A. Donohue-Rolfe, M. P. Jackson, S. Olsnes, K. Sandvig, A. A. Lindberg, and G. T. Keusch.** 1992. Shiga toxin: biochemistry, genetics, mode of action, and role in pathogenesis. *Curr. Top. Microbiol. Immunol.* **180**:65–94.

70. **Oh, P., D. P. McIntosh, and J. E. Schnitzer.** 1998. Dynamin at the neck of caveolae mediates their budding to form transport vesicles by GTP-driven fission from the plasma membrane of endothelium. *J. Cell Biol.* **141**:101–114.

71. **Orlandi, P. A.** 1997. Protein-disulfide isomerase-mediated reduction of the A subunit of cholera toxin in a human intestinal cell line. *J. Biol. Chem.* **272**:4591–4599.

72. **Orlandi, P. A., P. K. Curran, and P. H. Fishman.** 1993. Brefeldin A blocks the response of cultured cells to cholera toxin: implications for intracellular trafficking in toxin action. *J. Biol. Chem.* **268**:12010–12016.

73. **Orlandi, P. A., and P. H. Fishman.** 1998. Filipin-dependent inhibition of cholera toxin: evidence for toxin internalization and activation through caveolae-like domains. *J. Cell Biol.* **141**: 905–915.

74. **Parton, R. G.** 1996. Caveolae and caveolins. *Cur. Opin. Cell Biol.* **8**:542–548.

75. **Parton, R. G.** 1994. Ultrastructural localization of gangliosides; GM1 is concentrated in caveolae. *J. Histo. Chem. Cytochem.* **42**:155–166.

76. **Parton, R. G., and K. Simons.** 1995. Digging into caveolae. *Science* **269**:1398–1399.

77. **Pelham, H. R. B.** 1990. The retention signal for soluble proteins of the endoplasmic reticulum. *Trends Biochem. Sci.* **15**:483–486.

78. **Pelham, H. R. B., L. M. Roberts, and M. Lord.** 1992. Toxin entry: how reversible is the secretory pathway. *Trends Cell Biol.* **2**:183–185.

79. **Pizza, M., M. Domenighini, W. Hol, V. Giannelli, M. R. Fontana, M. M. Giuliani, C. Magagnoli, S. Peppoloni, R. Manetti, and R. Rappuoli.** 1994. Probing the structure-activity relationship of *Escherichia coli* LT-A by site-directed mutagenesis. *Mol. Microbiol.* **14**:51–60.

80. **Ramegowda, B., and V. L. Tesh.** 1996. Differentiation-associated toxin receptor modulation, cytokine production, and sensitivity to Shiga-like toxins in human monocytes and monocytic cell lines. *Infect. Immun.* **64**:1173–1180.

81. **Rodighiero, C., A. T. Aman, M. J. Kenny, J. Moss, W. I. Lencer, and T. R. Hirst.** 1999. Structural basis for the differential toxicity of cholera toxin and *Escherichia coli* heat-labile enterotoxin. Construction of hybrid toxins identifies the A2-domain as the determinant of differential toxicity. *J. Biol. Chem.* **274**:3962–3969.

82. **Rodighiero, C., Y. Fujinaga, T. R. Hirst, and W. I. Lencer.** 2001. A cholera toxin B-subunit variant that binds ganglioside G(M1) but fails to induce toxicity. *J. Biol. Chem.* **276**:36939–36945.

83. **Ruddock, L. W., S. P. Ruston, S. M. Kelly, N. C. Price, R. B. Freedman, and T. R. Hirst.** 1995. Kinetics of acid-mediated disassembly of the B subunit pentamer of *Escherichia coli* heat-labile enterotoxin. Molecular basis of pH stability. *J. Biol. Chem.* **270**:29953–29958.

84. **Sandvig, K., Ø. Garred, K. Prydz, J. V. Kozlov, S. H. Hansen, and B. van Deurs.** 1992. Retrograde transport of endocytosed Shiga toxin to the endoplasmic reticulum. *Nature* (London) **358**:510–511.

85. **Sandvig, K., K. Prydz, S. H. Hansen, and B. van Deurs.** 1991. Ricin transport in brefeldin A-treated cells: correlation between Golgi structure and toxic effect. *J. Cell Biol.* **115**:971–981.

86. **Sandvig, K., M. Ryd, Ø. Garred, E. Schweda, P. K. Holm, and B. van Deurs.** 1994. Retrograde transport from the Golgi complex to the ER of both Shiga toxin and the nontoxic Shiga B-fragment is regulated by buteric acid and cAMP. *J. Cell Biol.* **126**:53–64.

87. **Sandvig, K., and B. van Deurs.** 1996. Endocytosis, intracellular transport, and cytotoxic action of Shiga toxin and ricin. *Physiol. Rev.* **76**: 949–966.

88. **Schmitz, A., H. Herrgen, A. Winkeler, and V. Herzog.** 2000. Cholera toxin is exported from microsomes by the sec61p complex. *J. Cell Biol.* **148**:1203–1212.

89. **Schnitzer, J. E., D. P. McIntosh, A. M. Dvorak, J. Liu, and P. Oh.** 1995. Separation of caveolae from associated microdomains of GPI-anchored proteins. *Science* **269**:1435–1439.

90. **Sears, C. L., and J. B. Kaper.** 1996. Enteric bacterial toxins: mechanisms of action and linkage to intestinal secretion. *Microbiol. Rev.* **60**:167–215.

91. **Simpson, J. C., L. M. Roberts, K. Romisch, J. Davey, D. H. Wolf, and J. M. Lord.**

1999. Ricin A chain utilises the endoplasmic reticulum-associated protein degradation pathway to enter the cytosol of yeast. *FEBS Lett.* **459:**80–84.

92. **Sixma, T. K., K. H. Kalk, B. A. van Zanten, Z. Dauter, J. Kingma, B. Witholt, and W. G. Hol.** 1993. Refined structure of *Escherichia coli* heat-labile enterotoxin, a close relative of cholera toxin. *J. Mol. Biol.* **230:**890–918.

93. **Sixma, T. K., S. E. Pronk, H. H. Kalk, E. S. Wartna, B. A. M. van Zanten, B. Witholt, and W. G. J. Hol.** 1991. Crystal structure of a cholera toxin-related heat-labile enterotoxin from *E. coli. Nature* **351:**371–377.

94. **Sixma, T. K., S. E. Pronk, K. H. Kalk, B. A. M. van Zanten, A. M. Berghuis, and W. G. J. Hol.** 1992. Lactose binding to heat-labile enterotoxin revealed by X-ray crystallography. *Nature* **355:**561–564.

95. **Spangler, B. D.** 1992. Structure and function of cholera toxin and the related *Escherichia coli* heat-labile enterotoxin. *Microb. Rev.* **56:**622–647.

96. **Tesh, V. L., B. Ramegowda, and J. E. Samuel.** 1994. Purified Shiga-like toxins induce expression of proinflammatory cytokines from murine peritoneal macrophages. *Infect. Immun.* **62:**5085–5094.

97. **Togawa, A., N. Morinaga, M. Ogasawara, J. Moss, and M. Vaughan.** 1999. Purification and cloning of a brefeldin A-inhibited guanine nucleotide-exchange protein for ADP-ribosylation factors. *J. Biol. Chem.* **274:**12308–12315.

98. **Townsley, F. M., D. W. Wilson, and H. R. Pelham.** 1993. Mutational analysis of the human KDEL receptor: distinct structural requirements for Golgi retention, ligand binding and retrograde transport. *EMBO J.* **12:**2821–2829.

99. **Tsai, B., C. Rodighiero, W. I. Lencer, and T. Rapoport.** 2001. Protein disulfide isomerase acts as a redox-dependent chaperone to unfold cholera toxin. *Cell* **104:**937–948.

100. **Tsuji, T., T. Honda, T. Miwatani, S. Wakabayashi, and H. Matsubara.** 1985. Analysis of receptor-binding site in *Escherichia coli* enterotoxin. *J. Biol. Chem.* **260:**8552–8558.

101. **Tsuji, T., M. Kato, H. Kawase, S. Imamura, H. Kamiya, Y. Ichinose, and A. Miyama.** 1997. *Escherichia coli* LT enterotoxin subunit A demonstrates partial toxicity independent of the nicking around Arg192. *Microbiology* **143:**1797–1804.

102. **van Setten, P. A., L. A. Monnens, R. G. Verstraten, L. P. van den Heuvel, and V. W. van Hinsbergh.** 1996. Effects of verocytotoxin-1 on nonadherent human monocytes: binding characteristics, protein synthesis, and induction of cytokine release. *Blood* **88:**174–183.

103. **Varma, R., and S. Mayor.** 1998. GPI-anchored proteins are organized in submicron domains at the cell surface. *Nature* **394:**798–801.

104. **Wilkinson, B. M., J. R. Tyson, P. J. Reid, and C. J. Stirling.** 2000. Distinct domains within yeast Sec61p involved in post-translational translocation and protein dislocation. *J. Biol. Chem.* **275:**521–529.

105. **Wilson, D. W., M. J. Lewis, and H. R. Pelham.** 1993. pH-dependent binding of KDEL to its receptor in vitro. *J. Biol. Chem.* **268:**7465–7468.

106. **Wimer-Mackin, S., R. K. Holmes, A. A. Wolf, W. I. Lencer, and M. G. Jobling.** 2001. Characterization of receptor-mediated signal transduction by *Escherichia coli* Type IIa heat-labile enterotoxin in the polarized human intestinal cell line T84. *Infect. Immun.* **69:**7205–7212.

107. **Wolf, A. A., Y. A. Fujinaga, and W. I. Lencer.** 2002. Uncoupling of the cholera toxin GM1 ganglioside-receptor complex from endocytosis, retrograde Golgi trafficking, and downstream signal transduction by depletion of membrane cholesterol. *J. Biol. Chem.* **277:**16249–16256.

108. **Wolf, A. A., M. G. Jobling, S. Wimer-Mackin, J. L. Madara, R. K. Holmes, and W. I. Lencer.** 1998. Ganglioside structure dictates signal transduction by cholera toxin in polarized epithelia and association with caveolae-like membrane domains. *J. Cell Biol.* **141:**917–927.

109. **Xuan-Cai, S. W., J. Q. Trojanowski, and J. O. Gonatas.** 1982. Cholera toxin and wheat germ agglutinin conjugates as neuroanatomical probes: their uptake and clearance, transganglionic and retrograde transport and sensitivity. *Brain Res.* **243:**215–224.

110. **Zeller, C. B., and R. B. Marchase.** 1992. Gangliosides as modulators of cell function. *Am. J. Physiol.* **262:**C1341–C1355.

111. **Zhang, R.-G., M. L. Westbrook, E. M. Westbrook, D. L. Scott, Z. Otwinowski, P. R. Maulik, R. A. Reed, and G. G. Shipley.** 1995. The 2.4 Å crystal structure of cholera toxin B subunit pentamer: choleragenoid. *J. Mol. Biol.* **251:**550–562.

TYPE III SECRETION SYSTEMS OF ENTERIC BACTERIAL PATHOGENS

Catherine A. Lee

22

Enteropathogenic *Escherichia coli* (EPEC), enterohemorrhagic *E. coli* (EHEC), *Salmonella enterica* serovars, and *Shigella* species are enteric bacterial pathogens that cause diarrhea, gastroenteritis, and/or dysentery. These gram-negative pathogens disrupt the normal physiology of the intestinal mucosa by inducing cytoskeletal rearrangements, proinflammatory responses, and/or cell death. Many of these cellular events are caused by bacterial effector proteins, which are delivered into intestinal cells and directly modulate the activities of host cell proteins (see chapters 20, 23, 24, and 25). The effector proteins are secreted and translocated into host cells via bacterial type III secretion systems (TTSSs).

Genetic and biochemical studies indicate that at least a dozen different proteins assemble to form a TTS apparatus, called a secreton, which mediates the secretion and translocation of effector proteins by making a direct connection between the bacteria and host cell. The Esc and Sep proteins that make up the EPEC and EHEC secretons are virtually identical. Phylogenetic studies indicate that EPEC

and EHEC strains evolved from common ancestors that acquired a bacteriophage containing the *esc/sep* TTS genes (26). The Esc/Sep secreton translocates Tir and Esp proteins into epithelial cells that allow EPEC and EHEC to form attaching and effacing lesions in the intestine (see chapter 23). *S. enterica* serovars have at least two different TTSSs. One TTSS is encoded on a genetic element called *Salmonella* pathogenicity island 1 (SPI1); another TTSS is encoded on SPI2. The SPI1 secreton is made up of Inv, Org, Prg, and Spa proteins. A large variety of effector proteins are translocated via the SPI1 TTSS into intestinal epithelial cells and macrophages. The SPI1 TTSS allows *S. enterica* serovars to infect the distal ileum, kill macrophages, and induce transepithelial neutrophil migration (see chapters 20 and 24). *Shigella flexneri* can secrete 25 different proteins via its secreton, which is made up of Mxi and Spa proteins (11). The Mxi/Spa secreton allows *Shigella* to enter and kill cells in the intestinal mucosa (see chapters 20 and 25). Phylogenetic studies indicate that all TTSSs were derived from a single ancestor. Such studies also suggest that the EPEC/EHEC secreton is distantly related to the *S. enterica* SPI2 secreton, while the *Shigella* Mxi/Spa and *Salmonella* SPI1 secretons diverged from a common derivative more recently (69).

Catherine A. Lee, Department of Microbiology and Molecular Genetics, Harvard Medical School, Boston, MA 02115.

Microbial Pathogenesis and the Intestinal Epithelial Cell, ed. by G. Hecht
© 2003 ASM Press, Washington, D.C.

This chapter covers what is known about how the EPEC/EHEC Esc/Sep, *S. enterica* serovar Typhimurium SPI1, and *S. flexneri* Mxi/Spa TTSSs secrete and translocate proteins into mammalian cells. Since studies of other TTSSs have guided our thinking about how the enteric TTSSs work, information about TTSSs in plant pathogens, the Ysc TTSS of *Yersinia* species, and the flagellar TTSS of *S. enterica* serovar Typhimurium is also discussed. Effectors delivered by the Ysc TTSS block the antimicrobial activities of macrophages, allowing *Yersinia* species to survive and grow in lymphoid tissues. Flagella are required for bacterial motility and induce inflammatory responses in intestinal epithelial cells (see chapter 9). Flagella are considered to represent a third TTSS in *S. enterica* serovar Typhimurium because at least seven components of the flagellar basal body (FBB) are homologous to a subset of components that make up the pathogenic TTSSs (Table 1). Components of the FBB mediate the secretion of flagellar subunits across the bacterial inner membrane. The mechanism by which TTSSs transport effector proteins across the bacterial inner membrane may have evolved from ancestral flagellar genes.

STRUCTURE AND FUNCTION OF TYPE III SECRETONS

The Esc/Sep, SPI1, and Mxi/Spa secretons of EPEC, *S. enterica* serovar Typhimurium, and *S. flexneri* have been visualized in bacterial cells by electron microscopy. These secreton complexes can also be extracted and purified from bacteria, allowing many structures to be visualized and modeled into two- and three-dimensional images (6, 8, 20, 48–51, 79, 83, 93). The base of these secretons resembles the FBB, with multiple rings located in different layers of the bacterial cell wall. But while flagella have a hook and flagellum, secretons have a straight needle-like structure protruding from the multiringed base (Fig. 1) (see chapter 25). Negative staining and cryoelectron microscopy of secreton structures indicate that the base and needle-like structures are hollow (8, 20, 50). It is thought that, similar to flagellar biosynthesis, protein subunits that make up the extracellular needle-like structure are secreted into the central channel at the base of the secreton and polymerize at the distal end of the secreton complex. Effector proteins are thought to be secreted via the same route. Visualization of Hrp and Avr proteins, newly secreted by the *Pseudomonas syringae* TTSS, indicates that these proteins exit from the tip of its needle-like structure (43). Thus, some components of the secreton are thought to play mainly structural roles, both constituting and anchoring the base and needle-like structures in the bacterial cell wall, while other components are thought to catalyze the secretion of proteins into the central channel.

The most comprehensive approaches to identify the proteins that make up the Esc/Sep, SPI1, and Mxi/Spa secretons have involved genomic and mutational studies. The genes encoding components of these secretons are clustered together in the genomes of these bacteria (69). These gene clusters appear to have been acquired intact via horizontal gene transfer and may have immediately conferred to the recipient the ability to secrete and translocate proteins into host cells. Sequence comparisons reveal that many of the gene products encoded by these clusters are highly conserved (Table 1). A comprehensive genetic study in *S. enterica* serovar Typhimurium showed that the conserved components encoded on SPI1 are required for bacterial invasion (Table 1) (82). Other studies have shown that many of these conserved components are required for effector secretion.

Structural Components

Most, if not all, of these conserved proteins are thought to be assembled into the functional secreton structure. PrgH, PrgK, and PrgI are present in purified preparations of the SPI1 secreton, and their homologues, MxiG, MxiJ, and MxiH, are found in preparations of the *S. flexneri* secreton (8, 48, 50, 51, 83). PrgI appears to form the needle of the SPI1 secreton (Fig. 1). Overexpression of the PrgI

TABLE 1 SPI1 secreton components conserved in other TTSSs

SPI1 Mutant Phenotypes			TTSSs				Proposed Role
Invasion	Needle	Base	SPI1	Mxi/Spa	Esc/Sep	FBB	
+/−	+/−	+/−	InvH	MxiM			Secretin assembly
−	−	−	InvG	MxiD	EscC		Secretin pore
−	+	+	InvE	MxiC			
−	−	+	InvA	MxiA	EscV	FlhA	Inner membrane secretion apparatus
−	−	+	InvC	SpaL	EscN	FliI	ATPase
−	−	+	SpaM	SpaM			
−	++	+	SpaN(InvJ)	SpaN(Spa32)		FliK	Regulator of secretion specificity
−	−	+	SpaO	SpaO(Spa33)		FliN	
−	−	+	SpaP	SpaP	EscR	FliP	Inner membrane secretion apparatus
−	−	+	SpaQ	SpaQ	EscS	FliQ	Inner membrane secretion apparatus
−	−	+	SpaR	SpaR	EscT	FliR	Inner membrane secretion apparatus
−	−	+	SpaS	SpaS	EscU	FlhB	Inner membrane secretion apparatus
−	−	−	PrgH	MxiG			Bottom inner membrane ring
−	−	+	PrgI	MxiH	EscF		Needle subunit
−	−	+	PrgJ	MxiI			
−	−	−	PrgK	MxiJ	EscJ	FliF	Top inner membrane ring; FBB MS ring
−	−	+	OrgA	MxiK	EscD	FliG	SPI2/Ysc/Psc TTSSs; cytoplasmic FBB C ring
−	−	+	OrgB	MxiN	EspA		Filamentous extension; not for secretion
					SepZ		
					SepQ		
					SepL		

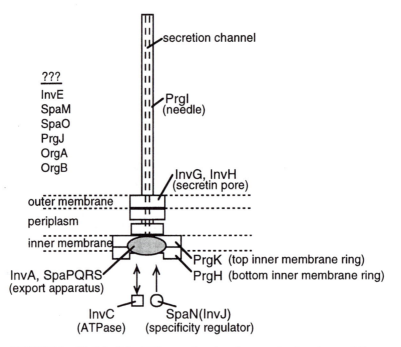

FIGURE 1 Model of the SPI1 secretion showing putative locations and functions of individual components

homologue, MxiH, in *S. flexneri* generates secretons with extremely long needle structures (83). PrgK and PrgH appear to form the rings of the SPI1 secreton that associate with the inner membrane (Fig. 1). Expression of *prgH* and *prgK* alone in *E. coli* K-12 is sufficient for assembly of a double-ringed structure (48). Mutations in *prgH* or *prgK* prevent the assembly of both the secreton base and needle structures. Thus, assembly of these rings in the inner membrane may be the first step required for assembly of the entire secreton structure. PrgK, MxiJ, and EscJ appear to be related to FliF, which makes up the flagellar MS ring in the inner membrane.

The composition of the inner membrane rings of the SPI1 and Mxi/Spa secretons appears to differ from that of the Esc/Sep secreton. The Esc/Sep TTSS does not have a PrgH/MxiG homologue. Instead, the EPEC/EHEC TTSSs have EscD, a homologue of FliG, which makes up part of the bottom C ring of the FBB. The SPI2, Ysc, and Psc TTSSs in *S. enterica* serovar Typhimurium,

Yersinia species, and *Pseudomonas aeruginosa*, respectively, also have EscD/FliG homologues, while the SPI1 and Mxi/Spa TTSSs apparently do not (Table 1). Future studies are needed to determine how these differences affect the structure and function of these TTSSs.

InvG and its homologues EscC and MxiD are also present in purified secretons (8, 50, 79, 83). These proteins are members of the secretin family, which form pores in the outer membrane (Fig. 1). Secretins function in different structural contexts to facilitate the transport of macromolecules across the outer membrane. Interestingly, PrgH, PrgK, and PrgI are still able to assemble into some sort of complex in an *S. enterica* serovar Typhimurium *invG* mutant, but no secreton structures can be visualized by electron microscopy (82). The secretins of TTSSs may be required for the proper assembly and stability of the secreton. Attempts to assemble the secreton needle in the periplasmic space of an *invG* mutant could indirectly disrupt the secreton structure. In addition, protein-protein interactions between InvG and other components of the SPI1 secreton could be required for the integrity and stability of the entire secreton structure. For example, InvG may interact with InvH and PrgK. InvH and MxiM are anchored in the outer membrane of *S. enterica* serovar Typhimurium and *S. flexneri*, respectively, and facilitate the assembly of their cognate secretin pores (18, 19, 77). PrgK and MxiJ are predicted to be in the *Salmonella* and *Shigella* inner membrane (2, 48). Both MxiM and MxiJ have been found to affect the stability of the MxiD secretin in *S. flexneri*, and both interact with MxiD (77). Interactions between MxiM-MxiD-MxiJ and InvH-InvG-PrgK might contribute to the integrity of the secreton base in *Shigella* spp. and *Salmonella* spp. by forming a structural connection between the outer and inner membranes.

Catalytic Components

Six secreton components are highly conserved and are homologous to the FBB components, FlhA, FliI, FliP, FliQ, FliR, and FlhB, which are required for formation of flagella (Table 1). *S. enterica* serovar Typhimurium mutants lacking the SPI1 homologues of these six proteins are still able to assemble the secreton base, but do not form the needle and cannot invade epithelial cells (82). Analogous to their flagellar homologues, these components likely mediate the secretion of needle subunits and effector proteins into the base of the secreton channel for subsequent assembly or secretion. Several of these conserved proteins are predicted to be integral membrane proteins. Macnab has proposed that they localize to a patch of inner membrane within the secreton base and facilitate protein secretion across this hydrophobic barrier (67).

FliI and its homologues have ATPase activity, which suggests that FliI and the hydrolysis of ATP energize the secretion process (27, 30). Models of TTSSs have commonly placed this ATPase component at the cytoplasmic face of the secreton structure, where it can facilitate protein secretion into the secreton base. However, FliI appears to shuttle between the cytoplasm, where its ATPase activ-

ity is inhibited by FliH, and the FBB, where it facilitates flagellar protein secretion (66). Thus, static diagrams of TTSSs could be misleading and FliI homologues may actually be cytoplasmic proteins that only transiently associate with the secreton (Fig. 1). Consistent with this idea, several TTSSs appear to have FliH homologues. The reversibility of the FliI-FBB interaction may provide a convenient regulatory target, and it is worth considering whether protein secretion by TTSSs can be modulated by FliH homologues or other factors that alter the association of the ATPase with the secreton.

Switch Components

An *S. enterica* serovar Typhimurium *spaN(invJ)* mutant cannot secrete effector proteins, but appears to make intact secreton structures (Table 1). However, the needles made by *S. enterica* serovar Typhimurium and *S. flexneri* *spaN(spa32)* mutants are not normal and can be extremely long (51, 82, 84). This phenotype resembles that of *S. enterica* serovar Typhimurium *fliK* mutants, which make extremely long flagellar hook structures. It has been proposed that FliK is needed to switch the specificity of the FBB from secreting hook subunits to secreting flagellin (59, 68). SpaN is weakly homologous to FliK and may be needed to switch secretons from secreting needle subunits to secreting effector proteins. Such a regulator of secretion specificity could be very important for the SPI1 and Mxi/Spa TTSSs. Since the needle structure is thought to contact and deliver effector proteins to adjacent host cells, it would be wasteful to have needleless secreton structures secrete effector proteins. SpaN may bind to completed secreton structures, which prevents them from secreting needle subunits and simultaneously permits them to secrete effector proteins (Fig. 1). Consistent with this idea, secretons lacking PrgI or MxiH, in *S. enterica* serovar Typhimurium or *S. flexneri*, are needleless and do not secrete effector proteins (8, 51).

Interestingly, FliK and SpaN are themselves secreted (17, 64, 84). It has been proposed that FliK is secreted by the FBB, but once the hook is complete, FliK is retained in the cytoplasm, where it interacts with and alters the secretion specificity of the FBB (64). Studies on the location and protein interaction partners of SpaN are needed to determine how it controls protein secretion. The Esc/Sep secreton appears to have an analogous secretion switch, since EPEC mutants lacking its needle homologue, EscF, do not secrete effector proteins (79, 93). However, the Esc/Sep secreton does not appear to have a SpaN homologue, so a different regulatory factor and mechanism seem to be involved.

As mentioned above, it is thought that several secreton components are directly involved in transporting proteins across the inner membrane and into the secreton channel. Unfortunately, since these components are required for secretion and assembly of the extracellular needle components, it is difficult to distinguish whether these components also facilitate effector secretion into the secreton channel. Mutants lacking these components may not be able to secrete effectors simply because the needle structure is missing. The complete secreton structure needs to be assembled before examining the importance of individual secreton components for effector secretion. For example, by allowing temperature-sensitive flagellar mutants to assemble flagella at the permissive temperature, before shifting them to the nonpermissive temperature, it was shown that FlhA, FlhB, FliH, and FliI are required for export and assembly of flagellin (65).

Filamentous Extensions

The needle structures of the purified SPI1 and Mxi/Spa secretons appear to have the same diameter along their entire lengths, presumably because they are polymers of a single protein, PrgI and MxiH, respectively. In contrast, electron micrographs show that the extracellular structure of the Esc/Sep secreton is composed of a long, thick filament that is attached to the secreton base via a short, thin segment (20, 79). The short segment appears to be composed of EscF, which is homologous to PrgI and MxiH, whereas the long filament is composed of EspA (93). Unlike EscF, EspA is not required for effector secretion and is required only for effector translocation (47, 49, 79). Effector proteins are thought to be delivered into the membrane and cytosol of adjacent epithelial cells through the hollow EspA filament. Interestingly, the extracellular portion of the EPEC/EHEC Esc/Sep secreton appears to retract or eject after interacting with the plasma membrane of epithelial cells (49). The EspA filament may span the mucus and glycocalyx layers to mediate direct contact between the bacteria and intestinal epithelial cells. Subsequent removal of the filament could be important to bring the bacterial and host cell surfaces together, so that attaching and effacing lesions can form (see chapter 23).

The SPI1 secreton may also have a filamentous extension. Scanning electron microscopy studies show that *S. enterica* serovar Typhimurium cells produce extracellular filamentous appendages soon after they adhere to epithelial cells. Interestingly, the filaments are not present after *S. enterica* serovar Typhimurium induces membrane ruffling and starts to enter the epithelial cells (34). It was speculated that these structures are part of the SPI1 secretion and translocation apparatus. In this case, these filaments could be analogous to the EPEC/EHEC EspA filament, which extends from the secreton needle and then is removed after facilitating effector secretion and translocation into epithelial cells. Interestingly, an *S. enterica* serovar Typhimurium *invE* mutant was reported to produce longer filaments that do not disappear and remain on the bacterial cells (34). InvE may affect the assembly and/ or disassembly of a filamentous extension on the SPI1 secreton that is formed only after bacterial contact with epithelial cells.

An *invE* mutant appears to make intact secreton structures with normal PrgI needles, yet cannot invade epithelial cells (Table 1). Unfortunately, it is not known if the *invE* mutant secretes effector proteins or not. If the mutant cannot secrete effector proteins, InvE may affect the secretion specificity of the SPI1 secreton, analogous to SpaN, switching the secreton from secreting components of the filament to secreting effector proteins. If an *invE* mutant is competent for secretion but cannot translocate effectors into epithelial cells, InvE may affect the structure and function of the filaments, which indirectly alters effector translocation into host cells. Unfortunately, nothing is known about the composition of these filamentous appendages. In addition, it is controversial as to whether or not they have anything to do with the SPI1 secreton. One study showed that *prgH* and *invG* mutants, which do not form SPI1 secretons, still produce filamentous appendages (74). However, *S. enterica* serovar Typhimurium might produce more than one type of filamentous appendage. Thus, further work is needed to investigate the intriguing possibility that, similar to the Esc/Sep secreton, the SPI1 secreton uses a filamentous extension to translocate effector proteins into host cells.

In summary, recent studies have revealed many interesting details about the structures and functions of the EPEC/EHEC, *Salmonella*, and *Shigella* secretons. Further work is needed to identify all the proteins, their stoichiometries, and locations in these structures. Micrographs of the purified complexes indicate that many are damaged and missing important substructures. Determining whether any of the purified complexes are functional secretons or whether all have lost essential components will require their reconstitution into lipid bilayers. In addition, more comprehensive studies need to be done in all three systems to identify the precise structural and functional roles each secreton component plays. We know virtually nothing about many secreton components. Some of these components appear to be uniquely present in SPI1 and Mxi/Spa secretons versus in the Esc/Sep secreton (Table 1). Comparisons of primary amino acid sequences may not be able to recognize that these components actually share ancestral origins and serve the same functions. Detailed information about their locations, structures, and functions could eventually match up some of these components. Alternatively, some of these components might have unique activities, which confer unique

mechanistic and biological features to the TTSSs.

TARGETING AND RECOGNITION OF TTS SUBSTRATES

Gram-negative bacteria secrete proteins onto their surface or into the culture supernatant via many different types of protein secretion systems. Proteins may be targeted to their cognate secretion system by specific interactions with a component of the secretion apparatus. Interestingly, unlike other types of protein secretion systems, TTSSs may be somewhat promiscuous, using common recognition signals to target proteins to more than one TTSS. For example, the *Yersinia* YopE protein can be secreted via the SPI1 secreton, and the *S. flexneri* IpaB protein can be secreted via the *Yersinia* Ysc TTSS, suggesting that the Ysc, SPI1, and Mxi/Spa secretons use the same mechanisms to recognize and target these effectors for secretion (75). The SPI1 and SPI2 secretons may also use common recognition mechanisms, since three *S. enterica* serovar Typhimurium proteins, SspH1, SlrP, and SipA(SspA), can be secreted via either secreton (10, 62; R. A. Murray, personal communication). However, other *S. enterica* serovar Typhimurium effectors appear to be preferentially secreted via SPI1 or SPI2, suggesting that these secretons also recognize unique targeting signals. Each TTSS might have more than one mechanism to target substrates for secretion. A single substrate may be able to use one, or more than one, of these mechanisms. Consistent with this idea, studies of TTSSs have derived three different targeting mechanisms for TTS substrates. By differentially regulating these targeting mechanisms, a bacterial pathogen could potentially secrete different subsets of effectors and alter different host cell activities at different times during infection.

Recognition of a Sequence or Structural Feature of the Protein Substrate

The N-terminal region of certain TTS substrates may facilitate their secretion. For example, deletion of the first 13 amino acids of

YopE, which is secreted by the Ysc TTSS, reduces its ability to be secreted by *Yersinia pseudotuberculosis*. However, Ysc-secreted proteins do not appear to contain a consensus amino acid sequence in this region. Instead, it has been proposed that any N-terminal sequence with amphipathic characteristics can be recognized by the Ysc secreton (57).

To identify regions of effectors sufficient for their secretion and translocation via the SPI1 and/or SPI2 secretons, Miller and coworkers fused N-terminal regions of six different *S. enterica* serovar Typhimurium effectors to the *Bordetella pertussis* adenylate cyclase toxin (CyaA) (62, 63). The delivery of these fusions from *S. enterica* serovar Typhimurium into the cytosol of macrophages is detected by an increase in intracellular cyclic AMP levels. Using this method, it was shown that the N-terminal 150 to 200 amino acids of these effectors, which are highly conserved, can mediate the secretion and translocation of the CyaA moiety through the SPI1 and/or SPI2 secreton. This conserved sequence appears to be important for SspH1 translocation via either the SPI1 or SPI2 secreton, since CyaA was not translocated into macrophages from *S. enterica* serovar Typhimurium expressing an SspH1-CyaA fusion containing a 4-amino-acid deletion in this region (62). However, it is not clear why some effectors that carry this sequence are translocated via both secretons while other effectors are preferentially translocated via the SPI2 secreton. Despite its apparent conservation, there could be differences in the sequence that determine whether an effector will be translocated via the SPI1 and/or SPI2 secreton. In addition, since these experiments measured effector delivery into macrophages, which requires both effector secretion from the bacterial cell and translocation of the effector across the host cell membrane, the 4-amino-acid deletion in this conserved sequence may affect translocation, not secretion, of SspH1. Further work is needed to determine whether the conserved sequence facilitates recognition of the effector for secretion into the base of the secreton and/

or facilitates translocation of the effector across the host cell membrane. Even if this conserved sequence is found to target these effectors to the SPI1 and/or SPI2 secreton, additional mechanisms must exist to target effectors to these two secretons since the sequence is not present on other SPI1- and SPI2-secreted effectors.

Similar to other TTSSs, the Mxi/Spa secreton appears to recognize the N-terminal region of at least one of its substrates, IpaC (72). To determine what components of the Mxi/Spa secreton might directly mediate substrate recognition and targeting, a yeast two-hybrid analysis was used to identify protein fragments encoded in the *S. flexneri mxi-spa* locus that bind to TTS proteins (71). Results from this analysis suggest that a component of the Mxi/Spa secreton, MxiK, binds to the secreted protein, IpaB, but, surprisingly, MxiK does not appear to interact with other TTS substrates. IpaB might be targeted to the Mxi/Spa secreton in a unique, MxiK-dependent manner. Alternatively, IpaB binding to MxiK may serve some other function. IpaB has been shown to inhibit the secretion of other proteins through the Mxi/Spa secreton (60), so its binding to MxiK may actually block, not facilitate, the secretion process.

Recognition of a Sequence or Structural Feature of the mRNA Encoding the Protein Substrate

It has been proposed that sequences present on the mRNA transcripts that encode TTS proteins can target the nascent polypeptide to the secreton. Since the targeting process would have to occur before the protein substrate detaches from the mRNA, translation may be inhibited until the mRNA-nascent polypeptide complex is properly localized at the secreton base.

This idea is supported by the finding that frameshift mutations that alter the N-terminal amino acid sequences of YopE, YopN, or YopQ(YopK) have no effect on their secretion in *Yersinia enterocolitica* (3, 4). In addition, translation of YopQ was shown to be inhibited in situations where *Y. enterocolitica* could not secrete it, consistent with the idea that the translation and secretion of YopQ are coupled (4). However, these results and conclusions have been controversial, partly because the 5′ frameshifted Yop sequences were fused to neomycin phosphotransferase (Npt). Random N-terminal sequences have been shown to direct the secretion of Npt from the flagellar TTSS in *S. enterica* serovar Typhimurium (15). In addition, Yops have been shown to be secreted from *Yersinia* sp. when expressed from transcripts in which the entire 5′ untranslated region of their mRNAs has been replaced by sequence from a gene encoding a nonsecreted protein (4, 57).

Still, it is difficult to eliminate the possibility that RNA sequences in the untranslated and/ or translated regions have targeting functions. The redundancy of targeting mechanisms may complicate these studies. It has been proposed that FlgM, which is secreted by the flagellar TTSS, and YopE possess both mRNA and protein-based targeting mechanisms (13, 45). So, simplistically, the idea that recognition of RNA, not protein, facilitates the targeting process may remain an intriguing possibility until a mutation in the mRNA sequence of a TTS substrate is identified that reduces its secretion but has no effect on its expression and amino acid sequence. Unfortunately, if translation is coupled to protein secretion such that translation of the nascent polypeptide pauses until the mRNA interacts with the secreton base, as has been proposed for YopQ, mutations that block mRNA recognition may also block translation. In fact, specific changes in the 5′ untranslated region of transcripts encoding Yop-Npt and FlgM prevent their translation (3, 45). Further studies of the regulation of translation might reveal whether mRNA targeting mechanisms exist that couple the secretion of certain TTS proteins to their translation.

The role of mRNA sequences in targeting proteins to the Esc/Sep, SPI1, or Mxi/Spa secretons has not been addressed in detail. Future studies will be guided by the results and controversies that have been generated by work on the *Yersinia* and flagellar TTSS.

Role of Chaperone Proteins in Protein Secretion

Cytoplasmic chaperone proteins have been identified that are required for the efficient secretion of certain TTS proteins (Table 2) (1, 5, 10, 23, 28, 29, 32, 45, 71, 87, 90). In general, these chaperone proteins are small (100 to 160 amino acids), acidic, and predicted to form α-helical domains. It has been proposed that chaperones bind directly to their cognate TTS substrates and deliver them to the secreton base for secretion. However, chaperones may actually be important for other processes that indirectly affect the secretion of TTS substrates.

Chaperones as Direct or Indirect Targeting Factors. Many studies have shown that secretion of TTS substrates is reduced in mutants lacking their cognate chaperone and/ or in mutants lacking the chaperone binding

TABLE 2 Chaperones and their cognate type III secreted proteins

TTS Protein	Chaperone	Substrate
SPI1	SicA	SipB
	SicA	SipC
	InvB	SipA
	SicP	SptP
	SigE	SigD(SopB)
Mxi/Spa	IpgC	IpaB
	IpgC	IpaC
	IpgE	IpgD
	SpaK?	IpaA?
Esc/Sep	CesD	EspB
	CesD	EspD
	CesF	EspF
	CesT	Tir
EBB	FlgN	FlgK
	FlgN	FlgL
	FlgN	FlgM
	FliT	FliD
	FliS	FliC

site on the TTS substrate. A simple explanation for these results is that some feature of the chaperone-TTS substrate complex is recognized and targets the substrate for secretion. The targeting feature could be on the TTS substrate, on the chaperone, or on both. For example, it has been proposed that the chaperone SycE(YerA) functions to recruit YopE to the secreton base, where the N terminus of YopE engages the protein secretion apparatus in the inner membrane (57). Unfortunately, using knockout mutants alone makes it extremely difficult to distinguish whether chaperones affect secretion because they mediate targeting or whether chaperones affect protein folding, protein-protein associations, and/or protein stability, which indirectly affect the secretion of their TTS substrates.

Chaperones as Antifolding Factors. It is thought that unfolded proteins cross the inner membrane and into the secreton base, analogous to the Sec-mediated protein secretion pathway. There are several ways by which protein folding might be prevented so that secretion can occur. Cotranslational secretion could totally prevent the folding of TTS substrates in the cytoplasm. Secreted proteins might inherently have slow rates of folding so that secretion could occur before they fold. Alternatively, chaperones may function to bind TTS substrates and prevent them from folding into their final conformation in the cytoplasm. In fact, X-ray crystallography of a StpP-SicP complex shows that a large domain of the StpP effector adopts an extended, unfolded conformation when bound to its SicP chaperone (81). Interestingly, cell fractionation studies indicate that a significant proportion of TTS substrates can remain in the cytoplasm and never be secreted. These cytoplasmic forms may represent folded, unsecretable proteins.

Unfortunately, nothing is known about the folding rates of TTS substrates that do and do not have chaperones, or the effect that chaperones may have on the folding of their cognate TTS substrates in vivo. In addition,

recent in vitro studies seem to contradict the idea that all chaperones prevent the folding of their substrates. Binding of the Tir and SigD(SopB) effectors to their chaperones, CesT and SigE, respectively, did not interfere with their ability to interact with other proteins or exhibit enzymatic activity (58). Thus, chaperone binding seems to cause minor or no unfolding of these effectors and other TTSS components may facilitate their unfolding during secretion.

Chaperones as Bodyguards. Many TTS proteins are destined to interact with each other after secretion. It is imagined that the premature association of TTS proteins with one another in the cytoplasm would prevent their subsequent secretion. Some chaperones appear to function to bind TTS substrates and act as bodyguards to block undesirable protein-protein interactions in the cytoplasm. For example, in the absence of the IpgC chaperone, IpaB and IpaC associate with one another and cannot be secreted by *S. flexneri* (61). However, other TTS substrates that have chaperones are not known to form protein-protein interactions with other TTS substrates, so the chaperones for these proteins may not function as bodyguards. In addition, IpgC seems to be both a bodyguard and an antidegradation factor for IpaB, since the stability of IpaB requires IpgC, even in the absence of IpaC (61).

Chaperones as Antidegradation Factors. Simplistically, if a chaperone directly facilitates the secretion of its cognate TTS substrate, the TTS substrate should accumulate in the bacterial cytoplasm in the absence of the chaperone. However, in many cases, loss of a chaperone actually reduces the level of its TTS substrate in whole cell samples. It has been proposed that chaperones protect their cognate TTS substrates from proteolysis in the bacterial cytoplasm. Consistent with this idea, the stability of SipA(SspA) appears to be significantly reduced in the cytoplasm of an *S. enterica* serovar Typhimurium mutant lacking its chaperone, InvB (10). Thus, chaperones may not be directly involved in secretion. The lower levels of a TTS substrate in the cytoplasm of a chaperone mutant could indirectly reduce its secretion. Unfortunately, most studies have not specifically measured the stability of TTS substrates in the cytoplasm and have looked only at whole cells. One approach would be to determine the effect of chaperones on TTS substrates in mutants lacking their cognate secreton, as was done for SipA(SspA) (10).

Chaperones as Translational Regulators. As discussed above, the secretion of certain TTS substrates may be cotranslational. In this case, chaperones might assist in coupling translation to secretion by binding and targeting the mRNA-nascent chain complex to the secreton. The case is strongest for FlgN, a flagellar chaperone, that mediates the secretion of FlgM via the flagellar TTSS. When the flagellar hook structure is incomplete, FlgM is not secreted and is retained in the cytoplasm, where it represses a subset of flagellar genes. However, upon completion of the hook, FlgM is secreted, which alleviates gene repression and allows for the production of functional flagella (46). Recent studies show that, when the hook is incomplete, FlgN is required for the translation of FlgM from one of two *flgM*-encoding transcripts (45). When the hook is completed, FlgM expressed from that same transcript appears to be preferentially secreted. It has been proposed that, upon hook completion, FlgN enhances the secretion of FlgM by recruiting nascent FlgM-mRNA complexes to the FBB. Since the regulation of flagellar gene regulation by FlgM occurs in the cytoplasm, it is not clear why *S. enterica* serovar Typhimurium would have a mechanism to synthesize FlgM proteins that are immediately destined to leave the bacterial cell. It is possible that FlgM has a noncytoplasmic role within the FBB or flagellar structure itself.

In summary, chaperones have different effects on their TTS substrates and may have more than one function. Unfortunately, this has left us with a chicken-and-egg dilemma, not knowing what are primary causes versus secondary events. Still, the idea that chaperones help target TTS substrates to be secreted and are themselves recognized by components of the secreton remains attractive. One particularly intriguing study showed that GST-SycE(YerA) fusions are not able to facilitate the secretion of YopE in *Y. enterocolitica*, but are still able to bind and stabilize it (14). The GST domain may disrupt an interaction between SycE(YerA) and the secreton base that is essential for YopE secretion. However, the idea that chaperones target their TTS substrates for cotranslational or posttranslational secretion will remain hypothetical until an interaction between a chaperone and a secreton component is shown to directly mediate the secretion of a TTS substrate.

Secretion by Alternate TTSSs

It is likely that many TTS substrates are targeted only to their cognate secretons. This would ensure their efficient secretion/translocation and may also prevent them from interfering with other TTSSs. However, as mentioned above, a few TTS substrates can be secreted from *S. enterica* serovar Typhimurium via either the SPI1 or SPI2 secreton. Since the SPI1 and SPI2 TTSSs are expressed during different stages of infection, the ability of TTS substrates to be recognized and secreted by both secretons might allow these effectors to contribute to multiple phases of pathogenesis. It is also possible that secretion/translocation of a TTS substrate via one versus another secreton could alter its effect on host cells. For example, the FBB TTSS appears to be capable of secreting SipA(SspA), when this SPI1 effector is overexpressed from a high-copy-number plasmid (R. A. Murray, personal communication). The delivery of SipA from *S. enterica* serovar Typhimurium into host cells allows it to interact with the actin cytoskeleton and affect bacterial invasion (96). In contrast, exposure of epithelial cells to extracellular purified SipA has been shown to activate a protein kinase C signal transduction pathway that ultimately stimulates transepithelial neutrophil migration (53) (see chapter 24). Since flagella would be predicted to secrete SipA to the extracellular milieu, rather than translocate it into epithelial cells, secretion of SipA via flagella may specifically promote the neutrophil transmigration response.

Much more work is needed to understand how and why certain TTS substrates can be secreted via alternate TTSSs. For bacterial pathogens such as *S. enterica* serovar Typhimurium that have more than one TTSS, it will be critical to investigate the relevance of such secretion routes by determining whether particular TTS substrates are ever expressed at the same time as alternate TTSSs during infection. In addition, although it is interesting to speculate that secretion via alternate TTSSs expands the utility of TTS substrates in vivo, studies must be done to test whether secretion of a TTS substrate via an alternate route has any effect on pathogenesis.

TRANSLOCATION OF TTS SUBSTRATES ACROSS THE MAMMALIAN CELL MEMBRANE

Secretons appear to act in conjunction with at least two other proteins to translocate effectors across the mammalian cell membrane. SipB and SipC, which are homologous to the IpaB and IpaC proteins of the Mxi/Spa TTSS, are required for the translocation of SPI1-secreted effectors into host cells (22). EspD and EspB appear to mediate the translocation of effectors secreted by the Esc/Sep TTSS (21, 94). These Sip, Ipa, and Esp proteins are not required for effector secretion and are themselves TTS substrates. The Sips, Ipas, and Esps have hydrophobic domains, and fractionation experiments indicate that they associate with the host cell membrane after bacterial-host cell contact (6, 41, 76, 80, 89, 94). In vitro studies of purified SipB, SipC, IpaB, and IpaC show that these translocation proteins have the intrinsic ability to associate with membranes (25, 37, 52, 70, 72, 85). SipB and SipC can form oligomers, and SipB may help SipC associate with mammalian membranes (37, 70, 76).

It is imagined that the Sips, Ipas, and Esps are secreted from their cognate secretons and form multimeric complexes in the host cell membrane, through which effectors are transported. Interestingly, some of these translocation proteins are also effectors (12, 37, 38, 52, 85, 86) (see chapter 20). Certain translocation proteins appear to span the mammalian membrane and alter cellular responses by interacting with host proteins at the cytosolic face of the host cell membrane. Other translocation proteins may have two conformations—one that localizes to the membrane bilayer and facilitates translocation versus one that is soluble and interacts with cytosolic host proteins.

The Sip, Ipa, and Esp proteins may mediate effector translocation by forming transmembrane pores in the host cell membrane. Transmembrane pores with an inner diameter of 3 to 5 nm have been seen in red blood cell (RBC) membranes after incubation with culture supernatants from a diffusely adhering (DA) EPEC strain (41). Other TTSSs also appear to form discrete transmembrane pores in mammalian cell membranes (6, 39, 80, 88, 91). However, instead of being induced by culture supernatants, pore formation in these other systems appears to require direct contact with bacterial cells. Interestingly, both active secretion and close contact with the target cells are required for *S. flexneri* to lyse RBCs (6). Active secretion and close contact are similarly required for *Y. enterocolitica* to damage HeLa cell membranes (39). The ability of *Shigella* and *Yersinia* translocation proteins to form pores in mammalian membranes may be coupled to their secretion.

Translocation proteins may even need to be physically attached to their cognate secreton structures for translocation to occur. Microscopy studies indicate that EPEC adhere to mammalian cells via the tips of their EspA filaments in an EspD-dependent manner (21, 49, 80). It has been proposed that binding of the EspA filament to mammalian membranes induces the secretion of EspD and EspB, which then attach the EspA filament to the membrane and direct the delivery of effectors into the host cell cytosol (36, 89, 94). *Y. enterocolitica* does not have an EspA-like filament and, instead, appears to use its YscF needle structure to insert a pore into mammalian membranes (39). It has even been proposed that the YscF needle itself is able to penetrate mammalian cell membranes and translocate effectors in the absence of the YopB and YopD translocation proteins (39, 55). However, further studies are needed to test this controversial proposal (7). In any case, the estimated diameters of the transmembrane channels formed by TTSSs suggest that effector proteins cross the mammalian membrane in an unfolded state.

If the secreton and translocation proteins form a contiguous channel that delivers effectors into the host cell cytosol, the cytopathic, transmembrane pores formed by TTSSs in vitro might represent nonfunctional translocation complexes. It has been proposed that movement of the host cell membrane breaks the attached Ysc TTSS needle, leaving behind a 1.2-to-3.5-nm translocation pore in the mammalian membrane (35, 88). *Y. pseudotuberculosis* apparently produces YopE or YopT to prevent localized cytoskeletal changes that would shear the Ysc TTS structure (88). For several TTSSs, hemolysis and pore formation require centrifugation of the bacteria with the RBCs. It is interesting to consider whether, in addition to promoting intimate contact between the secreton tip and the mammalian membrane, centrifugation may also produce a shearing force that helps break the TTS channel.

Although it is simplest to imagine that a direct connection between the secreton tip and a static transmembrane pore mediates effector translocation, it is possible that the translocation mechanism is more complicated. Translocation may involve an active transport process that uses energy and even protein factors from the host cell. Unfortunately, assays that detect transmembrane pores would not reveal such important mechanistic details. The use of hemolysis assays seems to be limiting in additional ways. The translocation proteins YopD, IpaC, and EspB are not essential for

Y. enterocolitica, S. flexneri, and EPEC, respectively, to lyse RBCs (6, 39, 80). Osmoprotection assays suggest that hemolysis induced by an *S. flexneri ipaC* mutant is not due to the formation of 2.6-nm pores produced by wide-type *S. flexneri* and may be nonspecific (6). Thus, much remains to be learned about how TTSSs induce hemolysis and whether this activity is relevant to effector translocation. If effector secretion is coupled to translocation, it will be extremely difficult to study the translocation process. In vitro reconstitution of translocation would first require the in vitro reconstitution of secretion. Detailed studies of protein localization and function in assays containing whole bacterial and host cells will be difficult to control for and interpret (7).

Although SipD and IpaD are required for effector translocation and are often called translocation proteins of the SPI1 and Mxi/Spa TTSSs, respectively, neither protein associates with mammalian membranes (6, 76). In addition, IpaD is not required for *S. flexneri*-induced hemolysis (6). SipD and IpaD appear to be involved in the regulation of protein secretion, such that loss of SipD or IpaD leads to hypersecretion of TTS substrates from serovar Typhimurium and *S. flexneri*, respectively (44, 60) (see below). The inability of *sipD* and *ipaD* mutants to translocate effectors into host cells may be indirectly due to the hypersecretion and depletion of the Sip and Ipa translocation proteins from the bacterial cells. Further studies are needed to address whether or not SipD and IpaD play a direct role in effector translocation.

REGULATION OF PROTEIN SECRETION BY TTSSs

Contact-Induced Protein Secretion

Contact with host cells has been shown to induce the secretion of translocation proteins and/or effector proteins from the Esc/Sep and Mxi/Spa secretons (60, 92, 94). It is believed that a signal at the host cell surface is sensed by these TTSSs, which upregulates a rate-limiting step in the protein secretion process. During infection, this regulatory mechanism could then limit the release of translocation/effector proteins to when *S. flexneri* and EPEC/EHEC are adjacent to a susceptible host cell.

Contact with host cells induces the secretion of SpaN(InvJ), a putative secretion specificity determinant of the SPI1 secreton (see below). However, surprisingly, even in the absence of host cells, *S. enterica* serovar Typhimurium secretes high levels of its SPI1 translocation/effector proteins into culture supernatants. It may not be important or desirable for this pathogen to limit the secretion of these proteins during infection. Alternatively, in vitro growth conditions could mimic an inducing signal, which artifactually leads to contact-independent secretion of the translocation/effector proteins by the SPI1 TTSS. Unfortunately, little is known about the signals at the host cell surface that stimulate secretion by TTSSs. Each TTSS may even respond to a different host cell signal, which determines the particular cell type that is targeted by these virulence systems in vivo.

Several secreted proteins have been identified that may modulate the activity of the SPI1 and Mxi/Spa secretons. SipD and IpaD seem to inhibit secretion through these TTSSs, since *S. enterica* serovar Typhimurium *sipD* and *S. flexneri* *ipaD* mutants secrete more effector proteins (44, 60). SipD and IpaD are thought to inhibit secretion by binding to the secreted translocation proteins, SipB and IpaB, respectively. Fractionation studies suggest that IpaB-IpaD complexes form in the *S. flexneri* outer membrane and inhibit the Mxi/Spa secreton (60). Contact with host cells stimulates the release of IpaB and IpaD, which may activate the Mxi/Spa TTSS (60, 92).

Both SpaO and SpaN may also be involved in regulating protein secretion from the SPI1 and Mxi/Spa secretons. But unlike SipD and IpaD, which inhibit secretion, SpaO and SpaN are required for protein secretion by these secretons (16, 78, 84). SpaO is itself secreted by *S. enterica* serovar Typhimurium (56). Interestingly, in *S. flexneri*, the localization of SpaO(Spa33) changes in response to

host cells, with SpaO(Spa33) becoming exposed at the bacterial surface and with IpaB and IpaC moving from the bacterial membrane fraction to the culture supernatant (78). In an *S. flexneri* *spaO(spa33)* mutant, the Ipas are not secreted and apparently remain associated with the bacterial inner membrane. These studies suggest that SpaO is more than just a static component of the SPI1 and Mxi/Spa secretons and plays a dynamic role in contact-induced activation of these TTSS.

SpaN(InvJ) is secreted by *S. enterica* serovar Typhimurium in response to contact with host cells (97). In *S. flexneri*, the relative stoichiometry of SpaN(Spa32) and SpaO(Spa33) appears to be critical for Ipa secretion, suggesting that these two proteins form a complex that controls Ipa secretion (78). As discussed previously, SpaN is required for effector secretion, but not needle assembly, and has been proposed to switch the specificity of the SPI1 and Mxi/Spa secretons from secreting needle subunits to effectors. In contrast to SpaN, SpaO may regulate a more general TTS function, because while serovar Typhimurium *spaN(invJ)* mutants make secretons with longer needles, *spaO* mutants make secretons lacking needles (82). Additional studies on how SpaN and SpaO affect secreton structures and activities are needed to understand how they might regulate secretion. If SpaN(InvJ) modulates secretion by the SPI1 secreton, it is not clear why SpaN(InvJ), but not the translocation/effector proteins, is secreted in response to host cell signals in vitro.

InvE and MxiC may also be involved in regulating the SPI1 and Mxi/Spa secretons, respectively. These proteins are weakly homologous to the *Yersinia* protein YopN(LcrE) (40). The *Yersinia* Ysc TTSS does not secrete any proteins unless the bacteria encounter a host cell signal. YopN(LcrE) and at least three other proteins, YopD, LcrQ(YscM1/2), and LcrV, appear to regulate the Ysc TTSS and are secreted by *Yersinia* in response to host cell contact (54, 73). These regulatory proteins seem to control the Ysc secreton via more than one mechanism. For example, genetic studies suggest that the regulatory effect of YopD is epistatic to that of YopN(LcrE) (54). In addition, the ability of LcrQ to inhibit Yop secretion appears to require the regulatory protein, LcrG, but not YopN(LcrE) (95). The ability of the Yop and Lcr regulatory factors to target multiple components and activities of the Ysc TTSS may account for the extremely tight, contact-dependent regulation of Yop secretion in *Yersinia*. It has been proposed that YopD inhibits YscY, which is a chaperone for an essential component of the Ysc secreton (24, 31, 42). LcrV is thought to control Yop secretion by interacting with LcrG at the cytoplasmic face of the Ysc secreton (73). YopN(LcrE) is proposed to block Yop secretion by binding to a more distal region of the Ysc secreton (73).

Many more studies are needed before we can even begin to understand how secretion by the enteric TTSSs is regulated by contact with host cells. However, it is likely that the mechanisms that regulate the enteric TTSSs are quite different from those that control the *Yersinia* system. The SPI1 and Mxi/Spa TTSSs do not appear to have homologues of LcrV, LcrG, or LcrQ. In addition, although the homology of InvE and MxiC with YopN(LcrE) is intriguing, it is not yet clear what these proteins do (see above). Even less is known about how the Esc/Sep TTSS is regulated. This system appears to lack the SpaN, SpaO, and InvE/MxiC proteins that are thought to regulate the SPI1 and Mxi/Spa TTSSs, suggesting that EPEC/EHEC uses totally different factors and mechanisms to regulate Esp secretion in response to host cells (Table 1).

Ordered Protein Secretion

In addition to secreting needle subunits first, the enteric TTSSs may secrete their other substrates in a hierarchical manner. For example, the discovery that two SPI1-secreted effectors, SopE and SptP, activate and inactivate Cdc42/Rac-1, respectively, suggests that these effectors are translocated in sequence into host cells: SopE first, followed by SptP (33). Recent studies suggest that the *Yersinia* Ysc TTSS secretes its effector proteins in a hierarchical fashion that is determined by competition between the Yops and/or their chaperones for recognition by the Ysc TTSS (9, 95). For example, in the absence of *yopH*, YopE appears to be secreted earlier and to higher levels (95). The binding of YopE to its chaperone, SycE, appears to increase its ability to compete with other Yop effectors for secretion and translocation by the Ysc TTSS (9). In addition, overexpression of the secreted, regulatory protein, LcrQ, and its chaperone, SycH, blocks the secretion of YopE and YopM, but not YopH (95).

Yersinia may also order the secretion of its translocation proteins versus its effector proteins. HeLa cell lysates have been shown to induce *Y. enterocolitica* to secrete its YopD translocation protein, but not its YopE effector (54). An additional signal, provided by contact with intact host cells, allows *Yersinia* to secrete its effectors, YopH and YopE (54, 73). The secretion of translocation proteins followed by effector proteins may ensure that effectors are not secreted until the TTSS is competent to translocate them into an adjacent host cell. It is not clear how the Ysc TTSS could be capable of secreting translocation proteins but incapable of secreting effectors (54). The Ysc secreton might have separate compartments that are capable of releasing different subsets of TTS substrates in response to specific host signals. Alternatively, the Ysc secreton may have two conformations—one that recognizes and secretes translocation proteins versus one that recognizes and secretes effectors.

Detailed kinetic studies may reveal that host cell signals trigger an ordered secretion of proteins from the Mxi/Spa and Esc/Sep TTSS. Unfortunately, similar analyses of the SPI1 TTSS will not be possible unless contact-induced secretion of the SPI1 translocation/effector proteins can be reproduced in vitro.

SUMMARY

Much has been learned about TTSS in enteric bacterial pathogens. Recent studies have shed light on the composition and structure of these TTSSs. Work has begun to reveal how effector proteins are targeted for secretion by these TTSS. Proteins required for effector translocation into host cells have been identified and characterized. Studies on the regulation of secretion by these TTSSs have begun. However, much remains unknown, and, despite their many structural and functional similarities, TTSSs exhibit clear differences. A better understanding of how each of the enteric TTSSs operates will be necessary to fully appreciate how these complex systems contribute to the pathogenesis of EPEC, EHEC, *Salmonella*, and *Shigella*.

ACKNOWLEDGMENTS

I thank many colleagues who generously provided reprints and preprints of their work, which helped me prepare this chapter. I thank J. Day, S. Jain, V. Lee, and R. Murray for helpful discussions and comments. I also thank the National Institutes of Health and the Funds for Discovery for supporting the work in my lab on the regulation of SPI1 TTS genes in *S. enterica* serovar Typhimurium.

REFERENCES

1. Abe, A., M. de Grado, R. A. Pfuetzner, C. Sánchez-SanMartín, R. DeVinney, J. L. Puente, N. C. J. Strynadka, and B. B. Finlay. 1999. Enteropathogenic *Escherichia coli* translocated intimin receptor, Tir, requires a specific chaperone for stable secretion. *Mol. Microbiol.* 33:1162–1175.

2. Allaoui, A., S. J. Sansonetti, and C. Parsot. 1992. MxiJ, a lipoprotein involved in secretion of *Shigella* Ipa invasins, is homologous to YscJ, a secretion factor of the *Yersinia* Yop proteins. *J. Bacteriol.* 174:7661–7669.

3. Anderson, D. M., and O. Schneewind. 1997. A mRNA signal for the type III secretion of Yop proteins by *Yersinia enterocolitica*. *Science* 278:1140–1143.

4. Anderson, D. M., and O. Schneewind. 1999. *Yersinia enterocolitica* type III secretion: an mRNA signal that couples translation and secretion of YopQ. *Mol. Microbiol.* 31:1139–1148.

5. Bennett, J. C. Q., and C. Hughes. 2000. From flagellum assembly to virulence: the extended family of type III export chaperones. *Trends Microbiol.* 8:202–204.

6. Blocker, A., P. Gounon, E. Larquet, K. Niebuhr, V. Cabiaux, C. Parsot, and P. San-

sonetti. 1999. The tripartite type III secreton of *Shigella flexneri* inserts IpaB and IpaC into host membranes. *J. Cell Biol.* 147:683–693.

7. Blocker, A., D. Holden, and G. Cornelis. 2000. Type III secretion systems: what is the translocator and what is the translocated? *Cell. Microbiol.* 2:387–390.

8. Blocker, A., N. Jouihri, E. Larquet, P. Gounon, F. Ebel, C. Parsot, P. Sansonetti, and A. Allaoui. 2001. Structure and composition of the *Shigella flexneri* "needle complex," a part of its type III secreton. *Mol. Microbiol.* 39:652–663.

9. Boyd, A. P., I. Lambermont, and G. R. Cornelis. 2000. Competition between the Yops of *Yersinia enterocolitica* for delivery into eukaryotic cells: role of the SycE chaperone binding domain of YopE. *J. Bacteriol.* 182:4811–4821.

10. Bronstein, P. A., E. A. Miao, and S. I. Miller. 2000. InvB is a type III chaperone specific for SspA. *J. Bacteriol.* 182:6638–6644.

11. Buchrieser, C., P. Glaser, C. Rusniok, H. Nedjari, H. d'Hauteville, F. Kunst, P. Sansonetti, and C. Parsot. 2000. The virulence plasmid pWR100 and the repertoire of proteins secreted by the type III secretion apparatus of *Shigella flexneri*. *Mol. Microbiol.* 38:760–771.

12. Chen, Y., M. R. Smith, K. Thirumalai, and A. Zychlinsky. 1996. A bacterial invasin induces macrophage apoptosis by binding directly to ICE. *EMBO J.* 15:3853–3860.

13. Cheng, L. W., D. M. Anderson, and O. Schneewind. 1997. Two independent type III secretion mechanisms for YopE in *Yersinia enterocolitica*. *Mol. Microbiol.* 24:757–765.

14. Cheng, L. W., and O. Schneewind. 1999. *Yersinia enterocolitica* type III secretion: on the role of SycE in targeting YopE into HeLa cells. *J. Biol. Chem.* 274:22102–22108.

15. Chilcott, G. S., and K. T. Hughes. 1998. The type III secretion determinants of the flagellar anti-transcription factor, FlgM, extend from the amino-terminus into the anti-$\sigma28$ domain. *Mol. Microbiol.* 30:1029–1040.

16. Collazo, C. M., and J. E. Galán. 1996. Requirement for exported proteins in secretion through the invasion-associated type III system of *Salmonella typhimurium*. *Infect. Immun.* 64:3524–3531.

17. Collazo, C. M., M. K. Zierler, and J. E. Galán. 1995. Functional analysis of the *Salmonella typhimurium* invasion genes *invI* and *invJ* and identification of a target of the protein secretion apparatus encoded in the *inv* locus. *Mol. Microbiol.* 15:25–38.

18. Crago, A. M., and V. Koronakis. 1998. *Salmonella* InvG forms a ring-like multimer that re-

quires InvH lipoprotein for outer membrane localization. *Mol. Microbiol.* **30:**47–56.

19. **Daefler, S., and M. Russel.** 1998. The *Salmonella typhimurium* InvH protein is an outer membrane lipoprotein required for the proper localization of InvG. *Mol. Microbiol.* **28:**1367–1380.

20. **Daniell, S., N. Takahashi, R. Wilson, D. Friedberg, I. Rosenshine, F. P. Booy, R. K. Shaw, S. Knutton, G. Frankel, and S.-I. Aizawa.** 2001. The filamentous type III secretion translocon of enteropathogenic *Escherichia coli*. *Cell. Microbiol.* **3:**865–871.

21. **Daniell, S. J., R. M. Delahay, R. K. Shaw, E. L. Hartland, M. J. Pallen, F. Booy, F. Ebel, S. Knutton, and G. Frankel.** 2001. Coiled-coil domain of enteropathogenic *Escherichia coli* type III secreted protein EspD is involved in EspA filament-mediated cell attachment and hemolysis. *Infect. Immun.* **69:**4055–4064.

22. **Darwin, K. H., and V. L. Miller.** 1999. Molecular basis of the interaction of *Salmonella* with the intestinal mucosa. *Clin. Microbiol. Rev.* **12:**405–428.

23. **Darwin, K. H., L. S. Robinson, and V. L. Miller.** 2001. SigE is a chaperone for the *Salmonella enterica* serovar Typhimurium invasion protein SigD. *J. Bacteriol.* **183:**1452–1454.

24. **Day, J. B., and G. V. Plano.** 2000. The *Yersinia pestis* YscY protein directly binds YscX, a secreted component of the type III secretion machine. *J. Bacteriol.* **182:**1834–1843.

25. **De Geyter, C., R. Wattiez, P. Sansonetti, P. Falmagne, J.-M. Ruysschaert, C. Parsot, and V. Cabiaux.** 2000. Characterization of the interaction of IpaB and IpaD, proteins required for entry of *Shigella flexneri* into epithelial cells, with a lipid membrane. *Eur. J. Biochem.* **267:**5769–5776.

26. **Donnenberg, M. S., and T. S. Whittam.** 2001. Pathogenesis and evolution of virulence in enteropathogenic and enterohemorrhagic *Escherichia coli*. *J. Clin. Invest.* **107:**539–548.

27. **Eichelberg, E., C. C. Ginocchio, and J. E. Galán.** 1994. Molecular and functional characterization of the *Salmonella typhimurium* invasion genes *invB* and *invC*: homology of InvC to the F_0F_1 ATPase family of proteins. *J. Bacteriol.* **176:**4501–4510.

28. **Elliot, S. J., S. W. Hutcheson, M. S. Dubois, J. L. Mellies, L. A. Wainwright, M. Batchelor, G. Frankel, S. Knutton, and J. B. Kaper.** 1999. Identification of CesT, a chaperone for the type III secretion of Tir in enteropathogenic *Escherichia coli*. *Mol. Microbiol.* **33:**1176–1189.

29. **Elliott, S. J., C. B. O'Connell, A. Koutsouris, C. Brinkley, M. S. Donnenberg, G. Hecht, and J. B. Kaper.** 2002. A gene from the locus of enterocyte effacement that is required for enteropathogenic *Escherichia coli* to increase tight-junction permeabiity encodes a chaperone for EspF. *Infect. Immun.* **70:**2271–2277.

30. **Fan, F., and R. M. Macnab.** 1996. Enzymatic characterization of FliI: an ATPase involved in flagellar assembly in *Salmonella typhimurium*. *J. Biol. Chem.* **271:**31981–31988.

31. **Francis, M. S., S. A. Lloyd, and H. Wolf-Watz.** 2001. The type III secretion chaperone LcrH co-operates with YopD to establish a negative regulatory loop for control of Yop synthesis in *Yersinia pseudotuberculosis*. *Mol. Microbiol.* **42:**1075–1093.

32. **Fu, Y., and J. E. Galán.** 1998. Identification of a specific chaperone for SptP, a substrate of the centisome 63 type III secretion system of *Salmonella typhimurium*. *J. Bacteriol.* **180:**3393–3399.

33. **Fu, Y., and J. E. Galán.** 1999. A *Salmonella* protein antagonizes Rac-1 and Cdc42 to mediate host-cell recovery after bacterial invasion. *Nature* **401:**293–297.

34. **Ginocchio, C. C., S. B. Olmsted, C. L. Wells, and J. E. Galán.** 1994. Contact with epithelial cells induces the formation of surface appendages on *Salmonella typhimurium*. *Cell* **76:**717–724.

35. **Håkansson, S., K. Schesser, C. Persson, E. E. Galyov, R. Rosqvist, F. Homble, and H. Wolf-Watz.** 1996. The YopB protein of *Yersinia pseudotuberculosis* is essential for the translocation of Yop effector proteins across the target cell plasma membrane and displays a contact-dependent membrane disrupting activity. *EMBO J.* **15:**5812–5823.

36. **Hartland, E. L., S. J. Daniell, R. M. Delahay, B. C. Neves, T. Wallis, R. K. Shaw, C. Hale, S. Knutton, and G. Frankel.** 2000. The type III protein translocation system of enteropathogenic *Escherichia coli* involves EspA-EspB protein interactions. *Mol. Microbiol.* **35:**1483–1492.

37. **Hayward, R. D., E. J. McGhie, and V. Koronakis.** 2000. Membrane fusion activity of purified SipB, a *Salmonella* surface protein essential for mammalian cell invasion. *Mol. Microbiol.* **37:**727–739.

38. **Hersh, D., D. M. Monack, M. R. Smith, N. Ghori, S. Falkow, and A. Zychlinsky.** 1999. The *Salmonella* invasin SipB induces macrophage apoptosis by binding to caspase-1. *Proc. Natl. Acad. Sci. USA* **96:**2396–2401.

39. **Hoiczyk, E., and G. Blobel.** 2001. Polymerization of a single protein of the pathogen *Yersinia enterocolitica* into needles punctures eukaryotic cells. *Proc. Natl. Acad. Sci. USA* **98:**4669–4674.

40. **Hueck, C. J.** 1998. Type III protein secretion systems in bacterial pathogens of animals and plants. *Microbiol. Molec. Biol. Rev.* **62**:379–433.

41. **Ide, T., S. Laarmann, L. Greune, H. Schillers, H. Oberleithner, and M. A. Schmidt.** 2001. Characterizaton of translocation pores inserted into plasma membranes by type III-secreted Esp proteins of enteropathogenic *Escherichia coli. Cell. Microbiol.* **3**:669–679.

42. **Iriarte, M., and G. R. Cornelis.** 1999. Identification of SycN, YscX, and YscY, three new elements of the *Yersinia* Yop virulon. *J. Bacteriol.* **181**:675–680.

43. **Jin, Q., and S.-Y. He.** 2001. Role of the Hrp pilus in type III secretion in *Pseudomonas syringae. Science* **294**:2556–2558.

44. **Kaniga, K., D. Trollinger, and J. E. Galán.** 1995. Identification of two targets of the type III protein secretion system encoded by the *inv* and *spa* loci of *Salmonella typhimurium* that have homology to the *Shigella* IpaD and IpaA proteins. *J. Bacteriol.* **177**:7078–7085.

45. **Karlinsey, J. E., J. Lonner, K. L. Brown, and K. T. Hughes.** 2000. Translation/secretion coupling by type III secretion systems. *Cell* **102**:487–497.

46. **Karlinsey, J. E., S. Tanaka, V. Bettenworth, S. Yamaguchi, W. Boos, S.-I. Aizawa, and K. T. Hughes.** 2000. Completion of the hook-basal body complex of the *Salmonella typhimurium* flagellum is coupled to FlgM secretion and *fliC* transcription. *Mol. Microbiol.* **37**:1220–1231.

47. **Kenny, B., L. C. Lai, B. B. Finlay, and M. S. Donnenberg.** 1996. EspA, a protein secreted by enteropathogenic *Escherichia coli*, is required to induce signals in epithelial cells. *Mol. Microbiol.* **20**:313–323.

48. **Kimbrough, T. G., and S. I. Miller.** 2000. Contribution of *Salmonella typhimurium* type III secretion components to needle complex formation. *Proc. Natl. Acad. Sci. USA* **97**:11008–11013.

49. **Knutton, S., I. Rosenshine, M. J. Pallen, I. Nisan, B. C. Neves, C. Bain, C. Wolff, G. Dougan, and G. Frankel.** 1998. A novel EspA-associated surface organelle of enteropathogenic *Escherichia coli* involved in protein translocation into epithelial cells. *EMBO J.* **17**:2166–2176.

50. **Kubori, T., Y. Matsushima, D. Nakamura, J. Uralil, M. Lara-Tejero, A. Sukhan, J. E. Galán, and S.-I. Aizawa.** 1998. Supramolecular structure of the *Salmonella typhimurium* type III protein secretion system. *Science* **280**:602–605.

51. **Kubori, T., A. Sukhan, S.-I. Aizawa, and J. E. Galán.** 2000. Molecular characterization and assembly of the needle complex of the *Salmonella typhimurium* type III protein secretion system. *Proc. Natl. Acad. Sci. USA* **97**:10225–10230.

52. **Kuwae, A., S. Yoshida, K. Tamano, H. Imuro, T. Suzuki, and C. Sasakawa.** 2001. *Shigella* invasion of macrophage requires the insertion of IpaC into the host plasma membrane. *J. Biol. Chem.* **276**:32230–32239.

53. **Lee, C. A., M. Silva, A. M. Siber, A. J. Kelly, E. Galyov, and B. A. McCormick.** 2000. A secreted *Salmonella* protein induces a proinflammatory response in epithelial cells, which promotes neutrophil migration. *Proc. Natl. Acad. Sci. USA* **97**:12283–12288.

54. **Lee, V. T., S. K. Mazmanian, and O. Schneewind.** 2001. A program of *Yersinia enterocolitica* type III secretion reactions is activated by specific signals. *J. Bacteriol.* **183**:4970–4978.

55. **Lee, V. T., and O. Schneewind.** 1999. Type III machines of pathogenic yersiniae secrete virulence factors into the extracellular milieu. *Mol. Microbiol.* **31**:1619–1629.

56. **Li, J., H. Ochman, E. A. Groisman, E. F. Boyd, F. Solomon, K. Nelson, and R. K. Selander.** 1995. Relationship between evolutionary rate and cellular location among the Inv/Spa invasion proteins of *Salmonella enterica. Proc. Natl. Acad. Sci. USA* **92**:7252–7256.

57. **Lloyd, S. A., M. Norman, R. Rosqvist, and H. Wolf-Watz.** 2001. *Yersinia* YopE is targeted for type III secretion by N-terminal, not mRNA, signals. *Mol. Microbiol.* **39**:520–531.

58. **Luo, Y., M. G. Bertero, E. A. Frey, R. A. Pfuetzner, M. R. Wenk, L. Creagh, S. L. Marcus, D. Lim, R. Sicheri, C. Kay, C. Haynes, B. B. Finlay, and N. C. Strynadka.** 2001. Structural and biochemical characterization of the type III secretion chaperones CesT and SigE. *Nat. Struct. Biol.* **8**:1031–1036.

59. **Makishima, S., K. Komoriya, S. Yamaguchi, and S.-I. Aizawa.** 2001. Length of the flagellar hook and the capacity of the type III export apparatus. *Science* **291**:2411–2413.

60. **Ménard, R., P. Sansonetti, and C. Parsot.** 1994. The secretion of the *Shigella flexneri* Ipa invasins is activated by epithelial cells and controlled by IpaB and IpaD. *EMBO J.* **13**:5293–5302.

61. **Ménard, R., P. Sansonetti, C. Parsot, and T. Vasselon.** 1994. Extracellular association and cytoplasmic partitioning of the IpaB and IpaC invasins of *S. flexneri. Cell* **79**:515–525.

62. **Miao, E. A., and S. I. Miller.** 2000. A conserved amino acid sequence directing intracellular type III secretion by *Salmonella typhimurium. Proc. Natl. Acad. Sci. USA* **97**:7539–7544.

63. **Miao, E. A., C. A. Scherer, R. M. Tsolis, R. A. Kingsley, L. G. Adams, A. J. Bäumler, and S. I. Miller.** 1999. *Salmonella typhimurium* leucine-rich repeat proteins are targeted to the

SPI1 and SPI2 type III secretion systems. *Mol. Microbiol.* **34:**850–864.

64. **Minamino, T., B. González-Pedrajo, K. Yamaguchi, S.-I. Aizawa, and R. M. Macnab.** 1999. FliK, the protein responsible for flagellar hook length control in *Salmonella*, is exported during hook assembly. *Mol. Microbiol.* **34:** 295–304.

65. **Minamino, T., and R. M. Macnab.** 1999. Components of the *Salmonella* flagellar export apparatus and classification of export substrates. *J. Bacteriol.* **181:**1388–1394.

66. **Minamino, T., and R. M. Macnab.** 2000. FliH, a soluble component of the type III flagellar export apparatus of *Salmonella*, forms a complex with FliI and inhibits its ATPase activity. *Mol. Microbiol.* **37:**1494–1503.

67. **Minamino, T., and R. M. Macnab.** 2000. Interactions among components of the *Salmonella* flagellar export apparatus and its substrates. *Mol. Microbiol.* **35:**1052–1064.

68. **Muramoto, K., S. Makishima, S.-I. Aizawa, and R. M. Macnab.** 1998. Effect of the cellular level of FliK on flagellar hook and filament assembly in *Salmonella typhimurium*. *J. Mol. Biol.* **277:**871–882.

69. **Nguyen, L., I. T. Paulsen, J. Tchieu, C. J. Hueck, and M. H. Saier, Jr.** 2000. Phylogenetic analyses of the constituents of type III protein secretion systems. *J. Mol. Microbiol. Biotechnol.* **2:**125–144.

70. **Osiecki, J. C., J. Barker, W. L. Picking, A. B. Serfis, E. Berring, S. Shah, A. Harrington, and W. D. Picking.** 2001. IpaC from *Shigella* and SipC from *Salmonella* possess similar biochemical properties but are functionally distinct. *Molec. Microbiol.* **42:**469–481.

71. **Page, A.-L., M. Fromont-Racine, P. Sansonetti, P. Legrain, and C. Parsot.** 2001. Characterization of the interaction partners of secreted proteins and chaperones of *Shigella flexneri*. *Mol. Microbiol.* **42:**1133–1145.

72. **Picking, W. L., L. Coye, J. C. Osiecki, A. B. Serfis, E. Schaper, and W. D. Picking.** 2001. Identification of functional regions within invasion plasmid antigen C (IpaC) of *Shigella flexneri*. *Mol. Microbiol.* **39:**100–111.

73. **Plano, G. V., J. B. Day, and F. Ferracci.** 2001. Type III export: new uses for an old pathway. *Mol. Microbiol.* **40:**284–293.

74. **Reed, K. A., M. A. Clark, T. A. Booth, C. J. Hueck, S. I. Miller, B. H. Hirst, and M. A. Jepson.** 1998. Cell-contact-stimulated formation of filamentous appendages by *Salmonella typhimurium* does not depend on the type III secretion system encoded by *Salmonella* pathogenicity island 1. *Infect. Immun.* **66:**2007–2017.

75. **Rosqvist, R., S. Håkansson, Å. Forsberg, and H. Wolf-Watz.** 1995. Functional conservation of the secretion and translocation machinery for virulence proteins of yersinia, salmonellae and shigellae. *EMBO J.* **14:**4187–4195.

76. **Scherer, C. A., E. Cooper, and S. I. Miller.** 2000. The *Salmonella* type III secretion translocon protein SspC is inserted into the epithelial cell plasma membrane upon infection. *Mol. Microbiol.* **37:**1133–1145.

77. **Schuch, R., and A. T. Maurelli.** 2001. MxiM and MxiJ, base elements of the Mxi-Spa type III secretion system of *Shigella*, interact with and stabilize the MxiD secretin in the cell envelope. *J. Bacteriol.* **183:**6991–6998.

78. **Schuch, R., and A. T. Maurelli.** 2001. Spa33, a cell surface-associated subunit of the Mxi-Spa type III secretory pathway of *Shigella flexneri*, regulates Ipa protein traffic. *Infect. Immun.* **69:**2180–2189.

79. **Sekiya, K., M. Ohishi, T. Ogino, K. Tamano, C. Sasakawa, and A. Abe.** 2001. Supermolecular structure of the enteropathogenic *Escherichia coli* type III secretion system and its direct interaction with the EspA-sheath-like structure. *Proc. Natl. Acad. Sci. USA* **98:**11638–11643.

80. **Shaw, R. K., S. Daniell, F. Ebel, G. Frankel, and S. Knutton.** 2001. EspA filament-mediated protein translocation into red blood cells. *Cell. Microbiol.* **3:**213–222.

81. **Stebbins, C. E., and J. E. Galán.** 2001. Maintenance of an unfolded polypeptide by a cognate chaperone in bacterial type III secretion. *Nature* **414:**77–81.

82. **Sukhan, A., T. Kubori, J. Wilson, and J. E. Galán.** 2001. Genetic analysis of assembly of the *Salmonella enterica* serovar Typhimurium type III secretion-associated needle complex. *J. Bacteriol.* **183:**1159–1167.

83. **Tamano, K., S.-I. Aizawa, E. Katayama, T. Nonaka, S. Imajoh-Ohmi, A. Kuwae, S. Nagai, and C. Sasakawa.** 2000. Supramolecular structure of the *Shigella* type III secretion machinery: the needle part is changeable in length and essential for delivery of effectors. *EMBO J.* **19:**3876–3887.

84. **Tamano, K., E. Katayama, T. Toyotome, and C. Sasakawa.** 2002. *Shigella* Spa32 is an essential secretory protein for functional type III secretion machinery and uniformity of its needle length. *J. Bacteriol.* **184:**1244–1252.

85. **Tran, N., A. B. Serfis, J. C. Osiecki, W. L. Picking, L. Coye, R. Davis, and W. D. Picking.** 2000. Interaction of *Shigella flexneri* IpaC with model membranes correlates with effects on cultured cells. *Infect. Immun.* **68:**3710–3715.

86. **Tran Van Nhieu, G., E. Caron, A. Hall, and P. J. Sansonetti.** 1999. IpaC induces actin polymerization and filopodia formation during *Shigella* entry into epithelial cells. *EMBO J.* **18:** 3249–3262.

87. **Tucker, S. C., and J. E. Galán.** 2000. Complex function for SicA, a *Salmonella enterica* serovar Typhimurium type III secretion-associated chaperone. *J. Bacteriol.* **182:**2262–2268.

88. **Viboud, G. I., and J. B. Bliska.** 2001. A bacterial type III secretion system inhibits actin polymerization to prevent pore formation in host cell membranes. *EMBO J.* **20:**5373–5382.

89. **Wachter, C., C. Beinke, M. Mattes, and M. A. Schmidt.** 1999. Insertion of EspD into epithelial target cell membranes by infecting enteropathogenic *Escherichia coli. Mol. Microbiol.* **31:** 1695–1707.

90. **Wainwright, L. A., and J. B. Kaper.** 1998. EspB and EspD require a specific chaperone for proper secretion from enteropathogenic *Escherichia coli. Mol. Microbiol.* **27:**1247–1260.

91. **Warawa, J., B. B. Finlay, and B. Kenny.** 1999. Type III secretion-dependent hemolytic activity of enteropathogenic *Escherichia coli. Infect. Immun.* **67:**5538–5540.

92. **Watarai, M., T. Tobe, M. Yoshikawa, and C. Sasakawa.** 1995. Contact of *Shigella* with host cells triggers release of Ipa invasins and is an essential function of invasiveness. *EMBO J.* **14:** 2461–2470.

93. **Wilson, R. K., R. K. Shaw, S. Danniell, S. Knutton, and G. Frankel.** 2001. Role of EscF, a putative needle complex protein, in the type III protein translocation system of enteropathogenic *Escherichia coli. Cell. Microbiol.* **3:**753–762.

94. **Wolff, C., I. Nisan, E. Hanski, G. Frankel, and I. Rosenshine.** 1998. Protein translocation into host epithelial cells by infecting enteropathogenic *Escherichia coli. Mol. Microbiol.* **28:**143–155.

95. **Wulff-Strobel, C. R., A. W. Williams, and S. C. Straley.** 2002. LcrQ and SycH function together at the Ysc type III secretion system in *Yersinia pestis* to impose a hierarchy of secretion. *Mol. Microbiol.* **43:**411–423.

96. **Zhou, D., M. S. Mooseker, and J. E. Galán.** 1999. An invasion-associated *Salmonella* protein modulates the actin-bundling activity of plastin. *Proc. Natl. Acad. Sci. USA* **96:**10176–10181.

97. **Zierler, M. K., and J. E. Galán.** 1995. Contact with cultured epithelial cells stimulates secretion of *Salmonella typhimurium* invasion protein InvJ. *Infect. Immun.* **63:**4024–4028.

HOW NONINVASIVE PATHOGENS INDUCE DISEASE: LESSONS FROM ENTEROPATHOGENIC AND ENTEROHEMORRHAGIC *ESCHERICHIA COLI*

Bruce A. Vallance, Crystal Chan, and B. Brett Finlay

23

In recent years, there has been a dramatic renewal of interest in the study of microbial pathogenesis. A novel focus of this work has been on defining the molecular and cellular mechanisms underlying the interactions between bacterial pathogens and host cells. In particular, an emerging theme has been the ability of many pathogens to hijack the host cell cytoskeleton and signal transduction pathways to colonize their hosts. Much of this research has examined bacterial pathogens that invade their hosts, such as *Salmonella* sp. and *Shigella* sp. In contrast, the extracellular bacterial pathogen enteropathogenic *Escherichia coli* (EPEC) has provided important lessons on the mechanisms used by noninvasive pathogens to cause disease. EPEC initially binds to the surface of intestinal epithelial cells and secretes virulence factors that are directly injected into the underlying cell through a type III secretion system (4). These translocated bacterial proteins ("effectors") interact with host cell components and signaling pathways, altering their function. These changes in host cell physiology, as well as the resulting host

inflammatory response, ultimately lead to diarrheal disease. As a result, EPEC is a serious and widespread cause of infantile diarrhea, particularly in developing countries (31, 36).

Using similar mechanisms, EPEC's more infamous relative enterohemorrhagic *E. coli* (EHEC), the causative agent of hamburger disease, inflicts diarrheal disease in adults as well as children and has been implicated in sporadic diarrheal outbreaks across North America. During infection, EPEC and EHEC induce a characteristic "attaching and effacing" (A/E) histopathology on gut enterocytes. A/E lesions are characterized by localized effacement of microvilli and intimate bacterial attachment to the underlying epithelial cells (31, 36). This is followed by changes in the cytoskeleton, with the most prominent being the accumulation of polymerized actin directly beneath the adherent bacteria. This actin reorganization forms a pedestal-like structure upon which the bacterium resides. A/E lesion formation thus firmly anchors the bacterium to the host cell and appears to be essential for EPEC pathogenicity.

Recent studies by our laboratory and others have radically altered our understanding of how EPEC and EHEC attach to host cells. These studies have been directed toward identifying the roles of many of EPEC's virulence

Bruce A. Vallance, Crystal Chan, and B. Brett Finlay, Biotechnology Laboratory, University of British Columbia, Vancouver, B.C., V6T 1Z3, Canada.

Microbial Pathogenesis and the Intestinal Epithelial Cell, ed. by G. Hecht factors in the regulation of host cytoskeletal rearrangements and altered host gene expression. These secreted bacterial proteins corrupt the normal function of host cell systems, redirecting the cells' own structural components to support the attachment of EPEC. These bacterial effectors also induce changes in host cell signaling pathways that not only contribute to pedestal formation, but also alter barrier function in a process that likely contributes to the diarrheal disease caused by EPEC infection. The key finding in this process was the discovery that EPEC inserts its own receptor (translocated intimin receptor [Tir]) into the membrane of host cells (25), rather than binding to a host receptor. Since this finding, a number of related A/E bacterial pathogens have also been shown to produce Tir homologues, including the hemolytic uremic syndrome causing EHEC, as well as animal pathogens such as rabbit enteropathogenic *E. coli* (REPEC) and the mouse pathogen *Citrobacter rodentium*. These findings indicate that the process of intimate attachment is conserved among this family of enteric pathogens. Since studies investigating the function of EPEC's virulence factors are the most advanced, in this chapter we consider EPEC as the prototype for the family of A/E-inducing pathogens.

DISEASE AND EPIDEMIOLOGY

EPEC is endemic in many parts of the world and is a well-established cause of diarrhea in young children, particularly in developing countries. Disease outbreaks in developed countries were still frequent until the 1940s and 1950s, but the incidence of EPEC infection in the United States and United Kingdom has since declined. Even so, EPEC is still responsible for occasional outbreaks in day care centers and pediatric wards. In contrast, EPEC has continued to remain an important cause of infant mortality in developing countries (31). Transmission is thought to occur through person to person contact, with recent outbreaks reporting mortality rates of up to 30%. EPEC infection is estimated to cause the

deaths of several hundred thousand children per year owing to dehydration and other complications (31). The hallmark of EPEC infection is the A/E histopathology (see Fig. 1) observed following the infection of epithelial cells in tissue culture and in small bowel biopsy specimens from infected patients. Infection generally causes profuse but acute watery diarrhea, but severe cases can lead to a protracted disease, resulting in chronic diarrhea. Aside from diarrhea, common symptoms of EPEC infection include vomiting and fever (31).

A more recently identified microbe, EHEC has in recent years eclipsed EPEC in notoriety as a pathogen in North America. First widely recognized as the causative agent of hamburger disease, EHEC is a zoonotic pathogen that appears to be asymptomatically carried by various ruminants. Cattle appear to be the major reservoir for this pathogen, with fecal contamination of meat or water supplies responsible for most outbreaks. Unlike EPEC, EHEC produces and releases Shiga toxin during infection, resulting in a worsening of dis-

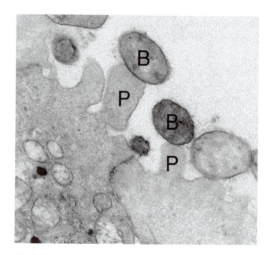

FIGURE 1 Transmission electron micrograph of A/E lesions in rabbit intestinal epithelial tissue (Peyer's patch) caused by the REPEC O103. Bacteria are labeled with "B"; pedestals are labeled with "P." (×20,000.) (Photograph courtesy of Ursula Heczko, Biotechnology Laboratory, University of British Columbia, modified with permission from reference 36.)

ease symptoms (31). As a result, infection can cause bloody diarrhea in both adults and children, and in severe cases, the toxin can shut down the kidneys, leading to hemolytic uremic syndrome and occasionally death. Based on the morbidity and mortality associated with these two microbes, both EPEC and EHEC strains are considered significant human health threats.

THE LOCUS OF ENTEROCYTE EFFACEMENT

All the genes necessary for EPEC to cause A/E lesions are contained within a 35-kb pathogenicity island called the locus of enterocyte effacement (LEE) (31, 36). The G+C content of the LEE is 38.4%, significantly lower than the 50% G+C composition of the surrounding E. coli chromosome. This difference in nucleotide content suggests that the LEE was inserted into the EPEC chromosome from a foreign source. The complete LEE region contains 41 genes that encode a type III secretion system, as well as other genes necessary for pedestal formation. These include several genes coding for type III-secreted proteins, termed Esps (EPEC-secreted proteins). Most of these proteins, including EspA, EspB, and EspD as well as an adhesin, intimin, and its translocated receptor Tir, are required for pedestal formation. However, there are other EPEC-secreted proteins such as EspF, EspG, and Orf19 (12, 24, 30) that, when mutated, have no effect on pedestal formation. The roles of these bacterial effectors in EPEC pathogenesis will be discussed in more detail later in the chapter.

Similar to other type III secretion systems, EPEC-secreted effector proteins require cytosolic chaperone proteins in order to be translocated. Two chaperones have been identified in the LEE, the CesD chaperone for EspB and EspD (36) and CesT, which chaperones Tir (28). Interestingly, the crystal structure of EHEC CesT was recently solved (28) and possesses similar structural characteristics to other type III chaperones. DNA sequences with a high degree of homology to the EPEC

LEE have been found in the other A/E lesion-causing bacteria, including EHEC, as well as the animal pathogens C. rodentium and REPEC. Examining the phylogeny of these various LEE sequences suggests that some pathogens acquired the LEE independently during their evolution (11). Despite these subtle differences, the similarity between LEEs suggests a common pathway underlying A/E lesion formation. This pathway is also self-contained, since the introduction of the cloned LEE of EPEC into a nonpathogenic E. coli strain was found to confer the ability to form A/E lesions.

LOCALIZED ADHERENCE OF EPEC TO EPITHELIAL CELLS

Infection of host cells by EPEC has been proposed to entail three distinct stages. The first stage involves the initial adherence of the bacterium to the host's intestinal epithelium. During this stage, EPEC form dense microcolonies on the surface of cells in a pattern known as localized adherence. A plasmid-encoded bundle-forming pilus (BFP) is thought to mediate localized adherence. Mutants lacking the BFP plasmid still attach to host cells, but do not form microcolonies and produce fewer A/E lesions than wild-type EPEC. Interestingly, BFP is an important virulence factor, since BFP mutant strains are severely impaired in causing diarrheal disease in human volunteers (31). Curiously, the mediators of this initial attachment vary among the family of A/E pathogens. For example, EHEC lacks BFP and, unlike EPEC, infects the colon rather than the ileum. Therefore, the site of bacterial colonization may be influenced by the expression of BFP and other adhesions such as fimbriae (29), as well as by environmental factors regulating the expression of other virulence factors.

EPEC-SECRETED PROTEINS

The second stage of EPEC pathogenesis involves the production and release of bacterial proteins, including the LEE pathogenicity island encoded Esps A-H. Also located within the LEE are the *esc* and *sep* genes that code for a type III secretion system that translocates these Esp proteins from the bacterial cytoplasm to the external environment. The supermolecular structure of EPEC's type III secretion machinery was recently characterized (34) and is thought to generate a pore in the host cell that allows this translocation. Much like the type III secretion systems used by *Yersinia* sp. and *Salmonella* sp., the type III secretion system in EPEC appears to enable virulence factors to be translocated directly from the bacterial cytoplasm to the host cell membrane or cytoplasm. Mutation of many of EPEC's secreted proteins abrogates A/E lesion formation. Despite this knowledge, the roles of these secreted proteins in EPEC pathogenesis are poorly defined. For example, EspA forms transient filamentous appendages on the bacterial surface (36). These filaments function as a physical bridge between the bacterium and the host cell that subsequently acts as a conduit for the translocation of bacterial effector proteins into the host cell. In contrast, EspB is directly translocated into the host membrane and cytosol by a process dependent on EspA (36), while EspD is also inserted into the host cell membrane. Based on their ability to lyse red blood cells and their sequence homology to previously characterized translocated *Yersinia* effector proteins, EspB and EspD are likely structural components of the translocation apparatus, forming a pore in the host membrane.

In the last few years, several new translocated effectors have been identified and studied. These include EspF and EspG, as well as Orf19, now termed mitochondrial-associated protein (MAP); however, probably other effectors remain to be identified with the LEE. Interestingly, mutation of these three genes appears to have no effect on pedestal formation by EPEC. In particular, the role of EspF in EPEC pathogenesis had been an unresolved question ever since its identification. In studies by Hecht, Donnenberg, and colleagues, EspF-adenylate cyclase fusions were shown to translocate into the host cell cytoplasm (30).

Studies looking at the effects of EPEC infection on barrier function in polarized intestinal epithelial cell monolayers found that EspF mutants were significantly impaired in their ability to disrupt barrier function compared to wild-type EPEC (30). Since impaired intestinal barrier function is a potential contributory factor to diarrheal disease, it has been proposed that EPEC translocates EspF into host cells to trigger the diarrhea associated with EPEC infection. Unfortunately, examination of the role of EspF in diarrheal disease in a relevant animal model has yet to be performed. Additional studies suggested a role for EspF in triggering apoptosis in host cells (5); however, it should be noted that the mode of host cell death induced by EPEC infection is a contentious issue, with studies in tissue culture difficult to interpret.

Two other EPEC effectors translocated into host cells are EspG and MAP. The loss of EspG, the homologue of *Shigella*'s VirA, causes no apparent defects in pedestal formation in tissue culture, but studies infecting rabbits with the RDEC-1 strain of REPEC, deficient in EspG, found delayed intestinal colonization (12). The exact role of EspG is unclear but may be related to the initial interactions between A/E lesion-causing pathogens and intestinal epithelium. Another recently described bacterial effector is MAP. As the name implies, following translocation into host cells, this effector is specifically targeted to the host cell mitochondria (24). The purpose of this interaction with the mitochondrion is still being studied, but MAP may interfere with the functions of this organelle by subverting energy production or allowing the bacterium to take control over host cell death.

INTIMATE ADHERENCE AND THE ROLE OF TIR

The third stage of EPEC infection is characterized by the effacement of microvilli, intimate attachment, and pedestal formation. The outer membrane protein, intimin, is an essential virulence factor required for the intimate attachment of the bacterium to the host cell. A 94-kDa protein encoded by the LEE *eae* gene, intimin mediates intimate attachment by binding to Tir following its translocation into the host membrane (25). Under sodium dodecyl sulfate-polyacrylamide gel electrophoresis (SDS-PAGE) analysis, the bacterial form of Tir migrates as 78 kDa, but following translocation into the host membrane, Tir undergoes phosphorylation on tyrosine, serine, and threonine residues (23). These modifications account for the apparent shift to 90 kDa for the membrane form of Tir. The crystal structures of the EPEC intimin carboxy-terminal fragment and the EPEC Tir intimin binding domain (IBD) have recently been described, providing insight into the molecular details of intimate adherence (27).

EPEC's delivery of Tir represents the first example of a pathogen injecting its own receptor into mammalian cells and has revised our concepts of how bacterial pathogens interact with and infect cells. By bypassing the usual dependence on a membrane-bound, host-derived receptor, EPEC can, at least in tissue culture, infect cells of most types and species. Based on its novel role in EPEC pathogenesis, Tir has undergone intense study since its identification. The transfer of Tir to the host cell requires the type III secretion system and those Esps required for A/E lesion formation. Tir has two predicted transmembrane domains and is proposed to adopt a hairpin-shaped conformation in the host membrane (27, 36). As predicted, the N- and C-terminal regions of Tir are located within the cell, while the intervening region between the transmembrane domains forms an extracellular loop. The transmembrane domains of Tir are critical for the translocation of Tir into the host membrane, while the extracellular loop (now termed the IBD) binds the C-terminal region of intimin. The Tir-intimin binding then leads to intimate attachment of EPEC to the surface of the host cell, and has been shown to be essential for pedestal formation and actin condensation (25, 29). Aside from acting as the receptor for intimin, Tir has

been implicated in several other processes, such as providing a link between the bacterium and the host-cell cytoskeleton, and triggering signaling events within the host cell. EPEC Tir undergoes several phosphorylation events in the host cell, with phosphorylation on tyrosine 474 being critical for pedestal formation. Interestingly, EPEC Tir does not undergo complete phosphorylation when delivered into host cells by EPEC-independent mechanisms. This suggests that other EPEC factors must be coexpressed with Tir for it to undergo full, functional modification inside the host. In contrast, EHEC Tir is not tyrosine phosphorylated inside the host and does not require tyrosine modification to orchestrate pedestal formation (10). In complementation studies, EHEC was able to form pedestals when its Tir was replaced by either wild-type EPEC Tir or the Y474F mutant. In contrast, EHEC Tir cannot functionally substitute for its homologue in EPEC (9, 22). These findings indicate that EPEC and EHEC Tir use different mechanisms and signaling pathways to mediate similar changes in the actin cytoskeleton.

Interestingly, intimin has been shown to bind in vitro to factors in host cells other than Tir through its C-terminal region (int280) (13). Such binding requires the cysteine 937 residue (13) and suggests that intimin may bind a host receptor on epithelial cells, as well as the bacterial-derived Tir. β1 integrins, along with other host proteins, have been proposed as the host cell factors mediating such binding. While integrins are not found on the apical surface of enterocytes, they are expressed on the apical surface of M cells overlying Peyer's patches, as well as by several types of immune cells (13). Indirect support for this concept comes from studies infecting mice with *C. rodentium* expressing its own intimin or that from EPEC. As expected, infection caused a strong immune response as well as colonic epithelial hyperplasia, but interestingly, an enema of formalin-fixed bacteria given to an ethanol-pretreated colon caused a similar host response, although an intimin substitution mutant for cysteine 937 failed to elicit this reaction (13, 20). Since Tir could not be delivered in this manner, these data suggest that intimin binding to a host cell receptor precipitates these events. An intriguing hypothesis would involve A/E pathogens directly interacting with mucosal T lymphocytes expressing β1 integrins to trigger the inflammation and intestinal pathology seen during infection. However, until such an interaction is demonstrated, the relevance of a host receptor for intimin will remain unclear.

STRUCTURE OF THE EPEC-INDUCED PEDESTAL

Immunofluorescence studies have shown that in addition to membrane-bound Tir, the tips of EPEC pedestals contain predominantly filamentous (F)-actin (Fig. 2), as well as talin, α-actinin, ezrin, and several other cytoskeletal proteins. As described by Goosney et al., these same proteins as well as other cytoskeletal and signaling proteins (16) accumulate along the length of the pedestal, with several thought to be involved in the cross-linking of actin microfilaments. Non-muscle myosin II and tropomyosin are also present, but at the base of the pedestal. While host cell cytoskeletal rearrangements are responsible for pedestal formation, they probably also mediate the effacement of microvilli seen in A/E lesions. It has been suggested that the loss of microvilli may result from a bacterial-triggered depolymerization of microvilli actin, which is then recruited to form pedestals. However, some proteins found in pedestals are not found in microvilli, suggesting a more complex process than a mere rebuilding of microvilli beneath the adherent bacteria. Interestingly, while EPEC- and EHEC-induced pedestals consist of many similar cytoskeletal proteins, some significant differences do exist; for example, the adaptor proteins Grb2 and CrkII are recruited to the EPEC but not the EHEC pedestal (16). It is unclear if the pathogen-specific recruitment results in any functional differences between EPEC- and EHEC-induced pedestals, since probably not all the cytoskel-

etal proteins identified within pedestals are essential for their formation.

Based on its location at the tip of the pedestal and its predicted structure, Tir is the best bacterial candidate to link EPEC to the host cytoskeleton and direct actin accumulation and pedestal formation. While the mechanism involved is still unclear, Tir may start this process by exploiting regulators of actin dynamics to initiate actin polymerization, such as the Rho family of small GTP-binding proteins. However, the Rac-, Rho-, and Cdc42-dependent pathways are not essential for pedestal formation. Instead, studies have implicated members of the Wiskott-Aldrich syndrome (WAS) family of proteins (WASP and N-WASP), as well as the actin nucleating heptameric Arp2/3 complex in pedestal formation (21). These factors are recruited to the tip of the pedestal (21) (Fig. 2), with recruitment dependent on Tir tyrosine 474 phosphorylation. Interestingly, mutation of the GTPase binding domain of WASP prevented both the recruitment of the Arp2/3 complex and pedestal formation. Thus, both WASP and Arp 2/3 appear to play key roles in the actin polymerization triggered by EPEC; however, a direct interaction between these factors and Tir was not shown (21). Recently, however, Gruenheid et al. demonstrated that the host adaptor protein Nck was required for the recruitment of N-WASP and Arp 2/3 to the pedestal (18). Furthermore, Nck was found to bind directly to phosphotyrosine 474 of EPEC Tir's intracellular carboxy-terminal domain. Mutation of this tyrosine or dephosphorylation prevented Nck from binding, explaining the requirement for this phosphotyrosine in pedestal formation. Fitting with the dispensability of tyrosine 474 phosphorylation in EHEC pathogenesis, EHEC uses a different mechanism and does not require Nck recruitment for pedestal formation (18); however, the factors used by EHEC to substitute for Nck remain to be determined.

Another two of the cytoskeletal proteins found at the tips of pedestals, α-actinin and talin, have also been found to bind directly to

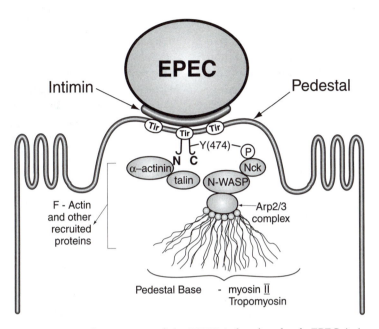

FIGURE 2 The structure of the EPEC-induced pedestal. EPEC intimately attaches to the host cell through intimin-Tir binding. Several cytoskeletal proteins including α-actinin, talin, and Nck are recruited to the tip of the pedestal. Talin binds to Tir, but to which region is unknown; however, α-actinin binds to the N terminus of Tir, while Nck binds to the phosphotyrosine 474 at the C terminus of Tir. Binding of Nck is required for the recruitment of N-WASP and the Arp 2/3 complex, resulting in the nucleation of actin. F-actin, as well as many other host proteins, is found along the length of the pedestal while non-muscle myosin II and tropomyosin are found at the pedestal base. (Modified with permission from reference 36.)

Tir. α-Actinin colocalizes with Tir in infected host cells and its recruitment to pedestals is Tir dependent (17); however, it is still undetermined if α-actinin recruitment is essential for pedestal formation. Binding of α-actinin occurs at the intracellular amino terminus of Tir, rather than the C terminus where Nck binds, and thus is independent of the phosphorylation of Tir's tyrosine 474. Talin also binds to Tir, and although the region that it binds to has not been identified, its recruitment was found to be necessary for pedestal formation (2). Thus, it appears that Tir mediates EPEC infection in at least three ways: (i) it mediates intimate binding between the host cell and bacterium via its intimin binding; (ii) it anchors to α-actinin and perhaps other proteins

through its amino terminus in a tyrosine phosphorylation-independent fashion; and (iii) it recruits other cytoskeletal proteins such as Nck through its carboxyl terminus in a tyrosine phosphorylation-dependent fashion, which then recruits N-WASP and Arp 2/3, resulting in actin polymerization.

SIGNAL TRANSDUCTION

While the cytoskeletal rearrangements that lead to pedestal formation are the most obvious form of EPEC's cellular exploitation, more subtle aspects involve the activation and/or subversion of host signaling pathways. One such pathway results in the tyrosine phosphorylation of substrates that colocalize with the accumulated actin beneath adherent bacteria. The major phosphorylation substrate detected in EPEC-infected cells is Tir (36). These phosphorylation events require both the type III secretion system and the Esps (36), suggesting that EPEC triggers these responses through bacterial effector molecules. Since phosphorylation occurs after Tir enters the host cell, tyrosine kinase activity must be recruited to the vicinity of Tir following its translocation. While its identity is unknown, the tyrosine kinase is probably of host origin and is recruited or activated by bacterial effector proteins, or by Tir mimicking an endogenous substrate. Alternatively, a bacterial effector with tyrosine kinase activity may be translocated into the host cell along with Tir. As previously described, the tyrosine phosphorylation event is critical for actin nucleation during EPEC infection, whereas EHEC O157:H7 Tir is not tyrosine phosphorylated (10), although both pathogens readily induce pedestal formation.

EPEC also induces inositol phosphate fluxes within the host cell, as well as the activation of protein kinase C (PKC), phospholipase-Cγ, and NF-κB (19, 36). Several groups have investigated the effect of EPEC infection on changes in intracellular calcium, but the results have been inconclusive. Crane and Oh measured PKC activity and found that membrane-associated PKC was enhanced, but such a response required intimate adherence, since intimin mutants had no such effect (5a). EPEC also induces the activation of NF-κB in intestinal epithelial cells, resulting in increased interleukin-8 (IL-8) production and the recruitment of polymorphonuclear cells (PMN) in a T84 cell culture model (19). While the importance of many of these signaling events in infection is demonstrated by their requirement for pedestal formation, these studies are preliminary and much further characterization is required. In fact, it remains unclear whether these responses are specifically triggered by bacterial effector proteins, or are a nonspecific consequence of EPEC infection and pedestal formation. In either case, changes in cell signaling likely play a major role in mediating changes in host epithelial cell function and in the resulting diarrhea.

MECHANISMS OF EHEC/EPEC-MEDIATED DIARRHEA

Diarrhea is undoubtedly the most prominent and widespread symptom associated with both EPEC and EHEC infection. Surprisingly, aside from the contributory role of Shiga toxin to EHEC-mediated diarrhea (as reviewed by Nataro and Kaper [31]), the mechanisms that mediate EPEC- and EHEC-induced diarrhea are still unclear. While diarrhea appears to be a stereotyped host response to enteric infections, EPEC may affect the onset or degree of diarrhea through the tissue damage caused by its intimate attachment or through the actions of specific virulence factors. For example, the dramatic loss of the absorptive microvilli in the A/E lesion could result in intestinal malabsorption and diarrhea. EPEC infection also reduces the integrity of tight junctions in epithelial cell monolayers, altering the distribution of tight junction proteins such as zonula occludens 1 (ZO-1) (19). Similarly, EPEC attachment triggers the phosphorylation of ezrin, followed by a significant increase in cytoskeleton-associated ezrin. Overexpression of dominant-negative ezrin in tissue culture cells attenuates the disruption of epithelial tight junctions during EPEC infection, linking ezrin recruitment to tight junction integrity (19). While the reduction in tight junction integrity could be an indirect result of cytoskeletal rearrangements, the EPEC-secreted protein EspF has been implicated in the increased monolayer permeability and altered distribution of the tight junction protein occludin (30) seen during EPEC infection. The possibility that tight junction integrity is specifically targeted by EPEC virulence factors is intriguing, but such a role will remain speculative until the role of EspF has been tested in vivo.

While cytoskeletal changes may contribute to EPEC-induced diarrhea, the observation in volunteer studies that ingestion of EPEC induces diarrhea in less than 4 h suggests the involvement of a more active secretory response. The most commonly described mechanism leading to infectious secretory diarrhea involves changes in chloride ion secretion (19). There have been reports that EPEC also alters chloride ion transport in intestinal epithelial cell monolayers mounted in Ussing chambers, resulting in a rapid but transient increase in short circuit current (Isc). These ionic changes were abrogated by mutation of *espB*, but not intimin (19). This agrees with volunteer infection studies, where EPEC intimin mutants, although less virulent than wild-type EPEC, still caused diarrhea in 4 out of 11 volunteers, suggesting other factors are involved in EPEC's ability to cause diarrhea. It should be noted that not all studies have supported a role for chloride ion secretion. Hecht and Koutsouris have implicated changes in bicarbonate (HCO_3^-) ion transport rather than chloride ions in the EPEC-mediated changes in intestinal ion transport (19).

EPEC-induced diarrhea may also reflect host factors beyond those present in epithelial cell cultures. The histology of infected tissues has shown a substantial recruitment of neutrophils and other PMN to the site of infection (36). The signals recruiting PMN may be from the infected epithelial cells, since EPEC infection activates NF-κB and induces IL-8 expression in tissue culture cells (19). Extracellular signal-regulated kinase (ERK)-1/2 is also activated in the host cell during EPEC infection and is required in this inflammatory response (6, 7, 33). The transmigration of PMN through epithelial cell monolayers results in increased paracellular permeability and chloride secretion, and thereby could contribute to EPEC-induced diarrhea (Fig. 3). Aside from the effects of transmigration, the recruitment of PMN and other inflammatory cells could alter epithelial cell function through the release of cytotoxic inflammatory mediators. Other inflammatory mediators present during infection, such as the cytokines gamma interferon (IFN-γ) and tumor necrosis factor alpha (TNF-α) have also been shown to directly alter epithelial cell function in tissue culture. Unfortunately, such an inflammatory response would take longer than 3 h to develop, suggesting that although it may contribute to the duration and severity of the diarrheal response, it is not the mechanism that initiates EPEC-mediated diarrhea. It should be noted that whether diarrhea is host or pathogen driven, its onset is probably beneficial to A/E lesion-causing bacteria. Particularly in the large bowel, these bacteria are in competition with normal enteric flora and even with other pathogens. Therefore, mechanisms such as diarrhea that disturb the normal host-prokaryote equilibrium should offer improved opportunities to colonize the intestinal mucosal surface. Through its intimate binding to the host's mucosal surface, EPEC can presumably remain attached to the host's intestinal surface, while other less adherent microbes are flushed away during the course of diarrhea.

EPEC'S INTERACTIONS WITH ITS HOST

While recent attention has focused on the molecular interactions between EPEC and the host cell, the determination of how EPEC causes disease has not been forthcoming. This is in part because EPEC infection and the resulting disease need to be considered in the context of the complexity of the host. Since EPEC is specifically a pediatric pathogen, ethical considerations have limited the number of studies examining naturally acquired infections. A few infection studies have been carried out using adult human volunteers given EPEC, and, while interesting, these studies have required the use of very large bacterial doses and thus represent an artificial situation. As a result, analysis of EPEC pathogenesis in vivo has recently focused on animal models. Since EPEC is human specific and does not infect most laboratory animal species, this has required the use of other members of the A/E family of enteric pathogens. This family includes bacterial pathogens capable of forming A/E lesions in rabbits as well as calves, sheep, pigs, dogs, and mice.

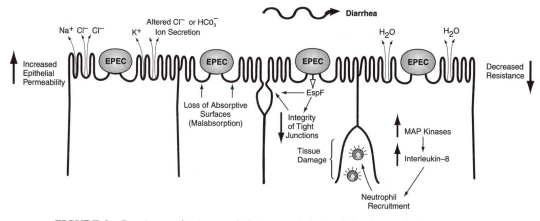

FIGURE 3 Putative mechanisms underlying EPEC-induced diarrhea include increased epithelial permeability and alterations in Cl⁻ and HCO₃⁻ ion secretion. Contributing structural changes include loss of absorptive surfaces, while the translocated EPEC effector EspF has been implicated in the loss of tight junction integrity. Signaling events within infected cells may also play a role in diarrhea, including increased MAP kinase activity and IL-8 production, causing the recruitment of neutrophils resulting in tissue damage. (Modified with permission from reference 36.)

The rabbit pathogen REPEC infects the small bowel of weanling rabbits, with infection resulting in both diarrhea and weight loss (1, 29). Despite the similarity to symptoms seen with EPEC infection, the model has limitations, including high mortality and the relative lack of genetic and immunological resources for rabbits. In this respect *C. rodentium* (formerly known as *Citrobacter freundii* biotype 4280) offers a comparative advantage. *C. rodentium* produces A/E lesions in mice, colonizing the large rather than the small bowel. This pathogen induces a strong T-helper cell 1 (Th1) immune response as well as colonic epithelial cell hyperplasia, but only mild diarrhea (20). Despite these differences, the basic mechanisms of A/E lesion formation, and the host response to infection, likely remain the same among EPEC, REPEC, and *C. rodentium*. The full *C. rodentium* LEE has recently been sequenced (8), and comparative analysis with the LEEs of EPEC, EHEC, and the rabbit diarrheagenic *E. coli* strain RDEC-1 shows high sequence similarities, with 41 common open reading frames (8). The wide array of reagents available for studying the

mouse, including antibodies, recombinant cytokines, and gene knockout strains, suggests *C. rodentium* will prove to be the most practical model in which to study the host response to infection.

Although most of EPEC's LEE-encoded genes have been assessed in vitro for their importance in A/E lesion formation (36), only a few have been assessed in vivo. Thus far, however, animal model studies have validated those findings made in tissue culture. Using the REPEC model, Abe and colleagues demonstrated that REPEC strains lacking either EspA or EspB lost the ability to form A/E lesions or cause diarrheal disease, although they were still able to locally adhere to the small bowel (1). Similarly, Tir and intimin were also found to be necessary for disease induction (29). The crucial role of EspB in the formation of A/E lesions has also been shown in the *C. rodentium* model in mice (32). Unfortunately, these studies demonstrate only that an effector protein is necessary for pedestal formation or diarrhea without identifying its actual role(s) in pathogenesis. As a result, only a few of EPEC's arsenal of effector proteins have been well characterized, and it is likely that even these factors have as yet unrecognized functions, as exemplified by the discovery by Higgins et al. of intimin's role in generating the immune response during *C. rodentium* infection (20). Interestingly, intimin expression on the surface of *C. rodentium* was found to be crucial for the development of both epithelial hyperplasia and Th1 immune responses during infection. Thus, characterizing the functions of EPEC's secreted and translocated effectors is the next step in the field of EPEC pathogenesis. In particular, the testing in animal models of EPEC effectors such as MAP and EspF, which have no apparent effect on pedestal formation in tissue culture, may well provide novel insights into EPEC pathogenesis. In vivo experiments have also proven to be valuable with respect to finding potential vaccine components.

While it is known that *C. rodentium*-infected mice develop acquired immunity and become resistant to reinfection, it was unclear whether the host response against bacterial surface components as well as type III secreted proteins is important for this resistance. A recent study found that EspA, EspB, Tir, and particularly intimin are targets of humoral immune responses in mice infected with *C. rodentium* (14). It was also shown that anti-intimin immune responses affected the outcome of infection by *C. rodentium*. These findings imply that intimin and type III secreted proteins could potentially be used as components in an EPEC or EHEC vaccine (14).

Another aspect that needs to be addressed using animal models is how EPEC interacts with and manipulates the wide array of cell types present within the intestine. The mammalian intestinal epithelium is a highly specialized tissue capable of maintaining complex and selective secretory and absorptive functions. Particularly in the colon, the epithelium exists within a diverse microfloral ecology, which contributes to and regulates the physiology of the lower gut. As a result, intestinal epithelial cells have evolved selective physical,

chemical, and immunological barriers that permit this mutually beneficial coexistence. The epithelial lining of the intestine is also a dynamic system, with epithelial cells being replaced every 3 to 4 days (36). As a result, the gut contains epithelial cells at varying stages of differentiation, ranging from immature crypt cells to mature enterocytes. As well, interspersed among the columnar epithelium are more specialized forms of epithelial cells, including Paneth cells, the mucus-secreting goblet cells, as well as the antigen-sampling M cells that overlie the gut-associated lymphoid tissues. At present, the questions of whether EPEC infects these cells and how their function might be altered during infection have yet to be addressed.

While most of EPEC's interactions with the host are with the intestinal epithelium, A/E lesion-causing bacteria also encounter inflammatory and immune cells in the infected gut. Histological examination of infected tissues has identified both neutrophils and macrophages as among the first cells responding to both EPEC and *C. rodentium* infection (20). This recruitment of inflammatory cells may be in response to signals sent by the infected epithelium, since epithelial cells in culture produce the neutrophil chemoattractant IL-8 in response to EPEC infection (19). In fact, as the host cells in most intimate contact with A/E lesion-causing pathogens, epithelial cells have great potential for playing an active role in host defense against these pathogens. Such a concept is not novel, as many studies have demonstrated that epithelial cells can secrete a number of proinflammatory and antimicrobial agents in response to bacterial infection or following immune stimulation (19). While the exact epithelial response elicited by these pathogens has yet to be determined, preliminary studies suggest that inducible nitric oxide synthase and antimicrobial peptides (defensins) are expressed by epithelial cells during *C. rodentium* infection (35). Studies of professional immune cells have shown that EPEC and EHEC infection in humans induces strong humoral and cellular immune responses. Similarly, studies examining the inflammatory milieu present during *C. rodentium* infection found the upregulation of IL-12 and IFN-γ expression, as well as other cytokines such as TNF-α (15, 35). Further studies found that TNF-α signaling was important in controlling the bacterial load found within the colonic lumen (15).

Interestingly, EPEC has evolved measures to counteract and subvert the host's immune response. EPEC uses a phosphatidylinositol 3-kinase-dependent mechanism to block its own uptake by professional phagocytes (3). This requires EPEC to possess a functioning type III secretion system and express EspA, EspB, and EspD, but not Tir. These requirements suggest that EPEC disrupts the phagocytic process through direct contact with macrophages, rather than through a soluble mediator. EPEC can also inhibit the host's acquired immune response, with Donnenberg and colleagues reporting that EPEC lysates contain a large toxin termed Lymphostatin that inhibits IL-2, IL-4, and IFN-γ production by both mucosal and splenic lymphocytes (26). This effect was not dependent on the type III secretion system. While it may seem incongruous that A/E lesion-causing bacteria would exert both proinflammatory and immunosuppressive effects on their hosts, these divergent immunomodulatory actions may be spatially targeted to stimulate diarrhea and disease within the host, yet suppress the responses of those cells the bacteria directly contact.

CONCLUSIONS AND PROSPECTS FOR THE FUTURE

As documented by this chapter, remarkable progress has been made in our understanding of the molecular mechanisms underlying EPEC pathogenesis. Approaches using molecular biology, genetics, and cell biology have provided many new insights into how EPEC and related pathogens interact with and exploit host cells during the course of infection and how this ultimately leads to disease. A much clearer view has been achieved of the strategies used by EPEC to anchor to host

cells, as well as the role of EPEC's bacterial effectors in the subversion of the host cell cytoskeleton. This research has identified features common to other enteric pathogens, as well as strategies apparently unique to A/E lesion-causing bacteria, such as the translocation of the bacterial receptor Tir into the host cell membrane. As a result, A/E lesion-causing pathogens have received much interest not only in the field of microbial pathogenesis, but from other fields as well. Cell biologists have identified EPEC as a useful tool to characterize the mechanisms underlying actin dynamics and cytoskeletal rearrangements, while immunologists and clinical gastroenterologists have approached EPEC as a model to study the mucosal immune system and intestinal inflammation.

Despite this progress, we still have much to learn about the complex interactions between A/E lesion-causing pathogens and their hosts that lead to infection and disease. This is true even about the mechanisms that mediate bacterial attachment to the host cell as well as the structure and function of pedestals. The differences in the structural components between EPEC- and EHEC-induced pedestals, as well as their divergence in Tir signaling requirements, suggest that subtle but important differences may exist between these two pathogens in their modes of pedestal formation. Additional studies are also needed to separate the effects of pedestal formation from other pathogenic actions of the bacteria during infection. In part, this would involve the continued characterization of EPEC's effector molecules, particularly those translocated effectors that have no obvious role in pedestal formation.

Future research avenues will undoubtedly focus more on pathogenic interactions within the intact host. For example, it still remains to be determined how these pathogens initially colonize their hosts and how they interact with the normal enteric flora. Since EPEC-induced diarrhea is probably multifactorial, both bacterial and host contributions need to be examined for their role in causing diarrhea and other aspects of EPEC-mediated disease. In addition, there may be genetic differences in host susceptibility to these infections that will be determined only in animal models. Better assessment of the host's innate mucosal defenses, as well as any active role played by intestinal epithelial cells during these infections, will aid in understanding how infection leads to intestinal pathology and diarrheal disease. Similarly, determining how hosts clear A/E pathogen infections and the mechanisms of acquired immunity that prevent reinfection will aid in the development of vaccines. Using our present knowledge of the factors that mediate bacterial adhesion to the host cell, and the demonstration that preventing bacterial adherence prevents most aspects of the disease, we have already identified potential targets for vaccination. A successful vaccination approach may target those factors found to be critically involved in bacterial adhesion, such as the components and effectors of the type III secretion machinery. Taken together, future studies integrating host genetics, physiology, and the immune system, all of which are critical determinants to the outcome of infection, should provide a better understanding of the pathogenesis of EPEC and other A/E pathogens, and together these developments may lead to new therapeutic strategies.

ACKNOWLEDGMENTS

We thank Wanyin Deng for helpful discussions and critical reading of this chapter and Ursula Heczko and Fern Ness for figures. Work in our laboratory is supported by operating grants from the Canadian Institutes of Health Research (CIHR), the Canadian Bacterial Diseases Network, the National Sciences and Engineering Research Council (NSERC), and the Howard Hughes Medical Institute (HHMI) International Scholars Program. B.A.V. is supported by a CIHR/Digestive Diseases Foundation Fellowship and is an honorary Isaak Walton Killam fellow. B.B.F. is a CIHR Distinguished Investigator and a Howard Hughes International Scholar.

REFERENCES

1. **Abe, A., U. Heczko, R. G. Hegele, and B. B. Finlay.** 1998. Two enteropathogenic *Escherichia coli* type III secreted proteins, EspA and EspB, are virulence factors. *J. Exp. Med.* **188:** 1907–1916.

2. **Cantarelli, V. V., A. Takahashi, I. Yanagihara, Y. Akeda, K. Imura, T. Kodoma, G. Kono, Y. Sato, and T. Honda.** 2001. Talin, a host cell protein, interacts directly with the translocated intimin receptor, Tir, of enteropathogenic *Escherichia coli*, and is essential for pedestal formation. *Cell. Microbiol.* **3:**745–751.

3. **Celli, J., M. Olivier, and B. B. Finlay.** 2001. Enteropathogenic *Escherichia coli* mediates antiphagocytosis through the inhibition of PI 3-kinase-dependent pathways. *EMBO J.* **20:**1245–1258.

4. **Cornelis, G. R., and F. Van Gijsegem.** 2000. Assembly and function of type III secretory systems. *Annu. Rev. Microbiol.* **54:**735–774.

5. **Crane, J. K., B. P. McNamara, and M. S. Donnenberg.** 2001. Role of EspF in host cell death induced by enteropathogenic *Escherichia coli*. *Cell. Microbiol.* **2:**197–211.

5a.**Crane, J. K., and J. S. Oh.** 1997. Activation of host cell protein kinase C by enteropathogenic *Escherichia coli*. *Infect. Immun.* **65:**3277–3285.

6. **Czerucka, D., S. Dahan, B. Mograbi, B. Rossi, and P. Rampal.** 2001. Implication of mitogen-activated protein kinases in T84 cell responses to enteropathogenic *Escherichia coli* infection. *Infect. Immun.* **69:**1298–1305.

7. **de Grado, M., C. M. Rosenberger, A. Gauthier, B. A. Vallance, and B. B. Finlay.** 2001. Enteropathogenic *Escherichia coli* infection induces expression of the early growth response factor by activating mitogen-activated protein kinase cascades in epithelial cells. *Infect. Immun.* **69:**6217–6224.

8. **Deng, W., Y. Li, B. A. Vallance, and B. B. Finlay.** 2001. Locus of enterocyte effacement from *Citrobacter rodentium*: sequence analysis and evidence for horizontal transfer among attaching and effacing pathogens. *Infect. Immun.* **69:**6323–6335.

9. **DeVinney, R., J. L. Puente, A. Gauthier, D. Goosney, and B. B. Finlay.** 2001. Enterohaemorrhagic *Escherichia coli* use a different Tir-based mechanism for pedestal formation. *Mol. Microbiol.* **41:**1445–1458.

10. **DeVinney, R., M. Stein, D. Reinscheid, A. Abe, S. Ruschkowski, and B. B. Finlay.** 1999. Enterohemorrhagic *Escherichia coli* O157: H7 produces Tir, which is translocated to the host cell membrane but is not tyrosine phosphorylated. *Infect. Immun.* **67:**2389–2398.

11. **Donnenberg, M. S., and T. S. Whittam.** 2001. Pathogenesis and evolution of virulence in

enteropathogenic and enterohemorrhagic *Escherichia coli. J. Clin. Invest.* **107:**539–548.

12. **Elliott, S. J., E. O. Krejany, J. L. Mellies, R. M. Robins-Browne, C. Sasakawa, and J. B. Kaper.** 2001. EspG, a novel type III system-secreted protein from enteropathogenic *Escherichia coli* with similarities to VirA of *Shigella flexneri. Infect. Immun.* **69:**4027–4033.

13. **Frankel, G., A. D. Philipps, L. R. Trabulsi, S. Knutton, G. Dougan, and S. Matthews.** 2001. Intimin and the host cell—is it bound to end in Tir(s)? *Trends Microbiol.* **9:**214–218.

14. **Ghaem-Maghami, M., C. P. Simmons, S. Daniell, M. Pizza, D. Lewis, G. Frankel, and G. Dougan.** 2001. Intimin-specific immune responses prevent bacterial colonization by the attaching-effacing pathogen *Citrobacter rodentium. Infect. Immun.* **69:**5597–5605.

15. **Goncalves, N. S., M. Ghaem-Maghami, G. Monteleone, G. Frankel, G. Dougan, D. J. Lewis, C. P. Simmons, and T. T. MacDonald.** 2001. Critical role for tumor necrosis factor alpha in controlling the number of lumenal pathogenic bacteria and immunopathology in infectious colitis. *Infect. Immun.* **69:**6651–6659.

16. **Goosney, D. L., R. DeVinney, and B. B. Finlay.** 2001. Recruitment of cytoskeletal and signaling proteins to enteropathogenic and enterohemorrhagic *Escherichia coli* pedestals. *Infect. Immun.* **69:**3315–3322.

17. **Goosney, D. L., R. DeVinney, R. A. Pfuetzner, E. A. Frey, N. C. Strynadka, and B. B. Finlay.** 2000. Enteropathogenic *E. coli* translocated intimin receptor, Tir, interacts directly with alpha actinin. *Curr. Biol.* **10:**735–738.

18. **Gruenheid, S., R. DeVinney, F. Bladt, D. Goosney, S. Gelkop, G. D. Gish, T. Pawson, and B. B. Finlay.** 2001. Enteropathogenic *E. coli* Tir binds Nck to initiate actin pedestal formation in host cells. *Nat. Cell. Biol.* **3:**856–859.

19. **Hecht, G.** 2001. Microbes and microbial toxins: paradigms for microbial-mucosal interactions. VII. Enteropathogenic *Escherichia coli*: physiological alterations from an extracellular position. *Am. J. Physiol. Gastrointest. Liver Physiol.* **281:**G1–G7.

20. **Higgins, L. M., G. Frankel, I. Connerton, N. S. Goncalves, G. Dougan, and T. T. MacDonald.** 1999. Role of bacterial intimin in colonic hyperplasia and inflammation. *Science* **285:**588–591.

21. **Kalman, D., O. D. Weiner, D. L. Goosney, J. W. Sedat, B. B. Finlay, A. Abe, and J. M. Bishop.** 1999. Enteropathogenic *E. coli* acts through WASP and Arp2/3 complex to form actin pedestals. *Nat. Cell. Biol.* **1:**389–391.

22. **Kenny, B.** 2001. The enterohaemorrhagic *Escherichia coli* (serotype O157:H7) Tir molecule is not functionally interchangeable for its enteropathogenic *E. coli* (serotype O127:H6) homologue. *Cell. Microbiol.* **3:**499–510.

23. **Kenny, B., and J. Warawa.** 2001. Enteropathogenic *Escherichia coli* (EPEC) Tir receptor molecule does not undergo full modification when introduced into host cells by EPEC-independent mechanisms. *Infect. Immun.* **69:** 1444–1453.

24. **Kenny, B., and M. Jepson.** 2000. Targeting of an enteropathogenic *Escherichia coli* (EPEC) effector protein to host mitochondria. *Cell. Microbiol.* **2:**579–590.

25. **Kenny, B., R. D. DeVinney, M. Stein, D. J. Reinscheid, E. A. Frey, and B. B. Finlay.** 1997. Enteropathogenic *E. coli* (EPEC) transfers its receptor for intimate adherence into mammalian cells. *Cell* **91:**511–520.

26. **Klapproth, J. M., I. C. Scaletsky, B. P. McNamara, L. C. Lai, C. Malstrom, S. P. James, and M. S. Donnenberg.** 2000. A large toxin from pathogenic *Escherichia coli* strains that inhibits lymphocyte activation. *Infect. Immun.* **68:** 2148–2155.

27. **Luo, Y., E. A. Frey, R. A. Pfuetzner, A. L. Creagh, D. G. Knoechel, C. A. Haynes, B. B. Finlay, and N. C. Strynadka.** 2000. Crystal structure of enteropathogenic *Escherichia coli* intimin-receptor complex. *Nature* **405:**1073–1077.

28. **Luo, Y., M. G. Bertero, E. A. Frey, R. A. Pfuetzner, M. R. Wenk, L. Creagh, S. L. Marcus, D. Lim, F. Sicheri, C. Kay, C. Haynes, B. B. Finlay, and N. C. Strynadka.** 2001. Structural and biochemical characterization of the type III secretion chaperones CesT and SigE. *Nat. Struct. Biol.* **8:**1031–1036.

29. **Marches, O., J. P. Nougayrede, S. Bouillier, J. Mainil, G. Charlier, I. Raymond, P. Pohl, M. Boury, J. De Rycke, A. Milon, and E. Oswald.** 2000. Role of Tir and intimin in the virulence of rabbit enteropathogenic *Escherichia coli* serotype O103:H2. *Infect. Immun.* **68:**2171–2182.

30. **McNamara, B. P., A. Koutsouris, C. B. O'Connell, J. P. Nougayrede, M. S. Donnenberg, and G. Hecht.** 2001. Translocated EspF protein from enteropathogenic *Escherichia coli* disrupts host intestinal barrier function. *J. Clin. Invest.* **107:**621–629.

31. **Nataro, J. P., and J. B. Kaper.** 1998. Diarrheagenic *Escherichia coli. Clin. Microbiol. Rev.* **11:** 142–201.

32. **Newman, J. V., B. A. Zabel, S. S. Jha, and D. B. Schauer.** 1999. *Citrobacter rodentium* espB

is necessary for signal transduction and for infection of laboratory mice. *Infect. Immun.* **67:**6019–6025.

33. **Savkovic, S. D., A. Ramaswamy, A. Koutsouris, and G. Hecht.** 2001. EPEC-activated ERK1/2 participate in inflammatory response but not tight junction barrier disruption. *Am. J. Physiol. Gastrointest. Liver Physiol.* **281:**G890–G898.

34. **Sekiya, K., M. Ohishi, T. Ogino, K. Tamano, C. Sasakawa, and A. Abe.** 2001. Supermolecular structure of the enteropathogenic *Escherichia coli* type III secretion system and its direct interaction with the EspA-sheath-like structure. *Proc. Natl. Acad. Sci. USA* **98:**11638–11643.

35. **Simmons, C. P., S. Clare, and G. Dougan.** 2001. Understanding mucosal responsiveness: lessons from enteric bacterial pathogens. *Semin. Immunol.* **13:**201–209.

36. **Vallance, B. A., and B. B. Finlay.** 2000. Exploitation of host cells by enteropathogenic *Escherichia coli. Proc. Natl. Acad. Sci. USA* **97:**8799–8806.

SALMONELLA SPP.: MASTERS OF INFLAMMATION

Beth A. McCormick

24

Epithelial cells that line mucosal surfaces are an important mechanical barrier separating the host's internal milieu from the external environment. In addition to barrier function, epithelial cells at different mucosal sites have specialized host adaptive functions. In the gastrointestinal tract, for example, epithelial cells have an important role in ion transport, fluid absorption, and secretion. For pathogens that invade the host, however, epithelial cells are the first sites of contact with the host. Infection of the intestinal mucosa with enteropathogenic *Salmonella* strains results in an intense inflammatory response consisting of polymorphonuclear leukocyte (PMN) migration toward and subsequently across the epithelial monolayer and into the lumenal compartment. To coordinate this inflammatory process, there is considerable communication between the cells of the intestinal epithelium and the underlying cells of the immune system. Further, there is communication between the host cells and pathogens that seek to breech the intestinal mucosa. Thus, insight into bacterial-epithelial-immune cell

interactions may likely contribute to an understanding of both pathogenesis and chronic inflammatory diseases of the intestine. This chapter highlights recent progress made toward understanding the molecular basis of *Salmonella*-induced enteritis.

PATHOPHYSIOLOGY OF NONTYPHOIDAL *SALMONELLA* INFECTION

Information is scarce on the specific course of events following nontyphoidal *Salmonella* infection in humans because most infected individuals are rarely hospitalized. As such, observations of nontyphoidal *Salmonella* infection have mostly come from patients admitted to the hospital with severe fatal infections. Case reports not only suggest that the colon is the primary site of bacterial colonization, but also indicate that the disease ranges in severity from slight to severe edema with subsequent PMN and neutrophil infiltration, lamina propria inflammation, mucosal degeneration, and PMN extravasation (8).

Instead, the majority of histological observations in vivo have come from studies employing animal model systems (5, 19, 24, 33, 42, 44, 56). In an elegant electron microscopic study, Takeuchi first described the events leading to *Salmonella enterica* serovar Typhi-

Beth A. McCormick, Department of Pediatric Gastroenterology and Nutrition, Massachusetts General Hospital and Harvard Medical School, Boston, MA 02129.

Microbial Pathogenesis and the Intestinal Epithelial Cell, ed. by G. Hecht
© 2003 ASM Press, Washington, D.C.

murium entry of intestinal enterocytes. Interactions between bacteria and intestinal tissue were examined in starved, opium-treated guinea pigs several hours after oral challenge with 10^8 invasive serovar Typhimurium (50). This study found that *Salmonella* closely contacts the epithelial cells lining the intestine, primarily the ileum, and thereafter elicits the local degeneration of filamentous actin in apical microvilli and the underlying terminal web. The morphology of other areas of the apical surface, either on the same cell or on adjacent enterocytes, remains unaffected. Subsequently, extruded membrane (described as "membrane ruffles") surrounds the bacteria and results in their internalization into vacuoles. Occasionally, several bacteria become engulfed simultaneously by one membrane projection. However, once the bacteria are internalized, the overlying apical membrane regains its microvillar morphology, and despite these drastic changes to the apical cytoarchitecture and the presence of intracellular bacteria, the infected enterocytes remain remarkably healthy. Interestingly, while some bacteria become internalized by enterocytes, the majority remain in the intestinal lumen (57). Similar observations have been reported in other animals, including calves, pigs, and primates, all of which present with diarrheal gastroenteritis in response to serovar Typhimurium and other related *Salmonella* strains (5, 44, 56).

A series of key experiments used the rhesus monkey to chronicle the disease course following orogastric administration of human-derived serovar Typhimurium strains (44). Conclusions from these studies revealed that at the height of clinical disease, viable counts of serovar Typhimurium in the lumen of the jejunum were low, but counts in both the ileal and colonic contents ranged from $10^{3.6}$ to $10^{5.5}$/g. In addition, monkeys with severe diarrhea had bacterial counts ranging as high as $10^{7.5}$/g. In these infected animals, increased severity of diarrhea was paralleled by increased bacterial invasion of the ileum and colon, and was accompanied by tissue damage and an acute inflammatory ileocolitis. Interestingly, the jejunal mucosa was undamaged. Moreover, all monkeys exhibiting diarrhea had inhibition of colonic water absorption or increased secretion. Mildly affected monkeys had jejunal secretion, with less markedly impaired ileal function, while in severely affected monkeys all three regions of the gut were in a secretory state. Thus, colonic and ileal fluid secretion in salmonellosis was associated with mucosal bacterial association and inflammation. Notably, these pathophysiologic findings in the rhesus monkey were comparable to those observed in infected human patients, postmortem (6).

Although the pathogenic mechanisms responsible for the onset of gastroenteritis are not as yet completely defined, the cellular events are clearly an interaction of nontyphoidal *Salmonella* with intestinal epithelial cells followed by a massive efflux of neutrophils. Following exposure to serovar Typhimurium and other gastroenteritis-causing strains of *Salmonella* sp., the intestinal epithelium generates an intense inflammatory response, characterized by fluid secretion and the recruitment of PMN to the infected epithelium. Villi on the surface of the epithelium become blunted and swollen with fluid, and this is typically accompanied by occasional blebbing of dead cells from the villus tip (25). Some but not all strains of serovar Typhimurium induce the formation of abscesses in the crypt area of the epithelium, where many PMN are observed. However, in contrast to the extensive mucosal damage directly caused by bacterial pathogens such as *Shigella* sp. and *Listeria* sp., the epithelium remains mostly intact during initial *Salmonella* infection.

MODEL SYSTEMS TO STUDY *SALMONELLA* ENTEROPATHOGENICITY

Over the last several decades, in vivo model systems for examining *Salmonella*-induced inflammation have been developed using ligated ileal loops in rabbits, calves, and other animals that present with gastroenteritis (19, 25). Although murine ligated loops have also been used to study the interactions of *Salmonella* sp. with intestinal mucosa, it is not possible to correlate results from this model to *Salmonella*-induced enteritis, as mice do not ordinarily develop overt signs of diarrhea. Furthermore, not all mutations that influence systemic virulence in mice influence the induction of enteritis in other animal species (59) and vice versa (61). However, in rabbit ileal loops, only *Salmonella* strains that caused enteritis in primates induced enteropathogenic responses such as fluid secretion, intestinal inflammation, and mucosal damage (25, 44, 53).

More recently, studies have turned to the use of cattle to model the pathophysiology of *Salmonella*-induced enteritis in humans (51, 56). Cattle are particularly useful for studying *Salmonella*-induced enteropathogenicity, since these animals are not only a natural target species for *Salmonella* sp. but also present with a disease profile similar to that seen in humans. For instance, after oral challenge with virulent serovar Typhimurium or *Salmonella enterica* serovar Dublin, calves exhibit a pyrexial response along with a mucopurulent diarrheal disease. In addition, this model system is predictive of human disease, since *Salmonella* strains with reduced enteropathogenicity were attenuated in calves following oral challenge (58), whereas mutations that did not reduce enteropathogenesis in loops did not affect the severity of the enteritis in orally infected calves (55, 59). Therefore, since this infection method can model the natural route of infection, the role of different virulence factors can be assessed through the use of strains containing defined mutations. The severity of the disease can also be semiquantified using a clinical scoring system.

In vitro model systems have also been developed to assess the mechanisms underlying *Salmonella* enteropathogenicity. A polarized intestinal organ culture model was originally designed to quantify the invasion capacity of different *Salmonella* strains into freshly isolated and functioning human gut tissue (3). This model system is an excellent indicator of *Sal-*

monella invasiveness of the intestinal mucosa; however, it is not particularly well suited for studying enteropathogenic potential. To evaluate enteropathogenicity in vitro, *Salmonella*-induced PMN transepithelial migration has been developed using human epithelial monolayers of T84 cells cultured on permeable supports to form monolayers (40). The T84 cells are a human-derived epithelial cell line with crypt-like features (10); they have been widely used as a relevant biological surface to integrate interactions between bacteria, the epithelial surface, and PMN. In this model system, the monolayers are infected with serovar Typhimurium on the apical membrane domain and primary peripheral human PMN are added to the basolateral epithelial membrane domain. *Salmonella*-induced PMN transmigration across the epithelial monolayer can subsequently be assessed. Such an established in vitro model system has become a valuable experimental tool since it serves to justify the use of transformed intestinal epithelia in models of PMN-epithelial interactions, and its simplicity allows one to unravel the molecular identity of agents potentially contributing to the course of enteropathophysiology.

SALMONELLA HOST CELL CROSS TALK AND THE INDUCTION OF ENTERITIS

Many microbial pathogens have evolved the capacity to engage their host cells in very complex interactions commonly involving the exchange of biochemical signals. Central to serovar Typhimurium enteropathogenicity is its ability to engage in host cell cross talk. As a consequence of this cross talk, a dedicated protein secretion system, termed type III, is activated in *Salmonella* spp. (18, 29). This protein secretion system directs the secretion and subsequent translocation into the host cell of a number of proteins that have the capacity to elicit host cell signaling pathways, which may lead to a multitude of responses, including cell invasion and induction of enteritis. The *Salmonella* pathogenicity island-1 (SPI-1) chromosomal region encodes more than 30 proteins, which include regulatory proteins and structural components of the type III secretion system (TTSS), along with TTSS-secreted proteins and their chaperones (18, 28, 29). An in-depth description of the TTSSs in enteric pathogens is discussed in chapter 22.

A set of at least nine different effector proteins are translocated into host cells and activate signaling cascades leading to a variety of responses. In addition to cell invasion, the TTSS-1 also plays a major role in the induction of intestinal inflammatory responses. Mutations in the genes that encode for the structural and regulatory proteins of the TTSS, such as HilA, InvH, or SirA, significantly attenuate induction of fluid secretion and the recruitment of PMN in bovine ligated ileal loops (1, 58). Likewise, *invH*, *hilA*, and *prgH* mutants markedly reduce the severity of enteritis in orally infected calves (51, 58), suggesting that mutations affecting entire TTSS functions almost invariably abrogate or greatly reduce enteropathogenicity. Some of the translocation and intracellular activities of translocated effector proteins are also thought to elicit a variety of pathogenic responses, ultimately leading to the onset of enteritis. Originally, these were designated Sop proteins, for *Salmonella* outer proteins (60). Genes encoding several Sops have been identified, including SopA, SopB, SopD, and SopE. These and other effector proteins that activate different aspects of *Salmonella* enteropathogenicity will be discussed in detail below.

SALMONELLA-INDUCED FLUID SECRETION

During the late 1970s, Gianella questioned whether the acute inflammatory reaction plays a role in the pathogenesis of *Salmonella*-induced secretion (25). To answer this question, Gianella used rabbit ileal loops to model *Salmonella*-induced enteritis. In this landmark study, two groups of rabbits were infected with serovar Typhimurium; one group represented the control and the other was the experimental group in which the rabbits were pretreated with nitrogen mustard. Nitrogen mustard was used to deplete the PMN pool to prevent the formation of an acute inflammatory response. Following nitrogen mustard administration, the rabbit ligated ileal loops were then infected with serovar Typhimurium for 72 h. Results from this study revealed that nitrogen mustard treatment markedly inhibited serovar Typhimurium-induced secretion. Additionally, ileal histology in normal loops infected with serovar Typhimurium revealed an intense acute inflammatory reaction, whereas in animals pretreated with nitrogen mustard, virtually no PMN were observed. These observations introduced the important concept that the mucosal inflammatory reaction induced by serovar Typhimurium may be essential to the pathogenesis of the *Salmonella* secretory process. This section will discuss three potential mechanisms by which nontyphoidal *Salmonella* sp. elicit intestinal fluid secretion. These mechanisms are highlighted in Fig. 1.

SopB

The watery diarrhea induced by serovar Typhimurium has been attributed to epithelial chloride (Cl^-) secretion into the lumen, followed by the net flow of water into the lumen to preserve isotonicity in the epithelium. Cl^- secretion is caused by the opening of chloride channels at the apical surface, which early in infection can be attributed to the SPI-1-secreted *Salmonella* protein SopB (or SigD) (26). SopB is translocated into eukaryotic cells via a Sip-dependent mechanism, and extracellular bacteria are able to mediate its translocation into the host cell (19). Even though inactivation of SopB in serovar Dublin greatly reduced fluid secretion into bovine-ligated ileal loops (19), this mutant failed to adversely influence the ability of the organism to invade the intestinal epithelium. It turns out that SopB is an inositol polyphosphate phosphatase, capable of hydrolyzing phosphates from both phosphoinositol-containing phospholipids and phosphorylated inositol sugars (43). These studies are consistent with the finding

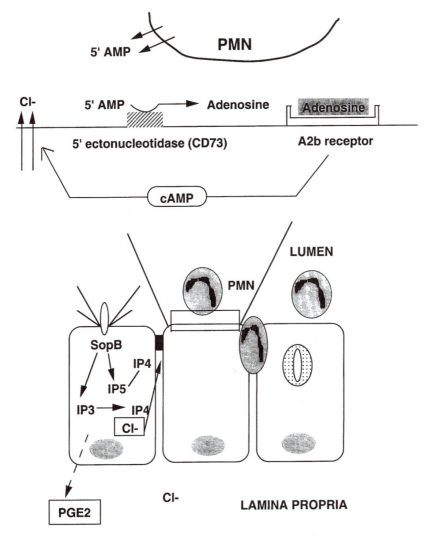

FIGURE 1 Cl^- secretory pathways induced by *Salmonella* during infection. The intracellular SopB protein affects inositol phosphate (IP) signaling events. One such event is the transient increase in IP_4, which antagonizes the closure of chloride channels influencing net electrolyte transport and, hence, fluid secretion. Infection of epithelial cells also results in the production of PGs such as PGE_2, which can further lead to Cl^- secretion. Finally, Cl^- release can be initiated by apically located and activated PMN. These PMN release 5'-AMP, which, through a series of steps, triggers signaling cascades involving cyclic AMP and thus promotes the opening of apical Cl^- channels.

that *Salmonella* infection of intestinal epithelial cells in vitro results in elevated cellular levels of the inositol sugar IP_4 (inositol-1,4,5,6-tetrakisphosphate) (14, 16, 43, 64). This is of particular interest since elevation of IP_4 in *Salmonella*-infected intestinal epithelial cells can promote Cl^- flux by antagonizing the signaling pathway activated by phosphatidyl-inositol-3 kinase pathway. This event prevents the closure of Cl^- channels. Therefore, it is possible that the increase in IP_4 levels in cells infected with *Salmonella* sp. could be directly or indirectly attributed to SopB production. In addition, SopB may have additional effects on the host cell because of its broad substrate specificity. For instance, SopB causes the phosphorylation and activation of the host protein kinase Akt, which elicits signals that promote cell survival (47).

Ectonucleotidase (CD73)

Cl^- release may also be potentiated later in the infection process by apically localized, activated PMNs. During states of intestinal inflammation, activated PMNs accumulate in the colonic crypts (the site of electro-genic chloride secretion). These transmigrated PMNs not only have direct access to the apical membrane domain but also release 5′-AMP, which is dephosphorylated by an ectonucleo-tidase (CD73) on the apical surface of enter-ocytes to adenosine (36). As shown in Fig. 1, adenosine release acts as an autocoid by inter-acting with the adenosine receptor, A_2b (49), which belongs to the family of seven trans-membrane G-protein-coupled cell surface re-ceptors. These G-protein-coupled adenosine receptors reside on the apical enterocyte membrane and are stimulated by the PMN-derived adenosine and, through intracellular signaling cascades involving cyclic AMP, pro-mote the opening of apical Cl^- channels and hence fluid secretion (36). Moreover, adeno-sine itself stimulates the epithelial expression of interleukin-6 (IL-6), which induces both the degranulation and activation of apically lo-calized PMN (45).

PGE$_2$

Prostaglandins (PGs) are important regulators of gastrointestinal fluid secretion (12). Fur-thermore, prostanoids are common mediators of diarrhea of different etiologies, ranging from radiation-induced diarrhea to diarrhea after bacterial infection. PGs are formed from free arachidonic acid through the conversion of arachidonic acid to prostaglandin H (PGH), which is catalyzed by the enzyme PGH syn-thase (PGHS). PGH is thereafter converted by specific synthases to PGE, PGF, thrombox-

anes, or prostacyclins (12, 46). Several studies have implicated PGs in *Salmonella*-induced enteropathogenic responses that may influence chloride secretory pathways. One study deter-mined that pretreatment of rabbits with in-domethacin, an inhibitor of PG biosynthesis, abolishes fluid secretion in ligated loops (54). Further, PGE_1 stimulates chloride secretion in polarized cells, and PGE analogues were found to induce diarrhea in vivo. Another study evaluated the role of the intestinal epithelium in the secretory response after infection with *Salmonella* sp. (15). In this investigation, infection of intestinal epithelial cells with *Salmonella* sp. resulted in a rapid upregulation in PGHS expression that subse-quently stimulated the production of PGE_2 and PGF_{2a} and, consequently, led to an in-crease in Cl^- secretion (15).

SALMONELLA-INDUCED ENTERITIS AND CELLULAR REGULATORS

The best characterized of the *Salmonella* spp. host responses is the dramatic rearrangement of the cytoskeleton and plasma membrane at the point of bacterial-host cell contact, exhib-ited by membrane ruffles, which leads to bac-terial internalization into the host cell (17, 50). However, a signature feature of serovar Typhimurium-induced pathology is the in-duction of an early inflammatory response characterized by infiltration of PMNs through the intestinal mucosa and into the lumen. This inflammatory response greatly contributes to the pathophysiology of the infection, exhib-ited by typical inflammatory diarrhea. Recent work has begun to disclose the molecular and cellular events involved in this complex phe-nomenon (5, 20, 38, 39, 55, 56, 58, 59). This work has led to the current paradigm that in-testinal epithelial cells respond to lumenal pathogens such as serovar Typhimurium by releasing distinctive proinflammatory chemo-attractants, which sequentially orchestrate PMN movement across the intestinal epithe-lium (illustrated in Fig. 2).

Serovar Typhimurium-intestinal epithelial cell interactions induce the epithelial synthesis

Intestinal Lumen

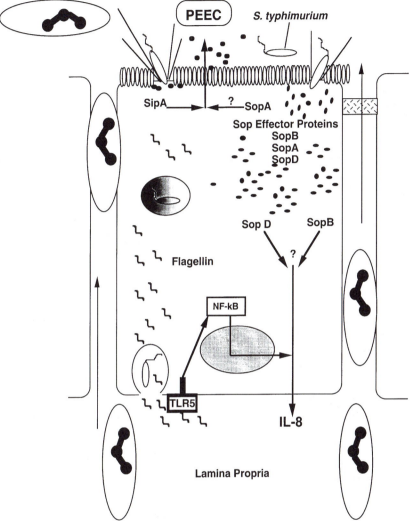

FIGURE 2 Model of proposed events affecting *Salmonella*-induced PMN transmigration across the intestinal epithelium. *Salmonella* spp. evoke a potent inflammatory response in the host, the hallmark of which is the migration of PMN across the intestinal mucosa. This process includes extravasation of circulating PMN from the microvasculature, passage of PMN across the lamina propria, and paracellular movement of PMN across the epithelium. PMN recruitment is coordinated by the release of proinflammatory cytokines, among which are IL-8 and PEEC. *Salmonella* interaction with enterocytes delivers Sop proteins into the cell cytoplasm via a TTS-dependent pathway. These Sop proteins play a role in enteropathogenic responses in the intestinal mucosa. Intracellular bacteria reside within membrane-bound vesicles and possibly continue to translocate TTSS-1-secreted effectors. By an unknown mechanism, *Salmonella* invasion also causes the transcellular transport of flagellin to the basolateral membrane domain, where it promotes the release of IL-8 by interacting with TLR-5. Concurrently, the *Salmonella* TTSS-1 product, SipA, was found to be both necessary and sufficient for induction of PMN transmigration across model intestinal epithelia in a PKC-dependent manner.

and polarized basolateral release of the potent PMN chemokine IL-8 (20, 38, 39, 40). Such a basolateral release of IL-8 imprints subepithelial matrices with long-lived haptotactic gradients that function to guide PMN through the lamina propria and to a subepithelial position (38). However, basolateral release of this chemokine is insufficient to induce migration of PMN across the intestinal epithelium, suggesting that the production of other inflammatory mediator(s), whose release would be polarized apically, is important for the execution of this step in the inflammatory pathway. Recently, the first such proinflammatory mediator has been characterized: pathogen-elicited epithelial chemoattractant (PEEC) (41). As the ability of bacteria to induce PEEC secretion from the intestinal epithelia appears to correlate well with their ability to cause enteritis in humans, secretion of this mediator is likely an important proinflammatory event. The specific roles of IL-8 and PEEC with respect to their contribution in the molecular basis of *Salmonella*-induced enteropathogenicity will be discussed below.

IL-8

The primary role for the basolateral secretion of IL-8 by epithelia is recruitment of neutrophils through the matrix of the lamina propria and into a subepithelial space (20). Epithelial-derived IL-8 exhibits many properties that would make this chemokine well suited for this purpose. One important property is that IL-8 is extremely resistant to inactivation. Thus, once present in the inflamed tissue, this chemokine is likely to retain its biological activity for several hours, as shown by local intradermal administration in animals and humans (4). Further, IL-8 is highly cationic and thus binds avidly to glycosaminoglycans of the tissue matrix (4). This combination of characteristics makes such bound IL-8 gradients particularly resistant to the sweeping away effects of fluid flow.

Activation of the IL-8 promoter during *Salmonella* invasion of cultured epithelial cells is primarily dependent upon the transcription factor NF-κB (27). Upregulation of IL-8 during *Salmonella* invasion requires both p38 mitogen-activated protein kinase activity and an increase in intracellular calcium, which is necessary for degradation of the NF-κB inhibitor IκBα and consequent nuclear translocation of the transcription factor (21, 27). In addition, Madara and colleagues found that the apical invasion of T84 cells with serovar Typhimurium caused the release of a bacterial factor into the basolateral medium that, when added to uninfected epithelial monolayers, could recapitulate the IL-8 induction caused by whole bacteria (23). Upon purification, this protein was identified as flagellin, the functional component of *Salmonella* flagella (23). Concurrently, flagellin was also found to promote the release of IL-8 in response to enteroaggregative *Escherichia coli* and to cause degradation of IκBα and increase the inducible nitric oxide synthase expression in response to serovar Dublin (11, 26, 48). As illustrated in Fig. 2, flagellin from these different bacteria may activate proinflammatory cascades by binding to Toll-like receptor 5 (TLR-5), one of a family of pattern recognition receptors involved in the innate immune response (22, 26). The flagella export apparatus and the TTs apparatus share structural as well as functional similarities (37), and some SPI-1 products can be secreted via the flagellar export apparatus (30, 63). This proinflammatory event is further discussed in chapter 9.

PEEC

Although IL-8 is required for recruitment of PMNs to the basal aspect of epithelial cells, an additional chemoattractant, PEEC, guides PMN movement across the intestinal epithelium (40, 41). This apically secreted chemoattractant is highly efficient in driving PMN transmigration across the epithelium (the final step of transepithelial migration). The PEEC bioactivity harbors properties that appear to set it apart from other known peptide- or lipid-based PMN chemoattractants. The distinguishing features of PEEC indicate that it is relatively small (<1 kDa), stable, and not highly hydrophobic, and it does not appear to signal via the *n*-formyl peptide or the IL-8 receptors. Like most neutrophil chemoattractants, PEEC induces a PMN signal transduction cascade involving a GTP binding protein ($G_{\alpha i}$) that also elicits a rise in $[Ca^{2+}]_i$. In addition, bioassays reveal that PEEC directly signals PMNs, but unlike known chemoattractants, PMNs respond to PEEC with essentially a purely chemotactic response in which degranulation or superoxide generation is virtually not detectable, even at saturating concentrations of PEEC bioactivity. Thus, PEEC appears to exhibit characteristics that are even distinct from "pure" PMN chemoattractants. Therefore, in the final step of transepithelial migration, subepithelial PMNs would be ideally positioned to traffic across the monolayer in response to secreted PEEC activity. It is possible that interference with a PEEC-based signaling pathway may provide a potentially important new therapeutic target for treatment of acute inflammatory diseases of intestinal mucosal surfaces.

Other Cytokines

Different studies have also shown that stimulation of human intestinal epithelial cells with serovar Typhimurium evokes the increased expression and secretion of a number of other cytokines with chemoattractant and proinflammatory functions. For instance, stimulated epithelial cells express and secrete the chemokines GRO α, β, γ, and ENA-78 (13, 32). Like IL-8, these cytokines belong to the CXC family of chemokines and are characterized by their ability to chemoattract and activate PMN, suggesting an important secondary (redundant) function of intestinal epithelial cells to initiate the mucosal influx of PMN. In addition, *Salmonella*-infected human intestinal epithelial cells express and secrete other proinflammatory cytokines, including tumor necrosis factor-alpha, granulocyte-macrophage colony-stimulating factor, and IL-1α and β, although expression of these cytokines is generally much lower (orders of magnitude) than that observed for chemokines (13, 32). Fur-

ther, intestinal epithelial cells do not appear to express a number of cytokines such as IL-2, IL-4, IL-5, IL-12, or gamma interferon that are more commonly associated with antigen-specific acquired immune responses (13, 32). These findings indicate that such cytokines secreted by intestinal epithelial cells are likely to play a more important role in initiating and regulating the innate mucosal inflammatory response rather than the antigen-specific mucosal immune response.

THE ROLE OF SipA IN *SALMONELLA*-INDUCED ENTERITIS

Although it is generally accepted that *Salmonella* invasiveness is essential for virulence, the actual requirement for intestinal invasion for the induction of enteritis is not clear. Several lines of evidence support this predication. First, in orally infected calves, extracellular bacteria reside in the intestinal lumen in high numbers. Likewise, in bovine ligated ileal loops, more than 90% of the inoculum is gentamicin sensitive, suggesting that bacteria are localized primarily in an extracellular niche (57). Second, extracellular bacteria are able to translocate effector proteins into epithelial cells in the absence of invasion, and these effector proteins are required for induction of enteritis (19). Third, independent investigations have revealed that different serotypes of *Salmonella* sp. that equally invade intestinal epithelial cells induce different levels of enteropathogenic responses, implying there is no direct correlation between the magnitudes of invasion and enteropathogenicity (20, 39, 57, 58). Consistent with these studies, invasion of epithelial cells has been uncoupled from *Salmonella*-induced PMN transmigration in vitro. Thus, these observations question whether invasion of the intestinal mucosa by *Salmonella* sp. is required for the induction of enteritis.

Supporting this concept, release of PEEC requires the SPI-1 secretion apparatus but does not require bacterial entry or bacterial protein synthesis (after *Salmonella*-epithelial interactions have been established) (39). These results implicate the existence of *Salmonella* SPI-1-

secreted proteins that specifically direct PMN without affecting bacterial entry. In a recent study, we screened isogenic strains of serovar Typhimurium deficient in various SPI-1 effectors to identify a gene product necessary for PMN transmigration across model intestinal epithelia but dispensable for bacterial internalization (or vice versa). We determined the molecular basis of this requirement by showing that a serovar Typhimurium *sipA* mutant failed to induce PMN transepithelial migration but was still able to enter intestinal epithelial cells (34). In the same study, we also found that purified serovar Typhimurium SipA protein can trigger the PMN migration response in the absence of TTs and translocation factors, such as SipB and SipD (34). Thus, SipA is not only necessary but sufficient to activate signaling pathways and promote PMN transepithelial migration. Additionally, these results indicate that SipA may act differently from other SPI-1-secreted proteins (such as SopE or SopB), which must enter the cytosol to modify their targets. Thus, this observation puts into question the long-held view that serovar Typhimurium effector proteins must be delivered into host cells by a TTs and translocation system.

These features identify SipA as an important mediator of the inflammatory response. The fact that purified SipA in contact with the apical epithelial surface directly activates the signal transduction pathway governing PMN transepithelial migration favors the idea that SipA may not need to enter the cell cytosol to stimulate this proinflammatory event but rather may engage a host surface receptor. Furthermore, PMN transmigration occurs only following apical but not basolateral exposure to serovar Typhimurium, which implies that host factors functioning at the apical domain of epithelial cells may also assist in the modulation of this event (39). While it is also conceivable that SipA may translocate into the host cell by a process independent of the TTSS, this appears less likely considering our recent advances toward understanding the molecular basis of this process.

Our recent findings provide evidence for the regulation of serovar Typhimurium-PMN transmigration by a novel mechanism involving the GTPase ADP-ribosylation factor 6 (ARF6) (7), which is illustrated in Fig. 3. In this model, serovar Typhimurium contacting the apical surface of polarized epithelial cells elicits a signal through the bacterial effector, SipA, that recruits an ARF6 guanine exchange factor (such as ARNO) to the apical plasma membrane. ARNO facilitates ARF6 activation at the apical membrane, which in turn stimulates phospholipase D (PLD) recruitment to and activity at this site. The PLD product phosphatidic acid (PA) is metabolized by a phosphohydrolase into diacylglycerol (DAG), which recruits cytosolic protein kinase C (PKC) to the apical membrane. Activated PKC phosphorylates downstream targets that are responsible for the production and apical release of PEEC, which drives transepithelial PMN movement. At present, ARF6 is the first example of a "molecular switch" specifically modulating the PMN transmigration aspect of serovar Typhimurium pathogenesis, independently of bacterial internalization or the release of other proinflammatory mediators such as IL-8.

ARF6 is a member of the Arf subgroup of GTPases of the Ras superfamily, which were first defined as cofactors necessary for the cholera toxin-catalyzed ADP ribosylation of the α_s subunit of the heterotrimeric G proteins. ARF6, the only class III ARF, is novel in its localization to the plasma membrane and endosomal structures in nonpolarized cells (10), and is highly expressed in polarized cells where it localizes primarily to the apical brush border and apical early endosomes (2, 35). Although ARF6 was initially identified as a modulator of vesicular traffic and of cortical actin cytoarchitecture, recent evidence suggests that ARF6 is also a regulator of signal transduction cascades initiated by a variety of external stimuli, and appears to be a key signal transducer downstream of G-protein-coupled receptors (52). Even though the identity of the cellular "receptor" for *Salmonella* sp. and/or its

MEMBRANE

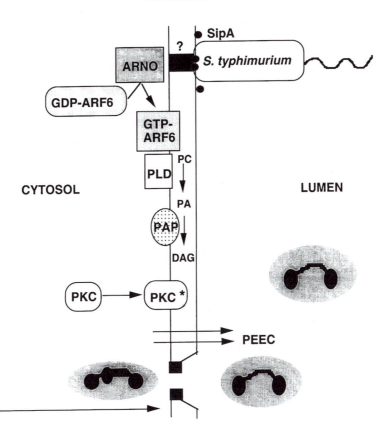

FIGURE 3 Model of *S. enterica* serovar Typhimurium-induced signaling in epithelial cells by the *Salmonella*-secreted protein SipA. Interaction of the serovar Typhimurium-secreted effector protein SipA with the apical domain of polarized epithelial cells leads to activation of ARF6 (GTP-ARF6) at the apical membrane, most likely through the mammalian guanine exchange factor (GEF) ARNO. This leads to an increase in PLD activity and local production of PA, which is metabolized to DAG by PA phosphohydrolase (PAP). Generation of DAG recruits PKC to the apical membrane. Activation of PKC at this site (PKC★) is necessary for the apical release of the chemokine PEEC and subsequent basolateral-to-apical PMN transmigration.

effector SipA is not known, our observations would suggest that bacterial adherence to the apical membrane of polarized epithelial cells promotes ARF6 in an analogous manner.

OTHER *SALMONELLA* GENES THAT REGULATE PMN TRANSEPITHELIAL MIGRATION

Some of the translocation and intracellular activities of other translocated *Salmonella* effector proteins also elicit a variety of pathogenic re-

sponses ultimately leading to the onset of enteritis. Although SopB is the best studied to date, other secreted and translocated effector proteins are also involved in the induction of enteritis. This has been shown to be the case for the SopD protein. Mutation of *sopD* has an additive effect in relation to the SopB mutation (31) and implies that secreted effector proteins of *Salmonella* sp. can act in concert to induce enteritis. Furthermore, other secreted effector proteins also have a role in the induction of enteropathogenic responses. Thus, in addition to SopB and SopD, SopA contributes to enteropathogenicity (62). However, in contrast to SopB, the biochemical functions of the SopA and SopD enteropathogenicity effectors remain obscure.

Since the interaction of *Salmonella* sp. with epithelial cells results in the production of a set of inflammatory regulators by epithelial cells, it is likely that some Sops may be needed for the release of signals leading to the attraction of PMNs from the peripheral blood into the lamina propria, whereas others might be involved in orchestrating the migration of PMNs across the monolayer. Indeed, in both the bovine ligated ileal loop and the T84 intestinal cell model, a *Salmonella sopA* mutant failed to successfully induce the proinflammatory event of PMN transepithelial migration when compared to the wild-type strain (62). Interestingly, this was in contrast to the effects elicited by a double *sopB/sopD* mutant of *Salmonella* sp. The *sopB/sopD* mutant strain was as efficient as the wild type at recruiting PMNs across the model epithelial monolayer despite being affected in enteropathogenicity in vivo in bovine ligated ileal loops (31, 62). These data argue that different Sops may be involved in the control of different stages of PMN influx. In this regard, it is possible that SopB and SopD may be needed for the release of signals leading to the attraction of PMNs from the peripheral blood into the lamina propria, whereas SopA may be involved in orchestrating the migration of PMNs directly across the epithelial monolayer.

In addition to TTSS-1-associated genes, several other genes affecting *Salmonella* enteropathogenicity are currently being investigated. The Pip pathogenicity island (SPI-5) was identified while mapping the location of SopB on the *Salmonella* chromosome (62). This locus is conserved in *Salmonella* sp. and maps approximately at 20 centrisomes of the serovar Typhimurium chromosome. Sequence analysis revealed that this *Salmonella*-specific DNA fragment is flanked by DNA sequences with significant sequence similarity

to the *E. coli* genes; *serT* on one side and *copS/copR* on the other. SerT in *Pseudomonas aeruginosa* is a site of integration of the cytotoxin-converting phage CTX and indicates the presence of horizontally acquired virulence-associated sequences at this locus. SPI-5 harbors five novel genes, *pipA*, *pipB*, *pipD* (pathogenicity island-encoded proteins), and *orfX*, in addition to *sopB*. The effect of the mutations in SPI-5-encoded genes on the induction of intestinal secretory and inflammatory responses by *Salmonella* sp. was assessed in bovine ligated ileal loops. The magnitude of the secretory and inflammatory responses elicited by *Salmonella* strains carrying a mutation in *pipD*, *pipB*, or *pipA* was significantly reduced compared to that of the wild-type strain; however, there was no effect on systemic virulence in mice (29).

Apart from *pipC*, which encodes a specific SopB chaperone (62), the function and sites of action of other Pips are unknown. Although no homologies have been found for the Sops, the gene products of *pipB* and *pipD* have structural similarities to proteins from other bacterial species; thus, the observed sequence similarities may indicate putative functions for these SPI-5-encoded proteins. For example, PipB is similar to the HglK protein from *Anabaena* and *Synechocystis* spp., and therefore PipB may have a structural role in glycolipid biogenesis. PipD, on the other hand, is structurally similar to dipeptidases from *Lactobacillus* spp., and thus, this may imply that PipD is a secreted peptidase of *Salmonella* sp. with its target on the surface or within host cells.

REFERENCES

1. **Ahmer, B. M., J. van Reeuwijk, P. R. Watson, T. S. Wallis, and F. Heffron.** 1999. *Salmonella* SirA is a global regulator of genes mediating enteropathogenesis. *Mol. Microbiol.* **31:** 971–982.

2. **Altschuler, Y., S. Liu, L. Katz, K. Tang, S. Hardy, F. Brodsky, G. Apodacca, and K. Mostov.** 1999. ADP-ribosylation factor 6 and endocytosis at the apical surface of Madin-Darby canine kidney cells. *J. Cell Biol.* **147:**7–12.

3. **Amin, B. M., G. R. Douce, M. P. Osborne, and J. Stephen.** 1994. Quantitative studies of invasion of rabbit ileal mucosa by *Salmonella typhimurium* strain which differ in virulence in model gastroenteritis. *Infect. Immun.* **62:**569–578.

4. **Baggiolini, M., B. Dewald, and A. Walz.** 1992. Interleukin-8 and related cytokines, p. 247–263. *In* J. I. Gallin, I. M. Golstein, and R. Snyderman (ed.), *Inflammation: Basic Principles and Clinical Correlates*, 2nd ed. Raven Press, New York, N.Y.

5. **Bolton, A. J., M. P. Osborne, T. S. Wallis, and J. Stephen.** 1999. Interaction of *Salmonella cholersuis, Salmonella dublin,* and *Salmonella typhimurium* with porcine and bovine terminal ileum in vivo. *Microbiology* **145:**2431–2441.

6. **Boyd, J. E.** 1985. Pathology of the alimentary tract in *Salmonella typhimurium* food poisoning. *Gut* **26:**935–944.

7. **Criss, A. K., M. Silva, J. E. Casanova, and B. A. McCormick.** 2001. Regulation of *Salmonella*-induced neutrophil transmigration by epithelial ADP-ribosylation factor 6. *J. Biol. Chem.* **276:**48431–48439.

8. **Day, D. W., B. K. Mandal, and B. C. Morson.** 1978. The rectal biopsy appearances in *Salmonella* colitis. *Histopathology* **2:**117–131.

9. **Dharmsathaphorn, K., and J. L. Madara.** 1990. Established intestinal cell lines as model systems for electrolyte transport studies. *Methods Enzymol.* **192:**354–389.

10. **D'Souza-Shorey, C., G. Li, M. I. Colombo, and P. D. Stahl.** 1995. A regulatory role for ARF6 in receptor-mediated endocytosis. *Science* **267:**1175–1178.

11. **Eaves-Pyles, T., K. Murthy, L. Liaudet, L. Virag, G. Ross, F. G. Soriano, C. Szabo, and A. L. Salzman.** 2001. Flagellin, a novel mediator of *Salmonella*-induced epithelial activation and systemic inflammation: I kappa B alpha degradation, induction of nitric oxide synthase, induction of proinflammatory mediators, and cardiovascular dysfunction. *J. Immunol.* **166:**1248–1260.

12. **Eberhart, C. E., and R. N. DuBois.** 1995. Eicosanoids and the gastrointestinal tract. *Gastroenterology* **109:**285–301.

13. **Eckmann, L., H.-C. Jung, C.-C. Schuerer-Maly, A. Panja, E. Morzycka-Wroblewska, and M. F. Kagnoff.** 1993. Differential cytokine expression by human intestinal epithelial cell lines: regulated expression of interleukin-8. *Gastroenterology* **105:**1689–1697.

14. **Eckmann, L., M. T. Rudolf, A. Ptasznik, C. Schultz, T. Jiang, N. Wolfson, R. Tsein, J. Fierer, S. Shears, M. F. Kagnoff, and A. E. Traynor-Kaplan.** 1997. D-Myo-inositol 1,4,5,6-tetrakisphosphate produced in human intestinal epithelial cells in response to *Salmonella* invasion inhibits phosphoinositide 3-kinase signaling pathways. *Proc. Natl. Acad. Sci. USA* **94:**14456–14460.

15. **Eckmann, L., W. F. Stenson, T. C. Savidge, D. C. Lowe, K. E. Barrett, J. Fierer, J. R. Smith, and M. F. Kagnoff.** 1997. Role of intestinal epithelial cells in the host secretory response to infection by invasive bacteria. *J. Clin. Investig.* **100:**296–309.

16. **Feng, Y., S. R. Wente, and P. W. Majerus.** 2001. Overexpression of the inositol phosphate SopB in human 293 cells stimulates cellular chloride influx and inhibits nuclear mRNA export. *Proc. Natl. Acad. Sci. USA* **98:**875–879.

17. **Finlay, B. B., S. Ruschkowski, and S. Dedhar.** 1991. Cytoskeletal arrangements accompanying *Salmonella* entry into epithelial cells. *J. Cell Sci.* **99:**283–296.

18. **Galan, J. E.** 1996. Molecular genetic bases of *Salmonella* entry into host cells. *Mol. Microbiol.* **20:**263–271.

19. **Galyov, E. G., M. W. Wood, R. Rosqvist, P. B. Mullan, P. R. Watson, S. Hedges, and T. S. Wallis.** 1997. A secreted effector protein of *Salmonella dublin* is translocated into eucaryotic cells and mediates inflammation and fluid secretion in infected ileal mucosa. *Mol. Microbiol.* **25:**903–912.

20. **Gewirtz, A. T., A. M. Siber, J. L. Madara, and B. A. McCormick.** 1999. Orchestration of neutrophil movement by intestinal epithelial cells in response to *Salmonella typhimurium* can be uncoupled from bacterial internalization. *Infect. Immun.* **67:**608–617.

21. **Gewirtz, A. T., A. S. Rao, P. O. Simon, D. Merlin, D. Carnes, J. L. Madara, and A. S. Neish.** 2000. *Salmonella typhimurium* induces epithelial IL-8 expression via Ca^{2+}-mediated activation of the NF-κB pathway. *J. Clin. Investig.* **105:**79–92.

22. **Gewirtz, A. T., A. T. Navas, S. Lyons, P. J. Godowski, and J. L. Madara.** 2001. Bacterial flagella activates basolaterally expressed TLR5 to induce epithelial proinflammatory gene expression. *J. Immunol.* **167:**1882–1885.

23. **Gewirtz, A. T., P. O. Simon, C. K. Schmitt, L. J. Taylor, C. H. Hagedorn, A. D. O'Brien, A. S. Neish, and J. L. Madara.** 2001. *Salmonella typhimurium* translocates flagellin across intestinal epithelia, inducing a proinflammatory response. *J. Clin. Investig.* **107:**99–109.

24. **Gianella, R. A., S. B. Formal, G. J. Dammin, and H. Collins.** 1973. Pathogenesis of salmonellosis: studies of fluid secretion, mucosal

invasion, and morphologic reaction in the rabbit ileum. *J. Clin. Investig.* **52:**441–453.

25. Gianella, R. A. 1979. Importance of intestinal inflammatory reaction in *Salmonella*-mediated intestinal secretion. *Infect. Immun.* **23:**140–145.

26. Hayashi, F., K. D. Smith, A. Ozinsky, T. R. Hawn, E. C. Yi, D. R. Goodlett, J. K. Eng, S. Akira, D. M. Underhill, and A. Aderem. 2001. The innate immune response to bacterial flagellin is mediated by Toll-like receptor 5. *Nature* **410:**1099–1103.

27. Hobbie, S., L. M. Chen, R. J. Davis, and J. E. Galan. 1997. Involvement of mitogen-activated protein kinase pathways in the nuclear responses and cytokine production induced by *Salmonella typhimurium* in cultured epithelial cells. *J. Immunol.* **159:**5550–5559.

28. Hong, K. H., and V. L. Miller. 1998. Identification of a novel *Salmonella* invasion locus homologous to *Shigella ipgDE*. *J. Bacteriol.* **180:**1793–1802.

29. Hueck, C. J. 1998. Type III secretion systems in bacterial pathogens of animals and plants. *Microbiol. Mol. Biol. Rev.* **62:**379–433.

30. Iyoda, S., T. Kamidoi, K. Hirose, K. Kutsukake, and H. Watanabe. 2001. A flagellar gene *fliz* regulates the expression of invasion genes and virulence phenotype in *Salmonella enterica* serovar Typhimurium. *Microb. Pathog.* **30:**81–90.

31. Jones, M. A., M. W. Wood, P. B. Mullan, P. R. Watson, T. S. Watson, and E. E. Galyov. 1998. Secreted effector proteins of *Salmonella dublin* act in concert to induce enteritis. *Infect. Immun.* **66:**5799–5804.

32. Jung, H. C., L. Eckmann, S.-K. Yang, A. Panja, J. Fierer, E. Morzycka-Wroblewska, and M. F. Kagnoff. 1995. A distinct array of proinflammatory cytokines is expressed in human colon epithelial cells in response to bacterial invasion. *J. Clin. Investig.* **95:**55–65.

33. Kumar, N. B., T. T. Nostrant, and H. D. Appelman. 1982. The histopathologic spectrum of acute self-limited colitis (acute infectious type colitis). *Am. J. Surg. Pathol.* **6:**523–529.

34. Lee, C. A., M. Silva, A. M. Siber, A. J. Kelly, E. Galyov, and B. A. McCormick. 2000. A secreted *Salmonella* protein induces a proinflammatory response in epithelial cells, which promotes neutrophil migration. *Proc. Natl. Acad. Sci. USA* **97:**12283–12288.

35. Londono, I., V. Marshansky, S. Bourgoin, P. Vinay, and M. Bendayan. 1999. Expression and distribution of adenosine diphosphate ribosylation factors in the rat kidney. *Kidney Int.* **55:**1407–1416.

36. Madara, J. L., T. W. Patapoff, B. Gillece-Castro, S. P. Colgan, C. A. Parkos, C. Delp, and R. J. Mrsny. 1993. 5′-Adenosine monophosphate is the neutrophil-derived paracrine factor that elicits chloride secretion from T84 intestinal epithelial cell monolayers. *J. Clin. Investig.* **91:**2320–2325.

37. Makishima, S., K. Komoriya, S. Yamaguchi, and S. I. Aizawa. 2001. Length of the flagella hook and the capacity of the type III export apparatus. *Science* **291:**2411–2413.

38. McCormick, B., P. Hofman, J. Kim, D. Carnes, S. Miller, and J. Madara. 1995. Surface attachment of *Salmonella typhimurium* to intestinal epithelia imprints the subepithelial matrix with gradients chemotactic for neutrophils. *J. Cell Biol.* **131:**1599–1608.

39. McCormick, B., S. Miller, D. Carnes, and J. Madara. 1995. Transepithelial signaling to neutrophils by *Salmonellae*: a novel virulence mechanism for gastroenteritis. *Infect. Immun.* **63:**2302–2309.

40. McCormick, B. A., S. P. Colgan, C. D. Archer, S. I. Miller, and J. L. Madara. 1993. *Salmonella typhimurium* attachment to human intestinal epithelial monolayers: transcellular signalling to subepithelial neutrophils. *J. Cell Biol.* **123:**895–907.

41. McCormick, B. A., C. A. Parkos, S. P. Colgan, D. K. Carnes, and J. L. Madara. 1998. Apical secretion of a pathogen-elicited epithelial chemoattractant (PEEC) activity in response to surface colonization of intestinal epithelia by *Salmonella typhimurium*. *J. Immunol.* **160:**455–466.

42. McGovern, V. J., and L. J. Slavutin. 1979. Pathology of *Salmonella* colitis. *Am. J. Surg. Pathol.* **3:**483–490.

43. Norris, A. F., M. P. Wilson, T. S. Wallis, E. E. Galyov, and P. W. Majerus. 1998. SopB, a protein required for virulence of *Salmonella dublin*, is an inositol phosphate phosphatase. *Proc. Natl. Acad. Sci. USA* **95:**14057–14059.

44. Rout, W. R., S. B. Formal, G. J. Dammin, and R. A. Giannella. 1974. Pathophysiology of *Salmonella* diarrhea in the rhesus monkey: intestinal transport, morphological and bacteriological studies. *Gastroenterology* **67:**59–70.

45. Sitaraman, S. V., D. Merlin, L. Wang, M. Wong, A. T. Gewirtz, M. Si-Tahar, and J. L. Madara. 2001. Neutrophil–epithelial cross-talk at the intestinal lumenal surface mediated by reciprocal secretion of adenosine and IL-6. *J. Clin. Investig.* **107:**861–869.

46. Smith, W. L., and D. L. DeWitt. 1996. Prostaglandin endoperoxidase H synthase-1 and -2. *Adv. Immunol.* **62:**167–215.

47. **Steele-Mortimer, O., S. Meresse, J. P. Gorval, B. H. Toh, and B. B. Finlay.** 1999. Biogenesis of *Salmonella typhimurium*-containing vacuoles in epithelial cells involves interaction with the early endocytic pathway. *Cell Microbiol.* **1:**33–49.

48. **Steiner, T. S., J. P. Nataro, C. E. Poteet-Smith, J. A. Smith, and R. L. Guerrant.** 2000. Enteroaggregative *Escherichia coli* expresses a novel flagellin that causes IL-8 release from intestinal epithelial cells. *J. Clin. Investig.* **105:**1769–1777.

49. **Strohmeier, G. R., S. M. Reppert, W. L. Lencer, and J. L. Madara.** 1995. The A_{2b} adenosine receptor mediates cAMP responses to adenosine receptor agonists in human intestinal epithelia. *J. Biol. Chem.* **270:**2387–2394.

50. **Takeuchi, A.** 1967. Electron microscope studies of experimental *Salmonella* infection. *Am. J. Pathol.* **50:**109–119.

51. **Tsolis, R. M., G. Adams, T. A. Ficht, and A. J. Baumler.** 1999. Contribution of *Salmonella typhimurium* virulence factors to diarrheal disease in calves. *Infect. Immun.* **67:**4879–4885.

52. **Venkateswarlu, K., and P. J. Cullen.** 2000. Signalling via ADP-ribosylation factor 6 lies downstream of phosphatidylinositide 3–kinase. *Biochem. J.* **345:**719–724.

53. **Wallis, T. S., W. G. Starkey, J. Stephen, M. P. Osborne, and D. C. A. Candy.** 1986. The nature and role of mucosal damage in relation to *Salmonella typhimurium*-induced fluid secretion in the rabbit ileum. *J. Med. Microbiol.* **22:**39–49.

54. **Wallis, T. S., A. T. M. Vaughan, G. J. Clarke, G.-M. Qi, K. J. Woron, D. C. A. Candy, M. P. Osborne, and J. Stephen.** 1990. The role of leucocytes in the induction of fluid secretion by *Salmonella typhimurium*. *J. Med. Microbiol.* **31:**27–35.

55. **Wallis, T. S., S. M. Paulin, J. S. Plested, P. R. Watson, and P. W. Jones.** 1995. The *Salmonella dublin* virulence plasmid mediates systemic but not enteric phases of salmonellosis in cattle. *Infect. Immun.* **63:**2755–2761.

56. **Wallis, T. S., and E. E. Galyov.** 2000. Molecular basis of *Salmonella*-induced enteritis. *Mol. Microbiol.* **36:**997–1005.

57. **Watson, P. R., S. M. Paulin, A. P. Bland, P. W. Jones, and T. S. Wallis.** 1995. Characterization of intestinal invasion by *Salmonella typhimurium* and *Salmonella dublin* and effect of a mutation in the *invH* gene. *Infect. Immun.* **63:**2743–2754.

58. **Watson, P. R., E. E. Galyov, S. M. Paulin, P. W. Jones, and T. S. Wallis.** 1998. Mutation of *invH*, but not *stn*, reduces *Salmonella*-induced enteritis in cattle. *Infect. Immun.* **66:**1432–1438.

59. **Watson, P. R., S. M. Paulin, A. P. Bland, P. W. Jones, and T. S. Wallis.** 1999. Differential regulation of enteric and systemic salmonellosis by slyA. *Infect. Immun.* **67:**4950–4954.

60. **Wood, M. W., R. Rosqvist, P. B. Mullan, M. H. Edwards, and E. E. Galyov.** 1996. SopE, a secreted protein of *Salmonella dublin*, is translocated into the target eukaryotic cell via a sip-dependent mechanism and promotes bacterial entry. *Mol. Microbiol.* **22:**327–338.

61. **Wood, M. W., M. A. Jones, P. R. Watson, S. Hedges, T. S. Wallis, and E. E. Galyov.** 1998. Identification of a pathogenicity island required for *Salmonella* enteropathogenicity. *Mol. Microbiol.* **29:**883–892.

62. **Wood, M. W., M. A. Jones, P. R. Watson, A. M. Siber, B. A. McCormick, S. Hedges, R. Rosqvist, T. S. Wallis, and E. E. Galyov.** 2000. The secreted effector protein of *Salmonella dublin*, SopA, is translocated into eukaryotic cells and influences the induction of enteritis. *Cell Microbiol.* **2:**293–303.

63. **Young, G. M., D. H. Schiel, and V. L. Miller.** 1999. A new pathway for the secretion of virulence factors by bacteria: the flagellar export apparatus functions as a protein secretion system. *Proc. Natl. Acad. Sci. USA* **96:**6456–6461.

64. **Zhou, D., L. M. Chen, L. Hernandez, S. B. Shears, and J. E. Galan.** 2001. A *Salmonella* inositol polyphosphate acts in conjunction with other bacterial effectors to promote host cell actin cytoskeleton rearrangements and bacterial internalization. *Mol. Microbiol.* **39:**248–259.

EFFECTOR MOLECULES OF *SHIGELLA* PATHOGENESIS AND HOST RESPONSES

M. Isabel Fernandez and Philippe J. Sansonetti

25

Microbial pathogens have evolved different ways of interacting with their hosts and possess a great array of virulence factors that interfere with or stimulate a variety of host-cell physiological responses. This interaction between bacteria and host cells is not unidirectional; rather, both pathogens and host cells engage in a signaling cross talk that leads to several responses. For example, in a variety of gram-negative bacteria, activating signals for the secretion of proteins by the type III secretion apparatus result from the interaction between bacteria and their host cells (40).

Shigellae are gram-negative, nonsporulating, facultative anaerobic bacilli belonging to the family *Enterobacteriaceae*. Infection by *Shigella* spp. causes bacillary dysentery or shigellosis in humans, an acute inflammatory colonic disease characterized by fever, intestinal cramps, and discharge of mucopurulent and bloody feces. Histological studies of colonic biopsies from patients with shigellosis show inflammatory cell infiltration into the epithelial layer, tissue edema, and eroded areas of the colonic epithelium (72).

The genus *Shigella* comprises four different species. *Shigella flexneri*, with six serotypes, and *Shigella sonnei*, with one serotype, account for the endemic form of the disease. *Shigella dysenteriae*, with 16 serotypes including *S. dysenteriae* serotype 1, accounts for deadly epidemics in developing countries, largely because of its capacity to produce Shiga toxin, a potent cytotoxin. Finally, *Shigella boydii*, with eight serotypes, is observed only on the Indian subcontinent.

In 1999, the World Health Organization attributed an estimated 1.1 million deaths per year to shigellosis (60). Shigellosis is endemic throughout the world, but 99% of the cases occur in the developing world. Moreover, shigellosis is mostly a pediatric disease, since more than 60% of cases occur in children between 1 and 5 years old. Because the disease is transmitted by person-to-person contact or by contaminated water or food, lack of hygiene is one of the most important factors contributing to the frequent occurrence of shigellosis in developing countries. Moreover, the public health burden of shigellosis is aggravated by the prevalence of antibiotic resistance in both endemic and epidemic areas; the cost of treating the disease with antibiotics, especially in developing countries; and the severity of such acute complications as

M. Isabel Fernandez and Philippe J. Sansonetti, Unité de Pathogénie Microbienne Moléculaire, INSERM U389, Institut Pasteur, Rue du Dr Roux 28, 75724 Paris Cedex 15, France.

Microbial Pathogenesis and the Intestinal Epithelial Cell, ed. by G. Hecht
© 2003 ASM Press, Washington, D.C.

hypoglycemia, intestinal perforations, peritonitis, septicemia, or hemolytic-uremic syndrome (119). Unfortunately, no vaccine is currently available that provides adequate protection against the many prevalent species and serotypes of *Shigella*.

Epithelial cells at mucosal surfaces constitute the first line of defense against microbial pathogens. In the colon, epithelial cells are in constant contact with bacteria and bacterial products. In fact, these cells are now considered to be major sentinels of host defense. Under normal conditions, colonic epithelial cells do not respond to the lumenal contents, as induction of an inflammatory response would be detrimental to the host. In contrast, epithelial cells are able to discriminate between pathogenic bacteria and resident flora (57). This ability might be, in part, based on the intracellular localization of recognition systems that would be induced if bacteria adhered to the cell surface, entered into the cell, or gained access to the basolateral compartment of the epithelium. Many pathogens, such as *Shigella*, possess a specific set of virulence factors that affect the host, in addition to the ability to invade epithelial cells. As a consequence, the host develops specialized strategies to resist such infections. This cross talk between enteric pathogens and their intestinal host allows the induction of inflammation and the development of the disease. The ability of *Shigella* to invade and colonize the intestinal epithelium, in association with an intense inflammatory response leading to the destruction of the colonic mucosa, is a key determinant in the establishment of the disease. Understanding the cellular and molecular mechanisms by which bacteria invade and destroy the intestinal barrier is essential to improve our knowledge of the pathogenesis of shigellosis, to develop new therapeutic strategies, and to design innovative vaccines for the prevention of the disease. This chapter outlines our current understanding of the expression of the *Shigella* invasive phenotype, as well as the effector molecules required and their unique modes of action. The features of the disease involve specific interactions of *Shigella*

with different cell populations, particularly intestinal epithelial cells, resident macrophages, and polymorphonuclear leukocytes (PMN). These interactions between invasive bacteria and the host cell initiate diverse responses, leading to rupture, invasion, dissemination, and inflammatory destruction of the intestinal barrier.

PATHOGENESIS OF SHIGELLOSIS: A GENERAL OVERVIEW OF THE INFECTIOUS PROCESS

Shigella sp. is highly infectious, with ingestion of as few as 100 microorganisms resulting in disease (33). Bacteria invade and disrupt the rectal and/or colonic mucosae leading to tissue destruction, although the basis for this tissue specificity is not yet understood. The disease remains essentially limited to the intestinal mucosa, and the effectors of innate immunity that eradicate the bacteria, thus preventing their systemic dissemination, have been the focus of intense research. As a consequence of the development of an acute inflammatory response, the intestinal tissue is destroyed. Therefore, shigellosis is considered to be a disease resulting from an imbalance in the host mechanisms that regulate inflammation in the presence of an invading microorganism.

M cells in the follicle-associated epithelium (FAE), which overlie lymphoid tissue within the colonic epithelium, are specialized in sampling and transport of luminal antigens. These cells are characterized by their poorly organized brush border, absence of glycocalix, high endocytic activity, and basolateral lymphocyte-containing pocket. Several microorganisms, including *S. flexneri*, *Salmonella enterica* serovar Typhimurium, *Salmonella enterica* serovar Typhi, *Yersinia enterocolitica*, *Yersinia pseudotuberculosis*, and *Campylobacter jejuni* (109), use M cells to cross the epithelial barrier of the gut, taking advantage of this unique portal of entry. On the other hand, M cells form a pocket filled with lymphocytes, macrophages, and dendritic cells, thereby providing direct contact between the intestinal microbial flora and the mucosal immune system (125). *Shigella* is not able to invade epithelial cells from the apical pole and exploits M cells to enter into the colonic epithelium, a process that requires the expression of the *Shigella* invasive phenotype (117). After crossing of the FAE, bacteria reach the dome area of the lymphoid follicle, where they are phagocytosed by macrophages. *Shigella* kills macrophages essentially by apoptosis (167), then escapes to the subepithelial tissue and invades the epithelial lining by the basolateral surface. The infected macrophages release the proinflammatory cytokine interleukin 1 beta (IL-1β) through direct activation of caspase-1 by *Shigella* (24). As a consequence, PMN are recruited, which then infiltrate the infected site and destabilize the epithelium (127). The destruction of the epithelial barrier permits more bacteria to traverse into the subepithelial space, providing easy access to the basolateral side of epithelial cells where bacteria can invade epithelial cells. At the same time, bacteria disseminate throughout the epithelium by spreading from cell to cell. Infected epithelial cells release proinflammatory chemokines such as IL-8, which then contribute to the exacerbation of inflammation (121).

BACTERIAL DETERMINANTS

Virulence Plasmid

In *Shigella* a large 213-kb virulence plasmid contains most of the genes required to express the invasive phenotype, and the expression of

this invasive phenotype is dependent upon the host cellular target (122, 123, 129, 158). Sequencing of the virulence plasmid of *S. flexneri* M90T 5a pWR100, composed of 213,494 bp, has permitted the identification of genes encoding approximately 25 proteins secreted by the type III secretion apparatus (20).

A 31-kb segment of the virulence plasmid, known as the *ipa/mxi-spa* locus or entry region, is necessary and sufficient for entry of bacteria into epithelial cells, macrophage apoptotic death, and activation of PMN (58, 73, 76, 128–130) (Fig. 1). This segment is organized in two operons transcribed divergently. On one hand, it contains genes that encode for proteins composing the type III secretion apparatus, which is a flagella-like structure involved in translocation of *Shigella* effector molecules from the bacterial cytoplasm to the membrane and cytoplasm of the host cell. On the other hand, this fragment also contains the *ipaA-D* genes, *ipgB1*, and *ipgD* encoding proteins secreted by this secretion system, and the genes encoding the cytoplasmic chaperones, IpgC and IpgE. The *virB* gene codes for the activator required for transcription of these operons (3).

Three genes have been implicated in *Shigella*'s ability to move within the cytoplasm of infected cells: (i) the *icsA*(*virG*) encoding the outer membrane protein directly responsible for the motility of bacteria within the host cytoplasm (15, 35, 46, 65, 69); (ii) *virK* encoding

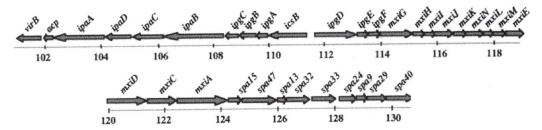

FIGURE 1 Genetic map of the 30-kg *ipa/mxi-spa* locus or entry region of the *S. flexneri* 5a virulence plasmid pWR100. On the top, the *ipa* operon, which encodes the secreted entry effectors, is hatched, and genes that encode for chaperones are indicated in black. At the bottom, the *mxi* and *spa* operons, which encode the type III secretion apparatus components, are shown in gray. The *virB* gene codes for the activator required for transcription. Courtesy of C. Parsot (Institut Pasteur, Paris, France).

a protein required for a proper production or localization of IcsA(VirG) (85); and (iii) icsP(sopA) encoding an outer membrane protease implicated in cleavage of IcsA (34, 138). Expression of icsA and virB is controlled by VirF, a transcriptional activator of the AraC family (134, 147).

The virulence plasmid also carries five ipaH genes whose specific functions have not yet been identified. Recently, Fernandez-Prada et al. (37) described a role of IpaH7.8 in the escape of Shigella from the phagosome in macrophages. Furthermore, the IpaH9.8 can be transported into the host cell nucleus and stimulate protein secretion from Shigella (148). In addition, other genes have been identified in pWR100, such as sepA encoding a protein with proteolytic activity whose inactivation leads to an attenuation of virulence (13, 14),

the multigene osp family (outer membrane proteins) with unknown functions, and mvpT and mvpA genes encoding a toxin and an antidote, respectively (102).

Type III Secretion Apparatus: Secreted Proteins and Chaperones

Type III secretons are found in many pathogenic gram-negative bacterial species, and their major function is to translocate proteins from the bacterial cytoplasm into the host cell upon contact (27, 41). The type III secretion apparatus of Shigella spp., similar to Salmonella spp., is composed of approximately 20 proteins that assemble into a structure spanning both the inner and outer bacterial membranes, and extend into the external milieu (16, 61) (Fig. 2). As a consequence of contact between bacteria and host cell, IpaB and IpaC are in-

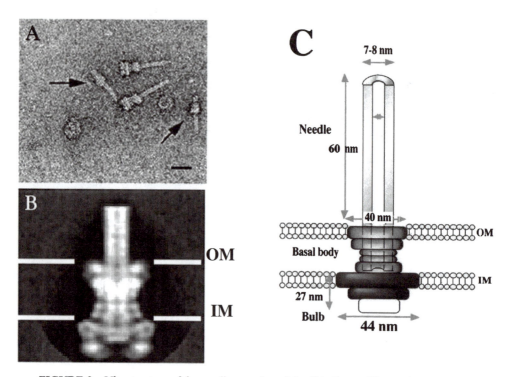

FIGURE 2 Ultrastructure of the needle complex of the *Shigella* type III secretion apparatus. (A) Negative staining of the isolated needle complex (arrows) by transmission electron microscopy (courtesy of A. Blocker, P. Gounon, and E. Larquet, Institut Pasteur, Paris, France) and (B and C) representation of the structure of the needle complex. OM and IM, outer and inner bacterial membrane, respectively. Scale bar, 100 nm.

serted into the host membrane and form a 25Å pore that is used to transport the other invasins into the cell cytoplasm. The IpaB and IpaC proteins interact to form a large protein complex that is required for the formation of this pore (16).

The ultrastructure of the needle complex of the type III secretion apparatus can be subdivided into three parts (Fig. 2C): (i) an external needle, (ii) an upper ring doublet that is the transmembrane neck domain, and (iii) a triangular base resembling a large proximal bulb (17). This complex is composed of six proteins encoded within the virulence plasmid of *Shigella*: MxiD, MxiG, MxiJ, MxiH, MxiM, and MxiI (6, 93, 131). MxiD probably constitutes the upper ring doublet and part of the periplasmic needle shaft. MxiM interacts with MxiD in the cell envelope, influencing both MxiD stability and multimerization. MxiJ also interacts with MxiD. MxiM/MxiD/MxiJ can form a transmembrane structure required for the process of needle complex assembly (132). MxiG likely forms part of the triangular base, and MxiH and MxiI are needle components that are required for needle assembly (17). Recently, Schuch and Maurelli (133) showed that the Spa33 protein, a protein encoded by the virulence plasmid, is an essential subunit of the *Shigella* type III secretion system and indispensable for Ipa protein secretion. After induction of secretion, Spa33 is mobilized in conjunction with another outer membrane-associated mobile element (Spa32) to the bacterial surface, driving Ipa invasin translocation from the internal membrane toward the outer bacterial membrane (157). Moreover, Spa32 is involved in the control of needle length (145).

Storage of some of the effector proteins in the bacterial cytoplasm requires a specific chaperone (159, 160). So far, three chaperones have been described in *Shigella* spp. In the bacterial cytoplasm, IpaB and IpaC bind independently to a common chaperone, IpgC, whereas, upon secretion, these invasins form a complex (77). It has been shown that in addition to stabilizing IpaB and IpaC, IpgC also appears to be involved in lysis of the cell

membranes that surround bacteria in protrusions during intercellular spread (91, 108). IpgD is associated in the bacterial cytoplasm with another chaperone, IpgE, and upon secretion IpgD interacts with IpaA (86). Finally, it has been recently described that the chaperone Spa15 is able to associate with three proteins in the cytoplasm of *S. flexneri*, IpgB1, IpaA, and OspC3, and possibly with OspC2/3 and OspB. This newly characterized chaperone is necessary for IpgB1 stability and for the secretion of IpaA molecules stored in the cytoplasm (92).

The regulation of the Mxi-Spa secretion apparatus occurs in response to external signals, including contact with the host cell, exposure to artificial compounds such as the dye Congo red, inactivation of *ipaB* or *ipaD*, and alterations in the growth environment (8, 78, 93, 158). At this point, it should be mentioned that certain chaperones could also be involved in the regulation of gene expression in response to external signals. Thus, it has been shown that the presence of MxiE and IpgC chaperone in the bacterial cytoplasm is required for transcription of some genes (74). In summary, in response to an external signal, IpaB and IpaC are secreted. As consequence of this active secretion, IpgC becomes free in the cytoplasm and may associate with MxiE, which then activates the transcription of genes such as *virA* and *ipaH*.

SHIGELLA AND EPITHELIAL CELLS

How Does *Shigella* Invade Epithelial Cells?

The ability of *Shigella* spp. to invade and colonize the colonic epithelium is a key determinant in the establishment of disease (118). *Shigella* entry into epithelial cells is a complex process that involves the coordinated action of numerous bacterial effectors. Because of this, numerous in vitro studies using epithelioid cell lines have been used to identify different steps controlling the entry process. Upon contact with nonpolarized cultured epithelial cells, for example, HeLa cells, *Shigella* induces the formation of cellular extensions at the point of the bacterial interaction with the host cell membrane (Fig. 3A). By using this strategy of membrane ruffle formation, *Shigella* provokes its internalization by the epithelial cell in a macropinocytic-like process (Fig. 3B). Actin polymerization is likely to provide the force responsible for the formation of these cellular protrusions, and numerous cytoskeletal actin-associated proteins are recruited, such as plastin, α-actinin, and cortactin, as well as ezrin, a protein that cross-links the plasma membrane and the subcortical cytoskeleton, and focal adhesion components such as vinculin and talin (87, 136, 150). For *Shigella* entry, Ipa invasins are critical since these proteins orchestrate the cytoskeletal rearrangements necessary for bacterial invasion (78, 94, 150, 156). In contrast, when epithelial cells are polarized and grow to form a confluent monolayer, *Shigella* is able only to invade by the basolateral side of the epithelial cells (83). This finding illustrates that more complex in vitro

systems and/or in vivo studies are required to more closely approximate the invasion process.

Surface Receptor of Epithelial Cells

In contrast to other invasive pathogens, *Shigella* shows little cell binding ability. However, bacteria may bind transiently to the host cell surface and induce the formation of cellular extensions that engulf the bacterium and enclose it into a large vacuole (1, 81). In cultured epithelial cells, the IpaB/C complex secreted by *Shigella* has been shown to bind the $\alpha_5\beta_1$ integrin, the receptor of fibronectin. Moreover, *Shigella* entry induces the phosphorylation of p125^{FAK}, a tyrosine kinase activated upon integrin engagement by extracellular matrix components (156). IpaB/C complex binding to β_1 integrins may induce the formation of cellular structures similar to focal adhesions with the concomitant reorganization of the actin cytoskeleton. In fact, several studies pointed to focal adhesion components as important players of *Shigella* entry (2, 157).

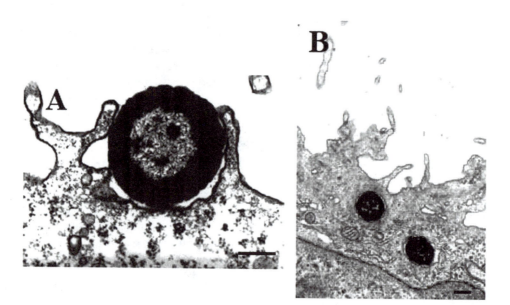

FIGURE 3 Transmission electron microscopy images of *S. flexneri* entry into epithelial (HeLa) cells (P. Gounon and P. J. Sansonetti, Institut Pasteur, Paris, France). Note in (A) the formation of cellular extensions on the host cell that will engulf the bacteria. In (B), two bacteria are inside the epithelial cell that shows multiple cellular extensions. Scale bars, 1 μm.

Integrins do not appear to be exclusive receptors for the IpaB/C complex. During *Shigella* entry, a functional role for CD44, the receptor for hyaluronic acid, has been observed. IpaB can bind to this receptor in epithelial cells (136), leading to local recruitment and possibly to activation of ezrin. Engagement of CD44 by IpaB involves Rho activation (143). The CD44 and/or integrin interactions with the Ipa complex may contribute to an adherence step, representing an early step in the entry process. This step may be involved in triggering the secretion of bacterial proteins by the Mxi-Spa secretion system or may aid in the proper folding of the Ipa complex within the host cell membrane. Alternatively, engagement of these receptors could mediate signals that may act in concert with those signals sent by effectors translocated through the type III secretion apparatus. Then, although not essential, these receptors could contribute to more efficient bacterial entry (151).

Rho GTPases, Src Tyrosine Kinase, and *Shigella* Entry

The Rho family of GTPases, a subset of the Ras superfamily, modulates multiple membrane traffic events, as well as actin polymerization and morphology of cellular extensions. These small GTPases may also play important roles in the establishment and/or maintenance of epithelial cell polarity (153). The Rho family in mammals comprises more than 10 members, including Rho (A, B, C, and D), Rac, RhoG, and Cdc42. Cdc42 is implicated in the formation of filopodial extensions or microspikes, whereas Rac is involved in the formation of lamellipodia and membrane leaflets (47). Both GTPases, Cdc42 and Rac, have been shown to induce actin polymerization in their activated GTP-bound form through the activation of N-WASP and the Arp2/3 complex (164). Rho, on the other hand, induces the formation of actin stress fibers and focal adhesions through the activation of myosin (21, 62).

It has been shown that Cdc42, Rac, and Rho are essential for *Shigella* uptake by cultured epithelial cells, being implicated in bacteria-induced cytoskeletal rearrangements (2, 82, 156) (Fig. 4). The use of the Rho inhibitor, clostridial C3 chimeric toxin, demonstrated that *Shigella*-induced actin rearrangements, but not actin nucleation, are dependent upon Rho activation (2). During entry, Cdc42 and Rac1 are recruited to the entry focus and are associated with the cytoskeletal projections that support the structure. RhoA, in contrast, is associated with the membrane of the phagosome containing the bacteria. Both Cdc42 and Rac1 are involved in actin polymerization and in the formation of microspikes and lamellipodia during bacterial entry. After this initial step, RhoA is likely activated to remodel the entry foci and recruit ezrin, leading to the final formation of a focal adhesion-like structure involved in bacterial uptake (151) (Fig. 4).

The expression of a kinase-negative form of the tyrosine kinase Src leads to inhibition of foci formation and bacterial uptake (31). Src appears to play a double role during the process of *Shigella* entry, since on the one hand, it is involved in the formation of the entry foci, while on the other, it appears to be involved in the downregulation of the process. One possible explanation for this duality may be that during bacterial entry, Src activity is regulated by the recruitment of several substrates at the entry foci. Src might up- or downregulate foci formation through the phosphorylation of a different set of substrates (31).

Cross talk between Rho and Src-mediated responses is also evident during the *Shigella* entry process. Rho activation is necessary for the recruitment of Src, which, in turn, modulates and downregulates Rho-dependent responses. Duménil et al. (32) analyzed the relation between Src and Rho GTPases during *Shigella* entry: whereas Rho is necessary for ezrin recruitment at the level of the foci, an event that occurs at the very early stage of foci development (136), Src has the opposite effect,

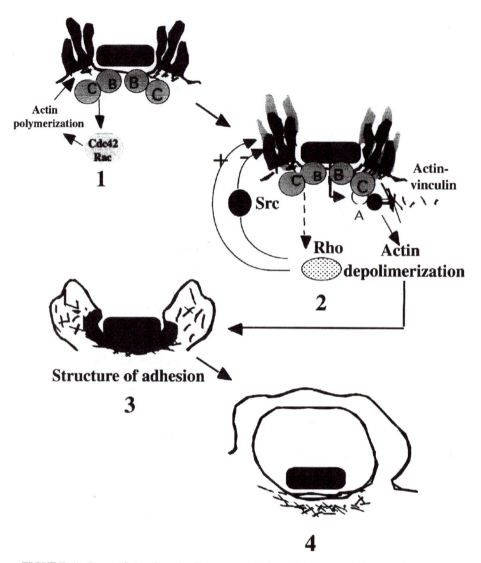

FIGURE 4 Bacterial signals and cell responses during *Shigella* entry. (1) Intracellular IpaC induces actin polymerization by activation of Cdc42 and Rac, and filopodial extensions are formed. (2) Translocated IpaA binds to vinculin, and this complex allows the formation of an adhesive structure at the site of bacterial contact with the host cell membrane. (3) Filopodial extensions are transformed into leaflet structures. (4) Finally, *Shigella* is internalized in a vacuole. Courtesy of G. Tran Van Nhieu (Institut Pasteur, Paris, France).

since it leads to a decrease of ezrin recruitment resulting from a decrease in Rho activity. In conclusion, *Shigella* entry requires two distinct steps: (i) an induction of actin polymerization depending upon the coordinated activities of Src, Rac, and Cdc42 and (ii) organization of actin filaments and recruitment of ezrin coordinated by Src and Rho (Fig. 4).

Shigella Effectors Implicated in the Entry Process

Actin polymerization at the point of bacterial contact with the epithelial cell is dependent on IpaB and IpaC invasins. As described earlier, IpaB and IpaC associate in the extracellular medium to form a complex that might bind to cell surface receptors (77, 94, 136,

156). However, the IpaB/C complex is not sufficient to trigger cytoskeletal rearrangements induced by *Shigella* spp. during entry. These cytoskeletal modifications could then be induced by intracytosolic IpaB and IpaC proteins either directly or through other *Shigella* effectors whose translocation is in turn dependent on the IpaB/C complex translocation (152).

IpaC translocated into the host cell cytosol acts as a direct effector for *Shigella*-induced actin polymerization, induces formation of filopodial and lamellipodial extensions dependent on Cdc42 and Rac GTPases (152), and promotes the uptake of an *ipaC* null mutant of *S. flexneri* by cultured cells (28, 71, 151) (Fig. 4). In addition, not only translocated IpaC, but extracellular IpaC as well, is able to induce actin polymerization in Henle407 cells (149). This direct effect occurs via the interaction of extracellular IpaC with $\alpha_5\beta_1$ integrin, as previously reported (156). Recently, Picking et al. (100) characterized three different functional regions of IpaC respectively involved in the secretion of IpaC, in IpaC-phospholipid membrane interactions, and possibly in the signaling to the host cell. It is possible that whereas extracellular IpaC can interact with phospholipid membranes, active insertion of IpaC into the host cell by the type III secretion apparatus may increase the efficiency of the process (16, 100). The role of IpaB during this process needs to be determined, although it has been suggested that IpaB may influence the ability of IpaC to penetrate phospholipid membranes (149).

Following IpaB/C-induced actin polymerization required in the initial step of *Shigella* internalization, the IpaA protein, which is also translocated into the host cytoplasm, is implicated in the organization of polymerized actin to create a structure adequate for bacterial entry (Fig. 4). IpaA directly binds vinculin and controls those cytoskeletal rearrangements (150). Although the molecular mechanism is not clear, it has been shown that IpaA binding to vinculin promotes the association of vinculin with F-actin and induces F-actin depolymerization. As a consequence, the formation

of new projections that could repel the bacterium away from the host cell surface could be regulated. It is also possible that the activation of vinculin by IpaA allows the recruitment of focal adhesion components, such as α-actinin, cytoskeletal proteins, and tyrosine kinases implicated in the recruitment of signaling molecules (18). Moreover, the IpgD protein associates with IpaA after bacterial secretion and contributes to the formation of the entry focus (86).

Shigella Inside Epithelial Cells: Vacuole Disruption and Intra- and Intercellular Spreading

After entry, the bacterium is surrounded by a vacuole that, within a few minutes, is disrupted. In this way, *Shigella* enters the host cytoplasm, where bacteria can proliferate and spread intracellularly (15, 69), and to neighboring cells by way of finger-like protrusions that extend from the cell surface (29, 45) (Fig. 5). Engulfment of these protrusions by adjacent cells and lysis of the cellular membranes allow *Shigella* to gain access to the cytoplasm of new cells without release into the extracellular environment (5). The IpaB and IpaC invasins are necessary to induce escape from the phagocytic vacuole. IpaC is directly involved (9), whereas the role of IpaB remains to be determined. The *Shigella* capacity to invade host cells, to escape from the phagosome, and to spread are essential for leading to shigellosis; in this way, loss of the ability of *S. flexneri* to efficiently lyse the membrane of the vacuole and/or to spread has been correlated with a reduction of the inflammatory response induced by *Shigella* (36).

The actin-based motility of *Shigella* spp. is dependent on IcsA(VirG) encoded by the *icsA(virG)* gene. The IcsA(VirG) protein is essential for intracellular movement by inducing actin nucleation and polymerization at the bacterial surface (15, 65). It has been described that invaded cells may limit bacterial spread by phosphorylating IcsA in vivo (30). Phosphorylation could thus represent a mechanism of epithelial cell defense. The IcsA protein can be divided into three portions: (i) the signal

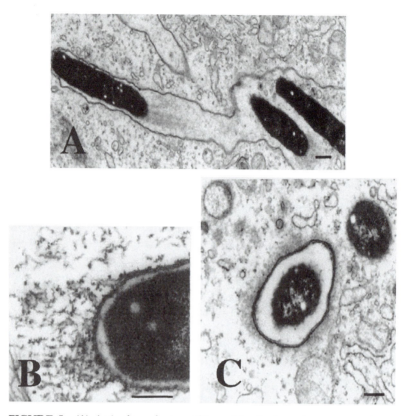

FIGURE 5 (A) Actin-dependent motility enables the bacterium to move intracellularly and invade adjacent cells. (B) S1 myosin fragments decorate short actin filaments nucleated, elongated, and assembled at the pole of a bacterium. (C) Bacterium enclosed by a double membrane after invasion of an adjacent cell. (P. Gounon and P. J. Sansonetti, Institut Pasteur, Paris, France.) Scale bars, 1 μm.

peptide, (ii) the central domain IcsA$_\alpha$, and (iii) the C-terminal domain IcsA$_\beta$. Motility is enabled by the accumulation of short actin filaments at one pole to form a tail that propels the bacterium (Fig. 5A and 5B). This unipolar distribution may occur by delivering IcsA strictly to one pole of the bacterium and lateral diffusion of the protein controlled by membrane fluidity. Finally, IcsA is cleaved by a bacterial serine protease IcsP(SopA), leading to IcsA$_\alpha$ secretion (29, 111, 138). IcsP(SopA), a homologue of OmpT and OmpP, outer membrane proteases of *Escherichia coli*, is thus essential for polar localization of IcsA and for actin-based motility (34).

Unipolar distribution of IcsA at the bacterial surface requires intact lipopolysaccharide (LPS). Several genes involved in LPS synthesis affect IcsA localization (102, 114, 115). Moreover, virulence plasmid determinants are not implicated in the correct positioning of IcsA (116). Recently, Mogull et al. (80) identified *dksA* as being required for the intracellular spread of *S. flexneri*, influencing the polar localization of IcsA in the bacteria. However, the specific mechanism responsible for this effect has not yet been elucidated.

Vinculin and N-WASP interact with IcsA (140, 142). Although IcsA-vinculin interaction is not necessary for *Shigella* intracellular movement (44), it may contribute to actin assembly induced by *Shigella* (64). Also, existing actin filaments already bound by vinculin at the bacterial surface may contribute to actin nucleation (141). N-WASP is a member of the WASP family of proteins, with the particularity of containing a consensus CRIB motif for Cdc42 binding (79), and it is essential for *Shigella*-induced actin nucleation (Fig. 6) (64, 137). On the other hand, Arp2/3, which induces actin nucleation, is activated by N-WASP; activation can be enhanced by Cdc42 (79, 112). The *Shigella* IcsA protein mimics Cdc42, and three of the six glycine-rich repeats contained in a region in IcsA$_\alpha$ are required for the interaction with N-WASP (C. Egile and P. J. Sansonetti, submitted). Moreover, IcsA increases the affinity of N-WASP for the Arp2/3 complex. As a conse-

quence, an IcsA/N-WASP/Arp2/3 complex binds to the bacterial surface, inducing efficient actin assembly (Fig. 6). Cdc42, although essential for *Shigella* entry, does not seem to be required for bacterial motility, as evidenced by the fact that Cdc42 is not accumulated on motile *Shigella* with a formed actin tail (68, 139) and that *Shigella* motility is not affected in Cdc42-deficient cells (135). In addition, actin depolymerization factor/cofilin, capping protein, and profilin are also involved in the stabilization of the actin tail (67).

When bacteria reach the inner face of the host cell membrane, a finger-like protrusion is formed that is phagocytosed by the adjacent

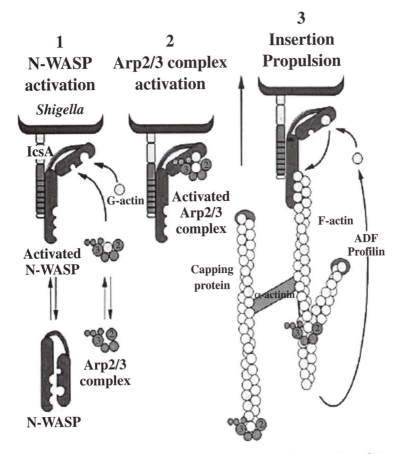

FIGURE 6 Model for actin-based movement of *Shigella*. (1) Binding of N-WASP to IcsA at *Shigella* surface activates the connector. Arp2/3 is activated and binds to G-actin. (2) Interaction of VCA domain of N-WASP with activated Arp2/3-G-actin complex. (3) The VCA domain shuttles G-actin subunits to the growing barbed end.

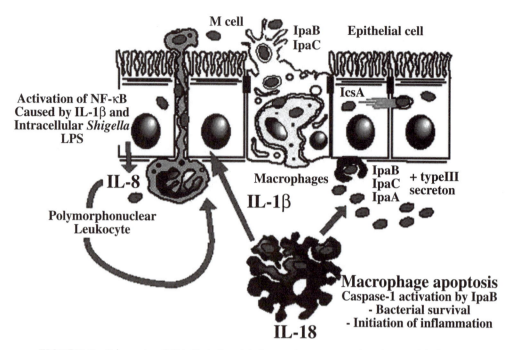

FIGURE 7 Schematic of *Shigella*-induced inflammation: rupture, invasion, and inflammatory destruction of the intestinal barrier.

cell, thus causing cell-to-cell spread (101, 124) (Fig. 5A). E-cadherin, a protein involved in intercellular adhesion and localized in intermediate junctions, is an important cellular component involved in the intercellular spread of *Shigella* (124, 154). In addition, components of the intermediate junction, such as α-catenin, β-catenin, α-actinin, and vinculin, colocalize with the bacterial protrusions (124). Once endocytosed by the adjacent cell, bacteria are enclosed inside a vacuole surrounded by a double membrane (Fig. 5C). The expression of IpgC, IpaB, and IpaC proteins is required for cell-to-cell spread, being probably implicated in lysis of the cell membranes in protrusions (91). By this mechanism, bacteria gain access to the cell cytoplasm.

HOST DEFENSE: THE INNATE IMMUNE RESPONSE

Inflammation is a nonspecific response to various tissue injuries, including infection. In shigellosis, acute inflammation is the cost for

rapid eradication of the invading bacteria. Paradoxically, inflammation causes severe damage to the colonic mucosa and allows further bacterial invasion (95, 96) (Fig. 7). The acute inflammatory response generated by *Shigella* infection is characterized by diffuse erythema and swelling of the mucosa, focal hemorrhages, and a mucopurulent exudate. At the later stages of shigellosis, the histopathological lesions cannot be differentiated from those observed in acute ulcerative colitis. Probably, as with other enteropathogens, *Shigella* sp. has developed strategies to upregulate proinflammatory signals and downregulate antiinflammatory signals.

In shigellosis, several lines of evidence indicate that cytokines and chemokines are mediators of tissue damage. In patients in the acute and convalescent stages of *S. flexneri* and *S. dysenteriae* 1 infection, immunohistochemistry of rectal samples shows a pattern of IL-1, IL-4, IL-6, IL-8, tumor necrosis factor alpha (TNF-α), and gamma interferon (IFN-

γ) production (104, 107). Severe disease is associated with increased IL-1β, IL-6, TNF-α, and IFN-γ expression. IL-1 is essentially produced by monocytes/macrophages, whereas IL-6 and IL-8 are produced by epithelial cells (107).

Shigella Invades and Induces Apoptosis of Macrophages

The initial step of tissue invasion of *Shigella* is association with the FAE, where bacteria cross the epithelial barrier via M cells (Fig. 7). Early during infection, macrophages, the resident phagocyte population, phagocytose *Shigella*. Recently, Sasakawa's group (63) showed for the first time that the central hydrophobic portion of IpaC, the membrane-spanning domain, is critical for entry of *Shigella* into macrophages. As in the case of epithelial cells, *Shigella* initiates its internalization into macrophages using IpaC. Although the global mechanism has not yet been elucidated, surface receptors, such as Mac-1 ($\alpha_M\beta_2$ integrin), and an integrin-mediated adhesion process have been implicated. Moreover, paxillin and c-Cbl, involved in the interaction with Src family kinases, are so far the only proteins tyrosine-phosphorylated in the macrophage cell line J774, contributing to *Shigella* invasion of macrophages.

It has been shown that several pathogens, such as *Listeria monocytogenes*, *S. flexneri*, or *Salmonella* spp., can induce apoptosis in host cells (24). In vitro, shigellae phagocytosed by macrophages are able to escape from the phagosome and, following their release into the cytoplasm, induce macrophage apoptosis (167, 168) (Fig. 8). Furthermore, clinical isolates of *Shigella* spp. induce apoptosis, a process of programmed cell death that appears to be increased in the rectal mucosa of patients with shigellosis (56). By use of this mechanism, *Shigella* not only defends itself from killing, but also ensures an important inflammatory response, since apoptotic macrophages secrete the inflammatory cytokines IL-1β and IL-18, which trigger the acute inflammation characteristic of shigellosis. For instance, this inflam-

matory cascade allows *Shigella* to invade new cells and finally to colonize the entire colonic epithelium (25, 126, 166) (Fig. 7). During the course of experimental shigellosis in the rabbit ligated loop model, the balance between IL-1 receptor antagonist (IL-1ra) and IL-1 is severely impaired at the early stage of bacterial challenge. Futhermore, administration of IL-1ra decreased inflammation as well as bacterial invasion, confirming that early inflammation is important in disrupting epithelial permeability and facilitating invasion of the mucosa (7, 120).

Macrophage apoptosis occurs after 1 to 2 h postinfection. IpaB secreted by the type III secretion apparatus within the macrophage cytoplasm induces macrophage apoptosis (24, 49, 166) by binding to IL-1β-converting enzyme or caspase-1, a cysteine protease with the capacity to cleave the proinflammatory cytokine IL-1β and IL-18 into its mature form (49, 126). Using an in vivo murine model of pulmonary infection (96), IL-1β has been shown to be responsible for the intensity of the acute inflammation associated with *Shigella* infection, whereas IL-18 is implicated in induction of an effective inflammatory response capable of eradicating the bacteria (126). Caspase-11 has been shown to regulate caspase-1 activation (155). However, *Shigella*-induced apoptosis can be considered unique, since it is dependent only on caspase-1 activation and occurs independently of caspase-11. In this model, caspase-1 can be considered as a component of the innate immune response that coordinates the use of an apoptotic pathway to release mature cytokines and to induce an inflammatory response.

The signal pathway for *Shigella*-induced apoptosis of macrophages is being elucidated. In addition to caspase-1, another endogenous protease, the cytoplasmic serine protease tripeptidyl peptidase II, has recently been identified as a component of the apoptotic pathway induced by *S. flexneri* and located upstream of caspase-1 (50). In addition and as for other pathogens, it is known that *Shigella*-induced apoptosis is a downstream event fol-

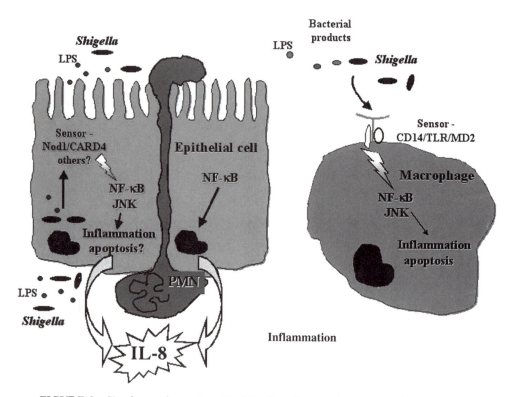

FIGURE 8 Signaling pathways in epithelial cells and macrophages induced by *Shigella* infection, *Shigella* LPS, and/or bacterial products.

lowing stimulation of Toll-like receptor 2 (TLR2) by bacterial lipoproteins (4), suggesting that programmed cell death may also be induced through the activation of TLRs (Fig. 8). TLRs, therefore, are important components of the innate immune system for sensing microbes and their products. In fact, the induction of cell death appears to be an evolutionarily conserved response to pathogens across the animal and plant kingdoms (98).

Proinflammatory Molecules Produced by Epithelial Cells

In response to bacterial infection, intestinal epithelial cells can provide important signals for the initiation and amplification of an acute mucosal inflammatory response (48) (Fig. 7 and 8). After bacterial infection, colonic epithelial cells, which are the first barrier against the pathogen, express a large array of proin-

flammatory molecules, particularly IL-8. This cytokine can be considered the most important chemoattractant for PMN (57), although it is not responsible for their transepithelial migration (75). IL-8 also induces degranulation, respiratory burst, and leukotriene B_4 (LTB_4) release by PMN. IL-8 causes PMN-mediated arrest of *Shigella* translocation through the intestinal epithelium into the lamina propria at the cost of massive epithelial destruction (121).

In vitro, LPS released from *S. flexneri* at the apical side of epithelial cells can be internalized and transported to their basolateral side without detoxification. TLR4 receptor has been described recently as the main mediator of innate immune responses to LPS (23, 103, 144). Cario et al. (22) showed a subcellular redistribution of TLR4 receptor in differentiated T84 cells in response to LPS stimulation. After apical exposure of T84 cells with LPS in the presence of serum, in addition to an apical accumulation of TLR4 receptors, both LPS and TLR4 are localized intracellularly in vesicular structures resembling multivesicular lysosomes and endosomes. Moreover, bacterial internalization also allows presentation of LPS into the intracellular compartment. The transcellular routing of LPS in polarized epithelial cells has been elucidated and described (10). In in vitro studies (11, 99), it has been shown that intracellular *Shigella* LPS induced IL-8 production in amounts sufficient to direct neutrophils to a subepithelial location. However, LPS alone is not able to induce the paracellular movement during transepithelial migration of PMN. Thus, other *Shigella* determinants would be the mediators of paracellular PMN movement (11). However, it is clear that epithelial cells can initiate specific defense responses against invasive enteropathogens or their determinants, implicating a major role of these cells in the host immune response.

Philpott et al. (99) linked the *S. flexneri* LPS intracellular signaling and the subsequent initiation of the inflammatory response with NF-κB activation (Fig. 8). NF-κB is an important transcription factor implicated in the regulation of several genes whose expression is involved in the inflammatory response, including IL-8. In nonstimulated conditions, NF-κB is held latent in the cytoplasm through its binding to inhibitory proteins called IκBs. After activation, IκBs are phosphorylated and subsequently ubiquitinated and degraded. NF-κB becomes free in the cytoplasm, and then is translocated to the nucleus where it binds to κB elements in the promoter region of responsive genes (19, 42). The activation of the transcription factor by intracellular LPS leads to an induction of the IL-8 secretion. Thus, NF-κB may play an important role in modulating the immune response during infection in vivo. *S. flexneri* invasion and intracellular LPS can also activate c-Jun N-terminal kinase (JNK), a kinase implicated in the stress response (43). JNK phosphorylates c-Jun, which is a component of the transcription factor AP-1, also considered to be an important regulator

of the inflammatory response (38). Importantly, both responses are mediated by Nod1, a cytosolic protein analogue of plant resistance proteins (43, 53, 54). Ogura et al. (90) also proposed Nod2 as a macrophage-specific sensing molecule for LPS. Activation of NF-κB through Nod proteins is mediated through RICK, a serine/threonine kinase that interacts with the IκB kinase complex. A mutation in the *nod2* gene located on chromosome 16 has been associated with susceptibility to Crohn's disease. As Nod proteins act as receptors of microbial components, it is possible to link the innate immune response to bacterial components and the development of inflammatory disease (52, 90).

PMN

Recruitment and activation of monocytes and PMN is observed during shigellosis. PMN transmigrate and disturb the epithelium, opening a way for bacterial invasion at the basolateral membrane domain (95) (Fig. 7). Thus, recruitment of PMN is advantageous to the bacteria. On the other hand, the efficient killing of *Shigella* by PMN has been reported (70, 110, 165). Thus, although PMN may initially contribute to the severe tissue damage, they are ultimately involved in clearance and resolution of infection. This is illustrative of the dual role that innate immune responses may play throughout the course of infection.

Signals that induce the transmigration of neutrophils are dependent on basolateral membrane-*Shigella* interactions, and require genes encoded by the virulence plasmid as well as a functional type III secretion apparatus (76). However, many questions have to be resolved to completely understand the nature of the intracellular signaling cascade that is directly involved in the induction of the PMM transepithelial migration during progress of the disease.

Shigella can directly activate PMN and induce strong PMN adherence and degranulation, and finally neutrophil necrosis. Entry and the subsequent necrosis event of PMN depend on a functional type III secretion apparatus and the IpaB and IpaC proteins (39). PMN necrosis also contributes to the establishment of inflammation, since necrosis is characterized by the release of granular proteins that can damage the tissue. For example, PMN contain several cytotoxic polypeptides and proteolytic enzymes. Of these, one of the most injurious enzymes is elastase, a serine proteinase capable of inducing epithelial cell lysis (84).

IFN-γ and IL-10

In patients with shigellosis, the expression of IFN-γ increases by twofold during convalescence compared to the acute stage (105, 106). Experimental studies showed that NK cell-mediated IFN-γ production is essential to host resistance following primary Shigella infection (161) and promotes the killing of Shigella by isolated primary macrophages and macrophage and fibroblastic cell lines. Similarly, Shigella is not cleared from the lungs of IFN-γ-deficient mice. In conclusion, the protective role of IFN-γ is to promote the clearance of intracellular Shigella (161). In addition to IFN-γ, IL-10 production is induced in mononuclear cells in response to bacterial inoculation, as well as to purified recombinant Shigella invasins IpaC and IpaD (113). The role of IL-10 may be to limit the inflammatory response by inhibition of both T and NK cell responses (12, 51), and by decreasing the induction of IL-1 (120).

CELLULAR AND HUMORAL IMMUNE RESPONSES

The adaptative immune response is essential for recovery of a second infection and might also contribute to the recovery from primary infection. Both humoral and cellular immune responses are elicited in natural or experimental infections. Although rare data are available on cell-mediated immunity, it might be induced in response to Shigella infection and thus may eventually play a role in protection. The polysaccharide portion of the homologous LPS molecule stimulates lymphocyte proliferation (55). However, induction of specific cytotoxic T lymphocytes and their protective role of killing infected enterocytes has not been documented so far. Protection against S. flexneri 2a in the mouse bronchopulmonary model is independent of T lymphocytes, even if T-cell responses to Shigella antigens occur (163). NK cells are activated against infected HeLa cells by S. flexneri (59), but the relevance of this mechanism has not yet been established in vivo. Furthermore, it has been shown that IFN-γ, essential for innate immunity to Shigella infection, is not essential for acquired protection (161).

Serum immunoglobulin G (IgG), and systemic and mucosal IgA antibodies following Shigella infection are directed primarily to Shigella LPS, together with a response against Ipa invasins (66, 88, 113). Epidemiological studies have indicated that the LPS O-antigen may be associated with protective immunity against shigellosis (26, 146). In shigellosis, mucosal immunity does play a major role, since Shigella infection remains mainly localized at the colonic mucosal level. Phalipon et al. (96a) analyzed the role of the humoral mucosal immune response in passive protection against shigellosis. Using the murine pulmonary infection model that mimics the lesions occurring in natural infection, they showed that mucosal IgA antibodies specific for a serotype determinant on the polysaccharide part of Shigella LPS are sufficient to confer protection. Recently, using the same in vivo model, Phalipon et al. (96a) showed that this protection is more efficient when IgA is presented as secretory IgA (SIgA), that is, the two monomeric IgA molecules, covalently linked through the J chain and secretory component (SC). In fact, SIgA is the main antibody in mucous membrane secretions and essential in protecting mucosal surfaces. Thus, SC through its glycosylated residues improves the protective capacity of IgA by immune exclusion. In contrast, Way et al. (162), using the same murine model, have suggested that IgA is not required for active adaptive immunity, and that IgM or IgG may be the protective antibody isotype. In this study, vaccinated mice that lack IgA have no increase in susceptibility against bacterial challenge.

Infected individuals also produce antibodies to IpaB and IpaC, and at a lower frequency, to IpaA, IpaD, and IcsA. Although the role of anti-Ipa antibodies is much more difficult to assess, sIgAs against Ipa proteins have been related with a decrease in the duration of the disease (89). However, a direct effect of anti-Ipa immunity in protection has not yet been established. Actually, several IgG monoclonal antibodies specific for IpaB or IpaC, either alone or combined, failed to protect animals against *Shigella* infection (Phalipon, personal communication).

HOST CELL-*SHIGELLA* INTERACTION: A RELATIONSHIP NOT YET COMPLETELY UNDERSTOOD

In recent years, studies have focused on the molecular mechanisms of the interactions between bacteria, the intestinal epithelium, and the immune system. Essential virulence gene products and cellular components have been identified. Elucidation of different mechanisms implicated in the recognition of bacteria and bacterial determinants, as well as the response triggered by these factors, will improve our understanding of both the immunology of mucosal surfaces and bacterial pathogenesis. So far, many questions have been left unanswered. It is difficult to assess which bacterial components can be sensed by the cells. In fact, although LPS undoubtedly plays an essential role, it is not unique and other bacterial determinants may have the ability to trigger a response, which could occur through the same pathway used by LPS. However, the existence of different signaling pathways should not be discarded. Another important question is whether different Nod-like proteins recognize distinct bacterial products.

In relation to *Shigella* spp., it will be important (i) to elucidate their human colonic specificity, (ii) to confirm whether bacterial translocation through M cells in vivo is the unique way to invade the colon, (iii) to proceed to exhaustive identification of the signaling pathways that lead to severe inflammation characteristic of shigellosis, and (iv) to improve our understanding regarding the bases of immune protection against the disease. Shigellae are among the most important etiologic agents causing endemic diarrheal disease; however, an efficient vaccine is not yet available. Thus, it is necessary to develop new experimental models, particularly in vivo, that closely mimic the disease in humans. Such studies should be directed to the improvement of treatments and to the development of new vaccine candidates for the prevention of shigellosis.

ACKNOWLEDGMENTS

We are grateful to M. Mavris, A. Phalipon, and D. Philpott for careful review of the manuscript and for helpful discussion. We also thank members of the P. J. Sansonetti laboratory, past and present, whose work was discussed in this chapter. P.J.S. is a Howard Hughes Medical Institute Scholar. M.I.F. is supported by the Fondation pour la Recherche Médicale.

REFERENCES

1. **Adam, T., M. Arpin, M. C. Prevost, P. Gounon, and P. J. Sansonetti.** 1995. Cytoskeletal rearrangements and the functional role of T-plastin during entry of *Shigella flexneri* into HeLa cells. *J. Cell. Biol.* **129:**367–381.
2. **Adam, T., M. Giry, P. Boquet, and P. Sansonetti.** 1996. Rho-dependent membrane folding causes *Shigella* entry into epithelial cells. *EMBO J.* **15:**3315–3321.
3. **Adler, B., C. Sasakawa, T. Tobe, S. Makino, K. Komatsu, and M. Yoshikawa.** 1989. A dual transcriptional activation system for the 230 kb plasmid genes coding for virulence-associated antigens of *Shigella flexneri*. *Mol. Microbiol.* **3:**627–635.
4. **Aliprantis, A. O., D. S. Weiss, J. D. Radolf, and A. Zychlinsky.** 2001. Release of Toll-like receptor-2-activating bacterial lipoproteins in *Shigella flexneri* culture supernatants. *Infect. Immun.* **69:**6248–6255.
5. **Allaoui, A., J. Mounier, M. C. Prevost, P. J. Sansonetti, and C. Parsot.** 1992. icsB: a *Shigella flexneri* virulence gene necessary for the lysis of

protrusions during intercellular spread. *Mol. Microbiol.* **6:**1605–1616.

6. **Allaoui, A., P. J. Sansonetti, R. Menard, S. Barzu, J. Mounier, A. Phalipon, and C. Parsot.** 1995. MxiG, a membrane protein required for secretion of *Shigella* spp. Ipa invasins: involvement in entry into epithelial cells and in intercellular dissemination. *Mol. Microbiol.* **17:**461–470.

7. **Arondel, J., M. Singer, A. Matsukawa, A. Zychlinsky, and P. J. Sansonetti.** 1999. Increased interleukin-1 (Il-1) and imbalance between IL-1 and IL-1 receptor antagonist during acute inflammation in experimental Shigellosis. *Infect. Immun.* **67:**6056–6066.

8. **Bahrani, F. K., P. J. Sansonetti, and C. Parsot.** 1997. Secretion of Ipa proteins by *Shigella flexneri*: inducer molecules and kinetics of activation. *Infect. Immun.* **65:**4005–4010.

9. **Barzu, S., Z. Benjelloun-Touimi, A. Phalipon, P. Sansonetti, and C. Parsot.** 1997. Functional analysis of the *Shigella flexneri* IpaC invasin by insertional mutagenesis. *Infect. Immun.* **65:**1599–1605.

10. **Beatty, W. L., S. Meresse, P. Gounon, J. Davoust, J. Mounier, P. J. Sansonetti, and J. P. Gorvel.** 1999. Trafficking of *Shigella* lipopolysaccharide in polarized intestinal epithelial cells. *J. Cell Biol.* **145:**689–698.

11. **Beatty, W. L., and P. J. Sansonetti.** 1997. Role of lipopolysaccharide in signaling to subepithlial polymorphonuclear leukocytes. *Infect. Immun.* **65:**4395–4404.

12. **Benjamin, D., T. J. Knobloch, and M. A. Dayton.** 1993. Human B-cell interleukin-10: B-cell lines derived from patients with acquired immunodeficiency syndrome and Burkitt's lymphoma constitutively secrete large quantities of interleukin-10. *Blood* **80:**1289–1298.

13. **Benjelloun-Touimi, Z., P. J. Sansonetti, and C. Parsot.** 1995. SepA, the major extracellular protein of *Shigella flexneri*: autonomous secretion and involvement in tissue invasion. *Mol. Microbiol.* **17:**123–135.

14. **Benjelloun-Touimi, Z., M. S. Tahar, C. Montecucco, P. J. Sansonetti, and C. Parsot.** 1998. SepA, the 110 kDa protein secreted by *Shigella flexneri*: two-domain structure and proteolytic activity. *Microbiology* **144:**1815–1822.

15. **Bernardini, M. L., J. Mounier, H. d'Hauteville, M. Coquis-Rondon, and P. J. Sansonetti.** 1989. Identification of *icsA*, a plasmid locus of *Shigella flexneri* that governs bacterial intra- and intercellular spread through interaction with F-actin. *Proc. Natl. Acad. Sci. USA* **86:**3867–3871.

16. **Blocker, A., P. Gounon, E. Larquet, K. Niebuhr, V. Cabiaux, C. Parsot, and P. Sansonetti.** 1999. The tripartite type III secreton of *Shigella flexneri* inserts IpaB and IpaC into host membranes. *J. Cell Biol.* **147:**683–693.

17. **Blocker, A., N. Jouihri, E. Larquet, P. Gounon, F. Ebel, C. Parsot, P. Sansonetti, and A. Allaoui.** 2001. Structure and composition of the *Shigella flexneri* "needle complex," a part of its type III secreton. *Mol. Microbiol.* **39:**652–663.

18. **Bourdet-Sicard, R., M. Rudiger, B. M. Jockusch, P. Gounon, P. J. Sansonetti, and G. T. Nhieu.** 1999. Binding of the *Shigella* protein IpaA to vinculin induces F-actin depolymerization. *EMBO J.* **18:**5853–5862.

19. **Brown, K., S. Gerstberger, L. Carlson, G. Franzoso, and U. Siebenlist.** 1995. Control of I kappa B-alpha proteolysis by site-specific, signal-induced phosphorylation. *Science* **267:**1485–1488.

20. **Buchrieser, C., P. Glaser, C. Rusniok, H. Nedjari, H. D'Hauteville, F. Kunst, P. Sansonetti, and C. Parsot.** 2000. The virulence plasmid pWR100 and the repertoire of proteins secreted by the type III secretion apparatus of *Shigella flexneri*. *Mol. Microbiol.* **38:**760–771.

21. **Burridge, K., K. Fath, T. Kelly, G. Nuckolls, and C. Turner.** 1988. Focal adhesions: transmembrane junctions between the extracellular matrix and the cytoskeleton. *Annu. Rev. Cell. Biol.* **4:**487–525.

22. **Cario, E., D. Brown, M. McKee, K. Lynch-Devaney, G. Gerken, and D. K. Podolsky.** 2002. Commensal-associated molecular patterns induce selective Toll-like receptor-trafficking from apical membrane to cytoplasmic compartments to polarized intestinal epithelium. *Am. J. Pathol.* **160:**1665–1673.

23. **Cario, E., and D. K. Podolsky.** 2000. Differential alteration in intestinal epithelial cell expression of Toll-like receptor 3 (TLR3) and TLR4 in inflammatory bowel disease. *Infect. Immun.* **68:**7010–7017.

24. **Chen, Y., M. R. Smith, K. Thirumalai, and A. Zychlinsky.** 1996. A bacterial invasin induces macrophage apoptosis by binding directly to ICE. *EMBO J.* **15:**3853–3860.

25. **Chen, Y., and A. Zychlinsky.** 1994. Apoptosis induced by bacterial pathogens. *Microb. Pathog.* **17:**203–212.

26. **Cohen, D., M. S. Green, C. Block, R. Slepon, and Y. Lerman.** 1992. Natural immunity to shigellosis in two groups with different previous risks of exposure to *Shigella* is only partly expressed by serum antibodies to lipopolysaccharide. *J. Infect. Dis.* **165:**785–787.

27. **Cornelis, G. R., and H. Wolf-Watz.** 1997. The *Yersinia* Yop virulon: a bacterial system for subverting eukaryotic cells. *Mol. Microbiol.* **23:** 861–867.

28. **Davis, R., M. E. Marquart, D. Lucius, and W. D. Picking.** 1998. Protein-protein interactions in the assembly of *Shigella flexneri* invasion plasmid antigens IpaB and IpaC into protein complexes. *Biochim. Biophys. Acta* **1429:**45–56.

29. **d'Hauteville, H., R. Dufourcq Lagelouse, F. Nato, and P. J. Sansonetti.** 1996. Lack of cleavage of IcsA in *Shigella flexneri* causes aberrant movement and allows demonstration of a cross-reactive eukaryotic protein. *Infect. Immun.* **64:** 511–517.

30. **d'Hauteville, H., and P. J. Sansonetti.** 1992. Phosphorylation of IcsA by cAMP-dependent protein kinase and its effect on intracellular spread of *Shigella flexneri*. *Mol. Microbiol.* **6:**833–841.

31. **Dumenil, G., J. C. Olivo, S. Pellegrini, M. Fellous, P. J. Sansonetti, and G. T. Nhieu.** 1998. Interferon alpha inhibits a Src-mediated pathway necessary for *Shigella*-induced cytoskeletal rearrangements in epithelial cells. *J. Cell Biol.* **143:**1003–1012.

32. **Dumenil, G., P. Sansonetti, and G. Tran Van Nheiu.** 2000. Src tyrosine kinase activity down-regulates Rho-dependent responses during *Shigella* entry into epithelial cells and stress fibre formation. *J. Cell Sci.* **113:**71–80.

33. **DuPont, H. L., M. M. Levine, R. B. Hornick, and S. B. Formal.** 1989. Inoculum size in shigellosis and implications for expected mode of transmission. *J. Infect. Dis.* **159:**1126–1128.

34. **Egile, C., H. d'Hauteville, C. Parsot, and P. J. Sansonetti.** 1997. SopA, the outer membrane protease responsible for polar localization of IcsA in *Shigella flexneri*. *Mol. Microbiol.* **23:**1063–1073.

35. **Egile, C., T. P. Loisel, V. Laurent, R. Li, D. Pantaloni, P. J. Sansonetti, and M. F. Carlier.** 1999. Activation of the CDC42 effector N-WASP by the *Shigella flexneri* IcsA protein promotes actin nucleation by Arp2/3 complex and bacterial actin-based motility. *J. Cell Biol.* **146:**1319–1332.

36. **Fernandez, I. M., M. Silva, R. Schuch, W. A. Walker, A. M. Siber, A. T. Maurelli, and B. A. McCormick.** 2001. Cadaverine prevents the escape of *Shigella flexneri* from the phagolysosome: a connection between bacterial dissemination and neutrophil transepithelial signaling. *J. Infect. Dis.* **184:**743–753.

37. **Fernandez-Prada, C. M., D. L. Hoover, B. D. Tall, A. B. Hartman, J. Kopelowitz, and M. M. Venkatesan.** 2000. *Shigella flexneri* IpaH(7.8) facilitates escape of virulent bacteria from the endocytic vacuoles of mouse and human macrophages. *Infect. Immunol.* **68:**3608–3619.

38. **Foletta, V. C., D. H. Segal, and D. R. Cohen.** 1998. Transcriptional regulation in the immune system: all roads lead to AP-1. *J. Leukoc. Biol.* **63:**139–152.

39. **Francois, M., V. Le Cabec, M. A. Dupont, P. J. Sansonetti, and I. Maridonneau-Parini.** 2000. Induction of necrosis in human neutrophils by *Shigella flexneri* requires type III secretion, IpaB and IpaC invasins, and actin polymerization. *Infect. Immun.* **68:**1289–1296.

40. **Galan, J. E., and J. B. Bliska.** 1996. Cross-talk between bacterial pathogens and their host cells. *Annu. Rev. Dev. Biol.* **12:**221–255.

41. **Galan, J. E., and A. Collmer.** 1999. Type III secretion machines: bacterial devices for protein delivery into host cells. *Science* **284:**1322–1328.

42. **Ghosh, S., M. J. May, and E. B. Kopp.** 1998. NF-kappa B and Rel proteins: evolutionarily conserved mediators of immune responses. *Annu. Rev. Immunol.* **16:**225–260.

43. **Girardin, S. E., R. Tournebize, M. Mavris, A. L. Page, X. Li, G. R. Stark, J. Bertin, P. S. DiStefano, M. Yaniv, P. J. Sansonetti, and D. J. Philpott.** 2001. CARD4/Nod1 mediates NF-kappaB and JNK activation by invasive *Shigella flexneri*. *EMBO Rep.* **2:**736–742.

44. **Goldberg, M. B.** 1997. *Shigella* actin-based motility in the absence of vinculin. *Cell. Motil. Cytoskel.* **37:**44–53.

45. **Goldberg, M. B., O. Barzu, C. Parsot, and P. J. Sansonetti.** 1993. Unipolar localization and ATPase activity of IcsA, a *Shigella flexneri* protein involved in intracellular movement. *Infect. Agents Dis.* **2:**210–211.

46. **Goldberg, M. B., and J. A. Theriot.** 1995. *Shigella flexneri* surface protein IcsA is sufficient to direct actin-based motility. *Proc. Natl. Acad. Sci. USA* **92:**6572–6576.

47. **Hall, A.** 1998. Rho GTPases and the actin cytoskeleton. *Science* **279:**509–514.

48. **Hedges, S. R., W. W. Agace, and C. Svanborg.** 1995. Epithelial cytokine responses and mucosal cytokine networks. *Trends Microbiol.* **3:** 266–270.

49. **Hilbi, H., J. E. Moss, D. Hersh, Y. Chen, J. Arondel, S. Banerjee, R. A. Flavell, J. Yuan, P. J. Sansonetti, and A. Zychlinsky.** 1998. *Shigella*-induced apoptosis is dependent on caspase-1 which binds to IpaB. *J. Biol. Chem.* **273:**32895–32900.

50. **Hilbi, H., R. J. Puro, and A. Zychlinsky.** 2000. Tripeptidyl peptidase II promotes maturation of caspase-1 in *Shigella flexneri*-induced macrophage apoptosis. *Infect. Immun.* **68:**5502–5508.

51. Hsu, D. H., K. W. Moore, and H. Spits. 1992. Differential effects of IL-4 and IL-10 on IL-2-induced IFN-gamma synthesis and lymphokine-activated killer activity. *Int. Immunol.* **4**:563–569.

52. Hugot, J. P., M. Chamaillard, H. Zouali, S. Lesage, J. P. Cezard, J. Belaiche, S. Almer, C. Tysk, C. A. O'Morain, M. Gassull, V. Binder, Y. Finkel, A. Cortot, R. Modigliani, P. Laurent-Puig, C. Gower-Rousseau, J. Macry, J. F. Colombel, M. Sahbatou, and G. Thomas. 2001. Association of NOD2 leucine-rich repeat variants with susceptibility to Crohn's disease. *Nature* **411**:599–603.

53. Inohara, N., T. Koseki, L. del Peso, Y. Hu, C. Yee, S. Chen, R. Carrio, J. Merino, D. Liu, J. Ni, and G. Nunez. 1999. Nod1, an Apaf-1-like activator of caspase-9 and nuclear factor-kappaB. *J. Biol. Chem.* **274**:14560–14567.

54. Inohara, N., Y. Ogura, F. F. Chen, A. Muto, and G. Nunez. 2001. Human Nod1 confers responsiveness to bacterial lipopolysaccharides. *J. Biol. Chem.* **276**:2551–2554.

55. Islam, D., P. K. Bardhan, A. A. Lindberg, and B. Christensson. 1995. *Shigella* infection induces cellular activation of T and B cells and distinct species-related changes in peripheral blood lymphocyte subsets during the course of the disease. *Infect. Immun.* **63**:2941–2949.

56. Islam, D., B. Veress, P. K. Bardhan, A. A. Lindberg, and B. Christensson. 1997. In situ characterization of inflammatory responses in the rectal mucosae of patients with shigellosis. *Infect. Immun.* **65**:739–749.

57. Jung, H. C., L. Eckmann, S. K. Yang, A. Panja, J. Fierer, E. Morzycka-Wroblewska, and M. F. Kagnoff. 1995. A distinct array of proinflammatory cytokines is expressed in human epithelial cells in response to bacterial invasion. *J. Clin. Invest.* **95**:55–62.

58. Kato, J., K. Ito, A. Nakamura, and H. Watanabe. 1989. Cloning of regions required for contact hemolysis and entry into LLC-MK2 cells from *Shigella sonnei* form I plasmid: *virF* is a positive regulator gene for these phenotypes. *Infect. Immun.* **57**:1391–1398.

59. Klimpel, G. R., D. W. Niesel, and K. D. Klimpel. 1986. Natural cytotoxic effector cell activity against *Shigella flexneri*-infected HeLa cells. *J. Immunol.* **136**:1081–1086.

60. Kotloff, K. L., J. P. Winickoff, B. Ivanoff, J. D. Clemens, D. L. Swerdlow, P. J. Sansonetti, G. K. Adak, and M. M. Levine. 1999. Global burden of *Shigella* infections: implications for vaccine development and implementation of control strategies. *Bull. W. H. O.* **77**:651–666.

61. Kubori, T., Y. Matsushima, D. Nakamura, J. Uralil, M. Lara-Tejero, A. Sukhan, J. E. Galan, and S. I. Aizawa. 1998. Supramolecular structure of the *Salmonella typhimurium* type III protein secretion system. *Science* **280**:602–605.

62. Kureishi, Y., S. Kobayashi, M. Amano, K. Kimura, H. Kanaide, T. Nakano, K. Kaibuchi, and M. Ito. 1997. Rho-associated kinase directly induces smooth muscle contraction through myosin light chain phosphorylation. *J. Biol. Chem.* **272**:12257–12260.

63. Kuwae, A., S. Yoshida, K. Tamano, H. Mimuro, T. Suzuki, and C. Sasakawa. 2001. *Shigella* invasion of macrophage requires the insertion of IpaC into the host plasma membrane. Functional analysis of IpaC. *J. Biol. Chem.* **276**:32230–32239.

64. Laine, R. O., W. Zeile, F. Kang, D. L. Purich, and F. S. Southwick. 1997. Vinculin proteolysis unmasks an ActA homolog for actin-based *Shigella* motility. *J. Cell. Biol.* **138**:1255–1264.

65. Lett, M. C., C. Sasakawa, N. Okada, T. Sakai, S. Makino, M. Yamada, K. Komatsu, and M. Yoshikawa. 1989. *virG*, a plasmid-coded virulence gene of *Shigella flexneri*: identification of the VirG protein and determination of the complete coding sequence. *J. Bacteriol.* **171**:353–359.

66. Li, A., T. Pal, U. Forsum, and A. A. Lindberg. 1992. Safety and immunogenicity of the live oral auxotrophic *Shigella flexneri* SFL124 in volunteers. *Vaccine* **10**:395–404.

67. Loisel, T. P., R. Boujemaa, D. Pantaloni, and M. F. Carlier. 1999. Reconstitution of actin-based motility of *Listeria* and *Shigella* using pure proteins. *Nature* **401**:613–616.

68. Lommel, S., S. Benesch, K. Rottner, T. Franz, J. Wehland, and R. Kuhn. 2001. Actin pedestal formation by enteropathogenic *Escherichia coli* and intracellular motility of *Shigella flexneri* are abolished in N-WASP-defective cells. *EMBO Rep.* **2**:850–857.

69. Makino, S., C. Sasakawa, K. Kamata, T. Kurata, and M. Yoshikawa. 1986. A genetic determinant required for continuous reinfection of adjacent cells on large plasmid in *S. flexneri* 2a. *Cell* **46**:551–555.

70. Mandic-Mulec, I., J. Weiss, and A. Zychlinsky. 1997. *Shigella flexneri* is trapped in polymorphonuclear leukocyte vacuoles and efficiently killed. *Infect. Immun.* **65**:110–115.

71. Marquart, M. E., W. L. Picking, and W. D. Picking. 1996. Soluble invasion plasmid antigen C (IpaC) from *Shigella flexneri* elicits epithelial cell responses related to pathogen invasion. *Infect. Immun.* **64**:4182–4187.

72. **Mathan, M. M., and V. I. Mathan.** 1991. Morphology of rectal mucosa of patients with shigellosis. *Rev. Infect. Dis.* **13:**S314–S318.

73. **Maurelli, A. T., B. Baudry, H. d'Hauteville, T. L. Hale, and P. J. Sansonetti.** 1985. Cloning of plasmid DNA sequences involved in invasion of HeLa cells by *Shigella flexneri. Infect. Immun.* **49:**164–171.

74. **Mavris, M., A. L. Page, R. Tournebize, B. Demers, P. J. Sansonetti, and C. Parsot.** 2002. Regulation of transcription by the activity of the *Shigella flexneri* type III secretion apparatus. *Mol. Microbiol.* **43:**1543–1553.

75. **McCormick, B. A., S. I. Miller, D. Carnes, and J. L. Madara.** 1995. Transepithelial signaling to neutrophils by salmonellae: a novel virulence mechanism for gastroenteritis. *Infect. Immun.* **63:**2302–2309.

76. **McCormick, B. A., A. M. Siber, and A. T. Maurelli.** 1998. Requirement of the *Shigella flexneri* virulence plasmid in the ability to induce trafficking of neutrophils across polarized monolayers of the intestinal epithelium. *Infect. Immun.* **66:**4237–4243.

77. **Menard, R., P. Sansonetti, C. Parsot, and T. Vasselon.** 1994. Extracellular association and cytoplasmic partitioning of the IpaB and IpaC invasins of *S. flexneri. Cell* **79:**515–525.

78. **Menard, R., P. J. Sansonetti, and C. Parsot.** 1993. Nonpolar mutagenesis of the *ipa* genes defines IpaB, IpaC, and IpaD as effectors of *Shigella flexneri* entry into epithelial cells. *J. Bacteriol.* **175:**5899–5906.

79. **Miki, H., T. Sasaki, Y. Takai, and T. Takenawa.** 1998. Induction of filopodium formation by a WASP-related actin-depolymerizing protein N-WASP. *Nature* **391:**93–96.

80. **Mogull, S. A., L. J. Runyen-Janecky, M. Hong, and S. M. Payne.** 2001. *dksA* is required for intercellular spread of *Shigella flexneri* via an RpoS-independent mechanism. *Infect. Immun.* **69:**5742–5751.

81. **Mounier, J., F. K. Bahrani, and P. J. Sansonetti.** 1997. Secretion of *Shigella flexneri* Ipa invasins on contact with epithelial cells and subsequent entry of the bacterium into cells are growth stage dependent. *Infect. Immun.* **65:**774–782.

82. **Mounier, J., V. Laurent, A. Hall, P. Fort, M. F. Carlier, P. J. Sansonetti, and C. Egile.** 1999. Rho family GTPases control entry of *Shigella flexneri* into epithelial cells but not intracellular motility. *J. Cell Sci.* **112:**2069–2080.

83. **Mounier, J., T. Vasselon, R. Hellio, M. Lesourd, and P. J. Sansonetti.** 1992. *Shigella flexneri* enters human colonic Caco-2 epithelial cells through the basolateral pole. *Infect. Immun.* **60:**237–248.

84. **Nahori, M. A., P. Renesto, B. B. Vargaftig, and M. Chignard.** 1992. Activation and damage of cultured airway epithelial cells by human elastase and cathepsin G. *Eur. J. Pharmacol.* **228:**213–218.

85. **Nakata, N., C. Sasakawa, N. Okada, T. Tobe, I. Fukuda, T. Suzuki, K. Komatsu, and M. Yoshikawa.** 1992. Identification and characterization of *virK*, a virulence-associated large plasmid gene essential for intercellular spreading of *Shigella flexneri. Mol. Microbiol.* **6:**2387–2395.

86. **Niebuhr, K., N. Jouihri, A. Allaoui, P. Gounon, P. J. Sansonetti, and C. Parsot.** 2000. IpgD, a protein secreted by the type III secretion machinery of *Shigella flexneri*, is chaperoned by IpgE and implicated in entry focus formation. *Mol. Microbiol.* **38:**8–19.

87. **Nobes, C. D., and A. Hall.** 1995. Rho, rac, and cdc42 GTPases regulate the assembly of multimolecular focal complexes associated with actin stress fibers, lamellipodia, and filopodia. *Cell* **81:**53–62.

88. **Oaks, E. V., T. L. Hale, and S. B. Formal.** 1986. Serum immune response to *Shigella* protein antigens in rhesus monkeys and humans infected with *Shigella* spp. *Infect. Immun.* **53:**57–63.

89. **Oberhelman, R. A., D. J. Kopecko, E. Salazar-Lindo, E. Gotuzzo, J. M. Buysse, M. M. Venkatesan, A. Yi, C. Fernandez-Prada, M. Guzman, R. León-Barúa, and R. Bradley Sack.** 1991. Prospective study of systemic and mucosal immune responses in dysenteric patients to specific *Shigella* invasion plasmid antigens and lipopolysaccharides. *Infect. Immun.* **59:**2341–2350.

90. **Ogura, Y., D. K. Bonen, N. Inohara, D. L. Nicolae, F. F. Chen, R. Ramos, H. Britton, T. Moran, R. Karaliuskas, R. H. Duerr, J. P. Achkar, S. R. Brant, T. M. Bayless, B. S. Kirschner, S. B. Hanauer, G. Nunez, and J. H. Cho.** 2001. A frameshift mutation in NOD2 associated with susceptibility to Crohn's disease. *Nature* **411:**603–606.

91. **Page, A. L., H. Ohayon, P. J. Sansonetti, and C. Parsot.** 1999. The secreted IpaB and IpaC invasins and their cytoplasmic chaperone IpgC are required for intercellular dissemination of *Shigella flexneri. Cell. Microbiol.* **1:**183–193.

92. **Page, A. L., P. J. Sansonetti, and C. Parsot.** 2002. Spa15 of *Shigella flexneri*, a third type of chaperone in the type III secretion pathway. *Mol. Microbiol.* **43:**1533–1542.

93. **Parsot, C., R. Menard, P. Gounon, and P. J. Sansonetti.** 1995. Enhanced secretion through

the *Shigella flexneri* Mxi-Spa translocon leads to assembly of extracellular proteins into macromolecular structures. *Mol. Microbiol.* **16:**291–300.

94. **Parsot, C., and P. J. Sansonetti.** 1996. Invasion and the pathogenesis of *Shigella* infections. *Curr. Top. Microbiol. Immunol.* **209:**25–42.

95. **Perdomo, J. J., P. Gounon, and P. J. Sansonetti.** 1994. Polymorphonuclear leukocyte transmigration promotes invasion of colonic epithelial monolayer by *Shigella flexneri. J. Clin. Invest.* **93:**633–643.

96. **Perdomo, O. J., J. M. Cavaillon, M. Huerre, H. Ohayon, P. Gounon, and P. J. Sansonetti.** 1994. Acute inflammation causes epithelial invasion and mucosal destruction in experimental shigellosis. *J. Exp. Med.* **180:**1307–1319.

96a.**Phalipon, A., A. Cardona, J. P. Kraehenbuhl, L. Edelman, P. J. Sansonetti, and B. Corthesy.** 2002. Secretory component: a new role in secretory IgA-mediated immune exclusion in vivo. *Immunity* **17:**107–115.

97. **Phalipon, A., M. Kaufmann, P. Michetti, J. M. Cavaillon, M. Huerre, P. Sansonetti, and J. P. Kraehenbuhl.** 1995. Monoclonal immunoglobulin A antibody directed against serotype-specific epitope of *Shigella flexneri* lipopolysaccharide protects against murine experimental shigellosis. *J. Exp. Med.* **182:**769–778.

98. **Philpott, D. J., S. E. Girardin, and P. J. Sansonetti.** 2001. Innate immune responses of epithelial cells following infection with bacterial pathogens. *Curr. Opin. Immunol.* **13:**410–416.

99. **Philpott, D. J., S. Yamaoka, A. Israel, and P. J. Sansonetti.** 2000. Invasive *Shigella flexneri* activates NF-kappa B through a lipopolysaccharide-dependent innate intracellular response and leads to IL-8 expression in epithelial cells. *J. Immunol.* **165:**903–914.

100. **Picking, W. L., L. Coye, J. C. Osiecki, A. Barnoski Serfis, E. Schaper, and W. D. Picking.** 2001. Identification of functional regions within invasion plasmid antigen C (IpaC) of *Shigella flexneri. Mol. Microbiol.* **39:**100–111.

101. **Prevost, M. C., M. Lesourd, M. Arpin, F. Vernel, J. Mounier, R. Hellio, and P. J. Sansonetti.** 1992. Unipolar reorganization of F-actin layer at bacterial division and bundling of actin filaments by plastin correlate with movement of *Shigella flexneri* within HeLa cells. *Infect. Immun.* **60:**4088–4099.

102. **Radnedge, L., M. A. Davis, B. Youngren, and S. J. Austin.** 1997. Plasmid maintenance functions of the large virulence plasmid of *Shigella flexneri. J. Bacteriol.* **179:**3670–3675.

103. **Rajakumar, K., B. H. Jost, C. Sasakawa, N. Okada, M. Yoshikawa, and B. Adler.** 1994. Nucleotide sequence of the rhamnose biosynthetic operon of *Shigella flexneri* 2a and role of lipopolysaccharide in virulence. *J. Bacteriol.* **176:**2362–2373.

104. **Raqib, R., A. A. Lindberg, B. Wretlind, P. K. Bardhan, U. Andersson, and J. Andersson.** 1995. Persistence of local cytokine production in shigellosis in acute and convalescent stages. *Infect. Immun.* **63:**289–296.

105. **Raqib, R., A. Ljungdahl, A. A. Lindberg, U. Andersson, and J. Andersson.** 1996. Local entrapment of interferon gamma in the recovery from *Shigella dysenteriae* type 1 infection. *Gut* **38:**328–336.

106. **Raqib, R., A. Ljungdahl, A. A. Lindberg, B. Wretlind, U. Andersson, and J. Andersson.** 1996. Dissociation between cytokine mRNA expression and protein production in shigellosis. *Eur. J. Immunol.* **26:**1130–1138.

107. **Raqib, R., B. Wretlind, J. Andersson, and A. A. Lindberg.** 1995. Cytokine secretion in acute shigellosis is correlated to disease activity and directed more to stool than to plasma. *J. Infect. Dis.* **171:**376–384.

108. **Rathman, M., N. Jouirhi, A. Allaoui, P. Sansonetti, C. Parsot, and G. Tran Van Nhieu.** 2000. The development of a FACS-based strategy for the isolation of *Shigella flexneri* mutants that are deficient in intercellular spread. *Mol. Microbiol.* **35:**974–990.

109. **Raupach, B., J. Mecsus, U. Heczko, S. Flakow, and B. B. Finlay.** 1999. Bacterial epithelial cell cross talk. *Curr. Top. Microbiol. Immunol.* **236:**137–161.

110. **Renesto, P., J. Mounier, and P. J. Sansonetti.** 1996. Induction of adherence and degranulation of polymorphonuclear leukocytes: a new expression of the invasive phenotype of *Shigella flexneri. Infect. Immun.* **64:**719–723.

111. **Robbins, J. R., D. Monack, S. J. McCallun, A. Vegas, E. Pham, M. B. Goldberg, and J. A. Theriot.** 2001. The making of a gradient: IcsA (VirG) polarity in *Shigella flexneri. Mol. Microbiol.* **41:**861–872.

112. **Rohatgi, R., L. Ma, H. Miki, M. Lopez, T. Kirchhausen, T. Takenawa, and M. W. Kirschner.** 1999. The interaction between N-WASP and the Arp2/3 complex links Cdc42-dependent signals to actin assembly. *Cell* **97:**221–231.

113. **Samandari, T., K. L. Kotloff, G. A. Losonsky, W. D. Picking, P. J. Sansonetti, M. M. Levine, and M. B. Sztein.** 2000. Production of IFN-gamma and IL-10 to *Shigella* invasins by mononuclear cells from volunteers orally inoc-

ulated with a Shiga toxin-deleted *Shigella dysenteriae* type 1 strain. *J. Immunol.* **164:**2221–2232.

114. **Sandlin, R. C., M. B. Goldberg, and A. T. Maurelli.** 1996. Effect of O side-chain length and composition on the virulence of *Shigella flexneri* 2a. *Mol. Microbiol.* **22:**63–73.

115. **Sandlin, R. C., K. A. Lampel, S. P. Keasler, M. B. Goldberg, A. L. Stolzer, and A. T. Maurelli.** 1995. Avirulence of rough mutants of *Shigella flexneri*: requirement of O antigen for correct unipolar localization of IcsA in the bacterial outer membrane. *Infect. Immun.* **63:**229–237.

116. **Sandlin, R. C., and A. T. Maurelli.** 1999. Establishment of unipolar localization of IcsA in *Shigella flexneri* 2a is not dependent on virulence plasmid determinants. *Infect. Immun.* **67:**350–356.

117. **Sansonetti, P., and A. Phalipon.** 1996. Shigellosis: from molecular pathogenesis of infection to protective immunity and vaccine development. *Res. Immunol.* **147:**595–602.

118. **Sansonetti, P. J.** 1993. Molecular mechanisms of cell and tissue invasion by *Shigella flexneri*. *Infect. Agents Dis.* **2:**201–206.

119. **Sansonetti, P. J.** 1998. Pathogenesis of shigellosis: from molecular and cellular biology of epithelial cell invasion to tissue inflammation and vaccine development. *Jpn. J. Med. Sci. Biol.* **51:**S69–S80.

120. **Sansonetti, P. J., J. Arondel, J. M. Cavaillon, and M. Huerre.** 1995. Role of interleukin-1 in the pathogenesis of experimental shigellosis. *J. Clin. Invest.* **96:**884–892.

121. **Sansonetti, P. J., J. Arondel, M. Huerre, A. Harada, and K. Katsushima.** 1999. Interleukin-8 controls bacterial transepithelial translocation at the cost of epithelial destruction in experimental shigellosis. *Infect. Immun.* **67:**1471–1480.

122. **Sansonetti, P. J., H. d'Hauteville, C. Ecobichon, and C. Pourcel.** 1983. Molecular comparison of virulence plasmids in *Shigella* and enteroinvasive *Escherichia coli*. *Ann. Microbiol.* (*Paris*) **134A:**295–318.

123. **Sansonetti, P. J., D. J. Kopecko, and S. B. Formal.** 1982. Involvement of a plasmid in the invasive ability of *Shigella flexneri*. *Infect. Immun.* **35:**852–860.

124. **Sansonetti, P. J., J. Mounier, M. C. Prevost, and R. M. Mege.** 1994. Cadherin expression is required for the spread of *Shigella flexneri* between epithelial cells. *Cell* **76:**829–839.

125. **Sansonetti, P. J., and A. Phalipon.** 1999. M cells as ports of entry for enteroinvasive pathogens: mechanisms of interaction, consequences

126. **Sansonetti, P. J., A. Phalipon, J. Arondel, K. Thirumalai, S. Banerjee, S. Akira, K. Takeda, and A. Zychlinsky.** 2000. Caspase-1 activation of IL-1beta and IL-18 are essential for *Shigella flexneri*-induced inflammation. *Immunity* **12:**581–590.

127. **Sansonetti, P. J., G. Tran Van Nhieu, and C. Egile.** 1999. Rupture of the intestinal epithelial barrier and mucosal invasion by *Shigella flexneri*. *Clin. Infect. Dis.* **28:**466–475.

128. **Sasakawa, C., K. Kamata, T. Sakai, S. Makino, M. Yamada, N. Okada, and M. Yoshikawa.** 1988. Virulence-associated genetic regions comprising 31 kilobases of the 230-kilobase plasmid in *Shigella flexneri* 2a. *J. Bacteriol.* **170:**2480–2484.

129. **Sasakawa, C., K. Komatsu, T. Tobe, T. Suzuki, and M. Yoshikawa.** 1993. Eight genes in region 5 that form an operon are essential for invasion of epithelial cells by *Shigella flexneri* 2a. *J. Bacteriol.* **175:**2334–2346.

130. **Sasakawa, C., S. Makino, K. Kamata, and M. Yoshikawa.** 1986. Isolation, characterization, and mapping of Tn5 insertions into the 140-megadalton invasion plasmid defective in the mouse Sereny test in *Shigella flexneri* 2a. *Infect. Immun.* **54:**32–36.

131. **Schuch, R., and A. T. Maurelli.** 1999. The Mxi-Spa type III secretory pathway of *Shigella flexneri* requires an outer membrane lipoprotein, MxiM, for invasin translocation. *Infect. Immun.* **67:**1982–1991.

132. **Schuch, R., and A. T. Maurelli.** 2001. MxiM and MxiJ, base elements of the Mxi-Spa type III secretion system of *Shigella*, interact with and stabilize the MxiD secretin in the cell envelope. *J. Bacteriol.* **183:**6991–6998.

133. **Schuch, R., and A. T. Maurelli.** 2001. Spa33, a cell surface-associated subunit of the Mxi-Spa type III secretory pathway of *Shigella flexneri*, regulates Ipa protein traffic. *Infect. Immun.* **69:**2180–2189.

134. **Schuch, R., R. C. Sandlin, and A. T. Maurelli.** 1999. A system for identifying post-invasion functions of invasion genes: requirements for the Mxi-Spa type III secretion pathway of *Shigella flexneri* in intercellular dissemination. *Mol. Microbiol.* **34:**675–689.

135. **Shibata, T., F. Takeshima, F. Chen, F. W. Alt, and S. B. Snapper.** 2002. Cdc42 facilitates invasion but not the actin-based motility of *Shigella*. *Curr. Biol.* **12:**341–345.

136. **Skoudy, A., G. T. Nhieu, N. Mantis, M. Arpin, J. Mounier, P. Gounon, and P. Sansonetti.** 1999. A functional role for ezrin during

Shigella flexneri entry into epithelial cells. *J. Cell Sci.* **112:**2059–2068.

137. **Snapper, S. B., F. Takeshima, I. Anton, C. H. Liu, S. M. Thomas, D. Nguyen, D. Dudley, H. Fraser, D. Purcich, M. Lopez-Ilasaca, C. Klein, L. Davidson, R. Bronson, R. C. Mulligan, F. Southwick, R. Geha, M. B. Goldberg, F. S. Rosen, J. H. Hartwig, and F. W. Alt.** 2001. N-WASP deficiency reveals distinct pathways for cell surface projections and microbiol actin-based motility. *Nat. Cell Biol.* **3:**897–904.

138. **Steinhauer, J., R. Agha, T. Pham, A. W. Varga, and M. B. Goldberg.** 1999. The unipolar *Shigella* surface protein IcsA is targeted directly to the bacterial old pole: IcsP cleavage of IcsA occurs over the entire bacterial surface. *Mol. Microbiol.* **32:**367–377.

139. **Suzuki, T., H. Mimuro, H. Miki, T. Takenawa, T. Sasaki, H. Nakanishi, Y. Takai, and C. Sasakawa.** 2000. Rho family GTPase Cdc42 is essential for the actin-based motility of *Shigella* in mammalian cells. *J. Exp. Med.* **191:**1905–1920.

140. **Suzuki, T., S. Saga, and C. Sasakawa.** 1996. Functional analysis of *Shigella* VirG domains essential for interaction with vinculin and actin-based motility. *J. Biol. Chem.* **271:**21878–21885.

141. **Suzuki, T., and C. Sasakawa.** 2001. Molecular basis of the intracellular spreading of *Shigella. Infect. Immun.* **69:**5959–5966.

142. **Suzuki, T., and C. Sasakawa.** 1998. N-WASP is an important protein for the actin-based motility of *Shigella flexneri* in the infected epithelial cells. *Jpn. J. Med. Sci. Biol.* **51:**S63–S68.

143. **Takahashi, K., T. Sasaki, A. Mammoto, K. Takaishi, T. Kameyama, S. Tsukita, and Y. Takai.** 1997. Direct interaction of the Rho GDP dissociation inhibitor with ezrin/radixin/moesin initiates the activation of the Rho small G protein. *J. Biol. Chem.* **272:**23371–23375.

144. **Takeuchi, O., K. Hoshino, T. Kawai, H. Sanjo, H. Takada, T. Ogawa, K. Takeda, and S. Akira.** 1999. Differential roles of TLR2 and TLR4 in recognition of gram-negative and gram-positive bacterial cell wall components. *Immunity* **11:**443–451.

145. **Tamano, K., S. Aizawa, E. Katayama, T. Nonaka, S. Imajoh-Ohmi, A. Kuwae, S. Nagai, and C. Sasakawa.** 2002. Supramolecular structure of the *Shigella* type III secretion machinery: the needle part is changeable in length and essential for delivery of effectors. *EMBO J.* **19:**3876–3887.

146. **Taylor, D. N., A. C. Trofa, J. Sadoff, C. Chu, D. Bryla, J. Shiloach, D. Cohen, S. Ashkenazi, Y. Lerman, W. Egan, R. Schneerson, and J. B. Robbins.** 1993. Synthesis, characterization, and clinical evaluation of conjugate vaccines composed of the O-specific polysaccharides of *Shigella dysenteriae* type 1, *Shigella flexneri* type 2a, and *Shigella sonnei* (*Plesiomonas shigelloides*) bound to bacterial toxoids. *Infect. Immun.* **61:**3678–3687.

147. **Tobe, T., M. Yoshikawa, T. Mizuno, and C. Sasakawa.** 1993. Transcriptional control of the invasion regulatory gene *virB* of *Shigella flexneri*: activation by *virF* and repression by H-NS. *J. Bacteriol.* **175:**6142–6149.

148. **Toyotome, T., T. Suzuki, A. Kuwae, T. Nonaka, H. Fukuda, S. Imajoh-Ohmi, T. Toyofuku, M. Hori, and C. Sasakawa.** 2001. *Shigella* protein IpaH(9.8) is secreted from bacteria within mammalian cells and transported to the nucleus. *J. Biol. Chem.* **276:**32071–32079.

149. **Trans, N., A. B. Berfis, J. C. Osiecki, W. L. Picking, L. Coye, R. Davis, and W. D. Picking.** 2000. Interaction of *Shigella flexneri* IpaC with model membranes correlates with effects on cultured cells. *Infect. Immun.* **68:**3710–3715.

150. **Tran Van Nhieu, G., A Ben-Ze'ev, and P. J. Sansonetti.** 1997. Modulation of bacterial entry into epithelial cells by association between vinculin and the *Shigella* IpaA invasin. *EMBO J.* **16:**2717–2729.

151. **Tran Van Nhieu, G., R. Bourdet-Sicard, G. Dumenil, A. Blocker, and P. J. Sansonetti.** 2000. Bacterial signals and cell responses during *Shigella* entry into epithelial cells. *Cell. Microbiol.* **2:**187–193.

152. **Tran Van Nhieu, G., E. Caron, A. Hall, and P. J. Sansonetti.** 1999. IpaC induces actin polymerization and filopodia formation during *Shigella* entry into epithelial cells. *EMBO J.* **18:**3249–3262.

153. **Van Aelst, L., and C. D'Souza-Schorey.** 1997. Rho GTPases and signaling networks. *Genes Dev.* **11:**2295–2322.

154. **Vasselon, T., J. Mounier, R. Hellio, and P. J. Sansonetti.** 1992. Movement along actin filaments of the perijunctional area and de novo polymerization of cellular actin are required for *Shigella flexneri* colonization of epithelial Caco-2 cell monolayers. *Infect. Immun.* **60:**1031–1040.

155. **Wang, S., M. Miura, Y. K. Jung, H. Zhu, E. Li, and J. Yuan.** 1998. Murine caspase-11, an ICE-interacting protease, is essential for the activation of ICE. *Cell* **92:**501–509.

156. **Watarai, M., S. Funato, and C. Sasakawa.** 1996. Interaction of Ipa proteins of *Shigella flexneri* with alpha5beta1 integrin promotes entry of the bacteria into mammalian cells. *J. Exp. Med.* **183**:991–999.

157. **Watarai, M., Y. Kamata, S. Kozaki, and C. Sasakawa.** 1997. Rho, a small GTP-binding protein, is essential for *Shigella* invasion of epithelial cells, *J. Exp. Med.* **185**:281–292.

158. **Watarai, M., T. Tobe, M. Yoshikawa, and C. Sasakawa.** 1995. Contact of *Shigella* with host cells triggers release of Ipa invasins and is an essential function of invasiveness. *EMBO J.* **14**:2461–2470.

159. **Wattiau, P., B. Bernier, P. Deslee, T. Michiels, and G. R. Cornelis.** 1994. Individual chaperones required for Yop secretion by *Yersinia. Proc. Natl. Acad. Sci. USA* **91**:10493–10497.

160. **Wattiau, P., S. Woestyn, and G. R. Cornelis.** 1996. Customized secretion chaperones in pathogenic bacteria. *Mol. Microbiol.* **20**:255–262.

161. **Way, S. S., A. C. Borczuk, R. Dominitz, and M. B. Goldberg.** 1998. An essential role for gamma interferon in innate resistance to *Shigella flexneri* infection. *Infect. Immun.* **66**:1342–1348.

162. **Way, S. S., A. C. Borczuk, and M. B. Goldberg.** 1999. Adaptive immune response to *Shigella flexneri* 2a cydC in immunocompetent mice and mice lacking immunoglobulin A. *Infect. Immun.* **67**:2001–2004.

163. **Way, S. S., A. C. Borczuk, and M. B. Goldberg.** 1999. Thymic independence of adaptive immunity to the intracellular pathogen *Shigella flexneri* serotype 2a. *Infect. Immun.* **67**:3970–3979.

164. **Welch, M. D.** 1999. The world according to Arp: regulation of actin nucleation by the Arp2/3 complex. *Trends Cell. Biol.* **9**:423–427.

165. **Zhang, Z., L. Jin, G. Champion, K. B. Seydel, and S. L. J. Stanley.** 2001. *Shigella* infection in a SCID mouse-human intestinal xenograft model: role for neutrophils in containing bacterial dissemination in human intestine. *Infect. Immun.* **69**:3240–3247.

166. **Zychlinsky, A., J. J. Perdomo, and P. J. Sansonetti.** 1994. Molecular and cellular mechanisms of tissue invasion by *Shigella flexneri. Ann. N. Y. Acad. Sci.* **730**:197–208.

167. **Zychlinksy, A., M. C. Provost, and P. J. Sansonetti.** 1992. *Shigella flexneri* induces apoptosis in infected macrophages. *Nature* **358**:167–169.

168. **Zychlinksy, A., K. Thirumalai, J. Arondel, J. R. Cantey, A. O. Aliprantis, and P. J. Sansonetti.** 1996. In vivo apoptosis in *Shigella flexneri* infections. *Infect. Immun.* **64**:5357–5365.

TOXINS OF *VIBRIO CHOLERAE*: CONSENSUS AND CONTROVERSY

Karla Jean Fullner

26

At first glance, the molecular basis of cholera disease seemed quite simple. The bacterial agent of disease, *Vibrio cholerae*, was presumed to require only two virulence factors: toxin-coregulated pili (TCP) to colonize the human intestinal epithelium and cholera toxin (CT) to elicit diarrhea. However, JBK70, a CT⁻, TCP⁺ variant of the *V. cholerae* O1 El Tor strain N16961, was pathogenic in human volunteers. The volunteers succumbed to mild diarrhea, fever, cramps, emesis, and anorexia, symptoms collectively called "reactogenicity." The severity of symptoms portrayed by these volunteers suggested that other virulence factors beyond colonization and CT contribute to *V. cholerae*-associated enteric disease (60). A search for the virulence factors responsible for residual symptoms in the absence of CT has led to the discovery of new cytotoxins and a reemerging interest in previously identified toxins. In addition, the role of CT itself in disease is being revised.

Understanding the role of these toxins in cholera disease is important to the challenge of protecting susceptible populations from dis-

ease. Despite years of research, a safe live attenuated vaccine for protection of indigenous populations against cholera is still not available (115). Identification and characterization of virulence factors beyond CT and elimination of these factors from candidate strains are essential to the improved safety of these vaccines.

This review covers each of the known cytotoxins of *V. cholerae* in a separate section. The discussion focuses on recent research and aspects of the toxins that may not be covered in other reviews. In particular, where discord in the interpretation of data is obvious, both sides of the controversy are presented, although the bias of the author in these disputes is evident.

CT

Intestinal Secretion
It is incontrovertible that CT is the most important virulence factor of *V. cholerae*. CT is an A-B subunit toxin composed of five copies of CtxB in a pentameric ring and one copy of the catalytic subunit CtxA. The CtxB proteins bind to GM_1-ganglioside in lipid rafts at the luminal surface of intestinal cells, and the toxin subsequently enters cells by endocytosis. Upon entry, the holotoxin undergoes retrograde

Karla Jean Fullner, Department of Microbiology-Immunology, Northwestern University Medical School, 303 E. Chicago Avenue, Morton 6-626, Chicago, IL 60611.

Microbial Pathogenesis and the Intestinal Epithelial Cell, ed. by G. Hecht
© 2003 ASM Press, Washington, D.C.

transport through the *trans*-Golgi network, the Golgi apparatus, and the endoplasmic reticulum, where CtxA is translocated to the cytoplasm. The catalytically active CtxA ADP-ribosylates the heterotrimeric GTPase Gsα, resulting in constitutive activation of the host adenylate cyclase. The resulting increased concentration of intracellular cyclic AMP (cAMP) alters membrane channel activity, resulting in a net efflux of Cl$^-$ and water from the cells to the lumen. The resulting massive diarrhea eventually leads to the death of the cholera victim by secondary dehydration (for a more detailed review, see reference 59 and chapter 21).

Suppression of Inflammation

This massive fluid secretion induced by the action of CT is the prevailing characteristic of cholera disease. A second major characteristic of *V. cholerae* infection is the apparent lack of a host inflammatory immune response. Hence, cholera is considered the classic example of noninflammatory toxigenic diarrhea (64). Biopsies taken from cholera patients indicate that the intestinal epithelium remains intact during the infectious stage, although abnormal distention of the apical intracellular junctions has been observed (reference 70 and references therein). A massive recruitment of inflammatory cells to the site of infection is not apparent in the intestines of cholera victims (70). In contrast, naturally occurring *V. cholerae* strains that do not produce CT and vaccine strains genetically modified to delete genes for CT show a marked increase in the inflammatory component of the host immune response (85, 86). This alteration in the immune response to *V. cholerae* has been linked directly to immunomodulatory action by CT, suggesting that control of the host immune response may be a significant component of the role of CT in disease.

CT has been demonstrated to inhibit virtually every stage in the development of the proinflammatory immune response (Fig. 1). During the initial stages of infection, the innate immune response to a gram-negative bacterial infection is typically signaled by lipopolysaccharide (LPS), which is recognized by surface Toll-like receptors on resident macrophages and monocyte-derived dendritic cells (1). *V. cholerae* is known to be translocated across M cells both in vitro and in vivo, indicating that these immune cells present in the lymphatic tissue below the intestinal barrier would detect *V. cholerae* antigens (55, 89). In vitro experiments have demonstrated that isolated bone marrow macrophages stimulated with LPS will secrete tumor necrosis factor alpha (TNF-α) and interleukin-1 (IL-1), but costimulation with CT will inhibit production of these cytokines (18). In the host, expression of TNF-α and IL-1 would normally act on local endothelial cells that in turn would produce chemokines to signal for recruitment and translocation of neutrophils to the site of infection (1). Thus, CT could block recruitment of neutrophils at the earliest stage of infection by inhibiting production of TNF-α and IL-1.

Macrophages stimulated by LPS also secrete IL-12 (1). This cytokine acts on many types of immune cells to stimulate the proinflammatory response. At the earliest stages, IL-12 signals local natural killer (NK) cells to release gamma interferon (IFN-γ) that in turn signals macrophage activation by amplifying the LPS signal. In addition, IL-12 will signal NK cells to kill bacteria directly by releasing toxic granules (1). However, macrophages stimulated by LPS, but also treated with CT, produce IL-10 instead of IL-12 (18). IL-10 acts on the stimulated macrophage itself to downregulate IL-12 production, thereby blocking stimulation of the NK cells and other cells of the proinflammatory immune response (1). In the bone marrow macrophages, CT will also inhibit production of nitric oxide (NO) by downregulating the synthesis of inducible nitric oxide synthase (iNOS) (18). Decreased NO will result in reduced bacterial killing by activated oxygen radicals and loss of protection against tissue-damaging toxins (1, 118). Similar results on cytokine and NO production have been obtained with other types of antigen-presenting cells, including peripheral blood

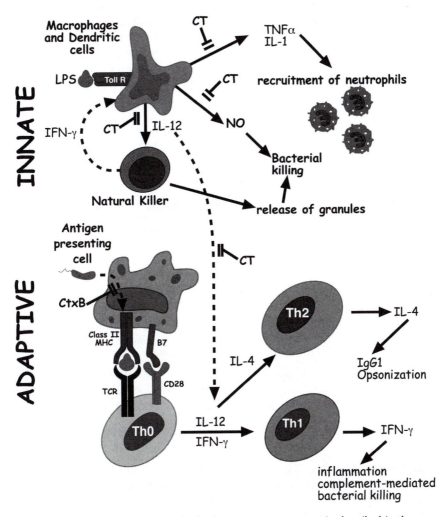

FIGURE 1 CT blocks innate and adaptive immune responses. As described in the text, CT or the subunit CtxB blocks multiple stages of the immune response during *V. cholerae* infection. The production of cytokines and NO by antigen-presenting cells downregulates the innate response. Antigen processing and the development of a Th1 adaptive immune response are inhibited. Evidence suggests that CtxB stimulates a Th2-type response.

mononuclear cells (PBMC), dendritic cells, and mast cells (41, 57, 68). Hence, CT may block three key branches of the innate immune response—recruitment of neutrophils, activation of NK cells, and NO-mediated bacterial killing—by inhibiting production of iNOS and the proinflammatory cytokines by antigen-presenting cells.

CT can also alter development of the adaptive immune response. During infection, ac-tivated macrophages that take up *V. cholerae* bacteria by phagocytosis present antigenic peptides to naive T cells on major histocom-patibility complex (MHC) class II. In the pres-ence of IL-12 and IFN-γ, these activated T cells will differentiate to Th1 cells that then amplify the inflammatory response through production of IFN-γ. The Th1 adaptive immune response includes activation of macrophages, recruitment of neutrophils, stimulation of NK cells, and maturation of B cells to produce immunoglobulin G1 (IgG1) for complement-mediated killing of bacteria (1). However, uptake of CtxB has been demonstrated to block class II antigen processing and presentation by cultured J774.2 macrophages, although the inhibition is much weaker than the block introduced by EtxB, the B-subunit of the related heat-labile toxin of enterotoxigenic *Escherichia coli* (75). This block in antigen presentation to naive T cells, in conjunction with the downregulation of IL-12 and IFN-γ during early infection, could effectively eliminate the development of the Th1 inflammatory response, accounting for the noninflammatory diarrhea observed during *V. cholerae* infection.

A significant role of CtxB in the inhibition of Th1 responses has been verified in vivo by investigators studying oral tolerance and autoimmunity (111). For example, experimental autoimmune encephalomyelitis (EAE), a model for the human Th1-mediated autoimmune disease multiple sclerosis, can be induced in rats by inoculation with myelin basic protein (MyBP). However, oral feeding of MyBP conjugated to CtxB protected experimental animals from developing paralysis by decreasing infiltration of leukocytes into the spinal cord (96). Similarly, EAE induced in C57BL/6 mice by inoculation of myelin oligodendricyte glycoprotein (MOG) was suppressed by nasal administration of CT (122). Thus, CT, and particularly CtxB, blocked development of the Th1-mediated autoimmune disease to a model antigen.

This downregulation of the Th1 response may in turn enhance the development of a Th2 response (41, 120). CtxB is known to act as a potent adjuvant enhancing mucosal immune responses to intranasally administered antigens (23). For example, CT promotes the development of serum antibodies against tetanus toxoid and ovalbumin (OVA) peptide after intranasal immunization (87, 120). A particularly strong stimulation of the IgG1, IgG2, and IgG3 subclasses of antibodies as well as stimulation of IgE was noted when CtxB

was used as the adjuvant, indicating initiation of both Th1- and Th2-mediated protection against administered antigen (87, 120). The stimulation of antibody production coincided with the stimulation of a Th2-type cytokine profile including IL-4, IL-5, IL-6, and IL-10 (120). Thus, the role of CT as a serum adjuvant is partially linked to the ability to direct an immune response toward a Th2 response.

Apoptosis of CD8+ T Cells

A final role for CT in immune suppression may be to deplete the population of CD8+ T cells that would normally eliminate infected cells. CD8+ T cells respond to presentation of cytosolic antigens on MHC class I (1). In the case of *V. cholerae*, these antigens could be derived from toxins, including CT itself or other toxins, that act in the cytosol. Treatment of mesenteric lymph node cells with CtxB for 48 h triggers apoptosis of about 75% of the CD8+ T-cell population, a reaction that may occur through signaling by c-Myc based on observations with the related protein EtxB (5, 92). Thus, CT would effectively inhibit the destruction of epithelial cells that it has entered by concurrently eliminating cell-mediated killing by CD8+ T cells.

Primary Role in Pathogenesis

From the patient's perspective, the most important aspect of cholera disease is the profuse diarrhea that leads to death. Thus, classic paradigms of *V. cholerae* pathogenesis suggest that the selective advantage for *V. cholerae* that acquires genes for CT is the ability to induce massive diarrhea, presumably allowing for rapid dissemination through a population. However, it is increasingly evident that CT plays an important role in modulating the host immune system at many levels, including suppression of innate immunity, alteration of adaptive immunity to a more tolerant Th2 response, and signaling apoptosis of CD8+ T cells. Therefore, from the bacterial point of view, the most important selective advantage for the gain of CT may be to evade the proinflammatory immune response and persist within the nutrient-rich intestine for a longer period of time. When the immune system does successfully clear the infection, the concurrent dissemination by induction of diarrhea would be a secondary strategy allowing survival of the entire species. Thus, resolution of any controversy over the primary function of CT in cholera disease may depend on whether one looks from the perspective of the bacterium rather than the view of the cholera victim.

ZONULA OCCLUDENS TOXIN

Effect on Intestinal Tight Junctions
In the preceding section, it was noted that ultrastructural studies of intestinal biopsies from cholera patients revealed abnormalities in the apical intercellular junctional complexes (70). In some cases, the zonula occludens or tight junction, the most apical region of the intercellular junctional complex, was distorted and often S-shaped, and the subjacent zonula adherens was widened (70). Distortion of the zonula occludens also occurred when rabbit ileal tissue mounted in Ussing chambers was treated with filtered supernatant fluid from *V. cholerae* cultures, indicating the presence of a secreted factor that affects intestinal tight junctions (29). The ultrastructural change in the ileal tissue correlates with an increase in transcellular conductance that is reversible when the culture media are replaced (29). The protein responsible for this toxic activity is encoded by the gene *zot* (for zonula occludens toxin) found immediately adjacent to the *ctxAB* genes that encode CT (8).

The mechanism of action against intestinal tight junctions has been investigated using Zot protein purified from *E. coli*. Within 60 min of addition of picomolar concentrations of purified Zot protein, a 20% decrease in transepithelial resistance is observed (33). This decrease in electrical resistance is likely due to changes in paracellular permeability, since the rate of passive transport of radiolabeled insulin, immunoglobulin G (IgG), and polyethylene glycol 4000 (PEG) across tissue mounted in

the Ussing chamber is increased 1.5- to 2-fold by the addition of Zot (32, 33). Perfusion of Zot into a rabbit jejunum or ileum correlated with increased secretion of water and Cl^- into the intestine and with enhanced translocation of PEG or insulin from the lumen into the bloodstream (33). Likewise, polarized Caco-2 intestinal epithelial cells treated with 80 nM Zot show a two- to fourfold increase in the flux rate of mannitol or insulin after 2 h (19). Together, these data indicate that Zot increases the permeability of the tight junctions in the ileum and jejunum both in vitro and in vivo. However, the slight nature of the effects induced by Zot has led to a controversy over whether the activity of Zot is important in cholera disease.

Proposed Mode of Action
Assuming that the slight activity attributed to Zot is clinically relevant, the proposed mode of action is quite interesting (28). The current model suggests that Zot binds and activates cell signal pathways via a surface receptor for a host regulatory protein called zonulin, a factor proposed to modulate fluid secretion through the paracellular junctions during the acute phase of celiac disease (31, 108). Attempts to identify this surface receptor have not been successful. Binding of Zot to cultured intestinal cells is weak and dependent upon permeabilization of fixed cells, suggesting that the receptor is not surface exposed (24, 63, 104). Purified Zot-binding proteins purported to be the receptor for Zot and zonulin include proteins with peptide sequences that best match human serum albumin and β-tubulin, indicating that the true receptor has not been identified by this approach (see references 63 and 104) and PSI-BLAST [4] searches performed for this chapter). Downstream of receptor binding, it is proposed that Zot leads to the rearrangement of filamentous (F)-actin dependent upon signaling through protein kinase C (30). However, the rearrangement of F-actin has not been demonstrated using purified protein, a considerable distinction since other proteins found in *V.*

cholerae supernatant fluids are implicated in alterations to the structure of F-actin, including the RTX toxin and hemagglutinin/protease (see below).

Thus, Zot is proposed to alter the permeability of tight junctions by interaction with a host receptor followed by initiating a signal cascade, resulting in a rearrangement of F-actin that maintains the integrity of the tight junction. Clearly, identification of the surface receptor and further analysis of the signal cascade will be essential to proving the validity of this model.

CTXΦ Filamentous Phage Assembly

Additional controversy concerning the role of Zot in pathogenesis has arisen from the demonstration that Zot is essential for a function unrelated to toxinogenesis. A number of filamentous phages produced by the *Vibrio* spp. have been identified both by electron microscopy and by sequence analysis (25, 52, 106; N. Basu and R. K. Ghosh, unpublished data; Genbank accession no. AF453500). One of these, the CTXΦ phage, carries the CT structural genes *ctxAB* (105). In the sequenced genome of the O1 El Tor strain N16961, CTXΦ occurs as a single copy integrated into one of the two circular chromosomes, although some *V. cholerae* isolates have multiple copies of CTXΦ inserted in one or both chromosomes (7, 50, 72). An internal deletion within the *zot* gene on the replicative form of CTXΦ completely blocks production of transducing phage particles, implicating the *zot* gene in CTXΦ phage biology rather than toxicity (105).

Enterobacteriophage f1 of *E. coli* is the best-characterized filamentous phage and will be used as a comparison for the gene products of the CTXΦ phage (for reviews, see references 69 and 82). The virion particle of f1 is composed of the single-stranded phage DNA encased by five proteins: the major coat protein pVIII and minor virion proteins pIII, pVI, pVII, and pIX. Assembly and export of f1 across the bacterial inner and outer membranes require three proteins (34, 46, 67). pI and pXI are encoded by the same gene, with

pXI arising from an internal translational start site within gene I, creating a protein that is identical in sequence to the last 108 amino acids of pI (45). Both proteins are integral inner membrane proteins essential for assembly of the virion particle possibly by interacting with the single-stranded DNA (ssDNA) packaging signal or the major coat protein (34, 46). The assembling f1 filamentous phage is extruded from the bacterial cell through an outer membrane aqueous channel formed by oligomerization of pIV, also referred to as "secretin" (66, 67). Assembly and extrusion of f1 bacteriophage may involve binding of nucleotides since a consensus nucleotide binding site (NBS) is present on the cytoplasmic-exposed N terminus of pI (82).

A schematic diagram of the gene arrangement of CTXΦ is shown in Fig. 2. A colinear gene arrangement with f1 is apparent. At the left end of CTXΦ, the *rstA* and *rstB* genes are necessary for phage replication and integration, respectively, under the control of a repressor encoded by *rstR* (106). Proteins for replication of f1, pII, pX, and pV, are encoded at a similar locus (82). The virion particle proteins are encoded next on the f1 phage. The first two genes encode pIX and pVII, which are assembled at the leading tip of the viral particle; the third gene encodes the major coat protein pVIII, followed by the genes for pIII and pVI, which are attached to the end of the virion particle that is released last from the bacterium (82). Previous annotation of the CTXΦ genome identified genes for only three putative virion coat proteins, Cep, OrfU, and Ace, paralogs of pVIII, pIII, and pVI, respectively (105). An open reading frame analysis done for this chapter identified a small open reading frame between *rstB* and *cep* that encodes a protein similar in size to pIX and pVII with hydrophobic stretches similar to those found in all filamentous phage coat proteins (69). These data indicate that four virion-associated proteins may encase the CTXΦ ssDNA.

Based on the colinear arrangement, *zot* would be predicted to encode the equivalent of the f1 phage assembly protein pI. A BLAST

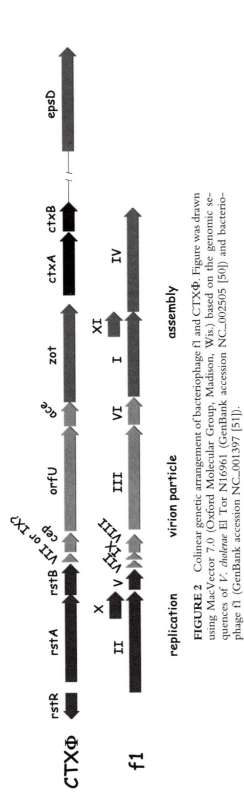

FIGURE 2 Colinear genetic arrangement of bacteriophage f1 and CTXΦ. Figure was drawn using MacVector 7.0 (Oxford Molecular Group, Madison, Wis.) based on the genomic sequences of *V. cholerae* El Tor N16961 (GenBank accession NC_002505 [50]) and bacteriophage f1 (GenBank accession NC_001397 [51]).

2 alignment (98) of the amino acid sequence of pI and Zot revealed little sequence similarity, although both proteins have the characteristic nucleotide binding site at amino acids 8 to 15 (Fig. 3). The structural genes for CT, *ctxAB,* are apparently substituted at the expected location of the secretin gene. Recent data support that the secretin protein EpsD, previously known to be essential for CT secretion, may be coopted by the CTXΦ phage to associate with Zot to create a complete phage assembly apparatus (22, 84).

Dual Function for Zot?

To reconcile the controversy over whether Zot is a toxin or a phage assembly protein, a dual function model has been proposed (24). Although an inner membrane localization would be predicted for Zot based on the need for the NBS to be exposed to ATP or GTP in the cytoplasm, immunolocalization studies using anti–Zot antibodies detect both a 45-kDa form (Zotp45) and a 33-kDa (Zotp33) form in the *V. cholerae* bacterial outer membrane (103). Zotp33 maintained an N-terminal polyhistidine tag, indicating that processing by an endopeptidase releases a 12-kDa subfragment from the C terminus, presumably to the extracellular environment (103). Structure-function analysis of purified Zot localized the portion of the protein able to induce a drop in resistance to the C terminus (24). This active subfragment would correspond to the segment of Zot released by proteolytic processing. Therefore, the dual function model suggests that the Zotp33 subfragment functions in phage assembly and the Zotp12 subfragment is the cytotoxin. However, the secreted Zotp12 fragment has not as yet been detected in supernatant fluids, even though the activity is present (24, 103). Identification of this active polypeptide and demonstration of its activity against intestinal epithelium are imperative to the justification of this model.

Given the currently available information, it is impossible to distinguish the primary role of Zot. The slight nature of the intestinal response needs to be revisited in a more sensitive

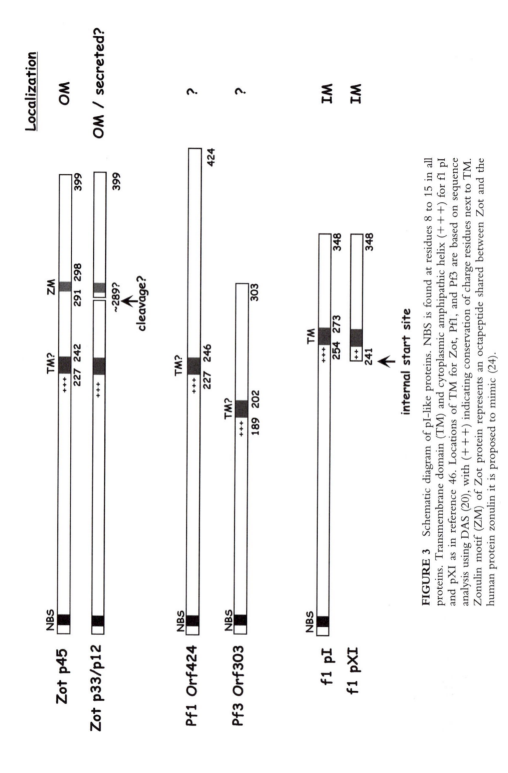

FIGURE 3 Schematic diagram of pI-like proteins. NBS is found at residues 8 to 15 in all proteins. Transmembrane domain (TM) and cytoplasmic amphipathic helix (+++) for f1 pI and pXI as in reference 46. Locations of TM for Zot, Pf1, and Pf3 are based on sequence analysis using DAS (20), with (+++) indicating conservation of charge residues next to TM. Zonulin motif (ZM) of Zot protein represents an octapeptide shared between Zot and the human protein zonulin it is proposed to mimic (24).

model using physiologically relevant concentrations. On the other hand, there are no data on the exact role of Zot in phage biology beyond analogy to other filamentous phages, and it is conceivable that Zot could be a bifunctional protein. As the research progresses, it is intriguing to consider that *V. cholerae* could be incredibly thrifty to use a byproduct of phage assembly, Zotp12, as a modulator of intestinal permeability to increase diarrhea during infection by mimicking a host regulator of fluid secretion.

ACCESSORY CHOLERA ENTEROTOXIN

Calcium-Dependent Channel Agonist

Similar to Zot, the controversy surrounding accessory cholera enterotoxin (Ace) derives from its dual characterization. Ace was first described as a protein that stimulates an increase in short-circuit current (I_{sc}) across rabbit ileal tissue mounted in Ussing chambers (102). Supernatant fluids from a core deletion *V. cholerae* strain (deleted in genes VII/IX to *ctxB* in Fig. 2) did not demonstrate the increase in I_{sc}, indicating the gene encoding the activity is present on integrated CTXΦ phage DNA. In *trans* complementation studies revealed the activity is not due to CT or Zot but to a third CTXΦ-encoded enterotoxin, the product of the gene *ace* (102). Ace protein purified both from concentrated *V. cholerae* culture supernatant fluid and from the yeast *Pichia pastoris* stimulated I_{sc} by 10 to 25 $\mu A/cm^2$ in a dosage-dependent manner when applied to the apical side of rabbit ileal tissue and to polarized T84 intestinal epithelial cells (100, 101). Although the toxin was purified as an 18-kDa dimer, the 9-kDa monomer form is more active against T84 cells (101). Pharmacological studies indicate that the stimulation of I_{sc} from T84 cells results from Ace functioning as an agonist of L-type voltage-gated Ca^{2+} channels. The resulting change in electrical current derives from the secretion of Cl^- and HCO_3^- from the cells. Similar to the action of CT, secreted anions would be cotransported with water, leading to a net efflux of water and diarrhea (101).

CTXΦ Minor Virion Coat Protein

A role of Ace in phage biology has never been tested experimentally, but comparison to bacteriophage f1 and the more closely related Pf1 indicates that Ace could be a structural protein of the CTXΦ phage particle, engaging in a function similar to that of pVI of f1. As shown in Fig. 2, the gene *ace* is similar in size to gene VI of f1 and is found in the same location on the colinear gene arrangement of CTXΦ and f1. Although there is no amino acid sequence similarity between Ace and pVI, Ace is 49% similar to the pVI-like protein of *Pseudomonas* bacteriophage Pf1 (BLAST 2 algorithm [98]). All three proteins differ in length, but a secondary structure analysis (94, 95, 110) revealed a common structure of alpha helices with alternating buried and exposed residues typical of channel-forming proteins.

pVI of f1 and Pf1 are minor virion proteins found in three to five copies at the terminal end of the assembled phage in a complex with the adsorption protein pIII (80). In the core deletion strain used for studies of Ace toxicity, Ace would not be associated with a phage particle in the supernatant fluids because other phage genes *cep*, *orfU*, and *zot* are deleted. Thus, it is surprising that Ace is found in supernatant fluids in these strains (100). Prior to assembly into the phage particle, all coat proteins of f1, including pVI, are inserted into the inner membrane and are retained as integral membrane proteins until the coat proteins are attached to the ssDNA (26). Interestingly, the presence of pVI in the inner membrane is unstable when pIII is absent (80). This observation has been attributed to rapid degradation of pVI unless it is complexed with pIII. However, it is conceivable that the instability of pVI in the membrane results from export of pVI to supernatant fluids. By comparison, in the absence of OrfU to stabilize localization of Ace in the inner membrane, Ace would be secreted. Thus, although Ace is likely to be primarily a phage particle protein, it could be present as a soluble protein in supernatant fluids of the core deletion strains used for cytotoxicity studies. The alteration of channel activity due to Ace would then be consistent with self-insertion of the purified protein into the eukaryotic membrane.

Dual Function or Artifact?

Although purified Ace has cytotoxic activity, it is unlikely that Ace is naturally present as a soluble exported protein. A molecular analysis of clinical and environmental isolates of *V. cholerae* revealed only one strain in which *ace* occurred in the absence of *zot* (90). Although this study did not examine the coincident gain of all CTXΦ genes, the data point toward a conclusion that Ace may not be generally found in nature unassociated with assembled phage particles. It would thus be interesting to consider whether Ace is part of the CTXΦ particle and whether Ace presented on the phage particle has cytotoxic activity. If this were the case, Ace could have a dual function. However, until conclusive experiments are performed, it seems likely that Ace has in vitro biological effects that may not translate to in vivo effects since Ace protein expressed by *V. cholerae* may not be normally exposed to the intestinal epithelium.

HEMAGGLUTININ/PROTEASE

Discovery and Rediscovery

In 1947, a mucinase activity of *V. cholerae* was reported that induced desquamation of epithelial tissue (13). This activity has been recently revisited as an activity of hemagglutinin/protease (HA/P) (36). HA/P is a zinc-metalloprotease synthesized as a 47-kDa precursor that is processed to the mature 32- to 34-kDa form (49). It is exported from *V. cholerae* to supernatant fluids by the same type II secretion apparatus that exports CT (79, 84). Production of HA/P by *V. cholerae* requires cAMP-cAMP receptor protein (CRP) complexes as opposed to expression of CT, which is repressed by cAMP-CRP (10, 91).

HA/P has both hemagglutinating and proteolytic activity (48). It is a nonspecific protease implicated in the digestion of fibronectin, ovomucin, bovine serum albumin, gelatin, and nonfat milk (36, 79, 116). In addition, HA/P inactivates CTXΦ transducing particles, presumably by degrading the major and minor coat proteins (56). HA/P can also activate CT by nicking CtxA, although HA/P is apparently not the only protease with this activity since *hapA* mutants produce active CT (12, 38).

When applied to adherent cells grown in culture, HA/P behaves similarly to trypsin, causing rounding and detachment of cells from the tissue culture dish as the surface attachment proteins are degraded (116) (Fig. 4). The 33-kDa non-membrane-damaging cytotoxin and the WO7 toxin also cause cell rounding and detachment and share similar physical properties with HA/P, suggesting that these proposed novel cytotoxins are either HA/P or close relatives (83, 107). Thus, the characterization of HA/P as a cytotoxin that degrades cell surface proteins leading to cell rounding has been repeatedly rediscovered and reported.

Degradation of Occludin in Tight Junctions

Although HA/P is a generalized protease, it may make a specific contribution to diarrheal disease. When supernatant fluid or purified HA/P is added to polarized T84 intestinal cells or Madin Darby canine kidney (MDCK-I) cells, a sharp drop in the transepithelial electrical resistant is observed. Unlike the modest effect attributed to Zot, HA/P will cause a complete loss of paracellular integrity, measured as a 90 to 100% loss of transepithelial electrical resistance (TER) within 1 h (73, 116). This loss of integrity of paracellular tight junctions is evident in the redistribution of F-actin and the widening of the intercellular tight junction observed by a more diffuse staining of ZO-1, a eukaryotic peripheral membrane protein associated with tight junc-

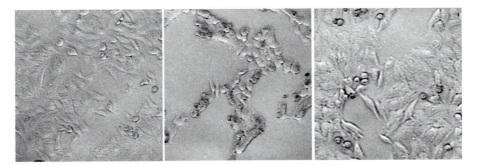

FIGURE 4   HA/P causes rounding and detachment of HEp-2 cells. Phase-images of 70% confluent monolayers of HEp-2 epithelial cells treated for 60 min with phosphate-buffered saline (left) or ammonium sulfate-precipitated supernatant fluids from a HA/P$^+$ strain (middle) and an isogenic HA/P$^-$ strain (right). Data previously presented as data not shown (73).

tions (116). Redistribution of F-actin and ZO-1 is enhanced when MDCK-1 cells are pretreated with an inhibitor of NO production, suggesting that NO protects cells from the damaging effects of HA/P (118).

At the membrane, ZO-1 interacts with the cytoplasmic domains of the transmembrane proteins claudin and occludin that extend from the cell to contact the neighboring cells (76). When HA/P is applied to the apical surface of polarized MDCK cells, occludin is degraded, thus contributing to the complete loss of the barrier function of the epithelial layer. Occludin is not degraded by trypsin and ZO-1 is not degraded by HA/P, demonstrating that the proteolysis of occludin is specific to HA/P and works only against exposed protein (117). It is not yet clear if the action of HA/P against occludin is substrate specific or if HA/P could degrade all proteins that extend from the cell to form the tight junctions, including the claudins and junction adhesion molecule.

In Vivo Activities

Increased permeability across the tight junctions and destruction of tissue by HA/P cause leakage of fluid into the intestinal lumen. Rabbit ligated loops inoculated with an attenuated *V. cholerae* strain that does not produce either CT or HA/P accumulate 36% less fluid than loops inoculated with the parent strain deleted of only CT (9). In addition, the 50% lethal dose (LD$_{50}$) in infant mice increases 10-fold when the gene for HA/P is deleted in addition to CT (9). If it is presumed that the purified WO7 toxin is also HA/P, then inoculation of purified HA/P to rabbit ligated loops also increases fluid secretion to the lumen (107).

HA/P may also contribute to stimulation of the proinflammatory response when CT is not present. HT29-18N2 intestinal epithelial cells exposed to *V. cholerae* will secrete CXCL8 (81), a chemokine produced by endothelial and epithelial cells to signal recruitment of neutrophils to the site of infection (1). This stimulation of CXCL8 is reduced when cells are exposed to isogenic strains deleted of HA/P, suggesting that HA/P may contribute to recruitment of neutrophils (81). In all, these data suggest that tissue destruction by HA/P digestion of surface-exposed proteins may stimulate proinflammatory responses and fluid leakage.

HEMOLYSIN

Pore Formation

Hemolytic *V. cholerae*, called biotype El Tor, was first isolated in Indonesia in 1937 associated with a mild cholera-like disease outbreak

(6). Since 1961, the O1 El Tor biotype has emerged as the predominant agent of epidemic cholera (114). Hemolytic activity is no longer strictly linked with biotype El Tor since nonhemolytic El Tor strains have been isolated and hemolysis is associated with isolates from serotypes other than O1 (90).

The hemolysin protein, HlyA, is translated as an 84-kDa propolypeptide that is translocated to the periplasm where the 25-amino-acid signal sequence is cleaved (47, 119). This form is secreted from the periplasm to the extracellular medium by HlyB (2). HlyA is then activated by a second proteolytic processing to remove a 15-kDa amino-terminal fragment, resulting in the active cytolytic molecule of 60 to 65 kDa (47, 119).

Similar to HA/P, HlyA has been discovered by numerous approaches such that the same protein has been characterized as a β-hemolysin, cytolysin, and vacuolating toxin (3, 17, 35, 43, 44, 65, 77, 125). Within membranes, HlyA monomers assemble to form a pentameric pore about 1.2 nm in diameter and 12 nm in length (121, 126). An early report using culture supernatant fluids concluded that HlyA could assemble to form an ion-permeable channel in any lipid bilayer (74). More recent studies have concluded that the addition of cholesterol and ceramide enhances pore formation and subsequent leakage of chemical compounds from liposomes (53, 123, 126). The requirement for cholesterol and sphingolipids could suggest that HlyA spontaneously inserts into lipid rafts (124). These rigid microdomains of lipid bilayers accumulate on the apical surface of polarized epithelial cells and are rich in cholesterol and glycosphingolipids (88).

Cell Vacuolation

Although originally identified as a hemolysin, HlyA also has cytotoxic activity against intestinal epithelial cells (125). HEp-2 epithelial cells treated with HlyA-containing supernatant fluids lyse and release [51]Cr (3). At more moderate dosages of HlyA, pore formation

does not cause severe membrane damage, as indicated by exclusion of trypan blue and propidium iodide, but does cause a depletion in ATP (125). Incubation of diluted HlyA-containing supernatant fluids with green monkey kidney fibroblasts (Vero) or HeLa epithelial cells induces the formation of large, mildly acidic vacuoles within the cell (17, 35, 77). These vacuoles appear as early as 2 h post-inoculation and fully develop 24 h later (17). They remain for up to 48 h until the cells lyse (77). Vacuolation requires HlyA in the supernatant fluids, and the addition of 50 ng/ml purified HlyA gave rise to the same vacuoles (17). Unlike the cytological effects of VacA, the vacuolating toxin of *Helicobacter pylori*, vacuoles due to HlyA do not take up neutral red rapidly and some vacuoles do not take up the stain at all (35). These vacuoles are insensitive to the inhibitors of vacuolar-type proton pumps, such as bafilomycin A or concanamycin (Fig. 5), and do not swell in response to exogenous ammonia (17, 35). These data all indicate that the HlyA vacuoles are less acidic than VacA-induced vacuoles. Exclusion of endocytosed horseradish peroxidase from HlyA-generated vacuoles indicates that these vacuoles are not part of the normal endocytic

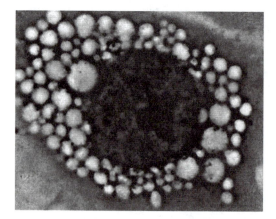

FIGURE 5 Vacuolation of Vero cells treated for 2 h with HlyA-producing culture supernatant fluid in the presence of 100 nM concanamycin. Reproduced from reference 35 with permission.

circuit, unlike the VacA-generated vacuoles. These data predict that the mechanism of HlyA-induced vacuolation is distinct from the VacA mechanism.

The variation in cytolytic activities associated with HlyA may result from polymorphisms in the sequence of HlyA, leading to altered membrane specificity. Supernatant fluids from wild-type non-O1 strain 52201, isolated in Oaxaca, Mexico, has strong vacuolating activity, but the strain is nonhemolytic, suggesting that its affinity for erythrocytes is lost (35). On the other hand, hemolytic El Tor strains such as E7946 and P27459 have been characterized as nonvacuolating (17). This absence of vacuolating activity may not reflect variations in HlyA affinity or activity but rather differences in gene regulation. Wild-type non-O1 strain 52453 is weakly hemolytic and does not cause vacuolation. However, high titers of vacuolation are observed when the *hlyA* gene of strain 52453 is cloned and expressed in *E. coli* (35). Thus, the difference in the sequence of *hlyA* and variations in expression may result in a range of pathological effects during a *V. cholerae* infection.

In Vivo Activities

Loss of the *hlyA* gene may reduce the virulence of *V. cholerae* in infant mice. HlyU is a transcriptional regulator of the *hlyA* gene (115). Deletion of *hlyU* resulted in a 100-fold decrease in LD_{50} of infant mice, suggesting that HlyA contributes to virulence, although HlyU might regulate other factors (112). Mice orally inoculated with mutants with an insertion in *hlyA* do survive longer and show less swelling of intestinal villi than the isogenic parent strains (3). The increased virulence associated with HlyA is probably not due to diarrhea since fluid accumulation in rabbit ileal loops is not significantly affected by the absence of *hlyA*, although the fluid is reported to be less viscous with less free hemoglobin than observed for the isogenic parent strains (3).

Enzymatic Genes Linked to *hlyA*

Other extracellular enzymes are encoded on the small chromosome linked to *hlyA*, suggesting that the *hlyA* gene is part of a "pathogenicity island." These activities include a lipase (*lipA*), a lecithinase (*lec*), and a metalloprotease (*prtV*) (78). Lipase has also been characterized as an extracellular CHO cell-elongation factor (71). Mutation of *lipA* or *prtV* had no effect on the LD_{50} or colonization of an infant mouse (15, 78), and mutation of *lec* had no effect on fluid accumulation in a rabbit ileum (37). Purified lipase does increase fluid accumulation in a sealed infant mouse, although fluid secretion in the model barely rose above buffer controls, even when CT was inoculated (71).

It is conceivable that all of the genes of the *hly* locus contribute to pathogenesis, although only the HlyA pore-forming toxin has any substantial data linking it to virulence. Even the role of HlyA could be deemed controversial. However, variation in observations linking HlyA to virulence may reflect differences in gene expression such that HlyA has a major contribution in some strains, with minimal or no contribution in others.

THE RTX TOXIN

Discovery and Epidemiology

The latest entry into the field of alternate toxins of *V. cholerae* is the RTX toxin. This toxin is extremely large—the single polypeptide transcript is predicted to be more than 450 kDa in size. It is also extremely cytotoxic, causing all cell types to round up within 60 min of exposure to bacteria that produce the toxin (40, 62).

Several factors likely account for the lag in discovery of this potent toxin. First, most studies of *V. cholerae* have been done with classical O1 strains since CT and TCP production are easily controlled (42). These classical strains have a natural deletion in the *rtx* locus that eliminates the RTX toxin activity (62). In addition, the toxin is apparently expressed only in early log phase and is completely absent by both Western blotting and activity, during the stationary phase (40). Overnight cultures have generally been used for purification of HlyA, HA/P, and other extracellular cytotoxins, explaining the failure to detect this novel activity in supernatant fluids.

Given that the presence of this toxin was obscured for so long, it is a wonder that three different approaches discovered the RTX toxin almost simultaneously. Progress on the genome sequence of El Tor N16961 revealed the presence of a very large open reading frame tightly linked to the *ctx* genes (50). The deduced protein sequence had several features of the RTX family of pore-forming toxins including "RTX repeats" at the C terminus (62). However, these repeats are different from the normal nonapeptide repeats in that they occur within an 18- to 20-amino-acid repeat. Structural analysis has revealed that this more unusual RTX repeat would still bind Ca^{2+} (109). The gene is found in an operon with a putative cytolysin-activation gene and adjacent to an operon for a type I secretion apparatus, accessory genes essential for activation and secretion of all known members of the RTX family of toxin (62, 109). The type I secretion apparatus is essential for RTX secretion, as is an unlinked *tolC* gene (see reference 11 and our unpublished data). Interestingly, a mutation in the secretion gene *rtxB* inhibited *in vivo* expression of the *ctxAB* genes, suggesting the *rtx* and *ctx* loci are coordinately regulated during infection (58).

As Lin and Mekalanos were completing annotation of the *rtx* locus, Calderwood and colleagues were analyzing genes identified by representational difference analysis (RDA) that are present in the predominating El Tor strains but absent in the now extinct classical strains (14). The RDA study revealed a difference in the presence of *rtxC*, one of the genes lost in the deletion that inactivates the RTX toxin in classical strains (62). Mapping of their mutation against the genome revealed this important difference between the O1 El Tor and O1 classical strains.

Finally, the activity of the RTX toxin was observed in attempts by this author to establish an adherence assay for binding of N16961 and other El Tor strains to HEp-2 epithelial cells (39). This cell-rounding activity was missing in a subset of vaccine strains, indicating that the toxic factor was linked to the *ctx* genes. A defined insertion in the neighboring *rtxA* eliminated cell rounding, indicating that the RTX toxin causes cell rounding (62).

The three approaches were synergistic, and the findings were rapidly published in a joint manuscript in 1999 (62). It is now recognized that active RTX toxin is produced by all isolates of *V. cholerae* that have been tested, except the classical strains, including both environmental and clinical isolates (16, 21). An epidemiological survey of 300 strains representing every known serotype of *V. cholerae* revealed that all isolates have the genes for the RTX toxin (61). This conservation of the RTX toxin implies there is incredible evolutionary pressure to maintain the genes for this very large toxin. Its role in pathogenesis or in the environment has not yet been elucidated, but the gene is apparently important to the persistence of the organism.

Actin Cross-Linking Activity

Cell lysis studies demonstrated that the *V. cholerae* RTX is not a cytolytic, pore-forming toxin and does not cause the release of ^{51}Cr from cells (40). Indeed, cell rounding is generally indicative of toxins that affect the cytoskeleton. Many of these toxins target the regulators of actin polymerization, the Rho family GTPases, while others directly target actin (93). Unlike any other known toxin, the RTX toxin causes a very dramatic change in the structure of the cellular actin: all the actin is covalently cross-linked together to form first dimers, then trimers, and eventually a dense aggregate of inactivated actin (40). The covalent cross-linking of actin leads to the disassembly of the actin cytoskeleton (Fig. 6). We propose that this occurs by depleting the pool of freely soluble G (globular) actin to disrupt the equilibrium between polymerized F-

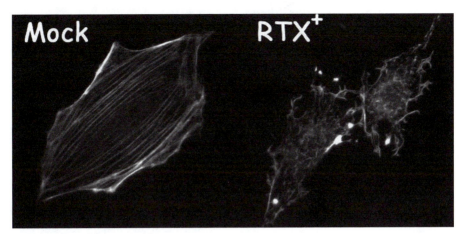

FIGURE 6 Depolymerization of F-actin by RTX toxin. PtK2 cells were either treated for 60 min with phosphate-buffered saline (mock) or incubated with *V. cholerae* secreting RTX toxin. Cells were fixed and stained with fluorescently labeled phalloidin to visualize polymerized F-actin. Data previously reported as data not shown (40).

actin and free G-actin. The depolymerization of actin would result in the observed cell rounding (40).

The net effect of depolymerization of actin on intestinal epithelial cells may be to open the paracellular tight junctions. Bacteria added to the apical or basolateral surfaces of polarized epithelial cells will express the RTX toxin. After a 45-min delay, the integrity of the tight junction is lost and the flux rate of 3,000-Da dextran across the monolayer increases sixfold (38). The monolayers do maintain some stability, showing a consistent 80% loss in TER, suggesting that the monolayer does not fully collapse as occurs from HA/P exposure (38, 73). Cumulatively, these data suggest that the RTX toxin leads to a controlled depolymerization of the actin cytoskeleton, resulting in a loss of the integrity of the tight junctions. Given the dramatic loss of TER and the increased flux rate compared to results using Zot toxin (19, 38), could RTX actually be the toxin responsible for the distortion of zonula occludens observed in intestinal biopsies (70) or the extensive tissue destruction in the absence of CT (85)? In vivo data comparing the contribution of these toxins to pathology, fluid accumulation, and the proinflammatory

response will be needed before the important factors for these symptoms of disease can be fully elucidated.

Contribution to Disease?

Efforts to connect the *in vitro* activity of actin cross-linking and disruption of tight junctions with in vivo effects on the intestines have not yet been successful. The *rtxA* gene is not essential for colonization of an infant mouse (11). In addition, neither the RTX⁺ Bah1 nor the RTX⁻ Bah2 strains induced significant fluid secretion in rabbit ligated loops (27). This failure to demonstrate in vivo secretion has led some to suggest that the *rtx* locus is strongly conserved because it is essential for environmental survival.

A recent study of the histopathology of lung tissue following intranasal inoculation of adult mice with *V. cholerae* revealed that there is less epithelial damage and improved health of the mice when the *rtxA* gene is deleted in combination with *ctxAB*, compared to a *ctxAB* deletion alone. Such improvement was not noted when the genes for HA/P or HlyA were deleted (37a). Although these data may indicate an important role for RTX toxin in epithelial layer damage, a contribution to tissue damage in the intestine has yet to be demonstrated. However, the mouse results suggest the contribution of RTX disease is more likely to be apparent in pathology rather than in effects on colonization or fluid secretion. Clearly, more advanced studies using purified toxin and analysis of intestinal tissue damage will be important to further link the potent activity of the RTX toxin with cholera pathogenesis.

LIVE ATTENUATED VACCINES AND REACTOGENICITY

The greatest impact of the study of toxins in *V. cholerae* is likely to be on the development of safe, live attenuated vaccines for protection against natural infection. All of the aforementioned toxins—Zot, Ace, HA/P, HlyA, and RTX—have been deleted from potential vaccine candidate strains in combination with CT and tested for reactogenic symptoms.

El Tor vaccine candidate strain CVD110 bears the core deletion eliminating *ctxA*, *zot*, and *ace* with a gene interruption in *hlyA*, but *rtxA* and *hapA* remain intact. Eight of 10 volunteers given this strain had adverse reactions (97). In addition, neutrophil transmigration to the lumen was high in these volunteers, suggesting residual stimulation of the proinflammatory response (86). Thus, loss of HlyA does not obviate reactogenicity.

In another El Tor vaccine candidate, strain 638, the core region is deleted to eliminate *ctxAB*, *zot*, and *ace* and *hapA* is disrupted, but *rtxA* and *hlyA* are presumably intact. Of 42 volunteers given this strain, 9.5% still had mild diarrhea and as many as 25% had other reactogenic symptoms including abdominal cramps and vomiting (9). Although less reactogenic than CVD110, the *hapA⁻* strain 638 is still slightly virulent.

El Tor vaccine candidate strains Bah-3 and Peru-3 bear a large deletion, eliminating the entire integrated CTXΦ phage and a part of *rtxA*, but have an intact *hlyA* gene and still express HA/P (73, 99). Volunteers given these strains reported mild to moderate diarrhea and

abdominal cramping (99). This result indicates that absence of the RTX toxin alone does not eliminate reactogenicity. A nonmotile derivative of Peru-3, known as Peru-15, is tolerated well by vaccinees even though it still expresses HA/P (54, 73). Ten of 11 vaccinees showed no reactogenic symptoms, and all but one developed vibriocidal antibody (54). This result suggests that the loss of motility may affect delivery of reactogenic factors to the appropriate tissue.

We propose that a multitoxin mutant would be even safer than the uncharacterized, nonmotile strain that could easily revert to motility and enhanced virulence. Recently, the author's laboratory has been investigating multitoxin mutants deleted of all the primary toxins discussed above including CT, Zot, Ace, HlyA, HA/P, and RTX. Our results in animal models indicate that these strains still colonize but are significantly attenuated for virulence and stimulation of proinflammatory responses (37a). Characterization of such strains is continuing, and we hope that future studies will answer the question of how various toxins are working together to contribute to cholera-induced diseases.

ACKNOWLEDGMENTS

I thank Stephen Miller of Northwestern University for assistance on the immunology portions of this manuscript. K.J.F. is supported by the Biomedical Research Support Program of the Howard Hughes Medical Institute.

REFERENCES

1. **Abbas, A. K., and A. H. Lichtman.** 2001. *Basic Immunology: Functions and Disorders of the Immune System.* The W. B. Saunders Company, Philadelphia, Pa.
2. **Alm, R. A., and P. A. Manning.** 1990. Characterization of the *hlyB* gene and its role in the production of the El Tor haemolysin of *Vibrio cholerae* O1. *Mol. Microbiol.* **4:**413–425.
3. **Alm, R. A., G. Mayrhofer, I. Kotlarski, and P. A. Manning.** 1991. Amino-terminal domain of the El Tor haemolysin of *Vibrio cholerae* O1 is expressed in classical strains and is cytotoxic. *Vaccine* **9:**588–594.
4. **Altschul, S. F., T. L. Madden, A. A. Schaffer, J. Zhang, Z. Zhang, W. Miller, and**

D. J. Lipman. 1997. Gapped BLAST and PSI-BLAST: a new generation of protein database search programs. *Nucleic Acids Res.* **25:**3389–3402.

5. Aman, A. T., S. Fraser, E. A. Merritt, C. Rodigherio, M. Kenny, M. Ahn, W. G. Hol, N. A. Williams, W. I. Lencer, and T. R. Hirst. 2001. A mutant cholera toxin B subunit that binds GM1- ganglioside but lacks immunomodulatory or toxic activity. *Proc. Natl. Acad. Sci. USA* **98:**8536–8541.

6. Barua, D. 1992. History of cholera, p. 1–36. *In* D. Barua and W. B. Greenough (ed.), *Cholera.* Plenum Medical Book Co., New York, N.Y.

7. Basu, A., A. K. Mukhopadhyay, P. Garg, S. Chakraborty, T. Ramamurthy, S. Yamasaki, Y. Takeda, and G. B. Nair. 2000. Diversity in the arrangement of the CTX prophages in classical strains of *Vibrio cholerae* O1. *FEMS Microbiol. Lett.* **182:**35–40.

8. Baudry, B., A. Fasano, J. Ketley, and J. B. Kaper. 1992. Cloning of a gene (*zot*) encoding a new toxin produced by *Vibrio cholerae*. *Infect. Immun.* **60:**428–434.

9. Benítez, J. A., L. García, A. Silva, H. García, R. Fando, B. Cedré, A. Pérez, J. Campos, B. L. Rodríguez, J. L. Pérez, T. Valmaseda, O. Pérez, A. Pérez, M. Ramírez, T. Ledón, M. D. Jidy, M. Lastre, L. Bravo, and G. Sierra. 1999. Preliminary assessment of the safety and immunogenicity of a new CTXF-negative, hemagglutinin/protease-defective El Tor strain as a cholera vaccine candidate. *Infect. Immun.* **67:**539–545.

10. Benitez, J. A., A. J. Silva, and R. A. Finkelstein. 2001. Environmental signals controlling production of hemagglutinin/protease in *Vibrio cholerae*. *Infect. Immun.* **69:**6549–6553.

11. Bina, J., and J. J. Mekalanos. 2001. *Vibrio cholerae tolC* is required for bile resistance and colonization. *Infect. Immun.* **69:**4681–4685.

12. Booth, B. A., M. Boesman-Finkelstein, and R. A. Finkelstein. 1984. *Vibrio cholerae* hemagglutinin/protease nicks cholera enterotoxin. *Infect. Immun.* **45:**558–560.

13. Burnet, F. M., and J. D. Stone. 1947. Desquamation of intestinal epithelium *in vitro* by *V. cholerae* filtrates: characterization of mucinase and tissue disintegrating enzymes. *Austr. J. Exp. Biol. Med. Sci.* **25:**219–226.

14. Calia, K. E., M. K. Waldor, and S. B. Calderwood. 1998. Use of representational difference analysis to identify genomic differences between pathogenic strains of *Vibrio cholerae*. *Infect. Immun.* **66:**849–852.

15. Camilli, A., and J. J. Mekalanos. 1995. Use of recombinase gene fusions to identify *Vibrio cholerae* genes induced during infection. *Mol. Microbiol.* **18:**671–683.

16. Chow, K. H., T. K. Ng, K. Y. Yuen, and W. C. Yam. 2001. Detection of RTX toxin gene in *Vibrio cholerae* by PCR. *J. Clin. Microbiol.* **39:**2594–2597.

17. Coelho, A., J. R. C. Andrade, A. C. P. Vicente, and V. J. DiRita. 2000. Cytotoxic cell vacuolating activity from *Vibrio cholerae* hemolysin. *Infect. Immun.* **68:**1700–1705.

18. Cong, Y., A. O. Oliver, and C. O. Elson. 2001. Effects of cholera toxin on macrophage production of co-stimulatory cytokines. *Eur. J. Immunol.* **31:**64–71.

19. Cox, D. S., H. Gao, S. Raje, K. R. Scott, and N. D. Eddington. 2001. Enhancing the permeation of marker compounds and enaminone anticonvulsants across Caco-2 monolayers by modulating tight junctions using zonula occludens toxin. *Eur. J. Pharm. Biopharm.* **52:**145–150.

20. Cserzo, M., E. Wallin, I. Simon, G. von Heijne, and A. Elofsson. 1997. Prediction of transmembrane alpha-helices in prokaryotic membrane proteins: the dense alignment surface method. *Protein Eng.* **10:**673–676.

21. Dalsgaard, A., O. Serichantalergs, A. Forslund, W. Lin, J. Mekalanos, E. Mintz, T. Shimada, and J. G. Wells. 2001. Clinical and environmental isolates of *Vibrio cholerae* serogroup O141 carry the CTX phage and the genes encoding the toxin-coregulated pili. *J. Clin. Microbiol.* **39:**4086–4092.

22. Davis, B. M., E. H. Lawson, M. Sandkvist, A. Ali, S. Sozhamannan, and M. K. Waldor. 2000. Convergence of the secretory pathways for cholera toxin and the filamentous phage, CTXΦ. *Science* **288:**333–335.

23. Del Giudice, G., and R. Rappuoli. 1999. Genetically derived toxoids for use as vaccines and adjuvants. *Vaccine* **17**(Suppl. 2):S44–S52.

24. Di Pierro, M., R. Lu, S. Uzzau, W. Wang, K. Margaretten, C. Pazzani, F. Maimone, and A. Fasano. 2001. Zonula occludens toxin structure-function analysis. Identification of the fragment biologically active on tight junctions and of the zonulin receptor binding domain. *J. Biol. Chem.* **276:**19160–19165.

25. Ehara, M., S. Shimodori, F. Kojima, Y. Ichinose, T. Hirayama, M. J. Albert, K. Supawat, Y. Honma, M. Iwanaga, and K. Amako. 1997. Characterization of filamentous phages of *Vibrio cholerae* O139 and O1. *FEMS Microbiol. Lett.* **154:**293–301.

26. Endemann, H., and P. Model. 1995. Location of filamentous phage minor coat proteins in

phage and in infected cells. *J. Mol. Biol.* **250**:496–506.

27. **Faruque, S. M., M. M. Rahman, A. K. Hasan, G. B. Nair, J. J. Mekalanos, and D. A. Sack.** 2001. Diminished diarrheal response to *Vibrio cholerae* strains carrying the replicative form of the CTXF genome instead of CTXF lysogens in adult rabbits. *Infect. Immun.* **69**:6084–6090.

28. **Fasano, A.** 2000. Regulation of intercellular tight junctions by zonula occludens toxin and its eukaryotic analogue zonulin. *Ann. N.Y. Acad. Sci.* **915**:214–222.

29. **Fasano, A., B. Baudry, D. W. Pumplin, S. S. Wasserman, B. D. Tall, J. M. Ketley, and J. B. Kaper.** 1991. *Vibrio cholerae* produces a second enterotoxin, which affects intestinal tight junctions. *Proc. Natl. Acad. Sci. USA* **88**: 5242–5246.

30. **Fasano, A., C. Fiorentini, G. Donelli, S. Uzzau, J. B. Kaper, K. Margaretten, X. Ding, S. Guandalini, L. Comstock, and S. E. Goldblum.** 1995. Zonula occludens toxin modulates tight junctions through protein kinase C-dependent actin reorganization, in vitro. *J. Clin. Invest.* **96**:710–720.

31. **Fasano, A., T. Not, W. Wang, S. Uzzau, I. Berti, A. Tommasini, and S. E. Goldblum.** 2000. Zonulin, a newly discovered modulator of intestinal permeability, and its expression in coeliac disease. *Lancet* **355**:1518–1519.

32. **Fasano, A., and S. Uzzau.** 1997. Modulation of intestinal tight junctions by zonula occludens toxin permits enteral administration of insulin and other macromolecules in an animal model. *J. Clin. Invest.* **99**:1158–1164.

33. **Fasano, A., S. Uzzau, C. Fiore, and K. Margaretten.** 1997. The enterotoxic effect of zonula occludens toxin on rabbit small intestine involves the paracellular pathway. *Gastroenterology* **112**: 839–846.

34. **Feng, J. N., P. Model, and M. Russel.** 1999. A *trans*-envelope protein complex needed for filamentous phage assembly and export. *Mol. Microbiol.* **34**:745–755.

35. **Figueroa-Arredondo, P., J. E. Heuser, N. S. Akopyants, J. H. Morisaki, S. Giono-Cerezo, F. Enriquez-Rincon, and D. E. Berg.** 2001. Cell vacuolation caused by *Vibrio cholerae* hemolysin. *Infect. Immun.* **69**:1613–1624.

36. **Finkelstein, R. A., M. Boesman-Finkelstein, and P. Holt.** 1983. *Vibrio cholerae* hemagglutinin/lectin/protease hydrolyzes fibronectin and ovomucin: F.M. Burnet revisited. *Proc. Natl. Acad. Sci. USA* **80**:1092–1095.

37. **Fiore, A. E., J. M. Michalski, R. G. Russell, C. L. Sears, and J. B. Kaper.** 1997. Cloning, characterization, and chromosomal mapping of a phospholipase (lecithinase) produced by *Vibrio cholerae*. *Infect. Immun.* **65**:3112–3117.

37a.**Fullner, K. J., J. C. Boucher, M. A. Hanes, G. K. Haines 3rd, B. M. Meehan, C. Walchle, P. J. Sansonetti, and J. J. Mekalanos.** 2002. The contribution of accessory toxins of *Vibrio cholerae* O1 El Tor to the proinflammatory response in a murine pulmonary cholera model. *J. Exp. Med.* **195**:1455–1462.

38. **Fullner, K. J., W. I. Lencer, and J. J. Mekalanos.** 2001. *Vibrio cholerae*-induced cellular responses of polarized T84 intestinal epithelial cells dependent of production of cholera toxin and the RTX toxin. *Infect. Immun.* **69**:6310–6317.

39. **Fullner, K. J., and J. J. Mekalanos.** 1999. Genetic characterization of a new type IV pilus gene cluster found in both classical and El Tor biotypes of *Vibrio cholerae*. *Infect. Immun.* **67**:1393–1404.

40. **Fullner, K. J., and J. J. Mekalanos.** 2000. *In vivo* covalent crosslinking of actin by the RTX toxin of *Vibrio cholerae*. *EMBO J.* **19**:5315–5323.

41. **Gagliardi, M. C., F. Sallusto, M. Marinaro, A. Langenkamp, A. Lanzavecchia, and M. T. De Magistris.** 2000. Cholera toxin induces maturation of human dendritic cells and licenses them for Th2 priming. *Eur. J. Immunol.* **30**:2394–2403.

42. **Gardel, C. L., and J. J. Mekalanos.** 1994. Regulation of cholera toxin by temperature, pH, and osmolarity. *Methods Enzymol.* **235**:517–526.

43. **Goldberg, S. L., and J. R. Murphy.** 1985. Cloning and characterization of the hemolysin determinants from *Vibrio cholerae* RV79(Hly$^+$), RV79(Hly$^-$), and 569B. *J. Bacteriol.* **162**:35–41.

44. **Goldberg, S. L., and J. R. Murphy.** 1984. Molecular cloning of the hemolysin determinant from *Vibrio cholerae* El Tor. *J. Bacteriol.* **160**:239–244.

45. **Guy-Caffey, J. K., M. P. Rapoza, K. A. Jolley, and R. E. Webster.** 1992. Membrane localization and topology of a viral assembly protein. *J. Bacteriol.* **174**:2460–2465.

46. **Haigh, N. G., and R. E. Webster.** 1999. The pI and pXI assembly proteins serve separate and essential roles in filamentous phage assembly. *J. Mol. Biol.* **293**:1017–1027.

47. **Hall, R. H., and B. S. Drasar.** 1990. *Vibrio cholerae* HlyA hemolysin is processed by proteolysis. *Infect. Immun.* **58**:3375–3379.

48. **Häse, C. C., and R. A. Finkelstein.** 1993. Bacterial extracellular zinc-containing metalloproteases. *Microbiol. Rev.* **57**:823–837.

49. **Häse, C. C., and R. A. Finkelstein.** 1991. Cloning and nucleotide sequence of the *Vibrio cholerae* hemagglutinin/protease (HA/protease)

gene and construction of an HA/protease-negative strain. *J. Bacteriol.* **173:**3311–3317.

50. **Heidelberg, J. F., J. A. Eisen, W. C. Nelson, R. A. Clayton, M. L. Gwinn, R. J. Dodson, D. H. Haft, E. K. Hickey, J. D. Peterson, L. Umayam, S. R. Gill, K. E. Nelson, T. D. Read, H. Tettelin, D. Richardson, M. D. Ermolaeva, J. Vamathevan, S. Bass, H. Qin, I. Dragoi, P. Sellers, L. McDonald, T. Utterback, R. D. Fleishmann, W. C. Nierman, O. White, S. L. Salzberg, H. O. Smith, R. R. Colwell, J. J. Mekalanos, J. C. Venter, and C. M. Fraser.** 2000. DNA sequence of both chromosomes of the cholera pathogen *Vibrio cholerae*. *Nature* **406:**477–484.

51. **Hill, D. F., and G. B. Petersen.** 1982. Nucleotide sequence of bacteriophage f1 DNA. *J. Virol.* **44:**32–46.

52. **Ikema, M., and Y. Honma.** 1998. A novel filamentous phage, fs-2, of *Vibrio cholerae* O139. *Microbiology* **144:**1901–1906.

53. **Ikigai, H., A. Akatsuka, H. Tsujiyama, T. Nakae, and T. Shimamura.** 1996. Mechanism of membrane damage by El Tor hemolysin of *Vibrio cholerae* O1. *Infect. Immun.* **64:**2968–2973.

54. **Kenner, J. R., T. S. Coster, D. N. Taylor, A. F. Trofa, M. Barrera-Oro, T. Hyman, J. M. Adams, D. T. Beattie, K. P. Killeen, D. R. Spriggs, J. J. Mekalanos, and J. C. Sadoff.** 1995. Peru-15, an improved live attenuated oral vaccine candidate for *Vibrio cholerae* O1. *J. Infect. Dis.* **172:**1126–1129.

55. **Kerneis, S., A. Bogdanova, J. P. Kraehenbuhl, and E. Pringault.** 1997. Conversion by Peyer's patch lymphocytes of human enterocytes into M cells that transport bacteria. *Science* **277:**949–952.

56. **Kimsey, H. H., and M. K. Waldor.** 1998. *Vibrio cholerae* hemagglutinin/protease inactivates CTXΦ. *Infect. Immun.* **66:**4025–4029.

57. **Leal-Berumen, I., D. P. Snider, C. Barajas-Lopez, and J. S. Marshall.** 1996. Cholera toxin increases IL-6 synthesis and decreases TNF-α production by rat peritoneal mast cells. *J. Immunol.* **156:**316–321.

58. **Lee, S. H., S. M. Butler, and A. Camilli.** 2001. Selection for in vivo regulators of bacterial virulence. *Proc. Natl. Acad. Sci. USA* **98:**6889–6894.

59. **Lencer, W. I.** 2001. Microbes and microbial toxins: paradigms for microbial-mucosal interactions. V. Cholera: invasion of the intestinal epithelial barrier by a stably folded protein toxin. *Am. J. Physiol. Gastrointest. Liver Physiol.* **280:**G781–G786.

60. **Levine, M. M., J. B. Kaper, D. Herrington, G. Losonsky, J. G. Morris, M. L. Clements, R. E. Black, B. Tall, and R. Hall.** 1988. Volunteer studies of deletion mutants of *Vibrio cholerae* O1 prepared by recombinant techniques. *Infect. Immun.* **56:**161–167.

61. **Li, M., T. Shimada, J. G. Morris, Jr., A. Sulakvelidze, and S. Sozhamannan.** 2002. Evidence for the emergence of non-O1/non-O139 *Vibrio cholerae* strains with pathogenic potential by exchange of O-antigen biosynthesis regions. *Infect. Immun.* **70:**2441–2453.

62. **Lin, W., K. J. Fullner, R. Clayton, J. A. Sexton, M. B. Rogers, K. E. Calia, S. B. Calderwood, C. Fraser, and J. J. Mekalanos.** 1999. Identification of a *Vibrio cholerae* RTX toxin gene cluster that is tightly linked to the cholera toxin prophage. *Proc. Natl. Acad. Sci. USA* **96:**1071–1076.

63. **Lu, R., W. Wang, S. Uzzau, R. Vigorito, H. R. Zielke, and A. Fasano.** 2000. Affinity purification and partial characterization of the zonulin/zonula occludens toxin (Zot) receptor from human brain. *J. Neurochem.* **74:**320–326.

64. **Mandell, G. L., J. E. Bennett, and R. Dolin (ed.).** 1995. *Principles and Practices of Infectious Diseases*, vol. 2. Churchill Livingstone, New York, N.Y.

65. **Manning, P. A., M. H. Brown, and M. W. Heuzenroeder.** 1984. Cloning of the structural gene (hly) for the haemolysin of *Vibrio cholerae* El Tor strain 017. *Gene* **31:**225–231.

66. **Marciano, D. K., M. Russel, and S. M. Simon.** 1999. An aqueous channel for filamentous phage export. *Science* **284:**1516–1519.

67. **Marciano, D. K., M. Russel, and S. M. Simon.** 2001. Assembling filamentous phage occlude pIV channels. *Proc. Natl. Acad. Sci. USA* **98:**9359–9364.

68. **Martin, M., D. J. Metzger, S. M. Michalek, T. D. Connell, and M. W. Russell.** 2001. Distinct cytokine regulation by cholera toxin and type II heat-labile toxins involves differential regulation of CD40 ligand on CD4(+) T cells. *Infect. Immun.* **69:**4486–4492.

69. **Marvin, D. A.** 1998. Filamentous phage structure, infection and assembly. *Curr. Opin. Struct. Biol.* **8:**150–158.

70. **Mathan, M. M., G. Chandy, and V. I. Mathan.** 1995. Ultrastructural changes in the upper small intestinal mucosa in patients with cholera. *Gastroenterology* **109:**422–430.

71. **McCardell, B. A., M. H. Kothary, R. H. Hall, and V. Sathyamoorthy.** 2000. Identification of a CHO cell-elongating factor produced by *Vibrio cholerae* O1. *Microb. Pathog.* **29:**1–8.

72. **Mekalanos, J. J.** 1983. Duplication and amplification of toxin genes in *Vibrio cholerae*. *Cell* **35:**252–263.

73. **Mel, S. F., K. J. Fullner, S. Wimer-Mackin, W. I. Lencer, and J. J. Mekalanos.** 2000. Association of protease activity in *Vibrio cholerae* vaccine strains with decreases in transcellular epithelial resistance of polarized T84 intestinal cells. *Infect. Immun.* **67:**1393–1404.

74. **Menzl, K., E. Maier, T. Chakraborty, and R. Benz.** 1996. HlyA hemolysin of *Vibrio cholerae* O1 biotype El Tor. Identification of the hemolytic complex and evidence for the formation of anion-selective ion-permeable channels. *Eur. J. Biochem.* **240:**646–654.

75. **Millar, D. G., and T. R. Hirst.** 2001. Cholera toxin and *Escherichia coli* enterotoxin B-subunits inhibit macrophage-mediated antigen processing and presentation: evidence for antigen persistence in non-acidic recycling endosomal compartments. *Cell. Microbiol.* **3:**311–329.

76. **Mitic, L. L., C. M. Van Itallie, and J. M. Anderson.** 2000. Molecular physiology and pathophysiology of tight junctions. I. Tight junction structure and function: lessons from mutant animals and proteins. *Am. J. Physiol. Gastrointest. Liver Physiol.* **279:**G250–G254.

77. **Mitra, R., P. Figueroa, A. K. Mukhopadhyay, T. Shimada, Y. Takeda, D. E. Berg, and G. B. Nair.** 2000. Cell vacuolation, a manifestation of the El Tor hemolysin of *Vibrio cholerae.* *Infect. Immun.* **68:**1928–1933.

78. **Ogierman, M. A., A. Fallarino, T. Riess, S. G. Williams, S. R. Attridge, and P. A. Manning.** 1997. Characterization of the *Vibrio cholerae* El Tor lipase operon *lipAB* and a protease gene downstream of the *hly* region. *J. Bacteriol.* **179:**7072–7080.

79. **Overbye, L. J., M. Sandkvist, and M. Bagdasarian.** 1993. Genes required for extracellular secretion of enterotoxin are clustered in *Vibrio cholerae.* *Gene* **132:**101–106.

80. **Rakonjac, J., and P. Model.** 1998. Roles of pIII in filamentous phage assembly. *J. Mol. Biol.* **282:**25–41.

81. **Rodriguez, B. L., A. Rojas, J. Campos, T. Ledon, E. Valle, W. Toledo, and R. Fando.** 2001. Differential interleukin-8 response of intestinal epithelial cell line to reactogenic and nonreactogenic candidate vaccine strains of *Vibrio cholerae.* *Infect. Immun.* **69:**613–616.

82. **Russel, M., N. A. Linderoth, and A. Sali.** 1997. Filamentous phage assembly: variation on a protein export theme. *Gene* **192:**23–32.

83. **Saha, P. K., H. Koley, and G. B. Nair.** 1996. Purification and characterization of an extracellular secretogenic non-membrane damaging cytotoxin produced by clinical strains of *Vibrio cholerae* non-O1. *Infect. Immun.* **64:**3101–3108.

84. **Sandkvist, M., L. O. Michel, L. P. Hough, V. M. Morales, M. Bagdasarian, M. Koomey, V. J. DiRita, and M. Bagdasarian.** 1997. General secretion pathway (*eps*) genes required for toxin secretion and outer membrane biogenesis in *Vibrio cholerae.* *J. Bacteriol.* **179:**6994–7003.

85. **Shuangshoti, S., and S. Reinprayoon.** 1995. Pathologic changes of gut in non-O1 *Vibrio cholerae* infection. *J. Med. Assoc. Thai.* **78:**204–209.

86. **Silva, T. M. J., M. A. Schuleupner, C. O. Tacket, T. S. Steiner, J. B. Kaper, R. Edelman, and R. L. Guerrant.** 1996. New evidence for an inflammatory component in diarrhea caused by selected new, live attenuated cholerae vaccines and by El Tor and O139 *Vibrio cholerae.* *Infect. Immun.* **64:**2362–2364.

87. **Simecka, J. W., R. J. Jackson, H. Kiyono, and J. R. McGhee.** 2000. Mucosally induced immunoglobulin E-associated inflammation in the respiratory tract. *Infect. Immun.* **68:**672–679.

88. **Simons, K., and D. Toomre.** 2000. Lipid rafts and signal transduction. *Nat. Rev. Mol. Cell. Biol.* **1:**31–39.

89. **Sincharoenkul, R., W. Chaicumpa, E. Pongponratn, R. Limpananont, P. Tapchaisri, T. Kalambaheti, and M. Chongsanguan.** 1993. Localization of *Vibrio cholerae* O1 in the intestinal tissue. *Asian Pac. J. Allergy Immunol.* **11:**155–165.

90. **Singh, D. V., M. H. Matte, G. R. Matte, S. Jiang, F. Sabeena, B. N. Shukla, S. C. Sanyal, A. Huq, and R. R. Colwell.** 2001. Molecular analysis of *Vibrio cholerae* O1, O139, non-O1, and non-O139 strains: clonal relationships between clinical and environmental isolates. *Appl. Environ. Microbiol.* **67:**910–921.

91. **Skorupski, K., and R. K. Taylor.** 1997. Control of the ToxR virulence regulon in *Vibrio cholerae* by environmental stimuli. *Mol. Microbiol.* **25:**1003–1009.

92. **Soriani, M., N. A. Williams, and T. R. Hirst.** 2001. *Escherichia coli* enterotoxin B subunit triggers apoptosis of CD8$^+$ T cells by activating transcription factor c-Myc. *Infect. Immun.* **69:**4923–4930.

93. **Steele-Mortimer, O., L. A. Knodler, and B. B. Finlay.** 2000. Poisons, ruffles and rockets: bacterial pathogens and the host cell cytoskeleton. *Traffic* **1:**107–118.

94. **Stultz, C. M., R. Nambudripad, R. H. Lathrop, and J. V. White.** 1997. Predicting protein structure with probabilistic models. *Adv. Mol. Cell Biol.* **22B:**447–506.

95. **Stultz, C. M., J. V. White, and T. F. Smith.** 1993. Structural analysis based on state-space modeling. *Protein Science* **2:**305–314.

96. Sun, J.-B., C. Rask, T. Olsson, J. Holm-gren, and C. Czerkinsky. 1996. Treatment of experimental autoimmune encephalomyelitis by feeding myelin basic protein conjugated to cholera toxin B subunit. *Proc. Natl. Acad. Sci. USA* **93:**7196–7201.

97. Tacket, C. O., G. Losonsky, J. P. Nataro, S. J. Cryz, R. Edelman, A. Fasano, J. Michalski, J. B. Kaper, and M. M. Levine. 1993. Safety and immunogenicity of live oral cholera vaccine candidate CVD110, a Δ*ctxA* Δ*zot* Δ*ace* derivative of El Tor Ogawa *Vibrio cholerae*. *J. Infect. Dis.* **168:**1536–1540.

98. Tatusova, T. A., and T. L. Madden. 1999. BLAST 2 sequences—a new tool for comparing protein and nucleotide sequences. *FEMS Microbiol. Lett.* **174:**247–250.

99. Taylor, D. N., K. P. Killeen, D. C. Hack, J. R. Kenner, T. S. Coster, D. T. Beattie, J. Ezzell, T. Hyman, A. Trofa, M. H. Sjogren, A. Friedlander, J. J. Mekalanos, and J. C. Sadoff. 1994. Development of a live, oral, attenuated vaccine against El Tor cholera. *J. Infect. Dis.* **170:**1518–1523.

100. Trucksis, M., T. L. Conn, A. Fasano, and J. B. Kaper. 1997. Production of *Vibrio cholerae* accessory cholera enterotoxin (Ace) in the yeast *Pichia pastoris*. *Infect. Immun.* **65:**4984–4988.

101. Trucksis, M., T. L. Conn, S. S. Wasserman, and C. L. Sears. 2000. *Vibrio cholerae* ACE stimulates Ca^{2+}-dependent Cl^-/HCO_3^- secretion in T84 cells in vitro. *Am. J. Physiol. Cell. Physiol.* **279:**C567–C577.

102. Trucksis, M., J. E. Galen, J. Michalski, A. Fasano, and J. B. Kaper. 1993. Accessory cholera enterotoxin (Ace), the third toxin of a *Vibrio cholerae* virulence cassette. *Proc. Natl. Acad. Sci. USA* **90:**5267–5271.

103. Uzzau, S., P. Cappuccinelli, and A. Fasano. 1999. Expression of *Vibrio cholerae* zonula occludens toxin and analysis of its subcellular localization. *Microb. Pathog.* **27:**377–385.

104. Uzzau, S., R. Lu, W. Wang, C. Fiore, and A. Fasano. 2001. Purification and preliminary characterization of the zonula occludens toxin receptor from human (CaCo2) and murine (IEC6) intestinal cell lines. *FEMS Microbiol. Lett.* **194:**1–5.

105. Waldor, M. K., and J. J. Mekalanos. 1996. Lysogenic conversion by a filamentous phage encoding cholera toxin. *Science* **272:**1910–1914.

106. Waldor, M. K., E. J. Rubin, G. D. N. Pearson, H. Kimsey, and J. J. Mekalanos. 1997. Regulation, replication and integration functions of the *Vibrio cholerae* CTXφ are encoded by region RS2. *Mol. Microbiol.* **24:**917–926.

107. Walia, K., S. Ghosh, H. Singh, G. B. Nair, A. Ghosh, G. Sahni, H. Vohra, and N. K. Ganguly. 1999. Purification and characterization of novel toxin produced by *Vibrio cholerae* O1. *Infect. Immun.* **67:**5215–5222.

108. Wang, W., S. Uzzau, S. E. Goldblum, and A. Fasano. 2000. Human zonulin, a potential modulator of intestinal tight junctions. *J. Cell Sci.* **113**(Part 2):4435–4440.

109. Welch, R. A. 2001. RTX toxin structure and function: a story of numerous anomalies and few analogies in toxin biology. *Curr. Top. Microbiol. Immunol.* **257:**85–111.

110. White, J. V., C. M. Stultz, and T. F. Smith. 1994. Protein classification by stochastic modeling and optimal filtering of amino-acid sequences. *Math. Biosci.* **119:**35–75.

111. Williams, N. A., T. R. Hirst, and T. O. Nashar. 1999. Immune modulation by the cholera-like enterotoxins: from adjuvant to therapeutic. *Immunol. Today* **20:**95–101.

112. Williams, S. G., S. R. Attridge, and P. A. Manning. 1993. The transcriptional activator HlyU of *Vibrio cholerae*: nucleotide sequence and role in virulence gene expression. *Mol. Microbiol.* **9:**751–760.

113. Williams, S. G., and P. A. Manning. 1991. Transcription of the *Vibrio cholerae* haemolysin gene, *hlyA*, and cloning of a positive regulatory locus, *hlyU*. *Mol. Microbiol.* **5:**2031–2038.

114. World Health Organization. 2001. Cholera, 2000. *Wkly Epid. Rec.* **76:**233–240.

115. World Health Organization. 2001. Cholera vaccines: WHO position paper. *Wkly. Epid. Rep.* **76:**117–124.

116. Wu, Z., D. Milton, P. Nybom, A. Sjö, and K.-E. Magnusson. 1996. *Vibrio cholerae* hemagglutinin/protease (HA/protease) causes morphological changes in cultured epithelial cells and perturbs their paracellular barrier function. *Microb. Pathog.* **21:**111–123.

117. Wu, Z., P. Nybom, and K.-E. Magnusson. 2000. Distinct effects of the *Vibrio cholerae* haemagglutinin/protease on the structure and localization of the tight junction-associated proteins occludin and ZO-1. *Cell. Microbiol.* **2:**11–18.

118. Wu, Z., P. Nybom, T. Sudqvist, and K.-E. Magnusson. 1998. Endogenous nitric oxide in MDCK-I cells modulates the *Vibrio cholerae* haemagglutinin/protease (HA/P)-mediated cytotoxicity. *Microb. Pathog.* **24:**321–326.

119. Yamamoto, K., Y. Ichinose, H. Shinagawa, K. Makino, A. Nakata, M. Iwanaga, T. Honda, and T. Miwatani. 1990. Two-step processing for activation of the cytolysin/

hemolysin of *Vibrio cholerae* O1 biotype El Tor: nucleotide sequence of the structural gene (*hlyA*) and characterization of the processed products. *Infect. Immun.* **58:**4106–4116.

120. **Yamamoto, S., H. Kiyono, M. Yamamoto, K. Imaoka, K. Fujihashi, F. W. Van Ginkel, M. Noda, Y. Takeda, and J. R. McGhee.** 1997. A nontoxic mutant of cholera toxin elicits Th2-type responses for enhanced mucosal immunity. *Proc. Natl. Acad. Sci. USA* **94:**5267–5272.

121. **Yuldasheva, L. N., P. G. Merzlyak, A. O. Zitzer, C. G. Rodrigues, S. Bhakdi, and O. V. Krasilnikov.** 2001. Lumen geometry of ion channels formed by *Vibrio cholerae* El Tor cytolysin elucidated by nonelectrolyte exclusion. *Biochim. Biophys. Acta* **1512:**53–63.

122. **Yura, M., I. Takahashi, S. Terawaki, T. Hiroi, M. N. Kweon, Y. Yuki, and H. Kiyono.** 2001. Nasal administration of cholera toxin (CT) suppresses clinical signs of experimental autoimmune encephalomyelitis (EAE). *Vaccine* **20:**134–139.

123. **Zitzer, A., R. Bittman, C. A. Verbicky, R. K. Erukulla, S. Bhakdi, S. Weis, A. Val-eva, and M. Palmer.** 2001. Coupling of cholesterol and cone-shaped lipids in bilayers augments membrane permeabilization by the cholesterol-specific toxins streptolysin O and *Vibrio cholerae* cytolysin. *J. Biol. Chem.* **276:**14628–14633.

124. **Zitzer, A., J. R. Harris, S. E. Kemminer, O. Zitzer, S. Bhakdi, J. Muething, and M. Palmer.** 2000. *Vibrio cholerae* cytolysin: assembly and membrane insertion of the oligomeric pore are tightly linked and are not detectably restricted by membrane fluidity. *Biochim. Biophys. Acta* **1509:**264–274.

125. **Zitzer, A., T. M. Wassenaar, I. Walev, and S. Bhakdi.** 1997. Potent membrane-permeabilizing and cytocidal action of *Vibrio cholerae* cytolysin on human intestinal cells. *Infect. Immun.* **65:**1293–1298.

126. **Zitzer, A., O. Zitzer, S. Bhakdi, and M. Palmer.** 1999. Oligomerization of *Vibrio cholerae* cytolysin yields a pentameric pore and has a dual specificity for cholesterol and sphingolipids in the target membrane. *J. Biol. Chem.* **274:**1375–1380.

PATHOGENICITY OF *CLOSTRIDIUM DIFFICILE* TOXINS

Michel Warny and Ciarán P. Kelly

27

Clostridium difficile is a gram–positive, spore-forming anaerobic bacillus. Pathogenic strains of *C. difficile* cause diarrhea and colitis in humans through the release of two protein exotoxins, toxin A and toxin B. This chapter reviews the mechanisms whereby these toxins exert their cytotoxic, enterotoxic, and pro-inflammatory effects. The role played by neuropeptides in mediating *C. difficile* toxin-induced diarrhea is reviewed in chapter 19.

C. DIFFICILE-ASSOCIATED DIARRHEA AND COLITIS IN HUMANS

C. difficile is now the most commonly diagnosed cause of infectious diarrhea in hospitalized patients in the developed world (58). This iatrogenic infection is associated with significant morbidity and mortality, with its annual cost exceeding $1.1 billion per year in the United States (51, 59). Antibiotic therapy is the main risk factor for *C. difficile* infection (Fig. 1). Antibiotics disrupt the colonization resistance conferred by the natural colonic microflora. Other host factors can also prevent *C. difficile* toxin-induced intestinal injury and inflammation since only a minority of individuals who are colonized with a toxigenic strain will develop symptoms (60, 75). The risk of developing symptomatic disease is increased by advanced age, severe or debilitating illness, and absence of a protective immune response to *C. difficile* toxin A (60, 61).

C. difficile infection is caused by ingestion of spores. Whereas vegetative forms are quickly killed by air exposure, *C. difficile* spores are highly resistant and persist in the environment. In hamsters, a single oral dose of clindamycin results in fatal *C. difficile*-induced ileocecitis if animals are also exposed to bacterial spores (53, 65). Infected patients disseminate spores into the hospital environment, resulting in endemic and epidemic cases of nosocomial *C. difficile* diarrhea.

C. difficile infection results in a broad spectrum of clinical manifestations ranging from asymptomatic carriage to severe, life-threatening pseudomembranous colitis (58). Intestinal injury and inflammation result from the effects of *C. difficile* toxins (90). In animal models, toxin A is enterotoxic, whereas toxin B is not (54, 67, 72, 78, 90, 105). However, there is evidence that toxin A and toxin B are both enterotoxic in the human colon (94). In

Michel Warny, Acambis, Inc., 38 Sidney Street, Cambridge, MA 02139. *Ciarán P. Kelly*, Gastroenterology Division, Dana 601, Beth Israel Deaconess Medical Center, 330 Brookline Avenue, Boston, MA 02215.

Microbial Pathogenesis and the Intestinal Epithelial Cell, ed. by G. Hecht
© 2003 ASM Press, Washington, D.C.

503

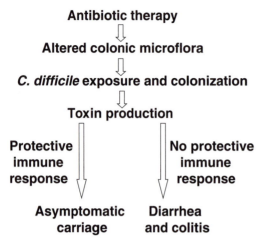

Antibiotic therapy
⇩
Altered colonic microflora
⇩
C. difficile **exposure and colonization**
⇩
Toxin production

| **Protective immune response** | **No protective immune response** |

Asymptomatic carriage   **Diarrhea and colitis**

FIGURE 1   Pathogenesis of *C. difficile*-associated diarrhea. The pathogenesis of *C. difficile*-associated diarrhea and colitis involves an initial disruption of the normal colonic bacterial flora by antibiotic treatment. This allows colonization with *C. difficile* if the individual is exposed to an environment where spores are sufficiently abundant. Pathogenic strains of *C. difficile* release toxins A and B, which cause colonic mucosal injury and inflammation. An early anamnestic immune response to toxin A can be detected in asymptomatic carriers but not in those who develop diarrhea and colitis. (From reference 58, with permission.)

most cases, diarrhea is of mild to moderate severity and the colonic mucosa appears relatively normal. In severe cases, systemic manifestations, including fever and an increase in peripheral blood neutrophil counts, are associated with colitis characterized by neutrophil infiltration of the colonic mucosa. If the colonic inflammation is severe, epithelial necrosis and ulcerations covered by pseudomembranes develop. These raised yellow structures are almost pathognomonic of *C. difficile* toxin-induced colonic injury and are composed of fibrin, cellular debris, and neutrophils (Fig. 2).

C. difficile-associated diarrhea and colitis are usually treated with oral metronidazole or vancomycin to eradicate vegetative forms of the bacterium. Despite a very high response rate, up to 25% of patients relapse after antibiotic therapy is discontinued. Non-antibiotic therapies are being developed to prevent and treat this frequent complication. Patients with

a single relapse are at increased risk for further recurrences. As discussed below, the presence or absence of a protective immune response to *C. difficile* toxins appears to play a central role in determining risk for recurrent *C. difficile* diarrhea.

THE PATHOGENICITY LOCUS OF *C. DIFFICILE*

The genes encoding toxin A and toxin B are part of a conserved chromosomal region of 19.6 kb called the *C. difficile* toxigenic element or pathogenicity locus (PaLoc) (34). PaLoc comprises five genes known as *tcdA–E*: four are transcribed in the same direction and include the genes encoding toxin A (*tcdA*) and toxin B (*tcdB*), whereas the fifth (*tcdC*) is oriented in the opposite direction and is downstream from the others (Fig. 3). The putative promoter regions of *tcdA* and *tcdB* show strong similarities. In toxigenic isolates, the gene structures and borders of the PaLoc are well conserved, whereas in nontoxigenic strains PaLoc is absent, replaced by a short segment of 115 to 127 bp. Thus, PaLoc appears as a coherent and stable genetic unit (7, 15, 34).

Most toxigenic strains produce both toxin A and toxin B. However, toxin production varies by several orders of magnitude among isolates, and toxin A yields consistently exceed those of toxin B. A number of environmental factors including amino acids and biotin have been shown to regulate toxin production in vitro (118). Moreover, exponential growth is associated with minimal toxin mRNA synthesis and protein production but with high levels of *tcdC* transcripts. By contrast, entry into the stationary phase is associated with low levels of *tcdC* transcripts; marked upregulation of *tcdA*, -*B*, -*D*, and -*E* expression; and toxin release. Rapidly metabolizable sugars inhibit stationary phase-associated toxin gene transcription (25). These observations suggest that *tcdC* might act as a repressor and that *tcdA* and *tcdB* expression may be controlled by common mechanisms.

In support of this model, *tcdD* (also known as *txeR*), which encodes a 22-kDa protein, was found to positively regulate transcription

A

B

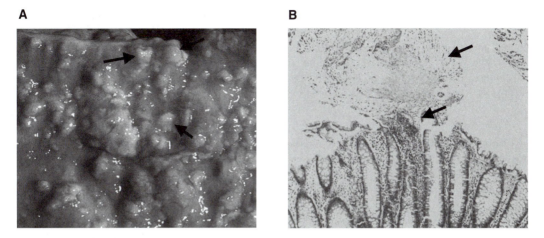

FIGURE 2 Pseudomembranous colitis. (A) The macroscopic features of pseudomembranous colitis, the most severe form of *C. difficile* infection, are shown in a colectomy specimen. The colonic mucosa is covered by characteristic yellow and raised pseudomembranes (arrows) containing fibrin, cellular debris, and neutrophils. These lesions have a patchy distribution but become confluent as the inflammation and ulceration progress in severity and extent. (B) Colonoscopic biopsy specimen from a patient with pseudomembranous colitis showing focal ulceration (lower arrow) surmounted by a "summit" or "volcano" lesion of pseudomembranous exudate (upper arrow). (Hematoxylin- and eosin-stained tissue section, original magnification ×55.) (From reference 51, with permission.)

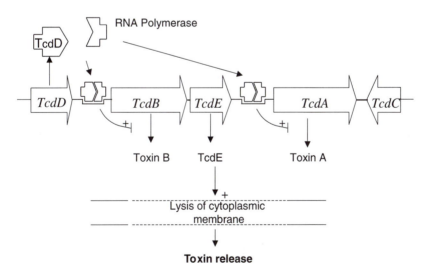

FIGURE 3 The *C. difficile* pathogenicity locus (PaLoc) is a 19.6-kb segment carrying five genes (*tcdA–E*) including the genes encoding toxin A (*tcdA*) and toxin B (*tcdB*). TcdD appears to activate toxin A and toxin B transcription by forming a complex with RNA polymerase that binds to *tcdA* and *tcdB* promoter regions. Whereas the function of TcdC is unknown, TcdE may regulate toxin release through its ability to disrupt the bacterial cytoplasmic membrane. (Figure based on data from references 7, 15, and 34.)

of both toxins. TcdD carries a potential helix-turn-helix DNA binding-motif and a structure similar to positive regulators of toxin genes such as the UV-inducible bacteriocin gene of *Clostridium perfringens*. When *tcdD* was expressed in *trans* with the toxin A or toxin B promoter fused to a *C. difficile* toxin DNA fragment, toxin expression was increased by 500 times or more (79). Furthermore, TcdD was reported to function as a sigma factor (74). In many bacteria, the RNA polymerase subunit sigma factor σ^{70} initiates transcription by binding to specific sequences near the -10 and the -35 positions in the promoter. Although these sequences do not exist on *C. difficile* toxin promoters, TcdD exhibits some structural similarities to RNA polymerase sigma factors. In gel shift experiments, recombinant TcdD bound to purified *C. difficile* RNA polymerase in the absence of toxin promoter DNA. TcdD did not bind directly to *C. difficile* toxin promoters but did allow RNA polymerase to bind these promoters. Based on these data, TcdD was proposed to regulate toxin gene expression by acting as an alternative sigma factor for RNA polymerase (Fig. 3) (74).

TcdE exhibits structural features similar to a family of bacteriophage-encoded proteins called holins (103). Holins accumulate and oligomerize to form a lesion that permeabilizes the plasma membrane of bacterial hosts (32). When expressed in *E. coli*, TcdE caused cell lysis, suggesting that TcdE is functionally similar to holins. This notion fits with the observation that toxin release in vitro peaks after 4 to 5 days of culture when most cells are lysed. Thus, TcdE may play an important role in controlling toxin release from *C. difficile* (Fig. 3).

STRUCTURE OF *C. DIFFICILE* TOXIN A AND TOXIN B

C. difficile toxin A and toxin B are the major known virulence factors of *C. difficile*. These AB-type toxins share similar domains including an N-terminal enzymatic domain responsible for the toxicity of the molecule and a C-terminal binding domain composed of repeating sequences. Toxin A and toxin B belong to the large clostridial cytotoxin (LCT) family. The LCT family also includes *Clostridium sordellii* hemorrhagic and lethal toxins and *Clostridium novyi* alpha toxin. LCTs share a number of features including (i) a high molecular weight, (ii) a carboxy-terminal domain carrying clostridial repetitive oligopeptides (CROPs), (iii) a central hydrophobic region, and (iv) an amino-terminal enzymatic domain that catalyzes the covalent modification of threonine 35/37 of small GTP-binding proteins (Fig. 4).

tcdA encodes a polypeptide of 2,710 amino acids (deduced molecular mass, 308,128 Da) whereas *tcdB* encodes a protein of 2,366 amino acids (269,711 Da) (5, 24). Both toxins were cloned from the reference strain VPI 10463. Toxin A and toxin B are 49% identical at the amino acid level, and an additional 14% of the residues are conservative substitutions (111).

Toxin A C terminus carries a total of 30 contiguous repeating units, or CROPs, that represent 31.5% of the molecule. These include a group of 7 homologous CROPs of 50 amino acids and 23 other CROPs of 21 amino acids that fall within four groups (111). Many of the CROPs are highly hydrophilic (24). Sequence similarity is high among units of the same group but low between groups. The monoclonal antibody PCG4, which neutralizes toxin A enterotoxicity (71), recognizes epitopes expressed in two regions of toxin A C terminus (residues 2097 through 2141 and residues 2355 through 2398) (Fig. 4) (29). By contrast, PCG4 does not prevent toxin A- or toxin B-induced cytotoxicity in cancer cell lines. Thus, toxin A enterotoxicity appears to require the interaction of the C terminus with a specific receptor that is expressed at the surface of the intestinal mucosa. Similarly, the toxin B C terminus carries 19 contiguous repeating sequences that encompass the last 515 residues. Toxin B CROPs include four segments of 50 amino acids and 12 CROPs of 21 amino acids that are similar to toxin A re-

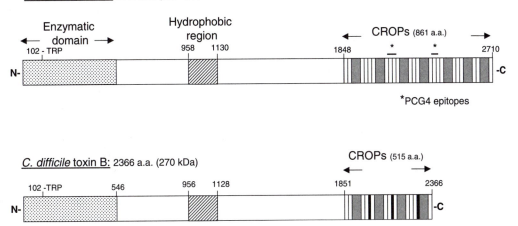

FIGURE 4 Structure of *C. difficile* toxins. Toxin A and toxin B are AB-type toxins and share three similar domains: (i) an N-terminal enzymatic domain responsible for cytotoxicity that carries a conserved tryptophan residue (Trp-102) probably involved in binding to UDP-glucose; (ii) a central, major hydrophobic region of 172 amino acids that is highly conserved and may act as a transmembrane domain to facilitate exit from endosomes; and (iii) a C-terminal binding domain composed of contiguous repeating units also known as CROPs. Toxin A carries 30 CROPs, whereas toxin B carries 19. They include sequences of 50 amino acids (represented in gray) and 21 amino acids (represented in white). The monoclonal antibody PCG4, which neutralizes toxin A enterotoxicity in animal models, recognizes epitopes on toxin A CROPs which are illustrated by horizontal bars.

peats. In addition, toxin B carries three peptides of 19 residues that are not present in toxin A (111).

Both toxins carry a major hydrophobic region of 172 amino acids that is highly conserved. Since *C. difficile* toxins appear to gain access to the cytosol via endocytosis (28), it is proposed that this region may act as a transmembrane domain during translocation of the enzymatic domain from an endocytosis vesicle to the cytosol.

Finally, the N-terminal portion of both toxins carries the enzymatic domain that is responsible for their cytotoxicity. In most cell lines, toxin A and toxin B induce cell rounding and retraction of the cell body as a result of collapse of the cytoskeleton. Toxin B is approximately 1,000-fold more cytotoxic than toxin A (the lowest cytotoxic concentrations in CHO cells are 30 pM for toxin A and 30 fM for toxin B). The cytotoxicity of toxin A and toxin B results from their ability to glu-

cosylate members of the Rho protein subfamily using UDP-glucose as substrate (46, 47, 110). A toxin B recombinant fragment encompassing the first 546 amino acids was cytotoxic following microinjection and glucosylated Rho proteins in vitro, as does native toxin B. By contrast, a slightly shorter fragment carrying the first 516 residues was almost inactive (41). The N-terminal domain carries a tryptophan residue (Trp-102) that is conserved among LCTs and is probably involved in binding to UDP-glucose (8) (Fig. 4).

BINDING AND INTERNALIZATION OF *C. DIFFICILE* TOXINS

Toxin A-Binding Polysaccharides and Their Carrier Molecules in Animal Models

The vast majority of studies aiming to identify *C. difficile* toxin receptors have focused on toxin A. Toxin A binds to carbohydrate moieties bearing a terminal α-linked or β-linked galactose. Krivan and coworkers have shown that toxin A binds to Galα1-3–Galβ4–GlcNAc, a trisaccharide also known as α-Gal epitope, which is abundant in various mammalian cells but not in humans (30, 56). The α-Gal epitope is expressed on hamster brush border membrane, rabbit erythrocytes, and calf thyroglobulin, all of which were bound by toxin A (56). Whereas in rabbit erythrocytes this polysaccharide is part of a membrane glycolipid (14), on hamster brush borders it is linked to a 164-kDa glycoprotein (95). The lectin-like properties of the α-Gal epitope are physiologically relevant, and in mouse teratocarcinoma cells, for instance, terminal α-linked galactose is abundant at the cell surface and promotes toxin A binding and internalization (106, 107). Furthermore, toxin A binding was inhibited in hamster intestine by pretreatment with α-galactosidase or the lectin *Bandereia simplicifolia* (BS-1), which also binds to α-Gal epitopes. Moreover, pretreatment of rat colonic loops with the lectin BS-1 inhibited toxin A-mediated enterotoxicity (90).

Pothoulakis et al. demonstrated that the brush border disaccharidase complex sucrase-isomaltase acts as a functional toxin A receptor in rabbit ileum (91). Toxin A bound purified sucrase-isomaltase, and this interaction was inhibited by α-galactosidase. Furthermore, intestinal inflammation induced by toxin A was inhibited by an antibody directed against sucrase-isomaltase. Although sucrase-isomaltase appears to be a receptor for toxin A in rabbit ileum, this cell surface digestive enzyme is not expressed in the human colon.

Human Toxin A-Binding Polysaccharides

The human intestinal receptor for toxin A is not known. Tucker and Wilkins reported that toxin A binds to several carbohydrates present in human colonic mucosa, including the antigens I, Lewis X, and Lewis Y (107). In other studies using purified human duodenal and colonic epithelial cells, radiolabeled toxin A specifically bound to a glycoprotein epithelial cell receptor, apparently through a β-galactose (102).

The observation that neonates and infants are frequently colonized by toxigenic *C. difficile* but remain asymptomatic suggests that the expression or glucosylation of human intestinal receptors for *C. difficile* toxins is not complete before the age of 2 years (64, 109). Newborn rabbits exhibit a similarly diminished intestinal biologic response to *C. difficile* toxin A as compared to adult animals (26). Binding studies indicated that intestinal toxin A receptor expression in rabbit ileum is age dependent and gradually increases from 5 days after birth onward. The reason(s) for this age-related reduction of toxin A binding sites in neonatal intestine is not known. Previous studies have shown that microsomal galactosyltransferase activity in rat colon is age dependent and increases gradually during neonatal life, reaching adult levels 2 weeks after birth (93). Thus, the age-dependent appearance of toxin A binding sites may reflect the developmental regulation of microsomal galactosyltransferase expression in enterocytes.

Toxin Internalization

The translocation of toxin A and toxin B into the cytosol is a prerequisite for their cytotoxic activity. Some bacterial toxins, including diphtheria toxin, translocate from the endosomal compartment to the cytosol following receptor-mediated endocytosis. This process involves acidification of the endosomal vesicle which is believed to trigger a conformational change resulting in the insertion of a hydrophobic toxin domain into the endosomal membrane. Early studies by Thelestam et al. showed that inhibition of endosomal acidification can prevent toxin B-induced cytopathic effect (28, 39). Bafilomycin A1, an inhibitor of endosomal acidification, also inhibited toxin B internalization (6, 92). Moreover, *C. difficile* toxin B appears to undergo structural changes at low pH. Using 2-(p-toluidinyl) naphthalene-6-sulfonic acid-mediated fluorescence, Qa'dan et al. demonstrated a reversible increase in hydrophobicity of toxin B at pH 5 or lower, without inhibition of cytotoxic activity (92). In addition, extracellular acidification (pH, ≤ 5.2) induced toxin B uptake into the cytosol despite the presence of bafilomycin A1. Moreover, toxin B was found to induce the formation of potassium-permeable channels at low pH (6). This observation was reproduced with a truncated toxin B fragment carrying amino acids 547 to 2366. Thus, these structural changes may contribute to membrane insertion, channel formation, and toxin translocation into the cytosol. Similarly, channel formation has been reported for several other protein toxins that are exported from endosomes (77).

MECHANISM OF ACTION OF *C. DIFFICILE* TOXINS: MONOGLUCOSYLATION AND INACTIVATION OF Rho GTPases

Rho Proteins Regulate Cytoskeletal Structure and Gene Expression

Rho proteins are intracellular proteins expressed in all eukaryotic cells and are a prime target for bacterial toxins. Rho proteins are small GTP-binding proteins (20 to 25 kDa) of the Ras superfamily. The Ras superfamily includes five subgroups based on their homology and functions: Ras, Rho (Ras homologue), Rab, Ran, and ARF. The Rho subfamily includes Rho (A, B, and C isoforms), Cdc42 (Cdc42 Hs and G25K isoforms), Rac (1 and 2 isoforms), Rho D, Rho E, and TC10. Rho, Cdc42, and Rac are substrates for *C. difficile* toxin A and toxin B. Rap, a member of the Ras subfamily, is a substrate for toxin A only.

Rho, Cdc42, and Rac have emerged as key regulators of the actin cytoskeleton. In Swiss 3T3 fibroblasts, Rho activation leads to the assembly of actin-myosin stress fibers and adhesion complexes. Rac regulates the formation of lamellipodial extensions that result from actin polymerization at the cell periphery. Cdc42 activation produces thin cytoplasmic extensions also known as filopodia or microspikes (33). These Rho proteins also regulate signaling pathways involved in cell cycle progression and gene transcription (73).

Rho Proteins Function as Molecular Switches

Rho GTPases shuttle between the cytosol and the membrane and function as molecular switches through a GTP-binding/GTPase cycle (Fig. 5 and 6). Three classes of proteins regulate this cycle: (i) guanine nucleotide exchange factors (GEFs), which stimulate the exchange of GTP for GDP; (ii) GTPase-activating proteins (GAPs), which activate the GTPase reaction; and (iii) guanine nucleotide dissociation inhibitors (GDIs), which have at least three functions—GDIs block the dissociation of GDP from Rho proteins, inhibit intrinsic and GAP-catalyzed GTP hydrolysis, and regulate the subcellular localization of Rho proteins. In the cytosol, Rho proteins are kept bound to GDI in the GDP-bound state. In response to an incoming signal, Rho is dissociated from GDI. The geranylgeranylated moiety of Rho, which was buried in a hydrophobic pocket of GDI, is inserted into the plasma membrane lipid bilayer, a step essential for Rho function. Moreover, a GEF catalyzes nucleotide exchange and activation. In its active membrane-associated state, Rho interacts with numerous target proteins to induce coordinated signals. Subsequently, GAPs interact with the GTPase-target complex and catalyze GTP hydrolysis. The GDP-bound form is then extracted from the membrane by Rho-GDI, and the cycle is complete.

C. difficile Toxins Glucosylate a Conserved Threonine Residue of Rho

Toxin A and toxin B are UDP-glucose hydrolases and glucosyltransferases; both hydrolyze UDP-glucose and catalyze the transfer of the glucose moiety to a conserved threonine residue (Thr-35 or Thr-37) of Rho proteins (46, 47). Rho, Cdc42, and Rac are substrates for both toxins, whereas Rap is a substrate for toxin A only (11). Both toxins glucosylate recombinant Rho proteins in vitro in the presence of UDP-glucose, but the toxin

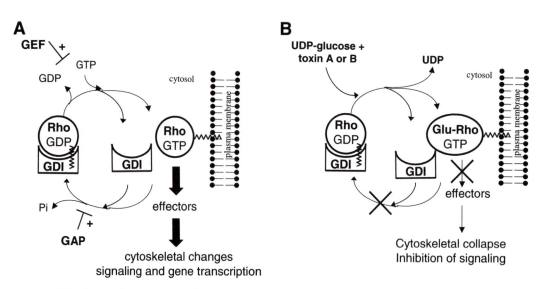

FIGURE 5 Rho protein cycle and the consequences of Rho glucosylation. (A) Rho proteins are signaling molecules that function as molecular switches. Rho GTPases function as a molecular switch through a GTP-binding/GTPase cycle regulated by three classes of proteins: (i) GEFs, which stimulate the exchange of GTP for GDP; (ii) GAPs, which catalyze GTP hydrolysis; and (iii) GDIs, which block the dissociation of GDP from Rho proteins, inhibit intrinsic and GAP-catalyzed GTP hydrolysis, and regulate the subcellular localization of Rho proteins. In the cytosol, Rho proteins are bound to GDI in the GDP-bound, inactive state. In response to upstream signals, Rho is dissociated from GDI. The geranylgeranylated moiety of Rho is then inserted into the plasma membrane lipid bilayer, a step essential for Rho function. Moreover, a GEF catalyzes nucleotide exchange and Rho activation. In its active membrane-associated state, Rho interacts with downstream effectors to induce coordinated signals that regulate cytoskeletal structure and gene transcription. Rho inactivation occurs as GAPs catalyze GTP hydrolysis. The GDP-bound form is then extracted from the membrane by Rho-GDI. (B) *C. difficile* toxin-induced glucosylation blocks Rho cycling, effector coupling, and downstream signaling. Toxins A and B are UDP-glucose hydrolases and glucosyltransferases. After hydrolyzing UDP-glucose, both toxins catalyze the transfer of the glucose moiety to a conserved threonine residue (Thr-35 or Thr-37) of Rho proteins when released from GDI. Since glucosylated Rho cannot bind GDI-1, glucosylated Rho cannot be extracted by GDI from the plasma membrane, and this interrupts Rho cycling. Furthermore, the glucose moiety prevents Rho interaction with downstream effectors, resulting in cytoskeleton collapse and inhibition of signaling.

concentrations that are required in vitro are much higher than those in a cell-based assay. In vitro, the toxins have similar Michaelis constants for UDP-glucose, but the maximal velocity of toxin B is about five times greater than that of toxin A (13). Moreover, microinjection studies have shown that toxin B enzymatic activity is approximately 100-fold greater than that of toxin A (11).

The threonine 37 of Rho and the corresponding threonine 35 of Cdc42 and Rac are located in the switch I domain of Rho. Originally observed on crystallized Ras, the switch I and switch II regions each contain a loop segment that undergoes conformational change during nucleotide exchange (76). These regions are exposed and form a continuous strip at the molecule surface. More importantly, the switch I region, which comprises residues 32 to 38, interacts with the downstream effectors (83). Thus, the threonine 37/35 is critically involved in Rho func-

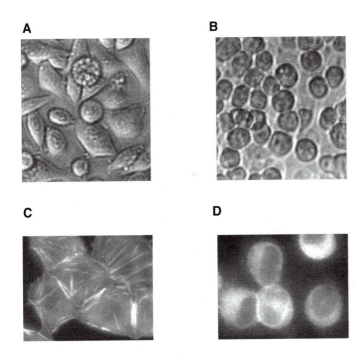

FIGURE 6 Morphological features of *C. difficile* toxin-induced cytotoxic effect in cultured cells. CHO cells were incubated overnight in the absence (A and C) or in the presence (B and D) of 30 fM *C. difficile* toxin B. (A and B) Cell morphology as observed by phase-contrast microscopy. Toxin exposure caused cell rounding and retraction of the cell body (B). (C and D) Cells were stained with fluorescein isothiocyanate-labeled phalloidin, which binds to actin microfilaments and reveals stress fibers. In toxin B-treated cells, the stress fibers have disaggregated (D). Toxin A causes identical effects (not shown).

tion, and its modification by *C. difficile* toxins will disrupt many steps of the Rho cycle.

Toxin-Induced Glucosylation Blocks Rho Cycling and Downstream Signaling

Rho glucosylation by *C. difficile* toxins or Ras glucosylation by *C. sordellii* toxins was found to decrease intrinsic GTPase activity and prevented GAP binding to Ras and stimulation of GTPase activity. In addition, Rho glucosylation inhibited Rho binding to protein kinase N, a downstream effector. Similarly, glucosylated Ras was unable to bind Raf, its main downstream effector, thereby inhibiting Ras signaling. Whereas Rho cannot be glucosylated by *C. difficile* toxins when bound to GDI-1, Rho becomes available for glucosylation upon its release from GDI induced by an upstream signal. In contrast to unmodified Rho, glucosylated Rho cannot bind GDI-1 and therefore cannot be extracted by GDI from the plasma membrane. Thus, upon release from GDI, monoglucosylation of threonine 37/35 by *C. difficile* toxins prevents

Rho from interacting with GAPs or GDIs and leads to its accumulation at the plasma membrane. This results in Rho cycle blockade and inhibition of downstream signaling (Fig. 5) (31, 40, 101).

INTESTINAL MECHANISMS OF *C. DIFFICILE* TOXINS

C. difficile is not an invasive bacterium. Its pathogenicity is mediated by the release of toxins that bind to their receptors located on the apical surface of enterocytes. Toxin-induced cytotoxic effects in intestinal epithelium are characterized by changes in tight junction structure and permeability, as discussed in detail below. In addition, *C. difficile* toxins trigger an inflammatory response orchestrated by lamina propria cells, including nerves, macrophages, and mast cells, that in turn stimulate neutrophil recruitment. Thus, *C. difficile* toxins are proinflammatory enterotoxins, in contrast to other enterotoxins such as cholera toxin that stimulate secretion and diarrhea in the absence of inflammation.

The early cytotoxic events and the mechanisms whereby *C. difficile* toxins trigger an acute inflammatory response are still poorly understood. Since toxins A and B are probably too large to reach the lamina propria and to directly activate subepithelial inflammatory cells, it is currently hypothesized that these cells are activated by cytokines or other mediators released by enterocytes. It is likewise unclear whether Rho inactivation is essential for cytokine release or whether Rho-independent mechanisms may trigger cell activation and inflammation.

In this section, we review growing evidence supporting the hypothesis that toxin B, which is not enterotoxic in animal models, is fully enterotoxic in humans. Next, the effect of toxins on intestinal epithelial cells is reviewed. The intestinal neuroimmune and inflammatory responses to *C. difficile* toxins are reviewed separately in chapter 19.

Are Both Toxin A and Toxin B Enterotoxic in Humans?

Toxin A is highly enterotoxic in animal models. When injected into the intestinal lumen, toxin A increases mucosal permeability and induces fluid secretion, acute neutrophil infiltration, and intestinal inflammation (90). Although toxin B is a more potent cytotoxin in cultured cells than toxin A, toxin B alone has no evident enterotoxic activity in animal intestine in vivo (72, 78, 105). Because of toxin B's lack of enterotoxic effect in animals, it was thought that it may not play a significant role in the pathogenesis of *C. difficile* diarrhea and colitis in humans. However, recent observations appear to contradict this hypothesis.

Lessons from Human Intestinal Studies. As discussed further below, the first indication that toxin B was enterotoxic in humans came from studies on human colonic strips (94). Toxin B was 10 times more potent than toxin A in inducing mucosal injury and in decreasing transepithelial electrical resistance. Moreover, the enterotoxicity of toxin B for human intestine was recently evaluated in severe combined immunodeficient (SCID) mice bearing subcutaneous human fetal intestinal

xenografts. In this model, toxin B caused acute mucosal inflammation, epithelial cell damage, interleukin-8 (IL-8) release, and neutrophil infiltration of the intestinal mucosa (100). Taken together, these data strongly suggest that toxin B is enterotoxic and proinflammatory in the human intestine.

Lessons from *C. difficile* variants. Additional evidence for the enterotoxicity of toxin B in humans comes from reports of the isolation of toxin A-negative/toxin B-positive strains of *C. difficile* from patients with antibiotic-associated diarrhea and colitis (44, 49, 57, 68, 80, 98, 99).

C. difficile exhibits a number of variations within its cell surface proteins and PaLoc. Fourteen serogroups were identified by agglutination and analysis of surface proteins by polyacrylamide gel electrophoresis (serogroups A–D, F–I, K, S1–4, and X). In addition, serogroup A contains another 20 subgroups as detected by polyacrylamide gel electrophoresis (21). Recently, 11 genotypic profiles, called toxinotypes (0 and I through X), have been identified by restriction fragment length polymorphism (RFLP) analysis of PCR fragments encompassing the PaLoc. The toxinotype of the reference *C. difficile* strain VPI 10463 (toxinotype 0) was found in 79% of a large pool of clinical isolates representing all serogroups (96). Moreover, toxinotype VIII was the most frequent variant and was characteristic of serogroup F, whose best-known representative is strain 1470.

Serogroup F strains are interesting from a pathophysiological standpoint for at least two reasons: (i) they appear to be pathogenic in humans but not in animal models and (ii) they do not make toxin A and produce a toxin B variant. In axenic mice, *C. difficile* 1470 did not cause diarrhea, although a cytotoxin recognized by toxin B antibodies was detected in the intestinal lumen (23). A series of polyclonal and monoclonal antibodies failed to detect any toxin A in vivo or in vitro. In fact, the toxin A-1470 gene carries at least two mutations: (i) a 1.7-kb deletion in the repeating units region that was found in virtually all toxin A-negative, toxin B-positive strains isolated from different continents (49, 80) and (ii) a nonsense mutation at the level of amino acid 47 found on all of a limited number of isolates. When expressed as a recombinant protein, toxin A-1470 repeats were also recognized by a monoclonal antibody that binds toxin A-10463 repeating units. Thus, the nonsense mutation was proposed to explain the lack of toxin A-1470 production (112).

Another feature of serogroup F is that toxin B-1470 appears to be a hybrid between toxin B-10463 and *C. sordellii* lethal toxin. The toxin B-1470 receptor-binding region is 99% identical to that of toxin B-10463, whereas the toxin B-1470 enzymatic domain is only 79% identical. Furthermore, toxin B-1470 glucosylates the same substrates as those modified by *C. sordellii* lethal toxin, including Ras, Rap, Rac, and RalA. By contrast, Rho and Rac are not glucosylated by toxin B-1470 (10, 89).

Although serogroup F or toxinotype VIII strains were initially isolated from asymptomatic infants (22), a number of recent reports implicate them in outbreaks of *C. difficile* diarrhea and in cases of pseudomembranous colitis (1, 44, 57, 68, 88, 98). In England and Wales, toxin A-negative/toxin B-positive strains account for 3% of clinical isolates referred to the Public Health Laboratory Service Anaerobic Reference Unit for typing. These clinical observations strongly support the hypothesis that toxin B-1470 is pathogenic in humans.

Toxin A and Toxin B Effects on Intestinal Epithelial Cells

Early studies in T84 human intestinal epithelial cells have shown that both toxin A and toxin B dramatically decrease transepithelial resistance and increase epithelial cell permeability (37, 38) (Fig. 7). These effects are associated with the appearance of discrete plaques of actin within the perijunctional ring, indicating F-actin reorganization. These responses were observed in the absence of cell damage or morphological evidence of tight junction alteration by electron microscopy (37, 38).

A recent study found that, in coordination with several other signaling pathways, protein kinase C (PKC) regulates ZO-1 assembly and transepithelial resistance. Toxin A activated PKCα and cytosolic PKCβ before Rho inactivation was detected. Furthermore, a PKCα/β antagonist inhibited Rho glucosylation, the decrease in transepithelial resistance, and ZO-1 translocation induced by toxin A (12, 48). These results suggest that early signaling events involving PKC are required for toxin-induced cytotoxic events.

In human colonic mucosal strips mounted in Ussing chambers, toxin A (32 nM) and toxin B (3 nM) caused rapid decreases in electrical resistance and an increase in [^{3}H]mannitol flux (94). In addition, both toxins caused condensation of F-actin and exfoliation of epithelial cells. These results indicate that purified toxin A and toxin B are highly cytotoxic in human colonic epithelial cells and that they disrupt tight junction integrity and function. The finding that toxin B is 10 times more potent than toxin A in causing colonic mucosal damage suggests that the pathogenic role of toxin B in human infection may be prominent or even preponderant (94).

The mechanism whereby *C. difficile* toxins disrupt tight junctions is only partially understood. There is strong but indirect evidence to support the hypothesis that *C. difficile* toxins modify F-actin tight junction and permeability through Rho glucosylation. First, Rho proteins have been implicated in the regulation of tight junction assembly and function. For instance, overexpression of RhoA or Rac mutants in Madin-Darby canine kidney cells modified the spatial organization of tight junction proteins and transepithelial electrical resistance (45). Second, in T84 cells, Rho inactivation by C3 exoenzyme (which catalyzes ADP-ribosylation of RhoA, B, and C) resulted in disassembly of perijunctional F-actin and in displacement of ZO-1 protein from its perijunctional membrane site, while

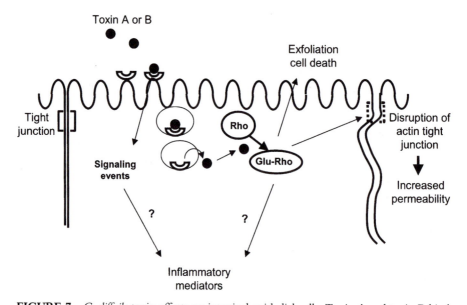

Toxin A or B

Exfoliation
cell death

Tight
junction

Rho

Disruption of
actin tight
junction

Signaling
events

Glu-Rho

Increased
permeability

?   ?

Inflammatory
mediators

FIGURE 7 *C. difficile* toxin effects on intestinal epithelial cells. Toxin A and toxin B bind to specific extracellular receptors expressed at the luminal surface of intestinal epithelial cells. After toxin internalization and transfer into the cytosol, the enzymatic domain catalyzes the glucosylation of Rho proteins. Inactivated Rho proteins cause perijunctional actin changes leading to loss of transepithelial electrical resistance and increased paracellular permeability. Toxin exposure also triggers the release of inflammatory mediators including IL-8 and reactive oxygen species that may in turn activate lamina propria cells. Whether this inflammatory response results from Rho glucosylation or Rho-independent mechanisms, such as receptor-mediated signaling, is not clear.

E-cadherin distribution remained unchanged (84). These molecular changes were associated with loss of transepithelial resistance to passive ion flow and increased permeability to 10-kDa dextran. Finally, in T84 cells, *C. difficile* toxin A and toxin B induced the rearrangement of apical F-actin and translocation of ZO-1 from the tight junction without modifying E-cadherin (85). In contrast to C3 exoenzyme, toxins A and B also caused disorganization of basal F-actin, a difference that can be explained by the ability of *C. difficile* toxins to glucosylate Rho family members such as CDC42 or Rac itself.

Taken together, these studies strongly support the hypothesis that *C. difficile*-induced perijunctional F-actin disassembly, displacement of ZO-1 protein, and loss of transepithelial electrical resistance result from Rho

glucosylation. Further studies are needed to clarify how glucosylated Rho disrupts tight junction permeability and to determine whether these events can trigger the release of inflammatory mediators.

PROINFLAMMATORY EFFECTS OF *C. DIFFICILE* TOXINS IN MONOCYTES
Neutrophil recruitment is an essential step in the pathogenesis of *C. difficile* toxin-induced intestinal injury. Biopsy specimens from patients with *C. difficile* colitis show striking vascular congestion and neutrophil infiltration of the lamina propria (58). In severe cases, a marked elevation of the peripheral blood neutrophil count with toxic granulations and band forms are common findings. In animal models, inhibition of neutrophil recruitment using neutralizing antibodies against the neutrophil

adhesion molecule CD18 or the neutrophil chemoattractant macrophage inflammatory protein-2 resulted in a marked reduction in fluid secretion, epithelial injury, and mucosal inflammation in toxin A-exposed intestinal loops (9, 50). Since neutrophils are instrumental in toxin-induced damage, it is important to understand the mechanisms whereby they are activated and recruited.

Several investigators have examined the effects of *C. difficile* toxins on peripheral blood leukocytes. Human neutrophils, lymphocytes, and basophils appeared relatively resistant to toxin A and toxin B, since no obvious signs of intoxication or activation were detected when exposed to toxin concentrations that cause cell rounding in cancer cell lines. For instance, these toxin concentrations did not inhibit neutrophil phagocytosis and viability (19), nor did they affect lymphocyte proliferation and viability (20, 27). Toxin A was shown to stimulate a rise in neutrophil cytosolic Ca^{2+} levels and a neutrophil chemotactic response, but the concentrations of toxin A needed to achieve these effects were high (10^{-7} M) (91a). Moreover, toxin A failed to activate $\beta 2$ integrins on neutrophils and did not activate histamine release from basophils (113). These data suggest that *C. difficile* toxins may induce neutrophil recruitment indirectly via the release of endogenous neutrophil activators and chemoattractants.

Toxin A and Toxin B Activate Proinflammatory Cytokine Release from Human Monocytes

In contrast to the high concentrations required for neutrophil activation, early studies found that lower, more physiologically relevant concentrations of *C. difficile* toxins have dramatic effects on human monocytes. Isolated monocytes pretreated with *C. difficile* toxins were unable to stimulate T-cell proliferation, whereas the toxins had no effect on IL-2-driven T-cell proliferation (20). Furthermore, Flegel et al. showed that toxin A at 10^{-9} M or toxin B at 10^{-12} M induced the release of

IL-1, tumor necrosis factor (TNF), and IL-6 release from human monocytes (27). Subsequently, we reported that similar concentrations of toxin A (10^{-10} M) or toxin B (10^{-12} M) induced a marked increase in production of the neutrophil chemoattractant IL-8 in monocytes (69). This was associated with activation of IL-8 gene expression, as demonstrated by an increase in monocyte IL-8 mRNA levels 3 h after toxin exposure. Thus, *C. difficile* toxins activate a strong proinflammatory response in human monocytes including the release of IL-8. This potent neutrophil chemoattractant may be instrumental in mediating neutrophil recruitment and intestinal inflammation in vivo.

C. difficile Toxins Cause Monocyte Necrosis and Release of IL-1β via Caspase-like Proteases

The dose-response curve of toxin-stimulated IL-8 release in monocytes was bell shaped, indicative of toxic effects at higher toxin concentrations (27, 69). In fact, both toxin A and toxin B were found to cause necrosis, and not apoptosis, in THP-1 monocytic cells and in primary monocytes (116). Human peripheral blood-derived monocytes underwent necrosis following exposure to 10^{-9} M toxin A or 10^{-12} M toxin B, whereas THP-1 cells were 100-fold more resistant. By contrast, neither human neutrophils nor lymphocytes showed any evidence of cell death or morphological evidence of toxicity when exposed to these toxin concentrations. Furthermore, *C. difficile* toxin-induced necrosis was associated with massive release of preformed IL-1β and shedding of CD14, the cell surface receptor for LPS. These effects were also associated with necrosis induced by other stimuli and were not specific for *C. difficile* toxins (116). Monocyte necrosis and IL-1β release were inhibited by the broad-spectrum caspase inhibitor z-VAD-fmk, suggesting that both events are mediated by activation of caspase-like proteases. Since macrophages are abundant within the colonic mucosa and are known to store large amounts of pro-IL-1, they may play a prominent role in mediating the intestinal inflammatory response to *C. difficile* toxins.

Signaling Mechanisms Involved in Monocyte Activation by *C. difficile* Toxins

The expression of chemokine and cytokine genes results from activation of a number of signaling cascades. The signaling mechanisms involved in toxin A-induced IL-8 gene expression in monocytes have recently been investigated. Using human monocytes, Jefferson et al. reported that IL-8 release induced by toxin A is inhibited by chelating intracellular and extracellular calcium or by using the calmodulin inhibitor W-7. (42). Furthermore, toxin A activated NF-κB, a transcription factor required for IL-8 gene expression (81). Interestingly, in CHO cells, toxin A causes severe mitochondrial dysfunction that is associated with ATP depletion and the generation of oxygen radicals (35). These mitochondrial events may be instrumental in toxin-mediated NF-κB activation and upregulation of IL-8 gene expression (36). We have investigated the role of mitogen-activated protein (MAP) kinases in toxin-mediated IL-8 gene expression in human monocytes (115). MAP kinases are a family of highly conserved, proline-directed kinases that regulate the transcription of inflammatory cytokines in response to various stress stimuli. Upon activation by upstream kinase(s), MAP kinases phosphorylate downstream kinases and transcription factors and transmit signals from the cell surface to the nucleus via three distinct but related pathways. These culminate in the selective activation of extracellular signal-related kinases (ERK), p38, and c-Jun N-terminal kinase (JNK) (63). Interestingly, the small GTP-binding proteins Rho, Cdc42, and Rac, which are substrates for toxin A and toxin B, are proinflammatory signaling intermediates acting upstream of the MAP kinases (62).

Toxin A (100 nM) activated the three main MAP kinase cascades in THP-1 monocytic cells within 1 to 2 min of exposure (115). Activation of p38 was sustained, whereas stimulation of ERK and JNK was transient. IL-8 gene expression was abrogated by the p38 inhibitor SB203580 or by dominant-negative mutants of the p38-activating kinases MKK3 and MKK6. Furthermore, SB203580 also blocked monocyte necrosis and IL-1β release caused by toxin A but not by other stimuli. Finally, in mouse ileum, SB203580 prevented toxin A-induced neutrophil recruitment, mucosal injury, and villus destruction. Taken together, these data indicate that p38 MAP kinase plays a critical role in the proinflammatory response to toxin A in the intestinal mucosa.

Role of Rho Glucosylation in Monocyte Activation

Whether Rho glucosylation is involved in monocyte activation has not been demonstrated as yet. It is known that, in addition to their role in the regulation of cytoskeletal structure and cell motility, Rho proteins are involved in signal transduction cascades that regulate activation of transcription factors. For instance, Rho, Cdc42, and Rac-1 activated NF-κB, a transcription factor required for the expression of a number of proinflammatory cytokine genes including IL-8 (87). In addition, Cdc42 and Rac activate the JNK and the p38 pathways (18, 73, 104). *C. difficile* toxin B (0.15 nM) has been shown to inhibit NF-κB activation induced by bradykinin, which depends on Rho proteins (86). This observation suggests that Rho glucosylation and inactivation can block Rho-dependent proinflammatory pathways. However, glucosylation of Rho, Cdc42, and/or Rac in monocytes might trigger a signaling cascade, leading to monocyte activation.

In support of this hypothesis, toxin B, which is 100-fold more potent than toxin A in glucosylating Rho proteins, is also more potent in inducing IL-8 release by monocytes (~1,000-fold) (11, 69). Recently, we obtained preliminary results supporting such a mechanism. A recombinant fragment of toxin B carrying the first 545 residues (which include the enzymatic domain) induced Rho glucosylation in THP-1 cells and primary monocytes. This fragment also induced IL-8 release in both cell types. By contrast, the same fragment rendered enzymatically inactive by mutation of the conserved tryptophan 102 (8) did not activate IL-8 release (Warny, unpublished data). Thus, Rho glucosylation by *C. difficile* toxins appears to be sufficient to trigger IL-8 release by monocytes. This is in agreement with the prior observation that toxin A is unable to activate IL-8 release by monocytes when immobilized on a plastic surface (42). Further studies are needed to elucidate the mechanisms whereby Rho glucosylation and inactivation by *C. difficile* toxins appear to activate proinflammatory pathways.

HUMORAL IMMUNE RESPONSES TO *C. DIFFICILE* TOXINS

C. difficile toxins are highly immunogenic in animals and humans. Recent studies in humans demonstrate that a defective antibody response to toxin A is associated with severe and recurrent forms of *C. difficile* infection.

Animal Studies of Immunity to *C. difficile* Toxins

It has long been known that passive or active immunization against *C. difficile* toxins can protect animals against *C. difficile*-induced enterocolitis (53, 54). Kim et al. found that immunization of hamsters with toxoid A alone was protective whereas toxoid B immunization was not (53, 54, 70). Immunized animals continue to be colonized by toxigenic *C. difficile*, indicating that protection probably results from toxin neutralization rather than prevention of colonization, a situation analogous to the asymptomatic carrier state in humans (60).

Parenteral passive immunotherapy is also effective in animals (2, 17). A monoclonal antibody against toxin A CROPs (carrying the putative receptor-binding region of toxin A) prevented lethal cecitis mediated by a toxigenic strain of *C. difficile*. This study demonstrates the ability of systemic anti-toxin A

antibodies to protect against toxin-induced intestinal disease and, along with other studies, indicates that in animals toxin A is a more important enterotoxin than toxin B (72, 78, 105).

Prevalence of Serum and Mucosal Antitoxin Antibodies in the General Population

Serum immunoglobulin G (IgG) and IgA to *C. difficile* toxins are found in the majority of healthy children and adults (3, 43, 52, 108, 117). The prevalence of antitoxin serum antibodies increases to 50 and 70% for toxin A and toxin B, respectively, during the first 10 years of life, but appears to decline in old age (4, 82, 108). This early seroconversion may be explained by the high colonization rates (25 to 80%) observed in infants and children up to the age of 2 years (64, 109). Mucosal secretory anti-toxin A antibody responses are also common. Human colonic aspirates frequently contain secretory IgA antibodies to toxin A, and these antibodies inhibit binding of the toxin to its intestinal receptors (52, 117).

A Serum Anti-Toxin A IgG Response Is Associated with a Favorable Clinical Outcome

Early studies found that many patients with *C. difficile* diarrhea mount a systemic antibody response to *C. difficile* toxins (3, 108). There is now growing evidence that a serum IgG response to toxin A is associated with immune protection against *C. difficile*-associated diarrhea and colitis. An association between recurrent *C. difficile* diarrhea and a defective immune response against *C. difficile* has been observed both in children (66) and in adults (3, 4, 117). Recently, we confirmed this association by prospectively studying a larger cohort of patients (61). We observed that patients with a single episode of *C. difficile* diarrhea had significantly higher levels of serum IgM against toxin A by day 3 of their illness and significantly higher serum levels of IgG against toxin A on day 12, compared to patients who later had recurrent diarrhea (Fig. 8). After adjusting for other risk factors, patients with *C. difficile* diarrhea and a low level of IgG against toxin A had a 48-fold greater risk of recurrence.

In another recent study we found that the risk of developing symptomatic infection is at least in part determined by the humoral immune response to *C. difficile* toxins (60). Although 15 to 31% of high-risk hospitalized patients are colonized with *C. difficile*, only a minority develop symptomatic infection (60, 75). In a cohort of 84 patients colonized with *C. difficile*, those who became asymptomatic carriers had higher serum IgG to toxin A within 3 days of colonization than those who developed diarrhea (Fig. 8). The absence of

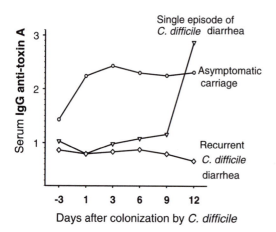

FIGURE 8 Serum IgG anti-toxin A antibody response and clinical outcome of infection. Patients with nosocomial *C. difficile* diarrhea were studied prospectively and serum IgG anti-toxin A antibody concentrations were measured by enzyme-linked immunosorbent assay at regular intervals. A correlation was observed between the IgG response and the clinical outcome of infection. Asymptomatic carriers mounted an early anamnestic response to toxin A. By contrast, no significant increase in serum IgG to toxin A was found in patients who suffered recurrent *C. difficile* diarrhea. In those who had a single episode of diarrhea, anti-toxin A IgG was generally increased on day 12 of their first episode. Thus, a serum antibody response to toxin A during *C. difficile* infection is associated with protection against symptoms or against recurrent diarrhea. (Figure based on data from references 60 and 61.)

this memory immune response to toxin A was associated with a 48-times-greater risk of diarrhea (60). Thus, two recent prospective studies strongly suggest that the strength and time course of IgG response to toxin A play an important role in determining the clinical outcome of *C. difficile* infection. Although the immune response to toxin B has not as yet been correlated as strongly with specific clinical outcomes, toxin B is clearly immunogenic in humans, and antibody responses to toxin B may also play a role in immune protection against *C. difficile*-associated diarrhea in humans.

Can Serum Anti-Toxin IgG Protect the Intestinal Mucosa?

Whether the association between a serum anti-toxin A IgG response and a favorable clinical outcome is a causal relationship has not been demonstrated. Since mucosal IgG concentration is normally very low, immune protection against *C. difficile* toxins might be mediated by an associated but undetected local response. However, some observations support the hypothesis that *C. difficile* toxin-induced mucosal inflammation provides access for serum IgG to mucosal and intraluminal compartments. In gnotobiotic mice, infection with a highly toxigenic *C. difficile* strain caused a 300-fold increase in intraluminal IgG concentration (16). In humans, a 740-fold increase in total IgG (from 1 to 740 μg/ml) was detected in feces containing anti-toxin A IgG from patients with *C. difficile* diarrhea (117). These data suggest that toxin-induced mucosal inflammation and epithelial permeability can result in substantial transfer of serum IgG into the intestinal mucosal and lumen. This mechanism would enable serum IgG to neutralize toxins in situ. If this model is correct, we can expect serum antibody-based therapeutic approaches to be effective in severe or recurrent forms of *C. difficile* infection.

Passive and Active Immunotherapy as Future Therapeutic Options

We have used passive immunotherapy with intravenous Ig (IVIG) to treat a small number of children and adult patients with recurrent or severe *C. difficile* diarrhea (66, 97, 114). Since healthy adults have serum IgG antibodies against *C. difficile* toxins (52, 108, 117), normal pooled human IVIG contains substantial amounts of IgG antitoxin (97). IVIG administration resulted in an increase in serum IgG antitoxin antibody levels and was also associated with resolution of recurrent *C. difficile* diarrhea. A *C. difficile* vaccine containing Formalin-inactivated toxins A and B has been developed and was highly immunogenic in humans (55). This vaccine will now be administered to professional plasma donors to produce hyperimmune human polyclonal IgG for passive immunotherapy. It will also be tested in clinical trials aimed at preventing primary and secondary *C. difficile* diarrhea.

CONCLUSION

Since *C. difficile* was recognized as an enteric pathogen in the late 1970s, we have learned a great deal regarding the epidemiology of *C. difficile* infection and about the molecular mechanisms underlying *C. difficile* toxin-induced intestinal injury and inflammation. Despite these advances, *C. difficile* remains the most common cause of nosocomial infectious diarrhea in developed countries and effective means to prevent and control outbreaks are still lacking. Clearly, additional research is needed to translate our knowledge of the pathophysiologic mechanisms that mediate *C. difficile* toxin-induced intestinal injury into novel and effective preventive and therapeutic interventions.

REFERENCES

1. **Alfa, M. J., A. Kabani, D. Lyerly, S. Moncrief, L. M. Neville, A. Al-Barrak, G. K. Harding, B. Dyck, K. Olekson, and J. M. Embil.** 2000. Characterization of a toxin A-negative, toxin B-positive strain of *Clostridium difficile* responsible for a nosocomial outbreak of *Clostridium difficile*-associated diarrhea. *J. Clin. Microbiol.* **38:**2706-2714.
2. **Allo, M., J. Silva, Jr., R. Fekety, G. D. Rifkin, and H. Waskin.** 1979. Prevention of clindamycin-induced colitis in hamsters by *Clostridium sordellii* antitoxin. *Gastroenterology* **76:**351-355.
3. **Aronsson, B., M. Grantsrom, R. Mollby, and C. E. Nord.** 1985. Serum antibody response to *Clostridium difficile* toxins in patients with *Clostridium difficile* diarrhoea. *Infection* **13:**97-101.
4. **Bacon, A. E., 3rd, and R. Fekety.** 1994. Immunoglobulin G directed against toxins A and B of *Clostridium difficile* in the general population and in patients with antibiotic-associated diarrhea. *Diagn. Microbiol. Infect. Dis.* **18:**205-209.
5. **Barroso, L. A., S. Z. Wang, C. J. Phelps, J. L. Johnson, and T. D. Wilkins.** 1990. Nucleotide sequence of *Clostridium difficile* toxin B gene. *Nucleic Acids Res.* **18:**4004.
6. **Barth, H., G. Pfeifer, F. Hofmann, E. Maier, R. Benz, and K. Aktories.** 2001. Low pH-induced formation of ion channels by *Clostridium difficile* toxin B in target cells. *J. Biol. Chem.* **276:**10670-10676.
7. **Braun, V., T. Hundsberger, P. Leukel, M. Sauerborn, and C. von Eichel-Streiber.** 1996. Definition of the single integration site of the pathogenicity locus in *Clostridium difficile*. *Gene* **181:**29-38.
8. **Busch, C., F. Hofmann, R. Gerhard, and K. Aktories.** 2000. Involvement of a conserved tryptophan residue in the UDP-glucose binding of large clostridial cytotoxin glycosyltransferases. *J. Biol. Chem.* **275:**13228-13234.
9. **Castagliuolo, I., A. C. Keates, C. C. Wang, A. Pasha, L. Valenick, C. P. Kelly, S. T. Nikulasson, J. T. LaMont, and C. Pothoulakis.** 1998. *Clostridium difficile* toxin A stimulates macrophage-inflammatory protein-2 production in rat intestinal epithelial cells. *J. Immunol.* **160:**6039-6045.
10. **Chaves-Olarte, E., P. Low, E. Freer, T. Norlin, M. Weidmann, C. von Eichel-Streiber, and M. Thelestam.** 1999. A novel cytotoxin from *Clostridium difficile* serogroup F is a functional hybrid between two other large clostridial cytotoxins. *J. Biol. Chem.* **274:**11046-11052.
11. **Chaves-Olarte, E., M. Weidmann, C. von Eichel-Streiber, and M. Thelestam.** 1997. Toxin A and B from *Clostridium difficile* differ with respect to enzymatic potencies, cellular substrate specificities and surface binding to cultured cells. *J. Clin. Invest.* **100:**1734-1741.
12. **Chen, M. L., C. Pothoulakis, and J. T. LaMont.** 2002. Protein kinase C signaling regulates ZO-1 translocation and increased paracellular flux of T84 colonocytes exposed to *Clostridium difficile* toxin A. *J. Biol. Chem.* **277:**4247-4254.

13. **Ciesla, W. P., Jr., and D. A. Bobak.** 1998. *Clostridium difficile* toxins A and B are cation-dependent UDP-glucose hydrolases with differing catalytic activities. *J. Biol. Chem.* **273:**16021–16026.

14. **Clark, G. F., N. C. Krivan, T. D. Wilkins, and B. F. Smith.** 1987. Toxin A from *Clostridium difficile* binds to rabbit erythrocyte glycolipids with terminal Galα1-3Galβ1-4GlcNAc sequences. *Arch. Biochem. Biophys.* **257:**217–229.

15. **Cohen, S. H., Y. J. Tang, and J. Silva, Jr.** 2000. Analysis of the pathogenicity locus in *Clostridium difficile* strains. *J. Infect. Dis.* **181:**659–663.

16. **Corthier, G., M. C. Muller, G. W. Elmer, F. Lucas, and F. Dubos-Ramare.** 1989. Interrelationships between digestive proteolytic activities and production and quantitation of toxins in pseudomembranous colitis induced by *Clostridium difficile* in gnotobiotic mice. *Infect. Immun.* **57:**3922–3927.

17. **Corthier, G., M. C. Muller, T. D. Wilkins, D. Lyerly, and R. L'Haridon.** 1991. Protection against experimental pseudomembranous colitis in gnotobiotic mice by use of monoclonal antibodies against *Clostridium difficile* toxin A. *Infect. Immun.* **59:**1192–1195.

18. **Coso, O. A., M. Chiariello, J. C. Yu, H. Teramoto, P. Crespo, N. Xu, T. Miki, and J. S. Gutkind.** 1995. Small GTP-binding proteins Rac1 and Cdc42 regulate the activity of the JNK/SAPK signaling pathway. *Cell* **81:**1137–1146.

19. **Dailey, D. C., A. Kaiser, and R. H. Schloemer.** 1987. Factors influencing the phagocytosis of *Clostridium difficile* by human polymorphonuclear leukocytes. *Infect. Immun.* **55:**1541–1546.

20. **Daubener, W., E. Leiser, C. von Eichel-Streiber, and U. Hadding.** 1988. *Clostridium difficile* toxins A and B inhibit human immune response in vitro. *Infect. Immun.* **56:**1107–1112.

21. **Delmée, M., Y. Laroche, V. Avesani, and G. Cornelis.** 1986. Comparison of serogrouping and polyacrylamide gel electrophoresis for typing *Clostridium difficile. J. Clin. Microbiol.* **24:**991–994.

22. **Delmée, M., G. Verellen, V. Avesani, and G. Francois.** 1988. *Clostridium difficile* in neonates: serogrouping and epidemiology. *Eur. J. Pediatr.* **147:**36–40.

23. **Depitre, C., M. Delmée, V. Avesani, R. L'Haridon, A. Roels, M. Popoff, and G. Corthier.** 1993. Serogroup F strains of *Clostridium difficile* produce toxin B but not toxin A. *J. Med. Microbiol.* **38:**434–441.

24. **Dove, C. H., S. Z. Wang, S. B. Price, C. J. Phelps, D. M. Lyerly, T. D. Wilkins, and J. L. Johnson.** 1990. Molecular characterization of the *Clostridium difficile* toxin A gene. *Infect. Immun.* **58:**480–488.

25. **Dupuy, B., and A. L. Sonenshein.** 1998. Regulated transcription of *Clostridium difficile* toxin genes. *Mol. Microbiol.* **27:**107–120.

26. **Eglow, R., C. Pothoulakis, S. Itzkowitz, E. J. Israel, C. J. O'Keane, D. Gong, N. Gao, Y. L. Xu, W. A. Walker, and J. T. LaMont.** 1992. Diminished *Clostridium difficile* toxin A sensitivity in newborn rabbit ileum is associated with decreased toxin A receptor. *J. Clin. Invest.* **90:**822–829.

27. **Flegel, W. A., F. Muller, W. Daubener, H. G. Fisher, U. Hadding, and H. Northoff.** 1991. Cytokine response by human monocytes to *Clostridium difficile* toxin A and toxin B. *Infect. Immun.* **59:**3659–3666.

28. **Florin, I., and M. Thelestam.** 1986. Lysosomal involvement in cellular intoxication with *Clostridium difficile* toxin B. *Microb. Pathog.* **1:**373–385.

29. **Frey, S. M., and T. D. Wilkins.** 1992. Localization of two epitopes recognized by monoclonal antibody PCG-4 on *Clostridium difficile* toxin A. *Infect. Immun.* **60:**2488–2492.

30. **Galili, U., S. B. Shohet, E. Cobrin, C. L. Stults, and B. A. Macher.** 1988. Man, apes, and old world monkeys differ from other mammalians in the expression of α-galactosyl epitopes on nucleated cells. *J. Biol. Chem.* **263:**17755–17762.

31. **Genth, H., K. Aktories, and I. Just.** 1999. Monoglucosylation of RhoA at threonine 37 blocks cytosol-membrane cycling. *J. Biol. Chem.* **274:**29050–29056.

32. **Gründling, A., M. D. Manson, and R. Young.** 2001. Holins kill without warning. *Proc. Natl. Acad. Sci. USA* **98:**9348–9352.

33. **Hall, A.** 1998. Rho GTPases and the actin cytoskeleton. *Science* **279:**509–514.

34. **Hammond, G. A., and J. L. Johnson.** 1995. The toxigenic element of *Clostridium difficile* strain VPI 10463. *Microb. Pathol.* **19:**203–213.

35. **He, D., S. J. Hagen, C. Pothoulakis, M. Chen, N. D. Medina, M. Warny, and J. T. LaMont.** 2000. *Clostridium difficile* toxin A causes early damage to mitochondria in cultured cells. *Gastroenterology* **119:**139–150.

36. **He, D., S. Sougioultzis, S. Hagen, J. Liu, S. Keates, A. C. Keates, C. Pothoulakis, and J. T. LaMont.** 2002. *Clostridium difficile* toxin A triggers human colonocyte IL-8 release via mitochondrial oxygen radical generation. *Gastroenterology* **122:**1048–1057.

37. **Hecht, G., A. Koutsouris, C. Pothoulakis, J. T. LaMont, and J. L. Madara.** 1992. *Clostridium difficile* toxin B disrupts the barrier func-

tion of T84 monolayers. *Gastroenterology* **102:** 416–423.

38. **Hecht, G., C. Pothoulakis, J. T. LaMont, and J. L. Madara.** 1988. *Clostridium difficile* toxin A perturbs cytoskeletal structure and tight junction permeability of cultured human intestinal epithelial monolayers. *J. Clin. Invest.* **82:**1516–1524.

39. **Henriques, B., I. Florin, and M. Thelestam.** 1987. Cellular internalisation of *Clostridium difficile* toxin A. *Microb. Pathog.* **2:**455–463.

40. **Herrmann, C., M. R. Ahmadian, F. Hofmann, and I. Just.** 1998. Functional consequences of monoglucosylation of Ha-Ras at effector domain amino acid threonine 35. *J. Biol. Chem.* **273:**16134–16139.

41. **Hofmann, F., C. Bush, U. Prepens, I. Just, and K. Aktories.** 1997. Localization of the glycosyltransferase activity of *Clostridium difficile* toxin B to the N-terminal part of the holotoxin. *J. Biol. Chem.* **272:**11074–11078.

42. **Jefferson, K. K., M. F. Smith, Jr., and D. A. Bobak.** 1999. Roles of intracellular calcium and NF-kappa B in the *Clostridium difficile* toxin A-induced up-regulation and secretion of IL-8 from human monocytes. *J. Immunol.* **163:**5183–5191.

43. **Johnson, S., D. N. Gerding, and E. N. Janoff.** 1992. Systemic and mucosal antibody responses to toxin A in patients infected with *Clostridium difficile. J. Infect. Dis.* **166:**1287–1294.

44. **Johnson, S., S. A. Kent, K. J. O'Leary, M. M. Merrigan, S. P. Sambol, L. R. Peterson, and D. N. Gerding.** 2001. Fatal pseudomembranous colitis associated with a variant *Clostridium difficile* strain not detected by toxin A immunoassay. *Ann. Intern. Med.* **135:**434–438.

45. **Jou, T. S., E. E. Schneeberger, and W. J. Nelson.** 1998. Structural and functional regulation of tight junctions by RhoA and Rac1 small GTPases. *J. Cell Biol.* **142:**101–115.

46. **Just, I., J. Selzer, M. Wilm, C. von Eichel-Streiber, M. Mann, and K. Aktories.** 1995. Glucosylation of Rho proteins by *Clostridium difficile* toxin B. *Nature* **375:**500–503.

47. **Just, I., M. Wilm, J. Selzer, G. Rex, C. von Eichel-Streiber, M. Mann, and K. Aktories.** 1995. The enterotoxin from *Clostridium difficile* (ToxA) monoglucosylates the Rho proteins. *J. Biol. Chem.* **270:**13932–13936.

48. **Karczewski, J., and J. Groot.** 2000. Molecular physiology and pathophysiology of tight junctions. III. Tight junction regulation by intracellular messengers: differences in response within and between epithelia. *Am. J. Physiol. Gastrointest. Liver Physiol.* **279:**G660–G665.

49. **Kato, H., N. Kato, S. Katow, T. Maegawa, S. Nakamura, and D. M. Lyerly.** 1999. Deletions in the repeating sequences of the toxin A gene of toxin A-negative, toxin B-positive *Clostridium difficile* strains. *FEMS Microbiol. Lett.* **175:**197–203.

50. **Kelly, C. P., S. Becker, J. K. Linevsky, M. A. Joshi, J. Conor O'Keane, J. T. LaMont, and C. Pothoutakis.** 1994. Neutrophil recruitment in *Clostridium difficile* toxin A enteritis in the rabbit. *J. Clin. Invest.* **93:**1257–1265.

51. **Kelly, C. P., C. Pothoulakis, and J. T. LaMont.** 1994. *Clostridium difficile* colitis. *N. Engl. J. Med.* **330:**257–262.

52. **Kelly, C. P., C. Pothoulakis, J. Orellana, and J. T. LaMont.** 1992. Human colonic aspirates containing immunoglobulin A antibody to *Clostridium difficile* toxin A inhibit toxin A-receptor binding. *Gastroenterology* **102:**35–40.

53. **Kim, P. H., J. P. Iaconis, and R. D. Rolfe.** 1987. Immunization of adult hamsters against *Clostridium difficile*-associated ileocecitis and transfer of protection to infant hamsters. *Infect. Immun.* **55:**2984–2992.

54. **Kim, P. H., and R. D. Rolfe.** 1989. Characterization of protective antibodies in hamsters immunized against *Clostridium difficile* toxin A and B. *Microb. Ecol. Health Dis.* **2:**47–59.

55. **Kotloff, K. L., S. S. Wasserman, G. A. Losonsky, W. Thomas, Jr., R. Nichols, R. Edelman, M. Bridwell, and T. P. Monath.** 2001. Safety and immunogenicity of increasing doses of a *Clostridium difficile* toxoid vaccine administered to healthy adults. *Infect. Immun.* **69:** 988–995.

56. **Krivan, H. C., G. F. Clark, D. F. Smith, and T. D. Wilkins.** 1986. Cell surface binding site for *Clostridium difficile* enterotoxin: evidence for a glycoconjugate containing the sequence Gal alpha 1-3Gal beta-4GlcNAc. *Infect. Immun.* **53:** 573–581.

57. **Kuijper, E. J., J. de Weerdt, H. Kato, N. Kato, A. P. van Dam, E. R. van der Vorm, J. Weel, C. van Rheenen, and J. Dankert.** 2001. Nosocomial outbreak of *Clostridium difficile*-associated diarrhoea due to a clindamycin-resistant enterotoxin A-negative strain. *Eur. J. Clin. Microbiol. Infect. Dis.* **20:**528–534.

58. **Kyne, L., R. Farrell, and C. P. Kelly.** 2001. *Clostridium difficile. Gastroenterol. Clin. North Am.* **30:**753–777.

59. **Kyne, L., M. B. Hamel, R. Polavaram, and C. P. Kelly.** 2002. Health care costs and mortality associated with nosocomial diarrhea due to *Clostridium difficile. Clin. Infect. Dis.* **34:**346–353.

60. **Kyne, L., M. Warny, A. Qamar, and C. P. Kelly.** 2000. Asymptomatic carriage of *Clostridium difficile* and serum levels of IgG antibody against toxin A. *N. Engl. J. Med.* **342:**390–397.

61. **Kyne, L., M. Warny, A. Qamar, and C. P. Kelly.** 2001. Association between antibody response to toxin A and protection against recurrent *Clostridium difficile* diarrhoea. *Lancet* **357:**189–193.

62. **Kyriakis, J. M., and J. Avruch.** 1996. Sounding the alarm: protein kinase cascades activated by stress and inflammation. *J. Biol. Chem.* **271:**24313–24316.

63. **Kyriakis, J. M., P. Banerjee, E. Nikolakaki, T. Dai, E. A. Rubie, M. F. Ahmad, J. Avruch, and J. R. Woodgett.** 1994. The stress-activated protein kinase subfamily of c-Jun kinases. *Nature* **369:**156–160.

64. **Larson, H. E., F. E. Barclay, P. Honour, and I. D. Hill.** 1982. Epidemiology of *Clostridium difficile* in infants. *J. Infect. Dis.* **146:**727–733.

65. **Larson, H. E., A. B. Price, P. Honour, and S. P. Borriello.** 1978. *Clostridium difficile* and the aetiology of pseudomembranous colitis. *Lancet* **8073:**1063–1066.

66. **Leung, D. Y., C. P. Kelly, M. Boguniewicz, C. Pothoulakis, J. T. LaMont, and A. Flores.** 1991. Treatment with intravenously administered gamma globulin of chronic relapsing colitis induced by *Clostridium difficile* toxin. *J. Pediatr.* **118:**633–637.

67. **Libby, J. M., B. S. Jortner, and T. D. Wilkins.** 1982. Effects of the two toxins of *Clostridium difficile* in antibiotic-associated cecitis in hamsters. *Infect. Immun.* **36:**822–829.

68. **Limaye, A. P., D. K. Turgeon, B. T. Cookson, and T. R. Fritsche.** 2000. Pseudomembranous colitis caused by a toxin A(−) B(+) strain of *Clostridium difficile*. *J. Clin. Microbiol.* **38:**1696–1697.

69. **Linevsky, J., C. Pothoulakis, S. Keates, M. Warny, A. C. Keates, J. T. LaMont, and C. P. Kelly.** 1997. IL-8 release and neutrophil activation by *Clostridium difficile* toxin-exposed monocytes. *Am. J. Physiol.* **273:**G1333–G1340.

70. **Lyerly, D. M., J. L. Johnson, S. M. Frey, and T. D. Wilkins.** 1990. Vaccination against lethal *Clostridium difficile* enterocolitis with a nontoxic recombinant peptide of toxin A. *Curr. Microbiol.* **21:**29–32.

71. **Lyerly, D. M., C. J. Phelps, J. Toth, and T. D. Wilkins.** 1992. Characterization of toxins A and B of *Clostridium difficile* with monoclonal antibodies. *Infect. Immun.* **54:**70–76.

72. **Lyerly, D. M., K. E. Saum, D. K. MacDonald, and T. D. Wilkins.** 1985. Effects of *Clostridium difficile* toxins given intragastrically to animals. *Infect. Immun.* **47:**349–352.

73. **Mackay, D. J. G., and A. Hall.** 1998. Rho GTPases. *J. Biol. Chem.* **273:**20685–20688.

74. **Mani, N., and B. Dupuy.** 2001. Regulation of toxin synthesis in *Clostridium difficile* by an alternative RNA polymerase sigma factor. *Proc. Natl. Acad. Sci. USA* **98:**5844–5849.

75. **McFarland, L. V., M. E. Mulligan, R. Y. Kwok, and W. E. Stamm.** 1989. Nocosomial acquisition of *Clostridium difficile* infection. *N. Engl. J. Med.* **320:**204–210.

76. **Milburn, M. V., L. Tong, A. M. deVos, A. Brunger, Z. Yamaizumi, S. Nishimura, and S. H. Kim.** 1990. Molecular switch for signal transduction: structural differences between active and inactive forms of protooncogenic ras proteins. *Science* **247:**939–945.

77. **Milne, J. C., and R. J. Collier.** 1993. pH-dependent permeabilization of the plasma membrane of mammalian cells by anthrax protective antigen. *Mol. Microbiol.* **10:**647–653.

78. **Mitchell, T. J., J. M. Ketley, S. C. Haslam, J. Stephen, D. W. Burdon, D. C. Candy, and R. Daniel.** 1986. Effect of toxin A and B of *Clostridium difficile* on rabbit ileum and colon. *Gut* **27:**78–85.

79. **Moncrief, J. S., L. A. Barroso, and T. D. Wilkins.** 1997. Positive regulation of *Clostridium difficile* toxins. *Infect. Immun.* **65:**1105–1108.

80. **Moncrief, J. S., L. Zheng, L. M. Neville, and D. M. Lyerly.** 2000. Genetic characterization of toxin A-negative, toxin B-positive *Clostridium difficile* isolates by PCR. *J. Clin Microbiol.* **38:**3072–3075.

81. **Mukaida, N., Y. Mahe, and K. Matsushima.** 1990. Cooperative interaction of nuclear factor-kappa B- and cis-regulatory enhancer binding protein-like factor binding elements in activating the interleukin-8 gene by pro-inflammatory cytokines. *J. Biol. Chem.* **265:**21128–21133.

82. **Nakamura, S., M. Mikawa, S. Nakashio, M. Takabatake, I. Okado, K. Yamakawa, T. Serikawa, S. Okumura, and S. Nishida.** 1981. Isolation of *Clostridium difficile* from the feces and the antibody in sera of young and elderly adults. *Microbiol. Immunol.* **25:**345–351.

83. **Nassar, N., G. Horn, C. Herrmann, A. Scherer, F. McCormick, and A. Wittinghofer.** 1995. The 2.2 A crystal structure of the Ras-binding domain of the serine/threonine kinase c-Raf1 in complex with Rap1A and a GTP analogue. *Nature* **375:**554–560.

84. **Nusrat, A., M. Giry, J. R. Turner, S. P. Colgan, C. A. Parkos, D. Carnes, E. Lemichez, P. Boquet, and J. L. Madara.** 1995. Rho protein regulates tight junctions and perijunctional actin organization in polarized epithelia. *Proc. Natl. Acad. Sci. USA* **92:**10629–10633.

85. **Nusrat, A., C. von Eichel-Streiber, J. R. Turner, P. Verkade, J. L. Madara, and C. A.**

Parkos. 2001. *Clostridium difficile* toxins disrupt epithelial barrier function by altering membrane microdomain localization of tight junction proteins. *Infect. Immun.* **69:**1329–1336.

86. **Pan, Z. K., R. D. Ye, S. C. Christiansen, M. A. Jagels, G. M. Bokoch, and B. L. Zuraw.** 1998. Role of the Rho GTPase in bradykinin-stimulated nuclear factor-κB activation and IL-1beta gene expression in cultured human epithelial cells. *J. Immunol.* **160:**3038–3045.

87. **Perona, R., S. Montaner, L. Saniger, I. Sanchez-Perez, R. Bravo, and J. C. Lacal.** 1997. Activation of the nuclear factor-kB by Rho, CDC42 and Rac-1 proteins. *Gene Dev.* **11:** 463–475.

88. **Pituch, H., N. van den Braak, W. van Leeuwen, A. van Belkum, G. Martirosian, P. Obuch-Woszczatynski, M. Luczak, and F. Meisel-Mikolajczyk.** 2001. Clonal dissemination of a toxin-A-negative/toxin-B-positive *Clostridium difficile* strain from patients with antibiotic-associated diarrhea in Poland. *Clin. Microbiol. Infect.* **8:**442–446.

89. **Popoff, M. R., E. J. Rubin, D. M. Gill, and P. Boquet.** Actin-specific ADP-ribosyltransferase produced by a *Clostridium difficile* strain. *Infect. Immun.* **56:**2299–2306.

90. **Pothoulakis, C.** 1996. Pathogenesis of *Clostridium difficile*-associated diarrhea. *Eur. J. Gastroenterol. Hepatol.* **8:**1041–1047.

91. **Pothoulakis, C., R. J. Gilbert, C. Cladaras, I. Castagliuolo, G. Semenza, Y. Hitti, J. S. Moncrief, J. Linevski, C. P. Kelly, S. Nikulasson, H. P. Desai, T. D. Wilkins, and J. T. LaMont.** 1996. Rabbit sucrase-isomaltase contains a functional receptor for toxins A and B on rabbit ileum. *Gastroenterology* **93:**273–279.

91a. **Pothoulakis, C., R. Sullivan, D. A. Melnick, G. Triadafilopoulos, A.-S. Gadenne, T. Meshulam, and J. T. LaMont.** 1988. *Clostridium difficile* toxin A stimulates intracellular calcium release and chemotactic response in human granulocytes. *J. Clin. Invest.* **81:**1741–1745.

92. **Qa'Dan, M., L. M. Spyres, and J. D. Ballard.** 2000. pH-induced conformational changes in *Clostridium difficile* toxin B. *Infect. Immun.* **68:** 2470–2474.

93. **Rampal, P., J. T. LaMont, and J. C. Trier.** 1978. Differentiation of glycoprotein synthesis in fetal rat colon. *Am. J. Physiol.* **235:**E207–E212.

94. **Riegler, M., R. Sedivy, C. Pothoulakis, G. Hamilton, J. Zacherl, G. Bischof, E. Cosentini, W. Feil, R. Schiessel, J. T. LaMont, and E. Wenzl.** 1995. *Clostridium difficile* toxin B is more potent than toxin A in damaging human colonic epithelium *in vitro*. *J. Clin. Invest.* **95:** 2004–2011.

95. **Rolfe, D. F., and W. Song.** 1993. Purification of a functional receptor for *Clostridium difficile* toxin A from intestinal brush border membranes of infant hamsters. *Clin. Infect. Dis.* **16**(Suppl. 4)**:**S219–S227.

96. **Rupnik, M., V. Avesani, M. Janc, C. von Eichel-Streiber, and M. Delmée.** 1998. A novel toxinotyping scheme and correlation of toxinotypes with serogroups of *Clostridium difficile* isolates. *J. Clin. Microbiol.* **36:**2240–2247.

97. **Salcedo, J., S. Keates, C. Pothoulakis, M. Warny, I. Castagliuolo, J. T. LaMont, and C. P. Kelly.** 1997. Intravenous immunoglobulin therapy for severe *Clostridium difficile* colitis. *Gut* **41:**366–370.

98. **Sambol, S. P., M. M. Merrigan, D. Lyerly, D. N. Gerding, and S. Johnson.** 2000. Toxin gene analysis of a variant strain of *Clostridium difficile* that causes human clinical disease. *Infect. Immun.* **68:**5480–5487.

99. **Sambol, S. P., J. K. Tang, M. M. Merrigan, S. Johnson, and D. N. Gerding.** 2001. Infection of hamsters with epidemiologically important strains of *Clostridium difficile*. *J. Infect. Dis.* **183:**1760–1766.

100. **Savidge, T., W. Pan, P. Newman, M. O'Brien, and C. Pothoulakis.** 2002. *Clostridium difficile* toxin B is an enterotoxin for human intestine in vivo. *Gastroenterology* **122**(Suppl. 1)**:** A76.

101. **Sehr, P., G. Joseph, H. Genth, I. Just, E. Pick, and K. Aktories.** 1998. Glucosylation and ADP ribosylation of rho proteins: effects on nucleotide binding, GTPase activity, and effector coupling. *Biochemistry* **37:**5296–5304.

102. **Smith, J. A., D. L. Cooke, S. Hyde, S. P. Borriello, and R. G. Long.** 1997. *Clostridium difficile* toxin A binding to human intestinal epithelial cells. *J. Med. Microbiol.* **46:**953–958.

103. **Tan, K. S., B. Y. Wee, and K. P. Song.** 2001. Evidence for holin function of *tcdE* gene in the pathogenicity of *Clostridium difficile*. *J. Med. Microbiol.* **50:**613–619.

104. **Teramoto, H., P. Crespo, O. A. Coso, T. Igishi, N. Xu, and J. S. Gutkind.** 1996. The small GTP-binding protein rho activates c-Jun N-terminal kinases/stress-activated protein kinases in human kidney 293T cells. Evidence for a Pak-independent signaling pathway. *J. Biol. Chem.* **271:**25731–25734.

105. **Triadafilopoulos, G., C. Pothoulakis, M. J. O'Brien, and J. T. LaMont.** 1987. Differential effects of *Clostridium difficile* toxins A and B on rabbit ileum. *Gastroenterology* **93:**273–279.

106. **Tucker, K. D., P. F. Carring, and T. D. Wilkins.** 1990. Toxin A of *Clostridium difficile*

is a potent cytotoxin. *J. Clin. Microbiol.* **28:**869–871.

107. **Tucker, K. D., and T. C. Wilkins.** 1991. Toxin A of *Clostridium difficile* binds to the human carbohydrate antigens I, X, and Y. *Infect. Immun.* **59:**73–78.

108. **Viscidi, R., B. E. Laughon, R. Yolken, P. Bo-Linn, T. Moench, R. W. Ryder, and J. G. Bartlett.** 1983. Serum antibody response to toxins A and B of *Clostridium difficile. J. Infect. Dis.* **148:**93–100.

109. **Viscidi, R., S. Willey, and J. G. Bartlett.** 1981. Isolation rates and toxigenic potential of *Clostridium difficile* isolates from various patient populations. *Gastroenterology* **81:**5–9.

110. **von Eichel-Streiber, C., P. Boquet, M. Sauerborn, and M. Thelestam.** 1996. Large clostridial cytotoxins—a family of glycosyltransferases modifying small GTP-binding proteins. *Trends Microbiol.* **4:**375–382.

111. **von Eichel-Streiber, C., R. Laufenberg-Feldmann, S. Sartingen, J. Schulze, and M. Sauerborn.** 1992. Comparative sequence analysis of the *Clostridium difficile* toxins A and B. *Mol. Gen. Genet.* **233:**260–268.

112. **von Eichel-Streiber, C., I. Zec-Pirnat, M. Grabnar, and M. A. Rupnik.** 1999. A nonsense mutation abrogates production of a functional enterotoxin A in *Clostridium difficile* toxinotype VIII strains of serogroups F and X. *FEMS Microbiol. Lett.* **178:**163–168.

113. **Warny, M., B. Chatelain, and M. Delmee.** 1996. Effect of *Clostridium difficile* toxin A on CD11/CD18 expression *in vitro. Clin. Diagn. Lab. Immunol.* **3:**605–607.

114. **Warny, M., C. Denie, M. Delmee, and C. Lefebvre.** 1995. Gamma globulin administration in relapsing *Clostridium difficile*-induced pseudomembranous colitis with a defective antibody response to toxin A. *Acta Clin. Belg.* **50:**36–39.

115. **Warny, M., A. C. Keates, S. Keates, A. Qamar, I. Castagliuolo, J. Zacks, C. Pothoulakis, J. T. LaMont, and C. P. Kelly.** 2000. p38^{MAPK} activation by *Clostridium difficile* toxin A mediates monocyte necrosis, IL-8 production and enteritis. *J. Clin. Invest.* **105:**1147–1156.

116. **Warny, M., and C. P. Kelly.** 1999. Monocytic cell necrosis is mediated by potassium depletion and caspase-like proteases. *Am. J. Physiol.* **276:**C717–C724.

117. **Warny, M., J. P. Vaerman, V. Avesani, and M. Delmée.** 1994. Human antibody response to *Clostridium difficile* toxin A in relation to clinical course of infection. *Infect. Immun.* **62:**384–389.

118. **Yamakawa, K., T. Karasawa, T. Ohta, H. Hayashi, and S. Nakamura.** 1998. Inhibition of enhanced toxin production by *Clostridium difficile* in biotin-limited conditions. *J. Med. Microbiol.* **47:**767–771.

VIRAL PATHOGENS OF THE INTESTINE

Mary K. Estes and Robert L. Atmar

28

Viral infections of the gastrointestinal tract generally lead to acute gastroenteritis, a common illness that affects people and animals of all ages worldwide in both epidemic and endemic forms. Acute viral gastroenteritis is a major cause of infant morbidity and mortality in developed and developing countries, respectively. The outcome of infection frequently differs according to the country where such infections occur, with children in areas that lack access to medical treatment, such as developing countries, facing life-threatening dehydration and death. In the United States, viral gastroenteritis is second to respiratory diseases in frequency as a cause of acute illness. In the developing world, the impact of diarrheal diseases on infant mortality and malnutrition continues to be significant. Globally, dehydrating diarrhea caused by rotavirus infection is responsible for 6% of all deaths of children under the age of 5 years (77).

Several different viruses are now recognized to be etiologic agents of viral gastroenteritis in humans (Table 1). The agents (rotavirus, calicivirus, astrovirus, enteric adenovirus, Aichi virus [a picornavirus]) belong to distinct virus families, yet the clinical symptoms caused by these viruses are not sufficiently distinct to permit diagnosis based on symptoms alone (2, 26, 75). Instead, an examination of stools collected early after symptoms begin is needed to permit detection of viral particles by electron microscopy, of viral antigen by enzyme-linked immunoassays or latex agglutination, or of viral genome by reverse transcription PCR (RT-PCR) or PCR, to determine the specific etiologic agent causing disease.

Knowing the viral etiologic agent of cases of gastroenteritis can be important to rule out a bacterial cause of disease and to avoid unnecessary use of antibiotics, even though no specific therapies are currently available to treat virus-induced disease. Instead, supportive rehydration therapy will lead to recovery unless unexpected complications arise. The clinical severity of disease caused by, and the prevalence of, the gastroenteritis viruses make it important to understand how these viruses spread and cause disease, and argue for the development of vaccines against some of these agents.

Mary K. Estes, Departments of Molecular Virology and Microbiology and Medicine, Texas Gulf Coast Digestive Diseases Center, Baylor College of Medicine, 1 Baylor Plaza Mailstop BCM-385, Houston, TX 77030-3498. *Robert L. Atmar*, Departments of Medicine and Molecular Virology and Microbiology, Baylor College of Medicine, Houston, TX 77030-3498.

Microbial Pathogenesis and the Intestinal Epithelial Cell, ed. by G. Hecht
© 2003 ASM Press, Washington, D.C.

TABLE 1 Viral gastroenteritis in humans[a]

Characteristics	Etiological agent				
	Rotavirus	Calicivirus	Astrovirus	Enteric adenovirus	Aichi virus
Virus family	*Reoviridae*	*Caliciviridae*	*Astroviridae*	*Adenoviridae*	*Picornaviridae*
Genome	Segmented double-stranded RNA	Single-stranded RNA	Single-stranded RNA	Double-stranded DNA	Single-stranded RNA
Cultivable	Yes	No[b]	Yes	Yes	Yes
Symptoms					
Vomiting	80–100%	80–100%	80–100%	50–80%	Yes
Diarrhea	100% (moderate to severe)	50–60% (moderate to severe)	80–100% (mild)	80–100% (moderate)	Yes
Abdominal pain	Little	Severe	Moderate	Moderate	Yes
Fever	80–90%	Mild and rare	80–100%	Mild	Not reported
Respiratory symptoms	Common	Rare	Rare	Common	Detected
Age	6 months to 2 years[c]	All ages	Children < 5 years[d]	2 to 10 years	Children and adults
Antibody acquisition	100% by age 5	100% by age 5[e]	50 to 80% by age 5[f]	50% by age 4	>80% by age 35
Occurrence	Predominantly winter[g]	Endemic and epidemic	Endemic	Endemic	Not known
Duration of illness	3 to 7 days	24 to 48 h	2 to 3 days	Up to 25 days	2 to 3 days
Duration of shedding	Up to 15 days	>15 days			Not known
Dehydration	Common	Rare	Rare	Rare	Rare
Incubation period	12 to 96 h	12 to 36 h	3 to 5 days[h]	8 to 10 days	Not known
Transmission	Fecal-oral, fomites; water, nosocomial	Fecal-oral; water and food	Fecal-oral; water and food	Fecal-oral; nosocomial?	Fecal-oral; food (oysters)
Therapy	Oral rehydration	None or rare[i]	None or rare[i]	None[i]	None[i]

[a] All these viruses can cause chronic infections in immunocompromised individuals.
[b] Human caliciviruses remain noncultivatable. Some animal enteric caliciviruses are cultivatable under special conditions.
[c] Symptomatic infection in children, primarily of 6 months to 2 years of age, but infections can be asymptomatic in neonates or adults. Elderly may develop symptomatic infections.
[d] Adults may be infected later in life.
[e] Seroprevalence studies differ depending on type of study. Seroprevalence in developed countries may be lower (80% by age 20).
[f] Antibodies may wane late in life, making adults and the elderly susceptible to additional symptomatic infection.
[g] Rotavirus infections occur all year round in tropical countries. Rotavirus infection peaks in winter in developed countries but outbreaks may occur all year round.
[h] Incubation period in adult volunteers; incubation period in children may be only 1 to 2 days.
[i] Illness is generally self-limiting, but occasionally, oral rehydration is required.

526

Rotaviruses and caliciviruses are currently recognized as the etiologic agents of greatest medical and epidemiologic importance for humans (10), and this article summarizes current information on the epidemiology and consequences of infection with these viruses. Other viruses cause disease in animals (coronaviruses, picobirnaviruses, pestiviruses, toroviruses), but they have not yet been clearly associated with disease in humans and are not considered further in this chapter. Cytomegalovirus and the human immunodeficiency virus (HIV) (the cause of AIDS) can also infect cells in the intestine and lead to symptomatic infections. Although these infections can lead to severe, chronic diseases with both mucosal and systemic complications, they are not generally considered gastrointestinal (GI) viruses. The proceedings from a recent meeting on gastroenteritis viruses covers these and other GI viruses not discussed elsewhere in this chapter (6, 18).

Much of this chapter focuses on information about the pathophysiology of rotavirus-induced disease because this disease is the best understood at present. The reader should realize that lack of study of the other GI viruses does not imply that these pathogens do not cause important disease or serve as excellent models for understanding the unique aspects of virus-host intestinal cell interactions or the mechanisms of virus replication and pathogenesis.

ROTAVIRUS INFECTIONS OF THE INTESTINE

Epidemiology of Rotavirus Infections

Rotaviruses infect virtually every child in the world, illustrating that improvements in sanitation have not changed the risk to children of severe viral gastroenteritis. Newborns can be infected but rarely have disease, suggesting that maternally derived antibody offers protection against disease. The peak age of disease differs according to country, with children in developing countries generally becoming ill earlier, often between 3 and 6 months of age. In developed countries, children become ill later, frequently between 6 and 24 months of age. These differences in age of onset of disease may be important considerations in the development of vaccination strategies to induce protective immunity in different settings. Disease, including death, may be more severe in children in developing countries where they frequently suffer malnutrition and other concurrent infections, including HIV (16). More than 600,000 children are estimated to die annually worldwide from rotavirus infections. In the United States, it is estimated that 2% of infected children are hospitalized at a minimal cost of $1 billion annually.

Rotavirus Structure and Classification

Rotaviruses are large, complex viruses that consist of a nonenveloped protein capsid composed of three concentric protein shells, which surround the genome made up of 11 segments of double-stranded RNA (Color Plate 8). Each protein shell is composed of a single, distinct structural protein (called, respectively, viral protein VP2, VP6, and VP7). Dimeric spikes composed of the viral protein VP4 emanate from the surface of particles, and these spikes are the protein that initially binds to cells and that must be cleaved by trypsin to allow virus penetration into the cytoplasm of cells. The virus particle carries within it an RNA-dependent RNA polymerase (VP1) and a capping enzyme (VP3), located as complexes inside particles at the fivefold axes. Removal of the outer capsid layer occurs, in a poorly understood process, in conjunction with virus entry into cells and activates the endogenous polymerase that then synthesizes mRNAs copied from each genome segment (Color Plate 8, step e) to produce viral proteins. Expression of viral proteins leads to diverse virus-host protein interactions that affect cell function, including usurping of the cellular machinery to replicate the viral genome, translate viral proteins, and encapsidate newly made viral RNA into assembling viral particles. These events occur in an ordered cascade regulated by mechanisms that remain poorly understood.

Rotaviruses are genetically diverse viruses that are classified according to the antigenic properties of their capsid proteins or the sequences of the genes that code for these proteins. Rotaviruses are first classified into antigenic groups, and seven groups (A through G) have been described. Viruses within a group can undergo genetic exchange of genome segments. The group A rotaviruses are those that cause life-threatening disease in children and animals. This chapter considers information about group A rotaviruses. Rotavirus strains are further classified into serotypes according to the antigenic properties of the two outer capsid proteins. At present, 14 VP7 glycoprotein (G) serotypes and 20 P (protease-sensitive VP4) serotypes are known. Different properties of these outer capsid proteins are important and relevant to how a rotavirus initiates infection of epithelial cells.

Outcome of Rotavirus Infections

Clinical Course and Transmission of Rotavirus Infection. Rotavirus infection produces a spectrum of responses that vary from subclinical infection to mild diarrhea to severe, dehydrating diarrhea. The clinical signs of rotavirus infection include watery diarrhea, anorexia, depression, dehydration, and vomiting. The duration of illness ranges from 1 to 9 days. Deaths attributed to rotavirus infection result from severe dehydration secondary to the loss of fluids from diarrhea and vomiting. Diarrhea is observed in natural infections in most species, but is variable in animal models where heterologous virus infections, based on inoculating viruses isolated from one species into another species, are frequently studied. Other signs of infection include low-grade fever and abdominal distention. Respiratory symptoms are frequent in children, but these are likely caused by concurrent respiratory infections that occur commonly in children.

Respiratory symptoms have not been reported in animals infected with rotavirus. Failure to thrive is reported in children in developing countries where rotavirus infection may exacerbate malnutrition or be synergistic with other enteropathogens. Lack of weight gain has also been documented in domestic animals and in rotavirus-infected animal models (7, 84). The initial rotavirus infection is generally symptomatic, with subsequent infections being clinically less severe. Immunity develops with multiple infections, and most children with more than three infections are no longer susceptible to clinical disease, although reinfected children shed virus and can spread the infection and disease.

The incubation period of rotavirus infection varies from 12 h to several days. Virus particles are observed in stools or intestinal contents as early as 12 h postinfection and may persist or be shed for variable lengths of time (from 1 to 15 days). Virus can be shed in large amounts (up to 10^{10} particles per g of feces), and shedding can precede diarrhea or persist beyond the cessation of disease. Immunocompromised children or animals become chronically infected and shed virus for months. Frequently, the virus shed in such circumstances undergoes genetic alterations that can be detected by analysis of the migration of the 11 segments of double-stranded RNA following electrophoresis on polyacrylamide or agarose gels.

The capsid structure of rotavirus is stable, and large quantities of virions may contaminate the environment, leading to transmission. Infection is spread by direct fecal-oral contact or through fomites. Because high concentrations of virus are shed, and the minimal infectious dose is low (<1 to 100 tissue culture infectious units), minimal environmental contamination is able to transmit infection. Asymptomatic infections also occur frequently and likely contribute to transmission. Rotavirus infections frequently are acquired as nosocomial infections in children hospitalized for other reasons.

Tropisms and Pathologic Lesions in Rotavirus Infection. Rotaviruses replicate in the cytoplasm of non–dividing mature enterocytes of the villus epithelium of the small intestine (Fig. 1, left panel). This tropism suggests that differentiated enterocytes express factors required for efficient viral infection and replication. It is unknown whether differentiation of villus enterocytes results in expression of a viral receptor or other cell products that allow permissive replication.

Pathologic changes induced by rotavirus infections are almost exclusively limited to enterocytes in the small intestine. Cytolytic changes occur in infected villus enterocytes; in severe disease, sloughing of enterocytes may expose the basement membrane at the villus tips. Blunting and atrophy of villi are common, and villus fusion may occur in some species. In severe infection in some species (rabbits, piglets, possibly children), villi may be blunted with significant reductions in villus height and crypt cell ratios. This change results in a relative loss of absorptive cells and an increase in secretory cells, producing changes in gut homeostasis. A hallmark of viral infections of the intestine is that they do not produce a significant inflammatory response, and only mild mononuclear infiltration of the lamina propria is usually observed. Histopathologic changes typically appear within 24 h of infection and are maximal between 24 and 72 h postinfection. These pathologic lesions are generally first seen *after* diarrhea has begun, and similar pathologic lesions occur during subclinical infections, indicating that the observed pathology is not fully responsible for the diarrheal disease. In rodents, blunting of villi is not observed; instead, vacuolization of enterocytes is common.

The anatomic segment (duodenum> jejunum>ileum) of the small intestine affected by rotavirus infection varies between species and between homologous and heterologous infections. The significance of these differences is not understood. In pigs and lambs, the most pronounced lesions are seen in the distal intestine (jejunum, ileum), while the proximal intestine (duodenum, jejunum) is infected in calves, with changes being seen throughout the length of the small intestine. In mice, the most pronounced changes are in the proximal to middle small intestine, and lesions in rabbits are seen throughout the small intestine. In calves and mice, infection begins proximally and proceeds distally.

Rotavirus-induced lesions in the small intestine of some animals (piglets, calves, lambs, rabbits) appear to be the direct result of damage to epithelial cells caused by viral replication, because the sites of replication correlate with the sites of lesions. A correlation of replication sites with lesions in rodents (mice and rats) is less clear because the pathologic lesions and virus replication are limited. The virtual absence of histologic changes and evidence of viral replication by immunocytochemical staining or electron microscopy in the small intestine of mice (except for the appearance of vacuolated cells), in conjunction with frank, watery diarrhea in rodents, led to the recognition that mechanisms other than malabsorption are responsible for the diarrhea.

Rotavirus–Cell Interactions

Cultured Epithelial Cells. Initial information about rotavirus-cell interactions came from studies of viruses easily cultured in monkey kidney cells. These studies showed that rotaviruses replicate in the cell cytoplasm, infection shuts off host-protein synthesis, and production of maximum yields of virus requires the presence of trypsin in the medium of cells. Rotaviruses exhibit a unique process of morphogenesis, which involves budding of newly made virus particles into the lumen of the endoplasmic reticulum (ER) where further maturation results in the loss of a transient envelope and lysis of cells releases virus particles. The nonstructural protein NSP4 is important in this unique budding process. This process mimics what is seen in electron micrographs of thin sections of biopsies of enterocytes from

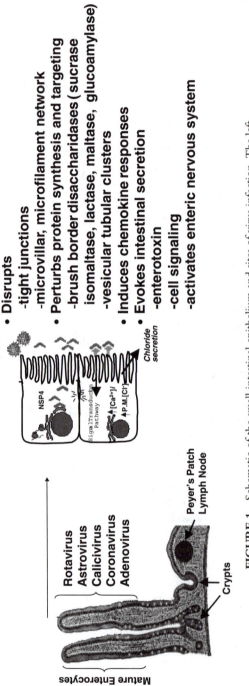

FIGURE 1 Schematic of the small intestinal epithelium and sites of virus infection. The left panel shows the locations of cells infected by specific GI viruses. The right panel shows the release of the viral enterotoxin from infected cells that can affect neighboring uninfected epithelial cells, and outlines the effects of rotavirus infection of mature enterocytes.

children with rotavirus-induced gastroenteritis, where the lumen of the ER is frequently expanded and full of enveloped and nonenveloped virus particles.

Recent studies have recognized that the large body of initial work on cultured rotaviruses examined a minority of rotaviruses that share a property of their spike protein, such that it possesses the ability to bind to neuraminidase-sensitive sialic acid (SA) molecules on cells. These neuraminidase-sensitive (previously called SA dependent) viruses grow readily in cell culture, and they may initiate infection by mechanisms that are distinct from the majority of rotaviruses, including all human rotaviruses, that are neuraminidase insensitive (previously called SA independent). Studies of replication of neuraminidase-insensitive rotaviruses are now being pursued, but such studies are more difficult because of lower virus yields.

The initial interaction of virus with cells requires the VP4 spike protein, and while virus binding does not require a cleaved VP4, penetration of virus into cells requires cleavage of this protein. Trypsin cleaves the spike protein into two cleavage products, an N-terminal fragment, VP8*, the hemagglutinin, and a C-terminal fragment, VP5*, which permeabilizes membranes in vitro; both VP5* and VP8* remain associated with the virus particle. Electron cryomicroscopy of trypsin-treated and untreated virions demonstrates that trypsinization confers icosahedral ordering to the spike (14), and biochemical studies show that cleavage induces a conformational change which induces dimerization of the VP5* region that may be needed for virus penetration into cells (20). Binding of neuraminidase-sensitive rotavirus strains to cells is initially mediated by VP8* through SA residues, and then by VP5*, whereas binding of neuraminidase-insensitive rotavirus strains is thought to be mediated directly by VP5* (82). The structure of VP8* from a neuraminidase-sensitive strain has been shown to possess a galectin fold in which the galectin binding site is blocked, and instead the molecule contains a novel carbohydrate binding site for SA binding (21). It is proposed that the rotavirus spike protein arose by the insertion of a host-derived, galectin-like carbohydrate binding domain into an ancestral membrane interaction protein, and these molecular events might have been accompanied by significant changes in viral tropism and pathogenicity (21). It remains to be seen if the structure of the spike of the neuraminidase-insensitive spikes is remarkably different, which might explain some of the distinct properties of replication of different rotavirus strains.

Polarized Epithelial Cells. In 1997, new ideas evolved about how rotavirus replicates in cells based on studies of virus infection of polarized intestinal epithelial cells grown on filters (42). Differential infection of these cells is observed depending on whether the infecting virus is neuraminidase sensitive or insensitive. Neuraminidase-sensitive viruses infect polarized cells through the apical surface while neuraminidase-insensitive strains infect cells through the apical or basolateral surfaces (9). All rotavirus strains tested are released from the apical plasma membrane, and, unexpectedly, virus release occurs prior to cell lysis by a nonclassical vesicular transport that bypasses the Golgi apparatus (42). The rotavirus spike protein VP4 has been shown to be targeted to the plasma membrane and becomes associated with membrane microdomains enriched in cholesterol and sphingolipids, also termed rafts, early after infection; other structural proteins are found in rafts within cells together with NSP4, the protein required for the final stage of virus assembly (71). Rafts contain infectious virus, and thus, a new model of rotavirus assembly is emerging that suggests that in polarized cells, final virus assembly may occur within rafts at the plasma membrane. It is possible that the VP8* lectin-like domain in the spike protein carries a raft-interacting function and that the cytoplasmic VP4 may follow a pathway to the plasma membrane, as does the cytosolic lectin, galectin 4 (36). The precise origin and properties of the cellular compartment that contains the rafts that will interact with VP4 and the ER, to accomplish the final assembly step, remain to be identified.

Infected epithelial cells respond to infection by changing their patterns of expressed genes. The cellular response to rotavirus infection has been studied by identifying changes in specific cellular proteins based on analyzing individual cellular proteins or mRNA levels and by using proteonomics. These first methods showed that rotavirus induces structural and functional alterations in the host cell, and some, but not all, responses require active viral replication. A reduction in cellular protein synthesis, changes in intracellular calcium homeostasis associated with virus maturation and possibly related to cell death, increases in the levels of two endoplasmic reticulum-resident chaperones (GRP78 and GRP94), changes in the organization of the cell cytoskeleton, structural and functional alternations in tight junctions, impaired targeting of some cellular plasma membrane proteins (such as sucrase isomaltase but not dipeptidyl peptidase IV), and induction of signaling pathways (including NF-κB involved in regulation of chemokines such as interleukin-8 [IL-8], interferons, and cytokines) have been reported (Fig. 1, right panel). Some of these cellular responses are thought to be important in pathogenesis, whereas others may be critical for the induction of host immune responses.

Microarray technology is beginning to be used to identify global changes in gene expression patterns in rotavirus-infected human intestinal epithelial cells (15). This first study examined gene regulation in Caco-2 cells in response to infection with a neuraminidase-sensitive rotavirus strain. Of more than 8,000 human transcripts in Caco-2 cells, 6.7% were regulated at 16 h postinfection, with the majority (74%) being upregulated genes. Several of these genes were expected on the basis of previous functional studies of cellular responses. Possible new insights from these studies are that rotavirus may have a specific viral mechanism to counter the interferon re-

sponse of the host cell, and upregulated cellular S100 proteins may participate in the Ca^{2+}-dependent disorganization of the cytoskeleton observed after virus infection. Future studies with other rotavirus neuraminidase-insensitive strains, with mutant virus strains, and with cells engineered to express specific viral genes should help delineate which components of the viral replication cycle (binding, entry, transcription and translation, assembly) are responsible for the observed cellular responses, which viral genes mediate these changes, and whether the transcriptional response program identified in cultured cells is representative of changes seen in the intestine in vivo.

Immune Cells. Rotavirus elicits protective immunity in children and most animal models in the absence of induction of intestinal inflammation. The lack of inflammation is a hallmark of most GI viral infections, and understanding the mechanisms that regulate the induction of such intestinal immunity is important for trying to induce protective mucosal immunity in general. In all models, the induction of intestinal antibody is a clear correlate of protective immunity. The mechanisms of protection differ according to whether one studies natural infection with replicating virus, where induction of intestinal immunoglobulin A (IgA) correlates with immunity, or vaccination with nonreplicating virus or virus-like particles, where induction of intestinal IgG occurs. The protein(s) targeted by protective intestinal antibody remains to be elucidated, and identifying such targets is a high priority since it should provide a clear correlate of protection that is needed to facilitate testing of new candidate vaccines.

Rotavirus-specific antibody can be induced in T-cell receptor-deficient mice that lack functional T cells, suggesting that rotavirus functions as a T-cell-independent antigen (25). Massive B-cell activation in gut-associated lymphoid tissues is an early cellular response to rotavirus infection, and this T-cell-independent response results in an early antibody response (4, 79). Identification of the virus proteins required to activate B cells and the cell signaling that leads to antibody induction without T cells could contribute to the development of vaccines against rotavirus and other viruses that infect across mucosal surfaces. The rotavirus spike protein has been shown to bind to cellular tumor necrosis factor receptor-associated factors and elicit NF-κB signaling (43). It remains unknown if this property is important as part of the epithelial cell response or induction of immunity, or both.

Pathophysiology of Rotaviral Gastroenteritis

Factors That Influence the Clinical Outcome of Rotavirus Infection. Variation in clinical outcome is associated with properties of both the host and a particular virus strain. There are several stages in enteric virus pathogenesis, including virus entry into the host, primary replication, local or disseminated host cellular responses (that may involve cell signaling), possible spread of virus locally or systemically, a host immune response that clears shed virus, and possible cell injury leading to pathology. For all species, some virus strains are found to be highly virulent while others cause less disease and are avirulent. Virulence has been associated with properties of several individual genes of the 11 genes of rotavirus (the genes that encode the structural proteins VP3, VP4, VP6, and VP7, and the genes that encode the nonstructural proteins NSP1, NSP2, NSP3, and NSP4), but the basis for these properties is understood for only some of the genes. Thus, VP4 is the spike protein that is needed for adsorption/penetration into cells. VP7 is a second outer capsid protein that also likely functions in virus entry into cells. The roles of most of the nonstructural proteins are not well understood, with the exception of the nonstructural glycoprotein NSP4. This protein is important for virus assembly and can function as an enterotoxin to stimulate diarrhea. The other nonstructural

proteins play a role in virus replication and likely affect the efficiency of virus replication or the host response to infection. NSP1 can interact with the interferon regulatory factor 3, and this may downregulate the host interferon response (26a).

The severity and location of rotavirus infection vary in different animal species and between studies (11, 30). These differences result from many factors, including the inoculum used (virus strain and dose), immune status of the host, host age at infection, and host intestinal physiology. In animal models where infection-naive animals can be infected, disease is age dependent. In small animals (mice, rats, rabbits), disease is restricted to infections that occur within the first 2 weeks of life. Infections occur throughout life. Disease is also age dependent in large animals (piglets and cows), and the peak of disease in children occurs between the ages of 6 months and 2 years. Studies in children are limited because of the difficulty and lack of clinical need to obtain biopsies from infants and small children and the inability to determine the exact time of natural infections. Rotavirus infections have been reported to occur repeatedly in humans from birth to old age, but the majority of infections after the first 2 years of life are asymptomatic or associated with mild disease. In humans, the age-related resistance to rotavirus-induced diarrhea is thought to be mediated by acquired immunity, but it is not possible to directly test whether humans also exhibit an age-dependent resistance to disease based on other cellular factors such as intestinal development and maturation. Currently, our best understanding of the pathophysiology comes from studies in animal models.

Mechanisms of Rotavirus-Induced Diarrhea

Rotaviruses cause disease by several mechanisms. Proposed mechanisms by which rotaviruses induce diarrhea include malabsorption secondary to enterocyte death, villus ischemia, the induction of secretion by the activity of a virus-encoded enterotoxin, and activation of the enteric nervous system. Diarrhea likely acts as a mechanism of host defense by the intestinal epithelium to "flush" organisms from the intestinal microenvironment. Alternatively, the induction of diarrhea by rotavirus is a survival mechanism exploited by the virus to assure escape from attack by the host and to ensure transmission of virus to new hosts. The relative importance of each of these mechanisms depends on a variety of viral and host factors.

Malabsorption. A number of studies have shown that rotavirus infection can lead to malabsorption due to destruction of enterocytes. This mechanism is based on the observation that histopathologic changes are seen in the intestines of rotavirus-infected animals and loss of enterocytes is associated with depressed levels of mucosal disaccharidases. In addition, diarrhea lessens if feeding of milk is stopped. While malabsorption clearly plays a role in rotavirus-induced diarrhea, it does not seem to be responsible for the initiation of disease, which occurs *prior* to any histologic changes in most animal models. Recently, rotavirus infection of cultured, polarized epithelial cells has been shown to inhibit the transport of disaccharidases to the cell surface in the absence of cell death (41), suggesting that mechanisms in addition to direct cell killing may play a role in malabsorption. Expression of the rotavirus enterotoxin alone in cultured cells can also inhibit cellular protein transport to the cell surface (78).

Diarrhea Resulting from Villus Ischemia. In mice, villus ischemia has been observed with rotavirus infection. Because of the lack of significant enterocyte damage, it was proposed that diarrhea might result from the virus-induced release of an unknown vasoactive substance from infected epithelial cells, causing local ischemia and subsequent functional damage to, but not loss of, enterocytes (57). The general significance of this observation is not known because ischemia has not been seen in other models. However, this

proposal has received renewed interest because of the description of a rotavirus-encoded enterotoxin.

Induction of Intestinal Secretion by Enterotoxin Action. The rotavirus enterotoxin was discovered by serendipity when investigators observed that mice get diarrhea after they are injected with a 22-amino-acid synthetic peptide from the nonstructural glycoprotein NSP4 of the simian rotavirus SA11 (3). This peptide and the full-length NSP4 protein can each induce age-dependent diarrhea in a dose-dependent manner in mice and rats, and chloride secretion is induced in intestinal mucosa as measured in classical electrophysiologic Ussing chamber experiments. The diarrhea mimics that seen following infection of mice with virulent, live rotavirus, and the enterotoxin activity of NSP4 from other rotavirus strains has been confirmed by others (35, 48). Recent data from in vivo and in vitro studies of NSP4 indicate that rotavirus replication in enterocytes produces and releases NSP4 from virus-infected cells (83). This extracellular NSP4 activates a signaling pathway that leads to chloride secretion by mobilization of intracellular calcium and regulation of a calcium-activated chloride channel (19, 23, 68). Extracellular or intracellular NSP4 may further contribute to diarrhea by affecting enterocyte function by altering paracellular permeability and intracellular actin distribution (73). NSP4 can also affect trafficking and functions of cellular proteins (34, 78). Antibody to NSP4 can reduce both the occurrence and the severity of virus-induced diarrhea in neonatal mice, confirming that this protein plays a significant role in the pathogenesis of the diarrhea (3, 80). Finally, NSP4 is a novel secretory agonist because it can cause diarrhea in cystic fibrosis transmembrane regulator (CFTR) knockout mice that do not respond to other classical c-AMP-mediated secretogogues, such as cholera toxin (49, 50). NSP4 appears to be a key component of the pathogenic process, because many of the properties of NSP4 mimic effects associated with rotavirus infection of polarized epithelial cells (5, 41, 55).

Induction of Intestinal Secretion by Activation of the Enteric Nervous System. Treatment of mice undergoing rotavirus-induced diarrhea with drugs that inhibit enteric nervous system functions has been shown to affect the secretory state of the infected mucosa (45). These results are of interest because they suggest that there may be common mechanisms of pathogenesis for viral and bacterial diarrheas (such as cholera) where the enteric nervous system has previously been shown to play a role. The studies in rotavirus-infected mice examined responses from tissues tested in Ussing chambers, and potential difference and net fluid transport were measured. The results showed that rotavirus increases fluid secretion, and this effect was significantly attenuated by pretreatment of the intestinal segments with tetrodotoxin, a blocker of sodium channels; lidocaine, a local anesthetic; or mesalamine, a ganglionic blocker. Rotavirus-induced diarrhea was also inhibited when lidocaine was given intraperitoneally in awake animals, confirming the in vitro effect of nerve blockers in this study. The tissues examined were from mice 48 to 60 h postinoculation, so the role of the enteric nervous system in the induction of the early diarrhea remains to be elucidated. Analysis of the data suggested that approximately two-thirds of the rotavirus-induced secretion could be attributed to enteric nerves. The mechanism of this response was not elucidated, so the mediators that activate the enteric nervous system in rotavirus-induced disease have yet to be identified.

Treatment and Control of Rotavirus-Induced Diarrhea

Current management of rotavirus-induced diarrhea is supportive, with rehydration therapy being the principal treatment. Oral rehydration therapy is usually sufficient, but intravenous rehydration produces more rapid responses. In some cases, oral Igs have been used for treatment, with good effects if preparations contain high antibody titers of specific neutralizing antibodies for rotavirus (31, 58). However, such treatments are expensive, reducing their general availability. Another, more affordable treatment option is the use of probiotics (65). The realization that rotavirus-induced diarrhea is caused by secretion in addition to malabsorption, and that altered paracellular pathways may contribute to pathogenesis, may alter future treatment strategies. Although the enterotoxin and enteric nervous system effects have not been definitively proven to participate in disease induction in children, successful treatment of children with racecadotril, an enkephalinase inhibitor with antisecretory and antidiarrheal actions, is consistent with the involvement of secretory pathways mediated by enterotoxins or neurotransmitters (70).

The impact of rotavirus disease on children in both developed and developing countries documents the need for development of an effective vaccine. After more than 15 years of development and clinical trials, a live-attenuated rhesus rotavirus-tetravalent vaccine called RotaShield (Wyeth Laboratories, Inc., Marietta, Pa.) was licensed in the United States in August 1998. Unfortunately, after more than 1 million doses had been administered, the vaccine was removed from the market because of the rare association of the vaccine with intussusception (a bowel obstruction in which one segment of the bowel becomes enfolded within another segment) (51, 66). It is not known whether intussusception is associated with natural rotavirus infections or if intussusception will be a problem with all live rotavirus vaccines. Nevertheless, live rotavirus vaccines based on different virus strains are continuing to be evaluated in field trials.

The occurrence of intussusception as a rare, temporally related event with the rotavirus vaccine has introduced new complications in the development of an effective vaccine for children, especially in the developing world where the vaccine is needed most to reduce high mortality rates. Future licensure of additional live candidate vaccines will require large field trials. Additionally, efficacy trials must be carried out simultaneously in developed and developing countries to permit the performance of risk-benefit analyses in different global settings.

Development of alternative vaccination strategies, e.g., virus-like particles (VLPs), vector-expressed proteins, and an enterotoxin vaccine, continues to be pursued. The strongest preclinical data involve VLPs because these nonreplicating particles are immunogenic and able to induce protective immunity in several animal models (8, 12, 13, 38, 46, 53, 54, 81). Phase 1 safety and immunogenicity studies of VLP vaccines should now proceed in humans.

Need for Further Understanding of Rotavirus-Induced Disease

The induction of intussusception by the tetravalent vaccine emphasizes the need to better understand the mechanisms of rotavirus pathogenesis, including details of the molecular interactions between rotavirus and epithelial and immune cells of the GI tract. A new animal model of intussusception suggests that rotavirus may be a cofactor in enhancing intussusception induced by lipopolysaccharide (LPS), and viral replication associated with induction of lymphoid hyperplasia is essential for this effect (K. L. Warfield, S. E. Blutt, S. E. Crawford, G. Kang, R. L. Ward, and M. E. Conner, submitted for publication). Understanding the molecules associated with the enhancement of LPS-induced intussusception in this model, and the determination of whether similar mechanisms occur in children with intussusception, may lead to new ways to evaluate and treat children with intussusception. New information is needed regarding the ways in which the rotaviruses affect intestinal epithelial cells and how epithelial and immune cell responses and signaling influence the outcome of an infection. Some of these responses are likely important for the induction of immunity, whereas others contribute to pathogenesis. Understanding these dynamic interactions should facilitate development of more effective and safer rotavirus vaccines and treatments.

CALICIVIRUS INFECTIONS OF THE INTESTINE

Epidemiology of Calicivirus Infections

Our understanding of the importance, epidemiology, and natural history of calicivirus infections has been changing rapidly since the genome of Norwalk virus was cloned (39). This accomplishment led to the cloning of other calicivirus genomes and resulted in the development of new, sensitive molecular diagnostic techniques able to be used to detect these viruses in large epidemiologic studies. This has resulted in the realization that the caliciviruses are "emerging viruses" that are genetically diverse, endemic worldwide pathogens that are the single most important cause of food-borne and waterborne outbreaks of viral gastroenteritis. In recent studies, the Norwalk-like viruses (noroviruses) have been associated with almost all (>95%) outbreaks of nonbacterial gastroenteritis in the United States and Europe (25, 77). These viruses cause occasional epidemic disease as well as international common-source outbreaks that are food and water related (52, 60, 63). Consumption of oysters is a common risk factor. Infections are more widespread than previously realized, with all age groups being susceptible. Norovirus disease has been associated with outbreaks in diverse settings, including schools and day care centers, vacation settings including camps and cruise ships, military ships and maneuvers, restaurants and catered meals, and hospitals and nursing homes. Outbreaks among the elderly in nursing homes can be life-threatening, and a recent study found noroviruses to be the principal cause of gastroenteritis in nursing homes (28). Asymptomatic infection and prolonged virus excretion (>2 to 3 weeks) occur more frequently than previously recognized, and asymptomatic shedders may be a source of widespread transmission (27, 56, 67). Animal caliciviruses that cause enteric disease have been found to be genetically related, but not (yet) identical, to human caliciviruses, raising the possibility that zoonotic transmission (animal to humans) occurs. This important possibility needs to be answered clearly, because zoonotic transmission will change our understanding of this pathogen's evolution and disease transmission.

Calicivirus Structure and Classification

Norwalk virus is the prototype human calicivirus in the *Caliciviridae*, a family of small, nonenveloped, icosahedral viruses that possess a genome of linear, positive-sense, single-stranded RNA. The Norwalk and related viruses have recently been assigned to a new genus, *Norovirus*, and these viruses have a genome that has three primary open reading frames (ORFs) (Fig. 2). The Norwalk virus genome is about 7.8 kb and is enclosed in a capsid composed of a single major structural protein and a few molecules of a second structural protein. The caliciviruses exhibit characteristic cup-shaped depressions on their surface (Color Plate 9), and the family name

is derived from the Latin word *calyx*, meaning cup, which refers to these surface depressions. A second genus, provisionally named *Sapovirus*, also contains human caliciviruses, but these viruses have a slightly different genome organization and their capsid structure frequently displays a more classical appearance similar to that of cultivatable animal caliciviruses. Within each of these two genera that contain human caliciviruses, there are many human virus strains that exhibit remarkable sequence diversity, and these strains are organized into genogroups and genetic clusters depending on the relatedness of their genomes. Currently, there are two genogroups, each with seven genetic clusters, in the noroviruses and two genogroups in the sapoviruses. The biological significance of these genogroups and clusters remains unclear due to the lack of cell culture systems for these human pathogens. Thus, it is not known if these genetic groupings represent distinct serotypes of virus or groupings of virus strains with other common biologic properties.

The Norwalk virus is a prototypical T=3 icosahedral virus, composed of 180 copies of

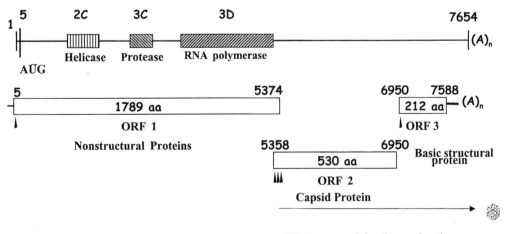

Expressed in baculovirus

FIGURE 2 Norwalk virus genome organization. The top line illustrates this nonenveloped virus's single-stranded RNA genome of ~7.7 kb. The lower boxes depict the three predicted ORFs encoded in the genome. ORF1 produces the nonstructural proteins, ORF2 is the major capsid protein, and ORF3 is a basic protein present as a few copies in virus particles. Expression of the 3′ end of the genome using recombinant baculoviruses results in the self-assembly of VLPs.

the major capsid protein organized into 90 dimers (Color Plate 9). The capsid protein self-assembles into VLPs that lack the viral genome when this protein, with or without the ORF3 protein, is produced in high yields in expression systems. These VLPs mimic the virus structure antigenically and morphologically. A 3.4-Å resolution structure of the capsid protein is known, and it folds into two principal domains: the S domain that forms the icosahedral shell and the P domain that forms the protrusions (64). A flexible hinge links the S and P domains. Current data indicate the protruding domains contain most of the biologically relevant properties, such as cell binding and neutralization epitopes.

Outcome of calicivirus infections

Clinical Course of Infections. Knowledge of the clinical course of disease caused by human caliciviruses comes from human volunteer studies performed since the 1970s, as well as from epidemiologic studies of outbreaks. The gastroenteritis is generally considered to be mild and self-limiting, although illness can last 24 to 48 h and be incapacitating during this time. Inoculation of nonselected, healthy adults with Norwalk virus results in clinical disease in approximately 50% of volunteers and asymptomatic infection occurs in at least 25% of volunteers (27). Early studies found that a spectrum of clinical manifestations occurs in adults given the same inoculum, with some adults having significant vomiting without diarrhea and others having diarrhea without vomiting. Parenteral fluid replacement therapy is required rarely, when vomiting is extensive. In a study of 51 volunteers, where 28 of 41 infected individuals were symptomatic, clinical symptoms included diarrhea (86%), vomiting (57%), nausea (96%), abdominal cramps (96%), headache/body ache (96%), chills (36%), and fever (32%). Bloody stools are not seen.

A series of challenges in volunteers found an unexpected apparent resistance of a subset of adults following inoculation with Norwalk virus (61). In these studies, some volunteers who did not become ill had little, if any, detectable antibody to Norwalk virus, suggesting that these individuals resisted infection because of other factors. It was suggested that a genetically determined variation in virus receptors in the intestinal tract might be responsible for resistance to challenge in the absence of detectable preexisting antibody (61). Recent studies have found a correlation with ABO histo-blood group and susceptibility to infection and disease caused by Norwalk virus (37); secretor status may further affect this susceptibility (J. LePendu, personal communication). It remains to be determined if histo-blood group phenotype will affect outcome with infections by other strains of human caliciviruses.

Studies of outbreaks have confirmed similar clinical outcomes for infections with noroviruses in adults. Children infected with noroviruses may exhibit more vomiting than diarrhea. Volunteer studies have not been performed with sapoviruses, but the clinical features of gastroenteritis in children in Finland suggested that the noroviruses cause more vomiting while the sapoviruses cause more diarrhea (59).

Tropisms, Pathologic Lesions, and Pathogenesis in Calicivirus Infection. All current information indicates that human caliciviruses exhibit a narrow species tropism; they cause disease only in humans, although they may also infect chimpanzees. No small-animal model of human calicivirus infection has been developed. Knowledge of the pathologic lesions caused by human caliciviruses comes from human volunteer studies performed since the 1970s. These experiments are limited, and available information comes from a relatively small number of small bowel biopsies obtained from infected volunteers. Viral infection was initiated by oral inoculation. The site of primary replication is assumed to be in the upper small intestine, because biopsies of the jejunum of volunteers who developed illness following oral administration of the Norwalk or Hawaii virus exhibit histopathologic lesions. Broadening and blunting of the villi of the proximal small intestine was observed, with the mucosa itself remaining histologically intact. Cytoplasmic vacuolization was also observed, as was some infiltration with mononuclear cells. Virus has not been detected by electron microscopy in epithelial cells of the mucosa, so the site of primary replication remains unknown. Of interest, the characteristic jejunal lesion was also observed in volunteers who were fed virus but who remained well, suggesting that these individuals were asymptomatically infected. Histologic lesions were not observed in the gastric fundus, antrum, or rectal mucosa of volunteers with Norwalk virus-induced illness.

The discovery of animal enteric caliciviruses that cause gastroenteritis in swine, calves, chickens, cats, dogs, and mink that are genetically related to human caliciviruses offers new animal models to study enteric calicivirus pathogenesis (17, 32, 44, 72). The pathogenesis of a porcine enteric calicivirus, which is genetically placed in the SLV genus (see below) of human caliciviruses, has been studied in gnotobiotic pigs, and unexpected new information was found (33). First, diarrhea induced in 4- to 6-day-old pigs persisted for 2 to 5 days, with fecal virus shedding for up to 7 days. Virus replication was detected in the proximal small intestine (duodenum and jejunum) and was accompanied by histologic lesions that included villus atrophy and fusion, crypt cell hyperplasia and reduction of villus/crypt ratios, cytoplasmic vacuolization, and infiltration of polymorphonuclear and mononuclear cells into the lamina propria. These results are striking because of their similarity to the lesions reported in volunteers given Norwalk virus. Virus was also detected in serum samples, and disease could be transmitted by intravenous inoculation of virus. Extraintestinal replication of other, nonenteric animal caliciviruses has been known, but this is the

first report of viremia with an enteric calicivirus. This is of particular interest because of new information that human caliciviruses can bind to red blood cells.

Knowledge of pathophysiologic mechanisms responsible for Norwalk virus-induced disease is limited, primarily because of the difficulty of having to obtain such information from human volunteer studies. A transient malabsorption of fat, D-xylose, and lactose has been reported, and levels of small intestinal brush border enzymes are decreased in Norwalk virus-infected individuals (1). Gastric emptying is delayed in infected volunteers who are ill, and this is proposed to be responsible for the nausea and vomiting associated with these viral agents (47). It is hoped that more information on pathophysiology of disease that is relevant to human disease may come from future physiology studies of animals infected with the animal enteric caliciviruses.

Calicivirus-Cell Interactions

The human caliciviruses have not been propagated in cell culture or organ cultures (29), so little information is known about calicivirus-cell interactions. In contrast, the porcine enteric calicivirus grows in cell culture, but only when cells are supplemented with a growth medium containing intestinal contents from uninfected, germfree piglets (62). The factor(s) in the intestinal cell preparations needed for virus growth remains to be identified.

Cloning of the Norwalk virus genome resulted in the discovery that expression of a subgenomic RNA that codes for the capsid protein of Norwalk virus will result in the protein's self-assembly into virus-like particles that lack the viral genome and are morphologically and antigenically similar to virus (40). VLPs have been used for many purposes, including as probes to identify cells that might bind and replicate virus. Binding studies with Norwalk virus VLPs found that all cells tested bind these particles, but the highest binding was to differentiated human intestinal Caco-2 cells (76). The observed binding to all cell lines suggests that an initial binding factor may be ubiquitous. In spite of these findings, attempts to grow Norwalk or other noroviruses in Caco-2 cells, a cell line able to support the growth of most other GI viruses, have failed.

Recently, the Norwalk virus VLPs have been shown to bind to human red blood cells, and this property led to the discovery that histo-blood group phenotype correlates with susceptibility of volunteers to infection and outcome of infection (37; unpublished data). The hemagglutination of human red blood cells, and not animal red blood cells, mimics the restricted host tropism for this virus and has led to the identification of the H antigen as the ligand that binds the VLPs (37a). This antigen is expressed on Caco-2 cells, so it may be the binding factor present on these cells, yet its presence is not sufficient for virus replication. The H antigen has also been shown to be a binding factor for the rabbit hemorrhagic disease virus, another noncultivatable animal calicivirus that causes a fatal hepatitis in rabbits (69). Other coreceptors or cellular factors must be needed for replication and responsible for the host restriction of these viruses. A protein of 105,000 molecular weight in the membranes of Caco-2 cells has been reported to bind VLPs, but the identity of this protein remains unknown and its presence on cells has also not resulted in a permissive cell culture system (74).

Treatment and Control of Calicivirus-Induced Diarrhea

Currently, there are no specific treatments for calicivirus-induced disease. Disease frequently resolves without complications, and oral fluid and electrolyte replacement therapy is normally sufficient to manage fluid loss. If severe vomiting or diarrhea occurs, parenteral administration of fluids may be needed. Hospitalization for severe dehydration is thought to be rare, although this possibility is being re-evaluated with new diagnostic assays, as it is possible that some patients, especially children, hospitalized for gastroenteritis of unknown etiology may have calicivirus disease. Oral administration of bismuth subsalicylate has somewhat reduced the severity and duration of symptoms in adults with Norwalk virus illness; its usefulness for infections with other caliciviruses is not known. Medications are not recommended for use in children.

Vaccines may be developed to prevent norovirus disease. VLP vaccines are available and have been shown to be safe and immunogenic in volunteers; their ability to induce either homotypic or heterotypic protective immunity remains to be evaluated by new challenge studies (22).

Needs for Further Understanding of Calicivirus-Induced Disease

Our understanding of the significance and epidemiology of calicivirus-induced disease is changing rapidly, and continued studies are needed to fully appreciate the spectrum of disease caused by these pathogens. It is likely that these viruses will be found to cause much more disease than previously appreciated. Based on persistent infections known to be caused by animal caliciviruses, it is possible that human caliciviruses will also be found to be associated with chronic diseases in humans. It is important to understand the molecular basis for the genetic diversity of human caliciviruses by asking the following questions. Does zoonotic transmission occur and do these viruses evolve based on high rates of recombination? If the latter is true, will this lead to changing tropisms? The availability of atomic resolution structures of caliciviruses offers the possibility of producing antivirals that could be useful for treating the elderly or others stricken by these incapacitating infections. Two major but related questions remain. Why do these viruses grow so well and cause disease easily in volunteers while remaining noncultivatable? What is the cellular basis of restriction for cultivation? Once these questions are answered, a molecular understanding of pathogenesis will be approachable, and new methods to treat and possibly prevent transmission can be developed. In particular, investigators will be able to determine the public health significance of detecting these viruses in food and water and of finding methods to inactivate infectivity.

SUMMARY AND FUTURE STUDIES

GI viruses cause significant human disease, and the use of new assays to detect these viruses indicates that the epidemiologic significance of these infections has been previously greatly underestimated and that infections with these viruses may be a particular concern in elderly residents in nursing homes. Even for the most intensively studied rotaviruses and caliciviruses, our knowledge of their epidemiology is changing. However, the high or increasing clinical significance of these two viruses indicates that vaccine development should be pursued.

The less-studied human GI viral pathogens, astroviruses, enteric adenoviruses, and Aichi viruses, remain a largely unmined resource to probe unique GI-host interactions and possible novel intestinal receptors. Astroviruses exhibit unusual mechanisms of gene expression for positive-strand RNA viruses, and Aichi viruses appear to have a unique mechanism of translational regulation. Most of these GI viruses induce protective immunity, and they may be exploited to develop new mucosal vectors. Understanding the intestinal immune response to these different GI viruses can be expected to lead to new insights into how to induce protective mucosal immunity. One interesting question raised by the association of intussusception with the now withdrawn live, attenuated rotavirus vaccine is, why was intussusception previously clearly associated only with respiratory but not enteric adenovirus infections? Is it possible this is due to a difference in receptor specificity for these viruses, with respiratory adenoviruses and rotaviruses sharing the ability to interact with integrins as postbinding receptors? What is the pathogenesis of intussusception, and is it possible that coinfections with bacteria or other environmental factors that affect intestinal permeability act as cofactors to trigger intussusception? Most GI viruses also cause more severe disease in malnourished children or animals, and the effects of diet on prevention and therapy remain to be fully understood and exploited for new therapies. A striking outcome of recent work on how GI viruses cause disease is the recognition that common mechanisms of pathogenesis may be shared by viruses and other intestinal microbes. This information is exciting because it suggests that common therapies might be able to be developed for these divergent pathogens that cause similar diseases.

REFERENCES

1. **Agus, S. G., R. Dolin, R. G. Wyatt, A. J. Tousimis, and R. S. Northrup.** 1973. Acute infectious nonbacterial gastroenteritis: intestinal histopathology. Histologic and enzymatic alterations during illness produced by the Norwalk agent in man. *Ann. Intern. Med.* **79:**18–25.
2. **Atmar, R. L., and M. K. Estes.** 2001. Diagnosis of noncultivatable gastroenteritis viruses, the human caliciviruses. *Clin. Microbiol. Rev.* **14:**15–37.
3. **Ball, J. M., P. Tian, C. Q. Zeng, A. P. Morris, and M. K. Estes.** 1996. Age-dependent diarrhea induced by a rotaviral nonstructural glycoprotein. *Science* **272:**101–104.
4. **Blutt, S. E., K. L. Warfield, D. E. Lewis, and M. E. Conner,** 2002. Early response to rotavirus infection involves massive B cell activation. *J. Immunol.* **168:**5716–5721.
5. **Brunet, J. P., J. Cotte-Laffitte, C. Linxe, A. M. Quero, M. Geniteau-Legendre, and A. Servin.** 2000. Rotavirus infection induces an increase in intracellular calcium concentration in human intestinal epithelial cells: role in microvillar actin alteration. *J. Virol.* **74:**2323–2332.
6. **Chadwick, D., and J. A. Goode.** 2001. *Novartis Foundation Symposium 238: Gastroenteritis Viruses.* John Wiley & Sons, Ltd., West Sussex, United Kingdom.
7. **Ciarlet, M., M. E. Conner, M. J. Finegold, and M. K. Estes.** 2002. Group A rotavirus infection and age-dependent diarrheal disease in rats: a new animal model to study the pathophysiology of rotavirus infection. *J. Virol.* **76:**41–57.
8. **Ciarlet, M., S. E. Crawford, C. Barone, A. Bertolotti-Ciarlet, M. K. Estes, and M. E. Conner.** 1998. Subunit rotavirus vaccine administered parenterally to rabbits induces protective immunity. *J. Virol.* **72:**9233–9246.

9. **Ciarlet, M., S. E. Crawford, and M. K. Estes.** 2001. Differential infection of polarized epithelial cell lines by sialic acid-dependent and sialic acid-independent rotavirus strains. *J. Virol.* **75:**11834–11850.

10. **Ciarlet, M., and M. K. Estes.** 2001. Rotavirus and calicivirus infections of the gastrointestinal tract. *Curr. Opin. Gastroenterol.* **17:**10–16.

11. **Conner, M. E., and R. F. Ramig.** 1997. Viral enteric diseases, p. 713–743. *In* N. Nathanson, R. Ahmed, F. Gonzalez-Scarano, D. E. Griffin, K. V. Holmes, F. A. Murphy, and H. L. Robinson (ed.), *Viral Pathogenesis.* Lippincott-Raven Publishers, Philadelphia, Pa.

12. **Coste, A., J. C. Sirard, K. Johansen, J. Cohen, and J. P. Kraehenbuhl.** 2000. Nasal immunization of mice with virus-like particles protects offspring against rotavirus diarrhea. *J. Virol.* **74:**8966–8971.

13. **Crawford, S. E., M. K. Estes, M. Ciarlet, C. Barone, C. M. O'Neal, J. Cohen, and M. E. Conner.** 1999. Heterotypic protection and induction of a broad heterotypic neutralization response by rotavirus-like particles. *J. Virol.* **73:**4813–4822.

15. **Crawford, S. E., A. K. Mukherjee, M. K. Estes, J. A. Lawton, A. L. Shaw, R. F. Ramig, and B. V. Prasad.** 2001. Trypsin cleavage stabilizes the rotavirus VP4 spike. *J. Virol.* **75:**6052–6061.

15. **Cuadras, M. A., D. A. Feigelstock, S. An, and H. B. Greenberg.** 2002. Gene expression pattern in Caco-2 cells following rotavirus infection. *J. Virol.* **76:**4467–4482.

16. **Cunliffe, N. A., J. S. Gondwe, C. D. Kirkwood, S. M. Graham, N. M. Nhlane, B. D. Thindwa, W. Dove, R. L. Broadhead, M. E. Molyneaux, and C. A. Hart.** 2001. Effect of concomitant HIV infection on presentation and outcome of rotavirus gastroenteritis in Malawian children. *Lancet* **358:**550–555.

17. **Dastjerdi, A. M., J. Green, C. I. Gallimore, D. W. Brown, and J. C. Bridger.** 1999. The bovine Newbury agent-2 is genetically more closely related to human SRSVs than to animal caliciviruses. *Virology* **254:**1–5.

18. **Desselberger, U., and J. J. Gray.** 2002. *Perspectives in Medical Virology: Viral Gastroenteritis.* Elsevier Science, Amsterdam, The Netherlands.

19. **Dong, Y., C. Q. Zeng, J. M. Ball, M. K. Estes, and A. P. Morris.** 1997. The rotavirus enterotoxin NSP4 mobilizes intracellular calcium in human intestinal cells by stimulating phospholipase C-mediated inositol 1,4,5-trisphosphate production. *Proc. Natl. Acad. Sci. USA* **94:**3960–3965.

20. **Dormitzer, P. R., H. B. Greenberg, and S. C. Harrison.** 2001. Proteolysis of monomeric recombinant rotavirus VP4 yields an oligomeric VP5★core. *J. Virol.* **75:**7739–7750.

21. **Dormitzer, P. R., Z. Y. Sun, G. Wagner, and S. C. Harrison.** 2002. The rhesus rotavirus VP4 sialic acid binding domain has a galectin fold with a novel carbohydrate binding site. *EMBO J.* **21:**885–897.

22. **Estes, M. K., J. M. Ball, R. A. Guerrero, A. R. Opekun, M. A. Gilger, S. S. Pacheco, and D. Y. Graham.** 2000. Norwalk virus vaccines: challenges and progress. *J. Infect. Dis.* **181:**S367–S373.

23. **Estes, M. K., and A. P. Morris.** 1999. A viral enterotoxin. A new mechanism of virus-induced pathogenesis. *Adv. Exp. Med. Biol.* **473:**73–82.

24. **Fankhauser, R. L., J. S. Noel, S. S. Monroe, T. Ando, and R. I. Glass.** 1998. Molecular epidemiology of "Norwalk-like viruses" in outbreaks of gastroenteritis in the United States. *J. Infect. Dis.* **178:**1571–1578.

25. **Franco, M. A., and H. B. Greenberg.** 1997. Immunity to rotavirus in T cell deficient mice. *Virology* **238:**169–179.

26. **Glass, R. I., P. E. Kilgore, R. C. Holman, S. Jin, J. C. Smith, P. A. Woods, M. J. Clarke, M. S. Ho, and J. R. Gentsch.** 1996. The epidemiology of rotavirus diarrhea in the United States: surveillance and estimates of disease burden. *J. Infect. Dis.* **174**(Suppl. 1):S5–S11.

26a. **Graff, J. W., D. N. Mitzel, C. M. Weisend, M. L. Flenniken, and M. E. Hardy.** 2002. Interferon regulatory factor 3 is a cellular partner of rotavirus NSP1. *J. Virol.* **76:**9545–9550.

27. **Graham, D. Y., X. Jiang, H. Tanaka, A. R. Opekun, H. P. Madore, and M. K. Estes.** 1994. Norwalk virus infection of volunteers: new insights based on improved assays. *J. Infect. Dis.* **170:**34–43.

28. **Green, K. Y., G. Belliot, J. L. Taylor, J. Valdesuso, J. F. Lew, A. Kapikian, and F. Y. Lin.** 2002. A predominant role for Norwalk-like viruses as agents of epidemic gastroenteritis in Maryland nursing homes for the elderly. *J. Infect. Dis.* **185:**133–146.

29. **Green, K. Y., R. M. Chanock, and A. Z. Kapikian.** 2001. Human caliciviruses, p. 841–874. *In* D. M. Knipe and P. M. Howley (ed.), *Fields Virology.* Lippincott Williams & Wilkins, Philadelphia, Pa.

30. **Greenberg, H. B., H. F. Clark, and P. A. Offit.** 1994. Rotavirus pathology and pathophysiology. *Curr. Top. Microbiol. Immunol.* **185:**255–283.

31. **Guarino, A., R. Berni Canani, and S. Russo.** 1994. Oral immunoglobulins for treatment of acute rotaviral gastroenteritis. *Pediatrics* **93:**12–16.

32. **Guo, M., K. O. Chang, M. E. Hardy, Q. Zhang, A. V. Parwani, and L. J. Saif.** 1999. Molecular characterization of a porcine calicivirus genetically related to Sapporo-like human viruses. *J. Virol.* **73:**9625–9631.

33. **Guo, M., J. Hayes, K. O. Cho, A. V. Parwani, L. M. Lucas, and L. J. Saif.** 2001. Comparative pathogenesis of tissue culture-adapted and wild-type Cowden porcine enteric calicivirus (PEC) in gnotobiotic pigs and induction of diarrhea by intravenous inoculaton of wild-type PEC. *J. Virol.* **75:**9239–9251.

34. **Halaihel, N., V. Lievin, J. M. Ball, M. K. Estes, F. Alvarado, and M. Vasseur.** 2000. Direct inhibitory effect of rotavirus NSP4 (114–135) peptide on the Na^+-D-glucose symporter of rabbit intestinal brush border membrane. *J. Virol.* **74:**9464–9470.

35. **Horie, Y., O. Nakagomi, Y. Koshimura, T. Nakagomi, Y. Suzuki, T. Oka, S. Sasaki, Y. Matsuda, and S. Watanabe.** 1999. Diarrhea induction by rotavirus NSP4 in the homologous mouse model system. *Virology* **262:**398–407.

36. **Hughes, R. C.** 1999. Secretion of the galectin family of mammalian carbohydrate-binding proteins. *Biochim. Biophys. Acta* **1473:**172–185.

37. **Hutson, A. M., R. L. Atmar, D. Y. Graham, and M. K. Estes.** 2002. Norwalk virus infection and disease is associated with ABO histo-blood group type. *J. Infect. Dis.* **185:**1335–1337.

37a. **Hutson, A. M., R. L. Atmar, D. M. Marcus, and M. K. Estes.** 2003. Norwalk virus-like particle hemagglutination by binding to H histo-blood group antigens. *J. Virol.* **77:**405–415.

38. **Jiang, B., C. Barone, V. Barniak, C. M. O'Neal, A. Ottaiano, H. P. Madore, M. K. Estes, and M. E. Conner.** 1999. Heterotypic protection against rotavirus infection in mice vaccinated with virus-like particles. *Vaccine* **17:**1005–1013.

39. **Jiang, X, D. Y. Graham, K. Wang, and M. K. Estes.** 1990. Norwalk virus genome: cloning and characterization. *Science* **250:**1580–1583.

40. **Jiang, X., M. Wang, D. Y. Graham, and M. K. Estes.** 1992. Expression, self-assembly, and antigenicity of the Norwalk virus capsid protein. *J. Virol.* **66:**6527–6532.

41. **Jourdan, N., J. P. Brunet, C. Sapin, A. Blais, J. Cotte-Laffitte, F. Forestier, A. M. Quero, G. Trugnan, and A. L. Servin.** 1998. Rotavirus infection reduces sucrase-isomaltase expression in human intestinal epithelial cells by perturbing protein targeting and organization of microvillar cytoskeleton. *J. Virol.* **72:**7228–7236.

42. **Jourdan, N., M. Maurice, D. Delautier, A. M. Quero, A. L. Servin, and G. Trugnan.** 1997. Rotavirus is released from the apical surface of cultured human intestinal cells through non-conventional vesicular transport that bypasses the Golgi apparatus. *J. Virol.* **71:**8268–8278.

43. **LaMonica, R., S. S. Kocer, J. Nazarova, W. Dowling, E. Geimonen, R. D. Shaw, and E. R. Mackow.** 2001. VP4 differentially regulates TRAF2 signaling, disengaging JNK activation while directing NF-kappa B to effect rotavirus specific cellular receptors. *J. Biol. Chem.* **276:**19889–19896.

44. **Liu, B. L., P. R. Lambden, H. Gunther, P. Otto, M. Elschner, and I. N. Clarke.** 1999. Molecular characterization of a bovine enteric calicivirus: relationship to the Norwalk-like viruses. *J. Virol.* **73:**818–825.

45. **Lundgren, O., A. T. Peregrin, K. Persson, S. Kordasti, I. Uhnoo, and L. Svensson.** 2000. Role of the enteric nervous system in the fluid and electrolyte secretion of rotavirus diarrhea. *Science* **287:**491–495.

46. **Madore, H. P., D. Zarley, B. Hu, S. Parsons, B. Jiang, B. Corsaro, S. E. Crawford, M. E. Conner, and M. K. Estes.** 1999. Biochemical and immunologic comparison of virus-like particles for a rotavirus subunit vaccine. *Vaccine* **17:**2461–2471.

47. **Meeroff, J. C., D. S. Schreiber, J. S. Trier, and N. R. Blacklow.** 1980. Abnormal gastric motor function in viral gastroenteritis. *Ann. Intern. Med.* **92:**370–373.

48. **Mori, Y., M. A. Borgan, N. Ito, M. Sugiyama, and N. Minamoto.** 2002. Diarrhea-inducing activity of avian rotavirus NSP4 glycoproteins, which differ greatly from mammalian rotavirus NSP4 glycoproteins in deduced amino acid sequence, in suckling mice. *J. Virol.* **76:**5829–5834.

49. **Morris, A. P., and M. K. Estes.** 2001. Microbes and microbial toxins: paradigms for microbial-mucosal interactions. VIII. Pathological consequences of rotavirus infection and its enterotoxin. *Am. J. Physiol. Gastrointest. Liver Physiol.* **281:**G303–G310.

50. **Morris, A. P., J. K. Scott, J. M. Ball, C. Q. Zeng, W. K. O'Neal, and M. K. Estes.** 1999. NSP4 elicits age-dependent diarrhea and $Ca(2+)$ mediated $I(-)$ influx into intestinal crypts of CF mice. *Am. J. Physiol.* **277:**G431–G444.

51. **Murphy, T. V., P. M. Gargiullo, M. S. Massoudi, D. B. Nelson, A. O. Jumaan, C. A. Okoro, L. R. Zanardi, S. Setia, E. Fair, C. W. LeBaron, M. Wharton, and J. R. Livingood.** 2001. Intussusception among infants given an oral rotavirus vaccine. *N. Engl. J. Med.* **344:**564–572.

52. **Noel, J. S., R. L. Fankhauser, T. Ando, S. S. Monroe, and R. I. Glass.** 1999. Identification of a distinct common strain of "Norwalk-like viruses" having a global distribution. *J. Infect. Dis.* **179:**1334–1344.

53. **O'Neal, C. M., J. D. Clements, M. K. Estes, and M. E. Conner.** 1998. Rotavirus 2/6 virus-like particles administered intranasally with cholera toxin, *Escherichia coli* heat-labile toxin (LT), and LT-R192G induce protection from rotavirus challenge. *J. Virol.* **72:**3390–3393.

54. **O'Neal, C. M., S. E. Crawford, M. K. Estes, and M. E. Conner.** 1997. Rotavirus virus-particles administered mucosally induce protective immunity. *J. Virol.* **71:**8707–8717.

55. **Obert, G., I. Peiffer, and A. L. Servin.** 2000. Rotavirus-induced structural and functional alterations in tight junctions of polarized intestinal Caco-2 cell monolayers *J. Virol.* **74:**4645–4651.

56. **Okhuysen, P. C., X. Jiang, L. Ye, P. C. Johnson, and M. K. Estes.** 1995. Viral shedding and fecal IgA response after Norwalk virus infection. *J. Infect. Dis.* **171:**566–569.

57. **Osborne, M. P., S. J. Haddon, A. J. Spencer, J. Collins, W. G. Starkey, T. S. Wallis, G. J. Clarke, K. J. Worton, D. C. Candy, and J. Stephen.** 1988. An electron microscopic investigation of time-related changes in the intestine of neonatal mice infected with murine rotavirus. *J. Pediatr. Gastroenterol. Nutr.* **7:**236–248.

58. **Pacyna, J., K. Siwek, S. J. Terry, E. S. Roberton, R. B. Johnson, and G. P. Davidson.** 2001. Survival of rotavirus antibody activity derived from bovine colostrum after passage through the human gastrointestinal tract. *J. Pediatr. Gastroenterol. Nutr.* **32:**162–167.

59. **Pang, X. L., S. Q. Zeng, S. Honma, S. Nakata, and T. Vesikari.** 2001. Effect of rotavirus vaccine on Sapporo virus gastroenteritis in Finnish infants. *Pediatr. Infec. Dis. J.* **20:**295–300.

60. **Parashar, U. D., and S. S. Monroe.** 2001. "Norwalk-like viruses" as a cause of foodborne disease outbreaks. *Rev. Med. Virol.* **11:**243–252.

61. **Parrino, T. A., D. S. Schreiber, J. S. Trier, A. Z. Kapikian, and N. R. Blacklow.** 1977. Clinical immunity in acute gastroenteritis caused by Norwalk agent. *N. Engl. J. Med.* **297:**86–89.

62. **Parwani, A. V., W. T. Flynn, K. L. Gadfield, and L. J. Saif.** 1991. Serial propagation of porcine enteric calicivirus in a continuous cell line. Effect of medium supplementation with intestinal contents or enzymes. *Arch. Virol.* **120:**115–122.

63. **Ponka, A., L. Maunula, C. H. Von Bonsdorf, and O. Lyytikainen.** 1999. An outbreak of calicivirus associated with consumption of frozen raspberries. *Epidemiol. Infect.* **123:**469–474.

64. **Prasad, B. V., M. E. Hardy, T. Dokland, J. Bella, M. G. Rossmann, and M. K. Estes.** 1999. X-ray crystallographic structure of the Norwalk virus capsid. *Science* **286:**287–290.

65. **Raza, S., S. M. Graham, S. J. Allen, S. Sultana, L. Cuevas, C. A. Hart, M. Kaila, E. Isolauri, and M. A. H. Saxelin.** 1995. *Lactobacillus GG* in acute diarrhea. *Indian J. Pediatr.* **32:**1140–1142.

66. **Rennels, M. B.** 2000. The rotavirus vaccine story: a clinical investigator's view. *Pediatrics* **106:**123–125.

67. **Rockx, B., M. de Wit, H. Vennema, J. Vinje, E. de Bruin, Y. van Duynhoven, and M. Koopmans.** 2002. Natural history of human calicivirus infection: a prospective cohort study. *Clin. Infect. Dis.* **35:**246–253.

68. **Ruiz, M. C., J. Cohen, and F. Michelangeli.** 2000. Role of Ca^{2+} in the replication and pathogenesis of rotavirus and other viral infections. *Cell Calcium* **28:**137–149.

69. **Ruveon-Clouet, N., D. Blanchard, G. Andre-Fontaine, and J. P. Ganiere.** 1995. Partial characterization of the human erythrocyte receptor for rabbit haemorrhagic disease virus. *Res. Virol.* **146:**33–41.

70. **Salazar-Lindo, E., J. Santisteban-Ponce, E. Chea-Woo, and M. Gutierrez.** 2000. Racecadotril in the treatment of acute watery diarrhea in children. *N. Engl. J. Med.* **343:**463–467.

71. **Sapin, C., O. Colard, O. Delmas, C. Tessier, M. Breton, V. Enouf, S. Chwetzoff, J. Ouanich, J. Cohen, C. Wolf, and G. Trugnan.** 2002. Rafts promote assembly and atypical targeting of a nonenveloped virus, rotavirus, in Caco-2 cells. *J. Virol.* **76:**4591–4602.

72. **Sugieda, M., H. Nagaoka, Y. Kakishima, T. Ohshita, S. Nakamuira, and S. Nakajama.** 1998. Detection of Norwalk-like virus genes in the caecum contents of pigs. *Arch. Virol.* **143:**1215–1221.

73. **Tafazoli, F., C. Q.-Y. Zeng, M. K. Estes, K. E. Magnusson, and L. Svensson.** 2001. The NSP4 enterotoxin of rotavirus induces paracellular leakage in polarized epithelial cells. *J. Virol.* **75:**1540–1546.

74. **Tamura, M., K. Natori, M. Kobayashi, T. Miyamura, and N. Takeda.** 2000. Interaction of recombinant Norwalk virus particles with the 105-kilodalton cellular binding protein, a candidate receptor molecule for virus attachment. *J. Virol.* **74:**11589–11597.

75. **Vinje, J., S. A. Altena, and M. P. Koopmans.** 1997. The incidence and genetic variability of small round-structured viruses in outbreaks of gastroenteritis in The Netherlands. *J. Infect. Dis.* **176:**1374–1378.

76. **White, L., J. M. Ball, M. E. Hardy, T. N. Tanaka, N. Kitamoto, and M. K. Estes.** 1996. Attachment and entry of recombinant Norwalk virus capsids to cultured human and animal cell lines. *J. Virol.* **70:**6589–6597.

77. **World Health Organization.** 1999. Rotavirus vaccines. *Wkly. Epidemiol. Rec.* **74:**33–38.

78. **Xu, A., A. R. Bellamy, and J. A. Taylor.** 2000. Immobilization of the early secretory pathway by a virus glycoprotein that binds to microtubules. *EMBO J.* **19:**6465–6474.

79. **Youngman, K. R., M. A. Franco, N. Kuklin, L. S. Rott, E. C. Butcher, and H. B. Greenberg.** 2002. Correlation of tissue distribution, developmental phenotype, and intestinal homing receptor expression of antigen-specific B cells during the murine anti-rotavirus immune response. *J. Immunol.* **68:**2173–2181.

80. **Yu, J., and W. H. Langridge.** 2001. A plant-based multicomponent vaccine protects mice from enteric diseases. *Nat. Biotechnol.* **19:**548–552.

81. **Yuan, L., A. Geyer, D. C. Hodgins, Z. Fan, Y. Qian, K. O. Chang, S. E. Crawford, V. Parreno, L. A. Ward, M. K. Estes, M. E. Conner, and L. J. Saif.** 2000. Intranasal administration of 2/6-rotavirus-like particles with mutant *Escherichia coli* heat-labile toxin (LT-R192G) induces antibody-secreting cell responses but not protective immunity in gnotobiotic pigs. *J. Virol.* **74:**8843–8853.

82. **Zarate, S., R. Espinosa, P. Romero, E. Mendez, C. F. Arias, and S. Lopez.** 2000. The VP5 domain of VP4 can mediate attachment of rotaviruses to cells. *J. Virol.* **74:**593–599.

83. **Zhang, M., C. Q.-Y. Zeng, A. P. Morris, and M. K. Estes.** 2000. A functional NSP4 enterotoxin peptide secreted from rotavirus-infected cells. *J. Virol.* **74:**11663–11670.

84. **Zijlstra, R. T., S. M. Donovan, J. Odle, H. B. Gelberg, B. W. Petschow, and H. R. Gaskins.** 1997. Protein-energy malnutrition delays small-intestinal recovery in neonatal pigs infected with rotavirus. *J. Nutr.* **127:**1118–1127.

INDEX

Complement system, immunoglobulin A interactions
with, 102, 103
Contiguous repeating units, *Clostridium difficile*
toxins, 506
Counterregulatory pathways, cytokines in, 70–71
Coxsackievirus and adenovirus receptor, 285–287,
294
Crohn's disease
colonic, 226–227
commensal bacteria response in, 230
mucosal defects causing, 232–233
Paneth cell defects and, 208
postoperative, 226–227
Crypt(s), 3–4
abscess of, 65–67
enteroendocrine cells in, 8–9
goblet cells in, 7–8
Paneth cells in, 9, 198, 208; *see also* Paneth cells
stem cells in, 10
undifferentiated enterocytes in, 6–7
Cryptdins
bactericidal activity of, 201
deficiency of, 209
distribution of, 200–201
genes of, 200–201
processing of, 202, 204
regulation of, 204
structures of, 200
Cryptococcus neoformans
defensin interactions with, 198
inflammation suppression by, 181
Cryptosporidium parvum
defense evasion by, 167
intestinal invasion of, 158
CSCR3, in intestinal immunity, 52
CXC chemokines, in innate immunity, 52, 162–
163, 167–168
Cyclic adenosine monophosphate (cAMP)
calcium interactions with, 258
in chloride secretion, 269–273
in ion transport, 256–258
Cyclic AMP response element binding protein, 68
Cyclic guanosine monophosphate (cGMP)
in chloride secretion, 274–276
in ion transport, 256–257
Cyclic nucleotides, in ion transport, 256–257
Cyclooxygenase, *Clostridium difficile* toxin and, 272
Cyclospora cayetanensis, phylogenetic analysis of, 117–
118
Cystic fibrosis transmembrane conductance regulator
function of, 250–251
in ion transport regulation, 256–257
mutations of, 269
Cytokines; *see also specific cytokines*
actions of, 61–62
in antigen processing and presentation, 64–65
autocrine activation pathways of, 67–70

in barrier function attenuation, 63
counterregulatory pathways of, 70–71
inhibition of, in *Yersinia* infections, 376–377
in innate immunity, 156
from intraepithelial lymphocytes, 54
in ion transport, 63–64
from lamina propria lymphocytes, 54–55
in NF-κB activation, 143
in oral tolerance, 46–47
paracrine activation pathways of, 63–67
in polymeric immunoglobulin receptor regulation,
97
in polymorphonuclear leukocyte trafficking, 65–
67
production of, ontogeny of, 337–338
receptors for, 62
response to, model for, 71–72
Cytoskeleton, 301–331
adherens junctions of, 308–309
contraction of
in pathogen interaction, 287–289
in tight junction regulation, 14
focal contacts of, 306–307
hemidesmosomes of, 306–307
purpose of, 301
regulation of, 309–311
structure of, 301, 304–306
tight junctions of, *see* Tight junctions
toxins affecting, 311–322; *see also specific organisms
and toxins*
actin, 311–312
cholera toxin, 322
protease, 319–321
Rho GTPases, 311–312
type III secretion effectors, 313–319
ZO toxin, 321–322
Cytosol, toxin translocation to, 395–396, 508–509

DC73 (ectonucleotidase), in chloride secretion, 444
Death receptors, in apoptosis, 368
Defensins, 161–162, 197–198
in chloride secretion, 280–281
family of, 192
genes of, 200
killing mechanisms of, 196
in Paneth cells, 198–200; *see also* Paneth cells
activation of, 204
antimicrobial activities of, 201
biosynthesis of, 200–201
processing of, 202–204
regulation of, 200–201
precursors of, 202
structures of, 192, 194–196, 198–200
Dendritic cells
in antigen capture, 28
in innate immunity, 163–165
in intestinal immunity, 52–53